PROCEEDINGS

OF THE

NAVC CONFERENCE

VOLUME 22

JANUARY 19-23, 2008

ORLANDO, FLORIDA

SMALL ANIMAL AND EXOTICS EDITION

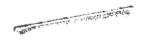

BOOK 2

The ideas, content and conclusions presented in these Proceedings are strictly those of the contributors and do not necessarily represent the viewpoint, position, or endorsement of the NAVC. The NAVC and the contributors do not take responsibility for information provided on dosages and methods of applications of drugs mentioned in these Proceedings. This information must be verified by the user from appropriate literature and/or additional sources.

While all contributors were invited to submit manuscripts for the general sessions, some chose not to do so. The NAVC regrets these omissions, but has done everything possible to ensure a comprehensive Proceedings for the NAVC Conference 2008.

"Special thanks for the assistance received from Robin Hipple, Medical Editor and Marcy Bryant, Layout."

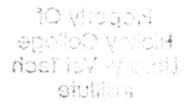

About the Cover: Jim Wilson's fascination with animals has influenced many aspects of his life including his career choice. A professional wildlife artist for over thirty five years, Jim spends many hours seeking out and researching his subjects for his detailed pen and ink drawings. He relies on reference material gathered from field work, museums, zoos, veterinary hospitals and rehabilitation facilities. His camera is a constant companion, providing a permanent collection of reference photos. Jim's work has been featured in a variety of NAVC material since 1992.

Larry G. Adams, DVM, PhD, DACVIM
Purdue University
School of Veterinary Medicine
625 Harrison Street
West Lafayette, IN 47907-2026
Pages: 721-732

Karin Allenspach, DMV, DECVIM-CA
Royal Veterinary College,
University of London
Hatfield, Hertfordshire
UNITED KINGDOM
Pages: 517-526

Fernando J. Alvarez, DVM
Olleros 3045
Conde 909
C.A. de Buenos Aires
ARGENTINA
Pages: 417-424

John C. Angus, DVM, DACVD
Southern Arizona Veterinary
Dermatology
2610 Lambert
Pasadena, CA 85705
Pages: 347-362; 1077-1080

P. Jane Armstrong, DVM, MS, MBA, DACVIM
University of Minnesota
College of Veterinary Medicine
1352 Boyd Avenue
St. Paul, MN 55108
Pages: 809-812

Clarke Atkins, DVM, DACVIM
North Carolina State University
College of Veterinary Medicine
4700 Hillsborough Street
Raleigh, NC 27606
Pages: 205-207

David Aucoin, DVM, DACVCP
1500 Olympic Blvd
Santa Monica, CA 90404
Pages: 667-668

Jean-Francois Bardet, DVM, MS, DECVS
32, rue Pierre
Neuilly Sur Seine 92200
FRANCE
Pages: 481-484; 639-641; 773-775; 963-967

Sharron Barnett, BS, MS
Novartis Animal Health
3200 Northline Ave
Ste 300
Greensboro, NC 27408
Pages: 1133-1134

Mary Battistella, DVM, CVA
Riverview Animal Clinic and
Kowaliga Whole Health Pet Resort
39 Alabama Drive
Alexander City, AL 35010
Pages: 1-4

Jim Baum
Matsco
710 Wyandotte Drive
Franklin Lakes, NJ 07417
Pages: 1167-1169

Matthew W. Beal, DVM, DACVECC
Michigan State University
College of Veterinary Medicine
East Lansing, MI 48824-1314
Pages: 183-185; 243-259

Brett Beckman, DVM, FAVD, DAVDC, DAAPM
Affiliated Veterinary Specialists
2607 Conway Blvd.
Port Charlotte, FL 33952
Pages: 329-335

Sagiv Ben-Yakir, DVM
Hod-Hasharon Veterinary Clinic
17 Gordon Street
Hod-Hasharon
ISRAEL
Pages: 5-22

Mark Bohling, DVM
University of Tennessee
College of Veterinary Medicine
C247 Vet Teaching Hospital
Knoxville, TN 37996
Pages: 1475-1476; 1601-1603; 1721-1723

Gregory D. Bossart, VMD, PhD
Harbor Branch Oceanographic Institution
5600 US 1 North
Ft. Pierce, FL 32968
Pages: 1613-1615

Dwight Bowman, BA, MS, PhD
Cornell University
College of Veterinary Medicine
Ithaca, NY 14853
Pages: 1135-1138

Edward B. Breitschwerdt, DVM, DACVIM
North Carolina State University
College of Veterinary Medicine
4700 Hillsborough Street
Raleigh, NC 27606
Pages: 669-684

Karla Brestle, DVM
Humane Alliance
231 Haywood Street
Asheville, NC
Pages: 1477-1478

Ronald Bright, DVM, MS, DACVS
VCA-Veterinary Specialists of
Northern Colorado
201 West 67th Court
Loveland, CO 80538
Pages: 1495-1509

Daniel J. Brockman, BVSc, CVR, CSAO, DACVS, ECVS, FHEA, MRCVS
University of London
Royal Veterinary College,
Hawkshead Lane, North Mymms
Hatfield, Hertfordshire AL9 7TA
UNITED KINGDOM
Pages: 1510-1525

Dennis Brooks, DVM, PhD, DACVO
University of Florida
College of Veterinary Medicine
2015 SW 16th Ave
Gainesville, FL 32608
Pages: 931-932

Scott A. Brown, VMD, PhD, DACVIM
University of Georgia
College of Veterinary Medicine
501 DW Brooks Drive
Athens, GA 30602
Pages: 733-735

Steven C. Budsberg, DVM, MS, DACVS
University of Georgia
College of Veterinary Medicine
501 DW Brooks Drive
Athens, GA 30602
Pages: 968

Steven J. Butterworth, MA, VetMB, CertVR, DSAO, MRCVS
Kemys Way
Swansea Enterprise Park
Swansea SA6 8QF
UNITED KINGDOM
Pages: 642-644; 969-978

Steve Callister, Ph.D.
Gundersen Lutheran Medical
Foundation
Gundersen Lutheran Medical Center
1300 Badger Street Room 5034
La Crosse, WI
Pages: 685-687

Sean Campbell
CMP, Inc
901 Lamberton Place, NE
Albuquerque, NM 87107
Pages: 589-599

Anthony P. Carr, Dr.med.vet, DACVIM
University of Saskatchewan
Western College of Veterinary Medicine
52 Campus Drive
Saskatoon   S7N 5B4
CANADA
Pages: 186-187

Sharon A. Center, DVM, DACVIM
Cornell University
College of Veterinary Medicine
Ithaca, NY 14853
Pages: 569-574

Daniel D. Chapel, AIA, NCARB
Chapel Associates Architects
8201 Cantrell Road, Suite 360
Little Rock, AR 72227
Pages: 600-611

Dennis Chew, DVM, DACVIM
The Ohio State University
College of Veterinary Medicine
601 Vernon L. Tharp Street
Columbus, OH 43210
Pages: 736-737

Alfonso C. Chico, M.V.M., Lic.VET
Director,
Veterinary Surgical Center
La Coruana
C/ Juan Florez, 91 Bajo
La Coruna   15005
SPAIN
Pages: 645; 979-987

Ross Clark, DVM
9400 South Union Avenue
Tulsa, OK 74132
Pages: 1170-1173

Leah Cohn, DVM, PhD, DACVIM
University of Missouri
900 E. Campus Drive
Clydesdale Hall
Columbia, MO 65211
Pages: 657-659; 1413-1415; 1446-1449

Rob Coke, DVM
San Antonio Zoo
3903 N St Marys Street
San Antonio, TX 78212
Pages: 1727-1742

Pamela Cole, CEO
Irvine Veterinary Services
5401 University Drive
Irvine, CA 92612
Pages: 1174-1175
B

Michael Conzemius, DVM, PhD, DACVS
University of Minnesota
College of Veterinary Medicine
1352 Boyd Avenue
Saint Paul, MN 50010
Pages: 1105-1107

John E. Cooper, DTVM, FRCPath, FIBiol, FRCVS, DECVP
The University of the West Indies
School of Veterinary Medicine
St Augustine, Trinidad & Tobago
WEST INDIES
Pages: 1903-1911

Margaret Cooper, LLB, FLS
The University of the West Indies
School of Veterinary Medicine
St Augustine, Trinidad and Tobago
WEST INDIES
Pages: 1724-1726

C. Guillermo Couto, DVM, DACVIM
The Ohio State University
College of Veterinary Medicine
601 Vernon L Tharp Street
Columbus, OH 43210
Pages: 425-432

Rick L. Cowell, DVM, MS, MRCVS, DACVP
1617 S. Hillside St.
Stillwater, OK 74074-2007
Pages: 299-302

Larry Cowgill, DVM, PhD, DACVIM
University of California-Davis
School of Veterinary Medicine
Davis, CA 95616
Pages: 738-741

Sharon Crowell-Davis, DVM, PhD, DACVB
University of Georgia
College of Veterinary Medicine
Athens, GA 30602-7382
Pages: 140

Mark W. Cunningham, DVM, MS
Florida Fish and Wildlife Conservation Commission
4005 South Main Street
Gainesville, FL 32601-9099
Pages: 1881-1883

Jenise C. Daigle, DVM, DACVD
10500 Avery Club Drive #25
Austin, TX 78717
Pages: 363-369; 1081-1083

Douglas J. DeBoer, DVM, DACVD
University of Wisconsin-Madison
School of Veterinary Medicine
2015 Linden Drive
Madison, WI 53706
Pages: 370-382; 411

Loic M. Dejardin, DVM, MS, DACVS
Michigan State University
College of Veterinary Medicine
East Lansing, MI 48824-1314
Pages: 988-999

Jennifer Demko, DVM
Mississippi State University
College of Veterinary Medicine
PO Box 6100
Mississippi State, MS 39762-6100
Pages: 1000-1002

Orlando Diaz-Figueroa, DVM, MS, DABVP
Lake Howell Animal Clinic
856 Lake Howell Rd
Maitland, FL 32708
Pages:1743-1751

Ray Dillon, DVM, MS, MBA, DACVIM
Auburn University
College of Veterinary Medicine
Auburn University, AL 36849
Pages: 1139-1145

Donna Dimski, DVM, MS, DACVIM
444 B Street
Springfield, OR 97477
Pages: 433-435; 527-530; 575-580; 873

Constance DiNatale, DVM
Veterinary Acupuncture and Complementary Therapy
742 Clay Street
Winter Park, FL 32789
Pages: 23-26

Johnathon Dodd, DVM, FAVD, DAVDC
Texas A&M University
College of Veterinary Medicine
4474 TAMU
College Station, TX 77845
Pages: 336-340

Amanda L. Donnelly, DVM, MBA
ALD Veterinary Consulting
1705 Curlew Court
Rockledge, FL 32955
Pages: 1184-1200

Tracy Dowdy, CVPM
Management Resource Group
704 Cabernet Court
Grapevine, TX 76051
Pages: 1201-1209

Louise Dunn
Snowgoose Veterinary Management
Consulting
12 Snowgoose Cove
Greensboro, NC 27455
Pages: 1170-1171; 1210-1211

**Janice A. Dye, DVM, MS, PhD,
DACVIM**
103 Ivy Hollow Ct.
Morrisville, NC 27560
Pages: 1416-1425

M. Scott Echols, DVM, DABVP
Westgate Pet and Bird Hospital
4534 Westgate Blvd, Suite 100
Austin, TX 78745
Pages: 1641-1659

**Christine Egger, DVM MVSc, CVA,
CVH, DACVA**
University of Tennessee
College of Veterinary Medicine
2407 River Road
Knoxville, TN 37996
Pages: 93-109

Erick Egger, DVM, DACVS
Colorado State University
College of Veterinary Medicine
Fort Collins, CO 80523
Pages: 1003-1015

Beate Egner, Dr. med. vet.
Poelser Str 10
Mainhausen D-63533
GERMANY
Pages: 188-191

Nicole Ehrhart, VMD, MS, DACVS
Colorado State University
Animal Cancer Center
300 W Drake Street
Fort Collins, CO 80528
Pages: 874-888

**Denise A. Elliott, BVSc, PhD,
DACVIM, DACVN**
Royal Canin USA
500 Fountain Lakes Blvd. Suite #100
St. Charles, MO 63301
Pages: 813-814

Gary Ellison, DVM, MS, DACVS
University of Florida
College of Veterinary Medicine
PO Box 100126
Gainesville, FL 32610
Pages: 815-817; 1526-1534

Christian Epe, Dr.med.vet., DEVPC
Novartis
Novartis Centre de Recherche
Sante Animale SA
Saint-Aubin FR CH - 1566
SWITZERLAND
Pages: 1146-1149

Donald Erceg
Vetmark
4240 SW Melville Ave
Portland, OR 97239
Pages: 1212-1227

Amara Estrada, DVM, DACVIM
University of Florida
College of Veterinary Medicine
Box 100126
Gainesville, FL 32610
Pages: 192-197

Valerie A. Fadok, DVM, PhD, DACVD
Gulf Coast Veterinary Dermatology and
Allergy
4402 Phil Street
Bellaire, TX 77401
Pages: 383-385

Byron S. Farquer, DVM
Simmons & Associates
11737 26 Mile Road
Oakdale, CA 95361
Pages: 1212-1227

**Andrea Fascetti, VMD, PhD, DACVIM,
DACVN**
University of California-Davis
Dept. of Molecular Biosciences
One Shields Ave.
Davis, CA 95616-8741
Pages: 818-821

Karen Faunt, DVM, MS, DACVIM
Banfield the Pet Hospital
8000 NE Tillamook
Portland, OR 97213
Pages: 110-113

**Karen E. Felsted, CPA, MS, DVM,
CVPM**
Gatto McFerson CPAs
528 Arizona Avenue, Suite 201
Santa Monica, CA 90401
Pages: 1228-1240

Brad Fenwick, DVM, PhD, DACVM
University of Tennessee
Vice Chancellor for Research
535 Andy Holt Tower
Knoxville, TN 24061
Pages: 1565-1567

Gregory J. Fleming, DVM, DACZM
Disney's Animal Kingdom
Veterinary Services
PO Box 10,000
Lake Buena Vista, FL 32830
Pages:1912-1913

**Neil A. Forbes, BVetMed, FRCVS,
DECAMS**
Great Western Referrals
Unit 10-14 Berkshire House
Country Park Estate, Shrivenham Rd
Swindon, Wilts SN1 2NR
UNITED KINGDOM
Pages: 1660-1674

**Richard B. Ford, DVM, MS,
CACVIM, DACVPM**
North Carolina State University
College of Veterinary Medicine
4700 Hillsborough Street
Raleigh, NC 27606
Pages: 649-656

**Barbara Fougere, BS, BVMS, BHSc,
MODT, MHSc, CVA, CVCP, CVBM**
All Natural Vet Care
292 Lyons Road
Russell Lea, NSW
AUSTRALIA
Pages: 27-50

**Philip R. Fox, DVM,
DACVIM/ECVIM, ACVECC**
Animal Medical Center
510 East 62nd Street
New York, NY 10021
Pages: 198-200

**Frederic P. Gaschen, PD,
Dr.Med.Vet, DACVIM, DECVIM-CA**
Louisiana State University
School of Veterinary Medicine
Baton Rouge, LA 70803-8410
Pages: 531-533

**James A. Gaynor, DVM, MS,
DACVA, DAAPM**
Animal Anesthesia and Pain
Management Center
5520 N Nevada Avenue
Suite 150
Colorado Springs, CO 80918
Pages: 1016; 1108-1112; 1568-1569

David B. Gerber, DVM, BA
Simmons & Associates Northwest
1040 N 23rd Street
Coeur d' Alene, ID 83814
Pages: 1241-1249

Alex German, BVSc, PhD, DECVIM
University of Liverpool
Small Animal Teaching Hospital
Chester High Road
Neston, Wirral, CH64 7TE   L7 7EX
UNITED KINGDOM
Pages: 822-825

Urs Giger, PD, Dr.med.vet, MS, DACVIM, DEVIM, DECVIM
University of Pennsylvania
School of Veterinary Medicine
3850 Spruce Street
Philadelphia, PA   19104-6010
Pages: 567-568

Kirsten Gilardi, DVM, DACZM
University of California-Davis
Wildlife Health Center
One Shields Avenue
Davis, CA   95616
Pages: 1884-1886

Gary I. Glassman, CPA
Burzenski & Company, P.C.
176 Bartlett Drive
Madison, CT   06512
Pages: 1250-1268

Richard E. Goldstein, DVM, DACVIM, DECVIM-CA
Cornell University
College of Veterinary Medicine
Ithaca, NY   14853
Pages: 688-690

Sonya G. Gordon, BSc, DVM, DVSc, DACVIM
Texas A&M University
College of Veterinary Medicine
College Station, TX   77843-4474
Pages: 201-204

Louis Gotthelf, DVM
Animal Hospital of Montgomery
3310 Atlanta Highway
Montgomery, AL   36109
Pages: 1084-1088

Greg Grauer, DVM, MS, DACVIM
Kansas State University
College of Veterinary Medicine
111B Mosier Hall
Manhattan, KS   66506
Pages: 205-207; 742-747

Thomas K. Graves, DVM, PhD, DACVIM
University of Illinois
College of Veterinary Medicine
1008 Hazelwood Drive
Urbana, IL   61801
Pages: 436-440

Deborah S. Greco, DVM, PhD, DACVIM
Nestle Purina PetCare
Checkerboard Square - 8T
St Louis, MO   63164
Pages: 441-444

Henry W. Green, III, DVM, DACVIM
Purdue University
School of Veterinary Medicine
625 Harrison Street
West Lafayette, IN   47907
Pages: 208-226

Lisa Greenhill, BA, MPA
Association of American Veterinary
Medical Colleges
101 Vermont Avenue, NW, Suite 301
Washington, DC   20005-3536
Pages: 621-626

Brenda Griffin, DVM, MS, DACVIM
Cornell University
College of Veterinary Medicine
Ithaca, NY   14850
Pages: 1479-1485

Gary Guccione
National Greyhound Assn.
P O Box 543
Abilene, KS   67410
Pages: 1570-1571

James E. Guenther, DVM, MBA, MHA, CVPM
Brakke Veterinary Practice Management
Group
P.O. Box 19642
Asheville, NC   28815
Pages: 1269-1275

Edward J. Guiducci, JD
Guiducci & Guiducci, PC
1623 Race Street
Denver, CO   80206
Pages: 1276-1289

Timothy Hackett, DVM, MS, DACVECC
Colorado State University
James L. Voss Veterinary
Medical Center
300 West Drake Road
Fort Collins, CO   80523
Pages: 260-267

John W. Harvey, DVM/PhD, DACVP
University of Florida
College of Veterinary Medicine
Box 100144
Gainesville, FL   32610
Pages: 303-310; 313-318

Eleanor C. Hawkins, DVM, DACVIM(SAIM)
North Carolina State University
College of Veterinary Medicine
4700 Hillsborough Street
Raleigh, NC   27606
Pages: 1413-1415; 1426-1449

Stephen J. Hernandez-Divers, BVetMed, DZooMed, MRCVS, DACZM
University of Georgia
College of Veterinary Medicine,
Athens, GA   30602
Pages: 1752-1776

Ian G. Holsworth, BSc, BVSc, MACVSc, DACVS
Veterinary Medical and
Surgical Group (VMSG)
2199 Sperry Avenue
Ventura, CA   93003
Pages: 1017-1022; 1572-1574

Debra Horwitz, DVM, DACVB
Veterinary Behavior Consultations
11469 Olive Blvd. #254
St. Louis, MO   63141-7108
Pages: 141-144

Kate F. Hurley, DVM, MPVM
704 Adeline Place
Davis, CA   95616
Pages: 691-693

Peter J. Ihrke, VMD, DACVD
University of California
School of Veterinary Medicine
One Shields Avenue
Davis, CA   95616-9737
Pages: 386-404

John F. Innes, BVSc, PhD, CertVR, DSAS, MRCVS
University of Liverpool
Small Animal Teaching Hospital,
Leahurst
Neston, Wirral   L7 7EX
UNITED KINGDOM
Pages: 1023-1039

Charles Innis, VMD
New England Aquarium
40 Woodridge Road
Milford, MA   01757
Pages: 1777-1792

Cathy A. Johnson-Delaney, BS, DVM, DABVP
Eastside Avian &
Exotic Animal Medical Center
13603 100th Avenue NE
Kirkland, WA   98034
Pages: 1809-1823

Russell Kelley, MS
6571 St. Rt. 503 N.
PO Box 189
Lewisburg, OH 45338
Pages: 1575-1576

Michael S. Kent, MAS, DVM, DACVIM, DACVR
University of California, Davis
Veterinary Medical Teaching Hosp
One Shields Avenue
Davis, CA 95616
Pages: 889-898

Kerry L. Ketring, DVM, DACVO
All Animal Eye Clinic
11913 Montgomery Road
Cincinnati, OH 45249
Pages: 933-944

David F. King, DVM, BS
Simmons Southcentral
9084 FM 2451
Scurry, TX 75158
Pages: 1241-1249

Claudia A. Kirk, DVM, PhD, DACVN, DACVIM
University of Tennessee
Deparatment of Small Animal
Clinical Sciences
2407 River Drive
Knoxville, TN 37996
Pages: 826-836

Kate Knutson, DVM
Pet Crossing Animal Hosp & Dental
Clinic
10861 Bloomington Ferry Road
Bloomington, MN 55438
Pages: 1174-1175

Sheryl G. Krohne, DVM, MS, DACVO
Purdue Veterinary Teaching Hospital
Purdue University - SVM
625 Harrison Street
West Lafayette, IN 47907
Pages: 945-948

Elise M. Lacher, CPA
Lacher, McDonald & Co., CPA
5666 Seminole Blvd
Seminole, FL 33772
Pages: 1170-1171; 1290-1299

Charlotte Lacroix, DVM, JD
Veterinary Business Advisors, Inc.
24 Coddington Road
Whitehouse Station, NJ 08889
Pages: 1293-1316

William R. Lance, DVM, MS, DACZM
Wildlife Pharmaceuticals Inc
PO Box 2023
Fort Collins, CO 80522
Pages: 1914-1917

Gary Landsberg, BSc, DVM, MRCVS, DACVB
Self employed - Doncaster Animal Clinic
99 Henderson Avenue
Thornhill, ON L3T 2K9
CANADA
Pages: 145-150

B. Duncan Lascelles, BSc, BVSc, PhD, MRCVS, CertVA, DSAS(ST), DECVS, ACVS
NCSU College of Veterinary Medicine
College of Veterinary Medicine
4700 Hillsborough Street
Raleigh, NC 27606
Pages: 1040; 1113-1124

Justine A. Lee, DVM, DACVECC
University of Minnesota
College of Veterinary Medicine
C339 VMC 1365 Gortner Avenue
St. Paul, MN 55108
Pages: 268-276

Angela M. Lennox, DVM, DABVP(Avian)
Avian and Exotic Animal
    Clinic of Indianapolis
9330 Waldemar Road
Indianapolis, IN 46268
Pages: 1824-1831; 1840-1850

Julie Levy, DVM, PhD, DACVIM
University of Florida
2015 SW 16th Ave
Gainesville, FL 32610
Pages: 1481-1487

Steven A. Levy, VMD
Durham Veterinary Hospital
Durham Veterinary Hospital
178 Parmelee Hill Road
Durham, CT 06422
Pages: 1150-1153

Marla Lichtenberger, DVM, DACVECC
Thousand Oaks Pet emregency clinic
11015 N Mequon Square Drive
Mequon, WI 53092
Pages: 1675-1684; 1832-1850

Susan E. Little, DVM, PhD, DEVPC
Oklahoma State University
Room 250 McElroy Hall
Oklahoma State University
Stillwater, OK 74078
Pages: 1154-1162

Meryl P. Littman, VMD, DACVIM
University of Pennsylvania
School of Veterinary Medicine
3900 Delancey St.
Philadelphia, PA 19104-6010
Pages: 319-328; 694-707

Heidi B. Lobprise, DVM, DAVDC
Pfizer Animal Health
851 Lake Carolyn Parkway #241
Irving, TX 75039
Pages: 341-346

Randall Lockwood, PhD
ASPCA
2214 Tulip Drive
Falls Church, VA 22046
Pages: 501-509

Jody P. Lulich, DVM, PhD, DACVIM
Dept of Veterinary Clinical Sciences
1352 Boyd Ave
University Of Minnesota
St. Paul, MN 55108
Pages: 748-753

Ron Lyman, DVM, DACVIM
Animal Emergency and Referral
Center
3984 South US 1
Ft Pierce, FL 34982
Pages: 711-715

Carlos Macias, LdoVet, DSAS, MRCVS, RCVS
Parque Empresarial Laurotorre 25
Alhaurin de la Torre
Malaga 29130
SPAIN
Pages: 1041-1048

Dennis W. Macy, DVM, MS, DACVIM
Colorado State University
A208 James L Voss - VTH
Fort Collins, CO 80523
Pages: 899-901

Denis Marcellin-Little, DEDV, DACVS, ECVS, CCRP
North Carolina State University
College of Veterinary Medicine
4700 Hillsborough St
Raleigh, NC 27606
Pages: 1049-1052

Stanley L. Marks, BVSc, PhD, DACVIM, DACVN
University of California, Davis
School of Veterinary Medicine
Dept. of Medicine & Epidemiology
Davis, CA 95616
Pages: 534-544; 837-839

Steven L. Marks, BVSc, MS, MRCVS, DACVIM
North Carolina State University
Dept. of Vet. Clinical Medicine
4700 Hillsborough
Raleigh, NC 27606
Pages: 277-279

Glenna E. Mauldin, DVM, MS, DACVIM, DACVN
Western Veterinary Specialist Centre
 Calgary, Alberta, Canada
1802-10th Avenue SW
Calgary, AB 70803
CANADA
Pages: 840-842; 902-911

Joerg Mayer, Drvetmed, MSc
Tufts University
Cummings School of Veterinary
Medicine
200 Westboro Road
North Grafton, MA 01536
Pages: 1851-1860

Laurie McCauley, DVM
TOPS Veterinary Rehabilitation
1440 E Belvidere Rd
Grayslake, AL 33414
Pages: 1577-1579

Ron McLaughlin, DVM, DVSc, DACVS
Mississippi State University
College of Veterinary Medicine
Mississippi State, MS 39762
Pages: 1580-1582

Richard Meadows, DVM, DABVP
University of Missouri
College of Veterinary Medicine
Clydesdale Hall 900 E Campus Drive
Columbia, MO 65211
Pages: 627-629

Lloyd S. Meisels, DVM
Hospital Director
Coral Springs Animal Hospital
1730 University Dr.
Coral Springs, FL 33071
Pages: 1317-1325

Patrick Melese, MA, DVM, DACVB
Veterinary Behavior Consultants
4824 Brookburn Drive
San Diego, CA 92130
Pages: 151-153

Melinda Merck, DVM
6175 Hickory Flat Hwy
Suite 110-233
Canton, GA 30115
Pages: 510-515

Christine Merle, DVM, MBA, CVPM
Brakke Consulting, Inc
9280 Greenthread Lane
Zionsville, IN 46077
Pages: 1326-1333

Lila T. Miller, BS, DVM
ASPCA
710 Riverside Dr. Apt. 3B
New York, NY 10031
Pages: 630-634

Darryl L. Millis, DVM, MS, DACVS, CCRP
8309 Birch Run Lane
Knoxville, TN 37919
Pages: 1053-1055; 1583-1585

Deborah Mitchell, DVM, MS
Knollwood Hospital for Pets
2237 W. Schaumburg Rd.
Schaumburg, IL 60194
Pages: 51-77

N. Sydney Moise, DVM, MS, DACVIM
Cornell University
College of Veterinary Medicine
Ithaca, NY 14853
Pages: 227-238

Eric Monnet, DVM, PhD, FAHA, DACVS, DECVS
Colorado State University
Department of Clinical Sciences
300 W. Drake Road
Fort Collins, CO 80523
Pages: 485-487; 843-845; 1535-1547

Claude T. Moorman, MD
Duke University
DUMC 3639
Durham, NC 27710
Pages: 1056-1057

James K. Morrisey, DVM, DABVP
Cornell University
College of Veterinary Medicine
Clinical Sciences
New York, NY 14853
Pages: 1861-1862

Wallace B. Morrison, DVM, MS, DACVIM
Purdue University
Lynn Hall, SVM, Room G-578
625 Harrison Street
West Lafayette, IN 47907-2026
Pages: 912-921

Ralf S. Mueller, DVM, PhD, FACVSc, DACVD, DECVD
Ludwig Maximilian University Munich
Veterinaestr. 13
Muenchen 80539
GERMANY
Pages: 405-412

Hayley Weston Murphy, DVM
Zoo New England
Zoo New England
1 Franklin Park Road
Boston, MA 02121
Pages: 1917-1927

Rafael Nickel, DVM, PhD, DECVS
Tierarztliche Klinik fur Kleintiere
Kabels Stieg 41
Nordstedt 22850
GERMANY
Pages: 754-760; 922

Will Novak, DVM, DABVP
Banfield, The Pet Hospital
8000 NE Tillamook
Portland, OR 97213
Pages: 114-119

James Noxon, DVM, DACVIM
Iowa State University
Veterinary Teaching Hospital
College of Veterinary Medicine, ISU
Ames, IA 50011
Pages: 1089-1092

James T. O'Connor, B.S., Marketing
Egan, Amato & O'Connor
2421 Atlantic Avenue
Manasquan, NJ 08736
Pages: 1334-1336

Gerhard U. Oechtering, Prof. Dr.vet.med, DECVAA
University of Leipzig
Department of Small Animal Medicine
University of Leipzig
Leipzig D-04103
GERMANY
Pages: 760; 1450-1455; 1548

Susan Orosz, PhD,DVM, DAPVP, DECAMS
Bird & Exotic Pet Wellness Center
5166 Monroe Street, #305
Toledo 43623
Pages: 1685; 1693-1698

Jerome S. Osteryoung, PhD
Florida State University
2912 Brandemere Drive
Tallahassee, FL 32306
Pages: 1336-1357

Karen Overall, MS, VMD, PhD, DACVB
Center for Neurobiology and Behavior
Penn Med - Psychiatry
10 County Lane
Center for Neurobiology and Behavior -
Penn Med; TRL; 125S
30th St., Philadelphia, PA 19104
Glen Mills, PA 19342
Pages: 154-169

Luisito S. Pablo, DVM, MS, DACVA
University of Florida
Department of Large Animal Clinical
 Sciences
Box 100136
Gainesville, FL 32610-0136
Pages: 1586-1591

Ross Palmer, DVM, MS, DACVS
Colorado State University
Vet Med Teaching Hospital
300 West Drake Rd
Fort Collins, CO 80523
Pages: 1058-1068; 1125

Mark G. Papich, DVM, MS, DACVCP
North Carolina State University
College of Veterinary Medicine
4700 Hillsborough Street
Raleigh, NC 27606
Pages: 657-659

R. Michael Peak, DVM, DAVDC
Tampa Bay Veterinary Dentistry, Inc.
1501-A Belcher Road S.
Largo, FL 33771
Pages: 1592-1595

Simon R. Platt, BVM&S, MRCVS, DACVIM
University of Georgia
College of Veterinary Medicine
Dept of Small Animal Med & Surgery
501 DW Brooks Drive
Athens, GA 30602-7390
Pages: 646-647; 776-791

Lysa Pam Posner, DVM, DACVA
North Carolina State University
4700 Hillsborough Street
College of Veterinary Medicine
Raleigh, NC 27606
Pages: 10-129; 1126-1128

Antonio Pozzi, DVM, MS, DACVS
University of Florida
2015 SW 16th Ave.
PO Box 100105
Gainesville, FL 32610
Pages: 1069-1073; 1596-1597

David T. Ramsey, DVM, DACVO
The Animal Ophthalmology Center
1300 W Grand River Avenue
Williamston, MI 48895
Pages: 949-958

Alan H. Rebar, DVM, PhD, DACVP
Purdue University
Discovery Park
Hovde Hall, 610 Purdue Mall
West Lafayette, IN 47907-2040
Pages: 311-318

Helen E. Roberts, DVM
5 Corners A H/Aquatic Veterinary Serv
2799 Southwestern Blvd, Suite 100
Orchard Park, NY 14127
Pages: 1616-1628

Sheilah Ann Robertson, BVMS, PhD
University of Florida
3522 NW 23rd Place
Gainesville, FL 32605
Pages: 1129-1131

Margo Roman, DVM
MASH Main St Animal Services of
 Hopkinton
72 West Street
Hopkinton, MA 01748
Pages: 78-80

John Rossmeisl, Jr., DVM, MS, DACVIM
VA-MD Regional College of Veterinary
Medicine
Department of Small Animal Clinical
Sciences
Blacksburg, VA 24061
Pages: 792-808

Rod A.W. Rosychuk, DVM, DACVIM
Colorado State University
Department of Clinical Sciences
300 W. Drake Road
Ft. Collins, CO 80523
Pages: 413-416; 1093-1104

Elizabeth Rozanski, DVM, DACVIM(SA), ACVECC
Tufts University
School of Veterinary Medicine
200 Westboro Road
North Grafton, MA 01536
Pages: 1456-1469

Karl R. Salzsieder, DVM, JD
Salzsieder Consulting and Legal SVC
611 Cowlitz Way W, Suite B
Kelso, WA 98626
Pages: 1358-1368

Sherry Lynn Sanderson, DVM, PhD, DACVIM, DACVN
University of Georgia
College of Veterinary Medicine
Athens, GA 30602
Pages: 846-848

Michael Schaer, DVM, DACVIM, DACVECC
University of Florida
College of Veterinary Medicine
Box 100126
Gainesville, FL 32610-0126
Pages: 280-299; 445-446; 660-662; 716-719

Margie Scherk, DVM, DABVP
Cats Only Veterinary Clinic
2578 Burrard Street
Vancouver, BC V6J 3J7
CANADA
Pages: 761-764

Nico J. Schoemaker, DVM, PhD, DECAMS, DABVP
Div. of Avian & Exotic Animals
Yalelaan 108
Utrecht 3584 CM
NETHERLANDS
Pages: 1863-1879

Rhonda L. Schulman, DVM, DACVIM
2610 Lambert Dr
Pasadena, CA 85718
Pages: 447-458; 765-767; 1470-1473

J. Catharine Scott-Moncrieff, MA, MS, VetMB, DACVIM, DECVIM
Purdue University
VCS, Lynn
625 Harrison Street
West Lafayette, IN 47907-2026
Pages: 459-476

Kersti Seksel, BVSc, MRCVS, MA, FACVSc, DACVB, CMAVA
Sydney Animal Behaviour Service
PO Box 276
Seaforth , NSW 2092
AUSTRALIA
Pages: 170-181

Margaret R. Slater, DVM, PhD
Texas A&M University
College of Veterinary Medicine
Department of Veterinary Integrative
 Biosciences
College Station, TX 77843
Pages: 1488-1490

Jonathan Sleeman, MA, VetMB, DACZM
Virginia Department of Game
4010 West Broad St.
Richmond, VA 23230
Pages: 1887-1898

Stephen A. Smith, MS, DVM, PhD
VMRCVM, Virginia Tech
Virginia-Maryland Regional
College of Veterinary Medicine
Duck Pond Drive, Virginia Tech (0442)
Pages: 1629-1640

Terry R. Spraker, DVM, PhD, DACVP
College of Veterinary Medicine
Diagnostic Laboratories
300 West Drake Road
Ft. Collins, CO 80523
Pages: 1899-1901

Jörg M. Steiner, DVM, PhD, DACVIM, DECVIM-CA
Texas A&M University
College of Vet Med & Biomedical
  and Biomedical Sciences
4474 TAMU
College Station, TX 77843
Pages: 545-552; 581-584

Rebecca L. Stepien, DVM. MS, DACVIM
University of Wisconsin
School of Veterinary Medicine
2015 Linden Drive West
Madison, WI 53706-1102
Pages: 239-241

Mark Stetter, DVM, DACZM
Disney's Animal Kingdom
PO Box 10000
Lake Buena Vista, FL 32830-1000
Pages: 1928-1929

Jean Stiles, MS, DVM, DACVO
Purdue University
School of Veterinary Sciences
625 Harrison Street
West Lafayette, IN 47907
Pages: 959-961

Steven F. Swaim, DVM, MS
Auburn University – Professor
Emeritus
1873 East 90th Street South
Geuda Springs, KS 67051
Pages: 1604-1608

John Symes, DVM
Beltline Animal Hospital
1212 W. I-65 Service Road South
Mobile, AL 36609
Pages: 81-90

Joseph Taboada, DVM, DACVIM
Louisiana State University
Office of Student & Academic Affairs
School of Veterinary Medicine
Baton Rouge, LA 70803
Pages: 477-480

Todd R. Tams, DVM, DACVIM
VCA Antech
12401 West Olympic Blvd
Los Angeles, CA 90064
Pages: 488-491; 553-554

Terry Terlep, DVM
13801 River Road
Fort Myers, FL 33905
Pages: 1598-1599

Mark Tetrick, DVM, PhD
The Iams Company
6571 State Route 503 N
Lewisburg, OH 45338
Page: 849

Carvel Tiekert, DVM
Abingdon Veterinary Clinic
2404 Laurel Bush Road
Abingdon, MD 21009
Pages: 91-92; 555-558

D. Michael Tillson, DVM, MS, DACVS
Auburn University
College of Veterinary Medicine
Department of Clinical Sciences
Hoerlein Hall, CVM
Auburn, AL 36849
Pages: 130-131; 1549-1563

Richard Timmins, DVM
University of California – Davis
School of Veterinary Medicine
P. O Box 72067
Davis, CA 95617
Pages: 35-637

Todd L. Towell, DVM, MS, DACVIM
Hill's Pet Nutrition, Inc
1452 Northridge Drive
Erie, CO 66601
Pages: 850-852

Amy Trejo, PhD
P&G Personal HealthCare
8700 Mason-Montgomery Road
DV3 - 3MI
Mason, OH 45240
Page: 853

Denise L. Tumblin, CPA
Wutchiett Tumblin and Associates
3200 Riverside Drive
Columbus, OH 43221
Pages: 1369-1385

David C. Twedt, DVM, DACVIM
Colorado State University
Dept. of Clinical Sciences
300 West Drake Road
Ft. Collins, CO 80523
Pages: 492-494; 585-587

Lee Tyner, MS, DVM
Mississippi State University
PO Box 6100
Mississippi State, MS 39762-6100
Pages: 132-139

David Vail, BSc, DVM, MS, DACVIM
University of Wisconsin-Madison
School of Veterinary Medicine
4270a Veterinary Med Bldg
2015 Linden Drive
Madison, WI 53706
Pages: 923-926

Laura Wade, DVM, DABVP
Broadway Veterinary Clinic, PC
5915 Broadway
Lancaster 14086
Pages: 1699-1719

Donald R. Waldron, DVM, DACVS, ABVP
Virginia Tech
VA-MD Regional College of VetMed
Blacksburg, VA
Pages: 1609-1612

Mark C. Walker, BVSc, MACVSc, DACVIM
North Florida Veterinary Specialists
1636 Challen Avenue
Jacksonville, FL 32073
Pages: 495-499

Ernest E. Ward, Jr., DVM
Seaside Animal Care, PA,
  E3 Management, Inc.
9256 Beach Drive SW
Calabash, NC 28467
Pages: 1074-1075; 1386-1397

Robert J. Washabau, VMD, PhD, DACVIM
University of Minnesota
1352 Boyd Avenue
College of Veterinary Medicine
St Paul, MN 55108
Pages: 559-561

David J. Waters, DVM, PhD, DACVS
Purdue University
G.P. Murphy Cancer Foundation
Gerald P Murphy Cancer Foundation
3000 Kent Ave., Suite E2-100
West Lafayette, IN 47906
Pages: 927-929

Alistair Webb, PhD, BVSc, FRCVS, DACVA
University of Florida
College of Veterinary Medicine
Box 100144
Gainesville, FL   32610-0144
Pages: 1163-1166

Jeffrey Werber, DVM
Century Veterinary Group
Pet Nation Pet Products
8750 Venice Blvd
Los Angeles, CA   90034
Pages 1398-1404

Jodi Westropp, DVM, PhD, DACVIM
University of California, Davis
School of Veterinary Medicine
Dept of Medicine & Epidemiology
3101 Tupper Hall
Davis, CA   95616
Pages: 768-71

Wendy Wheeler, MA
BDA Architecture, P.C.
901 Lamberton Place, NE
Albuquerque, NM   87107
Pages: 612-620

Christine Wilford, DVM
1) Feral Cat Spay/Neuter Project;
2) Cats Exclusive Veterinary Center
2609 NW 96th St.
Seattle, WA
Pages 1491-1493

Alice M. Wolf, DVM, DACVIM, DABVP
8232 McCarver Lane
Bryan, TX   77808
Pages: 663-665; 708-709

Hal F. (Fritz) Wood, BS, CPA, CFP®
H F Wood Consulting
520 Terrace Trail East
Lake Quivira, KS   66217
Pages: 1405-1411

Kevin Wright, DVM
Arizona Exotic Animal Hospital
1042 North Dresden Street
Mesa, AZ   85203
Pages: 1793-1808

Susan G. Wynn, DVM
University of Tennessee
334 Knollwood Lane
Woodstock, TN   30188
Pages: 854-866

Debra L. Zoran, DVM, PhD, DACVIM
Texas A&M University
3942 Parrot Cove
College Station, TX   77845-8181
Pages: 562-566; 867-871

TABLE OF CONTENTS
Small Animal Book 2: Pages 963-1930

i

BEHAVIOR

CARDIOLOGY

CRITICAL CARE

CYTOLOGY & DIAGNOSTICS

DENTISTRY

DERMATOLOGY

MISCELLANEOUS

NEPHROLOGY & UROLOGY

NEUROLOGY

ONCOLOGY

OPHTHALMOLOGY

OTITIS

PAIN MANAGEMENT

RESPIRATORY DISEASE

SHELTER MEDICINE

SOFT TISSUE SURGERY

EXOTICS

WILDLIFE

ZOOLOGICAL MEDICINE

HIP DYSPLASIA IN DOGS: WHAT IS THE BEST TREATMENT?

J.F. Bardet, DVM, MS, Diplomate ECVS
Small Animal Referral Center
Neuilly sur Seine, France

GENERAL CONSIDERATIONS

The causes of hip dysplasia are multifactorial; both hereditary and environmental factors play a part in the development of abnormal bone and soft tissue. However, hereditary factors are the primary determining factors. Rapid weight gain and growth through excessive nutritional intake may cause a disparity of development of supporting soft tissue, contributing to hip dysplasia.

Treatment depends on the patient's age and degree of discomfort, physical radiographic and arthroscopic findings and client's expectations and finances. Conservative and surgical options are available for juvenile and mature animals with hip pain secondary to hip dysplasia. Although early surgical intervention may increase the prognosis for long-term acceptable clinical function, approximately 50% of young patients treated conservatively return to acceptable clinical function with maturity. The remainder requires further medical or surgical management. Surgery is indicated in older patients when conservative treatment is not effective or when athletic performance is desired or the owner wishes to slow the progression of degenerative joint disease (DJD) and enhance the probability of good long-term limb function. However, the choice of the best treatment is based on the proper preoperative evaluation of the hip joint using the clinical examination as well as diagnostic, imaging and hip arthroscopy in immature animals.

DIAGNOSTIC IMAGING

The standard radiographic view for diagnosis of hip dysplasia is the ventrodorsal view of the pelvis with rear limbs extended symmetrically and rotated inward to center the patellae over the trochlear grooves. The dog must be heavily sedated or anesthetized for proper relaxation and positioning. Stress radiographs can be used to detect breed susceptibility to hip dysplasia as early as 4 months (Penn Hip). A distraction index is calculated from these views and is used to predict the likelihood of development of DJD secondary to hip laxity. Individual logistic regression curves that predict the risk of the development of DJD have been developed for different breeds because it appears that some breeds are more "laxity tolerant" than others. Older dogs with established DJD do not require perfect positioning or special studies for a diagnosis of hip dysplasia.

Arthroscopy

Arthroscopy of the coxofemoral joint is relatively simple technique in juvenile dogs with significant hip laxity. Arthroscopy of juvenile hip dysplasia has been reported. Arthroscopy permits direct visualization of cartilage damage, ligament tearing, and damage to the acetabular labrum. Assessment of arthroscopic findings may be of assistance in decision making relative to the appropriateness of triple pelvic osteotomy (TPO) to the treatment of juvenile hip dysplasia; arthroscopic evidence of moderate or severe cartilage damage worsens the prognosis for success of a TPO. Thorough knowledge of hip joint anatomy is important, providing few palpable landmarks for instrumentation of the joint. In most cases, a long 2.7-mm arthroscope is necessary to reach the joint.

MEDICAL MANAGEMENT

Conservative treatment is divided into short and long-term phases. Complete rest is mandatory and must be enforced for 10 to 14 days.

Adjunct physical rehabilitation is helpful in maintaining range of motion and providing comfort during this period. Physical rehabilitation should concentrate on strengthening periarticular structures. Anti-inflammatory drugs are indicated to relieve pain. Clients must be advised to continue the rest period even if the patient appears to have returned to normal function. Administering NSAIDs, begin with the lowest possible therapeutic dosage and administer with small amounts of food.

Long-term conservative treatment for pain associated with DJD includes application of the five principles of medical management of osteoarthritis. Weight management is the single most important aspect of these principles. The animal should be weighed weekly and its caloric intake determined. Feeding bulk diets low in fat and protein may be beneficial. Nutritional supplementation, including omega-3 fatty acids and glucosamine/chondroitin, may be of benefit in many cases. Exercise (eg, swimming and long walks) is important to maintain an appropriate weight. High-intensity activity should be allowed only for short durations after an adequate warm-up period. Anti-inflammatory drugs should be administered only as needed and should not take the place of weight control and a moderate exercise program. Physical rehabilitation may involve sit-to-stand exercises and aquatic therapy, specifically on an underwater treadmill.

SURGICAL TREATMENT

In puppies less than 20 weeks of age, **juvenile pubic symphysiodesis** (JPS) may be performed to alter growth of the pelvis and degree of ventroversion of the acetabulum. Most puppies of this age do not show clinical signs of hip dysplasia, so diagnosis depends upon use of a screening technique, such as Penn Hip, to determine which animals may be candidates for the procedure. Although specific criteria for application of JPS have not been developed, puppies under 20 weeks of age that have palpable and radiographic evidence of laxity on a hip distracted view should be considered for the procedure. Risks of complications with the procedure are low and failure of the procedure to reduce hip subluxation does not preclude further surgical treatment in the future.

In immature dogs, a decision must be made early to perform **pelvic osteotomy** for maximum benefits, but this decision must be balanced against the observation that many dogs diagnosed with hip dysplasia at a young age do not have clinical signs at long-term follow-up. Pelvic osteotomy is useful in younger patients to axially rotate and lateralize the acetabulum in an effort to increase dorsal coverage of the femoral head. This procedure is indicated in patients leading athletic lives (ie, working breeds) or when the client wants to arrest or slow the progress of osteoarthritis. The most favorable prognosis for public osteotomy is in patients with (1) radiographic evidence of hip subluxation with minimal degenerative changes in conjunction with; (2) an angle of reduction less than 30 degrees and an angle of subluxation less than 10 degrees; (3) a solid feeling of reduction of the femoral head into the acetabulum; and (4) minimal cartilage damage as visualized on hip arthroscopy.

A canine pelvic osteotomy plate is the most effective method of obtaining axial rotation and acetabular lateralization.

Femoral Neck Lengthening has been described to improve the hip joint stability in dogs with short femoral neck and weak hip muscles. In these patients, the author prefers the use of a total hip prosthesis directly because of the excellent prognosis even in young dogs.

Intertrochanteric Varus Osteotomy of Femur. The true angle of inclination of the canine femoral neck in relation to the diaphysis is about 146 degrees. In animals with hip dysplasia, this angle increases as much as 30 to 35 degrees, leading to the condition known as coxa valga. This is caused by subluxation of the hip joint and subsequent lack of normal stress on the femoral neck, which is necessary for development of the normal angle. This valgus angle of the head and neck contributes to further subluxation and instability, perpetuating a vicious cycle. In addition, the femoral neck inclines farther cranially (anteversion) from the normal angle of about 27 degrees and again contributes to subluxation and instability. This condition is rarely seen but most frequently in giant breed dogs such as Great Danes and Pyrenees.

The principle of varus derotation for treatment of congenital hip luxation and instability is well established. By making the femoral neck more perpendicular to the femoral shaft (varisation) and reducing anteversion, the femoral head can be placed more deeply within the acetabulum.

The purpose of intertrochanteric osteotomy is to improve the biomechanics of the hip and to reduce hip pain. It is more effective when done before DJD is present, between the ages of 4 and 10 months in most patients.

Total hip replacement (THR) is a highly advanced procedure and should be performed only by experienced surgeons trained in this technique. Most commonly, THR is performed when medical management of osteoarthritis of the hip can no longer maintain function of the limb and quality of life of the patient. Generally, the use of the five principles of medical management should be exhausted before electing THR because of the costs, risks and complications of the surgery. Traditionally, THR is done as late in life as possible. This philosophy is based on the concept that a prosthetic joint replacement is in a constant state of degeneration and placement as late in life as possible diminishes the potential need to revise or replace the original hip prosthesis. Some owners and surgeons may elect hip replacement instead of medical management for patients with significant complications from NSAIDs or for clients who are extremely concerned with potential complications from NSAIDs. The advent of cementless THRs has also altered the philosophy of when THR is indicated. Since cementless prostheses are much less inclined to loosen with time, their use in younger patients is more common and acceptable. Correction of body weight may eliminate or delay the need for THR and will decrease the risks of complications when THR is performed.

Contraindications to THR include septic arthritis and significant or progressive neurologic disease. Sepsis of the coxofemoral joint, although rare, is an absolute contraindication to cemented THR. Cementless THRs have been used for the revision of septic loosening of cemented THRs.

Femoral head and neck excision limits contact between the femoral head and acetabulum and allows formation of a fibrous false joint. This procedure can be used when conservative treatment has failed, and when financial, medical, or size constraints preclude alternative methods of surgical intervention. Caution should be used in treating juvenile animals with this procedure because a significant percentage of them improve with maturity. Because fibrous pseudoarthrosis is an unstable joint, clinical function postoperatively is unpredictable. For this reason, most surgeons consider femoral head and neck excision to be a salvage procedure. However, many patients with painful arthritic hips undergoing femoral head and neck excision have improved limb function and quality of life postoperatively.

There are no specific weight guidelines for the use of femoral head and neck ostectomy (FHO). Although smaller patients routinely have better results than larger patients, this procedure may yet be indicated in large- and giant-breed dogs in which other treatments have been ineffective or are not feasible.

Many other techniques have been described such as pectineal myectomy, denervation of the hip joint capsule, darplasty, muscle transposition associated with femoral head and neck excision and many others! However, our goal is to provide to our patients and owners the best clinical result in relation their activity, severity of the dysplasia and finances.

DISEASES OF THE SHOULDER IN THE DOG AND CAT

J.F. Bardet, DVM, MS, Diplomate ECVS
Small Animal Referral Center
Neuilly sur Seine, France

Shoulder pain is one of the common causes of lameness in companion animals. In the past, localizing the pain to the shoulder rarely led to making a precise etiological diagnosis. In the absence of a sufficiently precise diagnostic method and objective clinical signs, it was difficult to pinpoint the origin of signs, which were rather subjective. Many cases of shoulder pain were treated symptomatically with steroidal or nonsteroidal anti-inflammatory drugs (NSAIDs), implicating either degenerative joint disease (DJD) or tenosynovitis of the biceps tendon. Chronic biciptal tenosynovitis has been considered the most common shoulder disease in the dog.[1,2] Occasionally, other chronic diseases of the shoulder in the dog were recognized: medial, lateral or craniocaudal luxation of the shoulder, calcification of the infraspinatus tendon, calcifying tendinopathy of the biceps tendon, medial luxation of the biceps tendon in racing Greyhound, contracture of the infraspinatous muscle,[1] DJD of the shoulder, and osteochondritis dissecans (OCD) of the humeral head. Until most recently, the clinician had to rely on the history and signalment, physical examination, radiology with or without arthrography, and, as a last resort, exploratory arthrotomy of the shoulder in order to make a precise diagnosis. The goal of this article is to review the diagnostic and therapeutic strategies for chronic disorders of the shoulder.

DIAGNOSTIC STRATEGIES

The clinician has to differentiate between shoulder lameness that is due to shoulder pathology and lameness which is secondary from another source. The shoulder is often the seat of an early manifestation of systemic pain because of its role as principal link between trunk and cranial extremity and the proximity to major neurovascular structures. The improvement of diagnostic tests like synovial fluid analysis, electromyography, nerve fiber conduction velocity testing, arthroscopy and CT scanner (computed tomography) have facilitated diagnosis of shoulder disorders. These techniques moreover have improved our understanding of shoulder disorders and associated pathology. The diseases associated with shoulder pain have been artificially divided into disorders involving periarticular structures, disorders of the glenohumeral joint and local or regional pathologies (Table 1). The choice of a given diagnostic test has to be made in accordance with case history and physical, orthopedic and neurological examinations of the patient. The case history and orthopedic exam are the most important criteria in establishing the diagnosis of shoulder pain. Radiography remains the first-choice ancillary procedure for detecting disorders of the shoulder joint. Unfortunately, radiography is not as sensitive as more sophisticated tests, but it allows to identify degenerative changes of the joint, presence of tumors, fractures, luxation and OCD lesions. When there is an intra-articular lesion or when one is suspected, arthroscopy is the procedure of choice because it allows to confirm and, at the same time, treat a great number of intra-articular pathologies. CT scan, MRI, and ultrasonography are frequently used in human medicine, but they are not as commonly available in veterinary practices. When an evident joint lesion can be ruled out, other ancillary procedures are recommended such as synovial fluid analysis, electromyography, nerve fiber conduction velocity testing and, in some cases, myelography; these tests allow to differentiate between lesions affecting the joint and other sources of pain such as lesions of neurologic origin.

SHOULDER DISEASES

Among the disorders of the glenohumeral joint, three diseases predominate: instability of the shoulder; OCD of the humeral head, and rupture of the biceps tendon. The other disorders are seen more rarely, but they will be discussed as well (Table 2). Understanding of the origin of shoulder lameness has been developed with the used of shoulder arthroscopy.

Instability of the Shoulder

The advent of arthroscopy was most helpful in evaluating the signs of shoulder instability. Shoulder instability appears as the most common shoulder disease in dogs. Chronic front limb lameness, which can be permanent or intermittent, is the major sign of instability. Most of the animals presented with varying degrees of lameness of several weeks up to several years duration. Chronicity is associated with atrophy of the shoulder muscle. In some cases lameness is non-weight-bearing with the animal manifesting its pain spontaneously. Others are presented for herniated cervical disks. In all cases, the physical and orthopedic examinations reveal pain on hyperextension of the shoulder joint as well as, in 85% of cases, a positive biceps tendon test. Shoulder instability is characterized by a mediolateral or craniocaudal drawer sign. Craniocaudal and mediolateral radiographic views of the shoulder demonstrate the presence of DJD in 57% of cases.

The diagnosis of shoulder instability is based upon a complete patient history, physical examination, orthopedic examination, and the orthopedic examination repeated under anesthesia followed by arthroscopy. In case of DJD and in the presence of chronic lameness of the shoulder in an adult dog, instability appears to be the most probable diagnosis. DJD is not a primary disease of the shoulder, but it is rather secondary to an intra-articular abnormality, the nature of which has to be determined separately. This is why utilizing arthroscopy allows one to determine more precisely the direction of the instability and the importance of intra-articular changes. Shoulder instability is evaluated by looking at such arthroscopic landmarks as the synovial membrane, articular cartilages, glenohumeral ligaments, labrum, biceps tendon, subscapular muscle, and joint capsule. The synovial membrane may show more or less pronounced inflammation (synovitis). Cartilaginous lesions are not pathognomonic unlike those lesions involving the glenohumeral ligaments or the labrum. In case of mediolateral instability of the shoulder, the medial glenohumeral ligament is overstretched and inefficient, torn, vestigial, or even absent. Lateral and caudo-lateral instabilities are characterized by tears or avulsion of the labrum. In fact the subscapular muscle located in the craniomedial region of the shoulder has a tendon which partially inserts inside of the scapulo-humeral cavity. This tendon can be inflamed or even more or less completely torn. In this way, arthroscopy allows us to distinguish between different types of shoulder instability, which can be easily recognized once inside the joint.

In the past lameness caused by shoulder instability were most often classified as DJD of the shoulder or as bicipital tenosynovitis. As in humans, only by studying intra-articular structures in situ, using more sophisticated technological means and recording the lesions on video has it become possible to understand this disease.

Osteochondrosis of the Shoulder Joint

Osteochondrosis is the most common shoulder disease in young, growing, large to giant breed dogs. Most of the dogs are between the ages of 5 months and 1 year but are sometimes older. These dogs present with lameness which is not responsive to NSAIDs. The diagnosis is based on case history, physical examination, and radiographs. Radiographic signs of osteochondrosis can be recognized on the mediolateral view. Treatment may be either conservative or surgical. Rare are those who would challenge the view that surgery of some kind, either arthrotomy or arthroscopy, is indicated. The author excises all lesions due to osteochondrosis via arthroscopy. Lesions due to osteochondritis dissecans, or OCD, lesions are characterized either by a fragment which is still attached to the articular cartilage via a thin strip, by numerous broken-off articular fragments following detachment of the flap within the joint, or, more rarely, by the puffy aspect of the cartilage which has not yet detached from the articular surface and the subchondral bone. In all cases, treating the lesions of osteochondrosis via arthroscopy consists of complete removal of the main fragment and the associated fragments, or joint mice. The joint mice have to be removed from the caudal and medial recesses within the joint and from the biceps tendon sheath. Recovery is rapid and both shoulders may be operated on the same day.

Biceps Tendon Lesions

In humans, the biceps tendon was for a long time the proverbial stepchild of the shoulder. It is described in human medicine as something fairly Machiavellian, easy to inculpate, but difficult to condemn! Its functions have been misunderstood for a long time. The tendon has been tenodesed, translocated, reinserted through a hole in the humerus, or surgically debrided during arthroscopy. The recent veterinary literature mainly describes chronic bicipital tenosynovitis, luxation of the medial biceps tendon, and calicifying biceps tendinopathy.

A recent study dealing with the diagnosis and classification of biceps tendon lesions relates 25 cases of lesions in 23 dogs and 1 cat. Lesions of the biceps tendon constitute the third most common shoulder disease. In fact, the most common disorder affecting the biceps tendon is linked to a partial or complete tear occurring directly at the level of insertion at the supraglenoid tubercle. Tears represent 21 out of 25 cases, or 84% of biceps tendon lesions and are systematically located in the intra-articular portion of the shoulder. As such, they are for the most part inaccessible when exploring the bicipital groove via a craniolateral surgical approach. Sixteen out of 25 biceps tendon lesions occur in association with tendinitis. All of the lesions of the biceps tendon are localized close to the supraglenoid tubercle or the zone of insertion which is considered a relatively avascular zone and much more susceptible to tendinitis and tearing. Only direct examination of the biceps tendon in its intra-articular position allows one to tell the difference between one disorder and another and treat by addressing the primary cause.

The other disorders of the shoulder are much more rare. Among these diseases are the nonunion of the caudal ossification center of the glenoid, inflammatory arthropathies, fractures of the glenoid rim, trauma to the articular cartilage, septic arthritis, avulsion of the supraglenoid tubercle and biceps tenosynovitis (Table 2).

Other pathologies such as nonunion of the ossification center of the caudoventral angle of the scapula, immune-mediated inflammatory arthritides, medial and caudomedial glenoid rim fracture, subscapularis muscle tendon tear and tendinitis, and bicipital tenosynovitis will be discussed in the presentation.

In the past, the clinician did not have much choice when diagnosing the type of shoulder disease: in the absence of fractures, there was either a bicipital tenosynovitis, degenerative joint disease (DJD), or shoulder luxation. Today it is possible to differentiate between intra-articular, peri-articular, and local or regional diseases. Among intra-articular diseases, shoulder instability is the most common pathology. It affects adult dogs of all breeds. The second most common intra-articular shoulder disease is osteochondritis dissecans (OCD), seen especially in large growing dogs. The third most common lesion is associated with the biceps tendon.

BIBLIOGRAPHY
1. Bardet JF. Diagnosis of shoulder instability in dogs and cats : a retrospective study. J Am Anim Hosp Assoc. 1998;34:41-54.
2. Bardet JF. Shoulder diseases. Proc VOS, Val d'isère, France, 2000.

3. Bardet JF. Lesions of the biceps tendon diagnosis and classification. Vet Comp Orthop Traumatol. 1999;12:188-195.

4. Shepard S. Diagnosis Shoulder Diseases using MRI in dogs. Proc 2nd Advanced Arthroscopy and Orthopaedic Symposium. Naples. Florida, 2007.

Table 1. Common Causes of Shoulder Pain

Periarticular disorders:
- Tendinitis of the rotator cuff (supraspinatous, subscapular, infraspinatous, and terres minor muscles)
- Subscapular tendon mineralization
- Calcifying bicipital tendinopathy

Glenohumeral joint disorders
- Degenerative joint disease (DJD)
- Glenohumeral instability
- Luxations
- Tear in the glenoid labrum
- Tear of the biceps tendon
- Articular cartilage fracture
- Osteochondritis dissecans (OCD)
- Nonunion of the caudal ossification center of the glenoid
- Fractures
- Osteochondromatosis
- Septic arthritis

Local/regional disorders
- Cervical radiculopathy
- Brachial plexopathy
- Tumor of the brachial plexus
- Tumors
- Various:
  -intrathoracic tumors and other lesions
  -thoracic wall tumors and other lesions
  -tumors and other lesions at the thoracic inlet

Referred pain (thoracic and abdominal)

Table 2. Most Common Shoulder Pathologies in Dogs and Cats

- Instability
- Osteochondritis dissecans (OCD)
- Biceps tendon rupture
- Nonunion of the caudal ossification center of the glenoid
- Fracture of the glenoid cavity or lip
- Articular cartilage damage
- Inflammatory arthropathy
- Infraspinatus contracture
- Bicipital tenosynovitis
- Fracture of the supraglenoid tubercle
- Septic arthritis

A PRACTICAL APPROACH TO DIAGNOSING THE ARTHRITIC CAT

Steven C. Budsberg, DVM, MS Diplomate ACVS
College of Veterinary Medicine
University of Georgia, Athens, GA

Degenerative joint disease (DJD) is a syndrome affecting synovial joints that is characterized by pain and dysfunction, associated with degeneration of the articular cartilage and changes in the periarticular soft tissues. It occurs with varying degrees of severity, ranging from a mild, intermittent condition that causes mild discomfort and minimal disability, to a disease state characterized by constant pain along with severe functional disability. As such, it is often difficult to describe any single treatment that will cover the entire spectrum of change that may be present. In many species DJD and osteoarthritis (OA) are considered nearly synonymous; however this may not be true in cats. Thus in this article, we will use the term DJD. When DJD is found in cats, it is often not identified as a cause of significant clinical problems. This article will not focus on the immune-mediated erosive polyarthropathies.

CLINICAL PRESENTATION

There are several reasons for under appreciation of the clinical significance of DJD. First, the clinical manifestations of the problem in cats are more difficult to identify. Cats with DJD do not act like dogs affected by the same disease. Cats are not subject to the wide range of juvenile joint dysplasia conditions that result in a high occurrence of secondary osteoarthritis in young pure breed dogs, making this a very common finding in this species. Mobility disorders are much more readily identified in dogs where the owner is characteristically present while the animal is exercising and able to recognize lameness or changes in the activity pattern. Lastly, the radiographic appearance of an osteoarthritic joint in the cat is much more subtle than the dog with less obvious proliferative osteophyte formation. This may result in the problem being overlooked or dismissed as clinically insignificant.

Very little work on the assessment of DJD joint disease pain has been performed in cats. However it appears from early work that an approach similar to that in dogs is likely to be most successful. That is, owners need to be centrally involved in the process. The difficult part of assessment of DJD pain in cats is that the activities that are altered by osteoarthritis are less fully understood than in dogs. A recent study of 28 cats with osteoarthritis showed that overt lameness was not the most common clinical feature. Instead, features like jumping up, jumping down, height of the jump, general movement, "grumpiness" on handling, and seeking seclusion are likely to be activities and behaviors that should be followed.

DIAGNOSIS

Given the aforementioned discussion, how then do we develop a methodology to diagnose DJD in cats with high sensitivity and specificity? First, the possibility of the diagnosis must be on the rule-out list for any middle to older age cat presenting for nonspecific signs of changes or decreases in activity, or behavioral changes. Careful and complete history and physical examination must be done. These activities are time consuming and often overlooked in a busy day of seeing patients. If lameness or stiffness are noted, or it was reported that the cat has altered jumping activities (both height and frequency), then DJD must be very high up on the differential diagnosis list. On physical examination, pain or decreased range of motion in a joint are classic markers for DJD.

If there is suspicion of DJD, radiographs are the next diagnostic test to be considered. If no specific joint can be detected in the forelimb, consider taking films of the elbow first, then shoulder and finally the carpus. If no one joint can be singled out in the hind limb, consider taking films of the hips, followed by the tarsus and stifle. Also consider radiographs of the thoracolumbar spine. While the significance of radiographic findings of DJD has been questioned in the past because of the lack of associated signs, it should be argued that the lack of correlation is due to the inability of the clinician and owner to appreciate the signs being shown. While three different studies found low correlation, the reasons for this are most likely that feline gait/lameness and mobility dysfunction is much more difficult to identify and that either signs was overlooked in the retrospective populations or that overt lameness was not one of the main manifestations of the disease in cats. As owner assisted outcome measure tools become better defined and validated, it is very likely that the correlation between radiographic changes and clinical changes will dramatically improve.

EXTRACAPSULAR STABILIZATION OF THE STIFLE – TRICKS TO HELP, TRAPS TO AVOID

Steven J. Butterworth, MA, VetMB, CertVR, DSAO, MRCVS
Weighbridge Referral Centre
Swansea, Wales, United Kingdom

Cranial cruciate ligament (CCL) failure is considered to be the most common cause of "serious" hindlimb lameness affecting the adult dog. In the majority of cases, this failure is a result of degenerative pathology affecting the ligament, although the final breakdown and onset of lameness might be brought on by a minor injury. In the minority of cases, the ligament ruptures as a result of major injury and this failure might then be found in combination with rupture of other ligaments. The assessment of such multiple ligament injury needs to be made carefully and it must be remembered that in cases with cranial cruciate ligament failure in the absence of periarticular fibrosis the illusion of lateral collateral instability can be created by the increased internal rotation allowed by lack of constraint by the CCL. Collateral stability is best assessed with the stifle in full extension and it should be possible to show the deviation created on stressed radiographs.

The treatment of cruciate disease is, to say the least, controversial but it has been generally accepted for four decades that surgical intervention will lead to a more reliably favorable outcome. In terms of surgical technique, there is no currently accepted technique that is proven to be superior to the others but currently the general discussion lies between the use of fabellotibial sutures (DeAngelis sutures) or tibial plateau leveling/tibial tuberosity advancement.

SURGICAL TECHNIQUE FOR EXTRACAPSULAR STABILIZATION (FABELLOTIBIAL SUTURE TECHNIQUE)

- The skin incision begins near the distal limit of the tibial crest and ends proximal to the patella (Figure 1A).
- The fascial incision includes elevation of the cranial tibialis muscle from the lateral aspect of the tibial crest and release of the fascia from the proximal tibia (in the vicinity of the tubercle of Gerdi) (Figure 1B).
- A small area of periosteum is elevated from the medial aspect of the tibial crest and two transverse tunnels are drilled through the crest such that the drill bit emerges medially in the area exposed. The first tunnel is placed as proximal as possible, just cranial to the long digital extensor tendon, and the second tunnel is placed cranial and distal to this (Figure 1C). In small breeds of dog, one tunnel may be used with the suture passing under the patellar tendon.
- The lateral fascia is retracted sufficiently to allow palpation of the lateral fabella (Figure 1D).

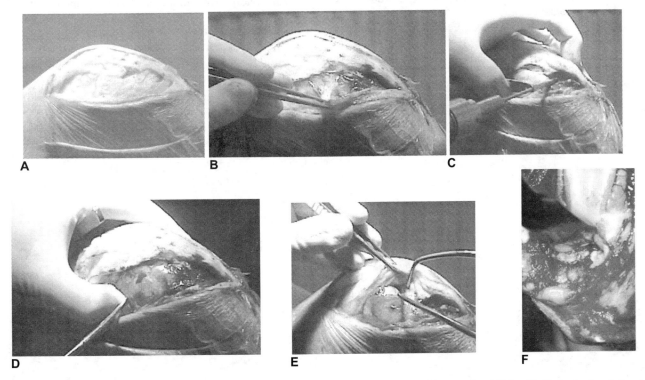

Figure 1. A, Skin incision. **B,** Reflection of lateral fascia. **C,** Tunnels created in proximal tibia. **D,** Palpate the lateral fabella. **E,** Mini lateral arthrotomy and expose menisci. **F,** lateral arthrotomy with reflection of the patella improves exposure.

- The joint capsule is then incised to allow evaluation of the intra-articular structures (Figure 1E). A lateral "mini" arthrotomy will suffice once experience has been gained and adequate exposure of the joint can easily be achieved by placement of a Gelpi retractor in a mediolateral direction and using a stifle joint distractor to separate the femoral condyles from the tibial plateau. In less experienced hands, or when the joint is very fibrotic, it may be better to extend the capsular incision proximally to allow luxation of the patella, which greatly improves visibility. Recognition of and dealing with meniscal pathology is a primary goal in management. Make the capsular incision a few millimeters away from the fascial edge. This will make closure far easier.
- Any remnants of the CCL are resected and the menisci are inspected.

MENISCAL EXAMINATION

Once exposed the menisci are examined with an instrument such as an arthroscopy probe or a Dandy nerve hook. It is worth probing the structures because some injuries are hidden on first appearance. As the tibia is drawn forward by a Hohmann retractor the medial meniscus tends to "buckle" and the surgeon must be aware that this is normal and not a sign of pathology. Remember to check both menisci because although injury is almost invariably to the medial one, it is only almost! The types of injury noted are classified as illustrated in Figure 2.

- Damaged portions of the menisci are treated by partial meniscectomy. In the case of longitudinal tears, the separated linear portion is removed by cutting each end. In the case of a folded caudal horn, it will be necessary to section the cranial attachment and the caudal meniscotibial ligament. An arthroscopy probe or Dandy nerve hook can be

helpful to stabilize the structure and sectioning can be achieved with a standard No 11 blade, a Beaver blade or an arthroscopy hook knife.

MENISCAL RELEASE

It has been suggested that the incidence of "late" meniscal injury in the cruciate-deficient stifle can be reduced by so-called meniscal release. This can be achieved in one of two ways. Firstly, the meniscus can be sectioned through its body or secondly, and perhaps less dramatically, the caudal meniscotibial ligament can be sectioned. The latter is aided by hooking the ligament with an instrument such as a Dandy nerve hook.

There is, however, some concern over the degree to which this procedure "protects" the meniscus from injury versus the potential long-term effect to the joint of destabilizing meniscal integrity. The jury is still out, so to speak, and meniscal release is, perhaps, something to try only if late meniscal injury is a common complication in your hands.

- The joint is flushed and the capsule closed with cruciate/crossed mattress sutures of polydioxanone (PDS, Ethicon).
- The lateral fascia is retracted sufficiently to allow palpation of the lateral fabella and a suture needle is passed around the fabella carrying an appropriate strand of Leader line (Figure 3A). A general guide would be: 50 lb Leader for small dogs and cats; 70 or 80 lb Leader for terriers to spaniel-sized dogs; and 100 lb Leader for dogs of >30 kg bodyweight. An alternative material that is increasing in popularity is Fibrewire or Orthowire;.5 metric material is the most commonly used
- The needle can usually be used to pass the material through one of the tibial tunnels and back through the other one to create a figure-of-eight pattern.

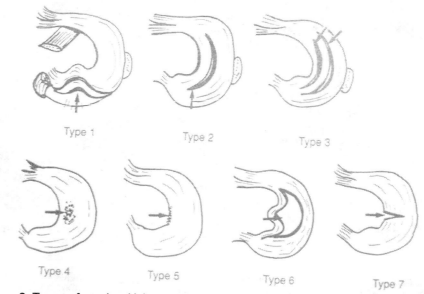

Figure 2. Types of meniscal injury.

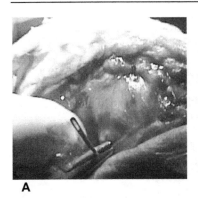
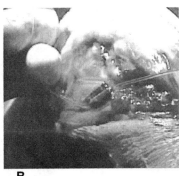
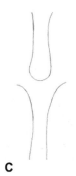
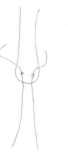
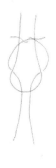

A B C

Figure 3. A, Needle being placed around lateral fabella. **B,** Crimps used to secure sutures. **C,** Self-locking knot.

- Either the suture material is then cut to produce two single strand sutures, which can be tightened and secured with crimps (Figure 3B), or the needle is cut off to leave one, double strand suture, which can be tied using a self-locking knot (Figure 3C). Such knots should, whenever possible, be "tied down" with PDS sutures so that the ends do not stand up and irritate the soft tissues.
- Closure. The periosteal flap on the medial aspect of the tibia is then reattached so as to cover the strands of nylon. The fascia of the cranial tibialis muscle is reattached with cruciate/crossed mattress sutures of the PDS. The lateral fascia is closed using PDS and an overlapping pattern achieved by placement of a row of Mayo mattress sutures followed by a simple, continuous suture along the remaining free edge. The remainder of closure is routine.

POSTOPERATIVE CARE

- **Analgesia** – Carprofen and pethidine are used perioperatively and a 3- to 5-day supply of carprofen is dispensed at the time of discharge.
- **Prophylactic use of antibiotics** – A broad-spectrum (marbofloxacin) intravenous antibiotic is given at induction and this is continued for 5 days post surgery.
- **Bandaging** – No bandage is applied. Ice packs are used only if swelling is considered excessive.
- **Sutures** – Removed after 10 days.
- **Exercise** – Limited to lead walks and room or pen rest for 3 months. The distance walked is governed only by what the dog can manage. No free access to stairs, gardens or furniture is allowed and the floor of the pen or small room in which the dog resides should not be slippery.
- **Physiotherapy** – Not routinely used unless an owner expresses a wish to be enrolled on a rehabilitation program. The owner will be encouraged to do so if a dog is not meeting expectations in progress during the recovery period and no other explanation for this can be found (see below).

After 3 months, if all is well, exercise can be gradually increased to normal over 4 to 6 weeks. Most dogs take between 4 and 6 months after surgery to reach their best. About 85% to 90% will achieve satisfactory function with about half of these being considered sound.

The main explanations for any continued lameness are:

- Meniscal injury
- Instability
- Infection
- Arthritis

If a dog is not making satisfactory progress then options to consider (depending on the clinical features) include:

- Joint tap to look for infection
- Arthrotomy/arthroscopy to re-inspect for meniscal injury
- Further surgery to stabilize the joint
- Physiotherapy
- Long-term management of OA

BACTERIAL INFECTIVE ARTHRITIS: DIAGNOSIS, MANAGEMENT, AND PREVENTION

Steven J. Butterworth, MA, VetMB, CertVR, DSAO, MRCVS
Weighbridge Referral Centre
Swansea, Wales, United Kingdom

A wide variety of infective agents can cause an inflammatory arthropathy. Bacteria, particularly *Streptococcus* spp and *Staphylococcus intermedius*, are the most common cause of infective arthritis in the dog.[1] In the cat, bite wounds are the most common cause, involving bacteria normally found in the mouth such as *Pasteurella multocida*, *Bacteroides* spp, and *Streptococcus* spp.

Bacterial arthritis may occur as a result of direct infection from a penetrating wound, as a complication of arthrotomy, by extension from a local purulent focus, or it may result from hematogenous spread. Although hematogenous spread of infection to joints is common in young farm animals, the condition is relatively uncommon in dogs. Infection tends to localize in joints that have already been damaged as a result of trauma or osteoarthritis.

DIAGNOSIS
History and Clinical Signs
Two syndromes are recognized, the classic acute onset case and those with a more chronic low grade infection. The condition occurs more commonly in large breeds of dog. The carpus is the joint most frequently affected joint but the shoulder, hip and stifle joints have also been implicated. Perhaps this is a result of an injury being more likely to penetrate a carpus than a more proximal joint. In the case of infection post surgery, the stifle joint (post cruciate surgery) is perhaps the most common one to be involved. Affected joints are swollen or thickened and painful. Lameness is often severe. Once infection is established in the joint there is rapid and extensive destruction of articular cartilage and subchondral bone but few cases show evidence of systemic illness.

RADIOLOGY
Radiographic changes will depend on the stage of the disease and the type of bacteria present. Initially, radiographic examination may reveal very little except for soft tissue swelling but later, destructive changes will be seen extending down into the subchondral bone and there will be varying degrees of periarticular new bone formation.

LABORATORY TESTS
Evidence of inflammation is not always consistent on hematologic and serologic tests. Although a neutrophilia, low grade anemia and mild thrombocytopenia are to be expected in positive cases, normal levels do not preclude a diagnosis of infective arthritis. Synovial fluid analysis will usually reveal the following:

- Increased volume
- Reduced viscosity
- Hemorrhagic or purulent appearance
- Increased turbidity and tendency to clot on exposure to air
- Elevated white cell count with polymorphonuclear leukocytes predominating
- Elevated protein levels
- Low blood glucose ratio

Synovial fluid or membrane may be submitted for bacteriology as culturing the infective agent from the joint leads to a definitive diagnosis. Swabs taken from synovial fluid should be plated out both on aerobic and anaerobic culture media. However, even when infection is present, culture of the organism is only successful in about 50% of cases.[3] Culture from synovial membrane biopsies is said to be more successful than direct culture from synovial fluid[4] but the results are not consistent. The most accurate and reliable method is to culture from synovial fluid following incubation in blood culture medium for 24 hours.[3] The most commonly isolated bacterial causes of infective arthritis are *Staphylococcus intermedius* and ß haemolytic *Streptococcus*.[1] Other bacteria which may be encountered include:

- Coliforms
- *Pasteurella multocida*
- *Pseudomonas aeruginosa*
- *Proteus* spp
- *Nocardia asteroides*
- *Brucella abortus*
- *Erysipelothrix rhusiopathiae*
- *Salmonella typhimurium*

MANAGEMENT
Cases of suspected infective arthritis require urgent treatment. A course of broad spectrum antibiotic such as amoxicillin and clavulanic acid, cephalosporin, or marbofloxacin should be initiated while the results of culture and sensitivity are awaited. An appropriate antibiotic should then be given for at least 3 weeks and it may be necessary to continue for 6 weeks or more before the infection is eradicated. The majority of cases, 88% according to Bennett & Taylor,[1] or 94% in a study conducted by Clements and others,[2] will have a satisfactory outcome provided treatment is started early, before extensive joint damage has occurred.

TREATMENT OF SEPTIC ARTHRITIS FOLLOWING JOINT SURGERY
In the acute case there is joint swelling, pain and pyrexia within a few days of surgery. Most cases, particularly those with low grade infection, will respond to antibiotic therapy, as discussed above. In addition to antibiotics, particularly if infection is thought to be severe, the joint should be flushed out with large quantities of sterile, lactated Ringer's solution. This can

be achieved using two needles or catheters introduced into the joint, one for ingress and the other for egress of fluid. Arthroscopy cannulas are particularly useful for this purpose. Pain relief is provided by the administration of a nonsteroidal anti-inflammatory drug and, when possible, joint immobilization using a Robert Jones bandage. If infection has been present for more than about 3 days then arthrotomy, rather than needle flushing, is necessary for removal of fibrin deposits, necrotic tissue, and purulent exudate. After the joint has been debrided and lavaged with Ringer's solution, the arthrotomy may be left open to granulate and heal by second intention or drains can be placed in the joint prior to wound closure. Irrigation and drainage is achieved by way of these for three to four days and then the drains are removed. The wound and drains (if used) must be carefully protected with sterile dressings to prevent interference from the patient and further contamination.

Chronic infections are seen most often following replacement of ligaments with synthetic materials such as braided nylon. If infection becomes established in a joint where such an implant has been used, eradication of the causal organism becomes impossible unless the implant is removed due to its capillary nature which harbors the infection. Lameness, which is often severe, persists for weeks or months following the initial surgery. The joint tends to be thickened and painful and sinus tracts appear over the region. Radiographic examination reveals soft tissue swelling, erosion of the articular surfaces, bone lysis around implants, and often extensive periarticular osteophyte formation. Treatment involves arthrotomy, removal of implanted material, debridement, synovectomy, lavage and irrigation drainage, together with prolonged antibiotic therapy. If culture and sensitivity results from an infected joint indicate the use of an antibiotic such as gentamicin, which can have toxic side effects if given systemically for long periods, then local administration may be achieved by using beads of polymethylmethacrylate impregnated with gentamicin (Septopal®). The beads are placed in the joint for up to 3 weeks and slowly release the gentamicin, providing good intra-articular levels of the antibiotic but very low systemic levels, thus minimizing the risk of toxic side effects.

PREVENTION

Strict asepsis is a prerequisite for successful joint surgery. Nevertheless, infections do occur occasionally and can usually be traced back to faults in asepsis, prolonged operating time or rough handling of tissues. Although the outcome of infection associated with joint surgery may be satisfactory, it is not always so and will definitely require more monitoring and cost than management of a similar case without infection. As a result, it is best to prevent wound contamination and/or infection becoming established.

The prevention of "iatrogenic" joint infection essentially comes down to good theater practice together with the administration of prophylactic antibiotics. Use of the latter, however, is not a substitute for aseptic technique. The fundamental principles of good theater technique can be summarized as:

- Operating theater
  - Clean environment
  - Minimize "theatre traffic"
  - Ventilation system (optimal is filtered, positive pressure system)
- Patient preparation
  - Clip adequate area
  - Thorough skin preparation
  - Draping of both the field and then the surgical wound (with either an adhesive film or by suturing/clipping the drape edge to the wound edge) using an impermeable material
- Surgeon preparation
  - Wear hat and mask
  - Adequate hand scrub
  - Wear long-sleeved, sterile gown and surgical gloves
- Surgical technique
  - Aseptic technique
  - Careful handling of soft tissues (to minimize further vascular damage)
  - Minimize operating time (wounds open for longer than one hour begin to show an exponential rise in the incidence of infection)—an assistant is useful in this respect

Although prophylactic antibiotics are justifiable as an *additional* measure to all of the above it is important that they are used peri-operatively rather than just post-operatively. Assuming that only the exceptional wound or operating environment will prevent all contamination, it is more effective for the antibiotic to be present when the contaminants arrive than after they are beginning to become established. Also, any postoperative hematoma will contain antibiotic if this is administered peri-operatively whereas diffusion of drugs administered postoperatively into the hematoma is less predictable. An intravenous bolus of antibiotic can be used just after induction of anesthesia or else systemic treatment can be introduced several hours before surgery. As far as choosing a prophylactic antibiotic, apart from it needing to be broad spectrum and bactericidal, this is based on surgeon's preference and experience of what works in that particular clinic. A scientifically based decision can be made by leaving agar plates out overnight and during use of the operating theater. Culture of these plates will help to establish the resident population in the environment and sensitivity tests will determine an appropriate choice of antibiotic. However, it is pertinent to remember that the source of many organisms causing joint infections post-surgery is the dog's own skin.

REFERENCES
1. Bennett D, Taylor DJ. Bacterial infective arthritis in the dog. J Small Anim Pract. 1988;29:207.
2. Clements DN, Owen MR, Mosley JR, et al. Retrospective study of bacterial infective arthritis in 31 dogs. J Small Anim Pract. 2005;46:171-176.

3. Montgomery RD, Long IR, Milton JL, et al. Comparison of aerobic culture from synovial membrane biopsy and blood culture medium in detection of canine bacterial arthritis. Vet Surg 1989;18: 300.

4. Sledge CB. Surgery in infectious arthritis. Clin Rheum Dis. 1978;4:149.

5. Walenkamp GHIM, Vree TM, Van Rens TJG. Clin Orthopaed Rel Res. 1996;205:171.

MEDICAL AND PHYSICAL MANAGEMENT OF OSTEOARTHRITIS

Steven J. Butterworth, MA, VetMB, CertVR, DSAO, MRCVS
Weighbridge Referral Centre
Swansea, Wales, United Kingdom

MEDICAL MANAGEMENT

Cases with osteoarthritis (OA) may show no lameness most of the time and then an acute flare-up as a consequence of a sprain-type injury to a sensitive joint. Such cases may respond to a restriction of exercise and a short course of nonsteroidal anti-inflammatory drugs (NSAIDs). In this discussion, we will concentrate on the more chronic cases that require ongoing management to control the clinical signs associated with OA.

There are a variety of approaches for medical treatment of OA but the aim generally revolves around pain management or trying to influence the progression of the disease process.

PAIN MANAGEMENT

Drugs used regularly for this purpose include:

- NSAIDs
- Acetaminophen (paracetamol)
- Corticosteroids
- Opiates (tramadol hydrochloride)
- Anticonvulsants and calcium channel blockers (gabapentin)

NSAIDs

NSAIDs are the mainstay of medical treatment of OA in small animal medicine. There are several NSAIDs licensed for use in the dog; these are mostly prostaglandin-blocking. Those licensed for long-term use include meloxicam (Metacam), carprofen (Rimadyl), tepoxalin (Zubrin), and firocoxib (Previcox – caution as only tested to 90 days).

There has been much debate on the effects NSAIDs have on cartilage. There is some evidence that certain of this group have a deleterious effect on cartilage when compared with others in the group; equally, some are heralded as chondroprotective. Much of this work has been carried out in vitro and extrapolation to the in vivo situation is difficult. The decrease in synovitis may be negated by the analgesic-induced overloading of a joint. Add to this the effect a drug may have on chondrocyte metabolism and clearly the situation is complex. However, the effects in the long term are generally felt to be minimal.

Several factors may influence the choice of drug :

- Clinical response
- Side effects (important if there is concurrent hepatic, gastrointestinal or renal disease)
- Cost
- Type of preparation (capsules, tablets, drops)
- Convenience of dosing regime.

It would seem unnecessary to consider the use of unlicensed products in the treatment of canine OA now that there is an adequate range of licensed drugs. NSAIDs available for use in humans without prescription, such as ibuprofen, should be avoided because their half-lives are much longer in dogs compared with humans, and so it is easy to overdose. Flurbiprofen should definitely not be used since it may lead to an idiosyncratic reaction and death.

All NSAIDs may cause gastrointestinal irritation resulting in vomiting or diarrhea (possibly with blood). If this occurs any more than occasionally, the drug should be withdrawn. To try to avoid such side effects these drugs are best given with some food. If such side effects result in withdrawal of a drug then, once the signs have settled down, another one may be tried. Particular dogs are often sensitive to certain agents. It may prove necessary in certain patients to consider the use of NSAIDs other than the ones mentioned above "off license..

"Trial and error" will determine a suitable drug for an individual dog.

Acetaminophen (Paracetamol, Pardale-V)

Acetaminophen is a centrally acting analgesic that can prove very useful in managing patients with chronic OA. Although its data sheet indicates it should not be combined with NSAIDs, the risk of side effects has to be considered less than if two NSAIDs were combined or used in conjunction with a corticosteroid.

Corticosteroids

The use of corticosteroids in the treatment of OA is a controversial area. Some work in experimental OA suggested that corticosteroids hasten the degeneration of cartilage and this evidence seemed to make the use of corticosteroids (particularly intra-articular use) contra-indicated. However, there is recent evidence that intra-articular (IA) methylprednisolone (Depo-Medrone V), at a dose of 20 mg for an average Labrador's shoulder or stifle, may have beneficial effects in canine OA. Certainly, there may be dramatic relief from clinical signs although the response is variable. Human rheumatologists may repeat IA injections up to three times a year. The response to IA corticosteroid seems to vary depending on the joint. It is probably important to rest the patient strictly for at least 2 days following the injection to encourage the drug to stay within the joint and limit the systemic effect. If corticosteroids are to be administered systemically, low-dose prednisolone (0.25-0.5 mg/kg once daily or every other day) is the preferred drug. A course of 2 to 3 weeks should be used initially.

Corticosteroids seem to be particularly helpful in certain situations, namely:

- When other medical treatments have failed and the dog's quality of life has declined
- In elderly dogs where there is concern over NSAID side effects

- After an acute flare-up of OA, which may be associated with a high level of polymorphs (15–30%) in synovial fluid
- In erosive OA

Opiates

Opiates are centrally acting agents that can be combined with NSAID therapy. They can prove very effective and their major draw back is the possibility of side effects such as sedation and nausea. Use of an opiate analogue such as tramadol hydrochloride at doses of 4 to 5 mg/kg orally 2 or 3 times daily seems to cause such side effects in dogs relatively infrequently.

Agents Acting Against Neuropathic Pain

It is now recognized that in conditions associated with chronic pain a situation may arise where constant stimulation of the pain pathways leads to a neuropathic element to the signs. Such an element will be almost completely unaffected by any medication aimed at the underlying primary condition. The use of certain drugs to help quash the neuropathic element of the pain can help. Such drugs include those used in humans for neuralgia, eg, gabapentin (5–10 mg/kg 2 or 3 times daily). Sedation may be seen but generally ceases with continued medication after a couple of weeks.

INFLUENCING THE PROGRESSION OF DISEASE
Slow-Acting Drugs in OA (SADOA)

The International League Against Rheumatism (ILAR) has proposed two categories in this group; disease-modifying OA drugs (DMOADS) and symptomatic slow-acting drugs in OA (SYSADOA). This classification aims to clearly define the concept of "chondroprotection" and distinguish drugs that have this property from those that merely give symptomatic relief. The concept of chondroprotection evolved from clinical trials of certain agents that appeared to retard the progression of OA. However, the pharmacology of these drugs could not be related to the pathology of OA and hence there is a need for a much tighter definition of "chondroprotective drugs."

There is some evidence that certain agents can alter the environment or activity of the chondrocyte in vitro such that the degeneration of cartilage is stopped or decreased. Unfortunately, although in vitro results may suggest that certain agents have these capabilities, in vivo work is hampered by the fact that there are, at present, no readily quantifiable criteria for measuring outcome of OA. This is even more applicable in clinical trials, many of which have been uncontrolled and poorly designed. Thus, there is much conflicting evidence in the literature.

At present, there is only one drug in this "class" licensed for use in the dog. This is sodium pentosan polysulfhate (PPS) (Cartrophen Vet), which is a polysaccharide sulfate ester prepared from beech hemicellulose. This drug has been shown to inhibit certain proteinases but it is structurally similar to heparin and so has anticoagulant properties. The mode of action in clinical cases is obscure and the recent studies suggest that the fibrinolytic action may shift microthrombi in the vascular supply of subchondral bone resulting in pain relief. Validated clinical trials with the drug are lacking but anecdotal evidence suggests that it can give impressive clinical results in certain cases. However, suitable case selection is a large stumbling block. An oral preparation of PPS has been used experimentally in dogs and is licensed in some countries.

More recently the terms "structure modifying" and "symptom modifying" drugs have been used to simplify the terminology whereby PPS would be viewed as an example of the former and a NSAID of the latter, although some NSAIDs are also claimed to have structure-modifying properties.

FUTURE POSSIBILITIES FOR DISEASE MODIFICATION

There are many avenues of research in treatment of OA. Certain forms of "treatment" have been around for some time but have yet to be proven useful. A good example of this would be polysulfated glycosaminoglycan preparations used for so-called *viscosupplementation*. These have been licensed, in various forms, for treatment of human and equine arthritis for some time (eg, Adequan®). Due to the difficulties in quantifying outcome in OA, their effectiveness in clinical trials is still variable. A recent study showed no difference between patients receiving intra-articular hyaluronic acid and those receiving intra-articular saline. The explanation for this might lie in reports on the usefulness of articular lavage in the symptomatic relief of OA in humans. Clearly, any preparation delivered after arthrocentesis would have to take this possible effect into account.

The theories of viscosupplementation revolve around improving the properties of the synovial fluid. This may have many effects such as decreasing abnormal load on cartilage or altering inflammatory mechanisms. There may be more efficacy in newer formulations of HA which have a high degree of cross linking which creates a very high molecular weight and improves the viscoelasticity.

Other medical developments are centered on attempting to *alter the activity of chondrocytes* by blocking the action of certain cytokines; for example, interleukin-1 (IL-1)-blocking agents are reaching the clinical trial stage. Cytokines, which stimulate synthetic activity of chondrocytes, have also received attention; for example, insulin-like growth factor-1 (IGF-1) has been used experimentally (in combination with PPS) and shown to have some promise in maintaining matrix integrity.

Gene therapy is a concept receiving attention throughout medicine. Recent experimental work has shown that the gene for IL-1ra can be implanted into synovial cells in joints and these cells will express this gene for several weeks. Clearly, there is exciting potential in such an approach to arthritis.

PHYSICAL MANAGEMENT

Managing a patient with OA is a long-term commitment but there are several aspects that may improve the quality of an afflicted dog.

Home Environment

The dog's bed should be warm, dry and well padded (or a waterbed). A blanket circulating warm water as a "base layer" is a very effective means of maintaining warmth and reducing morning stiffness. Avoid slippery floors, eg, laminate flooring; and avoid steps or provide ramps (with rubber surface).

Avoid over-exuberant activities with other pets although some play with others can be stimulating for them—in small doses.

Exercise

Reduce morning stiffness by providing appropriate bedding. Stretch exercises can be used for affected joints—but not beyond comfortable limits—15 to 20 slow repetitions.

Several short walks each day (at least three) with the time and length dictated by the patient and adjusted accordingly. Coats and/or leggings in cold weather. The aim is to provide a consistent amount of exercise each day – NOT more at weekends and little during the week!!

After exercise, massage affected joints +/- ice pack if painful.

Periods of Exacerbation

Exercise should be reduced, with focus on low-impact exercise. Any medication being used may need to be increased or augmented. Specific rehabilitation using hydrotherapy (swimming or walking on an underwater treadmill) may be required to restore the status quo. Other adjunct therapy involving the use of TENS (transcutaneous neuromuscular stimulation), ultrasound or acupuncture might assist recovery from this "acute" phase.

SURGICAL MANAGEMENT OF CARPAL AND TARSAL OSTEOARTHRITIS

Steven J. Butterworth, MA, VetMB, CertVR,
DSAO, MRCVS
Weighbridge Referral Centre
Swansea, Wales, United Kingdom

CARPUS

Osteoarthritis (OA) of the carpus can be secondary to a number of conditions, eg, previous trauma or developmental deformity. As a general rule all joints within the carpus will be involved and so the only surgical option for management of this situation is that of pancarpal arthrodesis. The principles of arthrodesis are:

- To remove "all" articular cartilage from the joint surfaces
- To compress the exposed subchondral bone surfaces and achieve rigid fixation to promote fusion
- To pack cancellous bone (or a synthetic substitute) into any gaps to aid and accelerate fusion

What varies is the means by which rigid fixation is achieved. Application of a dorsal plate to the distal radius, radial carpal bone and third metacarpal bone is, perhaps the commonest means of achieving this. Although plating on the palmar or medial surface would be mechanically superior it is anatomically more difficult and the success rate of dorsal plating limits the need for more complex surgery. External skeletal fixation can be used but the "hands on" aftercare tends to be more involved.

The main concern over dorsal plating is the need to protect the plate with a cast for about 2 months after surgery. This is generally not required in cases being treated because of OA because the palmar ligamentous support is intact. Furthermore, the risk of implant failure can be reduced by application of crossed-pins (to create a plate-rod situation) or use of a castless PCA plate (Orthomed). The latter are a little more difficult to apply that standard plates but they are mechanically superior and should not require external protection even in cases that lack any ligamentous support.

The results of treatment by pancarpal arthrodesis in a series of 40 dogs was published by Denny and Barr.[2] Seventy-four percent of the dogs regained full limb function. The most common complication of pancarpal arthrodesis was loosening of one or more of the distal screws. Other recognized complications of the procedure include fracture of the third metacarpal bone at a later date (8/64 arthrodeses reported by Whitelock and Houlton).[5] Plate removal was necessary in 8/43 arthrodeses reported by Denny and Barr[2] and 11/64 reported by Whitelock and Houlton.[5]

TARSUS

The commonest causes of clinical OA affecting the tarsus are probably previous injury or osteochondritis dissecans (OCD). In general the tarsocrural joint will be involved in a disease process and, as with the carpus, if arthrodesis is being considered then this will require a pantarsal approach. However, in cases where OCD is suspected as the primary disease process there is some merit in considering surgical debridement of the joint in an adult that has failed to respond to noninvasive options. Removal of intra-articular fragments in such an adult can lead to significant improvement and avoid the need for more radical surgery.

As with PCA, pantarsal arthrodesis (PTA) should follow the general guidelines for achieving arthrodesis and the differences arise in the method of fixation chosen. Dorsal plating is the favored option of the author as the approach allows for easy exposure of the joints for debridement, the application of a standard plate to the dorsal aspects of the distal tibia, tarsal bones and third metatarsal (precontoured to provide an appropriate standing angle of about 135 to 145 degrees), and access to the proximal tibia for harvesting a cancellous bone graft.

The arguments against this technique revolve around the plate being in a mechanically disadvantaged site, requiring protection within a cast for 2 months post-surgery. Use of tarsocrural pins to create a plate-rod construct has been advocated to reduce stress on the plate, but this may compromise plate screw placement. Most recently, it has been suggested that application of a customised plate to the medial (or lateral) aspect of the tarsus should be mechanically superior. However, external support is still provided for a period after surgery. As in the carpus, external skeletal fixation can be used but the "hands on" aftercare tends to be more involved.

DeCamp and others reported a satisfactory outcome in 10 of 10 dogs in which PTA was carried out using a dorsal plate.[1] However, 6 of the 10 plates ultimately broke or loosened and required removal. McKee and others reported a satisfactory outcome in 12 of 13 dogs in which PTA was promoted using a medial or lateral plate.[3] Four of the 13 showed complications relating to implant failure or loosening. In a more recent study that is in press (Roch and others, personal communication), the incidence of significant complications was 6 of 9 dogs in which PTA was promoted by medial plate application.

REFERENCES

1. DeCamp CE, Martinez SA, Johnston SA. Pantarsal arthrodesis in dogs and a cat: 11 cases (1983-1991).J Am Vet Med Assoc. 1993;203:1705-1707.
2. Denny HR, Barr ARS. Partial and pancarpal arthrodesis in the dog: A review of 50 cases. J Small Anim Pract. 1991;32:329-334
3. McKee WM, May C, Macias C, Lapish JP. Pantarsal arthrodesis with a customized medial or lateral bone plate in 13 dogs. Vet Rec. 2004;154:165-170
4. Parker RB, Brown SG, Wind AP. Pancarpal arthrodesis in the dog: A review of 45 cases. Vet Surg. 1981;10: 35-43
5. Whitelock RG, Houlton JEF. Pancarpal arthrodesis: Long term follow-up in 56 dogs. In: Clinical Research Abstracts for the 1998 BSAVA Congress, Birmingham, England, 1998, p 311

TREATMENT OPTIONS FOR ELBOW DYSPLASIA

Alfonso C. Chico, Lic. Vet, MVM
Veterinary Surgical Center
La Coruña, Spain

DEFINITION OF ELBOW DYSPLASIA

Elbow dysplasia has been described as "a polygenic, hereditary, developmental disease that results in the development of an ulnar trochlear notch that is too small in circumference to encompass the humeral trochlea, thus creating incongruity within the joint."

Depending partially on the breed of dog, the effect of this malformation on the elbow may result in one or several forms of dysplasia. These include ununited anconeal process (UAP), medial coronoid process disease (MCPD), osteochondritis dissecans (OCD) of the medial humeral condyle, or elbow incongruity (EI) (humero-radial or humero-ulnar).

Some authors recently have included other elbow conditions under the definition of elbow dysplasia, such as medial epicondylar disease (MED), or incomplete ossification of the humeral condyle (IOHC).

The end-stage situation of any form of dysplasia is degenerative joint disease. According to the International Elbow Working Group (IEWG), a finding of osteoarthrosis in the young dog, especially when it is bilateral, should be considered supportive of a diagnosis of elbow dysplasia, even when the primary cause has not been identified.

CONSERVATIVE TREATMENT OF ELBOW DYSPLASIA

Conservative treatment may play a role in the management of elbow dysplasia. All conservative management programs should take into account five principles:

1. Weight management;
2. Nutritional supplementation;
3. Exercise regulation;
4. Physical rehabilitation;
5. Anti-inflammatory drugs

Some authors demonstrated beneficial effects associated with implementation of a nonsurgical program. A prospective double-blinded study with a mean follow-up period of 66 weeks in 22 dogs with medial compartment disease compared conservative and surgical management (via arthrotomy) and found no difference in outcome in young dogs with mild lameness, whereas dogs with more significant lameness had a better outcome with surgical management.

Another randomized prospective clinical trial that compared surgical management (via arthrotomy) with conservative management (comprising only pentosan polysulfate) in 19 dogs with clinical, radiographic, and force plate follow-up up to 9 months found no significant difference between the two groups. The majority of dogs had improved lameness scores with progression of osteoarthritis.

Additional well-controlled clinical studies are needed to clarify the benefit and indications of conservative and surgical management in medial compartment disease. Given the ranges in disease severity, severity of clinical disease manifestation, conservative management options, owner compliance and surgical options available, evidence-based treatment protocols are difficult to establish.

UNUNITED ANCONEAL PROCESS

Ununited anconeal process is primarily a condition affecting young dogs between 5 and 9 months of age. It usually occurs in medium to large breeds of dog, most notably the German shepherd. The disorder also occurs in basset hounds and dachshunds, two chondrodystrophoid breeds with a marked incidence of dissimilar growth rates of the radius and ulna.

Ununited anconeal process occasionally is seen in older dogs, from 3 to 9 years of age, that present with an acute episode of severe forelimb lameness.

Fragment Removal

The anconeal process should be removed when it is osteolytic, malformed, sclerotic, or difficult to return to its normal anatomic position. In older dogs, the anconeal process may be removed if the surgeon is sure that it is causing a problem; however, the results of removal in older dogs (ie, over 3 years of age) have been much less rewarding than in younger dogs.

In a normal dog, the anconeal process locks into the olecranon fossa of the humerus when the elbow is in moderate to full extension. This locking tends to stop the medial and lateral motion of the elbow during weight bearing. Hence, removal of the anconeus may allow an instability ("wobbling") of the elbow.

A lateral approach to the caudolateral compartment of the elbow joint is performed. After dissection through the subcutaneous tissue, the lateral head of the triceps is elevated to expose the ancones muscle. A stab incision is made through it which then is extended dorsally and ventrally to allow visualization of the anconeal process. The anconeal fragment is grasped with bone-holding forceps. A scalpel is used to free the anconeal process from its fibrous attachments.

The long-term results of fragment removal have been disappointing and are currently a poor option for well-preserved anconeal fragments

Ulnar Osteotomy

A caudal approach is made to the proximal ulna. The periosteum of the bone is incised and the osteotomy line is directed cranially and distally in an approximate angle of 45° to the ulnar diaphysis. The results of this technique when used alone have been equivocal in the literature, with success rates ranging from 20% to 70%. It is currently believed that fusion of the anconeal process is only achieved when a strong band of fibrous tissue holds the fragment in place as healing proceeds.

Lag Screw Fixation and Ulnar Osteotomy

In many dogs, the anconeal process can be salvaged by reattaching it to the ulna, thus returning the elbow to as near-normal function as possible. This procedure does not produce the instability that results from removal of the anconeal process. Reattachment is indicated only when the anconeal process appears normal in size, shape, and density on both the radiographs and surgical evaluation and when the animal has limited secondary degenerative joint disease and osteophyte production.

A caudolateral approach is performed as described. The surfaces to be fixed are shaped and trimmed free of fibrous tissue to allow a precise contact of the anconeal process onto the ulna. The screw head must be placed on the caudodorsal aspect of the anconeal process so the screw head cannot contact the articular cartilage or interfere with the extension of the joint. The screw should pass in a 45° angle down the shaft of the ulna. The head of the screw may need to be countersunk gently into the anconeal process. Alternatively, the screw can be inserted from the caudal aspect of the ulna towards the anconeal process. The fixation is augmented with a   K-wire to prevent rotational movement around the screw. The ulnar osteotomy is then performed as described previously.

Currently, this is thought to be the best way to treat UAP. A recent report has shown the long-term results of the combination of theses two techniques. All patients had improved lameness scores, 95% achieved a complete fusion of the anconeal process, and in 70% of the dogs osteoarthrosis progression was halted.

Arthroscopy

Although arthroscopic removal of the anconeal process has been described, its main use in UAP is the examination of the medial compartment previous to fixation of the fragment or ulnar osteotomy. As has recently been demonstrated, up to 15% of the cases of UAP may have concurrently medial coronoid disease. If left untreated, that may account for some incomplete recoveries even though anconeal fragment fusion has been achieved.

FRAGMENTED MEDIAL CORONOID PROCESS

The abnormal development with fragmentation of the apex of the medial coronoid process is a common disease in the breeds affected. Radiological diagnosis only without advanced imaging techniques may be challenging for the inexperienced surgeon, and that may account for many undiagnosed cases.

Fragmented Coronoid Removal (Arthrotomy)

A medial approach to the elbow is begun by incising the fascia between the pronator teres and the flexor carpi radialis muscles. The joint capsule is identified and the arthrotomy performed. The incision must allow adequate visualization and inspection of the coronoid area. The opening of the joint is best achieved by using the edge of the table as a fulcrum.

The coronoid area must be inspected carefully for loose pieces or fissure lines through the cartilage. In many of these patients, a piece of FCP is still loosely attached to the remainder of the coronoid. Curettage, abrasion arthroplasty or micro-picking of that region can be subsequently performed.

Fragmented Coronoid Process Removal (Arthroscopy)

Studies comparing the results of treatment after arthroscopic versus conventional surgery are sparse, but they appear to be very promising. In a retrospective trial over eight years 518 joints from 421 dogs with fragmented medial coronoid process of the ulna (FCP) were included. 247 of the elbows were treated by arhtrotomy and 271 by arthroscopy. In the arthrotomy group, 42% of the dogs did not show any lameness, and 30% showed constant lameness. In the arthroscopy group, more than 60% of the dogs did not show any lameness and only 10% had constant lameness. It is generally agreed that, although the development of secondary arthrosis cannot be avoided by either method, arthroscopy gives better functional results than conventional arthrotomy.

Subtotal Coronoidectomy

This technique can be performed either through arthrotomy or arthroscopy, and is defined as the resection of a large triangular portion of the medial coronoid process including diseased cartilage and subchondral bone. A large prospective study on 389 elbows suggests that SCO is effective for the treatment of medial coronoid disease, ameliorating the cartilage abrasion of the opposing surface of the humeral condyle.

Clinical examination suggests that redistribution of load-bearing across the radial head does not induce clinically relevant collapse of the medial compartment or abnormal ulnar notch loading by 5 years postoperatively. SCO may have advantages over conventional procedures both in terms of improved lameness scores and progression of arthrosis in the short and medium term.

Dynamic Proximal Ulnar Osteotomy

The rationale of this treatment is to restore normal loading of the elbow joint, specifically the relationship between humero-ulnar and humero-radial loading.

Some authors report that clinically, all dogs did well after surgery and radiographically there was some evidence that proximal ulnar osteotomy can slow progression of osteoarthritis. Work in the laboratory demonstrated that proximal ulnar osteotomy can restore normal elbow joint contact patterns.

Several studies measuring the change in elbow contact patterns and medial joint load have been performed over the last years with different osteotomy types in the ulna. There has been no prospective, standardized study with control groups and force plate data that has looked at the effect of any of these procedures in clinically affected dogs. The decision to perform an osteotomy following arthroscopic debridement of the coronoid must therefore be made with little scientific data as support and with the knowledge that the technique has an inherently high morbidity. The association of ulnar osteotomy and fragment removal has been shown to increase functional and radiologic results in treating FCP.

Sliding Humeral Osteotomy

Humeral wedge and sliding humeral osteotomies have been recently proposed to shift weight-bearing from the medial to the lateral aspect of the elbow joint.

Although the long-term effects of osteotomies have yet to be clinically documented in statistically relevant numbers, they may have a role to play in the amelioration of joint pathology

ELBOW OCD

Two kinds of lesions affect the medial aspect of the humeral condyle. One is a frictional abrasion (the so-called kissing lesion), opposite the primary FMCP. The other is a true OCD lesion, with an ulcerated subchondral bone defect and associated cartilage flap. On CT scans, about 10% of elbows affected by FMCP had a concurrent OCD lesion.

Surgical treatment involves curetting the subchondral bed and removing the flap, either by arthrotomy or arthroscopy

JOINT INCONGRUENCY

Proximal ulnar osteotomy is the treatment of choice for perceived incongruency of the joint. The problem arises when trying to diagnose this condition since radiology, arthroscopy, and magnetic resonance have not proved useful to measure the amount of incogruency. Only CT has successfully been employed, although is not yet readily available. For that reason, it is difficult to evaluate surgical results or to measure the degree of incongruity to compare different techniques.

UNUNITED MEDIAL EPICONDYLE

Epicondylar lesions occur infrequently in the elbow joint, and can be divided into epicondylar spurring or calcification of the flexor tendons. Removal of the fragments or fixation with screws has resulted in good prognosis.

INCOMPLETE OSSIFICATION OF THE HUMERAL CONDYLE

This condition is diagnosed radiographically as a linear sagittal radiolucency in the region of the developmental cartilage zone separating the two condylar centres of ossification. It is usually treated with screw fixation with a good prognosis for resolution of lameness, although some dogs fail to show bony union on radiographs or CT scans.

REFERENCES

1. Morgan JP, Wind A, Davidson AP. Elbow dysplasia. In: Morgan JP, Wind A, Davidson AP (eds.): Hereditary Bone and Joint Diseases in the Dog, Hannover, Germany: Schlutersche, 2000.
2. Read RA, et al. Fragmentation of the medial coronoid process of the ulna in dogs: a study of
3. 109 cases. J.Small Anim Pract. 1990;31:330.
4. Bouck GR, et al. A comparison of surgical and medical treatment of fragmented coronoid process and osteochondritis dissecans of the canine elbow. Vet Comp Orth Traum. 1995, 177.
5. Meyer-Lindenberg A, Fehr M., Nolte I. Short and long-term results after surgical treatment of an ununited anconeal process in the dog. Vet Comp Orthop Traum. 2001;14:101-110.
6. Meyer-Lindenberg A, Fehr M, Nolte I. Co-existence of ununited anconeal process and fragmented medial coronoid process of the ulna in the dog. J Small Anim Pract. 2006;47(2):61–65.
7. Meyer-Lindenberg A, Langhamn A, Fehr M, Nolte I. Arthrotomy versus arthroscopy in the treatment of FMCP in 421 dogs. Vet Comp Orthop Traum. 2003; 16: 204-210.
8. Fitzpatrick N. Subtotal coroid ostectomy (SCO) for the treatment of FMCP:A prospective study of 389 elbows evaluating short and medium term outcome. Proceedings Autumn Scientific Meeting BVOA, Nov 2006, pp 22-29.
9. Ness MG. Evaluation of proximal ulnar osteotomy and concurrent fragment excision as a treatment for FCP. Proceedings ECVS Meeting, 1996, p 59.
10. Chico, AC. Screw fixation of an ununited medial epicondyle. Proceedings of ESVOT Congress, 2006, p 218.

STIFLE CONDITIONS IN THE IMMATURE DOG

Alfonso C. Chico, Lic Vet, MVM
Veterinary Surgical Center
La Coruña, Spain

Medial patellar luxation (MPL) is the most common orthopedic condition of the stifle in the immature dog. Small breed dogs are specially predisposed to be affected since the incidence of this pathology is two to four times greater than in large breed dogs. Up to 50% of the cases may have bilateral involvement.

MPL can be traumatic or congenital. The latter is by far the most common (more than 80% of the cases), and has a hereditary component, so affected individuals should not be used with breeding purposes. It has been estimated that MPL is one of the most common congenital defects, with an overall incidence of 7% (121/1679 animals affected in one large study).

The feline stifle can also be affected by patellar luxation. Medial luxation is most frequently encountered and 54% of the cases are bilateral.

CLINICAL SIGNS

It has been estimated that 95% of dogs with patellar luxation have some form of related structural deformity. Because of the wide range of deformities associated with patellar luxation, it is helpful to categorize the deformities into four grades for treatment and prognostic purposes.

Grade I. Intermittent patellar luxation results in the dog not bearing weight on the leg occasionally. With the joint in full extension, the patella can be manually luxated, but when released, it returns to the trochlea immediately. Rotation of the tibia and displacement of the tibial tuberosity is minimal.

Grade II. Frequent luxation occurs, which may last for long periods, causing disuse of the limb. The patella can be replaced either manually or by extension of the joint and derotation of the tibia, but reluxates easily when the tension is released. Pain and crepitus may be apparent during relocation and reluxation. The tibial tuberosity is rotated 30°. Mild angular and torsional changes may be present in the femur and tibia.

Grade III. The patella is permanently luxated with rotation of the tibia and tibial tuberosity from 30° to 60° Repositioning of the patella is possible with extension of the joint and derotation of the tibia, but reluxation occurs immediately. Although the luxation is permanent, many dogs use the limb in a semi-flexed position. There is angulation and torsion of the femur and tibia. The trochlea is shallow or flat.

Grade IV. The patella is permanently luxated with rotation of the tibia from 60° to 90°. Repositioning of the patella is impossible and extension of the stifle is limited by muscular contraction. The limb is non-weight-bearing, or if affected bilaterally, the animal moves in a crouched position with the limbs semi-flexed. The trochlea is flat or convex. Severe angular and torsional changes are present in the tibia and femur.

Radiographic, clinical, and gross anatomic observations of animals with medial patellar luxation reveal a wide range of pathologic changes. The number and severity of changes are related to the grade of the patellar luxation and the age of the animal at the time of luxation: Untreated patellar luxation in a young puppy is likely to result in progressive deformity. The reason is that the growth plate yields to abnormal pressure: Increased pressure parallel to the direction of the developing cartilage columns retards growth and decreased pressure accelerates growth, while forces at an angle to the direction of growth deflects the cartilage columns away from the force. The result, therefore, of linear and angular stress around an active epiphyseal growth plate is bending and torsional deformities of the bones. These pathologic changes appear to start in the hip and subsequently are reflected throughout the limb, resulting in the anatomic abnormalities listed below:

1. Retroversion of the femoral head and neck
2. Coxa vara
3. Medial displacement of the quadriceps muscle group and patella
4. Lateral bowing of the distal third of the femur
5. Shallow or flat trochlear groove
6. Lateral laxity of the stifle joint with increased internal rotation
7. Medial rotation of the tibial tuberosity medially and medial bowing of the proximal half of the tibia
8. Abduction of the hock joint

SURGICAL TREATMENT: WHAT TECHNIQUE(S) DOES THIS DOG NEED?

Procedure(s) selected for the surgical management of patellar luxation must specifically suit the individual needs of the patient. Careful preoperative assessment and decisions based on operative findings are needed to ensure that the correct procedures are selected in each case. Each case must be treated as an individual. Thus, one or several techniques of the following groups can be elected. A cardinal principle is that skeletal deformity, such as deviation of the tibial tuberosity and shallow trochlear sulcus, must be corrected by bone reconstruction techniques. Attempting to overcome such skeletal malformation by soft tissue reconstruction alone is the most frequent cause of failure. Soft tissue procedures, by themselves, must be limited to obvious grade I cases.

The clinician must be aware that internal rotation of the tibia and medial displacement of the quadriceps muscle results in overstretching of the lateral retinaculum, lateral joint capsule, and the lateral collateral ligament. Since the cranial cruciate ligament tries to compensate this abnormal movement, the end result in chronic cases is rupture of this ligament in up to 20 % of the cases.

How to Counteract Medial Periarticular Tension and Lateral Laxity

For lateral laxity, a lateral *capsular or retinacular overlap* is performed. The retinacular fascia and joint capsule are incised 3 to 5 mm from and parallel to the patella. Using nonabsorbable suture, the cut edge of the fascia attached to the patella is sutured beneath the more lateral fascia with several mattress sutures. The amount of tissue to imbricate depends on the laxity of the joint.

For medial tension, a *medial desmotomy* is a simple and effective technique. Desmotomy means a simple release incision of the contracted medial retinaculum that is usually left open.

How to Counteract the Shallow or Flat Trochlear Groove

Perhaps the most widely used technique of this type is *wedge recession sulcoplasty*. The purpose of the recession is to deepen the trochlear sulcus of the patellofemoral articulation while maintaining both a viable articular cartilage of the sulcus and the integrity of the medial trochlear ridge. The medial trochlear ridge acts as a buttress to prevent the patella from luxating medially.

A "V"-shaped wedge containing the trochlear groove is formed by two intersecting saw cuts that create an apex angle of 30 to 40°. This osteochondral piece is removed temporally. The resulting defect in the trochlea is widened by another saw cut on the lateral edge to remove a slice of bone. When the original bone wedge is replaced, it creates a new, deeper sulcus flatted with the original hyaline cartilage. This method is preferred in mature animals because of the risk of damaging the growth plate.

For dogs younger than 7 to 10 months, a *trochlear chondroplasty* is favoured: Through deep cuts in the trochlear cartilage and with the aid of a periosteal elevator, a flap of cartilage is raised from the subchondral bone, which is subsequently deepened and the flap replaced.

Another technique, *the trochlear block recession*, although technically demanding, seems to give better results than other methods.

How to Realign the Quadriceps Mechanism

Four different techniques can be used to realign the extensor mechanism of the stifle depending on the severity of the medial displacement.

Fibular head transposition. The fibular head is isolated from surrounding soft tissue attachments, displaced a few millimeters cranially and fixed with K-wires or cerclages. This produces tension on the collateral ligament that externally rotates the tibia.

Antirotational extra-articular sutures. A band of monofilament nonabsorvable suture is placed around the lateral fabella and passed through a bone tunnel transversal to the tibial tuberosity. The suture is then tightly tied to prevent tibial rotation. The fabella is the center of the arc of rotation of the patella; hence, the suture remains relatively taut during both flexion and extension of the stifle

Tibial crest transposition. In more severe cases of medial rotation of the tibial tuberosity, an osteotomy of a triangular portion of the proximal tibial crest with the patellar ligament attached is performed. The distal periosteal attachment is not transected to get a tension band wire effect. The cranial tibial muscle is elevated and retracted, and the cortex in a more lateral area is roughened with a chisel or curette in preparation for the graft. The fragment is transposed to this area and fixed with two K-wires.

Rectus femoris transposition. This is a recent technique developed to realign the quadriceps by transferring the insertion of the rectus femoris muscle from the ilium to the trochanter.

How to Correct Severe Conformational Defects

Oblique, wedge and rotational osteotomies must be used in deformities of the osseous structures in luxation grades III and IV. The timing of these corrections is essential since changes may become irreversible.

PROGNOSIS

Dogs with Grade I–III luxation have a good prognosis providing that a good combination of soft tissue and bone techniques have been elected. Prognosis for Grade IV luxations is fair and depends on the severity of the deformities and the age of the patient. Degenerative joint disease will progress irrespective of the method of treatment. Long-term follow up studies show an overall good surgical outcome of over 90% although a high incidence of patellar instability and reluxations can be expected frequently without clinical relevance.

STIFLE OCD

Osteochondritis dissecans is a well-recognized abnormality of endochondral ossification affecting young animals of different species, in which the cartilage of the epiphysis fails to form subchondral bone, leading to the formation of a focal area of thickened cartilage. Later in the course of the disease, fissures develop towards the underlying subchondral bone and a flap of cartilage is formed. The definition, etiology, and pathogenesis of OCD are not entirely understood and factors such as trauma within the joint, hormonal factors, nutritional factors, genetics, and ischemia have been implicated.

Stifle OCD is an uncommon cause of canine lameness. It only occurred in 7/1018 (0.7%) Labrador retriever dogs in one report.

In the canine stifle, OCD has been well described both as unilateral and bilateral lesions. The most typical clinical presentation is a gradual onset of lameness with stifle joint pain, synovial effusion, and possible crepitus and reduced range of motion in a 5- to 8-month-old male dog. This lesion typically affects the medial aspect of the lateral femoral condyle, although medial and bicondylar lesions have also been described. In the case of the distal femur, one of the main contributing causes to the development of OCD is the presence of conformational deformities, such as genu valgum and excessive loading of the lateral femoral condyle.

Surgical treatment involves removal of the offending osteochondral flap and curettage of the large subchondral bone defects that usually result. This can be done either through arthrotomy or arthroscopy.

Newer techniques utilize osteochondral bone graft harvesting devices to fill the defect in the femoral condyle.

Mild to severe degenerative joint disease may develop in these dogs irrespective of the method of treatment.

OCD IN OTHER LOCATIONS: TROCHLEAR GROOVE AND PATELLA

Reports on femoropatellar joint osteochondrosis are exceedingly rare. Three cases of osteochondral fragmentation of the patella were described in 1992, and in another report, OCD of the medial trochlear ridge was surgically treated in two bulldog siblings with a good outcome.

LATERAL PATELLAR LUXATION

Lateral patellar luxation (LPL) is far less common than MPL. It is occasionally seen in large dogs and is exceedingly rare in small dogs. As in MPL, the most common is the congenital form, and is usually associated with hip dysplasia, so correction of the quadriceps malalignment may eliminate the clinical signs, but may not correct the underlying problem. The osseous disorders associated with the disease are the opposite of those causing MPL, so most of the surgical techniques are similar but performed in the opposite aspect of the joint.

GENU VALGUM

This condition is often associated with hip dysplasia and LPL. Coxa valga with internal rotation and torsion of the distal femur are frequent features of the disease and lead to a "knock-knee" stance. In severe cases, the patellar luxation must be surgically reduced and corrective osteotomies of the femur performed.

AVULSION FRACTURES OF LIGAMENTS AND TENDONS

Avulsion of the origin of the cruciate ligaments or the tendon of the long digital extensor can occur in the immature stifle

OTHER CONGENITAL DEFECTS

Systemic diseases like congenital hypothyroidism or congenital agenesis of bone can result in stifle problems in puppies.

GROWTH PLATE ABNORMALITIES

Injury to the growth plate is a common disorder of the stifle in young dogs. Traumatic events are the most frequent cause, although developmental defects may take place.

REFERENCES

1. Alam MR, Lee JI, Kang HS, Kim IS, Park SY, Lee KC, Kim NS. Frequency and distribution of patellar luxation in dogs. 134 cases (2000 to 2005). Vet Comp Orthop Traumatol. 2007; 20(1):59-64.
2. Ruble RP, Hird DW. Congenital abnormalities in immature dogs from a pet store: 253 cases (1987-1988).J Am Vet Med Assoc. 1993;202(4):633-636.
3. Arthurs GI, Langley-Hobbs SJ. Complications associated with corrective surgery for patellar luxation in 109 dogs. Vet Surg. 2006;35(6):559-566.
4. Brinker, Piermattei DL, Flo GL. Patellar luxation. In: Piermattei, Flo (eds.): Handbook of Small Animal Orthopaedics and Fracture Repair. Philadelphia, WB Saunders, 1997, pp 516-534.
5. Johnson AL, Probst CW, Decamp CE, Rosenstein DS, Hauptman JG, Weaver BT, Kern TL. Comparison of trochlear block recession and trochlear wedge recession for canine patellar luxation using a cadaver model. Vet Surg. 2001;30(2):140-150.
6. Slocum B, Slocum TD. Rectus femoris transposition for medial patellar luxation. In: Bojrab JM (ed.): Current Techniques in Small Animal Surgery. Baltimore: Williams & Wilkins, 1998, pp 1234-1237.
7. Willauer CC, Vasseur PB. Clinical results of surgical correction of medial luxation of the patella in dogs. Vet Surg. 1987;16(1):31-36.
8. Morgan JP, Wind A, Davidson AP. Bone dysplasias in the Labrador retriever: a radiographic study. J Am Anim Hosp Assoc. 1999;35(4):332-340.
9. Shealy PM, Milton JL, Kincaid SA, Hathcock JT, Boosinger TR, Pernell RT. Osteochondral fragmentation (osteochondrosis) of the canine patella. Vet Comp Orth Traum. 1992; 5: 114-121.
10. Chico AC, Marti JM. OCD of the medial trochlear groove in two bulldog siblings Vet Comp Orthop Traum. 2003,4: 320-325.

COMMON SOFT TISSUE INJURIES OF THE TARSUS

Alfonso C. Chico, Lic Vet, MVM
Veterinary Surgical Center
La Coruña, Spain

BASIC ANATOMY OF THE TARSUS

The canine tarsus consists of seven bones arranged in three rows that define four clinically important horizontal joints: the tarsocrural, proximal intertarsal, distal intertarsal, and tarsometatarsal joints. The vertical joints between individual bones of the tarsus or intratarsal joints are very rigid and not prone to derangement. The tibial tarsal bone or talus is the only tarsal bone to articulate with the distal tibia and fibula, forming the tarsocrural joint.

The distal articulation of the calcaneus with the fourth tarsal bone (calcaneoquartal joint) joins the articulation of the talus with the central tarsal bone (talocalcaneoquartal joint), forming the proximal intertarsal joint. The central tarsal bone touches all of the other tarsal bones. Distally, it articulates with the first, second, and third tarsal bones, forming the distal intertarsal joint on the medial aspect of the tarsus. The first, second, and third tarsal bones articulate with the bases of metatarsals I to III, and the fourth tarsal with the bases of metatarsals IV to V, forming the tarsometatarsal joints.

The tarsus is supported by multiple soft tissue structures. The medial or tibial collateral ligament is divided into a long segment and two short segments. The lateral or fibular collateral ligament is also divided into a long and short component. In both cases, the long part stabilizes the joint in extension, whereas the short components act in flexion.

Dorsal ligamentous support is provided by many small intertarsal and tarsometatarsal ligaments. Proximal and distal transverse ligaments also exist. The plantar ligaments are heavier so that they can support tensile stresses placed on the join. The fibrous part of the tarsal joint capsule extends from the distal articular cartilage of the tibia and fibula to the bases of the metatarsal bones. On the plantar aspect of the tarsometatarsal joint the fibrous joint capsule is especially thick and fuses with the plantar ligaments to form the plantar tarsal fibrocartilage.

MALLEOLAR SHEARING INJURY

Shearing wounds of the tarsus are common in veterinary practice and most often result from road traffic accidents. Animals that sustain these injuries are dragged across a rough surface that avulses tissue and imbeds contaminated debris into the wound. The degree of tissue injury is variable, ranging from cutaneous laceration to severe soft tissue and bone loss.

Shearing wounds often disrupt the collateral ligaments and other supporting structures of the carpal and tarsal joints, leading to instability and loss of function. These wounds may exhibit both articular instability and severe soft-tissue injury. Initial treatment is directed at stabilization of the affected joint and concurrent wound management. Wet-to-dry saline dressings are commonly used to aid in debridement of devitalized soft tissues. The shearing wounds are covered with nonadherent dressings once granulation tissue has started to form. The goal of therapy at this stage is to induce growth of a viable granulation tissue layer on the exposed bone, which can function in wound contraction and over which epithelialization can occur or a skin graft may be applied. In many cases, slow wound healing over exposed bone delays the use of a skin graft and contributes to an extended period of open wound management. Bone perforation to enhance wound healing over exposed bone can be used in such cases.

Surgical Repair

The lateral side is less commonly involved and represents a less serious injury than a comparable injury on the medial side, owing to the fact that the dog normally stands with a few degrees of valgus deviation of the hindpaw, Prosthetic repair of the deficient collateral ligaments is the treatment of choice. Both the long and short functional components should be repaid to provide stabilization in flexion and extension.

The proximal screw is placed as distally in the tibia as possible, but the screw must not enter the joint. On the lateral side, the screw is placed more caudal, from the distal fibula into the tibia. The distal screws are placed to simulate the insertion points of the long and short parts of the collateral ligaments. Medially, both screws are placed in the talus, the proximal one in the body, and the distal screw in the head of the talus.

Laterally, the screws are similarly placed in the calcaneus. The proximal screw goes into the base of the coracoid process, and the distal is placed halfway between the coracoid process and the distal articular surface. Nonabsorbable suture material is then anchored to the screws and washers in a figure-of-8 pattern. The sutures are tied tightly enough to stabilize the joint, but motion without binding should still be possible. Adjunctive stabilization is provided, either with rigid coaptation or with transarticular external skeletal fixation.

More extensive wounds are best managed with external skeletal fixation until granulation tissue has covered the defect. Delayed primary closure or skin grafting is then appropriate. In some cases transarticular external skeletal fixation alone can permit adequate joint stabilisation by scar tissue formation.

Collateral ligament rupture which is not associated with shearing injury is less common. Despite the relatively mild talocrural laxity, severe lameness is evident. Radiography is indicated to rule out avulsion fracture. When there is adequate residual stability to prevent gross luxation, conservative management using coaptation may be considered. Most of the cases, however, will necessitate prosthetic reconstruction, as for shearing injury.

ARTHRODESIS

In extreme situations, the degree of tissue loss may be such that joint reconstruction is impossible. Acceptable options in these cases are limited to amputation or arthrodesis. Arthrodesis is usually utilized as a salvage procedure after other stabilization methods have failed, and it is frequently delayed until the local environment is improved. Alternatively, if joint stabilization could be performed early in the course of treatment (usually with external skeletal fixation) at the same time as soft-tissue debridement, the waiting period and staged approach could be eliminated, thereby simplifying overall case management.

Apart from severe shearing injury, other indications for arthrodesis of the hock joint are not uncommon in small animal practice:

- Degenerative joint disease (most commonly due to OCD, chronic instability or hyperextension).
- Comminuted intra-articular fractures.
- Calcanean tendon breakdown.
- Sciatic nerve palsy when combined with transposition of the long digital extensor tendon

Ideally the limb should be free of other orthopaedic disease, as proximal and distal joints will have to compensate for the loss of talocrural mobility, and the prognosis may be affected by the presence of contralateral hock pathology.

Talocrural Arthrodesis

There are three basic options for the fixation of talocrural arthrodesis: lag screw, bone plate and external skeletal fixation. In the majority of cases, a medial approach is made to the joint by medial collateral desmotomy, or malleolar osteotomy. The functional arthrodesis angle, typically between 135 and 145 degrees, is measured and the osteotomies are performed in distal tibia and fibula and trochlea of the astragalus. Two or more screws can be inserted from the distal tibia to the calcaneus and talus. This technique is usually reserved for small dogs and cats.

Bone plate fixation may be cranial or lateral. The cranial approach is most commonly used. However, the plate is on the compression aspect of the repair, and bone to plate contact is not always accurate. A lateral plate gives better resistance to bending forces. Use of a cuttable plate increases the number of screws per unit length of plate, and this aspect is critical because of the limitation of bone distal to the arthrodesis site. At least one screw should be inserted with lag effect to compress the arthrodesis site.

Although the use of external skeletal fixation alone is associated with the highest complication rate, open or shearing injury may dictate its use to allow adequate wound management. Curved connecting bars or acrylic cement constructs may facilitate pin placement. Because the talocrural joint is the site of highest motion in the tarsus, when it is fused the other joints are subjected to increased functional loads. Chronic sprain injury to the ligaments as well as degenerative joint disease may account for the functional problems observed when arthrodesing the tarsocrural joint. For this reason many authors recommend pantarsal arthrodesis as a better

solution to talocrural problems. Again, plate fixation, and to a lesser grade, external or circular ring fixators are the best choices. Historically plates were applied dorsally, although the use of custom-made, pre-bended plates for lateral placement are gaining popularity. Another recent development is the use of hybrid plates, with two different diameters of the holes, the smallest of which are used to engage the metatarsal bones.

INJURIES TO THE COMMON CALCANEAN TENDON

The common calcanean tendon, or Achilles mechanism, consists of three tendons that insert on the tuber calcanei of the talus: the gastrocnemius; the common tendon of the biceps femoris, semitendinosus, and gracilis muscles; and the tendon of the superficial digital flexor muscle. The gastrocnemius tendon is the largest of this group, and it can be damaged by a direct trauma (hunting injuries, cutting objects), or more frequently, during normal activity. Large middle-age dogs (particularly Doberman) are predisposed to this injury, and some authors suggest that degenerative changes in the tendon may play a part in the pathogenesis of this injury. According to the level of the injury within the Achilles mechanism, they can be divided as follows:

- Lesions of the muscle
- Lesions of the tendon
- Avulsion of the tendon from the tuber calcanei
- Luxation of the superficial flexor tendon
- Fractures of the calcaneus

The most common situations are the disruption of the tendon and the separation from the tuber calcanei. The animal is initially non-weight-bearing for several days, but later in the course of the disease they adopt the typical stance with the stifle slightly extended, the hock moderately flexed, and the digits flexed. Often, careful palpation will reveal the end of the tendon 2 to 3 cm proximal to the tuber calcanei. Eventually the gap between the tuber and the tendon becomes filled with fibrous tissue and gives the impression during palpation that the tendon is intact. In chronic cases, radiography reveals variable dystrophic calcification within the soft tissue, and proliferative new bone on the tuber calcanei.

Surgical Repair

A lateral paramedian approach is made over the distal tendon and tuber calcanei. In acute injuries, transverse tenotomy is performed to create a smooth end for suturing. In chronic cases considerable debridement is necessary to free the tendon and tuber from the fibroplasia. Bone tunnels can be drilled transversely through the calcaneus. Locking-loop sutures (monofilament nonabsorvable) are placed medially and laterally in the tendon. Flexion of the stifle and extension of the tarsus allow easier apposition of the tendon ends. To protect the reconstruction, hyperextension is maintained. A positional screw from calcaneus to tibia or a transarticular external skeletal fixator is left in place for 3 to 4 weeks.

PROXIMAL INTERTARSAL (CALCANEOQUARTAL) PLANTAR LUXATION

Intertarsal injuries almost exclusively involve the proximal intertarsal joint. This is expected since the fourth tarsal bone bridges the distal intertarsal joint forming a substantial buttress. Calcaneoquartal instability may be traumatic, with hyperextension of plantar ligaments or progressive, degenerative hyperextension of the joint. The latter is most commonly found, and two types of patients are seen: middle-aged, overweight dogs, especially of the collie or Shetland sheepdog breeds, and racing/coursing dogs.

Whether the cause is traumatic or degenerative, the patient presents with moderate to severe lameness and different degrees of plantigrade angulation at the tarsal joint. In chronic cases with significant plantigrade stance, the digital flexor tendons are placed under continual tension, which can result in hyperflexion of the digits. In some cases radiography will also demonstrate avulsed fragments of bone from the calcaneus or the fourth tarsal bone. Enthesiophyte formation in these bones can be seen in chronic cases.

Calcaneoquartal arthrodesis gives a good prognosis and is the preferred method of treatment. This can be easily accomplished with a figure-of-8 tension band wire. After articular cartilage is removed, transverse bone tunnels are drilled into the calcaneus and the plantar tubercle of the fourth tarsal bone.

A pilot hole for an intramedullary pin is drilled normograde into the calcaneus, preferably with a drill bit because of the extreme hardness and density of this bone. After the cancellous bone graft is packed around the arthrodesis site, the intramedulary pin is driven from the tuber calcanei to the distal end of the fourth tarsal bone. Finally, the cerclage wire is tightened to obtain the tension band principle.

PROXIMAL INTERTARSAL (CALCANEOQUARTAL) DORSAL LUXATION

This is a less common injury than the plantar luxation, and is associated with rupture of the small ligaments of the dorsal aspect of the proximal intertarsal joint, and sometimes, with tarsal bone fractures. It is associated with a traumatic incident. Medial or lateral instability is often present. In some cases, external coaptation can ameliorate the symptoms, although surgical stabilisation is favoured in larger dogs and if collateral instability is present. Dorsomedial instability is repaired by talocentral arthrodesis stabilised using a figure-of-8 wire about Talus and central tarsal bone screws. If there is significant lateral instability, a lateral calcaneoquartal tension band is added. In severe cases, external skeletal fixation or plate fixation can be used.

TALOCALCANEAL LUXATION

This is an uncommon injury in dogs and cats. It is associated with trauma and lameness can be serious. Rupture of the talocalcaneal ligaments resulting in dorsal displacement of the talar head with talocentral luxation, although plantar displacement has also been described. Talar neck fracture can be seen with this injury. If stable closed reduction is possible, coaptation fixation may suffice. Chronic luxations are very difficult to relocate due to fibrous infilling of the defect. Internal fixation using a positional screw from talus to calcaneus offers more rigid fixation and is the management of choice, offering a good prognosis.

DISTAL INTERTARSAL LUXATION (CENTRODISTAL LUXATION)

This injury can occur in isolation, but is more frequently seen as a complication of calcaneoquartal subluxation. Fourth tarsal bone is a frequent complication of the injury. Stress radiographs are useful in detecting the joints involved.

Centrodistal arthrodesis is indicated. Transverse screws are placed from Tc and T2 into T4. A figure-of-8 wire or monofilament suture is then looped around the washers. This repair may be combined with calcaneoquartal arthrodesis in the more complex injury.

TARSOMETATARSAL LUXATION

This is a less common injury than talocrural or proximal intertarsal luxation. Previous reports on relative frequency of tarsal joints show that 35% affect the intertarsal joint, 24 % the tarso crural joint, and only 12% of the times the injury occurs in the tarsometatarsal joint. As was the case with intertarsal injuries, subluxation with plantar instability is a more disabling injury than that which involves dorsal ligaments only. Cases of dorsal instability can be managed by coaptation, or simple cross pinning without tarsometatarsal arthrodesis. Any disruption which involves plantar ligament compromise is best managed by tarsometatarsal arthrodesis.

Several means of fixation have been described, including intramedullary pin and tension band wire; crossed Kirschner wires alone, an intramedullary pin, bone plate, and external skeletal fixation. Plate fixation is the preferred method for complicated cases, and is normally applied to the lateral aspect of the joint. Screws are purchased into metatarsal bones (ideally three screws), fourth tarsal bone, and lateral aspect of body and tuber calcanei. As with many surgical repairs in the tarsal region, care should be taken with skin closure over the implant and subsequent soft tissue management. Tarsometatarsal arthrodesis offers a good prognosis for return of normal function.

REFERENCES

1. Jaeger GH, Roe SC. Isometry of potential suture attachment sites for the medial aspect of the tibiotarsal joint. Vet Comp Orthop Traumatol. 2005;18(2):73-76.
2. Benson, JA, Budreau, RB. Severe carpal and tarsal shearing injuries treated with an immediate arthrodesis in seven dogs. J Am Anim Hosp Assoc. 2002;38:370.
3. Théoret MC, Moens NM. The use of veterinary cuttable plates for carpal and tarsal arthrodesis in small dogs and cats. Can Vet J. 2007; 48(2):165-168.
4. McKee WM, et al. Pantarsal arthrodesis with a customised medial or lateral bone plate in 13 dogs. Vet Rec. 2004;154(6):165-170.
5. Campbell JR, et al. Intertarsal and tarsometatrsal luxation in the dog. J Small Anim Pract. 1976;427-442.

MINIMALLY INVASIVE SURGERY IN ORTHOPEDICS

Loïc Déjardin, DVM, MS, Diplomate ACVS
College of Veterinary Medicine
Michigan State University, East Lansing, MI

Orthopedic surgeons have long attempted to obtain the maximal stability of their osteosynthesis repair while preserving the soft tissue environment of the fracture site. As an example, this philosophy has been the basis of the use of compression plating techniques after anatomical reduction and has proven clinically successful for decades. Of late, however, this approach has been critically evaluated. Starting in the mid 1980s, a better understanding of the crucial importance of gentle manipulation of soft tissues progressively led surgeons to increasingly rely on indirect reduction techniques during fracture treatment. The acceptance of these new techniques resulted in a paradigm shift, which became the foundation of a new concept known as "biological osteosynthesis." Adoption of biological osteosynthesis principles has been associated with several alterations of traditional plating techniques, which include the use of longer plates, a decrease in the number of plate screws and, more importantly, of interfragmentary reduction screws or cerclage wires. Other significant modifications include gentle manipulation of bone fragments using small fragment reduction forceps, no attempt at anatomical reduction and, last but not least, increasingly limited use of autogenous cancellous bone grafts. This evolution favors the preservation of a biological environment indispensable to bone healing and is further illustrated by the use of bridging plates, which bypass the fracture site altogether. The advantages of biological osteosynthesis have been experimentally demonstrated and validated in the dog and include faster bone healing and a decreased number of complications and failures when compared with traditional techniques.

A key factor in the success of biological osteosynthesis is the preservation of the blood supply to the fracture site. During the first week following the fracture, an inflammatory response, dominated by angiogenesis and controlled by key factors such hypoxemia resulting from local vascular damages takes place at the fracture site, leading to the formation of an early fibro-cartilaginous callus. The concept of minimally invasive surgery (MIS) techniques in the treatment of diaphyseal fractures aims at the preservation of this early callus, which has been demonstrated to be vitally important in optimizing bone healing. This next step in the evolution of the biological osteosynthesis philosophy led to the development of techniques that could avoid any manipulation of the fracture hematoma. In some instances, only limited "keyhole" incisions, remote to the fracture site, are used to slide a bone plate over the fracture (Figures 1 and 2). This sliding plate technique relies on the use of longer bone plates only anchored to the bone via a limited number of screws at each extremity. While this technique heavily relies on minimal disturbance of the biological environment to optimize bone healing, it results in mechanically weaker constructs and should only be used after careful case evaluation. Although clinically rewarding, this technique is technically more challenging. In addition, because the

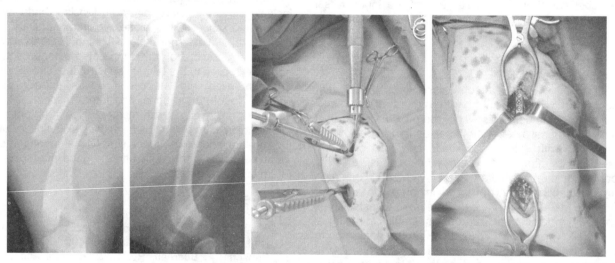

Figure 1. *Left two photographs:* Cranio-caudal and lateral preoperative radiographs of a femoral mid diaphyseal comminuted fracture from a 1-year-old, neutered male, 17 lb, mixed-breed dog. *Center:* Intraoperative photograph showing the small subtrochanteric and the distal periarticular "key hole" incisions used for reduction and fixation purposes. Two small bone reduction forceps are used to remotely reduce the fracture while an intramedullary pin is inserted in a normograde fashion. Although intraoperative fluoroscopy may be used to facilitate reduction and alignment of the fracture, clinical evaluation is often sufficient particularly in the treatment of mid-diaphyseal fractures. *Right:* Intraoperative photograph showing the bone plate affixed to the femur using three proximal and three distal bone screws. Note that the bone plate has been inserted percutaneously without exposure to the fracture site.

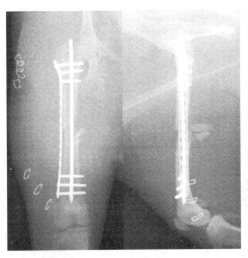
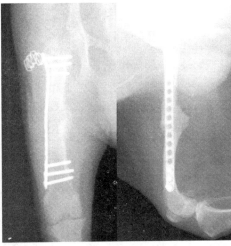

Figure 2. *Left:* Cranio-caudal and lateral postoperative radiographs showing restoration of limb alignment including length and fracture fixation using a combination of a bone plate and an intramedullary pin. Note that, in order to minimize surgical trauma, there has been no attempt at reducing the fracture fragments. The combination of a intramedullary pin and a bone plate is particularly advantageous when the transcortex is not reconstructed whether by choice (eg, biological osteosynthesis) or because it is not surgically feasible (eg, comminution with small fragments). *Right:* Cranio-caudal and lateral post-operative radiographs 6 weeks after surgery. Note that the fragments have been fully incorporated in the boney callus despite the absence of fracture reduction. The intramedullary pin has been removed to eliminate the risk of sciatic nerve damage secondary to migration.

fracture site cannot be visually controlled, a clear appreciation of the three-dimensional bone geometry as well as spatial limb alignment is indispensable

While the concept of MIS initially evolved from traditional plating techniques, other implants such as external skeletal fixators and interlocking nails are particularly well suited for this new therapeutic approach. Similarly, the use of MIS techniques in the treatment of diaphyseal fractures has been successfully expanded to the treatment of articular and periarticular fractures. In such cases, however, the orthopedic surgeon's reliance on intra-operative fluoroscopy becomes even more critical than it is in the treatment of diaphyseal fractures (Figures 3 and 4).

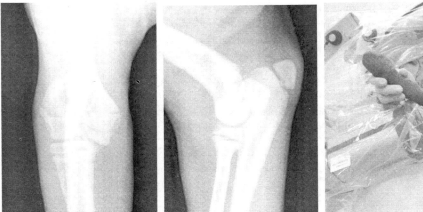
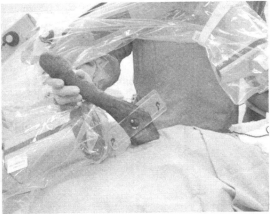

Figure 3. *Left:* Cranio-caudal and lateral pre-operative radiographs of a Salter and Harris type IV fracture of the distal humeral condyles in a 14-week-old female golden retriever. The fracture was externally reduced then temporally stabilized using a radiolucent condylar clamp (*right*). Anatomical reduction was ascertained via intraoperative fluoroscopy. Fixation was achieved by percutaneously inserting a temporary datum trans-condylar Kirschner wire from the medial epicondyle. Once proper position and orientation of the K-wire were verified, the K-wire was removed and replaced by a position trans-condylar bone screw inserted through a stab skin incision over the lateral epicondyle.

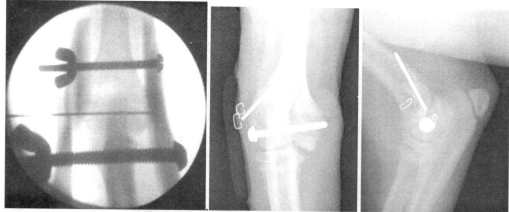

Figure 4. *Left:* Intraoperative fluoroscopic view of the reduced fracture seen through a radiolucent humeral condylar clamp. **Right:** Cranio-caudal and lateral postoperative radiographs showing anatomical alignment and fracture reduction. Stabilization was achieved using a trans-condylar position bone screw and a washer augmented with an anti-rotational Kirschner wire inserted in the lateral humeral epicondylar branch.

The concept of biological osteosynthesis has been further challenged in immature dogs by taking advantage of the rapid and extensive bone healing response. The concept of elastic fixation, which relies on the use of undersized plates and limited plate screws, is based on the premise that rapid bone healing will occur before implant failure and will be further stimulated by local micromotion of the fracture site. The success of such an approach however is dependent on the complete preservation of the fracture site, relying on either sliding plate or "Open-But-Do-Not-Touch" surgical techniques. Conversely, in adult dogs, a more rigid osteosynthesis is necessary. Towards that end, various implant combination techniques have been recommended (eg, plate-rod combination) in order to decrease the incidence of plate fatigue failure due to cyclic bending stresses.

Although biological osteosynthesis techniques do not seek anatomical reduction of the fracture, restoration of limb segment length and alignment in both frontal and sagittal planes, as well as in rotation, are crucial to functional recovery. Simple techniques such as plate pre-contouring using dry bones or contra-lateral radiographs are strongly recommended as is multiple, continuous intra-operative assessment of limb alignment. Finally, one must keep in mind that while striking a balance between biological and mechanical constraints is the basic principle governing biological synthesis, minimally invasive techniques are not applicable in all cases and are not meant as a substitute to more traditional fixation techniques with visual control of the fracture site and limb alignment.

SUGGESTED READINGS

1. Mast J. Planning and Reduction Technique in Fracture Surgery. Berlin: Springer-Verlag, 1989.
2. Johnson AL: Fragment reconstruction and bone plate fixation versus bridging plate fixation for treating highly comminuted femoral fractures in dogs: 35 cases. J Am Vet Med Assoc. 1998, 213(8):1157-1161.
3. Einhorn T. Fracture healing – 40 years after Schenk. AO Dialogue. 2004, 17(2):24-26
4. Krettek C. Concepts of minimally invasive plate osteosynthesis. Injury. 1997, 28S1:A1-2
5. Cabassu J. Elastic plate osteosynthesis of femoral shaft fractures in young dogs. Vet Comp Orthopaed Traumatol. 2001,14(1):40-45
6. Gerber A. Combined internal and external osteosynthesis a biological approach to the treatment of complex fractures of the proximal tibia. Injury. 1998, 29S3:C22-8
7. Hulse D. Reduction of plate strain by addition of an intramedullary pin. Vet Surg. 1997, 26:451-459

ARTHRODESES: INDICATIONS, CHALLENGES AND ALTERNATIVES

Loïc Déjardin, DVM, MS, Diplomate ACVS
College of Veterinary Medicine
Michigan State University, East Lansing, MI

Arthrodeses are surgical fusions of diarthrodial joints. These salvage procedures differ from an ankylosis, a pathological, often painful reduction in joint range of motion. The goal of arthrodeses is to improve overall limb function by eliminating painful motion of a diseased joint. Until joint replacements become readily available, arthrodeses are valuable alternatives to amputation for surgeons dealing with intractable joint conditions. This article addresses general indications, surgical principles, and postoperative care as well as specific challenges and complications associated with arthrodeses of the limb joints.

INDICATIONS

Arthrodeses are mainly indicated in the treatment of severe arthritis resulting in chronic pain not responding to medication. Other common indications include severe instability, secondary to acute or chronic luxations, irreparable intra-articular fractures and severe injury with significant loss of bone and/or articular surface, congenital defects, and malunions. Joint-specific indications consist of angular limb deformities, irreparable failure of the Achilles' mechanism, and motor nerve palsy. Ideally, arthrodesis of any joint should be limited to cases in which the remaining joints of the affected limb are able to withstand the additional stresses generated by the procedure.

SURGICAL PRINCIPLES

Successful arthrodeses require that, regardless of the joint, the following four basic principles be respected. Thorough **articular cartilage debridement** to the level of the subchondral bone or limited ostectomies are performed to favor bone union and to optimize bone contact between opposing surfaces. **Generous bone grafting**, preferably using autogenous cancellous bone is accomplished to enhance bone healing. As the time necessary to reach bone union is shortened, the risk of implant fatigue failure from cyclic bending decreases. This is critically important with carpal and tarsal arthrodeses where bone plates are routinely applied to the dorsal aspect of the bone (compression side of the joint) and are subjected to large bending moments. **Rigid and stable fixation** must be obtained through the application of an appropriate fixation device until clinical union is achieved. Poor postoperative stability will result in delayed or non-union and considerably increase the risk of implant failure. **Preservation or restoration of limb alignment** in three dimensions is critical to the success of the procedure. Indeed, any misalignment in valgus and varus as well as in internal and external rotation may result in alteration of the biomechanics of adjacent joints and therefore must be avoided to limit the risk of secondary degenerative joint disease of adjacent joints.

SURGICAL CONSIDERATIONS
Fixation Techniques

While transarticular pins, screws, and external skeletal fixators may be acceptable alone or in combination, the use of these fixation techniques has been associated with higher morbidity rates including implant failure in large and/or active dogs. External fixation (most often type II configuration) has been advocated to achieve distal joint panarthrodesis. When dealing with open fractures, luxations, and shearing injuries requiring daily wound management, the long-term use of external fixators is fraught with intrinsic postoperative morbidity including pin-tract infection, implant loosening, metacarpal or metatarsal bone fractures, and muscle trauma. Furthermore, suboptimal postoperative stability (compare with plate fixation) requires the use of cumbersome additional connecting bars spanning the joint cranially to overcome the intrinsic weakness of hinged or bent external fixator designs. Conversely, bone plates often represent a more effective alternative in providing immediate and long-term stability with minimal morbidity. Bone plates allow for compression of the surfaces, which in turn enhances frictional forces at the fusion site and therefore provides superior construct rigidity. When the ability to maintain postoperative stability is a concern, such as for carpal and tarsal arthrodeses, the combination of a bone plate with an intramedullary pin has been shown to significantly increase the stiffness of the constructs. Long-term postoperative immobilization (external coaptation) is often necessary to minimize the risk of implant failure, particularly with panarthrodesis of the carpus and tarsus.

Fusion Angles

The angle of fusion in the sagittal plane (flexion and extension) remains the focus of some debate. Although anatomic angles have been reported, substantial breed and individual variations may exist. Therefore, as a general rule, using the joint angle of the opposite limb, *measured under weight-bearing conditions*, is often considered optimal. Deviation from this rule *may be* necessary if the procedure requires resection of significant bone segments such as in arthrodesis of upper joints (shoulder, elbow, stifle). However, unlike humans, all major limb resting joint angles in companion animals are different from 180° (human knee) or 90° (human ankle). This particular feature provides animals with the unique ability to compensate for loss of length in a limb segment by altering the joint angles of that limb. While this ability may be overwhelmed in severe loss of length (eg, following gunshot injuries), the actual percentage of length loss beyond which compensation is impossible has not been determined. As a rule of thumb, however, one can consider that a 20% loss may jeopardize the efficiency of this compensatory mechanism. Because such a dramatic limb shortening is unlikely to result from most arthrodesis procedures, altering the fusion angle during surgery may not be necessary. Conversely, since during normal gait, flexion angles tend to increase during early swing phase, a mild reduction in overall limb length may actually be beneficial, helping to minimize secondary gait alterations such as circumduction, when performing arthrodesis of middle joints with high range of motions (elbow and stifle). Similarly, mild hyperextension (carpus) or hyperflexion (tarsus) likely lowers the risk of cutaneous abrasions as well as digital and/or tendinous injuries, secondary to hyperextension of the metacarpo-phalangeal or metatarsophalangeal joints.

POSTOPERATIVE CARE

Following distal joint arthrodeses, long-term external support is absolutely necessary to protect the implants from bending stresses and potential fatigue failure until radiographic evidence of bone fusion. Effective external coaptation is achieved using a generous even padding. To limit the risk of pressure sores over prominent anatomical structures (eg, over the accessory carpal pad), cast-padding material is added *around* the potential pressure point and applied parsimoniously over it. A bivalve fiber cast, spanning the carpus or tarsus is then applied for 6 to 8 weeks and activity is severely restricted until bone union. To further limit the risk formation of pressure sores, windows may be cut out over areas of concern. Since implant loosening/breakage is often seen following panarthrodeses, implants are routinely removed after complete bone healing. Continued restricted activity is highly recommended after implant removal to reduce the risk of secondary fracture of metacarpal or metatarsal bones weakened by the presence of empty screw holes.

Restricted postoperative activity is also paramount following arthrodesis of upper and middle joints since effective external coaptation is often more difficult. In such cases, although bone plates are often placed along the tensile side of the fusion site, and therefore are better protected against bending moments, restricted activity remains an integral and important part of the overall procedure. This is particularly true after shoulder arthrodesis because of the intrinsic fragility of the scapula.

CHALLENGES AND COMPLICATIONS

Along with general complications inherent to any surgery (eg,infection), arthrodeses are associated with specific complications induced by the profound alteration of the overall biomechanics of the operated limb.

Distal Joint Panarthrodeses

While numerous pancarpal and pantarsal arthrodesis techniques have been described, because of its ease of application, the most commonly performed procedure consists of application of a bone plate on the dorsal (compression) surface of these joints. This technique, however, is mechanically inferior to plate application on the plantar (tension) aspect of the joints. With a dorsal plate, weight-bearing forces will have several deleterious effects including increased inter-fragmentary motion and

poor inter-fragmentary compression, which in turn may delay proper bone healing or even result in nonunion. As a result, the plate becomes subjected to prolonged cyclic bending stresses, which will promote plate fatigue failure and/or implant loosening.

Additionally, a unique challenge to pantarsal arthrodesis is that the tarsus (and therefore the plate) are subjected to large bending moments inherent to the relatively small angle of tarsal fusion (135° to 145° in dogs and 100° to 115° in cats [compared with 170° in carpal arthrodesis]) and to the large lever arm provided by the tarsus-metatarsus-digits complex. Indeed, implant-related complications, including plate breakage and loosening, are common and failure rates of up to 50% have been reported following tibiotarsal arthrodesis. Interestingly, implant loosening often occurs after bony fusion has been achieved. This clinical observation suggests that healed constructs behave like composite materials with differential compliances between plate and bone. In response to cyclic bending and as a result of the relatively higher bone compliance (compared with that of the bone plate), continuous shear micromotion may occur at the bone plate interface progressively leading to implant loosening. Alternatively, repeated bending stresses may be placed on the bone plate leading to catastrophic failure over time.

In an effort to optimize surgical outcomes, long-term adjunctive external coaptation is mandatory to improve postoperative stability and spare the implant. However, because such approaches may result in increased morbidity and cost, the surgeon should strive to promote early bone healing and reduce the risk of implant failure by adhering to the previously described proper surgical principles. Specifically, the use of a tibio-calcaneal screw or the combination of plate fixation with intramedullary pinning has been recommended to reduce plate strain. Recently, a novel pantarsal arthrodesis plate applied over the medial surface of the tibio-tarsal joint has been designed. This plate features a reinforced 140° bend and is tapered in width and thickness from proximal to distal. The tibial segment of the plate accepts 3.5-mm screws while the thinner metatarsal segment receives 2.7-mm screws. A major potential advantage of this design results from its higher ability to resist bending stresses as the plate is bent on edge.

Pancarpal arthrodesis has been associated with additional specific complications. The poor soft tissue coverage of the dorsal aspect of the carpus often jeopardizes surgical closure with adequate plate protection. This in turn significantly increases the risk of postoperative dehiscence and pressure sores, particularly after long-term external coaptation and in thin skin breeds (Greyhounds). Furthermore, the use of conventional bone plates increases the risk of metacarpal fracture due to the relatively large size of the bone screw compared with that of the metacarpal bones. In an attempt to circumvent such complications, hybrid plates featuring a broad proximal segment and a tapered, thinner distal tip have been designed. Currently, 3.5/2.7 and 2.7/2.0 plates are available. While the use of such plates does facilitate skin closure over the metacarpus, postoperative stability may be compromised because of their lower structural properties, particularly with regard to bending. Recently, a new pancarpal arthrodesis plate has been designed to further reduce the risk of metacarpal fractures. The metacarpal segment of the plate features a triangular cross-section and pre-angled screw holes. This design allows the plate to be applied and anchored *between* metacarpal bones 3 *and* 4 rather than *over* metacarpal bone 3 *or* 4.

Proximal and Middle Joint Arthrodeses

Unlike arthrodesis of distal joints, fusion of the shoulder, elbow and stifle involves bone plates placed on the tensile side of the joint. This mechanically superior position promotes fragment compression and reduces plate stresses. However, fusion of proximal joints, endowed with intrinsically larger ranges of motion, results in the creation of long and rigid limb segments. These longer moment arms increase bending stresses on the adjacent bones and therefore the risk of secondary long bone fractures. The risk of fracture is particularly significant at the plate ends, which act as stress risers due to acute local changes in structural properties. It is important to understand that the risk of long bone fracture is not eliminated following bony union. The clinical relevance of this observation is that owners should be aware that the probability for a second surgery for implant removal might be higher than with plate fixation of long bone fractures. The risks of implant failure and bone fractures seem greater following shoulder arthrodesis (thin scapular bone) and stifle arthrodesis where both limb segments are inclined with respect to the vertical plane.

Arthrodeses of proximal joints also transfers compressive stresses and higher torques to the other joints of the operated limb. This "domino effect" may induce degenerative changes in the adjacent joints. The major complication following middle joint arthrodesis remains poor functional outcome despite successful bone healing. Indeed, since the elbow and the stifle provide most of the range of motion during gait, fusion of these joints often results in unacceptable gait alterations (circumduction), particularly at faster gaits.

Alternatives to Middle Joint Arthrodeses

Considering the questionable functional outcome of elbow and stifle arthrodeses, amputation may represent a viable alternative at least until total joint replacements become available. To date, both total elbow and total knee prostheses have been designed and are commercially available from BioMedtrix. While clinical feedback is encouraging, the use of such devices remains challenging and should be performed by experienced orthopedic surgeons.

CONCLUSION

As a general rule, functional limb recovery will improve with arthrodeses involving joints with limited physiologic range of motion during the gait cycle. Indeed, with regard to limb function, carpal and tarsal arthrodeses fare far better than elbow and stifle arthrodeses. Similarly, sparing the tibiotarsal joint by performing a partial tarsal arthrodesis yields a better clinical outcome than if a pantarsal arthrodesis must be performed.

HIGH TIBIAL OSTEOTOMIES FOR THE TREATMENT OF THE CRANIAL CRUCIATE DEFICIENT STIFLE

Loïc Déjardin, DVM, MS, Diplomate ACVS
College of Veterinary Medicine
Michigan State University, East Lansing, MI

In an attempt to circumvent the limitations of extra- and intra-articular techniques, two high tibial osteotomies (HTOs), namely the cranial tibial wedge osteotomy (CTWO) and the tibial plateau leveling osteotomy (TPLO), were introduced approximately 15 years ago. With these procedures, a new conceptual approach to cranial cruciate ligament (CrCL) rupture was proposed. Indeed, unlike previous approaches, HTOs do not attempt to stabilize the joint throughout its range of motion (ROM) but rather provide functional stability during weight bearing by reducing the cranial tibial thrust (CrTT). Since the introduction of the TPLO, several HTO procedures have been devised including the proximal tibial wedge osteotomy (PTWO), the tibial tuberosity advancement (TTA), and the dynamic tibial plateau leveling procedure (DTPLP). This article focuses on the TPLO, which has become the mainstream HTO and compares the TPLO to the above-mentioned procedures.

EFFECTS OF TIBIAL PLATEAU LEVELING ON STIFLE BIOMECHANICS

Rupture of the CrCL occurs when the tensile strength of the CrCL has been overcome as a result trauma and/or degenerative CrCL weakening. The stifle joint reaction force magnitude depends on the combination of ground reaction forces (GRF) and muscle forces generated during the gait cycle and largely exceeds body weight, thus inducing high stresses on passive restraints such as the CrCL. Because of the tibial plateau slope orientation, tibial compression (during weight bearing or tibial compression test) generates a cranially oriented shear force that induces cranial tibial translation in CrCL-deficient stifles. This shear force, the cranial tibial thrust (CrTT), is in part opposed by the CrCL. Accordingly, it has been suggested that CrTT magnitude depends on GRF magnitude and is likely amplified by greater tibial plateau slope angles (TPAs). The actual mechanism by which TPLO provides functional stifle stability under load was investigated in an in vitro study, which demonstrated that TPL consistently eliminates cranial tibial subluxation and also induces significant caudal tibial translation. This suggests that TPL stabilizes CrCL-deficient stifles by converting CrTT into caudal tibial thrust (CaTT). As a cranially oriented tibial thrust generates cranial tibial translation, in a like manner, the CaTT generates caudal tibial translation. Stifle stability then depends on the caudal cruciate ligament (CaCL) integrity. As increased tibial plateau angle has been clinically associated with CrCL rupture, similarly, increased CaCL strains have been shown to parallel experimental increases in the magnitude of the cranial tibial plateau slope angle, thus theoretically predisposing the CaCL to failure. True tibial plateau leveling (ie, reducing the TPA to 0°) is not necessary to provide functional stifle stability. Experimentally, a mean post-operative TPA of 6.5° is sufficient to restore stifle stability. This agrees with the clinical recommendation that the post-operative TPA should be 5° rather than 0° (true leveling). Because tibial plateau over-rotation increases CaCL stress, this smaller angle may represent the optimal angle of tibial plateau rotation providing joint stability in CrCL-deficient stifles, while sparing the CaCL from excessive strains. Clinically, while direct tibial translation can be manually induced, the tibial compression test should be negative after surgery.

Alternative high tibial osteotomies such as the CTWO, the PTWO and the TTA technically differ from the TPLO, their purpose however is similar, namely to reduce the cranial tibial thrust in order to eliminate the need for an intact cranial cruciate ligament. While this is allegedly accomplished through reduction of the TPA in the CTWO and PWTO, in contrast, the TTA relies on the surgical advancement of the tibia tuberosity until the patellar ligament becomes perpendicular to the TPS. The proposed net biomechanical effect is the elimination of the CrCL force, as the joint reaction force becomes a pure compressive force without a shear component. Although not an osteotomy procedure, the DTPLP has been devised to alter the slope of the tibial plateau in immature dogs. The alleged purpose of the DTPLP is to treat CrCL rupture in dogs with open physes (when performing a tibial osteotomy would be ill-advised) or even to prophylactically limit the incidence of CrCL rupture in dogs at high risk. The procedure induces premature closure of the cranial aspect of the tibial plateau growth plate via lag screw fixation. In turn, the unrestricted growth of the caudal aspect of the tibial plateau physis gradually reduces the tibial plateau slope as the dog ages.

SURGICAL TECHNIQUE
Tibial Plateau Leveling Osteotomy

Measurement of the tibial plateau angle (TPA) is performed preoperatively on lateral radiographs of the limb centered on the stifle joint. The TPA is the angle between the tibial slope and the perpendicular to the tibial functional axis. After routine anesthesia, joint exploration and meniscal and/or CrCL débridement is conducted via a limited arthrotomy or arthroscopy. When appropriate, medial meniscal release may be performed to prevent post-operative meniscal damage. The medial aspect of the proximal tibia is exposed and a proximal tibial circular osteotomy is performed using a specialized armamentarium. The magnitude of the tibial plateau rotation is based on preoperative TPA measurement and is such that the post-operative TPA is approximately 5°. After proper rotation of the tibial plateau the tibial fragments are stabilized in the desired relationship using specially designed bone plates. Routine closure in layers, including the arthrotomy, concludes the procedure.

Cranial Tibial Wedge Osteotomy

The procedure is conducted as described above, until the tibial osteotomy step. Using a protractor, a tibial wedge (opening cranially) is etched immediately below the medial aspect of the tibial crest and then removed with a bone saw. The wedge angle equals the preoperative TPA reduced by 5° or 6° (eg, ~ 20° for a preoperative TPA of 25°). The tibial fragments are then stabilized with a standard dynamic compression plate applied medially. Careful plate contouring and pre-stressing are necessary to ensure proper limb alignment and fragment compression. Routine closure in layers concludes the procedure. Although CTWO is meant to neutralize the CrTT, the relative effectiveness of this procedure vs. TPLO and its effect on CaCL stresses have yet to be reported.

Tibial Tuberosity Advancement

The initial steps of the TTA procedure are similar to those described above. The magnitude of the TTA is based on pre-operative radiographic evaluation and is such that with the stifle at ~ 135° the patellar ligament becomes approximately perpendicular to the medial tibial plateau. The tibial osteotomy is performed according to a protocol described by Montavon and requires the use of specialized equipment designed by Kyon (Zurich, Switzerland). Briefly, using an oscillating bone saw, a linear tibial crest osteotomy is performed between the tubercle of Gerdy proximally and the distal extent of the tibial crest. The proximal aspect of the tibial crest is then advanced cranially according to preoperative measurements and templates. The tibial crest is secured using a specially designed bone plate applied medially and a cage interposed between the crest and the tibia proximally. A bone graft is also used to fill the defect distal to the cage prior to routine closure in layers.

CLINICAL OUTCOME AND COMPLICATIONS

Patients are usually discharged within 24 hours of surgery and postoperative pain is managed with NSAIDS as needed. Strict in-house confinement, along with short leash walks, is recommended until radiographic evidence of clinical union. As with any other joint surgery, implementation of a controlled postoperative rehabilitation regimen is recommended to hasten recovery.

TPLO

The clinical outcome of the TPLO has been evaluated more thoroughly than that of other HTOs. To date, most reports have emphasized the rapid return to pre-injury limb function after TPLO. Based on subjective evaluations, functional recovery appears faster after TPLO than with other cruciate ligament procedures. Toe touching is usually observed within 1 to 2 weeks after surgery, followed by rapid improvement of limb function by 2 months. In a recent prospective clinical trial comparing TPLO and extra-articular techniques at 6 months, TPLO consistently yielded subjectively better outcomes for all parameters evaluated, including time to recovery, stifle range of motion, dog's ability to sit normally and postoperative complications. The effect of TPLO on limb function has been evaluated using force plate analysis. In contrast to previous clinical reports, no differences in peak vertical force (PVF) at 2 and 6 months were found between extra-articular and TPLO techniques, suggesting no clear superiority of any procedure in restoring limb function. However, the postoperative regimen of the group treated with an extra-articular procedure included controlled physical therapy while that of the TPLO treated dogs did not. Therefore, this report mainly emphasizes the importance of physical therapy in optimizing functional recovery after joint surgery. Reportedly, one of the most significant advantages of the TPLO procedure resides in its ability to control, unlike any other procedures before, the long-term progression of degenerative joint disease (DJD). Additional comparative clinical studies are needed to confirm this remarkable observation. While in vitro studies have suggested that meniscal release may have a deleterious effect on intra-articular stresses, a recent retrospective study reports that this procedure has no protective effect on secondary meniscal tears. Anecdotal reports also suggest that meniscal release has no negative impact on long-term clinical outcomes.

Inadequate tibial plateau correction may result from inaccurate radiographic measurement of the preoperative TPA or from poor intra-operative tibial correction. This should not be overlooked as it could potentially result in long-term complications. Indeed, while under-correction is unlikely to provide adequate postoperative joint stability, over-rotation may increase the risk of CaCL injury. Because such complications may be difficult to address, great attention should be paid to preoperative TPA measurement as well as to intra-operative technical details. As with any osteosynthesis, postoperative complications include implant failure, non-union or mal-union, and osteomyelitis. Other TPLO-related complications may be more challenging and include rotary instability, tibial crest fractures, patellar ligament desmitis, patellar fracture and luxation. The treatment of CrCL ligament stifle with excessive TPA (TPA>35°) is technically challenging and requires the combination of a TPLO and a CTWO. While the long-term outcome of this complex procedure is very good in most cases, the rate of significant complications remains high, including a ~28% risk for implant failure. In a recent clinical evaluation of this procedure, a second surgery (most often for implant removal) was necessary in ~30% of the cases and the mean time to clinical union was substantially longer that with a TPLO alone at ~18 weeks.

HTOs

The long-term clinical outcome of **CTWO** was recently evaluated. Interestingly, the percentage of good/excellent results was 86%, which compares only fairly with reported results of more traditional intra- or extra-articular procedures. Complications, however, were potentially more serious including tibial fracture and implant failure in 5% of the cases. One of the reported advantages of CTWO is faster return to weight bearing and performance despite a distinct tendency for postoperative stifle hyperextension. Unlike TPLO, the CTWO alters the normal femoro-patellar joint relationship, potentially causing patella baja unless the stifle is hyperextended. The clinical relevance of chronic stifle hyperextension after CWTO has yet to be determined. At Michigan State University, this procedure is rarely performed and is mainly reserved for the treatment of cases with a pathologically high TPA and associated patella alta.

While the **PTWO** initially appeared promising, this procedure is not recommended due to the unacceptable rate and severity of its postoperative complications. Shortly following the abandonment of the PTWO, the **TTA** was proposed as an alternative to the TPLO procedure. Today, only sparse reports evaluating the long-term outcome of this technique are available. The TTA is a derivation of the now defunct Maquet procedure (1960s) recommended in humans for the treatment of patellar chondromalacia. Based on a recent report, the TTA procedure seems to provide good to excellent results in a majority (~90%) of the cases. One force-plate analysis study reports that, by 4 months after surgery, the mean PVF of the operated limb reaches 64% of the dog's body weight (normal PVF = 75% BW). Thanks to iterations in the design of the original implants, the rate of implant failure has been reduced to approximately 6%. Although meniscal release is not recommended with this technique, the rate of late meniscal tear is approximately 10% in the absence of meniscal treatment. One of the limitations of the TTA is that, unlike the TPLO, its use in cases where the preoperative TPA is greater than 25° is associated with a potentially higher risk of complications. From a biomechanical and theoretical point of view, because the procedure is unlikely to control tibial internal rotation and allegedly reduces the femoro-patellar pressure, the risk of patellar luxation is potentially higher than with a TPLO. Therefore, large-scale objective studies are necessary to better evaluate the TTA procedure.

Control of the final tibial plateau angle with **DTPLP** remains unpredictable and is highly dependent on the age and breed of the patient. Potential complications include insufficient or excessive correction, with secondary failure of the CrCL or CaCL, respectively, as well as valgus or varus deformity. To date, the procedure remains experimental with ill-defined guidelines. Therefore, until publication of a standardized procedure and clinical results, this procedure should only be considered cautiously and should not be recommended as a reliable treatment modality for CCLR in juvenile patients.

CRANIAL CRUCIATE LIGAMENT RUPTURE: BIOMECHANICS, PATHOGENESIS, AND DIAGNOSIS

Loïc Déjardin, DVM, MS, Diplomate ACVS
College of Veterinary Medicine
Michigan State University, East Lansing, MI

Cranial cruciate ligament (CCL) rupture is the most common injury to the stifle joint of dogs and is the primary cause of degenerative arthritic changes diagnosed in that joint. As such, treatment of CCL injuries constitutes one of the preponderant activities of many small animal practices.

FUNCTIONAL STIFLE BIOMECHANICS
Relevant Stifle Anatomy
Cruciate and collateral ligaments are the major static stabilizers of the stifle although menisci, joint capsule, and peripheral musculature also contribute to joint stability. From its femoral origin to its tibial insertion, the CCL twists 90° on itself as it crosses the joint space in a cranio-medial direction. The CCL comprises two functionally distinct bands: the thin cranio-medial band taut throughout the range of motion (ROM) and the bulkier caudo-lateral band, which relaxes during stifle flexion. The CCL is an extra-synovial structure with a poorly vascularized central section.

Stifle Kinematics
Stifle motion can be described with respect to three mutually orthogonal axes. Rotation about and translation along each axis describe six basic movements, each of which, although present to some extent in normal motion, is limited by various ligamentous constraints. Normal stifle motion is a combination of flexion-extension about a medio-lateral axis with internal-external tibial rotation about a dorso-ventral axis. Hyperextension is prevented by the impingement of the CCL on the intercondylar notch (ICN) and to a lesser extent by the collateral ligaments. Internal tibial rotation occurs during flexion due to lateral collateral ligament relaxation. Excessive tibial internal rotation, however, is primarily prevented by the twisting of the cruciate ligaments about one another. Because of its spatial orientation and anatomical structure, the CCL also prevents cranial tibial translation throughout ROM. Accordingly, CCL failure allows for hyperextension, excessive tibial internal rotation and cranial tibial translation. Such abnormal movements cannot be limited by secondary constraints (collateral ligaments, menisci) and consequently often induces abnormal stresses to these structures eventually leading to secondary injuries such as meniscal tears.

Stifle Kinetics
Ground reaction forces (GRF) are external forces exerted by the ground against a body in reaction to gravity. For the rear legs, GRF approximate 40% of body weight (BW) at rest and increase with the velocity and acceleration of the body, reaching 70% BW at the trot and several times BW during jumping. To maintain equilibrium or generate motion, GRF must be counteracted by muscle forces; however, mechanical efficiency demands joint stability. The combination of GRF and muscle forces during physiological activity generates joint forces that largely exceed BW, which, in turn, may produce high stresses on passive restrains such as the CCL. For example, the resultant of GRF and extensor muscle forces during weight bearing generates compressive forces along the tibia. Because of the slope of the tibial plateau, tibial compression generates a cranially oriented shear force that induces cranial tibial translation in CCL-deficient stifles. The shear component of the compressive force at the knee, termed cranial tibial thrust (CTT), is opposed by the CCL. The magnitude of the CTT essentially depends on the magnitude of the GRF and extensor muscle forces (eg, walk vs. jump) and is likely amplified by greater tibial slope angles.

PATHOGENESIS
Rupture of the CCL occurs when the tensile strength of the ligament has been exceeded following acute severe trauma or more commonly because of chronic degenerative weakening. In the later case, even minor stresses during normal activity (running or jumping) may result in CCL rupture.

Traumatic CCL Rupture
Acute, traumatic ruptures of the CCL are uncommon and are generally observed in younger animals. The injury occurs as a result of specific, sudden stresses such as internal rotation and/or hyperextension of the limb and may show as mid-substance tears or avulsions. Major trauma (eg, hit by car) resulting in CCL rupture is commonly associated with concurrent ligamentous and/or meniscal injuries. More often, CCL weakening result from repetitive microtrauma because the poor blood supply of the CCL limits its healing potential. Such stress injuries may result from various conformational or anatomical causes. Increase in stifle angle (straight-legged dogs) results in continual relative stifle hyperextension, which may increase CCL stresses. Similarly, medial patellar luxation may increase the risk of CCL rupture by causing excessive tibial internal rotation and by compromising the cranial stability of the stifle. Congenital intercondylar notch (ICN) stenosis resulting in impingement of the CCL during motion has been proposed as a possible cause of CCL rupture in dogs. The impact of ICN stenosis on CCL rupture, however, is unclear, as it is a common consequence of degenerative joint disease secondary to CCL rupture. Because of the tibial plateau slope, the tibial condyles tend to slide cranially as the joint is loaded during stance phase. Cranial tibial translation, however, is primarily resisted by the CCL. Consequently, increases in tibial plateau slope angle could increase CCL stresses thus leading to fatigue failure. The relationship between tibial plateau slope angle and prevalence of CCL rupture, however, has yet to be determined. Finally, chronic joint overload resulting from obesity is a well-recognized contributing factor to further weakening of the CCL. The higher incidence of CCL rupture in spayed females has

been attributed to the excessive weight gain that frequently follows neutering.

CCL Degeneration

Most often, CCL weakening results from age-related degeneration. Indeed, by 5 years of age, the CCL consistently shows microscopic evidence of degeneration, which results in a significant deterioration of its material properties. Histologically, most changes occur within the poorly vascularized central third of the CCL and include loss of fibroblasts, chondroid metaplasia, decreased vascularity, and loss of the collagen crimping. CCL degeneration tends to occur later in life and to a lesser extent in smaller dogs (body weight <15 kg). Similarly, studies have demonstrated that decreased physiological stresses result in a rapid and significant decline in mechanical properties of tendons and ligaments. This may explain the frequency of CCL rupture in dogs having sedentary life styles.

Immune-mediated arthropathies such as rheumatoid arthritis have long been associated with CCL rupture. The immune-mediated origin of CCL rupture has been strengthened by the increasingly frequent diagnosis of lymphocytic plasmacytic synovitis, and finding of anticollagen antibodies against type I and II collagen in the serum and/or synovial fluid of dogs with CCL rupture. It is unclear, however, whether such immune reactions cause or follow CCL ruptures. The idea that an inflammatory process precedes CCL rupture is strengthened by the observation that bilateral DJD is often present with unilateral lesion and that the percentage of dogs who will rupture their opposite CCL within 18 month of diagnosis increases from 40% to 60% if degenerative joint disease is present at the time of initial diagnosis.

Tibial Plateau Slope

Clinical reports in dogs have suggested that increases in tibial plateau angle (TPA) predisposes to CCL rupture. While the mean TPA in dogs varies between 23° and 25°, a wide range of TPA has been reported (13° to 34°) in normal dogs. Read and Robins first described the correlation between CCL rupture and increases in tibial plateau slope (TPS) and suggested that a steep TPS places excessive stress on the CCL ultimately leading to its rupture. Although the correlation between CCL rupture and large increases in TPA (eg, secondary to growth plate injury) seems established, the association between TPA and CCL rupture in a normal canine population remains controversial. In two early reports, the mean TPA of dogs with CCL rupture was found to be significantly greater by as low as 2° or 5.7° than the mean TPA of dogs with intact CCL. Considering the wide variation in natural TPA in dogs (and humans), and the influence of radiographic technique in TPA measurements, further prospective studies are needed to confirm this data. The previous findings have not been supported by other studies. Comparing the TPA of breeds predisposed to CCL rupture (Labradors) and protected from it (Greyhounds), other authors report no significant differences in TPA (26° and 24.8°, respectively). Similarly, using age as a risk factor, it has been shown that the TPA of cruciate-deficient Labradors was not different from that of older Labradors with intact CCL (23.5° ± 3.1° and 23.6 ± 3.5°, respectively). Based on these findings, it appears that in dogs free of conformational abnormalities, there is little if any correlation between TPA and CCL rupture. Accordingly, TPA should not be used as predictor for CCL rupture in dogs.

Regardless of its cause, stifle instability following CCL rupture induces a consistent cascade of events, which include capsulitis, synovitis, articular cartilage degeneration, osteophytosis, bone sclerosis and meniscal injuries. Because of the severe morbidity associated with CCL rupture the ultimate therapeutic objective is to prevent or limit the progression of degenerative joint disease (DJD) through the appropriate combination of medical, surgical and post-operative treatments.

DIAGNOSIS

History

Acute, traumatic ruptures of the cranial cruciate ligament are diagnosed infrequently and most often are seen in young active animals. The injury, which may include the medial meniscus, occurs as a result of specific, sudden stresses such as internal rotation and/or hyperextension of the limb. In such cases, owners typically report an acute, short-lived (1 to 2 weeks), non-weight bearing lameness that often subsides to a mild limp over the following weeks to months as fibrous tissues partially stabilize the joint. Eventually, secondary meniscal tears and degenerative joint disease will result in a chronic, mild to moderate weight bearing lameness. Most often, ruptures of the CCL occur in middle age (5–8 years old), over weight, spayed females as a result of slow degeneration and weakening of the ligament. Degenerative ruptures have an ill-defined course and may show episodic, mild to moderate lameness for several weeks to months. The first episode of lameness may occur during normal daily activity. Lameness usually worsens with exercise. Dogs may also demonstrate difficulty rising as well as shifting weight from one leg to the other, particularly if both stifles are affected. Following partial functional recovery, the lameness becomes progressive as secondary arthritic degeneration develops. Dogs may become non-weight bearing, usually a sign of full rupture of the CCL (after an initial partial tear) or more often a sign of secondary meniscal damage. Several breeds (St Bernard, Rottweilers, Newfoundlands, Labradors) seem predisposed to rupture of the CCL. The differential diagnosis should include hip dysplasia, osteochondrosis and patellar luxation.

Clinical Examination

Upon presentation, clinical signs may include joint effusion with loss of palpable definition of the patellar ligament (acute cases), or gross enlargement of the joint due to thickening and fibrosis of the surrounding tissues particularly on the medial aspect of the joint (buttress sign evident in chronic cases). Palpation of the joint usually does not elicit a pain response except in very acute cases. Secondary meniscal tears often induce a "meniscal click" as the joint is put through a full range of motion. Definitive diagnosis is made by demonstrating the cranial drawer sign in which the tibia slides forward with respect to the femur. The drawer sign can be evidenced via direct cranio-caudal manipulation of the tibia with respect to the femur or indirectly using the tibial compression test during which the hock is flexed while the stifle flexion-extension angle is maintained at ~140°. The tibial compression test simulates a weight-bearing environment and is often better tolerated by the animal. The drawer sign is generally present in dogs with acute, complete tears of the cruciate ligament. In dogs with chronic lameness and/or partial cruciate tears, the drawer sign may be minimal or absent. For large dogs, apprehensive dogs, and those with chronic fibrosis, sedation may be necessary to overcome any muscle rigidity that might suppress the drawer sign. The drawer tests should be performed throughout stifle range of motion in order to detect partial rupture of the CCL. One should remember that immature animals might show a physiologic drawer characterized by a subtle cranio-caudal laxity and an abrupt stop of the tibia during a direct drawer test.

Radiographic Examination

The purpose of the radiographic examination is to confirm the clinical diagnosis and to rule out other causes of lameness such as osteochondrosis or tendon avulsion (long digital extensor or popliteal). In addition, radiographs can also provide prognostic information by demonstrating the degree of arthritic changes present. Finally, radiographs are used for preoperative planning when high tibial osteotomies, eg, tibial plateau leveling osteotomy (TPLO) or tibial tuberosity advancement (TTA) are considered. Radiographs will detect joint effusion but will not detect the ruptured ligament except in rare cases involving avulsion of the ligament with a detectable bony fragment.

In acute cases, joint effusion is seen on lateral radiographs as 1) a reduction in the size of the radiolucent fat pad (cranial compartment) and 2) a bulging of the caudal profile of the joint capsule between the fabellae and the tibial plateaus. This sign is characterized by a caudal displacement of the fatty interface between the joint capsule and the gastrocnemius. Within the following 3 weeks, osteophytes will appear at various locations including on lateral views 1) the distal pole of the patella, 2) the proximal aspect and the lateral surfaces of the femoral trochlea, 3) the lateral fabella, and 4) the caudal aspect of the medial tibial plateau. On cranio-caudal views, osteophytosis is most often seen as a narrowing of the intercondylar notch and a flare of the lateral aspect of the tibial plateau. In chronic cases, soft tissue thickening secondary to fibrosis of the medial aspect of the joint (medial buttress) is clearly visible on cranio-caudal views. The presence of joint effusion on the opposite stifle, even without clinical signs strongly suggests that rupture of the cruciate ligament is forthcoming (60% risk of CCL rupture within the following 12 months).

HOW DO JOINT PRESERVATION COMPOUNDS WORK AT THE CELLULAR LEVEL? MODE OF ACTION: GLUCOSAMINE, CHONDROITIN SULFATE AND AVOCADO SOYBEAN UNSAPONIFIABLES

Jennifer Demko, DVM
College of Veterinary Medicine
Mississippi State University, Mississippi State, MS

Clinical studies in humans and animals suffering from degenerative joint disease have documented the beneficial effect of glucosamine (Glu), chondroitin sulfate (CS), and avocado soybean unsaponifiables (ASU). Degenerative joint diseases, primarily osteoarthritis, are characterized by pain, immobility, and lameness in veterinary cases. The use of joint-preserving compounds (JPCs) such as Glu, CS, and ASU has been shown to relieve pain and improve joint movement in OA. Radiologic evidence in humans and in animals also suggests that these compounds may act as disease-modifying agents. Reports on the clinical benefits of Glu, CS and ASU in OA have prompted laboratory research to help clarify their mode of action. In vitro models using joint tissues and isolated cells have been instrumental in defining how these JPCs work at the cellular level.[1-6] Laboratory studies with in vitro models indicate that these JPCs exert anti-inflammatory and anti-catabolic activity. They also enhance production of cartilage matrix components indicating anabolic activity. More recent studies suggest that the combination of Glu, CS, and ASU may have more profound beneficial effects

ANTI-INFLAMMATORY AND ANTI-CATABOLIC ACTIVITY

OA is characterized by increased local production of pro-inflammatory mediators including cytokines, chemokines, nitric oxide (NO), reactive oxygen species (ROS), and products of arachidonic acid metabolism, such as prostaglandin (PGE_2) and leukotrienes.[1-7] These mediators have also been shown to induce production of metalloproteinases and aggrecanases that degrade cartilage. Studies support the critical role of these pro-inflammatory mediators and degradative enzymes in the pathogenesis of OA. The observation that Glu and CS inhibit production of nitric oxide, PGE_2, as well as expression of enzymes that regulate their synthesis may account for their clinical benefits.[8-12] These agents were reported to suppress expression of enzymes cyclo-oxygenase-2 (COX-2) and microsomal prostaglandin E synthase that control PGE_2 production.[1-5] Glu and CS were also documented to suppress inducible nitric oxide synthase (iNOS) expression. INOs is a critical enzyme that regulates NO production. Anti-inflammatory effects of ASU have also been documented in animal studies and in cell culture models.[9-12] In an ovine model of OA, ASU-treated animals showed a significant reduction in subchondral bone sclerosis. Treated animals also showed increased proteoglycan content and thickness in the articular knee joint. In an equine OA model, total gross examination of articular cartilage erosion and synovial membrane hemorrhage showed significant improvement in horses treated with ASU compared with placebo treatment. ASU also increased the production of transforming growth factor beta in the knee joint fluid of a canine model, suggesting increased synthesis of matrix components.[13] In human articular chondrocytes stimulated with IL-1β, ASU suppressed IL-6, IL-8, MIP-1α, PGE_2, and nitric oxide production.[14] Similar to Glu and CS, ASU reversed the catabolic effect of IL-1β in human fibroblasts by inducing a significant decrease in MMP-2, MMP-3, and TIMP-1.

Increased catabolic processes resulting in cartilage breakdown has been attributed to metalloproteinases (MMPs) and aggrecanases (ADAMTS). Increased levels of MMP isotypes including 1, 3, 13, and ADAMTS-4, 5 have been detected. In contrast, reduced levels of their natural inhibitors (TIMPS) were observed. Glu and CS inhibited the expression of these degradative enzymes.[15-17] Conversely, Glu and CS up-regulated the levels of TIMPS. Down-regulation of degradative enzymes while enhancing the expression of their inhibitors may attenuate cartilage breakdown in the arthritic joint. ASU also showed a similar inhibitory effect on the synthesis of these degradative enzymes.

ENHANCEMENT OF ANABOLIC ACTIVITY

Cell and tissue based studies have provided evidence that Glu and CS induce the synthesis of cartilage extracellular matrix components.[18-20] However, the mechanism by which these agents act as anabolic agents is still not defined. No compelling data show that they are directly incorporated into the matrix. Enhancement of proteoglycan and collagen synthesis has been attributed to indirect effects. By inhibiting pro-inflammatory mediators and enzymes that suppress de novo synthesis, Glu and CS are thought to enhance matrix synthesis. For example, nitric oxide is known to inhibit proteoglycan production. Suppression of NO production may thus promote proteoglycan synthesis. Similarly, studies suggest that ASU may have anabolic effects on cartilage metabolism. ASU restored aggrecan synthesis in IL-1β-stimulated chondrocytes and enhanced transforming growth factor-α and plasminogen activator inhibitor-1 expression in normal chondrocytes. In addition, ASU fully maintained aggrecan production and type II collagen expression in schondrocytes co-cultured with osteoarthritic subchondral osteoblasts. In a study utilizing an in vivo model of cartilage destruction, ASU preserved the glycosaminoglycan and hydroxyproline content in the cartilage tissue, demonstrating a possible chondroprotective effect on articular cartilage. These studies may help explain the observed clinical benefits such as pain relief and improved mobility.

CONCLUSION

Evidence drawn from studies using isolated cells and tissue explants indicate that Glu, CS, and ASU have chondroprotective effects. These agents reduce production of pro-inflammatory mediators and degradative enzymes while enhancing production of extracellular matrix components in arthritic joints. Recent data suggest that their anti-catabolic and pro-anabolic activities involve intricate cell signaling pathways. These pathways include down regulation of the I-kB-NF-kB inflammation loop via ERK–MAPK shown in Figure 1.[21-22].The potential mode of action of CS, Glu and ASU may simulate inhibition of many aspects of the inflammatory cascade and associated signaling pathways.

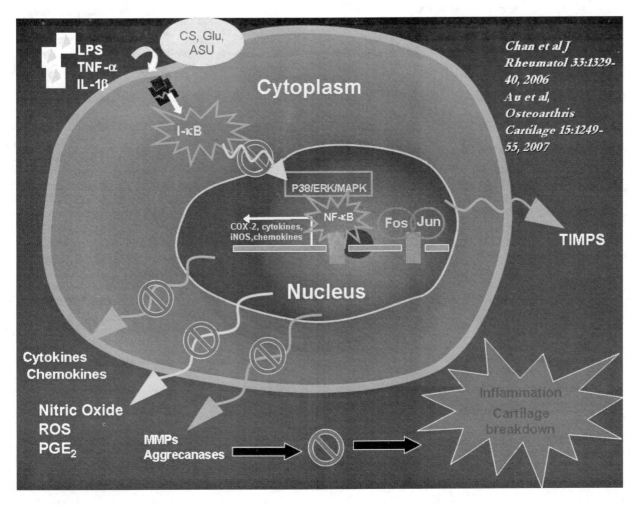

Figure 1. Mode of action of chondroitin sulfate (CS), glucosamine (Glu), and avocado soybean unsaponifiables (ASU) to preserve joint function..

REFERENCES

1. Chan PS, Caron JP, Orth MW. Short-term gene expression changes in cartilage explants stimulated with interleukin-1beta plus glucosamine and chondroitin sulfate. J Rheum. 2006;33:1329-1340.

2. Chan PS, Caron JP, Rosa GJ, et al. Glucosamine and chondroitin sulfate regulate gene expression and synthesis of nitric oxide and prostaglandin E(2) in articular cartilage explants. Osteoarthritis Cartilage. 2005;13:387-394.

3. Byron CR, Orth MW, Venta PJ, et al. Influence of glucosamine on matrix metalloproteinase expression and activity in lipopolysaccharide-stimulated equine chondrocytes. Am J Vet Res. 2003;64:666-671.

4. Meininger CJ, Kelly KA, Li H, et al. Glucosamine inhibits inducible nitric oxide synthesis. Biochem Biophys Res Commun. 2000;279:234-239.

5. Soeken KL. Selected CAM therapies for arthritis-related pain: the evidence from systematic reviews. Clin J Pain. 2004;20:13-18.

6. Reginster JY, Deroisy R, Rovati LC, et al. Long-term effects of glucosamine sulphate on osteoarthritis progression: a randomised, placebo-controlled clinical trial. Lancet. 2001;357:251-256.

7. Melchiorri C, Meliconi R, Frizziero L, et al. Enhanced and coordinated in vivo expression of inflammatory cytokines and nitric oxide synthase by chondrocytes from patients with osteoarthritis. Arthritis Rheum. 1998;41:2165-2174.

8. Kut-Lasserre C, Miller CC, Ejeil AL, et al. Effect of avocado and soybean unsaponifiables on gelatinase A (MMP-2), stromelysin 1 (MMP-3), and tissue inhibitors of matrix metalloproteinase (TIMP-1 and TIMP-2) secretion by human fibroblasts in culture. J Periodontol. 2001;72:1685-1694.

9. Henrotin YE, Sanchez C, Deberg MA, et al. Avocado/soybean unsaponifiables increase aggrecan synthesis and reduce catabolic and proinflammatory mediator production by human osteoarthritic chondrocytes. J Rheum. 2003;30: 1825-1834.

10. Kawcak CE, Frisbie DD, McIlwraith CW, et al: Evaluation of avocado and soybean unsaponifiable extracts for treatment of horses with experimentally induced osteoarthritis. Am J Vet Res. 2007;68:598-604.

11. Lippiello, L, Nardo, J, Harlan, R, et al. Metabolic effects of avocado/soy unsaponifiables on articular chondrocytes. ecam/nem132.3d; 2007.

12. Au RY, Al-Talib TK, Au AY, Phan PV, Frondoza CG. Avocado soybean unsaponifiables (ASU) suppress TNF-alpha, IL-1beta, COX-2, iNOS gene expression, and prostaglandin E(2) and nitric oxide production in articular chondrocytes and monocyte/macrophages. Osteoarthritis Cartilage. 2007; 15:1249-55.

13. Altinel L, Saritas ZK, Kose KC, Pamuk K, Aksoy Y, Serteser M. Treatment with unsaponifiable extracts of avocado and soybean increases TGF-beta1 and TGF-beta2 levels in canine joint fluid Tohoku J Exp Med. 2007;211:181-6.

14. Henrotin YE, Labasse AH, Jaspar JM, et al. Effects of three avocado/soybean unsaponifiable mixtures on metalloproteinases, cytokines and prostaglandin E2 production by human articular chondrocytes. Clin Rheum. 1998;17:31-39.

15. Chan PS, Caron JP, Orth MW. Effect of glucosamine and chondroitin sulfate on regulation of gene expression of proteolytic enzymes and their inhibitors in interleukin-1-challenged bovine articular cartilage explants. Am J Vet Res. 2005;66:1870-1876.

16. Nakamura H, Shibakawa A, Tanaka M, et al. Effects of glucosamine hydrochloride on the production of prostaglandin E2, nitric oxide and metalloproteases by chondrocytes and synoviocytes in osteoarthritis. Clin Exp Rheumatol. 2004;22:293-299.

17. Chan PS, Caron JP, Orth MW. The effects of glucosamine and chondroitin sulfate on cartilage explants cultured for 2 weeks. Am J Vet Res. 2007; 68;709-715.

18. Homandberg GA, Guo D, Ray LM, et al. Mixtures of glucosamine and chondroitin sulfate reverse fibronectin fragment mediated damage to cartilage more effectively than either agent alone. Osteoarthritis Cartilage. 2006; 14:793-806.

19. Lippiello L. Glucosamine and chondroitin sulfate: biological response modifiers of chondrocytes under simulated conditions of joint stress. Osteoarthritis Cartilage. 2003;11:335-342.

20. Lippiello L, Woodward J, Karpman R, et al. In vivo chondroprotection and metabolic synergy of glucosamine and chondroitin sulfate. Clin Orthop Rel Res. 2000;381:229-240.

21. Largo, R, Alvarez-Soria, MA, Diez-Ortego, I, et al. Glucosamine inhibits IL-1β-induced NFκB activation in human osteoarthritic chondrocytes. Osteoarthritis Cartilage. 2003;11:290-298

22. Holzmann, J, Brandi, N, Zemann, A, et al. Assorted effects of TGFβ and chondroitinsulfate on p38 and ERK 1/2 activation levels in human articular chondrocytes stimulated with LPS. Osteoarthritic Cartilage. 2006;14:519-525.

BASIC EXTERNAL FIXATION

Erick Egger, DVM, Diplomate ACVS
Veterinary Orthopedic Consultant
Colorado State University, Ft. Collins, CO

Any form of fixation must control disruptive forces at the fracture to be successful. The forces that will act at any given fracture are dependent on the location and pattern of that fracture. Bending is a force that must be controlled in nearly all fractures and can occur in all planes around the longitudinal axis. Experimental work has suggested that bending in the cranial-caudal plane is the most significant with walking. External fixators control bending well, particularly in the plane perpendicular to the fixation pins. Axial compression results from muscle pull and weight bearing. With oblique or comminuted fracture patterns, axial compression will result in fracture collapse or overriding unless adequately controlled. With simple more transverse fractures, axial compression will result in fracture impaction and increased fracture stability. The external fixator's ability to control axial compression is very dependent on the device's configuration. Torsion is the force that results in rotation if not controlled. While long oblique fractures tend to resist torsion, comminuted or transverse fractures tend to be unstable in torsion. Fixators are relatively good at controlling torsion. Tension is the force applied by a muscle or ligament to a bony avulsion fracture and will result in distraction of the fracture unless adequately controlled. Since tension tends to be applied to small avulsion fragments that limit fixation pin purchase, external fixation is a poor choice for controlling this disruptive force.

Once the disruptive forces acting at a fracture are determined, a configuration of external fixation can usually be designed or modified to control these forces consistent with anatomic and wound management.

BIOMECHANICS OF FIXATOR CONFIGURATION

The simplest configurations of external fixation use fixation pins, which pass through only one side of the limb and both bone cortices called "half pins." The pins are connected together on one side of the limb to form a type I (half pin) splint. Type I configurations can be used on the humerus or femur to avoid interfering with the body wall. They can also be positioned to avoid soft tissue injuries on the lower limbs. The original Kirschner-Ehmer apparatus copied the Anderson splint in using double connecting clamps and an additional connecting bar to connect individual half pin splints in each fragment. This avoided the need for linear fixation pin alignment and allowed significant adjustment of fracture reduction after fixation application. However clinical experience and biomechanical testing has shown that this double clamp type I configuration does not provide adequate resistance to weight bearing loads due to inherent weakness in the double clamp. Consequently its routine use for fracture treatment is not recommended and its usefulness is limited to very rapidly healing situations such as corrective osteotomies.

With proper application techniques, all the fixation pins can be attached to a single connecting bar. This type I single connecting bar configuration will provide adequate resistance to bending forces for treating most relatively stable simple fractures in smaller animals. Furthermore this configuration is lighter and requires less expensive equipment. For larger animals or less stable fractures that must be treated with a Type I configuration, a second connecting bar can be added to the same fixation pins, creating a double connecting bar design. This will nearly double the splint's resistance to compressive forces by converting the resulting bending force seen by a single connecting bar into compressive force on the inner bar and tensile force on the outer bar. Two half-pin splints can be applied oriented parallel and at 60 to 90 degrees of axial rotation to each other. The two splints can be linked to form a triangular cross section. The resulting biplanar type I configuration is more resistant to craniocaudal bending forces than even full pin uniplanar splints. More importantly, it can be applied to very proximal or distal fractures since fixation pins can be inserted from two planes.

"Full pins" pass through both sides of the limb and the bone. The pins can be connected together to form a type II (full pin) splint. Type II configurations are very resistant to compressive forces. Hence, they can be used on relatively unstable fractures. However, to avoid interference with the body wall, they are generally limited to use below the elbow or the stifle. Since it may be difficult to obtain perfect alignment of all full pins for attachment to connecting bars on both sides of the limb, many surgeons prefer to modify the type II splint by only using one full pin in each fragment with additional half-pins inserted from one or both bars for adequate stability. This not only greatly simplifies application but also increases the number of fixation pins, which can be used with the same number of clamps.

Combining a type I and type II splint will form a type III (trilateral) configuration which is the most rigid of currently used designs being roughly ten times as resistant to axial compression as type I splints. Consequently, they are used for highly unstable or infected fractures, nonunions, and arthrodesis where the need for prolonged rigid fixation is anticipated.

External fixators are most often used as the primary fracture fixation. Alternatively, an external fixator may be successfully used in conjunction with an intramedullary pin. The IM pin will control bending forces while the fixator controls torsional loads. Often the fixator can then be removed in 4 to 6 weeks once early callus formation has occurred. In order to increase the montague's bending strength and further reduce the incidence of post operative complications, the proximal end of the Type I fixator can be "tied-in" to the proximal end of an appropriately sized IM pin using an additional connecting bar and double connecting clamps.

EFFECT OF FIXATOR ARRANGEMENT ON BIOMECHANICS

The number of pins placed in each fragment affects the stiffness of the fixator. While the exact effect of pin number is dependent on a number of factors including fixator configuration and pin diameter, mechanical studies on a type II fixator found that increasing from two to three pins per fragment resulted in a 66% increase in axial stiffness, and increasing to four pins per fragment resulted in an additional 33% increase. Using more than four pins per fragment had relatively little effect on stiffness. More importantly for longevity of fixation, increasing the number of pins avoids overloading the bone surrounding each pin. Overloading causes microfractures of the bone and the subsequent resorption results in premature pin loosening. Consequently, we use a minimum of three and preferably four pins on each side of a fracture. The fixation pins are best spread over the length of the fractured bone to distribute the disruptive forces and maintain maximum fixator strength.

The diameter of the fixation pins is determined based on the diameter of the bone. If the pin diameter is too small, the pins will be too flexible and allow excessive motion with potential loss of fracture reduction. If the pin diameter is too large, the bone will be weakened and pinhole fracture may result. We compromise these factors and generally select a pin diameter about 20% of the bone diameter.

If all non-threaded fixation pins are used, at least two pins in each fragment should be placed at a divergent angle to each other to maintain a mechanical grip on the bone. An angle of 30 to 40 degrees between the outermost pins placed in each fragment has been suggested as offering the best compromise between pin strength and bone grip. The balance of the pins in the frame can be angled or perpendicular as most convenient. If threaded fixation pins are used they can be perpendicularly oriented to the bone. This will make pin placement easier, allow placing more pins in a shorter length without resulting in interference, and shorten the effective length of the pin (from bone to clamp) that will make the overall frame stiffer.

As the frame is constructed, the positioning of the connecting bar must be considered. Some distance must be provided between the skin and the bar to allow for swelling and callus formation without encroachment of skin on the clamps. However, increasing this distance significantly reduces the stiffness and strength of the frame. A good compromise appears to be about 2 to 3 cm for a medium-sized dog. Obviously this distance should be scaled to the size of the patient and the location of the device.

Traditionally non-threaded fixation pins were used with fixators. One Steinmann pin or double pointed Kirschner wire (for very small patients) could be cut in half to make two fixation pins. Much recent research has investigated the use of threaded fixation pins. Both clinically and experimentally, threaded pins offer a much better grip on the bone and increase stiffness of the fixator compared to non-threaded pins. While partially threaded (thread is cut into the pin shaft) Steinmann pins provide greater resistance to pin pull out, the stress collector effect at the threaded/non-threaded junction has often been the location of pin bending or breakage. One solution is the Ellis pin, which is threaded only a short distance (about three times the pin's diameter) from the tip so the pin will thread only into the far cortex, thus protecting the weak stress collector in the medullary canal. Alternatively, pin designs with a positive thread profile, where the inner thread diameter is that of the non-threaded shaft and the outer thread diameter is greater, have become available in sizes for veterinary application. Some clinicians suggest using a combination of non-threaded and threaded pins to minimize the post operative complications of pin loosening and pin tract drainage while maintaining good fixation pin strength at a reasonable cost. However, as the standard or care in veterinary medicine increases and the tolerance for morbidity and patient pain decrease, most specialty surgeons are using predominately positive profile threaded pins.

APPLICATION OF EXTERNAL FIXATORS

Erick Egger, DVM, Diplomate ACVS
Veterinary Orthopedic Consultant
Colorado State University, Ft. Collins, CO

External skeletal fixation is easy to use; however, close adherence to several principles of application will improve results and reduce the incidence of postoperative problems.

While the bulk of the external fixation is outside the body, the fixation pin to bone interface is usually the limiting factor in determining the longevity and stability of fixation. Consequently, the insertion of these pins must be done under the same aseptic conditions as would be used in placing any other orthopedic implant.

One of the most important advantages of external skeletal fixation is that it can be applied with little additional damage to vascularity, and hence, the healing process. Closed reduction of the fracture will minimize such damage. Consequently, some clinicians prefer this approach. However, closed reduction may not provide adequate fracture reduction or alignment, particularly with complex fractures or fractures located proximal to the elbow or stifle joint. Delayed, non-, or malunion can result. Consequently, the author generally prefers a limited open approach to achieve better overall fracture alignment and reduction. A limited open approach also allows the placement of autogenous cancellous bone graft into fracture defects. Using either open or closed reduction, the standard guideline for minimal acceptable reduction is at least 50% cortical contact on the worst of two cranial-caudal and medial-lateral radiographic projections.

As noted by Coombs "External fixation is only as effective as the pin contact with bone." Since premature loosening of fixation pins is the most common cause of postoperative problems, and even fixation failure, attention to pin application is essential.

The method of pin insertion is quite important. In the past, hand-chuck placement has been advocated to avoid thermal necrosis of bone from frictional heat. However, wobbling with a hand chuck can result in oversize pinholes and pin loosening. Furthermore, hand placement in cortical bone is very hard work, commonly resulting in less than the optimal number of pins being used. Consequently, direct power insertion is preferred. Research has shown that direct slow-speed (150 rpm or less) power drill placement does not result in significant temperature elevation or premature pin loosening in canine diaphyseal bone. However, excess pressure and high speed must be avoided. Pre-drilling the pin hole with a slightly smaller twist bit (about 90% pin diameter) is a commonly accepted technique in human orthopedics and should be considered in very dense bone such as the olecranon. Also, recent research has demonstrated that predrilling a slightly under sized pilot hole before pin insertion will result in "radial preload" of the surrounding bone that results in less pin loosening with cyclic pin loading as occurs with unstable fractures.

Before any pins are placed, the fracture should be approximately reduced so excessive skin tension does not develop against the pins when final reduction is achieved. When pins are inserted, they should be placed through small separate skin incisions. This decreases the tendency for soft tissues to wrap up around the rotating pin and subsequent skin necrosis. The pins should not be placed through the approach incisions because that makes closure very difficult. Where possible the fixation pins should avoid penetrating large muscle masses and areas of extensive soft tissue motion since this is a common cause of poor postoperative limb use and pin tract drainage. The pins should be placed through the widest diameter of the bone to provide the most strength and avoid cracking the bone. When applying a half pin splint, the pins need to be driven so the tip completely penetrates the far cortex. The triangular shape of the pin tip tends to make incompletely penetrating pins back out and loosen.

In certain oblique and comminuted fractures, interfragmentary fixation such as lag screws and cerclage wires can be used to achieve better reduction. However, the manipulation required to apply these devices may damage vascularity and slow healing. In addition, rigid interfragmentary devices should not be used with a flexible frame configuration, since they will have a stress concentrating effect. This may actually cause further fragmentation of the fracture. We prefer to use divergent Kirschner wires. These wires can be applied with minimal additional soft tissue damage, and they provide adequate stabilization without the stress concentrating effect.

GENERAL PROCEDURE FOR MECHANICAL (BAR AND CLAMP) TYPE FIXATOR APPLICATION

1. Fracture is approximately reduced by either closed manipulation or through a limited open approach minimizing soft tissue damage.
2. The most proximal and distal fixation pins are driven through small skin incisions into the two fragments at appropriate angles.
3. Connecting clamps and a connecting bar are slid onto the end pins with the anticipated number of "open" clamps in the middle of the bar.
4. The fracture is reduced. With an open approach, bone clamps can be used to facilitate manipulation and to maintain reduction. In selected comminuted or oblique fractures, interfragmentary fixation may be employed to hold fragments in place.
5. The connecting bar is positioned far enough from the body to allow for swelling and callous formation without encroachment of the skin on the clamps and the end clamps are tightened.
6. If a more rigid configuration is required, a second connecting bar can be "stacked" on top of the first to create a double connecting bar type I half pin splint. Distal to the elbow or stifle, the second bar can be added to the opposite end of full pins to form a type II configuration.

7. The remaining fixation pins are driven through the open clamps at appropriate angles, usually alternating sides of the fracture.
8. The clamps are tightened as each pin is placed and fracture reduction is rechecked.
9. Excessive fixation pin length is removed with a pin cutter.

USE OF ACRYLICS IN EXTERNAL FIXATORS

The first reports of acrylic-pin splints used Steinmann pins or very long orthopedic screws as fixation pins. The screws were inserted in the bones leaving the heads extended externally where they were connected with dental acrylic. Commercial kits have developed for acrylic-pin splints in human orthopedics because of their ability to provide maximum support of difficult fractures and ease of application with minimal cost. Use of these human devices for small animal fracture treatment has been reported, but their size and expense have limited widespread application. Homemade acrylic-pin splints are similarly constructed using methylmethacrylate, which is available as hoof repair or dental molding acrylic. Mechanical testing suggests a column diameter of 3/4" provides fixation stability similar or superior to the traditional device designs.

THE ACRYLIC-PIN EXTERNAL FIXATOR (APEF) SYSTEM

In order to improve consistency of results and convenience of application, we have developed the APEF system specifically for small animal veterinary use. The APEF base kit contains all material needed for construction of "standard" fixators comparable in size and strength to the medium Kirschner apparatus and "mini" fixators comparable in indication and strength to the small Kirschner.

TECHNIQUE FOR APEF SYSTEM APPLICATION

The APEF system is usually applied with a biphasic technique.

Stage I (Sterile)
1. Fixation pins (usually a combination of threaded pins for optimal bone-pin integrity, and non threaded pins for economy) are inserted in the bone fragments. Pin orientation is not restricted by frame alignment or clamp design. This allows the surgeon to design the frame configuration to best meet the mechanical needs of the fracture and minimize soft tissue tethering.
2. The APEF alignment frame is attached to pins on both sides of the fracture close to the skin level. The fracture is reduced (using closed manipulation or open reduction at the surgeons discretion), and the clamps are tightened to temporarily maintain reduction.
3. Open reduction approach incisions are closed or open wounds aseptically packed. Adequacy of closed reduction can be checked with radiographs.
4. Pins are cut off approximately 4 to 5 cm from the skin level.

5. The acrylic column molding tubes are "impaled" on the pin ends and the tubes are positioned adjacent to the alignment frame, parallel to the limb about 1/2 to 1 inch from the skin.
6. The most dependent end of each molding tube is plugged.

Stage II (Nonsterile)
1. Temporary divider is "popped" off the acrylic pack by pulling powder and liquid portion of bag in opposite directions
2. The acrylic is then mixed for 2 to 3 minutes to a smooth consistency, a corner of the bag is cut off with a scissors, and the acrylic is then poured into the open end of each tube.
3. The acrylic is allowed to cure (10 to 12 minutes).
4. The alignment frame, plugs and excess molding tube are removed.

Readjustment of a completed acrylic splint is more difficult in some respects than traditional linear devices, but does not require replacement of the fixation pins to correct rotational malalignments as they do. Splint adjustment requires removing a short segment of the acrylic column with a saw or cast cutter. The plastic molding tube is peeled back from each end and several holes drilled in the remaining acrylic to provide a base for the patch. A small amount of new acrylic is mixed and hand molded to fill the gap and overlap the existing column ends. The fracture is then manipulated into correct reduction and held while the acrylic cures. More fixation pins can be added to either replace existing pins or increase overall frame stability. The plastic molding tubing is removed from the existing acrylic column and several 1/8" diameter holes drilled in the acrylic adjacent to the proposed pin insertion site. After aseptically preparing the skin and acrylic column surface, the new fixation pin is inserted using appropriate technique. The free end of the pin is bent to contact or cross the column. A mini pack of APEF acrylic or other acrylic is mixed to dough consistency and molded around the new pin and existing column to incorporate it.

Acrylic splint removal is achieved by cutting each fixation pin between the skin and acrylic column. Each pin is then removed using a hand chuck or pliers. Alternatively, the acrylic connecting bar can be cut between pins and each pin removed.

Indications for acrylic splint use include routine fracture fixation. For highly unstable fractures, staged disassembly of an initially rigid configuration can be employed (by progressive removal of columns) to stimulate healing hypertrophy and remodeling while protecting from refractor. Acrylic splints are particularly useful for mandible fractures and transarticular application because the acrylic connecting columns are easily contoured to the shape of the body and joint angles. The acrylic used is radiolucent, which does not interfere with radiographic assessment of initial reduction or fracture healing.

ORIENTATION OF EXTERNAL FIXATORS ON SPECIFIC LONG BONES
Humerus

Application of external skeletal fixation to the humerus usually requires a minimal open approach to achieve adequate reduction. Type I splints are usually oriented laterally with the proximal pins placed cranial to the deltoid muscle while the distal pins can be placed through the condyle avoiding the supracondylar foramen and the radial nerve. Biplanar type I splints are oriented cranially and laterally.

Radius

The radius can be stabilized with external skeletal fixation after either open or closed reduction. Uniplanar type I splints are usually oriented laterally for proximal fractures, cranially for very small bones, or medially for distal fractures, although any of these orientations are acceptable to avoid penetrating and interfering with soft tissue injuries. Biplanar type I splints are oriented cranially and laterally for proximal fractures or cranially and medially for distal fractures. Type II splints are usually applied from medial to lateral.

Femur

Femoral fractures require an open approach to obtain adequate reduction. Only type I uniplanar splints applied from the lateral aspect should be used to avoid muscle entrapment and subsequent stifle joint stiffening. A second connecting bar can be applied to the half pins if needed for fixator strength.

Tibia

Tibial fractures can be reduced using open or closed methods. Uniplanar type I splints are best applied from the medial aspect to minimize soft tissue penetration but can be applied either cranially or laterally if necessary to avoid soft tissue wounds. Type II splints are placed from medial to lateral. Biplanar type I or type III splints use cranial and medial or lateral oriented pins. The proximal pins should be placed in the wider and stronger caudal aspect of the tibia.

INDICATIONS FOR EXTERNAL FIXATOR

Erick Egger, DVM, Diplomate ACVS
Veterinary Orthopedic Consultant
Colorado State University, Ft. Collins, CO

ADJUNCTIVE TO OTHER INTERNAL FIXATION

External skeletal fixation may be used for ancillary support of other forms of internal fixation. It can be effective in controlling axial rotation, and to some degree, axial collapse of the fracture site when used with intramedullary pins. Traditionally, a two-pin type I splint has been used for this purpose, although our experience suggests that using three pins, and better yet four pins, will significantly decrease the incidence of premature pin loosening and loss of fixation. Recently the concept of "Tie In" between an Intramedullary pin and the external fixator has been discussed in treating femoral fractures. This appears to not only increase the rigidity of the composite, but also decrease the incidence of IM pin migration. The supplementary external fixation can usually be removed in 3 to 5 weeks when the callus becomes sufficiently organized to control rotation.

SIMPLE FRACTURES

While simple fractures can be treated with many techniques, external fixation may be a good choice in certain instances. The patient with multiple fractures will become ambulatory much faster than with cooptation. The ease of implant removal and ability to avoid stress protection allows faster return to athletic function than plating. Finally, the clinician interested in developing the skills of external fixation will find starting with simple fractures to be more rewarding than developing experience on only "disaster" situations.

COMMINUTED FRACTURES

Severely comminuted fractures may be treated with external fixation when more exacting reconstruction is not possible. External fixation requires minimal bone for fixation and can span large defects. Care must be taken to avoid damage to osseous vascular since healing relies on early callous formation. Consequently, a closed reduction or limited open reduction with massive chancellors bone auto graft is necessary. Overall joint alignment, but not necessarily perfect fracture reduction, is sought. A relatively rigid configuration should be initially applied to neutralize disruptive forces. Destabilization after early fracture healing has occurred (6 to 10 weeks), should be considered in order to enhance callus hypertrophy and remodeling.

OPEN, GUNSHOT, AND INFECTED FRACTURES

External fixation has the advantage of not invading the fracture site and spreading contamination or infection. The fixation pins can usually be applied away from the affected area, lessening the chance of premature bone lysis and early implant failure, which could result in nonunion. External fixation is particularly useful for stabilizing severe open wound fractures because it will support the fracture and soft tissue vascular while preserving access to the traumatized area for continued treatment. Gunshot-induced fractures often combine the problems of severe combination and bone loss with significant contamination, and severe soft tissue vascular damage. Moderate debridement followed by rigid external fixation, cancellous bone autografting and packing the wound open is indicated. Repeated debridement may be required every 2 to 4 days as the healing process delineates viable from necrotic tissue. Treatment of fractures with established infections requires removal of unstable hardware, sequestra (necrotic, infected bone fragments), and infected proliferative scar tissue. A very rigid configuration of external fixation to allow revascularization is applied, avoiding the infected wound as much as possible. The wound is thoroughly lavaged and saucerized (packed open) to allow repeated lavage and debridement. Cancellous grafting may be delayed for 10 to 14 days to allow granulation tissue to cover the fracture ends and provide vascularity for the graft.

MANDIBULAR FRACTURES

External fixation has the advantage of being able to avoid the placement of implants in open wounds and infected alveolar sockets. Mandibular fractures are often very comminuted and open into the mouth. The use of external fixation allows the preservation of remaining vascular supply to the multiple small fragments. The acrylic-pin splint works very well, particularly for bilateral mandibular fractures.

NONUNIONS

Nonunions can be described as hypertrophic or atrophic. In hypertrophic nonunions, the bone is capable of biologic reaction (healing) when the proper environment exists. Stabilization is all that is usually necessary and can be provided in many cases with reduction and application of rigid fixation. Atrophic nonunions have lost the capacity of biologic reaction. This type is most commonly seen in fractures of hypovascular areas in miniature breeds, such as distal radius and ulna, that have poor leg use when treated with external coaptation or when a previous surgery has resulted in loss of fragment vascularity and fracture stability. Treatment requires open reduction, removal of unstable hardware, decortication of avascular bone, opening of the medullary canal, and packing with cancellous bone graft to stimulate vascular proliferation and allowing the bone stimulating stress of weight bearing

TRANSARTICULAR STABILIZATION

External fixation is being increasingly used for transarticular stabilization. This is ideal for cases of ligamentous rupture associated with adjacent, soft tissue injury. The ligament may be repaired or replaced with a prosthesis and protected by the external fixator while treatment of the open wound continues. A recent improvement involves bending the connecting bars to the desired joint angle. This facilitates fixator application, and minimizes frame bulk. The fixation is usually maintained for 3 to 6 weeks depending on the severity of injury. Ranges of motion exercises are recommended after fixator removal to restore joint motion.

Transarticular external fixation may be used to help protect articular or periarticular fractures from weight bearing forces. Note, however, that intra-articular fractures require anatomic reduction and fixation with an interfragmentary compression device such as a lag screw to avoid degenerative joint changes. Because of their metaphyseal location, such fractures tend to heal quickly so the transarticular portion of the fixator can usually be removed after 4 to 8 weeks. Physical therapy is needed to attain maximum joint function. External fixation may also be used for arthrodesing certain joints. It is especially useful in cases with severe soft tissue damage or infection where the use of internal fixation would be less desirable. The principles of arthrodesis should be followed as with any form of fixation. These include removal of articular cartilage, cancellous bone grafting, and prolonged fixation requiring multiple pins and a rigid configuration.

MALUNION AND DEFORMITY CORRECTION

External fixation is commonly used in the treatment of deformities created by prior inadequate fracture reduction or abnormal growth. The ability of the device to easily adjust in all three dimensions at once and provide adequate stability with minimal cortial bone contact facilitates this. Also the ability to provide multiplanar fixation allows adequate stabilization of very short segments as occurs with corrective osteotomies of the distal radius following premature close of the distal ulnar physis. By aligning the proximal and distal most pins with the adjacent joint, the pins can then be used as alignment handles as the realignment is achieved. The osteotomy can also often be created with a semi-closed approach minimizing biologic damage and optimizing healing.

EXOTIC PET AND AVIAN APPLICATION

We often use external fixation for stabilization of injuries in birds and particularly small exotic pets. The APEF concept is very light, inexpensive and easily adapted to many unique situations.

STAGED DISASSEMBLY

"Staged disassembly" or "destabilization" is the concept of initially applying very rigid fixation, which is converted to a less rigid form once early healing has occurred. The flexible frame allows enough stress of the fracture to stimulate optimal hypertrophy but protects the fracture from overloading that might be detrimental to healing. Our experimental studies have indicated that around 6 weeks after surgery is the optimal time for staged disassembly of fixates in dogs. Much earlier destabilization seems to result in excessive preinstall callus formation with poor fracture strength, much later had no positive effect when compared to continuously rigid fixation suggesting a limited "window of opportunity" for maximal effect. However factors that influence the biology of fracture healing such as the animal's age and general health, soft tissue damage and presence of infection at the fracture, and the addition of cancellous bone graft probably affects the optimal timing of destabilization. Unfortunately radiographic signs are rarely a good indicator for the timing of this approach since the biologic processes significantly precedes the passive mineralization apparent on radiographs. The technique is accomplished by removing the connecting bars and pins from one side of a type II or type III splint to form a type I splint. This type I configuration will be resistant enough to bending forces to prevent refracture, but flexible enough in axial compression to stimulate callus hypertrophy and bone remodeling. While both dynamization and induced micromotion require special fixator systems, staged disassembly is easily accomplished with any standard fixator device.

THE TPLO – WHY DOES IT WORK?

Erick L Egger, DVM, Diplomate ACVS
Veterinary Orthopedic Consultant
Colorado State University, Ft. Collins, CO

In larger dogs (greater than 15 kg), the results with nonsurgical management are reversed, with less then 20% of patients adequately recovering based on owner satisfaction. Since the criteria for a truly successful treatment is return to full function, the disruptive forces will return once the patient recovers. In the normal stifle, the cruciate cranial ligament acts to restrain the tibia from sliding forward as the foot pushes off. Disruption of the cruciate allows this sliding to occur during loading and has been described as "cranial tibial thrust" (CCT). This sliding results in a shearing force being applied parallel to the articular cartilage surface that appears to be very deleterious to cartilage health and results in the aggressive arthritis usually seen in larger dogs without

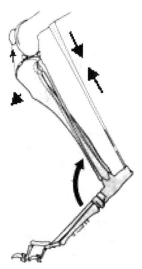

surgical stabilization. Conventional techniques for cruciate treatment attempt to replace the ligament's restraining function with another structure (ie, patellar ligament graft) or by temporarily stabilizing the stifle while joint capsule fibrosis develops (lateral retinacular sutures). While such techniques significantly improve results compared to no stabilization, the large shearing forces are still present. This commonly results in progressive arthritis and decreasing stifle flexibility. Traditionally a prognosis of 65% to 80% return to normal stifle function is given. Aggressive rehabilitation will significantly improve short-term results but long-term arthritis and stiffness are consistently seen.[3]

TIBIAL CLOSING WEDGE OSTEOTOMIES (TCWO)

Proximal tibial osteotomies were initially described to correct cranial bowing deformities thought to be associated with premature closure of the caudal aspect of the proximal tibial physis resulting in exaggerated tibial plateau angulation. It was noted in assessing many of these patients that the cranial cruciate ligament was ruptured resulting in the cranial tibial thrust (CCT)

previously described.[6] To correct the bowing, a cranial closing tibial wedge ostectomy was performed and interestingly the CCT resolved although the more traditional cranial drawer sign often remained. This technique was then described by Slocum (1984) for primary treatment of cruciate rupture though an additional conventional stabilization was recomended to control drawer.[7]

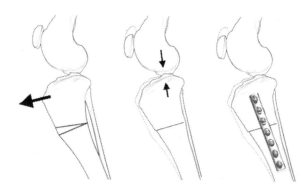

This converts the force seen by the articular surface from shear into compressive which is much better tolerated by the cartilage. By changing the slope of the tibial articular surface, forces generated by weight bearing makes the joint more dynamically stable with loading. More recent clinical studies[9] suggested the conventional drawer stabilization is not needed. The results reported were 86% excellent and good with rare complications of implant failure and osteotomy healing problems. Another found that more proximal placement of the wedge removal with alignment of the cranial cortices was more likely to achieve desired tibial plateau leveling and decreases cranial shifting of tibial long axis relative to more distal osteotomies.[2] Current research finds that a resected wedge angle resulting in a TPA angle of 5 degrees is required to stop the CCT.[1] Questions remain about the clinical effect of the relative distal displacement of the patella in the trochlear groove (patella baja).

TIBIAL PLATEAU LEVELING OSTEOTOMY (TPLO)

This technique has been developed by Dr. Barclay Slocum over the last 20 years.[8] Like the TCWO, the TPLO removes the need for the restraining effect of the cruciate ligament.

It is basically a very proximal "inverted dome" osteotomy that achieves tibial plateau level by rotation along the circumference of the cut instead of wedge removal. This provides a larger metaphyseal osteotomy interface that should reduce healing problems and not alter the patella postion relative to the trochlea. However, the surgical procedure of TPLO is technically demanding and specialized equipment is needed for performing and stabilizing the osteotomy. Clinical experience during the last decade suggest the initial recovery is faster with greater return to full stifle function then with conventional stabilization techniques. The standard TPLO can be performed on medium (45 lb) and larger dogs, and is particularly indicated in very active or giant breeds. New smaller saw blades and plates can be used in smaller highly athletic patients. The technique is used for both partial and complete, chronic and acute cruciate ruptures. Because the procedure apparently

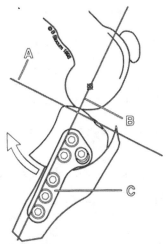

decreases stifle pain quickly, the most common problems have been related to excessive patient activity before healing is complete. Consequently, careful client education and strict patient compliance with a rehabilitation regime is recommended. Subjective opinion is that we see at least 90% of our patients obtain 90% desired function and most of the decrease is due to pre existing arthritis or meniscal injury. Clients should be warned that contra lateral cruciate disease is common and radiographic assessment is recommended. Complications can include routine surgical, post operative swelling, incisional concerns, and infection. Osteotomy healing routinely occurs over 6 to 8 weeks and minimal activity is advised during that time. Uncommon but significant problems include patellar tendonitis, tibial crest fracture or patellar fracture occurring as the patient activity increases. These appears to be related to poor placement of the osteotomy and possibily increased tension through the quadriceps mechanism secondary to the changed joint mechanics. Treatment of these complications are difficult, so we are currently researching this concern with the hope of optimizing surgical procedure and postoperative rehabilitation.

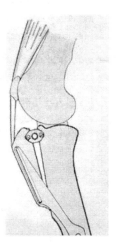

TIBIAL TUBEROSITY ADVANCEMENT (TTA)

TTA is a relatively new procedure developed by Dr. Pierre Montavon and Slobodan Tepic (a bioengineer) as a means of stabilizing the stifle after rupture of the cranial cruciate ligament. It is proposed to work by transfering the stabilizing influence from the cruciate ligament to the patellar tendon when that tendon is cranially advanced.

It is proposed to be less invasive and consequently have less potential for serious complications. In addition dogs are reported to recover faster than with other techniques so it may be useful in treating bilateral or otherwise difficult to rehabilitate patients. The goal of surgery is to create a right angle between the tibial plateau and the patellar tendon. This requires greater advancement with steeper tibial plateau slopes and may be a limitation in case selection. Also the procedure does not easily correct for internal rotational or distal femoral varus malalignment corrections. Consequently we are currently performing the procedure on carefully selected patients.

REFERENCES

1. Apelt D et al. Effect of tibial closing wedge angle on cranial tibial subluxation. Proc 32nd VOS Annu Conf. 3, 2005.
2. Bailey CJ et al. Geometric implications of tibial wedge osteotomies. Proc 30th VOS Annu Conf. 60, 2003.
3. Conzemius MG et al. Effect of surgical technique on limb function after surgery for rupture of the cranial cruciate ligament in dogs: J Am Vet Med Assoc. 2005;226:232.
4. Montavon P. Tibial Tuberosity Advancement: Biomechanics and Surgical Procedure. Proc 2005 ACVS Veterinary Symposium, 2005.
5. Pozzi A et al. In vitro effectt of meniscal release on tibial translation in stifles following tibial plateau leveling osteotomy. Proc 32nd VOS Annu Conf. 31, 2005.
6. Read RA, Robins GM. Deformity of the proximal tibia in dogs. Vet Rec. 1982;111:295.
7. Slocum B, Devine T. Cranial tibial wedge osteotomy: A technique for eliminating cranial tibial thrust in cranial cruciate ligament repair. J Am Vet Med Assoc. 1984;184:564.
8. Slocum B, Devine T. Tibial plateau leveling osteotomy for repair of cranial cruciate ligament rupture. Vet Clin North Am. 1993;23:777.
9. Watt PR et al. Tibial wedge osteotomy for treatment of cranial cruciate rupture. Vet Surg. 2000;29:478.

ACRYLIC-PIN EXTERNAL FIXATORS

Erick Egger, DVM, Diplomate ACVS
Veterinary Orthopedic Consultant
Colorado State University, Ft. Collins, CO

Acrylic-pin splints are external fixators in which the connecting clamps and rods have been replaced with moldable acrylic columns. This allows easily placing fixation pins in various orientations to best fit the fracture configuration and mechanical stabilization requirements while avoiding soft tissue injuries and important anatomy. This often leads to decreased morbidity in the post operative period. Positive profile pins can easily be placed using ideal pre-drilling pin placement technique at any position without the difficulties of passing through clamps. Indications for acrylic splint use include routine fracture fixation. For highly unstable fractures, staged disassembly of an initially rigid configuration can be employed (by progressive removal of columns) to stimulate healing hypertrophy and remodeling while protecting from re-fracture.

Acrylic splints are particularly useful for mandibular fractures and transarticular application because the acrylic connecting columns are easily contoured to the shape of the body and joint angles. The acrylic used is radiolucent, which does not interfere with radiographic assessment of initial reduction or fracture healing. The first reports of acrylic-pin splints used Steinmann pins or very long orthopedic screws as fixation pins. The screws were inserted in the bones leaving the heads extended externally where they were connected with dental acrylic. Homemade acrylic-pin splints are similarly constructed using methylmethacrylate that is available as hoof repair[a] or dental molding acrylic.[b] "Plumber's Epoxy" has also been described for this application.

TECHNIQUES FOR "HOMEMADE" ACRYLIC-PIN SPLINT APPLICATION

The appropriate number of fixation pins are inserted in the fragments using proper insertion technique. However, they are not required to be in planar alignment.

- One or more of the pins are bent to lie parallel with the bone an appropriate distance usually 3–4 cm) from the skin.
- For application after closed reduction, the nonsterile methyl methacrylate (dental molding or hoof repair) acrylic is mixed until it becomes doughy (3–4 minutes).
- The acrylic is molded to form a connecting column incorporating all pins.
- The fracture is then reduced and held until the acrylic sets (8–10 minutes).
- For open reduction, the fracture is temporarily stabilized with Kirschner type connecting clamps and bars placed further away from the skin on a few of the pins. The approach incision can then be closed and the fracture radiographed to assure adequate reduction.
- The acrylic is then mixed and molded to the pins as before. Once the methacrylate has set, the connecting clamps, bar, and excessive fixation pin length can be removed.

In order to improve consistency of results and convenience of application, the APEF system was developed specifically for small animal veterinary use. The APEF base kit contains all material needed for construction of "standard" fixators Mechanical testing suggests a column diameter of 22 mm provides similar fixation strength and greater stiffness than a 6.3 mm titanium rod. This is appropriate in size for use in medium and larger dogs. A 12.5-mm-diameter tube is available and suggested for small dogs and cats. Even smaller tubing is available for avian and other exotic applications. The acrylic has been designed to have optimal handling and curing characteristics, and is provided in a convenient "bipack" with appropriate premeasured liquid and powder amounts in a sealed mixing pack. This minimizes material waste, while decreasing the mess and odor of open mixing.

TECHNIQUE FOR APEF SYSTEM APPLICATION
Stage I (Sterile Phase)

1. Fixation pins are placed using appropriate insertion technique. Pin orientation and insertion order is not restricted by frame alignment or clamp design.

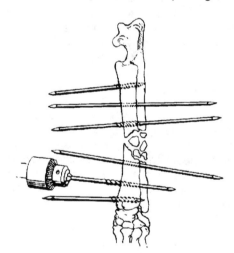

2. Alignment frame is attached to pins, the fracture reduced and clamps tightened to maintain reduction. Open reduction incisions are sutured, and pins are cut off one tube diameter away from clamps and pins "notched." Fracture alignment and reduction should be evaluated (radiographically if desired) at this time.

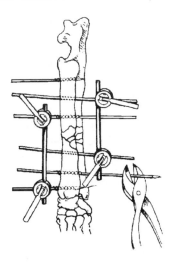

3. Sidebar tubing is "popped" on cut pin ends penetrating only one wall of the tubing. The dependent ends of tubes are plugged.

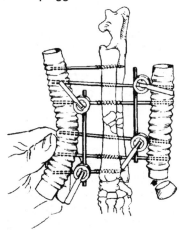

Stage II (Non-sterile)

4. Acrylic is mixed for 2 to 3 minutes after removing pack divider. Corner of bag is cut off and acrylic is poured into open ends of tubes.

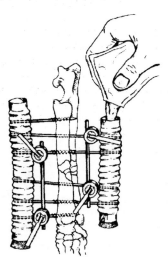

5. After acrylic hardens (10–12 minutes), the alignment frame is removed. Stoppers and excess tube length are cut away.

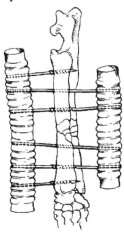

Readjustment of a completed acrylic splint is more difficult in some respects than clamp and bar type devices, but does not require replacement of the fixation pins to correct rotational malalignments as do the routine linear fixators. Splint adjustment requires removing a short segment of the acrylic column with a saw or cast cutter. The plastic molding tube is peeled back from each end and several holes drilled in the remaining acrylic to provide a base for the patch. A small amount of new acrylic is mixed and hand molded to fill the gap and overlap the existing column ends. The fracture is then manipulated into correct reduction and held while the acrylic cures. More fixation pins can be added to either replace existing pins or increase overall frame stability. The plastic molding tubing is removed from the existing acrylic column and several 1/8" diameter holes drilled in the acrylic adjacent to the proposed pin insertion site. After aseptically preparing the skin and acrylic column surface, the new fixation pin is inserted using appropriate technique. The free end of the pin is bent to contact or cross the column. A mini pack of APEF acrylic or other acrylic is mixed to dough consistency and molded around the new pin and existing column to incorporate it.

Acrylic splint removal is achieved by cutting each fixation pin between the skin and acrylic column. Each pin is then removed using a hand chuck or pliers. Alternatively, the acrylic connecting bar can be cut between pins and each pin removed using the small block of acrylic as a handle.

ADVANTAGES OF THE LOCKING PLATE

Erick Egger, DVM, Diplomate ACVS
Veterinary Orthopedic Consultant
Colorado State University, Ft. Collins, CO

Locking plates are implants with threaded screw holes that allow appropriate screws to thread and lock into the plate and function as a fixed-angle device. Many of these plates also have a mixture of normal or combination holes that also allow use of normal (non-locking) or lag screw placement. Locking plates were developed for use in human spinal and maxillofacial surgery and became available for general orthopedic use in the last 6 to 7 years. Veterinary interest in small animal application is just now developing.

LOCKING PLATE MECHANICS AND ADVANTAGES

Conventional plates create stability by compression the plate to the bone creating friction. This will impede blood flow to the bone and has been shown to negatively affect healing. The locking plate can provide stability with minimal bone contact and actually functions more like an external fixator. This induces minimal vascular damage and healing interference. This approach also is more consistent with the "minimally invasive" concepts now developing and several of the plate designs can be applied without exposure of the fracture particularly if fluoroscopic control is available.

Another major advantage of the locking plate concept is that exact contouring of the plate is not required to maintain desired reduction of the fracture as the screws are tightened. This is of particular concern in articular fractures such as acetabular were the anatomy is very complex and perfect conventional plate contouring is difficult and time consuming. Likewise, the locking plate concept is seeing increasing use in the stabilization of corrective and reconstructive osteotomies such as the TPLO, were complex geometries make conventional contouring difficult.

Biomechanically, the locking plate acts as the second strut of a ladder with the first cortex of the bone acting as the first. Consequently the screws can be applied as unicortical (particularly in the diaphyseal regions) and obtain adequate stability. This further reduces the need to traumatize the intrameduallary vascularity and biology resulting in optimal healing. Alternatively locking plates with unicortical screws can provide adequate stability if the plate is used in conjunction with an IM rod or to support an intramedullary prosthesis such as a total hip replacement femoral stem.

LOCKING PLATE SYSTEMS

Many companies now offer locking abilities in their products. Synthes developed the concept and provides the most complete line of devices. Their TPLO plate is particularly well designed and useful. The ALPS system from Kyon is relatively new and uses a more segmented plate shape that allows more contouring in the third dimension and is cuttable at surgery. It should be very adaptable in complex geometries much like reconstruction plates.

LOCKING PLATE DISADVANTAGES

The biggest disadvantage of locking plate systems is their expense. The manufacturing technique requires much more processing. The application process is also more exacting in requiring perfect threading of the screw head into the plate to avoid thread stripping or cold welding. Also, the concept of fixation with locking plates is somewhat different and must favor encouragement of rapid healing as opposed to overpowering the facture with stability. Plate and screw failures have been documented, so a thorough understanding of the concept's principles and technology is required

EARLY DIAGNOSIS AND TREATMENT OF CANINE HIP DYSPLASIA

Erick Egger DVM, Diplomate ACVS
Veterinary Orthopedic Consultant
Colorado State University, Ft. Collins, CO

PATHOGENESIS AND EARLY DIAGNOSIS OF HIP DYSPLASIA

Canine hip dysplasia is a developmental disorder with multifactor genetic origin and may be influenced by environmental conditions. In humans, "congenital hip luxation" is recognized in newborns based on palpation (the Ortoloni sign) and treated with corrective coaptation such as triple diapering to induce abduction, and cable bracing to induce femoral internal rotation. However, in the newborn puppy, hip laxity is commonly seen as demonstrated by either the Ortoloni or Barden's sign and yet clinical hip dysplasia and secondary arthritic changes do not develop. The Ortoloni sign demonstrates subluxation when the femoral head is pushed dorsally while the leg is held in adduction, then abduction results in a palpable "pop" as the femoral head reduces. Barden's sign is recognized as an increased lateral hip laxity but is more difficult to consistently demonstrate. Recent work by Gail Smith and the University of Pennsylvania group suggest this "puppy laxity" will be resolved by approximately 4 months of age and dogs still showing positive Ortoloni or demonstrating increased laxity on stress radiography (PennHIP views) will often develop clinical signs of dysplasia. Based on this understanding of dysplasia pathogenesis, we palpate for Ortoloni at our first puppy vaccination and wellness exam at roughly eight weeks of age. If Ortoloni is present, we imitate a discussion of the syndrome and encourage careful observation. If the instability is present at the 12-week second exam, we further discuss.

If instability persists at 16 weeks, the owners are advised that use for breeding is not recommended, stress radiography is suggested, and surgical intervention with juvenile pubic symphysiodesis (JPS) is discussed.

EARLY SURGICAL TREATMENT

Juvenile pubic symphysiodesis was developed with the goal of creating the same protective result as the triple pelvic osteotomy (TPO) without the deleterious side effects or high cost to owners associated with TPO. JPS is based on halting growth of the pubic physis (cranial half of the pelvic symphysis = pubic physis). JPS was originally performed in the immature guinea pig followed by canine studies where a similar coxofemoral conformational result was obtained with minimal clinical complications. Techniques originally used to perform JPS were 1) electrocautery of pubic physis, or removal of the pubic physis with placement of bone staples.

Currently we are using a modified technique combining the two options listed above. Following a routine approach to the cranial aspect of the pelvic symphysis, the pubic physis is identified by palpation of the pelvic symphysis and obturator foramen while also referring to preoperative radiographs. The pubic physis is then resected by use of rongeurs. The deep margin of the resection can readily be identified when pelvic fat falls into the resected area. Following physical removal of the pubic physis a gel-foam pad is placed into the resected space and is used to push the pelvic fat back into the pelvic canal. Finally, electrocautery is used to cauterize the margins of the pubic physis, ensuring cell death and cessation of pubic growth. Recognizing this is a genetically induced disease, we also insist on neutering the patient, and it can be completed at this time.

We have found this technique to be simple, fast, and provide the desired clinical effect when compared to the clinical results obtained by used of pubic physis resection and placement of bone staples. Additionally, we have also found that while JPS results in significantly improved acetabular coverage by the femoral head, it may not completely resolve the Ortoloni sign or preclude development of all arthritis, but obviously, the procedure's effectiveness will be severity and time dependent.

STEM CELL THERAPY FOR OSTEOARTHRITIS

James S. Gaynor, DVM, MS, Diplomate ACVA & AAPM
Animal Anesthesia and Pain Management Center
Colorado Springs, CO

Techniques for treatment of pain associated with osteoarthritis have varied over years. Currently, the most common approach to osteoarthritis is related to multimodal therapy including weight loss, nutritional support, analgesics including nonsteroidal anti-inflammatory drugs, and disease-modifying agents such as glucosamine/chondroitin supplements and injectable polysulfated glycosaminoglycans. A newer therapy which has both pain relieving and regenerative effects is stem cell therapy.

Stem cell therapy is considered a form of regenerative medicine because the therapeutic cells may actually differentiate into a number of different tissues including bone, cartilage, cardiac, nerve, muscle, blood vessels, fat, and liver tissue (Figure 1). This allows these adult stem cells to treat traumatic and degenerative diseases, including bowed tendons, ligament injuries, osteoarthritis, and osteochondral defects in horses and dogs.

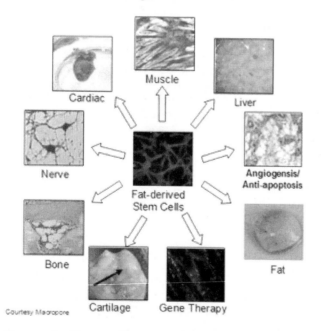

Figure 1. Stem cells can differentiate into various tissues..

A key concept is that this type of regenerative medicine utilizes ADULT stem cells. These adult stem cells are derived from adipose tissue from inguinal, caudal scapular or intra-abdominal areas, making them a readily available source, much easier to collect and much more plentiful than those derived from bone marrow. As mentioned above, these cells are able to differentiate into multiple lineages implicating their potential in bone, cartilage, and cardiac repair. Fractions isolated from adipose tissue contain a heterogeneous mixture of regenerative cells, including:

- Mesenchymal stem cells
- Endothelial progenitor cells
- Pericytes
- Immune cells
- Fibroblasts
- Other growth factor-secreting bioactive cells

There are multiple advantages of using stem cell regenerative medicine over a more traditional approach. The first is that stem cells do not rely on a single target receptor or a single pathway for their action. They can have very global effects. Additionally, the regenerative cell mixture is delivered either directly to the traumatic wound (e.g. tendonitis, desmitis, fracture) or is delivered systemically (e.g.: liver disease, renal disease). In the case of arthritis, stem cells are injected directly into two to four affected joints, or intra-articularly and intravenously to induce a more global effect. Once again the regenerative cells can differentiate into many tissue types, induce repair, and stimulate regeneration. They can also "communicate" with the cells of their local environment through paracrine and autocrine modalities, creating the optimal environment for natural healing. They also produce a variety of both secreted and cell surface substances that regulate tissue growth, integrity, and function.

Currently, over 200 dogs have been treated for osteoarthritis and orthopedic procedures. Most patients had elbow, hip, or knee problems. Initial studies demonstrate that intra-articular administration of regenerative stem cells significantly decreases pain and improves comfort in the majority of cases. Duration of the benefit from a single injection varies from several months to more than one year. The current indications for regenerative stem cell therapy in dogs include osteoarthritis and tendon and ligament injuries.

As more research is conducted, the likelihood of expanding the indications for stem therapy increases. Besides the overwhelming scientific data demonstrating the clinical efficacy of regenerative cellular therapy in animal models of osteoarthritis, osteochondral defects, tendon repair, and fractures, many additional studies demonstrate success in treating systemic disorders such as cerebral and myocardial infarction, muscular dystrophy, and immune-mediated disorders.

ARTICULAR & PERIARTICULAR FRACTURES

Ian G. Holsworth, BSc, BVSc (Hons), MACVSc
(Surgery), Diplomate ACVS
Veterinary Medical and Surgical Group, Ventura, CA

Fractures of the metaphysis, physis, and epiphysis of animals are common sequelae to traumatic injury. The specific anatomic location of the fracture, the severity of associated soft tissue trauma, the classification of the fractures as open or closed, and the involvement of the joint surface will dictate the diagnostic plan, the treatment strategy and the prognosis for successful return to normal activity.

Clinical evaluation of the neurovascular function in the affected leg and the degree of soft tissue damage at the fracture site is the initial step in fracture evaluation. Radiographic examination of the damaged joint area is essential to categorize the fracture type prior to surgical planning. Simultaneous assessment of ligamentous support structures is necessary to determine a complete treatment plan and will influence the prognosis for recovery. In severely injured patients diagnostically accurate radiographs are difficult to obtain and in the complex multiple bone joints of the carpus, tarsus, hip, elbow and stifle definitive localization of the fracture location and severity can be challenging. In human knee fracture patients the overall sensitivity of radiography was 83% and a negative radiograph was not reliable in ruling out a fracture. A significant improvement in diagnostic accuracy is seen when computer tomography is utilized in complex fracture cases and should be considered as part of the diagnostic plan if indicated.

In skeletally immature animals between 3 and 11 months of age physeal fractures are common and are classified according to the Salter-Harris scheme. The Type II fracture with metaphyseal involvement is the most common. Histologic examination of the physeal zone in clinical patients demonstrates considerable damage to the physeal cartilage; this may result in growth retardation in patients with bone length discrepancies or alignment abnormalities at maturity.

The primary goals of fracture repair are the preservation of the soft tissue envelope at the fracture site, provision of a stable fracture site construct able to support reasonable force transmission, uninterrupted bone healing, the re-alignment of the bone to restore the proximal and distal joint surfaces in functional anatomic position, and the reduction of disrupted articular surfaces to eliminate malarticualtion and a loss of joint congruity. In peri-articular fractures without articular surface disruption but a lack of bone stock with which to secure implants the circular external fixation frames in standard or hybrid configurations have greatly improved the ability of the surgeon to stabilize the fracture site and restore limb alignment. Good to excellent results have been achieved in 70% to 80% of canine and human patients with these apparatus types.

In articular fractures the major goals are accurate anatomic reconstruction of joint congruity and the provision of a stable fixation technique that prevents loss of fracture fragment alignment and the development of step or gap defects in the joint surface. Traditionally, bone screws placed in lag fashion with or without bone plate support have been utilized. The introduction of pre-contoured locking compression plates and minimally invasive placement techniques in human patients has improved success; however, results vary with outcomes correlated to the severity of the fracture, degree of anatomic reduction, adequate plate positioning, and concomitant injuries.

In dogs and cats the most commonly reported articular fractures in the literature are those of the humeral condyle. The fractures may either involve the lateral condyle, the medial condyle or both (Y-T fracture). Open arthrotomy and fixation with direct visualization of the joint surface reduction is the most common surgical technique utilised with a variety of approaches and implants. Closed reduction and fixation under fluoroscopic examination has also been successfully performed. In dogs with simple, lateral condyle fractures treated by open approach 80% were sound on re-examination, with 40% having radiographically apparent osteoarthritis. In the more complex Y-T fractures excellent limb function was seen in 40%, good in 50% and fair in 10% with major complications in 13%, the most common being infection and implant migration or failure. In human patients with distal humeral intra-articular fractures excellent results are seen in 20%, good in 45% to 60%, fair in 20% to 30%, and poor in 15% of cases. Re-operation rates are 25% to 35% and major complications include infection, implant migration/failure and nerve damage. A decrease in range of motion and muscle strength in the affected arm was common. The utilization of early, low impact physical therapy to maximize joint mobility and minimize disuse muscle atrophy but avoid bone-implant construct overload is highly recommended.

As the degree of soft tissue trauma increases around and within the traumatized joint the degree of surgical success also decreases. The presence of injuries to cartilage, ligament and skin, open fracture, closed soft tissue contusion and hemorrhage complicates surgical management and increases the type and severity of complications. In human patients with combined distal femoral and proximal tibial fractures the postoperative complications include malunion, nonunion, bony deformity, deep infection, persistent knee instability or severe loss of motion. The salvage procedures of arthrodesis and amputation for these patients are not uncommon and 60% of patients with knee fracture and dislocation have a poor result. Realistic goal setting for the veterinary client and surgical team initially is very important in small animals with similar injuries to prevent unrealistic expectations and disappointment when treating these very challenging cases.

REFERENCES

1. Mustonen AO, Koskinen SK, Kiuru MJ. Acute knee trauma: analysis of multidetector computed tomography findings and comparison with conventional radiography. Acta Radiol. 2005;

46(8):866-874.

2. Johnson JM, Johnson AL, Eurell JA. Histological appearance of naturally occurring canine physeal fractures. Vet Surg. 1994;23(2):81-86.

3. Anderson GM, Lewis DD, Radasch RM, et al. Circular external skeletal fixation stabilization of antebrachial and crural fractures in 25 dogs. J Am Anim Hosp Assoc. 2003;39(5):479-498.

4. Farese JP, Lewis DD, Cross AR, et al. Use of IMEX SK-circular external fixator hybrid constructs for fracture stabilization in dogs and cats. J Am Anim Hosp Assoc. 2002;38(3):279-289.

5. Rovesti GL, Bosio A, Marcellin-Little DJ. Management of 49 antebrachial and crural fractures in dogs using circular external fixators. J Small Anim Pract. 2007;48(4):194-200.

6. Ristiniemi J, Flinkkila T, Hyvonen P, Lakovaara M, Pakarinen H, Biancari F, Jalovaara P. Two-ring hybrid external fixation of distal tibial fractures: a review of 47 cases. J Trauma. 2007;62(1):174-183.

7. Hernanz Gonzalez Y, Diaz Martin A, Jara Sanchez F, Resines Erasun C. Early results with the new internal fixator systems LCP and LISS: a prospective study. Acta Orthop Belg. 2007;73(1):60-69.

8. McKee WM, Macias C, Innes JF. Bilateral fixation of Y-T humeral condyle fractures via medial and lateral approaches in 29 dogs. J Small Anim Pract. 2005;46(5):217-26.

9. Macias C, Gibbons SE, McKee WM. Y-T humeral fractures with supracondylar comminution in five cats. J Small Anim Pract. 2006;47(2):89-93.

10. Guille AE, Lewis DD, Anderson TP, et al. Evaluation of surgical repair of humeral condylar fractures using self-compressing orthofix pins in 23 dogs. Vet Surg. 2004;33(4):314-322.

11. Cook JL, Tomlinson JL, Reed AL. Fluoroscopically guided closed reduction and internal fixation of fractures of the lateral portion of the humeral condyle: prospective clinical study of the technique and results in ten dogs. Vet Surg. 1999;28(5):315-321.

12. Ozdemir H, Urguden M, Soyuncu Y, et al. Long-term functional results of adult intra-articular distal humeral fractures treated by open reduction and plate osteosynthesis. Acta Orthop Traumatol Turc. 2002;36(4):328-335.

13. Tyllianakis M, Panagopoulos A, Papadopoulos AX, Kaisidis A, Zouboulis P. Functional evaluation of comminuted intra-articular fractures of the distal humerus (AO type C). Long term results in twenty-six patients. Acta Orthop Belg. 2004;70(2):123-130.

14. McKee MD, Wilson TL, Winston L, Schemitsch EH, Richards RR. Functional outcome following surgical treatment of intra-articular distal humeral fractures through a posterior approach. J Bone Joint Surg Am. 2000;82(12):1701-1707.

15. Heckler MW, Hatic SO 2nd, DiCicco JD 3rd. Management of complications associated with fractures around the knee. J Knee Surg. 2007;20(1):78-87.

16. Sferopoulos NK. Concomitant physeal fractures of the distal femur and proximal tibia. Skeletal Radiol. 2005;34(7):427-430.

17. Krettek C, Schandelmaier P, Lobenhoffer P, et al. Complex trauma of the knee joint. Diagnosis-management-therapeutic principles. Unfallchirurg. 1996;99(9):616-627.

MULTIMODAL ARTHRITIS TREATMENT

Ian G. Holsworth, BSc, BVSc (Hons), MACVSc
(Surgery), Diplomate ACVS
Veterinary Medical and Surgical Group, Ventura, CA

Treatment of canine osteoarthritis is most successfully addressed by the implementation of a multi-modal treatment regime. The mainstays of that regime should include weight control, moderate exercise, nutraceuticals, chondroprotectives, and anti-inflammatories. Surgical treatment of arthritic patients includes intra-articular debridement of joint surfaces, stabilization and re-distribution of joint load, and salvage procedures to remove end-stage articular surfaces.

The anatomy, physiology, and biomechanics of the normal and arthritic articular joint are dramatically different and by targeting some of those differences with a treatment strategy a significant improvement in joint function and joint comfort may be obtained. Reduction and alteration of load across the joint, control of inflammation and improvement in metabolic function within the cartilage bed are the goals of treatment.

The cartilage bed is structured to maximize its resilience to compressive force by the organization of its collagen fibres, proteoglycan molecules and water content to allow flexibility and elasticity. The surface of the bed, although porous, restricts the entrance and exit of molecules to a very small size therefore limiting the entry and exit of both water and proteoglycans. Maintenance of the proteoglycan and water content within the bed is dependent upon the chondrocyte cells within the cartilage matrix. These cells must remain in sufficient numbers and in an anabolic state to produce the polysulfated glycosaminoglycans (PGAGs). These large chains, of which proteoglycans are a component, draw water to them via their hydrophilic charge. Disruption of the chondrocytes anabolic function by inflammatory enzymes derived from the joint capsule synoviocytes and vasculature induces catabolic alterations in the chondrocytes. The catabolic chondrocyte produces inflammatory enzymes such as the matrix metalloproteinases (MMPs) that actively destroy the PGAGs and therefore reduce the ability of the bed to retain water. The catabolic chondrocyte also decreases its proteoglycan production dramatically. With this reduction in water content in the cartilage matrix comes a reduction in elasticity and resilience to compression. The result is damage to the cartilage surface with chondromalacia, fibrillation and cleavage of the cartilage bed. The loss of the intact surface layer is irreversible and disastrous for the cartilage matrix as it no longer is able to withstand load, or retain water effectively and continued loss of matrix and exposure of the underlying subchondral bone is inevitable.

The inflammation within the joint capsule and the subsequent changes in the production of hyaluronic acid by the synoviocytes leads to loss of joint fluid viscosity and therefore its lubricant qualities. The volume of the joint fluid increases and the distension of the capsule is painful to the patient. The increase in prostaglandins within the joint lining increases the vascular permeability of the capsule and the inflammatory cycle proceeds unchecked with the deposition of collagen into the capsule structure from fibroblasts recruited to the inflammatory zone. The result of the fibroblastic response is a loss of capsule flexibility and a decrease in the affected joints range of motion. The stiff, distended joint is painful to use and the patient is forced to limit the load that is applied across the joint to limit the discomfort.

The most effective way to reduce the load that is applied across the arthritic joint surface is to decrease the weight of the patient. Maintaining an ideal body condition score delays the onset and progression of osteoarthritis. Research had demonstrated that bodyweight reduction of 15% in canine patients improves lameness scores significantly. The screening of the patient for concurrent medical conditions, the assessment of target weight, the calculation of the daily caloric requirement and the monitoring of the weight loss program should be performed by the veterinary practitioner in order to maximize program success. The concurrent implementation of a moderate exercise program allows improved muscle tone and mass, improved metabolic rate and an increase in the loss of stored body fat. These changes increase the efficacy of the weight loss program and improve the soft tissue support of the joints helping distribute load across the joints in a more balanced fashion.

Surgical therapy to improve joint stability and alter load across the unstable joint surface may also be very effective in improving joint function and limiting the rate of cartilage degeneration. This is the principle behind the triple pelvic osteotomy, tibial plateau levelling, tibial crest advancement, humeral osteotomy, and proximal and distal radial and ulna osteotomy. Salvage of an end-stage degenerative joint by joint replacement, joint fusion or joint surface removal may be very effective in controlling patient discomfort although avoiding post-surgical complications and maintaining normal limb function can be very challenging.

The limited scientific data presently available supporting the treatment efficacy of nutraceuticals compared with the massive quantity of these products that is presently consumed by veterinary and human patients, provides a treatment challenge to the veterinary practitioner. Cautious optimism regarding their use has prevailed although product quality is variable. A recent NIH-funded, multicenter, prospective, double-blind, placebo- and nonsteroidal anti-inflammatory-controlled study comparing placebo, oral glucosamine, oral chondroitin sulfate and NSAIDs in a human knee arthritis model found little statistical efficacy for the nutraceutical products in comparison to placebo in mildly to moderately affected patients. In more severely affected patients the glucosamine-chondroitin group had better improvement in pain scores than the NSAID and placebo groups. The very high positive placebo response seen with nutraceutical use complicates investigation of these products efficacy and the lack of positive treatment response in some trials makes administration of nutraceuticals equivocal. Although subjective opinions are strong on the use of these and other products the relatively small amount of scientific evidence, the lack of FDA regulation, and the enormous variation in manufacturer purities and price make recommending these products strongly to clients problematic.

The use of the chondroprotective PGAGs and hyaluronic acid medications is becoming more commonplace in several species including humans. There is an increasing amount of scientific literature that supports their use as part of a multimodal program. Although not complete and not available in a FDA-approved form for all veterinary patients their combination of anti-inflammatory and anabolic properties in the cartilage matrix and joint capsule are promising and should be considered when developing a treatment protocol.

Limiting inflammation and providing some local and central analgesia using nonsteroidal anti-inflammatory medications decreases a patient's pain status and encourages use of the arthritic joint. The decrease in painful sensation when the joint is loaded in turn allows a better range of active motion and active use of surrounding supportive musculature. Screening patients for pre-existing liver, kidney, and gastrointestinal dysfunction, monitoring for the development of these organ abnormalities and educating clients regarding their potential development is the responsibility of the prescribing practitioner.

The development of a multimodal medical and surgical treatment plan and the implementation of the program to the veterinary arthritis patient is the key to controlling our patients' comfort and maintaining functional use of their limbs. Attention to detail, continued supervision of the client, monitoring of the patient, introduction of new efficacious treatments as they become available, and the use of salvage procedures when debilitating, medically unresponsive joint pain is present are the keys to successful treatment.

REFERENCES

1. Smith GK, Paster ER, Powers MY, et al. Lifelong diet restriction and radiographic evidence of osteoarthritis of the hip joint in dogs. J Am Vet Med Assoc. 2006;229(5):690-693.
2. Impellizeri JA, Tetrick MA, Muir P. Effect of weight reduction on clinical signs of lameness in dogs with hip osteoarthritis. J Am Vet Med Assoc. 2000;216(7):1089-1091.
3. Mlacnik E, Bockstahler BA, Muller M, Tetrick MA, Nap RC, Zentek J. Effects of caloric restriction and a moderate or intense physiotherapy program for treatment of lameness in overweight dogs with osteoarthritis. J Am Vet Med Assoc. 2006;229(11):1756-1760.
4. McAlindon TE, LaValley MP, Gulin JP, et al. Glucosamine and chondroitin for treatment of osteoarthritis: a systematic quality assessment and meta-analysis. JAMA. 2000;283(11):1469-1475.
5. Clegg DO, Reda DJ, Harris CL, et al. Glucosamine, chondroitin sulfate, and the two in combination for painful knee osteoarthritis. N Engl J Med. 2006;354(8):795-808.
6. Cibere J, Kopec JA, Thorne A, et al. Randomized, double-blind, placebo-controlled glucosamine discontinuation trial in knee osteoarthritis. Arthritis Rheum. 2004;51(5):738-745.

JUVENILE HIP DYSPLASIA

Ian G. Holsworth, BSc, BVSc (Hons), MACVSc
(Surgery), Diplomate ACVS
Veterinary Medical and Surgical Group, Ventura, CA

Hip dysplasia is a developmental disorder of the coxofemoral (hip) joints. It is a disorder of complex inheritance profoundly influenced and confounded by environmental factors. Hip dysplasia expresses itself on a continuous scale from normal to severely abnormal. Clinical signs of the disease normally occur initially between four and fourteen months of age. Decreased activity and various degrees of joint pain are early manifestations. Young dogs can have a swaying and unsteady gait and the length of their hind leg stride is often reduced. When running both hind legs may move together in a hopping motion ('bunny-hopping'). Progression of the disease will cause difficulty in rising from a sitting or lying position and difficulty is experienced with stair climbing. Manipulation of the joint may cause a pain response particularly when the hind leg is extended rearwards. Following the initial appearance of clinical disease the patients will often improve clinically as the initial joint inflammation regresses and the microtrauma to the bony structures of the immature hip joint decreases. The reoccurrence of clinical signs may be anywhere from 2 to 9 years of age and are due to advanced degenerative changes in the hip joints associated with progressive osteoarthritis (OA).

Two primary criteria making up the diagnosis of canine hip dysplasia are subluxation (hip laxity) and radiographic evidence of OA. Subjective measurements of passive laxity are made through palpation (Bardens, Barlow, Ortolani, or subluxation/reduction methods) or ventrodorsal hip extended radiographs (OFA-style) of a non-ambulating dog under heavy sedation or anaesthesia. Significant variation in the subjective interpretation of these tests leads to wide variation in estimates of disease prevalence. Objective radiographic measurement of passive laxity with the hip joint in a laterally distracted or ventrally loaded position in juveniles improves the predictability of a particular dog developing progressive osteoarthritis but a 'gray zone' remains which makes decision-making about treatment and breeding strategies problematic

Functional hip laxity is the pathological form of laxity that occurs when the dog is weight bearing, and it is not measurable at the present. Other diagnostic modalities investigated include CT scanning, ultrasound, MRI, force plate, kinematic, and molecular studies. The absence of a definitive molecular genetic test and the limitations of present imaging techniques ensure that 'diseased' genes are passed to the next generation unless unrealistic breeding recommendations are implemented.

The goal in medical and surgical treatment of hip dysplasia is to relieve pain, and to return a patient to normal function and performance without untoward or harmful side effects. Along with those efforts is a requirement that any treatment modality is introduced under the tenet of evidence-based medicine. It is well recognized that a proportion of hip dysplasia patients will suffer persistent hip pain and lameness from their osteoarthritis, not respond to medical treatments, and require a salvage procedure. Retrospective evaluation of long-term management of dysplastic patients offers conflicting opinions on its effectiveness and persistence of clinical dysfunction. There is no data on the benefits of non-surgical vs. surgical treatments in dogs used for work or sport.

Without well-researched, non-biased, prospective, randomised studies with a control group it is very difficult to be conclusive about the benefits of any particular treatment as subjective bias prevails. Unfortunately over the past twenty years medical and surgical techniques have been introduced that purport to prevent hip osteoarthritis. No definitive data exists to support that any treatment technique in animal or man can prevent the development of hip osteoarthritis in hip dysplasia patients. What is unproven at this time is if the juvenile patients who are surgically treated early in the course of the disease process have a decrease in the progression and severity of their disease status and have a higher level of athletic function during their lifespan compared with medically treated patients.

Medical treatment consists of obtaining and maintaining an optimal body condition, encouraging routine moderate nonconcussive exercise, administering nutraceuticals, chondroprotectives and anti-inflammatory medications to help control signs of joint pain and maintain muscle mass and joint function. This may delay the onset of radiographic arthritis and clinical dysfunction; however, the degeneration of the joint structures and the progression of osteoarthritis continues in these patients.

Surgical management of juvenile dysplastic dogs by juvenile pubic symphysiodesis (JPS) and triple pelvic osteotomy (TPO) is controversial and the results are variable. The goal of both procedures is to improve the acetabular dysplasia present by encouraging the dorsal rotation of the acetabular cup to provide more normal acetabular configuration. JPS is performed between 15 and 20 weeks of age and may result in a significant improvement in hip joint conformation and hip laxity in dysplastic puppies treated. Although long-term follow-up is not available for this procedure (>2 years) JPS may be a promising treatment for hip dysplasia and is a safe and technically simple procedure to perform. Triple pelvic osteotomy is classically performed in dysplastic puppies from 5 months to 12 months old and requires careful assessment of the patient prior to surgery. The presence of radiographic osteoarthritis within the joint has precluded many surgeons from performing the procedure; however, the radiographic changes do not accurately reflect the degree of cartilaginous change within the dysplastic joint and a more complete examination via direct arthroscopic visualization may make surgical decision-making more accurate. Although some studies have found no improvement in hip laxity post procedure, there are others that purport an improvement in joint congruity and laxity post-TPO.

All hip dysplasia treatments have varying degrees of success and with all of them there are individual complications, which must be carefully considered by the practioner and discussed completely with the client prior to their initiation. The intended lifestyle of the patient, the goals of the clients in regards to their dog and the long-term reality of their dogs condition must be explored and discussed to allow the most appropriate treatment plan to be agreed upon.

REFERENCES

1. Corfield GS, Read RA, Eastley KA, et al. Assessment of the hip reduction angle for predicting osteoarthritis of the hip in the Labrador retriever. Aust Vet J. 2007;85(6):212-216.
2. Smith GK, et al. Between- and within-radiologist accuracy of subjective hip scoring of the ventro-dorsal hip-extended radiograph. Intl Symp Hip Dysplasia and OA in Dogs, Cornell University, Ithaca, NY, p 20, 1996.
3. Smith GK, et al. Coxofemoral joint laxity from distraction radiography and its contemporaneous and prospective correlation with laxity, subjective score, and evidence of degenerative joint disease from conventional hip-extended radiography in dogs. Am J Vet Res 1993;54:1021.
4. Farese JP, et al. Dorsolateral subluxation of hip joints in dogs measured in a weight-bearing position with radiography and computed tomography. Vet Surg. 1998;27:393.
5. Fluckiger MA, Friedrich GA, Binder H. A radiographic stress technique for evaluation of coxofemoral joint laxity in dogs. Vet Surg. 1999;28:1.
6. Todhunter RJ, Bertram JE, Smith S, et al. Effect of dorsal hip loading, sedation, and general anesthesia on the dorsolateral subluxation score in dogs. Vet Surg. 2003;32(3):196-205.
7. Rawson EA, Aronsohn MG, Burk RL. Simultaneous bilateral femoral head and neck ostectomy for the treatment of canine hip dysplasia. J Am Anim Hosp Assoc. 2005;41(3):166-170.
8. Barr ARS, Denny HR, Gibbs C. Clinical hip dysplasia in growing dogs: the long-term results of conservative management. J Small Anim Pract 1987;28:243.
9. Smith GK, Fordyce HH, Gregor TP. Non-surgical management of severe hip dysplasia: Long term results. Vet Orthop Soc Ann Mtg, Sun Valley, ID, p 12, 1999.
10. Farrell M, Clements DN, Mellor D, et al Retrospective evaluation of the long-term outcome of non-surgical management of 74 dogs with clinical hip dysplasia. Vet Rec. 2007;160(15):506-511.
11. Johnson AL, et al. Triple pelvic osteotomy: effect on limb function and progression of degenerative joint disease. J Am Anim Hosp Assoc, 1998;34:260.
12. Koch DA, et al. Radiographic evaluation and comparison of plate fixation after triple pelvic osteotomy in 32 dogs with hip dysplasia. Vet Comp Orthop Traumatol. 1993;6:9.
13. Rasmussen LM, Kramek BA, Lipowitz AJ. Preoperative variables affecting long-term outcome of triple pelvic osteotomy for treatment of naturally developing hip dysplasia in dogs. J Am Vet Med Assoc. 1998;213:80.
14. Tano CA, et al. Force plate analysis of dogs with bilateral hip dysplasia treated with a unilateral triple pelvic osteotomy: A long-term review of cases. Vet Comp Orthop Traumatol. 1998;11:85.
15. Manley PA, Adams WM, Danielson KC, et al. Long-term outcome of juvenile pubic symphysiodesis and triple pelvic osteotomy in dogs with hip dysplasia. J Am Vet Med Assoc. 2007;230(2):206-210.
16. Smith GK, Paster ER, Powers MY, et al. Lifelong diet restriction and radiographic evidence of osteoarthritis of the hip joint in dogs. J Am Vet Med Assoc. 2006;229(5):690-693.
17. Patricelli AJ, Dueland RT, Adams WM, et al. Juvenile pubic symphysiodesis in dysplastic puppies at 15 and 20 weeks of age. Vet Surg. 2002;31(5):435-444.
18. Holsworth IG, Schulz KS, Kass PH, et al. Comparison of arthroscopic and radiographic abnormalities in the hip joints of juvenile dogs with hip dysplasia. J Am Vet Med Assoc. 2005;227(7):1087-1094.
19. Hara Y, Harada Y, Fujita Y, et al. Changes of hip joint congruity after triple pelvic osteotomy in the dog with hip dysplasia. J Vet Med Sci. 2002;64(10):933-936.

PATELLAR LUXATION

John F. Innes, BVSc, PhD, CertVR, DSAS (Orth),
MRCVS
Faculty of Veterinary Science
University of Liverpool, Liverpool, UK

Patellar luxation is a common stifle condition in dogs that can result in pain, lameness, and osteoarthritis. The condition has traditionally been recognized in toy and miniature breeds; however, it is becoming an increasing problem in large-breed dogs, especially Labrador retrievers. Patellar luxation is most commonly a congenital disorder resulting from multiple anatomic abnormalities of the pelvic limb. Medial luxation is more frequently recognised than lateral luxation.

SIGNALMENT AND HISTORY

Medial patellar luxation is most commonly recognized in toy and miniature breeds, eg, Miniature Poodle and Yorkshire terrier. Also commonly presented are English and Staffordshire bull terriers and English bulldogs. Of the larger breeds the Labrador retriever, Mastiff, Akita, Flatcoat retriever, and Chow Chow are over-represented. Many dogs are presented when 6 to 12 months of age but in some mild cases lameness may only become a feature later in life or following cranial cruciate ligament rupture. Unilateral medial patellar luxation often presents as an intermittent lameness. Sudden luxation may result in acute lameness with non-weight bearing. The patella may spontaneously relocate and the lameness immediately resolve. Larger dogs should be considered carefully. Reports suggest a greater frequency of postoperative complications in larger breeds of dog.

CLINICAL FINDINGS

The clinical signs of medial patellar luxation vary according to the degree of deformity, duration of the condition and whether one or both stifles are affected. Genu varum or a "bow-legged" conformation is a feature in some dogs. The position of the tibial tuberosity should be assessed during weight bearing with the patella reduced. Tracking of the patella and the angle of the femorotibial joint when the patella luxates should be determined. Integrity of the cranial cruciate ligaments, evidence of femoropatellar crepitus or pain, and any reduced range of stifle extension should be noted.

Grading patellar luxations is useful for monitoring progression of the condition and response to surgery. The following clinical grades have been proposed:

Grade I – The patella can be manually luxated when the stifle is extended, however, when released it returns to the trochlea. Internal rotation of the tibia and displacement of the tibial tuberosity are minimal.

Grade II – The patella is frequently located medially with flexion of the stifle joint; however, it is easily reduced when the stifle is extended and the tibia externally rotated. The tibial tuberosity is displaced medially. Mild angular deformity of the femur and tibia may be present.

Grade III – The patella is permanently luxated. It may be reduced, however, luxation recurs immediately. Angular and rotational deformities of the femur and tibia are common. The trochlea is usually shallow or flat.

Grade IV – The patella is permanently luxated and it is not possible to manually reposition it in the trochlea. Muscle contracture reduces the range of stifle extension. Angular and rotational deformity of the femur and tibia are generally marked and the tibial tuberosity is displaced 60 to 90 degrees medially. Concurrent external rotation of the distal tibia may result in reasonable alignment of the hock and hind paw. The trochlea is flat or convex.

RADIOGRAPHY

Orthogonal view radiographs enable assessment of femoral and tibial deformity. Apparent angular and rotational deformities should be interpreted with caution since positioning may have a profound influence. Tangential ("skyline") views of the flexed stifle enable assessment of the femoral trochlea and femoropatellar congruence.

CT

For more complex cases, computed tomography can be indicated with subsequent 3-D rendered reconstruction of the whole pelvic limb. This allows an accurate assessment of femoral and tibial deformities and measurement of the angular and rotational deformities.

SYNOVIAL FLUID ANALYSIS – HOW, WHY, WHEN?

John F. Innes, BVSc, PhD, CertVR, DSAS(orth), MRCVS
Faculty of Veterinary Science
University of Liverpool, UK

The evaluation of joint fluid is an underused technique, and even when there are no overt clinical or radiological abnormalities within the joint, failure to examine joint fluid can result in important errors in case management. For example, cruciate ligament rupture can be diagnosed clinically but some cases are secondary to immune mediated polyarthritis, which can only be detected by synovial fluid analysis. Similarly, in a dog with chronic osteoarthritis presenting with an acute exacerbation of clinical signs, the signs might represent a "flare" of osteoarthritis, but could be due to haematogenous infective arthritis, or neoplasia.

INDICATIONS FOR ARTHROCENTESIS

The following are indications for synovial fluid analysis:

- Joint effusion
- Joint disease of unknown etiology
- Disease in multiple joints
- Suspected infective arthritis
- Pyrexia of unknown origin
- Monitoring response to therapy in infective arthritis and immune mediated polyarthritis

In suspect cases of polyarthritis, samples should be submitted from a minimum of three joints for cytology. Immune-mediated polyarthritis often affects the smaller joints (carpus and tarsus) and it can be difficult to obtain sufficient fluid from these: in this situation, sample other larger joints (shoulder, elbow, hip, stifle) as these will often also have inflammatory changes.

Sequential samples from the same joint may be required in some instances, such as monitoring treatment of infective or immune-mediated arthritis.

TECHNIQUE FOR ARTHROCENTESIS

Arthrocentesis in the dog is a simple procedure and can be performed under general anaesthesia or heavy sedation. The hair over the site should be clipped and the site aseptically prepared and if the operator wishes to palpate the insertion site, sterile gloves should be worn. If the operator is familiar with the insertion site landmarks, a "no touch" technique can be used as an alternative. The needle used should be of sufficient diameter to facilitate the flow of viscous synovial fluid (ie, 0.9 mm to 0.67 mm [20- to 23-gauge]) and be long enough to reach the joint cavity through the soft tissues. The length of the needle varies with the joint being sampled, with proximal joints requiring needles 25- to 63-mm (1–2.5 inches) long and distal joints requiring 16- to 25-mm (5/8–1 inch) needles. Typically, a 5-mL (or

2.5 mL in cats and small dogs) syringe is attached to the needle prior to insertion: this allows sufficient negative pressure to be produced (normal joints have a pressure below that of the atmosphere, so joint fluid generally requires aspiration). Once sufficient fluid has entered the syringe, negative pressure is released to avoid inadvert aspiration of blood, and the needle and syringe withdrawn. The fluid is then placed into appropriate sample tubes, usually EDTA and a blood culture bottle and squash smears should be made. Rapid air drying is useful to reduce cell shrinkage artefact and can be achieved by directing a hair dryer on warm setting at the back of the slide held at a distance of about 15 cm. If the sample is to be mailed to a laboratory it is important to make smears at the time of sampling and send these along with the sample tubes. Artefacts can develop in the cells in sample tubes; neutrophils may become lytic (mimicking degenerative change seen with infection) and synovial cells may become vacuolated (mimicking reactive change seen with osteoarthritis): these artefacts are avoided if smears are made immediately. If there is insufficient sample, then a direct smear can be made, although the examination of a direct smear alone is inferior without objective cell counts.

The volume of fluid aspirated is dependent on the size of the animal, the particular joint sampled, the health status of the joint, and the technique of the operator. However, normal joints in the dog generally only have 0.1 to 1.0 mL of clear, viscous synovial fluid.

EVALUATION OF SYNOVIAL FLUID
Gross Evaluation

Gross evaluation of synovial fluid can provide useful information but further analyses are generally required.

Normal Fluid

Synovial fluid is so named because of its similarity to egg white (syn-ovia) and this is how normal synovial fluid should appear in the dog and cat. The fluid should be a clear or slightly yellow in color, with a high viscosity and a non-Newtonian (viscoelastic) behavior. The viscosity of synovial fluid is provided by the high content of the long chain polysaccharide, hyaluronan.

Changes in Gross Appearance of Synovial Fluid

Blood contamination during arthrocentesis is usually recognised as a streak of blood running through an otherwise clear fluid, whereas in true hemarthrosis the fluid is uniformly discoloured. An increase in the volume of synovial fluid indicates effusion. This is often accompanied by a reduction in the apparent viscosity of the fluid. However, this may be caused primarily by a dilution of the hyaluronan by plasma dialysate. A true reduction in viscosity is caused by depolymerisation of the hyaluronan and is usually associated with inflammatory changes within the joint. A mucin clot test (q.v.) can be used to differentiate effusion from a true decrease in viscosity although, in reality, this is rarely necessary for clinical decision-making.

Changes in color can be associated with haemorrhage and inflammation. Recent hemorrhage within the joint (hemarthrosis) will produce a red color. Common causes of hemarthrosis are intra-articular injury (eg, fracture or ligament rupture), and recent surgery or arthrocentesis. Hemarthrosis is also seen less commonly in hemostatic disorders. After an isolated intra-articular hemorrhage, the hemoglobin is gradually removed over 2 to 4 weeks and the colour of the joint fluid may become more orange or yellow because of residual hemosiderin.

Changes in the transparency of synovial fluid generally indicate inflammatory change. The presence of high numbers of inflammatory cells will cause the fluid to become cloudy or turbid. The fluid may be white-yellow or gray-red in colour.

Cytology

Qualitative and quantitative cytological examination of synovial fluid is the most useful test to assist the clinician in classifying the disease process within the joint. Examination of a smear is useful, but the sensitivity, specificity and reliability of qualitative assessment is poor (Gibson, Carmichael et al, 1999; Gibson et al, 1999). Whenever possible, a total and differential cell count should be performed. Some laboratories will not perform a total cell count because the viscosity of synovial fluid can make this technically demanding. However, appropriate dilution of the sample should facilitate this and the clinician should use a laboratory that is prepared to perform these analyses. There is significant overlap in the cytologic changes between different articular disease processes, and cytologic results need to be interpreted in the light of patient history, clinical signs, and results of other diagnostic modalities.

It is generally possible to distinguish between "inflammatory" and "noninflammatory" joint disease on the basis of total cell count and the percentage of neutrophils, but there is considerable overlap between the inflammatory conditions (infective arthritis and immune-mediated disease) and the results must be interpreted in the light of other clinical information. As a general principle, if multiple joints show evidence of inflammatory change in a symmetric pattern with a predominance of neutrophils, the likely diagnosis is immune-mediated polyarthritis. Infective arthritis of multiple joints in dogs and cats is rare, particularly in adult animals, and is less likely to be symmetrical in distribution. The discussion below will briefly describe the cytologic features of the various arthropathies. Further summaries of the features of these diseases are detailed at the end of this chapter.

Normal Joint Fluid

Normal joint fluid has low cellularity (less than 1.5 x 10^9/L). On a squash smear this equates to </= 2 nucleated cells per x 40 field. Cells may be arranged in palisades or rows (windrowing) reflecting the viscous nature of the fluid. There is usually a prominent background staining consisting of pink granular material

(not to be confused with bacteria) caused by the glycosaminoglycans (mostly hyaluronan) in the fluid. Red cells are absent unless blood contamination occurred at sampling. Nucleated cells are a mixture of large mononuclear cells (synovial lining cells and macrophages 60% to 90% of cells) and lymphocytes (3% to 30% of cells) with < 5% neutrophils. Synovial lining cells are round cells with a single round nucleus and a moderate amount of basophilic cytoplasm. A small proportion of these may be activated with increased amounts of vacuolated cytoplasm appearing very similar to macrophages. It is not clinically important to distinguish synovial cells and macrophages and they are classified together as large mononuclear cells, although the proportion of vacuolated (reactive) cells is important and in normal joints is less than 10%.

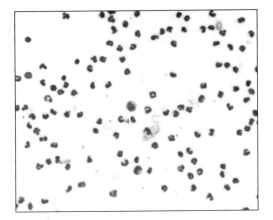

Figure 1. Cytology of normal synovial fluid.

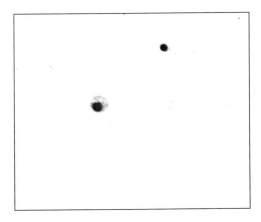

Figure 2. Cytology of synovial fluid in an infected joint.

NONINFLAMMATORY ARTHROPATHIES
Osteoarthritis

Cytologically, there is significant overlap with normal joints, as cell numbers are usually normal or very slightly raised (up to 5 x 10^9/L) with less than 2% to 4% neutrophils. Thus the majority of cells observed on cytology are large mononuclear cells, with >10% of these having abundant foamy/vacuolated or phagocytic cytoplasm. Occasionally, osteoarthritic joints have a moderately raised neutrophil count, accounting for up to 10% of cells. The reasons for this are often unclear but may involve recent joint trauma (sprain), crystal (hydroxyapatite) formation, or an idiopathic inflammatory "flare." A repeat sample 2 to 3 weeks later should usually see a return to more typical cytological features.

The diagnosis of osteoarthritis is supported by other diagnostic modalities, especially radiography (typical changes such as osteophyte and enthesophyte formation) and arthroscopy (articular cartilage fibrillation and loss).

Recent Joint Injury/Hemorrhage

Joint injury or hemorrhage will cause a hemarthrosis, reflected as large numbers of red cells. In acute hemarthrosis the differential nucleated cell count may be similar to that of peripheral blood and platelets may be present. With more long-standing hemorrhage there are increased numbers of neutrophils and macrophages and platelets are absent (these disintegrate rapidly within the fluid). Erythrophagocytosis and/or hemosiderin or hematoidin crystals in macrophages provide evidence of pre-existing hemorrhage into the joint; these features are not seen with iatrogenic blood contamination.

INFLAMMATORY ARTHROPATHIES

These can be divided into two main groups: immune-mediated and infective arthropathies. Both result in a moderate to marked increase in numbers of neutrophils with variable numbers of large mononuclear cells.

Immune-Mediated Polyarthritis (IMPA)

The synovial fluid cytology for all types of IMPA varies between joints and between patients. Typically, the white cell count is 20 to 90 x 10^9/L with 20% to 90% neutrophils (non-degenerate) and varying proportions of lymphocytes and large mononuclear cells. The proteinaceous background material seen in normal synovial fluid is usually present, although may be absent.

Infective Arthritis

Infective arthritis generally causes a large increase in neutrophils and these become the predominant cell type. Red cell counts may also be raised with associated hemorrhage. In acute infection, neutrophil counts are usually within the range of 95% to 98%. With more chronic disease (weeks), neutrophil counts may drop to the region of 70% to 95%. Neutrophils may appear degenerate and bacteria may be noted on cytologic inspection.

Bacterial Culture and Sensitivity

In cases of suspect infective arthritis, synovial fluid should be submitted for bacterial culture and sensitivity. However, not all synovial fluids from cases of infective arthritis will yield a positive culture, and the initial handling of the sample may influence this. There is evidence that placing the sample in a blood culture bottle, and initially incubating in this medium for 24 hours, can improve the sensitivity of synovial fluid culture and this is recommended. Culture of synovium obtained by needle biopsy, arthroscopy or arthrotomy is an alternative approach.

The common bacteria isolated from infected joints reflect the sources of infection. The most commonly identified organisms are *Staphlyococcus intermedius*, and β-hemolytic Streptococcus. Methicillin-resistant forms of *Staphylococcus aureus* (MRSA) have also been isolated from canine joints. Coliform and anaerobic organisms are less commonly involved, as are *Pseudomonas aeruginosa*, *Nocardia ateroides*, and *Bacillus* spp. In cats, *Pasteurella multocida*, *Bacteroides* spp. and *E. coli* are more commonly isolated as a result of bites from other cats.

Polymerase Chain Reaction for Infective Agents Associated with Joint Disease

While many organisms associated with infective arthritis can be cultured using traditional methods, some are more difficult to isolate. Some spirochetes have been linked to polyarthritis in dogs, most notably *Borrelia burgdorferi*, and these organisms cannot routinely be cultured. Culture of protozoal and other arthropod-borne organisms is also extremely difficult. Blood, urine, and synovial fluid may tested for the presence of DNA from these infective organisms using polymerase chain reaction (PCR). However, although a positive result is strong evidence for the presence of the organism within the sample, the relationship between the organism and the disease process may be complex. Recent investigations of synovial fluids of human patients with inflammatory polyarthritides have shown that PCR can detect bacterial DNA or rRNA from both organisms associated with arthritis and other skin and gut commensals in synovial fluid. It is suggested that there may be trafficking of organisms not involved in initiating the disease process to inflamed joints. Thus a positive PCR needs to be interpreted with caution.

Serology

Serology is used to aid the classification of immune-mediated polyarthritis (IMPA) and for detection of infectious agents (or antibodies to them).

Serology for Infectious Agents

Serology has also been used in the investigation of infectious diseases such as Lyme disease. The presence of antibody to *Borrelia burgdorferi* can support a diagnosis in the presence of other characteristic historical and clinical signs. However, since seroprevalance rates are often high in endemic areas, the value of such a test is limited. PCR is to be preferred in such instances, in an attempt to demonstrate the presence DNA from the relevant organism.

Serology for IMPA

Serology for IMPA is generally used to aid the classification of immune-mediated polyarthritis. It is important to note that serology cannot be used to diagnose immune-mediated polyarthritis—that requires synovial fluid analysis and confirmation of multi-joint inflammatory changes. However, serology is used to classify polyarthritis. For example, a positive titre for rheumatoid factor may help to support a diagnosis of rheumatoid arthritis but certain other criteria must be satisfied also. Similarly, anti-nuclear antibody (ANA) assay may support the diagnosis of systemic lupus erythematosus (SLE) but other criteria must be satisfied also. It should be remembered that chronic inflammation of any sort can cause positive results on these assays and thus the specificity of these tests is low.

The detection of rheumatoid factor (RF) is used as one of the diagnostic criteria for a canine rheumatoid arthritis. Readers are referred to veterinary rheumatology texts for more information on the diagnosis of this condition. Rheumatoid factor is an auto-antibody (anti-IgG immunoglobulin) and most assays will measure IgM RF, although the measurement of IgA RF has been reported in the dog, this does not seem to be used in diagnostic laboratories at present. Typically an ELISA assay is used and the concentration of RF determined by interpolation from a standard curve. Positive and negative controls should also be included. Because normal dogs and dogs with other arthritides will often have mild positive results for RF, assays are usually interpreted in the light of results from confirmed cases of rheumatoid arthritis and dogs with other arthritides. The laboratory performing the assay should be able to advise on what constitutes a positive result. Again, it should be stressed that a positive RF result does not constitute a diagnosis of rheumatoid arthritis; other diagnostic criteria must be satisfied.

Antinuclear antibody is antinuclear immunoglobulin and is associated with systemic lupus erythematosus (SLE). ANA may be detected in normal individuals as well as those with chronic inflammatory disease and so a positive ANA test result is not diagnostic of SLE. Compared with humans, dogs and cats generally have low titers of ANA, and there is a high prevalence of low ANA titers in the normal population, especially in cats. For example, cats with FeLV, FIV, and FIP infections can be positive for ANA and so it must be stressed that a positive ANA titer is only part of the diagnosis of SLE; typical clinical features must also be present and preferably evidence of immunologic disease mechanisms. The test for ANAs is the indirect immunofluorescence test using rat liver as substrate.

Synovial Fluid Biochemistry

Several simply measured biochemical parameters can be altered in synovial fluid during disease processes, eg, glucose can be lowered and protein elevated in bacterial infective arthritis. However, the usefulness of these tests is very limited and the results do not alter clinical decision-making.

There is much ongoing research on the measurement of various macromolecules ("biomarkers") in joint disease. These biomarkers are released from joint tissues (cartilage, bone or synovium) and are measured in synovial fluid (or possibly blood or urine) using a variety of techniques such as direct dye binding or enzyme-linked immunosorbent assay (ELISA). Typical markers are cartilage matrix molecules, or epitopes thereof, such as glycosaminoglycans, chondroitin sulfate (eg, epitopes with codenames such as "7D4," "3B3," "846"), keratan sulfate, and collagen. These markers remain to be validated and thus are confined to the clinical research arena.

Crystals

Crystal-induced arthropathies appear to be very rare in dogs and cats, although certain crystals have been reported in canine joint fluids. Crystals are identified in synovial fluid samples (in EDTA will suffice) using polarised light microscopy. Accurate identification requires skill and training and is based on morphology and birefringence characteristics. Staining with alizarin red can help detect calcium containing crystals. Basic calcium phosphate crystals such as hydroxyapatite crystals are often seen in canine joint fluid, particularly with osteoarthritis. However, the significance of these crystals is unknown. Synovitis associated with calcium pyrophosphate ("pseudogout") has been reported in two canine single case reports. Although the Dalmatian might be expected to be at risk of urate crystal arthropathy (gout), high renal excretion of uric acid appears to prevent urate crystal precipitation. Intra-articular corticosteroid therapy may also result in crystal formation in synovial fluid.

INVESTIGATION OF JOINT DISEASE IN SMALL ANIMALS

John F. Innes, BVSc, PhD, CertVR, DSAS (Orth), MRCVS
Faculty of Veterinary Science
University of Liverpool, Liverpool, UK

Joint disease is very common in small animals of all ages. This discussion outlines the basics of the various diagnostic aids and processes as they apply to joint diseases. Joint disease may present as lameness or in milder cases there may be stiffness following rest

CLINICAL EXAMINATION

Pain on manipulation of the joint is at the center of the clinical diagnosis. Flexion, extension, pronation, and supination should be performed and compared with the contralateral side. One must appreciate the nature of the patient and some dogs will react to the slightest manipulation whereas others may be very stoic. The range of movement may be decreased in chronic joint disease or there may be abnormal movement in the case of injury to supporting structures such as ligaments and tendons. The joint may be palpably enlarged due to joint effusion or chronic extracapsular fibrosis. Obviously this will not be detectable in the hip and shoulder. The stifle joint should be palpated with the forefinger and thumb either side of the patellar ligament. This should enable the edges of the ligament to be defined; effusion or fibrosis will make this less easy to feel. In the same way, one can palpate and displace synovial swellings in the carpus and hock. There may be heat in some acute inflammatory conditions.

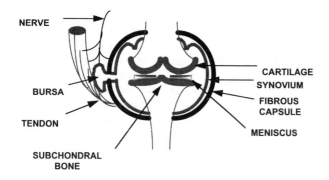

Figure 1. Diarthrodial joint.

RADIOGRAPHY

Radiography is the standard tool for initial investigation of joint disease. The changes seen in and around joints are listed below:

- Swelling of soft tissues
- Joint effusion
- Osteophytosis
- Enthesiophytosis
- Displacement of joint structures (eg, sesamoids, tibia with respect to femur)
- Fractures
- Intra-articular mineralization
- Joint mice
- Subchondral sclerosis
- Erosion
- Altered width of joint space
- Subchondral bone cysts

Two orthogonal views are the minimum requirement. Other more specialist views may be required in certain circumstances. Stressed views may be employed in certain situations such as carpal ligament injury. It is imperative that the radiographs are positioned correctly because otherwise features may be misinterpreted or pathology missed. Knowledge of normal variants should be acquired by reference to appropriate texts. Some common normal variations are listed below:

- Separate center of ossification at caudal aspect of glenoid
- Patella cubitae is a small sesamoid seen lateral to the elbow joint in some dogs
- The abductor pollicis longus has a small sesamoid medial to the carpus.
- The popliteal sesamoid may be seen at the caudal aspect of the stifle on a lateral view and superimposed on the medial joint space on the craniocaudal view.
- The fabellae may be multipartite or at different levels to each other
- The palmar sesamoids may be bipartite or multipartite

ARTHROGRAPHY

The use of positive contrast within joints may be employed when suspecting or investigating certain diseases. Arthrography can give information on:

- The articular surface
- Integrity of the synovial capsule
- Position of cartilaginous joint mice
- Adhesions in bursae

The shoulder joint is the most common site for the use of this procedure. Osteochondritis dissecans (OCD) of this joint may be delineated in this way annd information regarding the state of the bicipital bursa can be gained. To look at the articular surface, a low volume arthrogram is used (1–2 mL in a shoulder) but to look at the bicipital bursa a high volume (5–6 mL) is used to fill the bursa. Ionic water soluble agents are indicated.

A needle is placed as for arthrocentesis (q.v.) and synovial fluid aspirated. The contrast is injected, the needle removed and the joint manipulated. Radiographs should be taken immediately.

SCINTIGRAPHY

Nuclear imaging involves the systemic injection of a radionuclide, which in the case of bone scanning using 99m-technetium, binds to the hydroxyapatite of active bone. Thus joints with erosive, osteophytic, or sclerotic processes will be highlighted on the image obtained using a gamma camera. The technique is sensitive but non-specific.

ARTHROSCOPY

Arthroscopy is becoming increasingly common in small animal practice, particularly referral practice. Although arthroscopy can be used for operative procedures, it is also commonly used for diagnosis of intra-articular diseases. Arthroscopy is used mainly in the shoulder, elbow and stifle although the carpus, hip, and hock can also be examined.

MAGNETIC RESONANCE IMAGING

MRI is becoming more available for imaging the joints of small animals. However, the expense precludes the use of MRI in all but a few select cases and for research purposes. Probably the most common indications are for investigation of the internal structures of the stifle joint (menisci and cruciate ligaments) when the diagnosis is not clear, and for investigation of soft tissues in and around the shoulder joint.

ARTHROCENTESIS

The analysis of synovial fluid is probably under-used. It is in most cases a very straightforward procedure and may be carried out under heavy sedation for most joints, although the shoulder and hip may require general anaesthesia. The area for insertion of the needle should be clipped and washed with an antiseptic (eg, chlorhexidine) and sprayed with alcohol. If the area is to be handled, gloves should be worn. In most cases, 20- to 22-gauge 1-to 1.5-inch needles are used.

The most common problem with fluid aspiration is iatrogenic blood contamination. This is recognized as a "string" of blood within the fluid, whereas a joint with hemarthrosis will have sanguineous fluid, which is consistent in its color.

The handling of the sample will depend somewhat on the differential diagnosis and the volume available. A subjective assessment of color, turbidity, and viscosity can be made. Direct smears may be made for cytological assessment and a differential count and this should be done promptly.

A total cell count can be performed and the sample should be placed in an EDTA tube (since there may be fibrinogen present).

The viscosity of fluid may be assessed by the mucin clot test. This involves dropping some fluid into 5% acetic acid. Good viscosity produces a tight mucin clot whereas poor viscosity does not. The viscosity is a function of the length of the hyaluronic acid chains in the fluid. These are shorter than normal in inflammatory conditions such as infective arthritis or polyarthritis but near normal in osteoarthritis (OA). Effusion in OA may dilute the fluid and make it appear less viscus but the mucin clot test will be normal.

Table 1 summarizes the properties of normal and pathological synovial fluid. These are guidelines only.

Table 1. Properties of Normal and Pathological Fluid

	Normal	OA	Infective	Immune Mediated
Volume	0–0.75 mL	1–3 mL	1–4 mL	1–10 mL
Viscosity	High	High[1]	Low	Low
TCC (x10^9/L)	0.75	0.75–5.0	5.0–100+	5.0–90
PMNs (%)	0–1	1–5	95–98	20–80

IMMUNE-MEDIATED ARTHROPATHIES – WHY, WHEN, AND WHAT NOW?

John F. Innes, BVSc, PhD, CertVR, DSAS (Orth), MRCVS
Faculty of Veterinary Science
University of Liverpool, Liverpool, UK

INTRODUCTION AND PATHOGENESIS

Polyarthritides are an uncommon group of diseases that affect dogs and, to a lesser extent, cats. They are characterized by multiple, often symmetrical, joint swellings and effusions. There may be involvement of other body systems, particularly with diseases such as systemic lupus erythematosus. The etiology of these diseases is not known but it is clear that there are abnormalities of humoral and cell-mediated immunity.

Immune complexes are thought to form due to persistent foreign antigen or autoantibodies (eg, rheumatoid factor, which is anti-IgG IgM, or ANA). Immune complex deposition in the synovium is thought to fix complement and this may cause tissue damage and be chemotactic for polymorphonuclear cells (PMNs). PMNs phagocytose immune complexes and release degradative enzymes, causing further tissue damage. This process is continued if there is continued representation of antigen, failure to downregulate the immune response following elimination of the antigen, or autoantibody production as a result of tissue damage inciting antibody production to self antigens.

Abnormal cell-mediated immunity (CMI) responses are also thought to play a major role in these diseases. The synovium proliferates and is infiltrated with aggregates of lymphocytes and activated macrophages. Most of the lymphocytes are T cells but there may also be small "follicles" of B cells.

Macrophages and synovial cells release pro-inflammatory cytokines such as interleukin-1 (IL-1) and tumor necrosis factor α (TNF-α). These are the targets of revolutionary therapy for these diseases in humans. The action of these cytokines can be blocked with genetically engineered inhibitors or monoclonal antibodies. For example, anti-TNF-α antibodies have been used in clinical trials in humans and were associated with marked reduction in pain and swelling of joints. Interestingly, use of IL-1 receptor antagonist protein seems to help with reduction in disease progression in terms of cartilage erosion. This may say something with respect to the different roles of these cytokines in inflammatory joint diseases.

HISTORY

These cases often have histories involving stiffness and lameness but are occasionally nonambulatory. They are usually worse after rest and this often eases once they are moving although may last 20 to 30 minutes. They often have systemic signs such as depression and inappetence. In approximately 50% of cases, there may be other disease associated with the polyarthritis, eg, infection, neoplasia, or diarrhea.

CLINICAL EXAMINATION

The joints may show swelling and pain which is usually symmetrical. In addition, there may be joint instability or deformity. Because these may be multi-system diseases or be associated with other disease, one must be careful to examine everything (including eyes).

DIAGNOSIS

To begin, one would wish to confirm the diagnosis of polyarthritis and investigate if other body systems are affected. Thus arthrocentesis and routine hematology and biochemistry and urinalysis are first steps. Radiography should involve joints, chest, and abdomen. Echocardiogaphy is the most sensitive way to rule out

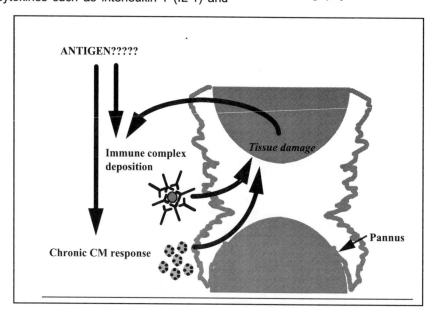

Figure 1. Proposed disease process in immune-mediated arthritis.

endocarditis. Arthrocentesis should involve four joints minimum. Once a diagnosis of polyarthritis has been established, one would wish to classify it further. In this respect one should perform serology (eg, rheumatoid factor, ANA, *Borrelia burgdorferi* antibody titer), blood culture, and synovial membrane biopsy.

Hematology and biochemistry and urinalysis may given an indication of other system disease, eg, liver, kidney, infection, anemia, thrombocytopenia, leukopenia/ leukocytosis, and proteinuria. Radiography of joints most often shows effusion and swelling. In addition, there may be osteophytosis or importantly, erosions. Chest and abdomen radiographs are taken to look for infection or neoplasia. Echocardiography if available is used to check for endocarditis—more sensitive than auscultation—by looking for vegetative lesions on valves.

Arthrocentesis is easy to perform. The animal should be heavily sedated or anesthetised. Aseptic technique is essential. A 20- to 21-gauge needle and usually a 5-mL syringe are used. The fluid is placed in an EDTA tube for total and differential counts. If one is concerned about bacterial infective arthritis, culture and sensitivity should be performed; a negative culture does <u>not</u> rule out infective arthritis but the clinical signs and SF cytology may. It is very rare for several joints to suffer bacteriologic infection in the dog. Infective arthritis is usually hematogenous in origin and can thus affect any joint.

Serology can be useful to classify the disease. Rheumatoid factor (anti-IgG IgM) supports, but does not provide, a diagnosis of rheumatoid arthritis. Equally antinuclear antibody (ANA) supports a diagnosis of systemic lupus erythematosus (SLE). Positive titers to *Borrelia burgdorferi* are not diagnostic of Lyme disease; a history of exposure to ticks, and rapid response to antibiotics must also be present. Thus a positive result to any of these tests does not constitute a diagnosis.

However, a positive titer may add to the diagnosis. Certainly ANA must be present for a diagnosis of SLE and RF for classical rheumatoid arthritis (RA). Be aware that these autoantibodies are not specific for these diseases. For example, they may be present in any chronic inflammatory disease state.

DISEASE GROUPS
Nonerosive Polyarthritides
Canine Idiopathic Polyarthritis
These are the most common group of polyarthritides and they are probably under diagnosed. Like most of the polyarthritides, the carpi and hocks are most commonly affected first. Some of these animals are thought to be early cases of RA since they will go on to develop erosive disease and are reclassified.

- Type I (50%); no associations
- Type II (reactive) (25%); chronic infection
- Type III (15%); gastrointestinal disease
- Type IV (10%); neoplasia

Systemic Lupus Erythematosus
Systemic lupus erythematosus (SLE) is a rare multisystem disease that is probably over-diagnosed. Presentation and clinical signs are variable, but most patients have pyrexia and symmetrical polyarthritis, and may also have hemolytic anemia, thrombocytopenia, leukopenia, glomerulonephritis, dermatitis, polymyositis, meningitis, pleuritis, or GI disease.

Criteria for diagnosis of SLE include:

- Involvement of more than one body system
- Significantly high titers of ANA in serum
- Evidence of immunopathologic mechanisms
- Antibodies to red cells, platelets, immunofluorescence of biopsy material (frozen sections)

Other Nonerosive Polyarthritides
Polyarthritis/Meningitis Syndrome
Sterile meningitis is a complicating factor.

Canine Polyarthritis/Polymyositis Syndrome
The reader is referred to Bennett and Kelly (Immune based non-erosive inflammatory joint disease of the dog 2. Polyarthritis/polymyositis syndrome. J Small Animal Pract. 1987;28:891) for information on this disease.

Lyme Disease
Caused by a spirochaete, *Borrelia burgdorferi,* which is carried by ticks (*Ixodes ricinus*), Lyme disease is strictly an infectious arthritis, although there may be an immune-mediated component. It is often monarticular or pauciarticular (up to five joints), and has received much attention in recent years but is probably very rare. Since up to 25% of dogs in endemic areas may have serological evidence of exposure to *Borrelia*, serology can only add weight to the diagnosis. Poylmerase chain reaction (PCR) testing for bacterial genomic DNA is recommended. The diagnosis is based on history of exposure to ticks, pyrexia and appropriate clinical signs, positive PCR, serology, and response to appropriate antibiotic therapy (eg, tetracyclines) for 3 weeks minimum.

Drug Reactions
Idiosyncratic drug reactions may occur at any time and can cause inflammatory arthritis. The most widely recognized is that in Doberman pinschers following sulfonamide treatment.

Erosive Arthritides (Causing Erosions of Bone)
Rheumatoid Arthritis (Canine)
Canine rheumatoid arthritis (CRA) is rare in dogs, and rheumatoid arthritis is very rare in cats. CRA is a chronic, progressive, destructive symmetrical polyarthritis. The criteria for diagnosis, based on ACR, include:

- Stiffness after rest
- Pain in motion of at least one joint
- Swelling of at least one joint

- Swelling of one other joint within 3-month period
- Symmetric joint swelling
- Subcutaneous nodules
- Radiographic evidence (erosions)(criteria = classic CRA)
- Rheumatoid factor in serum
- Abnormal synovial fluid
- Characteristic histopath in synovium
- Characteristic histopath in nodules

Other Erosive Polyarthritides

- Felty's syndrome
  - RA with spenomegaly and neutropaenia (caused by autoantibodies against WBCs)
- Periosteal proliferative polyarthritis of cats (and dogs)
  - Marked proliferation of periarticular new bone, especially hocks and carpi. May or may not be erosive and there may be erosions at the insertion of tendons and ligaments (erosive enthesitis).

TREATMENT OF POLYARTHRITIDES

Treat the initiating cause, whether remote infection, neoplasia, or drug reactions. Often these diseases will resolve if the primary trigger is removed.

If this cannot be achieved, relieve inflammation and suppress the immune response. This is usually achieved with prednisolone (2–4 mg/kg daily) initially and this should be gradually reduced after 2 to 3 weeks or when a clinical response is obtained. Some dogs can be weaned off treatment completely. One may need to cover with antibiotics during the high dose prednisolone period. Regular monitoring of hematology and biochemistry is good practice for those dogs on long-term treatment.

Cytotoxic drugs may be employed in refractory cases or in more aggressive disease such as SLE, Cyclophosphamide or azathioprine can be used in confirmed cases of CRA. Serious side effects can occur including renal failure, pulmonary fibrosis, bone marrow suppression, skin rashes, and corneal ulceration.

UNDERSTANDING OSTEOARTHRITIS AND NUTRITIONAL MANAGEMENT

John F. Innes, BVSc, PhD, CertVR, DSAS (Orth),
MRCVS
Faculty of Veterinary Science
University of Liverpool, Liverpool, UK

Osteoarthritis (OA) (osteoarthrosis or degenerative joint disease [DJD]) is a disease of synovial joints. While the apophyseal joints of the spine can also be affected, the association between OA of these joints, disk disease, and clinical signs is unclear. The following discussion will therefore be limited to the joints of the appendicular skeleton.

OA is the most common arthropathy of domestic species (and man) and the cause of much chronic suffering in elderly animals but it may also affect some young dogs. OA is a disease which mainly affects the articular cartilage but there are also changes in the synovium and subchondral bone. It is currently thought that the typical changes we see on a radiograph and call "osteoarthritis" simply represent the response of the joint to insult, ie, the final common pathway with a variety of initiating factors.

OA is a heterogeneous disease and assessment of the disorder is difficult. The poor correlation between radiographic and clinical data highlights this difficulty. The typical example of this, in dogs, is the dysplastic hip with secondary OA—severe radiographic changes may be present in a clinically silent joint. Expression of different facets of the disease seem to vary between individuals and even between different joints in the same individual. In small animal medicine, this is exemplified by differences in osteophyte expression which clearly do not tally with the clinical picture. This is a good example of the heterogeneity of OA that is particularly applicable to us as small animal clinicians. The current model of OA (Figure 1) attempts to incorporate the heterogeneic nature of OA and how various contributing factors may interact. It is thus helpful to think of OA as a disease process rather than a disease entity.

DISEASE MECHANISMS OF OA

It may not be long before there are new effective disease-modifying agents for treatment of OA. With this in mind, the following section of text aims to highlight some of the advances that have been made in the understanding of the pathogenesis of OA. In gaining a handle on the cellular and intercellular processes at work, we can understand how drugs might be designed to interrupt or slow down the destructive processes and/or stimulate repair mechanisms.

The main tissue affected in OA is the cartilage but the subchondral bone and synovium are also affected and indeed may be important in terms of disease progression. In the wake of improved understanding of the disease will undoubtedly come therapeutic agents. Some of these are reaching the clinical trial stage at the moment.

Basic Structure of Articular Cartilage

The mainstay of cartilage is the chondrocyte which produces the extracellular matrix. The matrix is composed of glycosaminoglycans (hyaluronic acid and proteoglycan) and collagens (mainly type II). The collagen forms a dense network that retains the proteoglycan. The proteoglycan is highly charged and attracts water into the tissue. Thus cartilage is 75% water. In normal cartilage there is a very slow turnover of collagens but the proteoglycan is constantly being renewed. The proteoglycans are aggregated into large molecules ("aggrecan") by means of a protein core. This core is in turn bound to hyaluronic acid chains with each chain containing many proteoglycan molecules.

Pathologic Changes of OA

The morphological changes seen in OA include;

- Cartilage loss, especially in areas of increased load
- Subchondral bone sclerosis
- Marginal osteophytosis
- Variable synovial inflammation

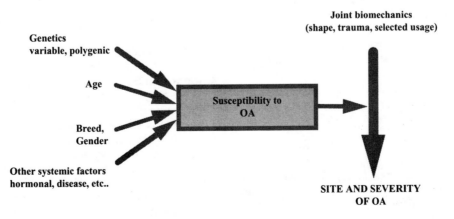

Figure 1. Current model of osteoarthritis (OA).

The biochemical changes in the cartilage include:

- Loss of proteoglycan,
- Upregulation in the degradative and synthetic activities of chondrocytes,
- Increase in space between collagen fibres
- Increase in water content

These changes reduce the elasticity of the cartilage leading to fibrillation and fissuring of the cartilage with eventual loss of tissue. If this continues eburnation of subchondral bone may result.

Intercellular Events in OA

The chondrocytes themselves are upregulated and the rates of proteoglycan synthesis and degradation are increased with the overall balance towards matrix depletion. It seems likely that the activity of the chondrocytes is increased following the binding of cytokines to the cell surface. Cytokines are cellular messengers produced locally in the tissues in response to various biological stimuli such as inflammation.

Cytokines responsible for stimulating cartilage degradation in OA are thought to be interleukins 1 and 6 (IL-1 and IL-6) and tumor necrosis factor-alpha (TNF-α). These are produced from chondrocytes, synovial cells, and activated monocytes. Binding of these cytokines to the chondrocyte stimulates the production of enzymes that have been shown to be capable of degrading all the components of the cartilage matrix. Synovial cells also release natural inhibitors of these cytokines such as IL-1 receptor antagonist (IL-1ra). There are also cytokines which stimulate synthesis of matrix and likely candidates for this include the insulin-like growth factors I and II (IGF-I and IGF-II) and transforming growth factor-β (TGF-β)

Cartilage Degradation

IL-1, IL-6, and TNF-alpha have been shown to stimulate the chondrocyte to produce enzymes that are capable of degrading all components of the matrix. The enzymes studied in most detail are the aggrecanases (ADAMTS-4 and -5) and matrix metalloproteinases (MMPs) (collagenases and stromelysins). Under normal circumstances the chondrocyte also produces a natural inhibitor of these enzymes known as tissue inhibitor of metalloproteinase (TIMP). TIMP production is decreased in OA.

CLASSIFICATION OF OA

At present OA is classified as idiopathic (primary) or secondary.

Idiopathic (Primary) OA

Idiopathic OA is not common in dogs and usually one can identify a causative disease, eg, osteochondritis dissecans (OCD) or cruciate deficiency. However, a generalized disease is occasionally seen in certain breeds such as the Chow Chow, Dalmatian, Labrador retriever, and spaniels. This is usually a symmetrical disease affecting both carpi, both stifles, or both elbows, for example.

Secondary OA

This would seem to be the most common form of OA in dogs. Common causes are listed below:

- Hip dysplasia
- Osteochondrosis
- Cruciate disease
- Collateral ligament damage
- Joint luxation
- Legg-Calvé-Perthes disease
- Articular fractures
- Other forms of arthritis

It may be that the OA is not the major consideration at the time of presentation and the primary disease may be more pressing (eg, cruciate disease) but there will be other cases where the contribution of the OA may be more important (eg, hip dysplasia with secondary change in a mature dog).

Basis of Conservative Management

There are several facets to conservative management. The activity of the dog will have an affect on the course of the disease. When acute flare-ups occur then complete rest for a period of 10 to 14 days seems to allow the majority of these to settle. The long-term activity of a dog with problematic OA will have to be altered. Short lead walks seem to be preferable with adequate periods of rest allowed should signs worsen. Obesity is to be avoided.

The tactical use of medical treatment is an important part of management of OA. In the earlier stages of the disease medical treatment may only be required occasionally but as the disease progresses maintenance therapy may be necessary.

NUTRITIONAL MANAGEMENT OF OA

Nutritional supplements and, more recently, functional foods, have become popular but controversial in the management of OA. Various supplements (nutraceuticals) are given either as capsules, pills or liquids, or are incorporated in to complete diets (functional foods).

Chondroitin Sulfate and Glucosamine

These agents are marketed as nutraceuticals and are often provided in combination. There are several preparations on the market and the constituents of these products can vary. Glycosaminoglycans (GAG) are unbranched polysaccharides with repeating subunits of an amino sugar and organic acid or sugar. Chondroitin sulfate (CS) is a constituent of GAG (aggrecan) of articular cartilage and has repeating subunits of glucuronic acid and N-acetyl galactosamine sulfate.

There has been much hype for these products as symptom-modifying and structure-modifying agents. To date, there is no clear answer as to their efficacy in either arena. Recent meta-analyses of glucosamine and

CS for treatment of human OA have failed to reach strong conclusions and indicated the need for further studies. However, it seems likely that both agents have weak to moderate pain-relieving effects. Two recent, as yet unpublished, studies have addressed the ability of glucosamine to act as a structure-modifying agent in OA of the human knee. Both studies appear to show some positive effect although until they are subject to peer review one must reserve judgement.

Chondroitin Sulfate

Studies of the distribution of CS in dogs have disagreed as to the fate of the molecule. Labeling with H^3 has demonstrated distribution to articular cartilage in dogs. However, labeling with C^{14} in a 3-month-old dog showed no distribution to articular cartilage although there was uptake in physeal cartilage. The implication from these results is that oral chondroitin sulphate may not reach the articular cartilage intact and there is some degree of depolymerization. Furthermore, 6 hours after oral administration of tritiated CS to rats, the majority of radioactivity in articular cartilage was from oligosaccharides, monomer and tritiated water.

The pharmacologic effects of CS have also been investigated. In vitro studies of the actions of CS on human neutrophils have been shown antichemotactic activity, a reduction in phagocytic activity, reduced lysosomal enzyme release, and reduced membrane damage. With respect to synovial tissues, CS has been shown to have a stimulatory effect on cultured human chondrocytes. It must be remembered that culture systems are models and very removed from the environment of the articular chondrocyte.

In experimental animals, CS has been demonstrated to have anti-inflammatory effects. In particular, CS was shown to reduce edema formation in a rat carrageenin model although this effect was not as potent as ibuprofen or indomethacin. CS was also shown to reduce neutrophil and macrophage infiltration. However, these experiments did not assess these activities in synovial joints but in soft tissues. Experiments in rabbits have shown that CS can stimulate hyaluronan synthesis by synoviocytes.

In human patients with OA of the knee, 10 days treatment with oral CS treatment resulted in an increase in synovial fluid hyaluronan concentration and decreased collagenolytic and phospholipase A2 activities. In an experimental study in dogs, treatment with oral CS (in combination with glucosamine and manganese) caused an elevation in expression of neo-epitopes of chondroitin sulfate in synovial fluid. However, this effect was demonstrated in synovial fluid from joints with induced OA (cruciate ligament transection) and contralateral control joints suggesting that this is a systemic effect. The meaning of these neo-epitopes is not clear but they are expressed in increased amounts following the induction of canine OA.

Glucosamine

Glucosamine has been used for the symptomatic relief of osteoarthritis for some time. Oral glucosamine sulfate is 90% absorbed and is a prodrug for glucosamine. In addition, it diffuses into articular tissues.

There are some data which suggest that glucosamine might influence chondrocyte metabolism. Exogenous glucosamine has been shown to stimulate proteoglycan synthesis in vitro. Specifically, glucosamine appears to stimulate the production of monomeric proteoglycan capable of assembling in to large PG aggregates. Glucosamine has also been demonstrated to increase aggrecan core protein mRNA. It has been suggested that glucosamine acts through increasing GAG synthesis which in turn stimulates proteoglycan core protein production. However, a recent study of canine chondrocytes in three dimensional culture demonstrated detrimental effects of glucosamine on cell viability and GAG production. Glucosamine has also been demonstrated to have weak anti-inflammatory effects in a variety of animal models of inflammation.

There have been several studies of the efficacy of glucosamine in the relief of pain and disability associated with OA. Most of these have been on human patients. The results of studies have varied and there have been problems with study design and size of patient groups. For example, one study showed treatment with glucosamine to be as effective as ibuprofen but another study showed no beneficial effect of glucosamine over placebo. Meta-analyses suggest that there may indeed be symptom-modification from use of glucosamine in human OA but there is general agreement that there is likely publication bias towards positive results and more studies are required to confirm therapeutic effects. There is a lack of controlled, randomised, blinded clinical trials of glucosamine in veterinary species.

Combination products of glucosamine and chondroitin sulfate are widely used in veterinary species. A randomized, controlled, comparator study was conducted in osteoarthritic dogs to compare NSAID treatments (meloxicam and carprofen) to a CS-G combination product. The primary outcome measure was peak vertical force as measured using a force platform. There was no measurable treatment effect from the G-CS combination product.

The NIH Glucosamine/Chondroitin Arthritis Intervention Trial (GAIT)

GAIT is the first, large-scale, multicenter clinical trial in the United States to test the effects of the dietary supplements glucosamine HCl and chondroitin sulfate for treatment of knee OA in humans. The study tested whether glucosamine and chondroitin sulfate used separately or in combination reduced pain in participants with knee OA. In GAIT, participants were randomly assigned to one of five treatment groups: (1) glucosamine alone, (2) chondroitin sulfate alone, (3) glucosamine and chondroitin sulfate in combination, (4) celecoxib, or (5) a placebo (an inactive substance that looks like the study substance). Glucosamine and chondroitin sulfate and their combination were compared with a placebo to evaluate whether these substances significantly improve joint pain. Celecoxib, which is a prescription drug effective in managing osteoarthritis pain, was also compared to placebo to validate the study design.

The study was double-blinded. Participants received treatment for 24 weeks. Participants were evaluated at the start of the study and at weeks 4, 8, 16, and 24 and closely monitored for improvement of their symptoms as well as for any possible adverse reactions to the study agents. Participants were also stratified into two pain subgroups—mild pain 1,229 participants (78%) and moderate-to-severe pain 354 participants (22%). The primary outcome of the study was defined as at least a 20% reduction in pain at 24 weeks. All participants had the option to use up to 4000 mg of acetaminophen, as needed, to control pain from OA throughout the study, except for the 24 hours prior to having their knee assessed.

The key results were that:

- Participants taking the positive control, celecoxib, experienced statistically significant pain relief versus placebo.
- Overall, there were no significant differences between the other treatments tested and placebo.
- For a subset of participants with moderate-to-severe pain, glucosamine combined with chondroitin sulfate provided statistically significant pain relief compared to placebo—about 79% had a 20% or greater reduction in pain versus about 54% for placebo. According to the researchers, because of the small size of this subgroup these findings should be considered preliminary and need to be confirmed in further studies.

- For participants in the mild pain subset, glucosamine and chondroitin sulfate together or alone did not provide statistically significant pain relief.

Essential Fatty Acids

Work from the author's laboratory in collaboration with the University of Cardiff indicated that the omega-3 EFA eicosapentaenoic acid (EPA) (but not other omega-3s tested) had an ability to reduce the activity of the aggrecanolytic enzyme, aggrecanase (ADAMTS-4). Further work at two US veterinary schools has suggested that EPA in a canine diet was able to reduce lameness in dogs with osteoarthritis as measured by a force platform. These data have resulted in the launch of a canine prescription diet for osteoarthritis.

Turmeric (Curcuminoids)

Curcuminoids, extracted from turmeric have some interesting anti-inflammatory effects in certain animal models and in vitro assays. Trials have been undertaken in human and canine OA. A randomized, double-blind, placebo-controlled trial in 58 dogs with elbow and hip OA failed to find a treatment effect using peak vertical force as the primary outcome variable although veterinary surgeon assessment of response to treatment was positive.

REFERENCES
1. Moreau M, Dupuis J, Bonneau NH, Desnoyers M. Clinical evaluation of a nutraceutical, carprofen and meloxicam for the treatment of dogs with osteoarthritis. Vet Rec. 2003;152:323.
2. Innes JF, Fuller CJ, Grover ER, Kelly AL, Burn JF: Randomised, double-blind, placebo-controlled parallel group study of P54FP for the treatment of dogs with osteoarthritis. Vet Rec. 2003;152:457-460.

SURGICAL MANAGEMENT OF ELBOW OSTEOARTHRITIS

John F. Innes, BVSc, PhD, CertVR, DSAS(Orth), MRCVS
Faculty of Veterinary Science
University of Liverpool, UK

Surgery for osteoarthritis of the elbow has limited forms. There are reported procedures that merely attempt to relieve pain (symptom-modifying procedures), such as debridement of osteophytes, proximal ulnar osteotomy, subtotal conroidectomy, and abrasion chondroplasty. In addition, there are salvage procedures such as excision arthroplasty and total elbow replacement.

SYMPTOM-MODIFYING PROCEDURES

Procedures aimed at relieving pain in the chronically osteoarthritic elbow joint are poorly documented in the veterinary literature but are sometimes reported at meetings. Debridement of osteophtyes is something that is sometimes performed in human elbow joints. Osteotomies of the ulna have been reported in young and older dogs but should be used with caution. Arthroscopic abrasion arthroplasty has also been reported anecdotally but evidence for efficacy is lacking.

SALVAGE PROCEDURES

Total Elbow Replacement (TER)

TER has been developed for the dog within the last decade by Conzemius and colleagues.[4,5] The success rate from a relatively small number of cases is estimated at 80%.

Indications for TER

Total elbow replacement is indicated for the intractably painful elbow in medium to large breed dogs. Elbow dysplasia and osteoarthritis are the most common indications although chronic or recurrent luxation or malunion of fractures of the humerus may also be an indication.

Dogs should have exhausted conservative measures in terms of weight control, exercise management, and medical treatments (NSAIDs and analgesia) to the point where quality of life is insufficient. The risk-benefit ratio of TER must be carefully contemplated in the light of the possible complications. If there is a complication with the procedure, necessitating implant removal, the function of the elbow is severely compromised; this risk is in the region of 20% and thus owners must be made fully aware of the possible complications as well as the potential benefits.

Contraindications for TER include:

- Persistent infection of another body system (e.g. severe skin, ear or dental disease)
- Debilitating musculoskeletal disease of the ipsilateral limb
- Dogs less than 10 to 12 months of age
- Dogs too small for the implant components
- (Debilitating musculoskeletal disease of other limbs)

Technique

A TER can be placed through a caudolateral approach to the elbow. The elbow is luxated following elevation of the lateral collateral ligament insertion on the radial head. The humeral shaft is drilled and the condylar cut is made using a guide. The radioulnar cut is then made with a guide that is linked to the placement of the humeral trial component to allow for alignment of the axis of rotation. The radial and ulnar canals are opened and the radioulnar trial placed. The trials are removed prior to cementing of the actual components. Bone graft is placed between the radius and ulna to encourage a synostosis. The elbow is reduced and the capsule sutured for stability (some surgeons place a collateral ligament prosthesis). A distal ulnar ostectomy is performed to limit radioulnar movement.

Complications

Complications include infection, luxation, femoral fracture, and aseptic loosening. These can result in the need for explantation followed by arthrodesis, or amputation or euthanasia.

Prognosis

Data suggest that recovery from this surgery takes 6 to 12 months. The author's data concur with published data on a gradual improvement of ground reaction forces in successful cases. Kinematic data suggest a normal range of motion during the gait cycle is achievable following TER in some dogs.

REFERENCES

1. Tsuge K, Mizuseki T. Debridement arthroplasty for advanced primary osteoarthritis of the elbow - Results of a new technique used for 29 elbows. J Bone Joint Surg [Br]. 1994;76B:641-646.
2. Ness MG. Treatment of fragmented coronoid process in young dogs by proximal ulnar osteotomy. J Small Anim Pract. 1998;39:15-18.
3. Bardet JF, Bureau S. Fragmentation of the coronoid process in dogs. A case-control study of 83 elbows treated by shortening osteotomy of the proximal ulna. Pratique Medicale Et Chirurgicale De L Animal De Compagnie. 1996;31:451-463.
4. Conzemius MG, Aper RL, Corti LB. Short-term outcome after total elbow arthroplasty in dogs with severe, naturally occurring osteoarthritis. Vet Surg. 2003;32:545-552.
5. Conzemius MG, Aper RL, Hill CM. Evaluation of a canine total-elbow arthroplasty system: A preliminary study in normal dogs. Vet Surg. 2001;30:11-20.

SURGICAL MANAGEMENT OF HIP OSTEOARTHRITIS

John F. Innes, BVSc, PhD, CertVR, DSAS(orth), MRCVS
Faculty of Veterinary Science
University of Liverpool, UK

Surgery for osteoarthritis of the hip has limited forms. There are reported procedures that merely attempt to relieve pain (symptom-modifying procedures), such as pectineal myectomy and hip joint denervation. In addition, there are salvage procedures such as excision arthroplasty and total hip replacement.

SYMPTOM-MODIFYING PROCEDURES

Pectineal myectomy is a procedure that was popularized some considerable time ago. It does not stop the progression of radiographic changes. It may reduce pain and it may do this through eliminating the biomechanical effect of the pectineus muscle, which is to cause adduction and consequent dorsal subluxation of the femoral head in a dysplastic hip. The other possibility is that the pectineus muscle is a source of pain itself in hip dysplasia/arthritis and removing the muscle may remove this source of pain. It is probably fair to say that it is a less popular technique that in the past.

Hip joint denervation is a newer concept with limited published information. It is suggested that a dorsolateral surgical approach to the hip can allow denervation of the capsule and subsequent pain relief. Uncontrolled clinical studies have been performed in an attempt to support this notion.

SALVAGE PROCEDURES

Total Hip Replacement (THR)

THR has been performed in dogs since the 1970s and is the treatment of choice for the intractably painful hip joint. Early systems (Richards) were two-component cemented systems with little accommodation for the variance in patient size and conformation. THR is now a routine procedure in orthopedic referral practice. Modular canine cemented and cementless systems are available from a variety of manufacturers. The success rate of the procedure is good (85%–95%).

Indications for THR

Total hip replacement is indicated for the intractably painful hip in medium to large breed dogs. Hip dysplasia and osteoarthritis are the most common indications although chronic or recurrent luxation or malunion of fractures of the femoral head or neck are also indications.

Dogs should have exhausted conservative measures in terms of weight control, exercise management and medical treatments (NSAIDs and analgesia) to the point where quality of life is insufficient. The risk-benefit ratio of THR must be contemplated. If there is a complication with the procedure, necessitating implant removal, the function of the hip is severely compromised; this risk is in the region of 5% to 10% and thus owners must be made fully aware of the possible complications as well as the potential benefits.

Contraindications for THR include:

- Persistent infection of another body system (eg, severe skin, ear or dental disease)
- Debilitating musculoskeletal disease of the ipsilateral limb
- Dogs less than 10 to 12 months of age (although there are exceptions to this)
- Dogs too small for the implant components (implants are now available for small dogs)
- (Debilitating musculoskeletal disease of other limbs)

Technique

A THR can be placed through a craniolateral approach to the hip. The femoral head is luxated and the head and neck cut using a template. The acetabulum is reamed and the acetabular component placed (cemented or non-cemented). The femur is then drilled and cancellous bone removed. The femoral component is placed and the appropriate femoral head applied to the femoral neck. The hip is reduced and the capsule sutured for stability.

Complications

Complications include infection, luxation, femoral fracture, and aseptic loosening.

Prognosis

The statistics from the US indicate that 85% of dogs only have one THR. Whether this is for clinical or economic reasons is unclear. There is likely to be significant clinical benefit for bilaterally affected dogs in that they can load the prosthetic hip to a greater degree and this might alleviate signs on the contralateral hip.

EXCISION ARTHROPLASTY

Femoral head and neck excision is a long-described technique for treating intractable pain of the canine hip joint. Care must be taken to remove all of the femoral neck so as not to leave a spur of bone. Although the technique may relieve pain, it is unlikely that it restores normal function even in small dogs.

REFERENCES

1. Bowen JM, Arnold RA, Wilson RC, Kneller SK, Lewis RE. Progression of hip dysplasia in German Shepherd dogs after unilateral pectineal myotomy. J Am Vet Med Assoc. 1972;161:899.
2. Bowen JM. Electromyographic analysis of reflex and spastic activities of canine pectineus muscles In presence and absence of hip dysplasia. Am J Vet Res. 1974;35:661-668.
3. Kinzel S, Fasselt R, Prescher A, Selzer C, von Keyserlingk DG, Kupper W. Innervation of the canine hip joint capsule. Tierarztliche Praxis Ausgabe Kleintiere Heimtiere. 1998;26:330-335.
4. Kinzel S, Von Scheven C, Buecker A, Stopinski T, Kupper W. Clinical evaluation of denervation of the

canine hip joint capsule: a retrospective study of 117 dogs. Vet Comp Orthop Traumatol. 2002;15:51-56.

5. Duff R, Campbell JR. Effects of experimental excision arthroplasty of hip-joint. Res Vet Sci. 1978;24:174-181.

6. Duff R, Campbell JR. Long-term results of excision arthroplasty of canine hip. Vet Rec. 1977;101:181-184.

7. Plante J, Dupuis J, Beauregard G, Bonneau NH, Breton L. Long-term results of conservative treatment, excision arthroplasty and triple pelvic osteotomy for the treatment of hip dysplasia in the immature dog. 2. Analysis of the ground reaction forces. Vet Comp Orthop Traumatol 1997;10:130-135.

FELINE OSTEOARTHRITIS

B. Duncan X. Lascelles, BSc, BVSC, PhD, MRCVS,
CertVA, DSAS(ST), Diplomate ECVS and ACVS
Director, Comparative Pain Research Laboratory
Director, Integrated Pain Management Service
College of Veterinary Medicine
North Carolina State University, Raleigh, NC

Appendicular joint osteoarthritis is considered to be present in approximately 25% to 30% of the canine population, and to be a potentially painful condition. However, little is known about the incidence of feline osteoarthritis or degenerative joint disease. It is assumed that osteoarthritis is the most common form of degenerative joint disease in cats, but this has not been fully evaluated. To date, the only studies performed have been retrospective evaluations of radiographs of cats taken for various reasons. One study found 64 of 100 cats (mean age 15 years) showed radiographic evidence of appendicular joint osteoarthritis. A similar study found that 22% of 262 cats had radiographic evidence of appendicular joint osteoarthritis, when at least one synovial joint was included on the radiograph, and a third study found that 16.5% of 218 cats had radiographic evidence of appendicular osteoarthritis. The most recent study evaluated a cohort of 28 cats in which osteoarthritis had been diagnosed (radiographically), and found the elbow and hip joints to be the most commonly affected. This is in line with a recent study by the author, where 19 cats with radiographic osteoarthritis were evaluated and a median of 4 appendicular joints in each cat had radiographic signs consistent with osteoarthritis, with hip (total of 16 joints affected) being the most commonly affected, followed by elbow (11 joints) and tarsus (11 joints), then stifle (10), shoulder (5) and carpus (2). All the cats but one had radiographic changes in the bones of the spinal column consisting of spondylosis deformans and/or radiographic signs consistent with intervertebral disk disease.

Despite the frequency of osteoarthritis in domesticated cats, very little is known about its association with pain, and indeed it has been suggested that feline osteoarthritis may not be painful, although most clinicians believe it can be associated with pain and impaired mobility.

Over the last year, the author, together with Dr. Wendy Simpson and Dr. Bernie Hansen, has been conducting a randomized, cross-sectional study of the incidence of feline degenerative joint disease in cats from 6 months to 20 years old. Cats were randomly picked from a first opinion practice and screened with radiographs of every appendicular joint and the axial skeleton. In addition, the radiographic changes seen have been correlated with clinical examination findings and owner observations. This information will be summarized during the presentation (currently data is still being processed at the time of writing, Aug 2007).

REFERENCES

1. Hedhammar A, Olsson SE, Andersson SA, et al. Canine hip dysplasia: study of heritability in 401 litters of German Shepherd dogs. J Am Vet Med Assoc. 1979; 174:1012-1016.
2. Johnson JA, Austin C, Breur GJ. Incidence of canine appendicular musculoskeletal disorders in 16 veterinary teaching hospitals from 1980 to 1989. Vet Comp Orthoped Traumatol. 1994; 7:56-69.
3. Moore GE, Burkman KD, Carter MN, et al. Causes of death or reasons for euthanasia in military working dogs: 927 cases (1993-1996). J Am Vet Med Assoc. 2001; 219:209-214.
4. Lascelles BD, Main DC. Surgical trauma and chronically painful conditions--within our comfort level but beyond theirs? J Am Vet Med Assoc. 2002; 221:215-222.
5. Hardie EM, Roe SC, Martin FR. Radiographic evidence of degenerative joint disease in geriatric cats: 100 cases (1994-1997). J Am Vet Med Assoc. 2002; 220:628-632.
6. Godfrey DR. Osteoarthritis in cats: a retrospective radiological study. J Small Anim Pract. 2005; 46:425-429.
7. Clarke SP, Mellor D, Clements DN, et al. Prevalence of radiographic signs of degenerative joint disease in a hospital population of cats. Vet Rec. 2005; 157:793-799.
8. Clarke SP, Bennett D. Feline osteoarthritis: a prospective study of 28 cases. J Small Anim Pract. 2006; 47:439-445.
9. Lascelles BD, Hansen B, Smith A, et al. Pilot evaluation of an activity monitor and client specific outcome measures for the measurement of pain relief in arthritic cats. In: 2nd World/33rd Annual Veterinary Orthopedic Society Conference, Keystone, CO, 2006, p 168.
10. Herzog W, Clark A, Longino D. Joint mechanics in osteoarthritis. Novartis Found Symp 2004; 260:79-95; discussion 95-79, 100-104, 277-109.
11. Hardie EM. Management of osteoarthritis in cats. Vet Clin North Am Small Anim Pract. 1997; 27:945-953.

INJURIES OF THE CANINE SHOULDER

Carlos Macias, Ldo Vet, DSAS(Orth), MRCVS,
RCVS, Specialist in Small Animal Orthopaedics
Bahia de Málaga Veterinary Referral Centre
Málaga, Spain

Shoulder injuries are responsible for many cases of forelimb lameness in the dog. Although there are still many unanswered questions, newer diagnostic tools such as arthroscopy and magnetic resonance imaging (MRI) are providing a novel approach to the investigation of shoulder conditions in the dog.

DIFFERENTIAL DIAGNOSIS OF SHOULDER INJURIES

Many conditions affecting the shoulder joint are recognized in the dog. The difficulties in achieving a diagnosis are due to the fact that these conditions are often present simultaneously. In addition, some can be present as incidental findings:

- Bicipital tenosynovitis
- Mineralization of the supraspinatus tendon
- Mineralization of the infraspinatus tendon
- Infraspinatus contracture
- Glenohumeral ligament rupture
- Subscapularis tendinopathy
- Teres minor myopathy

ETIOPATHOGENESIS

Several factors have been proposed in the etiopathogenesis of musculotendinous and ligamentous conditions affecting the shoulder in the dog. Most injuries are simple strain injuries, whether acute or in a chronic, repetitive manner, leading to complete or partial rupture and secondary changes including mineralisation of the damaged structure. Although active dogs are more commonly presented with such injures, unfit dogs and dogs with other orthopedic problems (eg, hip dysplasia) are also frequently presented.

Mineralization of the rotator cuff muscles is observed in humans. Local ischemia is thought to lead to fibrocartilaginous metaplasia and crystal deposition. The calcification itself is not painful, and symptoms, if presented, are thought to be due to vascular reaction and subsequent swelling and tension of the affected tendon.[19] This may also be true in dogs.[15]

Bicipital tenosynovitis has been described in young dogs secondary to osteochondrosis dissecans due to osteochondral fragments becoming trapped underneath the bicipital tendon.[9]

The concept of shoulder instability due to failure of passive or active restraining mechanisms is thought to be responsible for many of the shoulder conditions.[1] Although in vitro studies suggest that the joint capsule and glenohumeral ligaments are the main restraining mechanism in the dog,[21] it is likely that, as in humans, the muscles within the region of the shoulder play an important role in vivo, stabilizing the joint and preventing excessive strain injuries to specific muscle groups.[1]

HISTORY AND SIGNALMENT

Musculotendinous and ligamentous conditions of the shoulder typically affect middle aged dogs with the Labrador retriever, rottweiler and boxer being over-represented.[5,8,17,20] Most dogs with shoulder lameness will present with a history of chronic insidious, often progressive forelimb lameness of weeks to months duration. Occasionally a traumatic event will be recorded as the precipitant factor although in many cases, the onset of lameness is a vague event. The lameness usually worsens with exercise or after rest. An exception to this will be contracture of the infraspinatus muscle where a transient sudden onset of lameness may be recorded 4 to 6 weeks prior to the by loss of internal rotation of the shoulder.

CLINICAL FINDINGS

Clinical findings are often very subtle, sometimes reaching a presumptive diagnosis by exclusion of other problems elsewhere on the limb. Performing a flexion test (holding the shoulder in flexion for a minute or so) is a useful test as the lameness usually worsens when such procedure is performed.[17] Some degree of muscle atrophy, especially affecting the spinatus muscles group, is often noted. Pain on manipulation is not a constant feature although it is more readily elicited in cases of bicipital tenosynovitis if pressure is applied to the tendon of origin of the biceps tendon with the shoulder in full flexion with the elbow extended. In cases of contracture of the infraspinatus tendon, the limb is generally held in a permanently externally rotated position, as the dog is unable to internally rotate the limb. Circumduction of the limb is noted at the walk and trot.

A drawer test, similar to that performed to detect cranial cruciate ligament deficiency, has been described to detect shoulder instability associated with rupture of the glenohumeral ligaments.[1] Increased angle of abduction is also reported to be consistent with medial glenohumeral ligament ruptures[22]; however, these tests are difficult to demonstrate or to interpret.

ANCILLARY TESTS
Radiography

Standard orthogonal views are the minimal baseline projections of any shoulder investigation. Their usefulness is often limited to determine the presence of secondary changes within the joint. Periarticular new bone formation is commonly seen in the caudal aspect of the glenoid and humeral head. Multiple or, less commonly, single, smooth or irregular mineralized deposits in the region of insertion of the supraspinatus or infraspinatus tendons, if present, will be of diagnostic value. Sclerosis in the region of the bicipital grove can also be present, suggesting mineralisation of the biceps tendon. A useful view to investigate the bicipital grove is the cranio-proximal cranio-distal (CP-CD) skyline view.[5]

Synovial Fluid Analysis

Synovial fluid analysis should be routinely performed in the investigation of any joint disease, the shoulder being no exception.

Arthrography

Although largely superseded by arthroscopy, arthrography stills plays an important role, mainly to examine the distal aspect of the bicipital tendon sheath for the presence of joint mice which can not be visualised arthroscopically or to evaluate the possibility of tendon sheath tears.[6] A large volume of contrast (10–12 mL for a 30- to 40-kg dog) is recommended to achieve adequate distention and filling of the distal tendon sheath. Care must be taken to avoid the introduction of air bubbles.

Arthroscopy

Arthroscopy has become the gold standard in the investigation of shoulder lameness as it allows full inspection of all the intra-articular structures.

Ultrasonography and MRI

Ultrasonography has been described for the investigations of extra-articular conditions in the region of the shoulder joint (mineralization of the supraspinatus and infraspinatus tendon and teres myopathy) and for the evaluation of the bicipital tendon.[3,7] MRI offers a noninvasive alternative to arthroscopy in the evaluation of dogs with suspected shoulder injuries.

MANAGEMENT
Nonsurgical Management:

Conservative management should be attempted in all cases initially, as many dogs will respond favorably. One exception to this, where surgery is recommended first, is cases of infraspinatus contracture, Nonsurgical management is based on restricted activity for at least 3 months (client education is essential) and, if required, the use of systemic NSAIDs. Intra-articular injection of long acting glucocorticoids could be considered in the management of intra-articular shoulder conditions. Although there is lack of reliable data, empiric evidence suggests that this can be useful, probably more so in cases where there is evidence of intra-articular pathology (eg, bicipital tenosynovitis, glenohumeral ligament injuries).

Surgical Management

Surgery should be considered if there is a poor response to conservative management and significant lameness.

- Bicipital tenosynovitis: Bicipital tenodesis or tenotomy has been performed with success, although a worsening in lameness can be seen following surgery.[4,20] A craniomedial approach to the shoulder is performed. The tendon is sectioned form its origin and reattached to the proximal humerus with the use of staples or sutures drilled through the greater tubercle. If an osteochondral fragment is trapped underneath the tendon, removal of the fragment is indicated.[9]
- Mineralization within the insertion of the supraspinatus or infraspinatus tendon: Removal of the mineralized fragments with/without tenotomy is

advocated, with good long-term results despite the recurrence of the mineralization.[5,8,10,15] Care should be taken as the mineralization is often asymptomatic.
- Infraspinatus contracture: Surgery is always indicated. A tenotomy of the infraspinatus muscle and, if required, debridment of any adhesions to the joint capsule should restore normal shoulder movement intraoperatively. Early exercise should be encouraged to prevent adhesion formation that may otherwise compromise the generally excellent outcome (Brinker et al 1990).
- Teres myopathy: Resection of the teres minor muscle was used in the only case reported in the literature with good results.[3]
- Glenohumeral ligament ruptures: A ligament substitution suture has been described in one case of lateral glenohumeral ligament rupture.[14] Additional studies will be required to determine the usefulness of such procedure. Thermal shrinkage of the medial joint capsule has been recently described for the management of medial glenohumeral tears in one case although this technique remains very controversial.[18]

Prognosis

Good to excellent results are reported in most cases whether treated nonsurgically or surgically.[5,8,9,15] Complete resolution of lameness is, however, uncommon, with a significant proportion of dogs developing mild transient lameness after strenuous exercise.[4,11] This is of particular significance in the athletic dog if a return to normal activity is to be expected.

REFERENCES
1. Bardet JF. Diagnosis of shoulder instability in dogs and cats: a retrospective study. J Am Anim Hosp Assoc. 1998;34:42-54.
2. Bardet JF. Lesions of the biceps tendon: diagnosis and classification. A retrospective study of 25 cases in 23 dogs and one cat. Vet Comp Orthopaed Traumatol. 1999;12:188-195.
3. Bruce WJ, Spence S, Miller A. Teres minor myopathy as a cause of lameness in a dog. J Small Anim Pract. 1997;38:74-77.
4. Davidson EB, Griffey SM, Vasseur PB, Shields SL. Histopathological, radiographic, and arthrographic comparison of the biceps tendon in normal dogs and dogs with biceps tenosynovitis. J Am Anim Hosp Assoc. 2000;36, 522-530.
5. Flo GL, Middleton D. Mineralisation of the supraspinatus tendon in dogs. J Am Vet Med Assoc. 1990;1: 95-97.
6. Innes JF, Brown G. Rupture of the biceps brachii tendon sheath in two dogs. J Small Anim Pract. 2004;45:25-28.
7. Kramer M, Gerwing M, Sheppard C, Schimke E. Ultrasonography for the diagnosis of diseases of the tendon and tendon sheath of the biceps brachii muscle. Vet Surg. 2001;30:64-71.

8. Kriegleder H. Mineralisation of the supraspinatus tendon. Clinical observations in seven dogs. Vet Comp Orthopaed Traumatol. 1995;8:91-97.

9. La Hue TR, Brown SG, Roush JC, Ticer JW. Entrapment of joint mice in the bicipital tendon sheath as a sequela to osteochondrosis dissecans of the proximal humerus in dogs: A report of six cases. J Am Anim Hosp Assoc. 1998;24:99-105.

10. Laitinen OM, Flo GL. Mineralisation of the supraspinatus tendon in dogs: long-term follow-up. J Am Anim Hosp Assoc. 2000;36, 262-267.

11. Lincoln JD, Potter K. Tenosynovitis of the biceps brachii tendon in dogs. J Am Anim Hosp Assoc. 1984;20 385-391.

12. Long CD, Nyland TG. Ultrasonographic evaluation of the canine shoulder. Vet Radiol Ultrasound. 1999;4:372-379.

13. McKee WM, Macias C. Orthopaedic conditions of the shoulder in the dog. In Practice. 2004;26:118-129.

14. Mitchell RAS, Innes JF. Lateral glenohumeral ligament rupture in three dogs. J Small Anim Pract. 2001;41:511-514.

15. Muir P, Johnson KA, Cooley AJ, Manley PA. Force-plate analysis of gait before and after surgical excision of calcified lesions of the supraspinatus tendon in two dogs. Vet Rec. 1996;139: 137-139.

16. Muir P, Johnson KA. Supraspinatus and biceps brachii tendinopathy in dogs. J Small Anim Pract. 1994;35:239-243.

17. Muir P, Goldsmid SE, Rothwell TLW, Bellenger CR. Calcifying tendinopathy of the biceps brachii in a dog. J Am Vet Med Assoc. 1992;11:1747-1749.

18. O'Neill T, Innes JF. Treatment of shoulder instability caused by medial glenohumeral ligament rupture with thermal capsulorrhaphy. J Small Anim Pract. 2004;45(10): 521-524.

19. Solomon. The shoulder. In: Appley's System of Orthopaedic and Fractures. London: Arnold, 2001.

20. Stobie D, Wallace LJ, Lipowitz AJ, King V, Lund EM. Chronic bicipital tenosynovitis in dogs: 29 cases (1985-1992). J Am Vet Med Assoc. 1995;2:201-207.

21. Vasseur PB, Moore D, Brown SA, Eng D. (1982) Stability of the canine shoulder joint: an in vitro analysis. Am J Vet Res. 1982;2:352-355.

22. Cook JL, Renfro DC, Tomlinson JL, Sorenson JE. Measurement of angles of abduction for diagnosis of shoulder instability in dogs using goniometry and digital image analysis. Vet Surg. 2005;34(5):463-468.

THE CANINE HIP

Carlos Macias, Ldo Vet, DSAS(Orth), MRCVS, RCVS, Specialist in Small Animal Orthopaedics
Bahia de Málaga Veterinary Referral Centre
Málaga, Spain

HIP DYSPLASIA

Hip dysplasia is an inherited, developmental disease of the hip joint characterised by hip laxity and the development of osteoarthritis (Lust 1985, Smith et al, 1995). Hip dysplasia affects all breeds of dogs although the prevalence is higher in the large and giant breeds such as German shepherd dogs, Labrador retrievers, Golden retrievers, Rottweilers, English setters, American bulldogs, and Mastiffs. There is no sex predisposition.

Laxity of the hip joint is a constant feature of hip dysplasia. A direct correlation between laxity and the development of osteoarthritis has been demonstrated (Smith et al, 1995).

The clinical signs associated with hip dysplasia typically have a bimodal age distribution. Although clinical signs can appear at any age, many dogs under a year of age affected with hip dysplasia present with clinical signs related to hip instability and secondary synovitis. Older dogs present with clinical signs related to hip osteoarthritis.

Radiography is the standard method for the diagnosis of hip dysplasia. The ventrodorsal extended view remains the accepted position and is adequate for the diagnosis of hip dysplasia in symptomatic dogs.

In the young dog, secondary changes can be minimal, and therefore the diagnosis of hip dysplasia is based solely in the degree of femoral head subluxation. Mildly affected animals may appear normal or have a minimal degree of apparent laxity when evaluating the extended ventrodorsal projection due to self-tightening of the joint capsule (wind-up mechanism) (Adams et al, 2000).

The severity of secondary changes is very variable in dogs with hip dysplasia/osteoarthritis, from a very faint osteophyte in the area of joint capsule attachment to the femoral neck (Morgan's line or caudolateral curvilinear osteophyte) to severe remodelling of the femoral head, femoral neck, and acetabulum and marked osteophytosis.

The options available for the treatment of canine hip dysplasia can be broadly divided in conservative and surgical management options. The aim of any treatment is to alleviate pain, maintain or improve limb function, and whenever possible, reduce the progression of osteoarthritis. The decision as to which option is indicated should be made on an individual basis based on severity of clinical signs, age, dog's behaviour, and potential use as well as owners' considerations (eg, ability to provide adequate postoperative care, and financial constraints).

Conservative management of dogs with symptomatic hip dysplasia is indicated in all dogs with mild clinical signs regardless of age and should always be considered as the first line of treatment even for severely affected cases. Conservative management can produce very satisfactory long-term results regardless of the severity of the initial clinical signs.[1]

Conservative management can be broadly divided into three aspects, weight regulation exercise regimen, and the use of therapeutic drugs. These three aspects should be considered simultaneously if a successful outcome is to be achieved.

Surgical management is indicated in dogs with significant clinical signs that fail to respond to conservative management. Accepted surgical procedures available can be divided into "prophylactic procedures" in the young dog such as juvenile pubic symphysiodesis and triple pelvic osteotomy and "definitive procedures" such as total hip replacement and femoral head and neck excision arthroplasty.

LEGG-CALVE-PERTHES DISEASE

Legg-Calvé-Perthes disease is a developmental avascular necrosis of the femoral head that occurs in juvenile small dogs, particularly the terrier breeds. Commonly affected breeds included the Miniature poodle, West Highland white terrier, Cairn terrier, Manchester terrier and Yorkshire terrier.[10,11,13]

Affected dogs usually become lame when they are between four and 11 months of age. Animals present more commonly with a history of progressive lameness of one to two months' duration. Intermittent non-weight bearing lameness is often noted on visual inspection. Manipulation of the hip almost inevitably results in a marked pain response, especially when extension or abduction is attempted. A reduction in the range of motion and crepitus is often noted, especially in more chronic cases where there is established periarticular fibrosis. Varying degrees of gluteal muscle atrophy resulting in a prominent greater trochanter can also be detected.

Initial radiographic signs include areas of reduced radiodensity within the femoral head and neck and a widened, often irregular, joint space. Deformity of the epiphysis resulting in a grossly abnormal femoral head, sclerosis and thickening of the femoral neck as well as marked joint incongruency is noted in more advanced cases. These changes are almost pathognomonic. Femoral neck fractures, acetabular remodelling, flattening of the femoral head, and periarticular new bone formation can be detected in more chronic cases.

Conservative management is an option for dogs with very mild lameness and minimal radiographic changes and can result in an excellent functional outcome. Strict rest and the use of analgesics may allow a successful repair and the preservation of joint integrity. Surgical management by a femoral head and neck excision arthroplasty is recommended as the treatment of choice in dogs with marked lameness and advanced radiographic changes or in dogs that fail to respond to conservative treatment within the first 4 weeks.[13]

SLIPPED CAPITAL FEMORAL EPIPHYSIS

Spontaneous nontraumatic separation of the femoral epiphysis is recognised as a cause of lameness in young dogs and cats.[12] This condition has also been referred to as spontaneous femoral capital physeal fractures (McNicholas et al, 2002), and epiphyisiolysis.[6]

The disease is more frequently seen in neutered, young males less than 16 months of age. The condition appears more prevalent in Labradors. Obese animals appear to be predisposed.

Affected dogs usually present between the ages of six to 18 months with a history of moderate to severe, often non-weight bearing, and pelvic limb lameness. Other features include stiffness and difficulty rising and jumping, especially in bilaterally affected animals. A minor traumatic incident (eg, jumping from a bed) can usually be associated with the onset of lameness.

A ventrodorsal standard radiograph of the pelvis is usually diagnostic although a careful evaluation is required.

In the majority of cases, the secondary changes preclude surgical repair[12] and therefore surgical options are limited to salvage techniques such as total hip replacement or femoral head and neck excision arthroplasty.

ACETABULAR FRACTURES
Road traffic accidents are the most common cause. Isolated acetabular fractures are uncommon except in racing greyhounds or other very active breeds where non-traumatic, stress fractures of the acetabulum can occur.[15]

As with all articular fractures, accurate reconstruction and rigid fixation is recommended in the majority of acetabular fractures, especially those involving the cranial two thirds of the acetabulum. Conservative treatment can be adequate in many cases[4] although others authors advocate surgical management.[3]

LUXATIONS
Luxation of the coxofemoral joint is the most common luxation in dogs and cats.[9] Road traffic accidents are the most common cause although falls and a variety of other incidents have also been reported.[2] Affected animals are usually over one year of age. "Spontaneous," non-traumatic luxations can occur in dogs with hip dysplasia and marked joint laxity.[14] Bilateral luxations are uncommon.

The choice of treatment depends on the presence of pre-existing disease, duration of the luxation and other complicating factors such as concomitant orthopedic injuries. Management options can be divided into closed reduction +/- augmented stabilisation using an Ehmer sling, ischial-ilial pin or an external skeletal fixator, open reduction and stabilization techniques such as capsulorraphy, ilial-femoral suture, transarticular pinning, hip toggle, anchored extracapsular technique +/- distal transposition of the greater trochanter, triple pelvic osteotomy and salvage options such as femoral head and neck excision arthroplasty and total hip replacement.

Closed reduction should be attempted first in all cases of acute injury (less than 7 to 10 days old).

Success rates with closed reduction can be as high as 60%.[7]

Surgical management of coxofemoral luxations is indicated in noncomplicated cases where closed reduction has failed, chronic cases where closed reduction is not possible, unstable hips following closed reduction, or where concomitant orthopedic injuries are present. All surgical techniques reported can offer good functional results.[7]

Von WILLEBRAND HETEROTOPIC OSTEOCHONDROFIBROSIS
Von Willebrand heterotopic osteochondrofibrosis is an uncommon cause of lameness. It has been described predominantly in Dobermanns and has also been reported in the German shepherd dog and the St Bernard (Layton and Ferguson 1987).[5,8] Affected animals will present with a chronic, progressive, moderate to severe insidious onset pelvic limb lameness. Muscle atrophy is usually a feature. The range of hip extension is reduced and pain is usually detected on manipulation of the hip. A palpable mass is sometimes detected caudal and dorsal to the greater trochanter.

The disease is characterized by the development of a soft tissue mass (later calcified) involving the muscles caudal to the hip (mainly gemelli and internal and external obturator muscles). It is thought that minor trauma or spontaneous bleeding leads to focal myopathy. Chondro-osseous tissue is formed following initial fibrosis. Affected animals should test positive for Von Willebrand's disease.

REFERENCES
1. Barr ARS, Denny HR, Gibbs C. Clinical hip dysplasia in dogs: The long term results of conservative management. J Small Anim Pract. 1987;28:243-252.
2. Basher AWP, Walter MC, Newton CD (1986) Coxofemoral luxation in the dog and cat. Vet Surg. 1986;15(5):356-362.
3. Boudrieau RJ, Kleine LJ. Non-surgically managed caudal acetabular fractures in dogs: 15 cases (1979-1984). J Am Vet Med Assoc. 1988;193(6): 701-705.
4. Butterworth SJ, Gribben S, Skerry TM, Denny HR, Barr ARS, Gregory SP. Conservative and surgical treatment of canine acetabular fractures: A review of 34 cases. J Small Anim Pract. 1994;35: 139-143.
5. Dueland RT, Wagner SD, Parker RB. von Willebrand heterotopic osteochondrofibrosis in Doberman pinschers: five cases (1980-1987). J Am Vet Med Assoc. 1990;197(3):383-388.
6. Dupuis J, Breton L, Drolet R. Bilateral epiphysiolysis of the femoral heads in two dogs. J Am Vet Med Assoc. 1997;210(8):1162-1165.
7. Evers P, Johnston GR, Wallace LJ, Lipowitz AJ, King VL. Long-term results of treatment of traumatic coxofemoral joint dislocation in dogs: 64 cases (1973-1992). J Am Vet Med Assoc. 1997;210(1):59-64.

8. Janssens LAA, Ramon FA, De Schepper AMA, Van Bree H. A case of degenerative myopathy of the obturator externus muscle in a dog. Vet Comp Orthopaed Traumatol. 1993;6:66-69.

9. Johnston JA, Austin C, Breuer CJ. Incidence of canine appendicular musculoskeletal disorders in 126 veterinary teaching hospitals from 1980 through 1989. Vet Comp Orthopaed Traumatol. 1994;7: 56-59.

10. Lee R, Fry PD. Some observations in the occurrence of Legg-Calvé-Perthes disease (coxa plana) in the dog, and an evaluation of excision arthroplasty as a method of treatment. J Small Anim Pract. 1969;10:309.

11. Ljunggren GL. Legg-Perthes in the dog. Acta Orthopaed Scand. 1967;95, 1.

12. Moores AP, Owen MR, Fews D, Coe RJ, Brown PJ, Butterworth SJ. Slipped capital femoral epiphysis in dogs. J Small Anim Pract. 2004;45:602-608.

13. Piek CJ, Hazewinkel HA, Wolvekamp WT, Nap RC, Mey BP. Long-term follow-up of avascular necrosis of the femoral head in the dog. J Small Anim Pract. 1996;37(1):12-18.

14. Trostel CD, Peck JN, deHaan JJ. Spontaneous bilateral coxofemoral luxation in four dogs. J Am Anim Hosp Assoc. 2000;36(3):268-276.

15. Wendelburg K, Dee J, Kaderly R, Dee L, Eaton-Wells R. (1988) Stress fractures of the acetabulum in 26 racing Greyhounds. Vet Surg. 1988;17(3):128-134.

Additional references are available from the author upon request.

MANAGEMENT OF CHALLENGING LONG BONE FRACTURES IN DOGS AND CATS

Carlos Macias, Ldo Vet, DSAS(Orth), MRCVS,
RCVS, Specialist in Small Animal Orthopaedics
Bahia de Málaga Veterinary Referral Centre
Málaga, Spain

Fractures in long bones can be divided according to their location, such as diaphyseal, metaphyseal, or epiphyseal fractures; fracture configuration, such as transverse, oblique, spiral, comminuted, and segmented; and soft tissue integrity (open or closed). Although a classification has not been made according to easiness of repair or possible surgical complications, the experienced and non-experienced surgeon is presented on an almost daily basis with fractures than can represent a significant challenge to anyone, whether this has to do with the surgical approach required, size of patient, fracture configuration, or other factors that can make these cases difficult to manage, becoming those nightmare cases that one can remember by the name of the dog or even the name of owner. These cases usually have a significantly higher complication rate, whether it is a higher percentage of fracture non-union, whether they require second or third revision surgeries, or whether simply, the functional outcome is not what one expected. The fractures discussed in this article include supracondylar and Y-T fractures of the humerus, highly comminuted fractures of the femur, infected or non-healed chronic fractures, and those previously treated by another surgeon. I am going to highlight those fractures that I consider more challenging and discuss how I handle those situations. It is not the purpose of this article to offer a comprehensive review of the different methods of fracture repair as there as several excellent textbooks that already cover those aspects.

SUPRACONDYLAR AND "Y-T" HUMERAL FRACTURES

Y and T fractures constitute a significant proportion of the distal humeral fractures seen in practice. These fractures are surgical challenges, the aims of the repair being accurate fracture reduction, rigid fixation, and early weight bearing to achieve a return to full function.

In a similar manner to fractures of the medial and lateral aspects of the humeral condyle, excessive shear forces transmitted through the condyle can result in a Y or T fracture. Minimal or substantial trauma is required. The overrepresentation of spaniels and the prodromal lameness reported in one case suggests that incomplete ossification of the humeral condyle (IOHC) plays a role in the pathogenesis in many cases.

Adequate exposure to achieve fracture reduction and satisfactory implant positioning of surgical implants is required to achieve a successful outcome.

Several approaches and methods of repair are described in the literature including a single medial approach, caudal approach via transolecranon osteotomy, caudal approach via triceps tenotomy, and combined lateral and medial approaches. A single medial or lateral approach has been reported as insufficient to accurately reduce the fracture fragments and achieve adequate rigid fixation. Complications using the transolecranon approach included implant failure, malunion, and sepsis.

The combined medial and lateral approach is used routinely in the author's practice. In a review of consecutive series of 30 dogs and 5 cats excellent results were obtained in the majority of cases, with fewer complications than previously reported series.

The sequence of fracture fixation and thus the order of the surgical approaches is dictated by the configuration of the fracture fragments and the surgeon's preference for medial or lateral fixation. It is often preferable to reduce and stabilise the major fragments, with the exception of the lateral aspect of the humeral condyle, via a medial approach prior to reducing and stabilising the lateral aspect of the humeral condyle via a lateral approach. In this scenario the patient is positioned in dorsolateral recumbency with the affected limb down and the contralateral limb secured caudally. To assist repositioning the dog intraoperatively the affected limb is freely draped and the pelvis supported in dorsal recumbency in a trough.

A similar approach is taken with dealing with supracondylar fractures of the humeral condyle, whenever possible, a bilateral approach and the used of combined medially and laterally applied plates is preferred, especially for the giant dogs. In severely comminuted cases or in small size animals (cats and dogs under 10 kg body weight), the use of external fixators is recommended, using a full pin across the humeral condyle and a half pin in the epicondylar region but below the fracture line and three half pins in the proximal aspect, all linked with a lateral connecting bar and an angled medial to lateral second connecting bar. Whenever possible, additional stability is recommended with the use of an intramedullary pin (tied-in to the ESF [external skeletal fixator]) or by first applying cross pins to cross the fracture line. Occasionally, in very challenging cases where bone size limits implant application, I have combined a medially applied plate with a modified type I laterally applied ESF with excellent functional results.

HIGHLY COMMINUTED FEMORAL FRACTURES

These fractures are the result of a high-energy impact and are by definition associated with great deal of local and systemic injury to the surrounding soft tissues, often resulting in prolonged healing times. Some bone fragments can be devitalized and in addition, the fracture configuration makes accurate reconstruction not a viable possibility without further compromising the local blood supply and increasing the risk of infection due to prolonged surgical times if primary (anatomical) reconstruction is attempted. Thus, several minimally invasive strategies have been devised to minimize those risks and ensure a successful outcome. Surgical techniques reported will include lengthening plates, external skeletal fixators (with or without a tied-in pin), interlocking nails and plate-rod constructs.

I routinely used plate-rod constructs in order to deal with these fractures in both dogs and cats. Biomechanical studies have shown that an intramedullary pin reduces plate strain dramatically and therefore the combined use of a plate-rod can reduced the risk of cyclic implant loading and failure, commonly seen with these fractures when other methods of repair are used, mainly due to the prolonged healing times.

A lateral standard approach the femur is performed, the skin incision extending from proximal to the greater trochanter to the distal aspect of the patella. Without disturbing the osseous fragments, the proximal and distal aspect of the fracture are located and grasp with bone holding forceps. A pin that approximately equals half of the medullary cavity at this point is introduced in a normograde or retrograde fashion into the proximal femur. The pin is then blunted and introduced in the distal fragment initially without attempting any reconstruction or lengthening of the fracture. An adequately size plate of the size of the animal is pre contoured based on radiographs of the contralateral limb, allowing hopefully three screws to be placed proximally and distally in the metaphyseal regions. The pin is then used to restore bone length and then the plate is secured using plate holding forceps whilst one screw is placed at either end. Careful manipulation prior to screw placement should ensure adequate joint alignment is restored prior to screw placing. The pins should be cut to length to avoid injuries to the sciatic nerve. The remaining of the proximal and distal screws are then placed (it is important to secure the IM pin in its final position prior to place the screws as they can locked the IM pin in a manner that further manipulations are not possible. Bicortical screws are preferred in all positions and thus, the drill bit should be directed to avoid hitting the IM whenever possible. There are occasions when this is not possible and monocortical screws are then used.

Clinical outcomes are usually excellent; however, one should be aware of the possibly high complication rate encountered when dealing with highly comminuted fractures of the femoral diaphysis in cats. In a retrospective study of 18 cats with femoral fractures presented at the BSAVA 2005 Spring meeting, short-term complications recorded in seven cases included loosening of one screw (1), plate loosening due to screw pull out proximally (1) or distally (1), improper intramedullary pin positioning (2), sciatic neuropathy (1), and marked rotation of the distal femur (1). This unexpected high incidence of complications was attributed to the fracture configuration (highly comminuted in the majority of cases).

CHRONIC NON-HEALED FRACTURES

There are occasions when one encounters an untreated fracture that has been present in the animal for a long period of time, ranging from weeks to months. Despite commonly accepted beliefs, these fractures do not often healed. Although each fracture will require an initial assessment based on the location, size of patient, time lapse since the injury and degree of secondary changes affecting the area, they all have some similarities. First, there is a marked degree of soft tissue contracture leading to an inevitable shortening of the limb. This contracture makes reduction, even if this was possible based on the original fracture configuration a surgical challenge and many times becomes an impossible task and therefore one should adopt a different strategy than that used for fresh fracture repairs. Second, there is almost invariably a marked degree of fibrous tissue surrounding the fracture fragments, that comes from that produced in the initial stages of the repair. This fibrous tissue is often deprived of a good blood supply and covers the end of the fracture fragments. Surgical exposure is obviously difficult by this fibrous tissue, in addition, it act as a barrier for bone formation to occur. Third, local bone remodeling at the fracture lines has inevitably occurred and therefore normal bone apposition cannot be achieved.

My approach to these fractures is to reduce those difficulties previously highlighted by a careful surgical dissection to the fracture site, peeling off the evolving, nonfunctional soft tissue fibrous envelope, removing a portion of the fracture ends in order to be able to reduce the fracture (even if this requires shortening of the limb by several centimeters) and then placing a bone plate, combined or not with an intramedullary pin. A cancellous bone graft is applied from a previously prepared site prior to wound closure. Following radiographic assessment and once we are happy the fracture is stable and rigidly repaired, I commence a fairly intensive rehabilitation program in order to restore limb function as soon as possible.

REFERENCES

1. Coughlan A, Miller A. Manual of Small Animal Fracture Repair and Management. BSAVA Publications, Cheltenham, UK, 1998.
2. Macias C, et al. Plate-rod repair of comminuted femoral fractures. A retrospective study in 18 cats. BSAVA Clinical Research Abstracts, 2005.

Additional references are available from the author upon request.

PHYSICAL THERAPY: MINIMIZING THE CONSEQUENCES OF OSTEOARTHRITIS

Denis J. Marcellin-Little, DEDV, Diplomate ACVS and ECVS, CCRP
College of Veterinary Medicine
North Carolina State University, Raleigh, NC

The management of osteoarthritis (OA) is a lifelong commitment for the owner and clinician managing the arthritic patient. Osteoarthritis slowly progresses over a lifetime. Its progression rate is highly variable and dependent on the joint affected, the cause of osteoarthritis, the initial management or lack thereof, and the patient size and conformation. Some arthritic joints cause immediate problems due to joint subluxation, effusion, and pain during manipulation (eg, elbow or hip dysplasia at 4 to 5 months of age, osteochondritis of the talus at 6 months of age). Other arthritic joints cause minimal discomfort until the latter years of life (eg, osteoarthritis in the shoulder joints). Weight control is one of the few aspects of the management of OA that has a profound impact on its progression rate. In a group of Labradors retrievers followed for their lifetime, the OA rate in joints of overweight dogs was 5 to 8 times larger than the OA rate of non-overweight Labrador retrievers. It is therefore critically important to keep the weight of arthritic patients as low as possible over their lifetime.

THE CONSEQUENCES OF OSTEOARTHRITIS

Osteoarthritis impacts the quality of life and mobility of dogs because of four consequences: 1) OA hurts, 2) OA leads to a loss of limb strength, 3) OA potentially leads to a loss of fitness, and 4) OA often leads to a loss of joint motion. OA pain is well recognized. It has peripheral and central components. Both components are effectively targeted with nonsteroidal anti-inflammatory drugs (NSAIDs). Other medications or supplements (eg, tramadol, amantadine, eicosapentaenoic acid, glucosamine sulfate) are being investigated that may provide additional pain relief in painful OA joints that may not receive complete relief with NSAID use. Many physical therapy strategies (icing, heat, massage, transcutaneous electrical nerve stimulation, exercise) are also aimed at providing pain relief in patients with OA pain. Also, physical therapy includes a component of ergonomics and ambulation assistance that helps controlling the pain originating in arthritic joints

The loss of muscle strength in limbs with OA is multifactorial. A reflex inhibition of muscle contraction occurs when muscle contractions lead to joint pain. Also, OA patients naturally decrease their activity and exercise levels, leading to a loss of muscle mass. Strengthening through exercise and possibly through electrical stimulation will be one of the strategies used to combat the consequences of OA In companion animals. Loss of muscular and cardiovascular fitness is a common feature in older OA patients. Positively impacting fitness will be one of the key goals of the OA management strategies presented below.

Loss of joint motion is a common feature of OA in companion animals. Unfortunately, little has been written on this important aspect of OA. It appears that joints respond quite variably to the present of OA and that the loss of joint motion occurs unevenly for each joint. Subjectively, I have the impression that a loss of joint motion is more likely to occur in tight, intricate joints (elbow, tarsus) compared with looser joints (shoulder joint). Loss of joint motion is also more likely to occur for joint positions that are not used during locomotion, compared to joint positions that are used during locomotion. For example, a Labrador retriever with elbow OA is more prone to lose elbow flexion than elbow extension and a Labrador retriever with hip dysplasia is more likely to lose hip extension than hip flexion (Table 1). To make things more complicated, the loss of motion present in an individual arthritic joint may or may not lead to a significant loss of limb use or create pain. As a general rule, the joint motions that are used repeatedly throughout the day—the motion necessary to walk and to perform routine activities of daily living—are more important than the joint motions not routinely used. For example, for the walk, each joint is used through a different portion of its range of motion at a walk (Table 1). Overall, the clinician will need to assess the motion

Joint	Range of Motion (max)*	Range of Motion (walk)	Anticipated Change with OA
Shoulder joint	57 – 165°	88 – 125°	Loss of flexion
Elbow joint	36 – 165°	91 – 146°	Loss of flexion
Carpal joint	32 – 196°	128 – 239°	Loss of flexion
Coxofemoral joint	50 – 162°	111 – 147°	Loss of extension
Stifle joint	42 – 162°	111 – 146°	Loss of extension
Tarsal joint	39 – 164°	111 – 145°	Loss of flexion

Table 1. Joint Motion and Osteoarthritis

* Range of motion expressed as flexion–extension in Labrador retrievers. Sources: Jaegger et al. and Feeney et al. Abbreviations: max, maximal range of motion; OA, osteoarthritis

present in all joints with the use of a plastic goniometer and may design a specific strategy to avoid painful joint positions and to promote joint stretching during exercises.

PATIENT ASSESSMENT

Practically, the clinician will gather information about the impact of OA on the patient's daily activity, quality of life, and about the consequences of OA on joint pain, limb strength, joint motion, and fitness. This is achieved by gathering a complete medical history, by observing the patient at rest, during transitions between rest and stance, at a walk and trot, and by palpating the patient.

Collecting a complete medical history will ensure that metabolic and other systemic problems that may negatively impact a patient's mobility are accounted for. Collecting a history of the severity and progression of clinical signs is important. The clinical signs of OA vary widely over time with periods of relative calm separated by periods of more intense pain, called flares or flare-ups. Flare may be the consequence of excessive exercise (the 'weekend warrior' syndrome) or excessive stress placed on an arthritic joint (eg, a dog with elbow dysplasia steps in a hole while jogging outdoors). In humans, flares may also be the consequence of rapid change in temperature or barometric pressure. Over time, flares tend to become more common and more severe. When evaluating an arthritic dog, it is important to appreciate whether the patient is within or between flares.

The owner may be asked to fill a client-specific outcome measure questionnaire. This questionnaire includes approximately five questions that are time and space specific that relate to the patient's function and daily activities. These questions should relate to an activity that the dog could do in earlier times, when OA did not impact the dog's function and quality of life. For example, one may choose a question like: "How does he climb the steps to our bedroom at night?" or "How enthusiastic is he when walking around our neighborhood park in the morning?" The performance during these five activities may be graded as 'impossible,' 'possible with great difficulties,' 'possible with slight difficulty,' or 'done without difficulty.' When the patient is reevaluated, the client will have access to identical questions (but not their original grading) and will grade the patient's performance similarly to the initial assessment. By comparing the grades given over time, the clinician may assess the changes in patient's performance for activities that require strength and/or endurance and therefore judge the effectiveness of the OA management program.

Functional and pain-related information may be collected by observing the patient in the waiting room, in the examination room, and by taking a brief walk outside. Joint pain may be detected by observing an abnormal limb position at a rest, such as a forelimb that is excessively flexed and externally rotated because of pain perceived in the elbow joint or a pelvic limb that is excessively extended because of pain perceived in the stifle joint. Weight shifts at a stance should also be recorded; dogs with pain in one limb will shift weight away from that limb. Dogs with pain in both forelimbs or both pelvic limbs (or lower back) will shift weight back or forward, respectively. Weight shifts should also be recorded at a walk and trot. Weight shifts tend to be more significant when the patient is standing and walking slowly. At faster gaits, dogs do not have time to effectively shift weight. A dog's willingness and ability to trot should be assessed. Dogs with severe joint pain and dogs with severe loss of strength or fitness may not trot.

Palpation should include the neck, back, and limbs. It should be initiated while the dog is standing, with the clinician behind the patient. By running both hands simultaneously on the left and right sides of the patient, one can perceive differences in muscle mass, weight shifts, and tight muscles. The neck may be gently manipulated. Gentle finger pressure may be placed on or next to the dorsal spinous processes to detect spinal pain. Conscious proprioception and hopping may be tested at that time to make sure that the patient has appropriate postural reactions. If ataxia or a foot drop (dragging toes on the ground) was noted during gait observation or if the postural reactions are slow or asymmetric, a complete neurologic examination should be performed. While severe OA, a heavy weight, and older age may negatively impact the speed of a patient's postural reaction, they usually do not lead to clear ataxia. Palpation is continued with the patient in lateral recumbency. We prefer performing this palpation on a large 2-inch-thick (5-cm-thick) gymnastic mat. This is done awake for most patients. Aggressive, over-excitable, or poorly socialized dogs may be sedated. Performing palpation under sedation will decrease the clinician's ability to detect joint pain. The palpation focuses on the carpus, elbow, shoulder, tarsus, stifle and hip joint. For each of these 12 joints, crepitus, effusion, pain response during palpation, flexion, and extension are recorded. We prefer having a dedicated person who records this information as the patient is rapidly palpated. The clinician may report the findings as mild (1 out of 3), moderate (2/3), or severe (3/3). Mild crepitus represents barely detectable but repeatable roughness during joint motion, severe crepitus is a clear and unequivocal roughness during joint motion. Moderate crepitus is between mild and severe. Mild effusion is a barely detectable joint swelling, severe effusion is a clear and unequivocal swelling, primarily seen in early elbow dysplasia, osteochondritis dissecans, or acute damage to the cranial cruciate ligament. A mild pain response is a discreet objection to joint palpation such a repeatable movement of a rear foot during forelimb palpation or a change in breathing pattern or facial expression. Severe pain response is the presence of distress clearly associated with a specific joint position. Not all joint positions are equally painful in OA. For example pain response to palpation of a dysplastic hip joint is most likely to occur during extension, then during abduction, then during external rotation. By comparison, pain response during flexion of a dysplastic hip joint is very unusual. The information recorded about each joint may resemble the following: 39-154, C1 ext, E2, P3 ext. This information means that the joint has 39° of flexion, 154° of extension (measured with a goniometer). The mid-thigh circumference (girth) is assessed for both pelvic limbs. The circumference of other regions (ie, mid-crus, antebrachium, waist) may also be recorded if deemed necessary.

OA TREATMENT OPTIONS

Numerous treatment options have been proposed for the management OA in people and in dogs. Some options are 'passive' and do not require the patient's participation; other options are 'active.' Passive options include electrophysical modalities (ice, heat, sensory or motor electrical stimulation, electro-acupuncture) and manual therapy (massage, stretching, joint mobilization, acupressure). Cold therapy is achieved with a cold pack or gel pack placed directly on the skin. Superficial joints are effectively cooled in 10 to 15 minutes. Cold therapy is recommended when patients have flares or to cool joints after an exercise session. Low-level heat (ie, elevating tissue temperature by 1 to 2°C) is used in OA patients to increase the relaxation of tight muscle groups. This may be done with a microwaveable moist heat pack or a heating pad or bed. More vigorous heating (ie, elevating tissue temperature by 3 to 4°C) is used before and during stretching sessions. This is most often done under the supervision of a clinician but may be done by some owners after proper training. Trancutaneous electrical nerve stimulation (TENS) has been used in people to alleviate OA pain. TENS units are little device that deliver a low-intensity electrical current perceived as a tingling sensation. The current is delivered to affected areas using electrodes stuck on the skin. The optimal treatment time in people with OA pain is 40 minutes. While little is know about the use of TENS units in dogs with OA pain, the devices have proven efficacy in people. Neuromuscular electrical stimulation (NMES) has been used to strengthen muscles in limbs with severe OA. NMES relies on electrodes that are place across muscle groups (eg, hamstrings, quadriceps, antebrachial flexor or extensor muscles). NMES is to be considered when patients cannot perform therapeutic exercises because of the severity of their disease or other factors. TENS and NMES unfortunately require clipping to ensure proper electrical conduction.

Stretching may be critically important for patients with loss of range of motion. If proper limb use is present during specific exercises, these exercises may be used to stretch joints. Further stretching may be accomplished manually, in pre-heated joints. Little has been published regarding the optimal parameters of stretching programs in OA patients. Some suggest having stretching sessions with stretches sustained for 20 to 40 seconds repeated 10 to 15 times. Stretching sessions may be repeated several times daily, as needed. The anticipated gain in joint motion resulting from a stretching program is 3° to 5° per week. Joint mobilization, a specific low-velocity manual therapy used by physical therapists, has been shown to provide pain relief in OA joint in people, but not in dogs.

Therapeutic exercises are the cornerstone of the management of OA in companion animals. Exercises are in most cases active treatment options that require participation of the patient. The exercises should therefore be carefully chosen and introduced. Exercises achieve multiple goals: strengthening, stretching, increasing muscle and cardiovascular fitness, increasing proprioception, losing weight, and providing pain relief. Initiating the exercise program in the clinic with outpatient visits may be beneficial for dogs with severe OA or with lack of socialization or training. The fundamental exercise is a walk. Walking may be performed in many different ways in OA patients to achieve specific goals. The speed of the walk should be carefully chosen to make sure that the affected limbs are used well throughout the exercise session. Surprisingly, many owners do not appreciate the benefits of a leash walk or have not trained their dogs to be controlled during a walk. It may be beneficial to have a dedicated staff member fit the dog with a chest harness or other restraint device and to train the dog to walk at an even pace before the owner is asked to take these walks. Leash walk may be adapted to achieve further goals. Choosing a soft surface with good traction may be important. Speed should be adjusted over time as the dog's comfort, strength, and endurance increase. A speed that allows proper posture and limb use should be chosen. The duration of a walk is often dependent on owners' schedule and fitness goals. It is important, however, to walk for more than 10 minutes because that is the theoretically the shortest duration that allows muscle strengthening. Aquatic therapy should be considered in dogs with severe impairment that cannot be exercised effectively on land. While the primary goals of exercise are muscle strengthening, the relief of joint pain, and an increase in cardiovascular fitness, exercises may be used for stretching purposes. Climbing hills may be chosen to strengthen pelvic limbs and increase stifle and hip extension during exercise. Exercise may also be used to restore normal posture and increase proprioception. Exercises designed for these purposes promote slow and purposeful limb motion (eg, Cavaletti rails) and include rapid weigh shifts (eg, wobble or balance board, trampoline, walking on soft and uneven surfaces).

In people, arthritic joints and joints recovering from surgery or injury are often protected during exercise. Braces may be made of elastic tape, neoprene, or have a hinged metal frame. Protective braces for dogs are available but they tend to be cumbersome to use and have no proven efficacy at this point. It is very important to provide ambulation assistance to the most severely impaired patients because older dogs may be euthanatized after an OA flare limits their locomotion. Slings or even carts may be used to provide ambulation assistance to these severely affected OA patients. Aquatic exercises may greatly increase their comfort during exercise and may be used for a few weeks while the patients conditioning and limb strength increase and while their weight is managed, if deemed necessary. It may be acceptable to hospitalize a large, nonambulatory patient for a couple of weeks to allow him to have brief exercise sessions several times daily in a controlled environment and under specialized supervision. Adapting the home environment of patients with severe OA is recommended. Dogs with limited mobility should have easy access to water and food, possibly by using elevated bowls. A ramp may be used to facilitate ingress and egress from the house. Allowing dogs to sleep in a temperature controlled environment may limit OA flare, based on information available from people with OA.

Over time, the OA management program evolves based on the needs of the patient. Pharmacological (NSAID, supplements) and nonpharmacological (ice) pain management continues as needed. The weight and body condition are assessed regularly. Passive OA management measures and aquatic therapy are progressively discontinued as the patient becomes more independent. Home-based exercises increase and are sustained over time. Mildly affected patients with home-based exercise programs (aimed at maintaining muscle mass) may be reevaluated twice a year. Severely affected patients and patient with challenging exercise programs (aimed at increasing strength, stretching, eliminating weight shifts) or weight management programs should be check more regularly weekly or twice monthly. The success of an OA management program comes from having educated and dedicated owners having a strong bond with clinicians. The program should have medical, nutritional, environmental, and physical therapy aspects that are sustained and modified over time.

REFERENCES

1. Kealy RD, Lawler DF, Monti KL, et al. Effects of dietary electrolyte balance on subluxation of the femoral head in growing dogs. Am J Vet Res. 1993; 54:555-562.
2. Smith GK, Paster ER, Powers MY, et al. Lifelong diet restriction and radiographic evidence of osteoarthritis of the hip joint in dogs. J Am Vet Med Assoc. 2006; 229:690-693.
3. Ryan WG, Moldave K, Carithers D. Clinical effectiveness and safety of a new NSAID, firocoxib: a 1,000 dog study. Vet Therap. 2006; 7:119-126.
4. Jaegger G, Marcellin-Little DJ, Levine D. Reliability of goniometry in Labrador Retrievers. Am J Vet Res. 2002; 63:979-986.
5. Thomas TM, Marcellin-Little DJ, Roe SC, et al. Comparison of measurements obtained by use of an electrogoniometer and a universal plastic goniometer for the assessment of joint motion in dogs. Am J Vet Res. 2006; 67:1974-1979.

CURRENT CONCEPTS OF VETERINARY JOINT PRESERVATION THERAPY — USE IN CLINICAL CASES, POST-SURGICALLY, AND REHABILITATION THERAPY

Darryl Millis, MS, DVM, Diplomate ACVS, CCRP
College of Veterinary Medicine
University of Tennessee, Knoxville, TN

There has been much interest in treating joint disease in dogs, especially conditions that result in osteoarthritis (OA). OA is a progressive degenerative condition that affects synovial joints. Although it is traditionally considered a condition of articular cartilage, multiple structures and tissues are involved. OA may be thought of as a disease of an organ, affecting not only cartilage, but also bone, ligaments, tendons, muscles, joint capsule, blood vessels, and nerves. Patients with OA have restricted activity, limited ability to perform, muscle atrophy, pain and discomfort, decreased range of motion (ROM) and decreased quality of life.

As animals reduce their activity level, a vicious cycle of decreased flexibility, joint stiffness, and loss of strength occurs. There is increasing emphasis on early treatment of joint conditions because biochemical and biomechanical changes occur in cartilage before radiographic or gross changes occur in affected joints. By the time there is radiographic evidence of OA (subchondral sclerosis, osteophyte development, joint effusion); there is permanent damage to the articular cartilage. Therefore, if the disease process is to be attenuated, early treatment must be administered to help preserve as much normal cartilage as possible.

Disease-modifying osteoarthritis drugs (DMOADs) are thought to provide a healthy environment for cartilage and perhaps alter deleterious changes to it. The use of these agents may be considered in patients with existing OA and in patients following joint surgery and then rehabilitation from the injury. In addition, it is important to consider other treatments for joint preservation, including weight control, a therapeutic exercise program, and anti-inflammatory drugs. Unfortunately, nonsteroidal anti-inflammatory drugs (NSAIDs), which block cyclo-oxygenase enzymes, provide symptomatic relief but do not reverse the underlying disease process. Cartilage destruction can proceed unabated despite suppression of inflammation. Nevertheless, NSAIDs provide a valuable function in helping to relieve pain and inflammation, and may assist with weight loss and exercise.

Other forms of treatment include corrective osteotomies, modulation of biological processes, and cartilage grafting. The need for alternative modalities has encouraged the use of nutraceuticals and non-pharmacological agents for the management of veterinary joint disease. Such agents include glucosamine (Glu), chondroitin sulfate (CS), avocado-soybean unsaponifiables (ASU), and polysulfated glycosaminoglycans.

GLUCOSAMINE AND CHONDROITIN SULFATE

Glucosamine is a naturally occurring aminomonosaccharide in the body and is one of the principal substrates used in the synthesis of glycosaminoglycans, proteoglycans, and hyaluronan, all of which are components of articular cartilage. It has been shown to minimize deleterious subchondral bone change during the development of OA in a rabbit cruciate ligament transaction model. Glu administered early in the disease process suggested a preventive effect.

Chondroitin sulfate is a glycosaminoglycan found in the matrix of articular cartilage and was one of the first molecules to show a possible positive effect on chondrocytes. Chondroitin sulfate also improves chondrocyte repair in different experimental animal models of OA. The combination of Glu and CS has more dramatic effect than each agent alone. In a canine cranial cruciate ligament transection model with subsequent stifle stabilization, dogs treated with Glu and CS for 5 months had fewer clinical signs of OA and less periarticular fibrosis than controls. Furthermore, treated dogs had fewer histologic OA changes.

AVOCADO-SOYBEAN UNSAPONIFIABLES

Administration of ASU in a sheep meniscectomy model of OA and in human OA of the hip yielded clinical benefits. Moreover, data suggest that ASU may have DMOAD-like effects in the joint. Recent studies also indicated that ASU stimulated the production of transforming growth factor β-1 and -2 in joints of dogs, which may lead to production of cartilage matrix components.

POLYSULFATED GLYCOSAMINOGLYCAN

Polysulfated glycosaminoglycan (PSGAG) is a polysulfated chondroitin sulfate (ie, it has a higher sulfur content compared with chondroitin sulfate). It improves hyaluronan synthesis in human joints. This drug is anti-inflammatory and inhibits enzymes that degrade glycosaminoglycans (GAGs) and hyaluronic acid (HA) within the joint. It has a positive effect on HA and GAG synthesis in diseased joints. It is an FDA-approved drug, licensed as a disease-modifying osteoarthritis drug (DMOAD). PSGAG increases concentrations of synovial fluid HA, and inhibits metalloproteinases, complement activation, enzyme release from leukocytes, PGE-2, and toxic oxygen radical synthesis.

Support for the efficacy of PSGAG as a treatment for canine osteoarthritis was evaluated using a Pond-Nuki dog model. Treated dogs received 4 mg/kg PSGAG twice weekly for 4 weeks. The mean histologic scores of the operated control joints were significantly worse than in the operated PSGAG-treated joints. Total metalloproteinase activity in the operated PSGAG-treated joints was suppressed compared with the operated control joints. Similar results have been obtained in our laboratory.

PHYSICAL REHABILITATION MODALITIES

It is generally believed that mild to moderate exercise

and training in normal humans and dogs do not cause OA by themselves, but biochemical, histologic, and biomechanical changes do occur in articular cartilage. Most studies of moderate running exercise have indicated that this activity produces no injury to articular cartilage, assuming that there are no abnormal biomechanical stresses acting on the joints. Heavy training programs, however, may result in changes which predispose to the development of OA. The benefits of controlled exercise for patients with OA are also valuable but underutilized.

An exercise program must be tailored for the condition of each animal patient and to each owner. An improper program could hasten the progression of OA. Overloading joints should be minimized by performing activities such as walking and swimming until weight loss occurs. Unrealistic demands placed on the owner will likely decrease compliance, so it is important to consider the physical condition of the owner. Joint instability should be corrected before initiating an exercise program. Exercise programs must be tailored to account for the typical course of exacerbations and remissions of OA. The animal should not be forced to exercise during times of aggravation because inflammation may increase. In preparation for exercising, warming and stretching affected muscle groups and joints during a "warm-up" period is recommended. Tissue warming promotes blood flow to the area, promotes tissue and collagen extensibility, and decreases pain, muscle spasms and joint stiffness. Heat is contraindicated if swelling or edemas are present in the limb or joint. Heating agents such as moist or dry hot packs, circulating warm water blankets and warm baths typically heat the skin and subcutaneous tissues to a depth of 1 to 2 cm. Another physical agent used for heating is therapeutic ultrasound (US). Ultrasound frequencies of 1 and 3 MHz in continuous mode produce thermal and non-thermal effects. The effects are related to the treatment time, intensity, frequency, and area being treated. Tissue heating may penetrate up to 5 cm, much deeper than with superficial heating modalities. Non-thermal effects include increased cell membrane permeability, calcium transport across the cell membrane, removal of proteins and blood cells from the interstitial spaces, and nutrient exchange. Any stretching should be done during the latter part of warming or immediately after. Massage has been used to increase blood flow to muscles to "warm up" the area before activity, and to decrease stiffness after activity.

Controlled leash walking, walking on a treadmill, jogging, swimming, and going up and downstairs or ramp inclines, are excellent low-impact exercises. The length of the exercise should be titrated so there is no increased pain after activity. Also, it is better in the early phases of training to provide three 20-minute sessions than one 60-minute session. Walks should be brisk and purposeful, minimizing stopping. Avoiding sudden bursts of activity will help avoid acute inflammation of arthritic joints.

Swimming and walking in water are some of the best activities for dogs. The bouyancy of water is significant and limits the impact on the joint while promoting muscle strength and tone, and joint motion. Training in an underwater treadmill may increase peak weight bearing forces by 5% to 15%, which is comparable to achievements obtained using medication in many patients.

If joint pain is perceived to be greater after exercising, the length of the activity should be decreased by half. When stepping up the amount of activity, the increase should be approximately 20% and should not be stepped more than once each week. Ideally, anti-inflammatory drugs should not be administered immediately prior to stepping up activity because it is important to determine if the level of exercise is too great and causes pain. The exercise periods should be evenly spaced throughout each day and over the entire week. Training helps maintain an ideal body weight, improves ROM, and increases muscle strength and tone, which helps to stabilize joints.

Following exercise, a 10-minute warm down period allows muscles to cool down. A slower paced walk may be initiated for 5 minutes, followed by ROM and stretching exercises. A cool down massage may help decrease pain, swelling, and muscle spasms. Finally, cryotherapy (cold packs or ice wrapped in a towel) may be applied to painful areas for 15 to 20 minutes to control post-exercise inflammation. Application of cold packs decreases blood flow, inflammation, hemorrhage and metabolic rate.

OBESITY

Obesity is strongly associated with the development of OA in people and likely contributes to the progression of OA in dogs. For example, heavy people are 3.5 times more likely to develop OA than light people, and loss of 5 kg decreases the odds of developing OA by over 50%. Additionally, weight loss results in less joint pain and a decreased need for medication to treat OA. Weight reduction of 11% to 18% of the initial body weight of obese dogs resulted in significantly improved hind limb lameness associated with hip osteoarthritis in one study. In addition to restricting intake of the normal diet and eliminating treats, prescription diets are available that can dramatically assist in achieving and maintaining ideal body weight. In general, a goal is to reduce fat composition to 20% to 25% of an animal's total body weight. Clinically, the ribs should be easily palpable and there should be a "waist" when the animal is viewed from above.

NEW POTENTIAL TREATMENTS FOR IMPROVING JOINT HEALTH

Interleukin-1 receptor antagonist (IRAP) has been successfully used in horses with OA. The principle is to block the downstream biochemical events associated with IL-1 stimulation, and thereby alter the pathophysiological events associated with OA by competitively inhibiting the binding of IL-1. Gene therapy to promote the incorporation of anabolic genes, such as those that contribute to IGF-1 production, are being evaluated experimentally using viral vectors as a means to deliver genes to target joints. Stem cell therapy has recently become available for canine and equine use and utilizes adipose-derived mesenchymal stem cells to alter cell-to-cell signaling in the joint and reduce inflammation. Corrective osteotomies, such as sliding humeral osteotomy, are being developed to alter loading patterns in affected joints. Cartilage transplant procedures, such as osteochondral transplant have been used in people, horses, and dogs to provide articular cartilage to areas with severe cartilage erosion.

SUMMARY

Osteoarthritis is a common problem in dogs, and a great deal of effort and study has been devoted to preservation of articular cartilage following joint injury. Veterinarians are approached frequently to treat arthritic patients. Management of the arthritic patient involves a number of modalities and must be tailored to each patient and their owner. The main components for OA management are weight control, physical rehabilitation, medication, and also agents that maybe DMOADs. Cooperation among the veterinarian, therapist, veterinary technician, and owner are vital to carry out an appropriate management program. Regular monitoring of achievements is essential to help with decision-making for further treatment.

EXERCISE IN ARTHRITIS: CAUSE AND EFFECT?

Claude T. Moorman, III, MD
Duke University Medical Center
Durham, NC

There has been a considerable body of evidence to suggest the tremendous benefit of exercise on positively impacting mortality and quality of life (Figure 1). Blair et al have suggested cardiovascular mortality is inversely related to fitness. In Figure 1, both men and women who were in a high fitness group had significantly lower mortalities than those in a medium or low fitness category (Figure 1). We also know that fitness does not directly correlate with body composition (Figure 2). Lee et al have determined that even patients with a body fat percentage over 25% can have a lower mortality rate than patients under 16% provided that they are able to maintain their fitness profile as demonstrated on a maximal exercise test on a treadmill (Figure 2). In other words, it is possible to be fit but fat! This article will focus on the benefit of exercise on mortality as demonstrated in the recent literature. We will also focus on the effect of exercise on joint loading and arthritic progression. Finally, we will conclude with some emerging data related to low-impact exercise with the goal of better understanding how to educate our patients on the benefits of exercise in an environment that is joint preserving.

The health benefits of exercise have been recently analyzed in a meta-analysis looking at the effects of exercise on lipid profiles, which demonstrated an increase of 5% in the HDL, a 5% decrease of LDL, and a 3.7% decrease in triglycerides. There have been recent studies to demonstrate that there are further improvements in obesity, cardiovascular disease, diabetes, but also significant reductions in stress, improvement in depression, and improvement in the overall quality of life. Fortunately, the majority of Americans are well versed in the benefits of exercise and this has trickled down into common knowledge.

There has been more controversy and conflicting information related to the effect of exercise in causing and worsening preexisting arthritic conditions. A review of the literature suggests that in the absence of deformity and injury that exercise is not related to causing or worsening arthritis.[3,4] There is an evolving body of evidence that perhaps muscle dysfunction may be a more important factor in the development of osteoarthritis than joint loading.[3,4] It has also been shown that in women with isolated knee arthritis quadriceps weakness was present even where patients did not have pain, which may suggest that the quadriceps weakness actually precedes and may be more of the cause of arthritis than the joint destruction.

There has been an increased association with participation in power lifting and in soccer related to age match sedentary controls.[7] It has been felt that this is related to injury in the soccer players and a higher BMI in the weight lifters. In groups of runners and track and field athletes, there has not been any related increased risk of arthritic progression versus a control group. These findings suggest that injury is much more associated with arthritic development than exercise.

Among patients with preexisting arthritis, several studies have been performed to determine if this is worsened by continuing. Several systematic reviews have demonstrated that exercise is an effective therapy for patients with osteoarthritis of the hip and knee.[9,10] This would indicate that patients with preexisting osteoarthritis stand to benefit from continuing on with exercise in spite of the fact that they have joint damage.

A more difficult proposition has been to determine what exercises to recommend for patients with preexisting arthritis or those who are concerned with joint preservation. Recent efforts in the K-Lab at Duke University have focused on exercises to try to diminish joint reactive force while continuing to successfully activate muscle groups working towards an improvement in lean body mass. Principles of adherence to a low impact program of relatively high repetitions with low

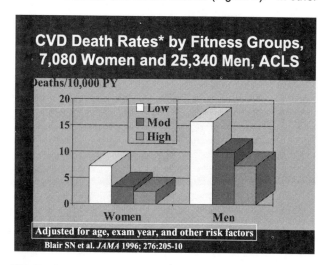

Figure 1.

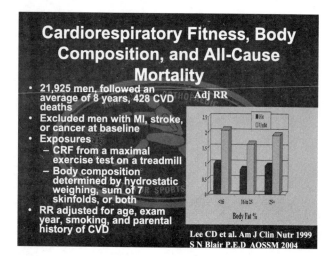

Figure 2.

weight have been a major component of this program. Additionally, a focus on close kinetic chain exercises for lower extremity and avoidance of extreme maneuvers in the upper extremity have been quite helpful. Finally, a core strengthening program which is sensitive to torques and bending moments on the lumbar sacral disc spaces has also been successful.

In summary, the benefits of exercise on overall cardiovascular, mental health, and mortality have been well documented. The more controversial areas of cause and effect as it relates to exercise and joint degeneration have suggested that the benefits of exercise programs far outweigh the risks. Muscle imbalances, joint mal alignment, and injury are the factors much more likely to predispose to or aggravate preexisting osteoarthritis. An approach to low impact weightlifting can help patients to achieve the goals of maintaining lean body mass, decreasing mortality, and increasing their quality of life.

REFERENCES

1. Leon AS, Sanchez OA. Response of blood lipids to exercise training alone or combined with dietary intervention. Med Sci Sports Exerc. 2001;44:S502-S515.
2. Paluska SA, Schwenk, TL. Physical Activity in Mental Health: Current Concepts. Sports Med. 2000; 29:167-180.
3. Hurley MV. The role of muscle weakness in the pathogenesis of osteaoarthritis. Rheum Dis Clin North Am. 1999;25(2):283-298.
4. Shrier I. Muscle dysfunction versus wear and tear as a cause of exercise-related osteoarthritis: An epidemiological update. Br J Sports Med. 2004;38(5):525-535.
5. Larsen MW, Kirkendall D, Garrett, WE. The relationship between exercise and osteoarthritis, unpublished manuscript, 2007.
6. Slemenda C, Brandt KD, Leilman DK, Mazzuca S, Braunstein EM, Katz BP, Wolinsky FD. Quadriceps weakness and osteoarthritis of the knee. Ann Intern Med. 1997;127:97-104.
7. Kujala UM, Kettunen J, Paananen H, et al. Knee osteoarthritis in former runners, soccer players, weight lifters, and shooters. Arthritis Rheum. 1995;38:539-46.
8. Kettunen JA, Kujala UM, Daprio J, et al. Lower-limb function among former elite male athletes. Am J Sports Med. 2001;29:2-8.
9. Roddy E, Zhang W, Doherty M, Arden NK, Barlow J, et al. Evidence-based recommendations for the role of exercise in the management of osteoarthritis of the hip or knee – the MOVE consensus. Rheumatology. 2005;44:67-73.
10. Jordan KM, Arden NK, Doherty M et al. EULAR recommendations 2003: An evidence-based approach to the management of knee osteoarthritis: report of a task force of the Standing Committee for International Clinical Studies Including Therapeutic Trials (ESCISIT). Ann Rheum Dis. 2003;62:1145-55.

WHERE CAN I SAFELY USE INTRAMEDULLARY PIN AND WIRE FIXATION?

Ross H. Palmer, DVM, MS, Diplomate ACVS
College of Veterinary Medicine & Biomedical Sciences
Colorado State University, Fort Collins, CO

The use of intramedullary (IM) pins and wires in the treatment of small animal fractures was first described in the 1940s. Use of IM pins and wires was the mainstay of small animal orthopedics for many years due in large part to their low cost, surgical ease/speed, and the minimal equipment investment needed. Today, IM pins and wires are probably both the most commonly used and mis-used fixation system available. IM pins and wires can be used to satisfy the goal of complete restoration of locomotor function, provided proper technique is used and the system's limitations are heeded. Limitations include the inability of IM pins to adequately control most disruptive forces acting on fractures. Failure to recognize these biomechanical limitations often leads to major postoperative complications.

PREOPERATIVE ASSESSMENT

Failure to recognize when not to use IM pin and wire fixation is the root cause of more complications than not knowing how to perform the techniques. Knowing when you can safely perform IM pin and wire fixation is the key to achieving consistent and predictable success with the modality. Probably the most common error is attempting to use IM pin and wire fixation in fractures where perfect anatomic reconstruction is not feasible. Perfect anatomic reconstruction of the bony column is required for safe use of IM pins and wire. Therefore, IM pin and wire fixation should only be considered for long oblique/spiral, reconstructable fracture configurations. Comminuted fractures with multiple, particularly small, butterfly fragments are prone to failure with IM pin and wire fixation.

Recognition of the proper fracture configurations in which to apply IM pin and wire fixation is only part of the challenge. Another common error with IM pin and wire fixation is failure to recognize that it is a relatively "weak" modality and that makes it a relatively "short term" fixation. That is to say, IM pin and wire fixation can only withstand relatively small loads and for a relatively short period of time. Thus, IM pin and wire fixation should typically be reserved for relatively "simple" scenarios such as a young, healthy animal with reasonable soft tissue health and three functional limbs. Conversely, IM pin and wire fixation should be avoided when mature patient age, questionable systemic/nutritional health, or extensive regional soft tissue injury suggest slow fracture healing is likely. Likewise, IM pin and wire fixation is best avoided when overload of the fixation is likely whether due to patient temperament, anticipated owner non-compliance, or mult-limb disability.

Preoperative IM Pin and Wire Checklist:
- Perfect anatomic reconstruction of a long oblique or spiral fracture can be achieved.
- Rapid fracture healing is very likely.
- The "other three limbs" are fully functional.
- Good owner/pet compliance is anticipated.

BASIC PINNING PRINCIPLES
Pin Insertion

IM pins can be inserted with a hand chuck or power drill. Care should be taken with hand chuck insertion to avoid creating an enlarged pin tract by wobbling the chuck during insertion. This may be less of a problem when the pin is first inserted through the fracture line (retrograde pinning) because the intramedullary canal "guides" the pin. However, this same "guiding effect" exerted by the intramedullary canal will influence where the pin exits the end of the bone. When using a power drill for insertion, slow speeds (<150 rpm) should be used to minimize the risk of excess heat buildup and resultant pin loosening due to thermal necrosis.

IM pins can be placed using either retrograde or normograde insertion techniques. *Normograde* technique is the insertion of the pin into either the proximal or the distal end of the bone, advancing it through the fracture zone and seating it into the cancellous bone at the opposite end. *Retrograde* technique is the insertion of the pin through the fracture zone, directly into the intramedullary canal of either the proximal or distal main bone segment. The retrograded pin is then advanced proximally or distal until the pin exits the end of the bone. The fracture is then reduced as the pin is advanced in the opposite direction across the fracture zone and seated into the cancellous bone at the opposite end of the bone. Retrograde insertion is easier to perform but may be more disruptive to the fracture zone. Retrograde insertion also allows less accurate control of the exit point of the pin from the bone which can result in damage to joint surfaces, nerves, or other soft tissue structures.

Pin Size

The size of the intramedullary pin selected has significant influence on the stability imparted. In theory, completely filling the intramedullary canal would offer at least three-point fixation (entrance point, endosteal contact at the isthmus, and pin seating point) and would allow use of maximal pin diameter. The resistance of a pin to bending is proportional to its radius raised to the 4th power. However, because bones are not perfectly cylindrical in shape, complete filling of the intramedullary canal and meaningful endosteal contact is difficult to accomplish without reaming the endosteal surface (which is not feasible in small animals due to the relatively thin cortical bone). Further, complete filling of the canal could disrupt the endosteal blood supply. In small animal practice, pins that occupy 60% to 75% of the intramedullary canal at the isthmus are typically selected. In these situations, two-point fixation (entrance point and seating point) is more accurately what occurs. In reconstructed fractures, these pins offer significant resistance to bending, but minimal resistance to rotational, tensile or shear forces acting upon the fracture. As a result, pin fixation as the primary stabilizer is most often performed in conjunction with supplemental cerclage wiring. Pins are also often used as the secondary stabilizer in conjunction with external skeletal fixation or bone plate fixation. Because of the inability of IM pins to significantly resist any forces other than bending, IM pins should not be used without appropriate supplemental fixation if rotational, shear, or tensile forces are anticipated to act upon the fracture zone during the healing period. Much discussion is given to interdigitation of fractured bone ends resisting rotation, but in reality this interdigitation is only able to resist rotation in the smallest of patients (example: some little < 2- to 3-pound kittens and puppies). Larger-sized animals generate too much rotational force at the fracture line to be resisted by bony interdigitation. Older animals do not heal generate callus quickly enough to support the fixation against the cyclic stresses of weight-bearing.

Supplemental Wire

Cerclage or hemi-cerclage wire is a supplemental fixation technique and should never be used as a primary method of fixation. Orthopedic wire is made from 316L stainless steel and readily available in 16, 18, 20 and 22 gauge; 18- and 20-gauge wires are the most frequently used in small animal orthopedics. Cerclage wires completely encircle the circumference of the bone and are most effectively used as supplemental fixation of long spiral or oblique fractures. Cerclage wires have also been used to reconstruct the bony column out of multiple bone fragments so that primary fixation can be applied; however, this is a common cause of fixation failure. When preoperative assessment has classified a fracture as "non-reconstructable" cerclage wires should not be used for fracture stabilization, but can be used to prevent propagation of fissures within a main bone segment.

Cerclage Wire Instrumentation and Application

Orthopedic wire is available on a spool or in individual preformed loops ("eyelet wires"). Either way, the wire is passed around the bone being careful not to entrap any soft tissue. A wire passer helps with safe passage of the wire. Spool wire is cut to the desired length and then secured by twisting the wire ends with pliers, needle holders or special twisting instruments. Firm, sustained even tension on the two wire ends during twisting ensures proper intertwining of the two wire ends rather than the twisting of one wire end around the circumference of the other. It is preferable not to bend the twist knot over because this causes a 30% loss of wire tension, but proximity of the protruding wire to neurovascular structures must be considered. The wire is usually cut at the 3rd or 4th twist. Preformed, or eyelet wires, are placed around the bone, then tightened and bent down flush with the bone surface using a special tightening instrument. Eyelet wires are simpler to properly tighten and have a lower profile into the surrounding soft tissues, but require a dedicated tightening instrument. Either twist knot or eyelet wires can be used with good clinical results if properly performed when indicated. Twist knotted wires provide greater resistance to knot failure than single-loop knotted eyelet wires, but final wire tension (thus compression) on the bone is greater with loop-knotted wire. A double-loop knotted wire provides greater final wire tension AND resistance to knot failure, but requires a dedicated tightening instrument.

Properly tightened and applied cerclage wires do not interfere with the blood supply to the underlying cortical bone. Likewise, cerclage wires can be placed around immature bone without disrupting bone growth. However, loose wires shift back and forth along the cortical bone and disrupt blood supply by shearing off developing periosteal vessels and compromising blood flow through the bony cortex.

Basic Principles of Cerclage Wiring for Fracture Stabilization

- Cerclage wires should only be used to stabilize *reconstructable* fractures (long oblique, long spiral, or single large butterfly fragment).
- Cerclage wires should only be used if the full cylinder of bone can be anatomically reconstructed. Wires should not be used if the bone is not cylindrical in shape.
- Sufficient strength wire should be used – 18- or 20-gauge most commonly; 22-gauge wire is only used for small puppies and kittens. Braided wire is never used.
- Wires should be placed ~ 0.5 bone diameter from the fragment ends and spaced ~ 1 bone diameter apart from one another.
- Minimum number of cerclage wires for fracture stabilization is 2.*
- Oblique fracture line length must be at least twice the diameter of the bone.
- On conical or tapered portions of the bone, wires should be secured by notching the cortex or by placing a small K-wire to prevent slipping of the cerclage wire down the bone.
- ALL wires should be tested and tight before closure.
- Wires should be perpendicular to the long axis of the bone.

SUMMARY

The primary goal of fracture fixation is complete restoration of locomotor function. When pin and wire fixation is applied using proper surgical techniques to appropriate fracture patients, this goal can be consistently realized. However, pin and wire fixation improperly applied or applied to inappropriate fracture patients is a leading cause of complications and patient morbidity in small animal orthopedics.

---

*Single cerclage wires can be used to prevent propagation of fissures in main fracture segments.

WHAT'S THE LATEST, GREATEST, AND HOTTEST TOPIC IN BONE PLATE FIXATION?

Ross H. Palmer, DVM, MS, Diplomate ACVS
College of Veterinary Medicine & Biomedical Sciences
Colorado State University, Fort Collins, CO

CONVENTIONAL BONE PLATING

Fracture healing requires that the fracture zone have adequate mechanical stability and biologic viability. Satisfying one condition, but not the other, leads to patient morbidity and nonunion of the fracture. For many years the primary challenge was to accomplish adequate fracture stability. One tremendous leap toward this goal was accomplished in 1965 when AO ASIF bone plating techniques were introduced to veterinary orthopedic surgery. The dynamic compression plate (DCP®, Synthes) was developed such that insertion of screws into the eccentric ends of the specially designed sloping, oval holes accomplished compression of transverse fractures. This era of bone plating focused on accomplishing rigid stability. Of course, not all fractures are of transverse configuration; therefore, anatomic reconstruction of the bony column is not always possible or desired. In fact, in an effort to achieve anatomic reconstruction of the highly comminuted bony column, tremendous disruption of fracture zone viability often contributed to nonunion. The concept of *biologic osteosynthesis* evolved in which highly comminuted fractures were spatially aligned rather than anatomically reduced in order to preserve fracture zone viability. In such instances, there is tremendous stress concentration at unfilled screw holes within the DCP. Further, the footprint of the plate against the surface of the bone disrupted cortical bone blood flow under the plate. Surgeons often desired to use plates in combination with intramedullary pins in order to extend the fatigue life of bone plates, but the screw hole configuration of these plates restricted screw angulation to a relatively narrow spectrum. The limited-contact dynamic compression plate (LC-DCP®, Synthes) was designed with a scalloped contour on its underneath surface such that the footprint of the plate upon the bony surface permits greater cortical blood flow (though this is also influenced by the contour and topography of the bony surface to which the plate is applied). The scalloped contour of the plate also reduces the stress concentrating effect of unfilled screw holes. Additionally, the screw holes of the LC-DCP are designed such that screws can be inserted at much greater angles than with the DCP. This feature permits screws to be more easily inserted at angles to avoid intramedullary devices.

Each of these evolutions of the bone plating utilizes tightening of conventional screws within the bone to firmly compress the bone plate to the surface of the bone. There is no rigid link between the bone plate and the screw such that construct rigidity is not achieved when the bone plate is not firmly compressed against the bone. The amount of compression between the plate and the bone surface is influenced by the number of screws inserted, thread diameter of screws, and bone quality. If patient loading of the limb induces forces in excess of the frictional hold at bone plate-bone interface there is a loss of stable fracture fixation. As a result, there is emphasis on screw tightening and maximizing the number of screws used to compress the plate against the bone. Screw tightening pulls underlying bone segments to the under side of the bone plate such that precise contouring of the plate to the contours of the normally shaped bone is required. When conventional screws are tightened through improperly contoured conventional bone plates a *primary loss of fracture reduction* is induced. Alternatively, premature screw loosening prior to fracture union causes a loss of stability and *secondary loss of fracture reduction* (Figure 1).

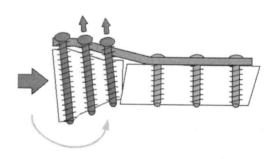

Figure 1. "Toggle" loosening of conventional screws from bone and DCP → secondary loss of fracture reduction.

LOCKING PLATE SYSTEMS

In this discussion, I will focus on the Locking Compression Plate® by Synthes Vet because this is the system with which I have the most clinical and research experience. There are other locking plate devices that are commercially available to the veterinary market including the SOP® and Kyon ALPS® devices. Each device has unique features that contribute to its own strengths and weaknesses. It is beyond the scope of this presentation to highlight each of these unique features. As a means of disclosure, Synthes Vet has provided me with LCP implants for use in my biomechanical research. I am not paid to promote their products and I pay for the implants that I use clinically.

The LCP is a dramatic shift from conventional bone plating. The LCP utilizes a specially designed locking screw that has a threaded, conical screw head that rigidly links to the bone plate through specially designed screw hole with matching thread form. The rigid link between the screws and the plate creates a fixed angle construct with dramatically different mechanical behavior than conventional bone plating. The rigid locking screw-LCP interface does not compress the LCP against the bone and maintains the fracture reduction present during plate application. This subtle evolution in bone plate design also alters the method of bone plate and screw application. The LCP is designed with combination-use screw holes (Combi-hole™) that accept traditional screws or locking screws (Figure 2). Different surgical techniques are used to apply *locking screw-LCP*

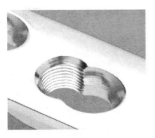

Figure 2. Combi-hole™ can accept conventional screws (right side of hole) or locking screws (left side of hole).

constructs as compared to combination locking screw/conventional screw-LCP constructs.

Locking screw-LCP constructs utilize exclusively locking screws throughout the construct and therefore do not require precise plate contouring. In selected instances the surgeon may elect not to contour the plate at all. This construct functions mechanically and biologically more as an internal fixator rather than as a conventional bone plate. The rigid locking screw-LCP interface ensures angular stability of the screws and prevents "toggle" loosening of the screws in the bone. The fracture must be reduced (or aligned) prior to plate application because this construct will not reduce (or align) the fracture as can be performed with conventional plating. Because the LCP is not compressed against the bony surface there is minimal disruption of cortical blood flow. This mode of application may be particularly advantageous in percutaneous plating where biologic osteosynthesis is indicated. However, one must be aware that construct stiffness is likely inversely proportional to the offset distance between the locking plate and the bone. Locking screws must be inserted in a fixed angle that is determined by drilling through a drill guide that is threaded into the locking screw hole. Care must be used to properly orient the bone plate because even minor angulations of locking screws to center them in the cross-sectional area of the bone are not possible. Locking screw-LCP constructs cannot be used to achieve dynamic compression because the screw heads of the locking screws do not slide within the contours of the screw holes.

In humans, unicortical placement of locking screws is more commonly employed than with conventional screws. Whereas bicortical placement helps eliminate toggle loosening of conventional screws, locking screws are not prone to toggle because they are stabilized by the bone on one end and the rigid link to the plate on the other end. All orthopedic constructs will fail at their "weak link" if fracture consolidation does not occur to protect the implant system. If the plate is the weak link (such as may occur when a screw hole is left unfilled over a non-load-sharing fracture), locking screw-LCP constructs fail similar to conventional screw-plate constructs. When the bone plate is not the weak link, locking screw-LCP constructs fail differently than conventional constructs. Conventional constructs often fail by screw loosening

that allows the screws to toggle free from the bone and bone plate. This mode of failure is particularly common in soft bone (growing dogs, flat bones, metaphyseal areas). Conversely, locking screw-LCP constructs are not prone to failure by screw loosening even in soft bone. Locking screw-LCP constructs may fail by catastrophic failure of the bone segment in which the screws are inserted or by fatigue failure of all screws within a cluster. Catastrophic failure of a bone segment may be more likely when unicortical locking screws are used in our small animal patients because they have relatively thin cortices as compared to humans and large animal patients.

Combination locking screw and conventional screw-LCP constructs are often employed to reduce implant costs, to accomplish dynamic fracture line compression or because surgeons are more comfortable with more traditional bone plating techniques. Surgeons must be cautious however, because surgical techniques for application of combination constructs are different from both conventional and locking constructs. LCPs applied as combination constructs must be precisely contoured to any surface of bone that will receive a conventional screw. Distortion of a screw hole during plate contouring will prevent application of a locking screw to that hole. It is important to place conventional screws into each bone segment prior to inserting locking screws – "lag before you lock" is a helpful reminder. If locking screws are placed first, subsequent placement conventional screws will attempt to compress the plate against the bone while the locking screws maintain the plate at a fixed position relative to the bone surface. Conventional screws can be used to achieve dynamic compression followed by insertion of locking screws to achieve a fixed angle construct. In selected instances, a locking screw-LCP cluster may be used in one bone segment for angular stability of screws in soft bone while a conventional screw-LCP cluster is used in the other bone segment to achieve dynamic compression (Figure 3).

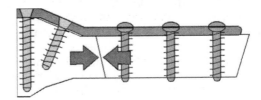

Figure 3. Locking screws (left) have angular stability in soft metaphyseal bone. Conventional screws (right) used to compress the fracture line.

SUMMARY

Locking plate systems are distinct and unique from traditional bone plates in their surgical application and biomechanical performance. Recognition of their unique features is foundational to their successful clinical application.

INTERLOCKING NAILS: THE GADGETRY AND SURGICAL METHODS

Ross H. Palmer, DVM, MS, Diplomate ACVS
College of Veterinary Medicine & Biomedical Sciences
Colorado State University, Fort Collins, CO

The interlocking nail system (ILN) for fracture fixation consists of an intramedullary nail with holes distributed over its length to accept interlocking screws or bolts. The most commonly employed ILN device in veterinary medicine in the United States is made by Innovative Animal Products and is the device discussed through the remainder of this monograph because it is the device with which I am most familiar. I am not paid to promote this device nor have I received support for my research from this company. The device utilizes a precision drill jig to aid the surgeon in accurate placement of the interlocking screws/bolts through the holes distributed in the nail without the need for intraoperative fluoroscopic guidance (Figure 1). Much of the instrumentation is to facilitate intramedullary placement of the nail and rigid, precise attachment of the drill jig so that a nicely engineered set of drill and tap guides direct accurate placement of the interlocking screws or bolts.

The ILN is available in 4.0, 4.7, 6.0, 8.0, and 10 mm diameters and is sold in four different sets. The **Model 22-6mm/8mm** set is an improved version of the original design. Now the instrumentation accommodates the 6-mm diameter nail with 2.7-mm holes, and the 8-mm diameter nail with 3.5-mm holes. Both the 6-mm and the 8-mm diameter nails in this set have an inter-hole spacing of 22.2 mm (Figure 2). The nails are available in 6 different lengths with either three or four interlock holes. This relatively wide spacing of the holes (compared to Model 11 sets) of the nails in this set, requires the nails of this set be used in fractures of the mid-shaft so that interlocking screws/bolts are not placed near or into fracture lines. The **Model 11-6mm/8mm** set is similar except that the nails have an inter-hole spacing of 11.1 mm distributed toward the ends of the nail and the corresponding instrumentation fosters accurate drilling and screw/bolt placement for this spacing. The tighter spacing of the holes at each end of these nails allows their use in fractures more widely distributed throughout the diaphysis. The **Model 11-4mm/4.7mm** is for smaller breeds of dogs and cats. Each of these nail sizes has 2.0-mm holes to accept 2.0-mm interlocking screws or bolts. The inter-hole spacing is 11.1mm and each diameter of nail is available in seven different lengths with either three or four screw holes. Within each of the three sets is instrumentation specific for placement of each diameter of nail and its corresponding interlocking screws or bolts. The most recently introduced nail is the **Model 11-10mm** for giant breeds of dogs. This nail accepts 4.5-mm screws/bolts.

Each ILN set consists of a series of nails of differing lengths and hole distributions. The appropriate size of nail (diameter and length) and hole distribution is selected by superimposing transparent templates on to

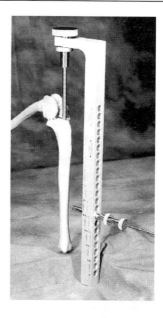

Figure 1. ILN extension/drilling guide unit (Model 11). Drill bit is inserted into drill guide resting within guide sleeve. The drilling guide aids the surgeon in accurate placement of interlocking screw through cannulations in the implanted nail. Note: Drilling guide is usually oriented such that drilling is directed within the medial–lateral plane.

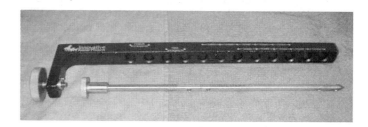

Figure 2. 8-mm (Model 22) nail with tibial (long) extension attached. Note the thumb screw at the top of the drilling jig. To couple the drilling jig to the extension/nail unit, the thumb screw is secured tightly into the extension.

radiographs of the fractured bone and the intact bone of the contralateral limb. The largest diameter of nail that can be safely inserted into the intramedullary cavity should be used. The nail should be long enough to ensure that the screw holes will not be positioned within or immediately adjacent to the fracture line. The nail should be shorter than the bone being stabilized such that its proximal end can be recessed below the bony surface following implantation. It is important to record the nail length and hole distribution prior to insertion as this information will be needed for accurate placement of the interlocking screws or bolts in later stages of the procedure. The distal end of the nails has a trocar point for cutting. The proximal end of the nail is hollow with a threaded inner surface and notched cut-out. This design is to accept an extension that is essentially a coupling device between the nail and subsequent applications of the nail *Insertion Tool* and, then, the *Drill Jig*. Each set contains extensions in two different lengths. The shorter *Femur Extension* is used for ILN applications to the femur and humerus. The longer *Tibia Extension* is used for tibial fractures because the longer length prevents the drill jig from interfering with the stifle. The selected extension has notched cut-out and coupling screw to correspond to that of the proximal end of the nail (Figure 3). The *Hex Driver* is used to firmly tighten the coupling screw of the extension as it is coupled to the proximal end of the nail such that the notched cut-outs of the nail and the extension rigidly interlock with one another.

Next, the *Insertion Tool* is attached to the extension/nail unit (Figure 4). The proximal end of the extension is engineered to receive the insertion tool. The insertion tool is firmly seated within the extension by way of a screw-in mechanism. Prior to insertion of the ILN, a reamer of corresponding size may be used to prepare the intramedullary cavity. Because dogs and cats have relatively thin cortices, the reamers are primarily used for reaming of trabecular bone rather than aggressive reaming of the endosteal surface of the cortex. When cortical reaming is indicated, it is important to use a sharp reamer with a delicate touch to decrease the risk of inducing cortical fracture lines. Once the intramedullary canal is prepared, the nail is placed as appropriate. Circumferential etched lines on the distal end of the extension allow the surgeon to monitor depth of insertion of the nail (Figure 3). Once the nail is

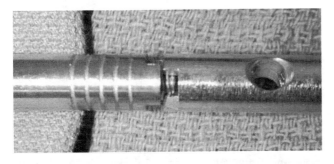

Figure 3. Extension (left) has a notched cut-out and coupling screw to correspond to that of the proximal end of the nail (right). Note the etched circumferential marks on the distal end of the extension that aid surgeons in judging the depth of nail insertion during implantation.

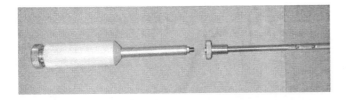

Figure 4. The proximal end of the extension (right) in preparation to receive the insertion tool (left). The knurled knob at the top of the insertion tool is used to firmly couple the insertion tool via a screw-in mechanism into the extension.

properly seated, the insertion tool is removed from the extension. It is prudent at this time to verify firm anchoring of the extension to the nail with the hex driver.

Next, the drill jig is firmly anchored to the extension (Figure 1). The drill jig lies outside the limb and allows the surgeon to locate and drill into the screw holes of the implanted ILN. The jig and extension have a peg-in-hole coupling that insures the drill jig is rotationally aligned on the nail such that subsequent drill holes in the bone will be accurately directed into the lumen of the corresponding holes in the nail. Once again, the drill jig must be firmly attached to the extension by way of an *Attachment Screw*. The knurled surface of the head of this screw allows for firm placement by hand. The drill jig/extension/nail unit is rotated to the orientation desired for screw/bolt placement (usually the medio-lateral plane). Proper rotational alignment of the long bone is confirmed. A scale is printed along the drill jig allowing the surgeon to know which holes along the jig arm correspond to the holes in the implanted nail.

Drilling for insertion of interlocking screws or bolts must be performed diligently to ensure accurate placement. It is important during all stages of drilling and screw/bolt placement to avoid applying pressure to the drill jig because even minor deformation of the jig can alter its position relative to the implanted nail resulting in misplaced screws. The most distal screw/bolt is usually placed first. First, the *Guide Sleeve* is placed in the appropriate hole of the drill jig. The sharp *Trocar* is passed through the guide sleeve to separate overlying soft tissues down to the bone. The sharp trocar tip is used to create a "dimple" in the bone's surface to help prevent migration of the drill bit. The guide sleeve is maintained within the drill jig and the trocar is removed. Next, the appropriate *Drill Guide* is placed within the guide sleeve. Extended length drill bits are needed to accommodate the drill jig/guide sleeve/drill guide. Care must be taken to prevent the drill bit from "walking along" the near-cortical surface before engaging the bone. Failure to prevent this is a common cause of mis-directed screws. Special "point tip" drill bits in extended lengths are now available from the manufacturer and these are extremely valuable in preventing this problem. A sharp, properly directed drill bit should smoothly penetrate the near-cortical surface, the transverse cannulation in the ILN, and the far-cortical surface. The drill bit and drill guide are removed leaving the tissue sleeve in place within the drill jig. The depth gauge is inserted into the guide sleeve and the hole-depth is measured. The depth gauge is removed from the guide sleeve and replaced with the *Tap Guide*. The hole is tapped routinely. The tap and tap guide are removed (Figure 5). If soft tissues are likely to obscure visualization of the hole, the screwdriver and screw can be inserted through the guide sleeve.

Interlocking bolts are available as an alternative to interlocking screws. The bolts consist of a solid shaft (as compared to the threaded shaft of screws) to impart greater resistance to screw bending (Figure 6). Immediately below the bolt head is a short threaded section to engage the near-cortical surface, preventing

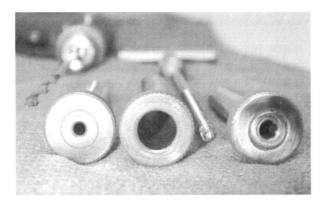

Figure 5. (Left to right) Drill bit, drill guide, guide sleeve, tap, tap guide. The guide sleeve accepts either the drill guide or the tap guide and is essential to ensure accurate guiding of the hole through the cannulation in the nail.

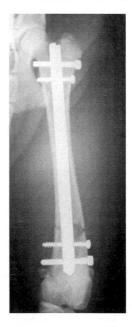

Figure 6. 8-mm Model 11 nail with 3.5-mm screws (adjacent to fracture line) and bolts (proximal and distal ends of the nail). Note that bolts have threads engaging the near cortex only and have a larger core diameter than corresponding screws.

bolt migration. Bolts are available in 2-mm, 2.7-mm, 3.5-mm, and 4.5-mm diameters and each are of fixed length that are cut with bolt cutters to appropriate length. Because the diameter of the bolt shaft is larger than the inner diameter of the threaded shaft of screws, drilling holes for their insertion is slightly different. For example, a 6mm ILN, which accepts a 2.7-mm bolt, should be drilled with a 2.7-mm drill bit, whereas a 2.0-mm hole should be drilled for a 2.7-mm screw. Holes do not need to be tapped for bolts.

Once the distal-most screw or bolt has been placed, the surgeon can rotate the jig/extension/nail unit to confirm proper placement of the interlock. Rotation of the jig should cause a palpable "stop" as walls of the transverse cannulation in the nail impinge on the interlocking screw/bolt. Additionally, rotation of the distal segment of bone should correspond to the degree of jig/extension/nail unit rotation. Proper axial alignment of the bone (rotation and length) should be reconfirmed and subsequent interlocking screws/bolts placed in a distal to proximal sequence. The heads of the interlocking screws/bolts, if properly inserted into the corresponding ILN cannulations, should be in line with one another. The drill guide is removed from the extension. The hex driver is used to uncouple the extension from the nail. Gentle tapping under the

collar of the extension may be required to pull the extension from the nail.

ILNs can be combined with external skeletal fixation (ESF). IMEX manufactures *Interlocking Nail Pins* for insertion into the cannulations of the ILN such that the ESF provides interlock within in the nail. These pins have smaller diameter smooth portion that functions as a "cut to length" interlocking bolt (2.0-, 2.7-, and 3.5-mm diameters). The ILN pin has a short threaded portion for engaging the near-cortical surface that tapers to larger diameter for gripping by the IMEX SK clamp. The 2-mm ILN pin adapts to 4-mm and 4.7-mm nails and Mini SK or Small SK Clamps. The 2.7-mm ILN pin adapts to 6mm nails and Small SK or Large SK clamps. The 3.5-mm ILN pin adapts to 8mm nails and Small SK or Large SK clamps. The addition of the ESF to the ILN improves its resistance to torsional moments.

MENISCAL VISUALIZATION: IF YOU CAN'T SEE IT, YOU CAN'T TREAT IT

Ross H. Palmer, DVM, MS, Diplomate ACVS
College of Veterinary Medicine & Biomedical Sciences
Colorado State University, Fort Collins, CO

ANATOMY

The lateral and medial menisci are semilunar fibrocartilage structures positioned between the articular surfaces of the femoral and tibial condyles (Figure 1). In cross section, the menisci are wedge shaped with the peripheral circumference being thicker and white in color, while the axial margins are very thin and almost translucent. The femoral surface of each meniscus is concave to receive the curved surface of the femoral condyle. The tibial surface is relatively flat. Each meniscus is anchored to the tibial plateau by cranial and caudal *menisco-tibial ligaments*. The cranial menisco-tibial ligaments are united by the *intermeniscal ligament*. This ligament is an important landmark because it borders the cranial margin of the tibial insertion of the cranial cruciate ligament (CrCL). In addition, the intermeniscal ligament is often used to anchor intracapsular grafts used for CrCL stabilization. The periphery of each meniscus is attached to the joint capsule. The attachment of the lateral meniscus differs from that of the medial meniscus in three distinct ways: (1) the caudal margin of the lateral meniscus is less firmly attached to the joint capsule, (2) the lateral meniscus is not attached to the lateral collateral ligament, but the medial meniscus is attached to the medial collateral ligament, and (3) the caudal margin of the lateral meniscus is also attached to the femur by way of the *menisco-femoral ligament*.

Only the peripheral 10% to 25% of the menisci is supplied by a vascular network and nervous innervation. The axial majority of the menisci is avascular and aneural and is nourished by diffusion of synovial fluid. The menisci have several important functions: (1) energy absorption and load distribution across the femoro-tibial joint, (2) stabilization of the joint by deepening the articular surfaces plateau – much like a "chock" behind a tire, (3) lubrication of the joint, (4) prevention of synovial membrane impingement between the femur and tibia, and (5) joint proprioception.

MENISCAL VISUALIZATION THROUGH AN OPEN ARTHROTOMY

Structures surrounding the menisci that must be protected from iatrogenic damage include the articular cartilage, caudal cruciate ligament (CdCL), medial collateral ligament, and popliteal artery. A suction unit with a fine suction tip is essential for precise visualization required for meniscal surgery. A headlight is very helpful in properly illuminating all pertinent structures. A surgical assistant is often times needed for at least a short time. A Senn retractor with sharp prongs on the fork end and a small Hohman retractor are required needed. Either a medial or a lateral parapatellar arthrotomy is performed and the patella is luxated accordingly. The forked end of

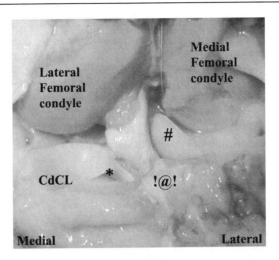

Figure. 1. Cadaveric dissection of left canine stifle (patella, patellar tendon and cranial cruciate ligament [!@!] have been excised) shows relationship of caudal cruciate ligament (CdCL) to medial menisco-tibial ligament (*) and lateral menisco-femoral ligament (#).

the Senn retractor is positioned on the proximal and caudal surfaces of the fat pad and it is retracted cranio-distally. Meniscal visualization is obscured by a healthy, intact CrCL; fortunately, meniscal pathology is most frequently encountered in conjunction with CrCL tears. The pathologic CrCL is debrided (if majority is still intact and healthy) or excised. Next, the tip of the Hohman retractor is placed caudal to the tibial plateau and is used to lever the tibial plateau cranially relative to the femur (Figure 2). Placement of the tip of the tip of the Hohman retractor between the CdCL's tibial insertion and the caudal horn of the medial meniscus effectively isolates the medial meniscus from the CdCL in most dogs.

Partial Meniscectomy - Clinical management of meniscal injuries is somewhat controversial. Major meniscal injuries, such as large bucket-handle tears, church-pew tears, caudal avulsion with cranial folding, and crushing injuries are undisputed sources of lameness and the damaged segment(s) should be excised. Excision of the damaged segment is termed, "partial meniscectomy". When bucket handle tears of the medial meniscal caudal body are encountered, a No. 11 blade is used to first transect the more cranial attachment of the bucket handle segment. A forceps can be applied to the segment to apply a craniomedially directed tension. The more caudal attachment of the bucket handle is then incised using caution to identify and protect the caudal cruciate ligament. After the bucket handle segment is excised, the remaining portions of the meniscus should be closely inspected for other tears that were hidden by the bucket handle segment. When the entire caudal body of the medial meniscus has been crushed, the caudal body is excised by transection along the cranial margin of the crushed zone. Typically, it is also necessary to incise the caudal menisco-tibial ligament (being sure to protect the CdCL with the Hohman retractor. Most of the time there are still some intact meniscal fibers along the peripheral margin of the medial mensical caudal body. Firm cranial tibial translation by a surgical assistant with the Hohman retractor is needed. Next, the surgeon uses a fine forcep in one hand to provide cranially-directed tension on the pathologic meniscal segment, while using a #11 blade to transect the remaining intact fibers along the meniscal periphery.

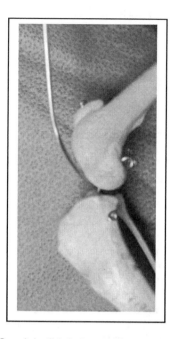

Figure 2. Cranial tibial translation with a Hohman retractor to improve meniscal visualization

PATELLAR LUXATION: NEW CONCEPTS IN DIAGNOSIS & TREATMENT

Ross H. Palmer, DVM, MS, Diplomate ACVS
College of Veterinary Medicine & Biomedical Sciences
Colorado State University, Fort Collins, CO

PELVIC LIMB ALIGNMENT AND PATELLAR LUXATION

Proper anatomic alignment of the quadriceps/patellar mechanism with the underlying skeleton promotes patellar stability. When the quadriceps muscle contracts, it seeks to form a straight line with the patella positioned between its origin and insertion (Figure 1A). If the long axis of the quadriceps is not centered over the trochlear sulcus, there is an imbalance in muscular forces favoring patellar luxation (PL). Excessive femoral varus and external femoral torsion are commonly associated with medial patellar luxation (MPL). Distal femoral varus moves the long axis of the quadriceps muscle medial to the trochlear sulcus (Figure 1B). This discrepancy causes a strong medial tension upon the patella during muscular contraction. The strength and length of the quadriceps muscle in large breed dogs amplifies this discrepancy as compared to small breeds of dogs. Femoral osteotomy is used to treat MPL complicated by excessive femoral varus (Figure 2).

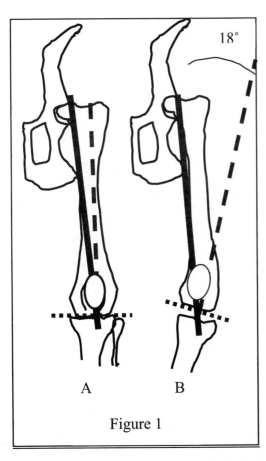

Figure 1

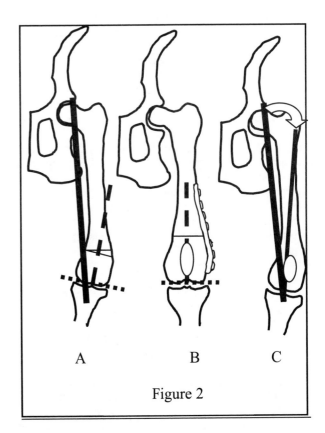

Figure 2

Figure 1. (A) Normal femoral anatomy. Solid black line shows long axis of rectus femoris muscle passing across center of trochlear sulcus. Dotted line is drawn across articular surface of femoral condyles. Dashed line is drawn perpendicular to dotted line. Perpendicular line within femoral shaft implies normal femoral varus/valgus. **(B)** Distal femoral varus. Note the long axis of rectus femoris (solid line) passes medial to center of trochlear sulcus creating a medially directed force upon the patella. Note the perpendicular (dashed line) extends laterally to the greater trochanter implying excessive distal femoral varus. Varus angle (18°) is formed between the perpendicular and the central axis of the proximal femur (long dash, dot dot line).

Figure 2. (A) Lateral closing wedge ostectomy for treatment of MPL complicated by femoral varus. **(B)** Completed lateral closing wedge ostectomy. Note the improved femoral alignment. **(C)** Rectus femoris transposition. The rectus femoris (RF) origin is transposed to the cervical tubercle of the greater trochanter. Note the improved alignment of long axis of the RF muscle over center of trochlear sulcus. In addition, the patellar position is made independent of external hip rotation, which can accentuate MPL.

RADIOGRAPHIC EVALUATION

To date, no radiographic method for measurement of femoral varus/valgus has been validated in dogs with patellar luxation. Work in our laboratory has shown radiographic measurement of canine femoral varus is repeatable within and between investigators, but is not statistically accurate in predicting true anatomic varus (at least in clinically normal large breed dogs). In that study, the femoral varus measurements in normal cadavers represent a small range of measurements in which to correlate radiographic femoral varus (RFV) with true anatomic femoral varus (AFV). Therefore, when dogs with excessive femoral varus are added into future study populations, the true accuracy of RFV in predicting AFV should be clarified.

The following reflects our current understanding and will likely be modified as ongoing investigations are completed. Accurate radiographic evaluation of limb alignment requires general anesthesia because subtle alterations in patient position induce markedly erroneous femoral alignment measurements. A craniocaudal (CrCd) radiograph from the hip to the proximal tibia is performed. The femur should be parallel to the spinal axis (neither abducted nor adducted) and to the radiographic cassette (maximal hip extension). In dogs with restricted hip extension proper CrCd positioning requires the patient's torso be lifted to sitting position. Alternatively, a horizontal beam method is used (when the radiography unit allows for movement of the radiographic tube). Without proper positioning the artifactual appearance of femoral varus is easily created. The most common errors in patient -positioning are external rotation and incomplete extension of the hip. Properly positioned radiographs show the tip of the lesser trochanter, the vertical walls of the intercondylar notch distinctly parallel and the fabellae split by the medial and lateral cortical margins of the femur.

Femoral varus is measured on CrCd radiographs by first drawing a line across the articular sufaces of the femoral condyle (Figure 1, dotted line). Next a perpendicular to this line is drawn, starting at the center of the intercondylar space (Figure 1, dashed line). To measure the femoral varus angle, a line is drawn down the central axis of the proximal femoral diaphysis by defining three center points along the cylindrical portions of the proximal femur between the lesser trochanter and the isthmus (Figure 1B, long dash, dot dot). Femoral varus is measured as the angle between the central axis of the proximal femur and the perpendicular to the femoral condyle (Figure 1B). Multiple properly positioned radiographs are advised to ensure repeatability of measurements because incomplete hip extension and/or external rotation of the hips commonly induce dramatic artifactual distal femoral varus measurement. Femoral torsion can be measured from an axial radiographic view.

CORRECTIVE FEMORAL OSTEOTOMY AND PATELLAR LUXATION

Although most veterinary surgeons agree that excessive femoral varus should be corrected, neither a validated imaging method nor an objective definition for "excessive" has been established. Recent work by Dudley suggests that mean RFV in a homogenous population of normal dogs is 7.4° Based upon this study, informal clinical surveys and extrapolation from several anatomic studies, I currently advise corrective osteotomy when MPL is accompanied by femoral varus exceeding 12°. Established breed-specific "normals" and an improved understanding of the biomechanical effects of femoral varus on the patello-femoral joint are sorely needed.

A laterally based closing wedge ostectomy is performed in most instances (Figures 2A, B). RFV is measured. The size and position of the wedge to be removed is determined from radiographs. In the laterally recumbent patient, a lateral parapatellar arthrotomy is made to allow medial displacement of the quadriceps/patella mechanism. A jig properly positioned on the cranial femoral surface helps maintain alignment during plate application. The proximal jig pin is placed within the anticipated span of the bone plate to reduce the risk of femoral fracture through the pin tract. A straight line is scored into the femur spanning the region of the planned osteotomy. In most instances, the ostectomy is 2 to 3 cm proximal to the lateral fabella. The wedge ostectomy is completed and the distal femoral segment is rotated about the distal jig pin into reduction. The femoral alignment is visualized by looking down its long axis. The previously etched line is used for reference in visualizing the varus correction and maintaining torsional alignment. Torsional manipulations can be made at this point if necessary. A bone plate is applied to the lateral aspect of the properly aligned femur with three screws planned for the distal segment and being careful to properly position the plate such that it will not be in contact with the parapatellar fibrocartilages during stifle range of motion. The jig is removed. Varus correction is confirmed visually. Necessary surgical treatments at the level of the stifle are performed. Corrective femoral osteotomy is typically delayed until skeletal maturity because of stress concentration created by the distal end of the plate near the distal femoral physis. This stress concentration effect combined with physeal weakening by the trochleoplasty may contribute to distal femoral physeal fracture in the early postoperative period.

NOTE: Corrective femoral osteotomy is a technically demanding procedure requiring knowledge of regional anatomy and substantial orthopedic surgical training, skill, and experience.

HIP DYSPLASIA: DECISION MAKING REGARDING SURGICAL OR MEDICAL MANAGEMENT

Antonio Pozzi, DVM, MS, Diplomate ACVS
College of Veterinary Medicine
University of Florida, Gainesville, FL

Hip dysplasia is an abnormal development or growth of the coxofemoral joint, characterized by subluxation or complete luxation in younger patients, and mild to severe degenerative joint disease (DJD) in older patients. Its incidence is greater in large breed dogs but is breed dependent. It is uncommon in toy breeds and cats.

Causes of hip dysplasia are multifactorial; both hereditary and environmental factors play a part in the development of abnormal bone and soft tissue. Hip dysplasia is a polygenetic trait which is further influenced by superimposed environmental factors. There is probably some disparity in the growth and development of soft tissues relative to bone such that the hip joint is lax. Soft tissue abnormalities result in skeletal developmental abnormalities of the acetabulum and femur. The physiological responses to joint laxity are thickening of the joint capsule and increased trabecular bone thickness. Erosion of the articular cartilage occurs due to abnormal articulation exposing the subchondral bone and its associated inflammatory and nociceptive properties. Pain is also seen in young animals before bony erosion. This may be due to capsular stretching and subchondral trabecular microfractures. Later the classic radiographic and gross signs of degenerative joint disease are evident.

A thorough physical examination including orthopedic and neurological evaluation is mandatory. Consistent clinical signs include pain on manipulation of the hip, particularly in extension, with a reduced range of hip motion, crepitus on hip manipulation, and atrophy of the pelvic musculature. Good quality radiographs including lateral pelvis and OFA-style hip-extended VD pelvis radiographs are required for diagnosis.

It is important to note that two distinct populations of animals with hip dysplasia are presented to veterinarians. First are dogs less than 12 months of age who have marked hip pain and palpable laxity. Radiographic signs of degenerative joint disease are usually not present. The goal of surgical treatment in these patients is to increase the congruency of the hip joint to avert later degenerative changes. Second are mature dogs, usually greater than 2 years of age with signs attributable to secondary degenerative joint disease. Laxity is usually not palpable. The goal of surgical therapy for this population is to relieve pain and restore function.

NONSURGICAL AND SURGICAL TREATMENT

Young animals typically respond to exercise restriction and non-steroidal antiinflammatory drugs (NSAIDs). Frequently, animals with only occasional bouts of hip pain will respond to therapy and be essentially normal in their young adult life. Medical treatment does not include the use of corticosteroids. Nutraceuticals and chondroprotective agents may be of benefit in these patients. Other animals may be best treated with surgical therapy early to prevent debilitating arthritis later in life. Early surgical treatments for hip dysplasia include triple pelvic osteotomy (TPO) and juvenile pubic symphysiodesis (JPS).

Triple pelvic osteotomy is a procedure to rotate the acetabulum over the femoral head to reestablish hip congruity. This procedure should also slow if not prevent the development of osteoarthritis secondary to hip dysplasia. It involves an osteotomy of the ilium, pubis, and ischium with reattachment of the ilium using an angled plate to achieve the acetabular rotation. Patient selection is critical for the success of this procedure. Animals should have little to no radiographic evidence of degenerative joint disease if this procedure is to be of benefit. Radiographic evidence of DJD progresses in most dogs; however, untreated dogs may have higher scores of DJD of the hip joint.

Juvenile pubic symphysiodesis procedure performed in immature dogs at risk for development of hip dysplasia. It is a technically simple, inexpensive, and effective treatment for hip dysplasia in the young dog. This method increases lateral acetabular coverage of the femoral head in dysplastic puppies through electrocautery-induced symphysiodesis of the pubic growth plate before 4 to 5 months of age.

There are no absolute criteria by which to separate animals that will become surgical candidates from animals that will essentially be normal in adult life. For this reason early surgical treatment of hip dysplasia remains controversial. General criteria for the selection of candidates for these surgeries include no evidence of DJD and young age. Dogs that are not lame should not be considered surgical candidates.

Older animals will respond to some degree to nonsurgical treatment of DJD. Spontaneous improvement in function of the limb has been reported to occur in the absence of surgical treatment in dogs as they mature. Nonsurgical management is a viable option to restore good to excellent, clinical, pet-quality performance even in the severe forms of hip dysplasia. Education about DJD should be the first form of "therapy." Education and non-surgical management techniques should be part of every treatment plan for every patient with DJD. Nonsurgical treatment of DJD is vital for any case of DJD and consists of three primary components: weight control, activity modification and medical therapy. Weight control is often the most challenging aspect of management of DJD. A clinical study investigating the effects of obesity on dogs with hip dysplasia reported that overweight dogs that achieved an 11% to 18% body weight reduction were significantly less lame compared with their lameness scores before weight reduction. Activity modification is very important because exercise is important for maintaining strength, stamina, joint range of motion and body conditions in patients with DJD. Low impact activities (walking and swimming) are favored over concussive activities.

Medication for DJD would relieve pain and inflammation. Combination of agents such as anti-inflammatory analgesics, opioids and NMDA antagonists may be used at different stages of DJD. Nutraceuticals (ie, glucosamine) have been also become commonplace in the treatment of DJD despite the paucity of scientific data confirming their clinical efficacy. Among the surgical treatments of DJD secondary to hip dysplasia in the adult dog, total hip replacement and femoral head and neck ostectomy are the most commonly performed.

Femoral head and neck ostectomy (FHO) will alleviate the pain caused by DJD and hip dysplasia. As this is an aggressive, permanent procedure with less than predictable outcome in all patients, it is not strongly recommended in young animals, as most will improve to some degree with nonsurgical therapy and time. An FHO can be performed at any time in the dog's adult life if indicated. Well-muscled, small to mid-size dogs are more likely to have the best outcome. Other factors that may affect the outcome include surgical technique, duration of injury, age of patient and underlying disease. The postoperative exercise protocol is critical for the success of this procedure. The patient should return to low-impact exercise soon after the surgery. Swimming and long leash walks are recommended for conserving joint range of motion and building musculature. The use of anti-inflammatory is recommended as needed to maintain the dog active and comfortable during recovery. Most animals do well with a correctly performed FHO and appropriate rehabilitation. Larger animals tend to have less predictable outcomes but many are successful.

Totoal hip replacement (THR) has proven to be a well-established and accepted surgical technique for management of hip dysplasia and other debilitating conditions of the coxofemoral joint. THR replaces the femoral head and neck with a prosthetic (cobalt chrome) component into the femoral canal, and a prosthetic cup into the acetabulum. Different techniques for placing the prosthetic components are used depending on the selection of the case: cemented fixation of the prosthesis, cementless fixation or a combination of the two techniques. Cemented implants are held in place by polymethylmethacrylate while cementless components are held by bone in-growth.

The selection of candidates for THR is very important for its success. There is a high expectation for the surgeon to deliver an excellent result. Consequently, it is mandatory that all candidates for THR be assessed critically. Ten months of age is the youngest routine age of THR implantation, but successful THR for the treatment of capital physeal fracture have been performed. In some selected cases, early evaluation may be indicated for the risk of losing bone stock from chronic subluxation. Typical history for hip dysplasia and DJD is of waxing/waning hindlimb stiffness or lameness, perhaps bilateral, with abnormal pelvic lateralization on hindlimb protraction extension. The degree of lameness in the majority of dogs with hip dysplasia is mild to moderate. The scope of the total hip prosthesis sizes allows inclusion of most medium-sized through giant breeds. Cocker spaniels, Shetland Sheepdogs are examples of the smaller breeds to be considered. Obesity is a complicating factor for THR and should be treated first. THR in dogs with a body condition score of 5/5 is technically more difficult, and the risk of complication during convalescence is increased.

Contraindications for THR include:

- Dysplastic but not clinical for the hip
- Satisfactory response to medical treatment
- Other significant orthopedic disease. The most common unrelated cause of hind lameness in the dysplastic dog is rupture of the cranial cruciate ligament. CCL repair is almost invariably the priority.
- Pyoderma or remote bacterial infection. Increased risk of peri-implant infection is reported in association with any concomitant infection. It should be noted that some dogs with recurrent pyoderma, perhaps underlain by atopy, would never be good candidates for THR.
- Neurological disease
- Myopathy
- Previous surgery. There is a fivefold increase in periprosthetic infection rate if prior hip surgery has been undertaken.
- Septic arthritis
- Immunosuppression
- Erosive arthropathy

PINS AND WIRES: DO'S AND DON'TS

Antonio Pozzi, DVM, MS, Diplomate ACVS
Collage of Veterinary Medicine
University of Florida, Gainesville, FL

Pin fixation is a common method of stabilizing long bone fracture in animals. Intramedullary pinning provides axial alignment and resist bending forces applied to the bone during weight bearing, but do not control shear and rotational forces at the fracture site. Additional stabilization must be provided in these cases by applying cerclage wires, external fixation or a bone plate to control these forces. Crossed pins may be used in selected metaphyseal fractures that can be anatomically reconstructed. In these cases, the interdigitation of the fragments and the crossing of the pins provide enough rotational stability to allow successful bone healing.

TYPES OF PINS

Pins are relatively inexpensive and are often easier to implant than other forms of fixation. The most common type of pin used in small animal orthopedics is the Steinmann pin. The stainless-steel pin is round (1/32 to 1/4) and has a trocar point at each end. Smaller versions are called Kirschner wires (K-wires). Because K-wires are quite flexible, they are rarely used as IM pins, except in small bone. Threaded pins are not routinely used because the stiffness of a threaded pin is equivalent only to that of a smooth pin of diameter equal to the root diameter of the threaded pin. Furthermore, the negative profile threaded pins are more likely to break at the end of the threads for a stress rising effect.

SIZE OF PINS

Selection of the appropriate pin depends on the size of the IM cavity, the bone being repaired, the fracture configuration and whether ancillary methods of fixation are to be used. Generally, when a single IM pin is used, it should be large enough to fill at least 60% to 70% of the medullary cavity at its narrowest point. In bone with large medullary cavities, two pins may be placed in the medullary cavity to provide stability ("stack pinning")

PIN INSERTION TECHNIQUES

Pins can be inserted in a close or open fashion. Closed pinning involves placing the pin without opening the fracture site and requires comprehensive knowledge of the bone and surrounding soft tissue anatomy to ensure proper pin placement and prevent damage to nerves and vessels. Intraoperative radiographs or fluoroscopy are necessary to confirm appropriate placement and fracture reduction.

Pins may be inserted in either a normograde or retrograde fashion. Normograde pinning is when the pin is started at one end of the bone and driven toward the other end. Retrograde pinning is when the pin is started at the fracture site and driven out one end of the one. Once the fracture is reduced, the pin direction is reversed, and the pin is driven into the opposite end of the bone. IM pins may be inserted with either a hand chuck or a power drill.

CERLAGE WIRE PRINCIPLES

- The cerclage wire should be tight and applied directly on bone.
- Appropriate size of the wire should be used.
- Twisted wires have at least three twists below the cut ends.
- Cerclage wires should be used in fixation of long oblique fractures.
- Wires are placed 5 mm from the end of the fracture, and spaced about 1 cm apart.
- Stability of cerclage wires requires that the tubular shape of the diaphysis be reconstructable, and that there are a maximum of three fragments included.

NUTS AND BOLTS OF IM PINNING

- Use large and long pins when possible. Small increases in pin radius will have a significant effect on rigidity of the fracture repair. Fill the isthmus of the medullary canal to increase contact interference and stability. The pins should engage proximal and distal metaphyseal/epiphyseal cancellous bone to increase bone purchase and stability.
- Plan preoperatively the size, position and indication for IM pinning. It may be impossible to use a straight pin to achieve anatomic reconstruction in a chondrodystrophic tibia. Cats have a straight femur and humerus and are good candidates for IM pinning. Radial fractures are poor candidate for IM pinning as pin insertion will be in the carpal or elbow joints. NEVER pin a radial fracture in toy breed dogs.
- In pediatric patients pins should smooth, inserted perpendicular to the physis, and should not occupy >25% physeal cross-sectional area to maintain the potential for growth.
- Normograde insertion is preferred to reduce complications associated with joint and soft tissue injury. Sciatic nerve damage is a common complication of retrograde femoral IM pinning.
- Countersink pins within joints using a nail punch. Check range of motion and limb alignment prior to closure.
- Consider auxiliary fixation if IM pin alone does not provide adequate stability. Choose IM pinning as a fixation mean only in cases with very good potential of healing (ie, young, healthy, mid-size dog).

EXPOSING THE MENISCUS DURING ARTHROTOMY

Antonio Pozzi, DMV, MS, Diplomate ACVS
College of Veterinary Medicine
University of Florida, Gainesville, FL

Meniscal injury in the dog is most commonly associated with ligament injury of the stifle joint. The reported incidence varies from 50% to 90%. Damage to the menisci can be either acute or degenerative and usually involves the caudal and medial portions of the medial meniscus. The medial meniscus is firmly attached to the tibia by the medial collateral ligament, the synovium, and the meniscal ligaments. As a result, during drawer movement and weight bearing the caudal pole may become entrapped between the femoral and the tibial condyle and therefore may tear due to the shear stress applied on the longitudinal and radial fibers.

MENISCAL TEARS CLASSIFICATION

Meniscal tears have been classified into five different types (see Figure 1A and 1B).

Vertical longitudinal tears include bucket handle tears, short vertical tears, and incomplete vertical tears. Incomplete vertical tears can be diagnosed only with careful probing. Bucket handle tears are the most common type of tear and may be seen as multiple tears in the same meniscus. Bucket handle tears may present displaced (see Fig. 1A) or minimally displaced (Fig. 1B).

Oblique or flap tears may be single or double, and include parrot beak tears. They usually start as vertical tears, become bucket handle tears, and then tear completely at either handle end and become a single or double flap (see Fig. 1C).

Radial tears more commonly occur in the lateral meniscus and they may propagate if left untreated (see Fig. 1D).

Horizontal or horizontal cleavage tears are less common than other tears. Incomplete horizontal tears can be difficult to diagnose (see Fig. 1E).

Degenerative tears are most commonly secondary to delayed treatment and chronic trauma from walking on injured menisci. Often they may present with the caudal pole folded cranially, after chronic femoro-tibial subluxation (see Fig. 1F).

DIAGNOSIS OF MENISCAL INJURIES BY ARTHROTOMY

Meniscal injuries are most commonly associated with CCL rupture in animals. The typical patient presenting with a meniscal tear is a large, overweight dog with a complete chronic CCL rupture, severe crepitus, effusion, and pain on palpation of the stifle joint.

Radiographic examination may help confirm the diagnosis of CCL rupture and meniscal tear by ruling out other stifle pathology and identifying characteristic osteoarthritic and soft tissue changes. If available, advanced diagnostic imaging techniques such as MRI or a CT may be used before performing surgery. However,

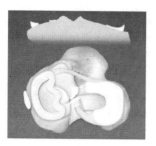

A, Bucket handle (BH) tear

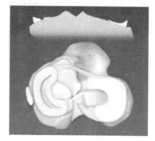

B, Minimally displaced BH tear

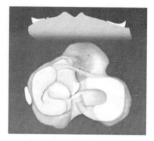

C, Flap tear

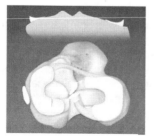

D, Radial tear

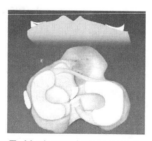

E, Horizontal cleavage tear

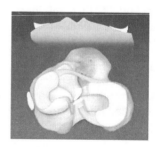

F, Folded caudal pole

Figure 1. Meniscal tears.

the most common ways to diagnose meniscal pathology are still arthrotomy and arthroscopy.

The medial meniscus may be exposed by arthrotomy through either a cranio-medial stifle approach or a caudomedial approach to the medial compartment of the stifle. Using a cranio-medial approach it is possible to examine the medial and lateral menisci, cranial and caudal cruciate ligaments and articular cartilage of the femoral and tibial condyles. A limited cranio-medial stifle approach may also be used to minimize soft tissue dissection.

Disadvantages of the cranio-medial approach include extensive soft tissue dissection and difficulty in visualization of the menisci in case of partial CCL rupture. The caudomedial approach to the stifle is used when there is a stable joint and the medial caudal pole of the meniscus is not visualized easily and if the surgeon does not suspect any other intra-articular pathology. Advantages of this technique include less tissue dissection and a better exposure of the caudal pole of the medial meniscus. On the other hand, the rest of the joint cannot be explored.

MENISCAL EVALUATION

1. *Exposure*: Initially the meniscus is exposed to evaluate its gross aspect. Exposure should be optimized using retractors, stifle distractor, flexion or extension and varus and valgus stresses as needed. In stable stifles with a partial CCL rupture the caudal pole of the meniscus may not be visualized with a cranio-medial arthrotomy. In case the caudal pole cannot be evaluated, the surgeon should debride the CCL or perform a caudomedial approach to the stifle. It should be emphasized that the caudal pole of the medial meniscus is the most common site of injury, thus should be evaluated carefully for the presence of tears.

2. *Meniscal Visualization/Evaluation*: The position of the meniscus is assessed. Commonly a portion or the entire caudal pole of the medial meniscus may be folded cranially, suggesting a displaced bucket handle, a flap or a peripheral detachment tear. Often degenerative tears may present with a folded caudal pole, suggesting chronic femoro-tibial subluxation.

The meniscus may be in its normal position and may look normal. However, careful probing should be performed to rule out vertical longitudinal tears.

3. *Meniscal Probing/Evaluation*: After visualization of the inner rim and femoral surface of the meniscus, probing should be performed to evaluate regions that cannot be visualized and to find non-displaced tears. The use of a probe (Figure 2) to palpate the meniscus increases the sensitivity for diagnosing meniscal pathology. The palpation with the probe should be performed to assess the integrity of both femoral and tibial surfaces and the meniscal attachments. Irregularities on the surface and hooking of the probe suggest an incomplete or non-displaced bucket handle tear. Hooking of the probe at the periphery of the meniscus should be interpreted carefully because the edge of the caudal pole is only loosely attached to the joint capsule. The probe is also used to evaluate the consistency of the meniscus. A soft meniscus may have a degenerative tear or a horizontal cleavage tear. After diagnosing a bucket handle tear, the rest of the meniscus should be evaluated for multiple tears that can be easily missed. This is important if a partial meniscectomy is performed.

KEY POINTS

- Improve the exposure of the meniscus using retractors, distractor, flexion and extension and varus and valgus stresses of the stifle joint as needed.
- Use a caudomedial approach to the stifle joint if the caudal pole cannot be visualized and evaluated with the cranio-medial arthrotomy.
- Carefully probe the meniscus to diagnose more challenging tears, including non-displaced or incomplete bucket handle tears and peripheral detachment.
- After debriding a bucket handle tear, reevaluate the meniscus with the probe to avoid missing a double bucket handle tear.

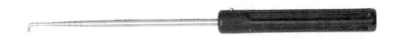

Figure 2. Meniscal probe

HOW DO I USE AND INTEGRATE JOINT PRESERVATION COMPOUNDS IN PRIVATE PRACTICE?

Ernest E. Ward, Jr., DVM
Seaside Animal Care, PA and E³ Management, Inc.
Calabash, NC

The use of nutritional supplements in medicine is as old as the practice itself. In reality, all medications were originally derived from natural substances such as plants, herbs, and other readily available natural and environmental sources. It is only in the past hundred years or so that the practice of medicine has distanced itself from the use of diet and natural substances in the prevention and treatment of disease. Today's physicians and veterinarians realize that in order to provide the highest standard of care for their patients they must be open to employing traditional medical and surgical methods while addressing each patient's nutritional and lifestyle concerns. If we focus solely on the medical and surgical treatments available and lose sight of the patient's entire lifestyle, we risk overlooking serious health threats that can lead to sub-optimal recovery and future relapses.

To this end, we must begin the transition from experts in disease treatment to disease prevention. While it is true that many conditions cannot be accurately predicted or even prevented, the majority of diseases and health threats are largely influenced by our lifestyle habits. Nutritional supplements such as glucosamine/chondroitin sulfate and the omega-3 fatty acids docosahexaenoic acif (DHA) and eicosapentaenoic acid (EPA) have a long history of benefiting the treatment of degenerative joint disease and osteoarthritis. Recent scientific studies over the past decade have identified the mechanisms by which these compounds aid in the prevention and treatment of joint disease. Armed with scientific data and the desire to proactively prevent disease as opposed to reactively treating disease, the use of diet, lifestyle management, and nutritional supplements in the practice of medicine becomes clear.

WHY SHOULD I RECOMMEND NUTRITIONAL SUPPLEMENTS?

The decision to recommend nutritional supplements, diet, and lifestyle changes to our clients and patients is as much a personal choice as a scientific one. At the core of this decision is the belief of the impact our actions have over disease processes. Some doctors and individuals believe that we have little control over the development of disease such as osteoarthritis, heart disease, cancer, and so on. They believe our lifestyle plays little, if any, role in our longevity and quality of life. Other people, including me, believe that our actions do have consequences and while we may not be able to prevent or lessen certain disease states, our lifestyle choices play a huge role not only in our longevity but, perhaps most importantly, in our quality of life. The emerging scientific research documents that what we eat, how we exercise and handle stress all have tremendous implications in our long-term well-being. Very few people would argue about the fact that being 100 pounds overweight will result in suboptimal health, the inability to perform at peak physical levels, and would place the individual at higher risk for developing obesity-associated conditions such as type 2 diabetes, osteoarthritis, and hypertension. Too often the people that agree with this example fail to recognize that their own negative lifestyle and habits are reducing their physical, intellectual, and emotional abilities.

It is into this arena that the decision to recommend nutritional supplements emerges. Doctors who are considering whether or not to suggest a supplement, lifestyle, or diet change should begin by becoming fully informed and convinced that their recommendation is sound and supported. Once a doctor becomes an advocate for a particular treatment, they should educate their staff. A doctor who believes in one manner coupled with staff who believes another will serve to confuse the client and result in impaired patient care. For any treatment, diagnostic, or patient care method to be completely successful, the entire staff must be in unison. Before discussing nutritional supplements with clients and patients, the doctor must first discuss it with their staff. It is during these training sessions that the doctor can fully develop their language and teaching points regarding a diet or supplement. The best arguments are those that originate with personal experience. A doctor who believes in a supplement or lifestyle and lives it speaks volumes to both staff and clients. When a doctor or staff member can tell a client that this is what they give their pet and why, clients are more fully engaged and interested.

Ultimately the decision to recommend nutritional supplements is a personal one. The decision should be individualized as opposed to generalized. For too long, physicians and veterinarians have simply ignored the science behind and swelling interest in disease prevention and optimization of health and the role diet, lifestyle, and natural supplements play in the pursuit of maintaining health. Each doctor must decide for themselves and then share their beliefs with their clients and patients.

WHICH BRAND SHOULD I RECOMMEND?

One of the most confounding aspects of integrating nutritional supplements and dietary recommendations into your practice is knowing which products to recommend. The choices are overwhelming with ever-increasing claims being made with each enhancement. Further complicating the issue is the potential risk to your professional reputation if you recommend a treatment that fails to provide the expected outcome. This has led many physicians and veterinarians to be reluctant to recommend a specific brand and simply suggest a class of nutritional supplements or dietary recommendations. This leads to clients and patients seeking specific recommendations from their pharmacist, the Internet, and even television infomercials. The result is that our clients and patients often receive inferior products or they become overwhelmed and intimidated by the plethora of choices and simply give up.

It is important that veterinarians research any nutritional supplements or diets they advise. In the absence of a specific recommendation, we force our clients to perform their own research and select products to comply with our recommendations. This is analogous to diagnosing a dog with a urinary tract infection and recommending that the patient should take a cephalosporin antibiotic for a short period of time—you can pick one out at your local pharmacy. While the example sounds ridiculous in that context, how far removed is it from advising your clients to select a glucosamine/chondroitin supplement for their dog's osteoarthritis? The concern that our recommendations may not work as we predict is the primary driver behind our reluctance to offer a specific product suggestion. If we look at the available options, dig deep into the manufacturing and processing procedures, and review scientific studies, we should be able to make accurate and reasonable conclusions. This is why it is important to not only understand our recommendations but what we are recommending.

When a doctor provides a patient or client with a specific recommendation backed by the evidence that supports his or her decision, the client and patient benefit maximally. The positive impact of stating a specific brand resonates with our clients. It demonstrates that we are knowledge in this area and have a very precise proposal for their pet. When we make generic recommendations, the client often interprets this as an optional treatment that doesn't necessarily affect their pet's condition or prevent disease. The more direct and specific a recommendation is, the more our clients will view it seriously.

If you are going to make dietary or nutritional supplement recommendations, be prepared to offer a specific product or brand you know your clients and patients can depend on. Research the compounds and claims, the companies and brands, and decide what is right for your patients. If you are unable to conclude that you trust a specific compound, brand or manufacturer, ask yourself if you should be making this recommendation at all. When you find a product leader supported by the most robust and generous research and sound manufacturing processes, the decision is an easy one.

WHAT SUPPLEMENTS SHOULD I RECOMMEND FOR JOINT HEALTH?

The number of choices for nutritional supplements for pets and people is staggering. The claims are even more overwhelming. What should you recommend, when should you recommend it and why? These are complex questions that each practitioner must answer before discussing them with their clients. Each doctor will have their own unique beliefs and philosophies that further make these issues individualized as opposed to generalized.

For optimal joint health, genetics, diet, exercise and lifestyle all interact to create a fully functional and pain-free joint. In the event that any single element is sub-optimal, the entire joint suffers. The current scientific literature fully supports the use of nutritional supplements to enhance joint health and reduce pain and inflammation. The leaders among recommended supplements to maintain a healthy joint environment are glucosamine/chondroitin sulfate and the omega-3 fatty acids DHA and EPA. In the face of degenerative joint disease (DJD) and osteoarthritis (OA), their use should be actively promoted. For most patients, the use of nutritional supplements prior to initiating nonsteroidal anti-inflammatory drugs (NSAIDs) is the preferred course. The concurrent use of glucosamine/chondroitin sulfate and DHA/EPA supplements with NSAIDs is perhaps the ideal treatment strategy for patients suffering from DJD and/or OA. In this scenario, we are using a prescription medication to reduce the damaging and eventually irreversible effects of DJD and OA while simultaneously promoting subchondral bone repair and synovial fluid production with glucosamine/chondroitin sulfate and reducing inflammation with DHA/EPA. The combination of these three treatments with weight reduction, exercise, and a healthy diet are the foundation for successfully managing DJD/OA.

Perhaps the most exciting use for glucosamine/chondroitin sulfate and DHA/EPA is in disease prevention or the extension of optimal joint health. While there is still debate on the full impact early use of these supplements has in the long-term health of joints, it is clear that prevention is preferable to treatment when it comes to joint pain. The use of nutritional supplements should be encouraged in all high-risk breeds for DJD/OA prior to the development of disease. Each client should be fully informed on the current state of our understanding of how these supplements may benefit their pet, the specific brand and dosing we recommend and why we believe this is of benefit to their pet. The client can then choose to follow our recommendation or consider it for later. It is important to consider nutritional supplements as just that—supplements to nutrition. Few pets or people will take in adequate much less optimal levels of these compounds in their regular diet. It is for this reason that supplementation becomes important, especially in at-risk individuals. As doctors, we should provide our clients with the latest information, articulate our best recommendation as effectively and compassionately as possible, and understand that they ultimately choose whether or not to adopt our suggestions.

PSEUDOMONAS OTITIS: WHAT TO DO WHEN NOTHING ELSE WORKS

John C. Angus, DVM, Diplomate ACVD
Animal Dermatology Clinic, Pasadena, CA

Clinically significant otitis externa occurs in 10% to 20% of the dog and cat population. The majority of cases result from common underlying problems, such as atopy, food allergy, or ectoparasites. Less commonly foreign objects, neoplasia, non-neoplastic masses, endocrinopathies, immune-mediated disorders are the primary cause. Bacteria and Malassezia overgrowth occur secondarily when normal local microenvironment is altered and passive immunity is disrupted. Overgrowth of resident organisms contributes directly to inflammation and perpetuation of clinical signs. Over time infection may extend to the middle ear or chronic physical changes alter the external canal, resulting in recurrence and increased severity of disease. Under appropriate conditions, opportunistic organisms such as *Pseudomonas aeruginosa*, *Proteus mirabilis*, *E. coli* and others replace resident organisms. Repeated exposure to antibiotics selects for resistant organisms. Although not the most common bacterial infection, *Pseudomonas aeruginosa* stands out as the most painful, smelly, frustrating, and difficult to manage. Frustration with *Pseudomonas* results from (1) severity of inflammatory response, (2) unpredictable antimicrobial susceptibility patterns, and (3) frequent treatment failure.

ROLE OF PSEUDOMONAS IN EAR DISEASE

Pseudomonas is an opportunistic bacteria found primarily in water, decaying vegetation, and only occasionally on or in animals. In order to colonize the ear canal or other animal tissues, *Pseudomonas* must first establish firm adhesion to epithelial cells. Under normal circumstances the adhesion points are occupied by the normal microflora, protected by passive immunity in the form of immunoglobulins and other antimicrobial peptides found in normal cerumen. For *Pseudomonas* to colonize the canine ear, two events are required: (1) presence of organism (water) and (2) disruption of normal microflora and healthy epithelial barrier. Once *Pseudomonas* has a foothold it is an excellent competitor, suppressing other bacteria and yeast, producing collagenases, protease, and exotoxins; which cause further disruption, eventually resulting in ulceration and tissue breakdown, including the tympanic membrane. To make matters worse the gram-negative cell wall and extracellular slime resists immune response. Vast numbers of neutrophils and macrophages are attracted to *Pseudomonas* infections. Although only partially effective against the bacteria, these WBC produce collagenases and proteases, which worsens tissue damage. In fact, serine proteases produced by neutrophils may actually enhance the ability of Pseudomonas to invade tissue. Clinically the result is an external ear canal characterized by severe inflammation, erythema, ulceration, pain, and large quantity of purulent exudate.

DIAGNOSIS

History is useful to help rank likely differential diagnoses for primary cause of otitis. For example, determine the "age of onset" of very first episode; if less than 1 year, parasites are most likely, but food allergy is also possible. If between 1 and 4 years of age, this is consistent with atopy, but any cause is possible. If older than 6 years of age, atopy is less likely, but any cause is possible. Seasonality strongly suggests atopy. Non-seasonal disease can be atopy or food allergy. If household affected or recently introduced, always consider parasites hypersensitivity, even if none are found on examination. Ask about prior medications. If the patient initially got better then suddenly worsened think about contact reactions. If current infection is of long duration (> 6 months) or more than three episodes a year then concurrent otitis media is very likely.

Physical Examination characterizes current state of infection and helps develop likely differential diagnoses for primary cause. A whole body dermatologic examination should be performed to find evidence of concurrent disease such as atopy, food allergy, parasites, pemphigus, hypothyroidism, etc. Begin with palpation of external canal and parotid region Record findings such as pain, edema, or soft-tissue swelling. Is the canal flexible or rigid due to fibrosis or mineralization? Is cerumen present on pinna? Normal clearance of debris should deposit this debris on the pinna. Absence of debris could indicate failure of epithelial migration. Excessive erythema, erosions, or pain could indicate contact reaction or more generalized dermatologic diseases. Finally, check the palpebral reflex. Reflex is diminished in some cases of otitis media cases or end-stage disease.

Otoscopy may be futile during initial examination of awake patient. The canal is often too painful, too ulcerated, or too full of pus to permit a satisfactory evaluation. Otoscopy should be attempted, however, to satisfy the owner's expectations and to evaluate for obvious problems such as a mass in the vertical canal. Recommend diagnostic evaluation under anesthesia, and combine with therapeutic flush to remove debris. If the canal is too edematous and stenotic to advance the scope into the vertical canal, then postpone. Treat with oral and topical steroids (prednisone 1–2 mg/kg/day) until edema is diminished. This will add value to the procedure.

Otic Cytology is a *mandatory* diagnostic test for every patient presenting with otitis. Cytology is necessary to characterize type and number of organisms seen. Mixed infections are common, with more than three species present in 30% to 60% of cases. Cytology allows you to identify current organisms, characterize the severity of disease, better interpret culture and susceptibility results, and make rational decisions regarding therapy. Use cytology to differentiate overgrowth from infection. Overgrowth occurs when native organisms take advantage of changes in the microenvironment. Overgrowth contributes to severity of disease, but is more easily managed with topical therapy alone. True infection results from either native or opportunistic organisms penetrating tissue, extending into middle ear, or creating severe inflammatory response resulting in purulent exudate. The presence of white blood cells almost always indicates true infection rather than overgrowth. Cytology is performed by direct smear and in-house stain, such as Diff-Quik. Examine on all objectives including oil immersion 100x. Be sure to record findings in the medical record for comparison with later cytology during re-evaluation: (1) Malassezia: presence/absence, estimated numbers; (2) Bacteria: presence/absence, rod or coccoid morphology, estimated number, phagocytosis by neutrophils; (3) White blood cells: presence/absence and which organisms are they targeting; and (4) Parasites: presence/absence.

Culture and Susceptibility testing of bacteria in otitis externa is of questionable value. Susceptibility breakpoints used by the laboratory do not correlate to achievable concentrations in external canal. Organisms present in the external ear canal are usually very different than those found in the tympanic cavity (89.5% of cases had different species or susceptibility patterns in one study). Laboratory results are not repeatable even when obtained from same ear canal collected submitted the same time. Variability between commercial laboratories methodology and reporting can yield very different results. Do not think of antibiotic susceptibility results as rock solid fact. Culture should never be used to monitor response to therapy. Culture only tells you presence or absence of organism, but provides little information regarding response to therapy, changing numbers, changing presence of white blood cells, etc. Culture and sensitivity is only indicated for antibiotic selection against bacteria with unpredictable susceptibility patterns, or if poor response to appropriate therapy.

Other Diagnostic Procedures

- **Food trial.** Eight weeks with provocative challenge at the end
- **Parasite treatment trial.** Eliminate the possibility of parasites with simple therapy.
  - Selemectin every 2 weeks for 3 treatments (95–100% effective)
  - Ivermectin 0.3 mg/kg weekly for 4 weeks (gradual step up to target dose in all breeds).
- **Allergy testing.** Intradermal Allergy Testing, Allergy serology
- **Thyroid profile.** T4, free T4; TSH is much better screen than T4 alone
- **Discontinue all prior topical or systemic therapies** in case of contact or adverse drug reaction

THERAPY

Specific therapy for the underlying primary disease is essential for long-term success. Simply chasing bacteria will ultimately result in treatment failure and progression to more severe disease. That said, anesthesia for otoscopy and deep ear flush is the most valuable diagnostic test and indispensable therapeutic procedure for *Pseudomonas* otitis. Flushing of mucopurulent, septic exudates from the middle ear is necessary for relief. Even the most spectacular antibiotic in the world cannot exceed the value of physical removal.

Preparation

You may need to postpone until there is a decrease in the inflammation in the canal. Prednisone 1.0 to 2.0 mg/kg/day for 4 to 7 days with a topical corticosteroid, such as flucinolone, is very useful prior to deep ear flush under anesthesia. The day of the procedure, be sure to collect a sample for cytology before flushing. Always, always, always use an endotracheal tube with a good cuff! Anesthestized or heavily sedated dogs lack a gag reflex and may aspirate irrigation fluid with microorganism and debris. The fluid can easily run through the ruptured tympanum, through the tympanic bulla, down the Eustachian tube, into the oropharynx, down the trachea and into the lower respiratory tract. Also, be sure to protect the eyes with excessive amounts of sterile lubricant. Tilt the head to prevent irritating irrigation fluids with debris, bacteria, and bacterial proteases from running over the eye and damaging the cornea. Finally, be sure to warm the sterile saline or other flush solution prior to cleaning. Large volumes of room temperature fluid should not to be used! You are very close to the brain and the brain is at body temperature. Cool or room temperature fluid will be very painful over time.

Procedure

Collect samples for cytology and culture prior to flush. If debris is thick and tenacious use a ceruminolytic to break up debris. Never leave ceruminolytics in the tympanic bulla, since they can damage the more sensitive respiratory epithelial lining. Only use ceruminolytics at the beginning to do the heavy lifting, then irrigate with warm water or sterile saline for the detail work and large volume flushing. You will finish with a drying agent so don't worry about leaving a wet canal at this stage. Bulb syringes, catheters, and 12-mL syringes or mechanical flush/suction devices are all useful. Use a lot of fluid, and keep flushing until debris is cleared. Use a buck curette to remove any adherent debris. Do not use cotton-tipped swabs.

Advantages of video-otoscopy versus standard operating head scopes include (1) superior optics provide significantly higher degree of magnification and detail resolution, (2) permits continuous viewing during irrigation, (3) avoids light reflecting off fluid interface, (4) decreases problem of blocking view by instrumentation, (5) increases precision, (6) decreases risk of injury to fragile structures, and (7) creates photographic record.

Assess the Tympanum

Otitis media may be present even if the tympanum appears intact. In one study, the tympanum appeared intact with standard hand-held operating head otoscope in 27 of 38 cases of otitis media. Video-otoscopy enhances opportunity for accurate diagnosis by increasing detail of image and permitting visualization under fluid. Hand-held otoscopes require suctioning of the ear canal. Typically the tympanum will appear opaque, sclerotic or discolored if the tympanic cavity contains fluid, mucus, or pus rather than air, or if healing from a prior rupture. Suspect otitis media if (1) large numbers of leukocytes on cytology, (2) characteristic changes in color or consistency of membrane, (3) vestibular signs, deafness, or Horner's syndrome, (4) poor palpebral or corneal reflex, (5) clinical signs of otitis externa for more than 6 months, (6) tympanum may be entirely absent, or (7) flush fluid is noticed emerging from the nostrils.

Flushing of the Tympanic Cavity

If the tympanum is ruptured and otitis media is present the cavity is often filled with purulent exudates. Any debris or infection is very irritating to the respiratory epithelium, which responds by producing more mucus and pus. Failure to adequately remove material during the flush will result in persistent otitis media, inability of the tympanic membrane to heal, and ultimately treatment failure regardless of follow-up. Warm sterile saline is excellent for breaking up mucus and is not ototoxic. Do not use ceruminolytics, chlorhexidine, or other ototoxic substances in this region. If using a catheter in the tympanic bulla, aim caudoventrally to avoid fragile structures such as the auditory ossicles, the corda tympani (a branch of the facial nerve), the round window and the oval window. Also, the largest portion of the tympanic bulla is ventral to the opening from the external canal. Be sure to avoid excessive pressure. Potential complications include: pain, vestibular signs, facial nerve injury, deafness, Horner's syndrome (cats in particular are predisposed). When flushing is complete suction the tympanic cavity as dry as possible. Rinse with drying agent or astringent that is "safe" in the tympanic cavity. (eg, Oticalm, Epiotic, Burotic-HC). Instill 50:50 mixture of Baytril injectable and Dexamethasone SP directly into the tympanic bulla. Steroid suppresses inflammation of respiratory epithelium and the injectable antibiotic should have a high enough concentration to overcome antibiotic resistance mechanisms. Dr. Craig Griffin reports success using amikacin and dexamethasone in this manner, without observing ototoxic reactions; however, aminoglycosides are reported as ototoxic agents, so proceed with caution unless peer-reviewed publications support usage of amikacin in this manner.

At-Home Therapy

Prescribe awake ear flush at home after patient has recovered. The goal is to remove debris, dry the canal, and kill microorganisms. Avoid irritating, ototoxic, or wet solutions. If the patient is too painful to permit at-home ear cleaning, treat with steroids and medicated drops only until able to tolerate cleaning. Product selection can be challenging. Recommend acidifying flushes for yeast infections to inhibit growth; however, in bacterial infections these products may decrease efficacy of topical antibiotics. Both fluoroquinolones and aminoglycosides function better at a neutral pH than acidic pH. Virtually any Pseudomonas can adapt to a constant acidic environment. TrisEDTA-containing products are the preferred solution for Pseudomonas or resistant bacteria. A pH of 8.0 is ideal for fluoroquinolones or aminoglycosides. The EDTA punches holes in the bacterial cell wall by chelating calcium and magnesium. In high concentrations and prolonged contact TrisEDTA is directly bactericidal. At a minimum, it is synergistic with antibiotics and may help to overcome many resistance mechanisms. Soak the ear for 10 minutes before topical antibiotic is applied.

Topical medication is typically prescribed to follow ear cleaning. In general thin liquids preferred over thick ointments. Several choices exist. Zymox is a gentle triple enzyme formulation that is very well tolerated by patients, even those with ulceration. Recent study in human burn patients demonstrated that lactoferrin inhibited binding of Pseudomonas to epithelium. This drug is my first choice if patient is too painful to tolerate anything else. Antibiotic/antifungal/steroid combinations are also a good choice. Fluoroquinolones are best if there is a lot of debris building up in the ear canal. Veterinary Baytril Otic™:(0.5% Baytril + 1% Silver Sulfadiazine) or the human product Cipro HC Otic can be used. A marbofloxacin otic formulation is available in Europe (Aurizon). A home-made solution of Baytril inj + + Dexamethasone SP in TrisEDTA–ketoconazole base in a 1:1:4 ratio can be useful. Aminoglycosides have excellent anti-Pseudomonas activity, but are inactive when large amounts of organic debris or in a low oxygen tension environment. Use only when after exudates are resolved. A home-made tobramycin solution combinines two 5ml bottles of tobramycin ophthalmic + 4 mL dexamethasone injectable. There is no commercial amikacin product; however, injectable amikacin + TrisEDTA or sterile saline with a target concentration of 30–50 mg/mL has been recommended. Gentamicin is available in many commercial ointments, but thickness of ointment may prevent penetration to deep canal. Ticarcillin and ticarcillin/clavunate have great anti-Pseudomonas activity. Unfortunately stability after reconstitution minimizes usefulness. If sending home, reconstitute with sterile saline, divide into aliquots, and keep frozen. The owner then thaws each aliquot prior to application. Ceftazidime has brilliant anti-Pseudomonas activity, but internists and criticalists will throttle anyone using ceftazidime for Pseudomonas otitis.

Systemic steroids are ESSENTIAL for managing severe Pseudomonas otitis. You must shut down neutrophils proteases, edema, and stenosis. The author recommends prednisone 1–2 mg/kg/day until recheck in 7 to 14 days combined with topical dexamethasone or flucinolone.

Systemic antibiotics are controversial. Resistance is high and concentration in the external canal is low. Use systemic antibiotic only for otitis media. There is a limited selection of effective antibiotics available for oral administration. Subcutaneous (SC) or intravenous (IV) administration of injectable antibiotics may not provide any substantial benefit and may select for resistance to drugs that should be preserved for use in dogs with life-threatening systemic infections (ie, don't use imipenem to treat ear disease). If using systemic antibiotics, ears require higher doses than other body systems because of difficulty penetrating into external and middle ear canal. As a general guideline use a dose and duration as if treating an osteomyelitis. Fluoroquinolones remain the best empirical choice for *Pseudomonas*; however, resistance is on the rise! With enrofloxacin 10% to 50% of isolates are susceptible; ciprofloxacin fares better at 75% to 90% susceptibility; with marbofloxacin more than 90% are susceptible. If using a fluoroquinolone aim for the highest achievable dosage: for enrofloxacin, the minimum acceptable dose is 15 mg/kg SID; for ciprofloxacin, there are limited studies in dogs but a suggested dose is 20 mg/kg BID; for marbofloxacin, 5 mg/kg SID. Combination therapy may be needed, since mixed infections with highly fluoroquinolone-resistant streptococcus, enterococcus, corynebacteria, or anaerobes are common. The author recommends marbofloxacin with clindamycin or Clavamox for mixed bacterial infections. Note: enrofloxacin and clindamycin have been shown to concentrate in WBC and therefore may be more effective in purulent otitis than other antibiotics. Treat for 6 to 12 weeks depending on severity of disease, the organism present, response to therapy, and healing of the ruptured tympanum.

Pain management is appropriate, since ear pain can be extreme in *Pseudomonas* otitis. Steroids decrease pain-causing events, but do not provide direct analgesic effects. Nonsteroidal anti-inflammatory drugs (NSAIDs) provide the best analgesia for ear pain, but cannot be used in conjunction with high dose prednisone. Opioid analgesics such as tramadol can be used in conjunction with steroids, but have more variable pain control.

Follow up to assess progress with physical examination and cytology. Cytology is the best method for monitoring response to therapy. Evaluate for decreasing numbers of organism, change in dominant organism, and change in WBC. Ideally at 2 weeks there are no WBC and substantial reduction of bacterial numbers. Repeat deep ear flush if significant mucopurulent exudate and debris remains. If responding continue with current course of therapy for additional 4 to 6 weeks, then recheck prior to discontinuation of therapy.

Long-term plan. Outline ideal management of primary disease (avoidance of food allergy, treating parasites, allergen-specific immunotherapy, cyclosporine, etc.). Keep ears dry. Flush with astringent ear solutions once or twice weekly; especially after swimming or bath. Avoid using water, dilute vinegar, or hydrogen peroxide. Monitor frequently for recurrence and treat all infections aggressively at the earliest sign. Surgical intervention with total ear canal ablation is appropriate for end-stage ears with chronic pain and no chance for response to medical management. Lateral ear canal resections except are of limited benefit and are not recommended.

SUGGESTED READING

1. Angus JC. Diseases of the Ear. In: Campbell KL, (ed.): Small Animal Dermatology Secrets. Philadelphia: Hanley & Belfus; 2004. pp. 364-384.
2. Gotthelf LN Small Animal Ear Diseases: An Illustrated Guide. 2nd ed. St. Louis, MO: Elsevier, 2005.
3. Matousek JL (ed): Ear Disease. Vet Clin North Am Small Anim Pract. March 2004.
4. Scott DW. External ear diseases. In Scott DW, Miller WH, Griffen CE (eds.): Muller and Kirk's Small Animal Dermatology, 6th ed. Philadelphia: WB Saunders, 2001, pp. 1203-1232.

TREATMENT OF CHRONIC OTITIS

Jenise C. Daigle, DVM, Diplomate ACVD
Austin Veterinary Dermatology & Allergy
Austin, TX

Otitis externa, which is inflammation of the epithelium that lines the external ear canal, is often difficult to diagnose because of the numerous agents that can be responsible for the development of the condition. Causes of otitis should be classified into predisposing, primary, secondary or perpetuating causes. Recognition of primary and perpetuating factors is **critical** to long-term control of chronic otitis. Bacterial culture and susceptibility is mandatory in chronic recurrent or unresponsive cases of otitis, when otitis media is confirmed or suspected, and when cytology reveals numerous rod-shaped bacteria.

PREDISPOSING FACTORS

Predisposing factors of otitis externa are those conditions or behavior that may result in ear problems, but by themselves do not actually cause inflammation of the ear canal. These factors facilitate the inflammation by permitting the external ear canal microenvironment to be altered allowing pathogenic or opportunistic bacteria to become established.

- **Conformation of the ear canal** can predispose an animal to otitis externa.
  - Pinnae (floppy versus erect ears): There is evidence that there is a higher prevalence of otitis externa in floppy versus erect ears.
  - Length and conformation of ear canals: Dogs of some breeds have very long and tortuous ear canals, which may restrict free airflow within the ear canal.
  - Stenosis or swelling of the opening of the external ear canal is a real problem in some breeds, such as the Chinese shar-pei. This lack of a significant opening into the canal may reduce air circulation in the external canal and also allows otic secretions to build up in the external ear can. The excess secretions provide a medium of growth for pathogenic bacteria.
- **Behavior**
  - Swimming: High moisture content of the ear canal can lead to maceration and disruption of the stratum corneum, predisposing to microbial colonization and infection.
- **Environmental factors:** Both heat and humidity will tend to make the microenvironment of the ear canal more suitable for bacterial and yeast growth.
- **Improper treatment**
  - Trauma to the ear canal during treatment of the ear canal, necessary or unnecessary, can damage the epithelial lining of the canal and predispose to infections.
  - The use of cotton-tipped applicators and excessive plucking of hair from the ear canal

are the most common examples and may lead to swelling and erosions of the epithelium.

PRIMARY FACTORS

Primary factors of otitis externa are those factors that actually cause or initiate the inflammatory process within the ear canal. In short, they are the reason that the problem begins.

- **Parasites**
  - Ectoparasites that cause inflammation of the ear include ear mites (*Otodectes cynotis*), various forms of mange (eg, sarcoptic mange, demodex mange), and ticks (eg, *Otobius,* the spinous ear tick).
  - Ear mites are the most common cause of otitis externa in cats!
- **Allergic skin disease**
  - Allergic skin diseases are the most common causes of persistent otitis externa in dogs!
  - Allergies include atopy, food allergy, and contact allergies.
- **Foreign bodies**
  - Many substances accidentally or otherwise end up in the external ear canals of dogs and cats. These result in irritation and inflammation. In some cases, the foreign object can damage or perforate the tympanic membrane and result in more serious damage.
  - The most common foreign bodies are plant materials, such as seeds or stickers from grasses or weeds. (eg, foxtails)
- **Keratinization disorders**
  - Keratinization disorders produce a ceruminous otitis externa. Primary idiopathic seborrhea and hypothyroidism may be associated with a ceruminous otitis externa.
- **Other dermatologic diseases**
  - Autoimmune diseases (eg, pemphigus foliaceus, discoid lupus erythematosus) can cause severe scaling, crusting and ulceration of the inner pinna and external ear canal.
  - Ear tumors and polyps can cause obstruction of the external ear canal, preventing removal of normal secretions.

PERPETUATING FACTORS

Perpetuating factors are those factors that allow the inflammation and irritation to continue, even if and when the primary factor is controlled. These factors prevent resolution or worsen an already present otitis externa. These are the factors we **must** control to prevent **chronic** otitis.

- **Bacterial and yeast infections**
  - Bacterial and yeast infections are the most common perpetuating factors.
  - The most common bacteria associated with ear infections are *Staphylococcus intermedius, Streptococcus* spp., *Proteus mirabilis, Pseudomonas aeruginosa, Enterococcus* spp.,

Corynebacteria spp., *and E. coli.* In the interpretation of ear cultures it should be remembered that a low number of commensals and potential pathogens is normal. Of the normal ears with positive cultures, the most frequent organisms isolated are *Staphylococcus intermedius,* coagulase-negative staphylococcus, and *Micrococcus* spp.

- Bacterial infections of the ear result in malodor, excessive production of exudate, and ulceration. They frequently make the ear extremely painful to any handling.

o *Malassezia pachydermatis* is the yeast found most frequently in association with otitis externa.

- *Malassezia* organisms are considered normal inhabitants of the ear canals, although in small numbers.
- *Malassezia* infections result in accumulation of a cream-to-dark waxy, odiferous discharge.
- *Malassezia* otitis is frequently associated with a generalized cutaneous infection by the same organism.

- **Otitis media**
  o Otitis media is inflammation of the middle ear.
  o Otitis media may result from trauma, neoplasia of the middle ear, or most commonly, by bacterial or fungal infections.

- **Chronic changes**
  o Repeated episodes of otitis externa and the development of scar tissue in the ear canal may cause hyperplasia of the ear canal. These changes may restrict the size of the ear canal.
  o Calcification of the cartilage of the ear canal results from chronic scarring and inflammation. It is irreversible and may lead to ear ablation as the only viable treatment option in some cases.

DIAGNOSIS

The following diagnostic tests are ***always*** useful to help diagnosis the causes of otitis externa:

- **Collection of the complete medical history**
- **A complete physical and dermatological examination** to evaluate other clinical signs of allergic skin disease
- **Otoscopic examination of the external ear canal**
  o This may require sedation if the ears are painful
- **Cytology of the ear canal**
  o A sample of exudate is taken from the ear and smeared onto a glass microscope slide, stained, and examined microscopically.
  o This test is necessary to identify perpetuating factors, such as bacterial or yeast infections.
  o The test is a MUST on follow-up examinations to determine the efficacy of treatment.

The following tests ***may*** be helpful and necessary to properly diagnose and treat:

- **Culture of the ear canal**
  o The test is performed by taking a sample of exudate from the ear as sterile as possible.
  o Culture is not necessary in all cases of otitis externa, but is indicated when cytology shows some types of bacteria (gram-negative rods) or when previous treatments have not been completely effective.
- **Radiography (x-rays)**
  o Bulla radiographs may be indicated when otitis media is suspected.
  o Heavy sedation or general anesthesia is generally required for this procedure.
- **Allergy tests**
  o These tests are indicated to identify the **primary** factors in otitis externa.
  o Remember allergies may be to molds or pollens, foods, or medications.
  o The history is the key to identifying possible allergies: season problems and otitis externa seen in conjunction with other signs of allergies.

TREATMENT
General Principles

Owners should be informed that management of chronic ear infections can not be done through the telephone or by the "smell" test. It is important to monitor patients treated for bacteria and/or yeast, preferably 2 to 3 weeks after initiating therapy. At that time, otic examination and microscopic examination of the ear exudate are repeated. If there has been no improvement and compliance has been good, a change in medications is indicated. The therapy should be continued until cytology and examination of the ears are that of what is considered normal.

Routine (I prefer weekly) ear cleaning at home by the owners is an essential component in the management of chronic otitis. It is also important that the veterinarian spend time with the owner showing the proper method of cleaning. Most cleaning products contain various types of acids often with a ceruminolytic or alcohol added.

Corticosteroids are important to use in the treatment of otitis externa to relieve the inflammation present (and its concurrent discomfort), especially if treating obstructive ear disease due to progressive pathologic change. Systemic steroids are usually indicated in severely stenotic, hyperplastic or erosive ear canals. I typically use systemic steroids in my gram negative otitis cases. I often use prednisone at 1 to 2 mg/kg (in the severely stenotic canals) daily for the first 7 days then taper. Topical steroids can be beneficial in the management of allergic otitis.

It is important to remember that otitis should be thought of as a symptom of an underlying disease and not a disease entity itself.

Management of *Malassezia* Otitis

Topical antifungal agents include nystatin, thiabendazole, clotrimazole, miconazole, and ketoconazole. Clotrimazole is available as a single agent (Clotrimazole Solution 1%, VET Solutions) and in combination with gentamicin and betamethasone valerate or mometasone (DVMax®, DVM Pharmaceuticals; Otomax®, Schering-Plough; Mometamax®, Schering-Plough) for mixed infections. Miconazole is most commonly used in the lotion formulation (Conofite® Lotion, Schering-Plough). Many self-formulated mixes are being used, especially for cases of *Malassezia* with concurrent hypersensitivity reactions in the ear canal. These types of patients usually have a primary allergy with secondary yeast otitis. These combinations include 1% clotrimazole solution and dexamethasone (2 mg/mL) mixed 1:1 and miconazole lotion and dexamethasone (2 mg/mlL mixed 1:1 and applied q12h

Management of Staphylococcal Otitis

For most cases of cocci (seen on microscopic examination of ear exudates), the following topicals are effective: Tresaderm® ((neomycin, thiabendazole and dexamethasone), Merial; Otomax® (gentamicin, betamethasone, and clotrimazole), Schering-Plough; Mometamax® (gentamicin, mometasone, and clotrimazole), Schering-Plough; Ear/Skin Cleanser® (boric acid, acetic acid), DermaPet.

Management of Gram-Negative Otitis

Gram-negative bacteria that are associated with purulent otitis include the following: *Pseudomonas aeruginosa, Proteus mirabilis, E. coli,* and *Klebsiella* spp. Gram-negative infections are associated with chronic and persistent infections due to multiple antibiotic resistance. The most common gram-negative bacteria associated with chronic otitis externa and/or media is *Pseudomonas aeruginosa.*

- **Tris-EDTA for treatment of gram-negative otitis**
  - o Cell surfaces of gram-negative bacteria are damaged by exposure of cells to ethylenediaminetetraacetic acid (EDTA). Tris buffer enhances the effects of EDTA. Gram-negative bacteria exposed to Tris-EDTA have increased permeability to extracellular solutes and leakage of intracellular solutes; are more sensitive to lyozyme, bactericides, and antibiotics.
  - o Two commercial veterinary preparations have been marketed (T8 Solution, DVM; TrizEDTA, DermaPet).
  - o Tris-EDTA in combination with benzoyl alcohol (T 8 solution,® DVM Pharmaceuticals) is effective against both gram-positive and gram-negative bacteria.
- **Treatment**
  - o 2–4 weeks of prednisone at 1–2 mg/kg.
  - o Deep ear flush preferably with a video-otoscope
  - o Twice daily flush with Tris-EDTA followed 15 minutes later with Baytril Otic (Bayer) or polymixin-containing ear drop. I prefer to use an "all in one" product of a Tris-EDTA product (4oz bottle) with 12 mL of LA Baytril = 10 mg/mL.
  - o Recheck every 7 days for 6 to 8 weeks for patency of ear canal, presence of exudate and cytologic evaluation of status of infection. During this period it would be good to evaluate for signs of allergy or other potential underlying cause of the severe otitis as well, as so that the work-up can begin in a timely fashion.

HOW TO APPROACH A CASE OF ACUTE OTITIS INCLUDING *MALASSEZIA*

Louis N. Gotthelf, DVM
Animal Hospital of Montgomery
Montgomery, AL

PRIMARY CAUSES OF EAR DISEASE

Pets with itchy ears may not have ear disease seen on otoscopic examination at all, but may be responding to a localized pruritus associated with an underlying pruritic disease. Since many diseases found in the ear arise as a result of an underlying skin disease, the veterinarian treating otitis externa should also do a careful evaluation of the pet's skin to determine the underlying etiology if possible. Often, diagnosis and treatment of the underlying skin disease diminishes the severity of ear disease.

Primary factors are those diseases of the skin that also have a direct effect on the skin that lines the ear canal. Diseases such as atopy, food hypersensitivity, parasites, foreign bodies, hypothyroidism, and keratinizing diseases frequently result in ear disease.

PREDISPOSING CAUSES OF EAR DISEASE

Predisposing factors are those things that directly change the microclimate in the ear canal. The microclimate changes include increased temperature from inflammation, increased humidity from poor ventilation and stenosis, and changes in the composition of the cerumen. Recent evidence has demonstrated that the superficial epithelial cells change their surface receptors increasing their affinity to bind to bacteria and yeasts. Certain breeds have more cerumen glands (Cockers, Labradors, and Springers) that favor yeast growth. Humid environments and excessive moisture in the ears from swimming or bathing promote bacterial growth. Excessive trauma to the ear canal resulting from exuberant ear cleaning or trauma from instruments used in the ear canal may allow bacterial colonization. Pathologic alterations to the ear canal epithelium such as fibrosis or tumors allow colonization of bacteria and yeasts along the increased surface area. These pathologic changes produce fissures and deep crevices where organisms are sequestered.

PERPETUATING FACTORS

Perpetuating factors are those things that prevent normal resolution of ear disease. Bacteria, yeasts, exudates and secretions from otitis media, and contact allergies from drugs such as neomycin keep the inflammatory process going. They are not the reason for the initial onset of otitis, but until they are dealt with, the ear disease will continue. Overtreatment of ear disease with ear cleaners keeps the epithelium moist and macerated. Too short a treatment duration may not rid the ear of organisms. Inappropriate antimicrobial therapy may be totally ineffective, such as treating an ear with yeasts by using an antibiotic.

To illustrate the interaction of these factors, consider a dog with atopy that may show inflammation of the ear canal resulting in redness, swelling, heat, and pain. The atopy is the **primary cause** of ear disease. In fact, almost 80% of atopic dogs have otitis externa. In a cylindrical cartilage tube, such as the ear canal, inflammation decreases the lumen diameter, which tends to decrease the ventilation and drying of the ear canal. Without ventilation, the humidity level of the ear canal increases. The resulting stenosis and increased humidity are **predisposing causes**. Humidity is a factor favorable for bacterial growth. The bacterial otitis externa then becomes a **perpetuating factor** and the symptoms of ear disease will not diminish until the bacterial component is removed. However, the underlying cause of the ear disease, atopy, remains in spite of the elimination of the bacterial infection.

Dermatologic conditions often affect the ear canal, making it susceptible to otitis externa. Examples of primary skin diseases that may also affect the ear canal include juvenille cellulitis, autoimmune diseases such as pemphigus and systemic lupus erythematosus, keratinization disorders, and erythema multiforme (a systemic drug reaction). The ear canal is an invagination of epidermis forming a hollow skin tube in the inside of the head which begins at the eardrum. Pathologic mechanisms affecting the skin of the animal have the same effect in the epithelial tube lining the ear canal. Not all cases of otitis externa are infected with bacteria or yeasts and it is a challenge for the clinician to seek out these cases and to treat them appropriately.

THE FOUR-STEP APPROACH TO OTITIS EXTERNA

1. Examination of Skin and Ears

It is always important to look at the overall patient. Checking the skin for problems may alert the clinician to potential primary causes for the ear disease. Classic signs of atopy may be noted or there may be symmetrical alopecia suggesting hypothyroidism. Then the ear canal should be examined for exudates, growths, or other pathological changes. The eardrum should always be evaluated because the choice of medications and flushing agents will depend on the integrity of the eardrum.

2. Cytologic Evaluation of Otic Exudate

The next step in approaching ear disease is examining a cytologic preparation of the otic exudate. Cytologic examination of every infected ear should be done routinely.

A sample is obtained with the use of a small-tipped cotton applicator. The swab is placed through a disinfected otoscope cone placed into the vertical ear canal near the junction with the horizontal canal. The swab is extended beyond the plastic cone and pressure is applied to the ear canal epithelium as the swab is withdrawn back through the cone. In this manner, packing of wax and exudate is minimal. Every attempt is made to sample only from the horizontal canal epithelium because the vertical canal is often contaminated with a number of commensal organisms unrelated to the ear disease.

The swab is then rolled onto a new, clean microscope slide by rolling the harvested material from the left ear on the left side of the slide and the swab from the right ear on the right side of the slide. The slide is labeled with the patient's name and the date of the sample. The slide is heat fixed and stained with blood stain (Diff-Quick or Wright-Giemsa). After the slide is dried, a drop of slide mounting medium (Cytoseal 60, Stephens Scientific) is applied and a coverslip placed over the material. In this manner a permanent slide is made. A drop of mineral oil can be spread on the stained slide if permanent slides are not desired. This standardized approach to making slides allows uniform identification of organisms from each ear and allows comparison of ear cytology from visit to visit.

To look for ear mites under the microscope, the ear swabs are rolled in a drop of mineral oil on a microscope slide and coverslipped. Low-power (40x–100x) examination reveals mites crawling across the field and/or the typical oblong dark brown *Otodectes* eggs may be seen.

Evaluation of slides should begin with a low-power (100x) overview of cell types. If there are large numbers of epithelial cells and few microorganisms, then noninfectious causes of otitis such as seborrheic diseases and hypothyroidism should be considered. Sheets of epithelial cells may indicate neoplasia as the cause of otitis externa and the presence of numerous intact nonstaining epithelial cells may indicate a seborrheic condition. Inflammatory cells and acantholytic cells may indicate autoimmune disease. High-power (400x) examination is needed to characterize bacteria and yeasts. Large numbers of bacteria and/or yeasts indicate secondary invaders. When neutrophils are seen in addition to bacteria or yeasts, deep infection must be considered. Ear mites are not often seen on stained ear swabs, but the eggs may be found on mineral oil preparations.

When infectious organisms are seen on high power (400x) cocci are usually staphylococci, and rods are usually *Pseudomonas* or *Proteus*. Budding yeasts of *Malassezia* may be seen individually in the background on a roll smear, but large numbers of yeasts colonizing on exfoliated epithelial cells are indicative of secondary yeast infection. Staphylococci and Malassezia are often found together in the same ear, and there is evidence to suggest that *Malassezia* growth is stimulated by staphylococci.

In ear disease, many antibiotics reported as sensitive may not penetrate into the ear when administered parenterally. Topical antibiotics can achieve significantly higher concentrations in the ear canal than the minimum inhibitory concentration (MIC). The high topical antibiotic concentration may actually be effective at killing a bacteria that was reported as resistant

3. Cleaning the Ears – See the following article in this proceedings for notes on ear cleaning techniques.

4. Guidelines for Treatment of Acute Otitis Externa

A treatment plan be formulated that is tailored specifically to the patient after the skin and ears are evaluated, the cytology is done, and the ear canal is cleansed.

Corticosteroids have a definite place in the treatment of otitis externa. Systemic corticosteroids reduce the intense pruritus associated with acute otitis externa and reduce the inflammation in the epithelium of the ear canal. Systemic high doses of corticosteroids (1 mg per pound prednisone orally daily) are used for several days to reduce the edema and stenosis that prevents adequate examination of the ear canal. Dexamethasone injection given at a dose of 0.1 mg per pound also helps decrease otic inflammation with fewer side effects. If the ear canal is patent, then a potent topical corticosteroid such as dexamethasone, betamethasone, or fluocinolone may be used to relieve the intense pain and itching. A relatively new corticosteroid, mometasone (Mometamax, Schering-Plough), has been introduced to decrease the systemic effects of topical otic corticosteroids.

As the otitis resolves, a less potent corticosteroid such as 1% hydrocortisone may be used in the ear to act as a preventative for inflammation in atopic dogs that may have recurrent otitis. Corticosteroids do not remove hyperplastic epithelium or glands, so if there is no response to high-dose corticosteroids after 7 to 10 days, the stenosis is probably the result of increased tissue growth rather than inflammation.

Antibiotics that kill staphylococci, *Pseudomonas,* and other gram-negative bacteria are used in many otic preparations. Although antimicrobial therapy may temporarily relieve the symptoms of otitis externa, the symptoms may recur unless the underlying disease is identified and treated as well. These infectious organisms are considered to be perpetuating factors in ear disease.

Topical otic formulations are made with combinations of pharmaceuticals such as antifungals, corticosteroids, insecticides, and topical anesthetics. First-line antibiotics such as gentamycin, amikacin, neomycin, and polymyxin B are potentially ototoxic, so if there is no tympanic membrane (TM), these antibiotics should be avoided. In addition, neomycin has been implicated as a sensitizer in contact dermatitis in the ear. If the ear becomes worse with neomycin treatment, the antibiotic should be stopped immediately. Tobramycin (0.3% ophthalmic drops) is safer to use instead of other topical aminoglycosides if the status of the TM is unknown. Ceftazidime (Fortaz, Sandoz) injectible (50 mg/mL) solution is safe and effective against a wide variety of bacteria

Baytril Otic (Bayer) has recently been introduced. It is a solution that contains 0.5% enrofloxacin and 1% silver sulfadiazine. The high concentration of enrofloxacin has been demonstrated in vitro to provide a high enough concentration to be effective against most bacteria. However, there are a number of fluoroquinolone-resistant *Pseudomonas* bacteria being found, and so this product is not recommended for first-line use in

Pseudomonas infections. Its use should be based on demonstration of susceptibility of the organism to enrofloxacin. Silver sulfadiazine may have some use against the yeasts in the ear.

Systemic antibiotics may be useful in some suppurative otitis externa cases as an adjunct to ear cleansing and topical antibiotic therapy. Culture and sensitivity should be reserved for those otitis cases that are unresponsive to topical therapy because the sensitivity results are often misleading, since they are based on BLOOD levels, not topical levels. If there is severe inflammation with inflammatory cells present on otic cytology, then using intracellular antibiotics like fluoroquinolones, azithromycin, or clindamycin may increase the success of systemic treatment.

Another useful compound as an adjunct in gram-negative ear infections is Tris-EDTA solution (TrizEDTA, DermaPet). EDTA chelates metal ions, such as calcium and magnesium, which are necessary to maintain the integrity of the cell membrane. The cell membrane of these bacteria becomes more porous so that the antibiotic can diffuse into the bacteria and kill it. Tris buffer keeps the ear canal at pH of 8.0, which is optimum for function of the aminoglycosides and fluoroquinolones. Tris-EDTA alone has been shown in vitro to have potent bactericidal effects. It has also been shown to irreversibly bind to the destructive elastase enzyme released from gram-negative bacteria. Clinically, Tris-EDTA is used as a pretreatment flush in the external ear 5 minutes prior to the instillation of topical antibiotics. Usually treatment is done on a twice-daily basis. Because of the high pH of Tris-EDTA, Malassezia infections may worsen when Tris-EDTA is inappropriately used in this infection.

Ear mite treatment can be done using selamectin (Revolution, Pfizer) twice a month or injectable cattle ivermectin (0.1 cc subcutaneously every 2 weeks). In young kittens otic 0.01% ivermectin (Acarexx, Idexx)) or 0.1% milbemycin (Milbemite, Novartis) are safe to use. Many topical ear mite drops containing insecticides are also available for ear mite treatment.

Alterations in cerumen lipid composition caused by underlying skin diseases such as food sensitivities, atopy, or hypothyroidism may play a role in Malassezia otitis externa. Low levels of free fatty acids in surface lipids coupled with increased levels of surface triglycerides favors Malassezia infection. Inflammatory diseases of the ear cause increases in the amount of sebaceous secretion and increases in the number and amount of lipid secretion from the apocrine (cerumen) glands. In addition to the liquid yellow-colored lipids secreted, an increased amount of humidity results. It has been shown that over 50% of atopic dogs have elevated Malassezia populations on their skin.

To remove these lipid substrates from the ear and to treat otitis externa complicated by Malassezia, the author prefers to clean the ear in the hospital first and then prescribes home use of an acetic acid/boric acid solution (Malacetic Otic, DermaPet). Acetic acid degreases the ear canal and boric acid keeps the epithelium relatively dehydrated. A topical solution of miconizole or clotrimizole may be used in the ear canal after cleaning. In addition to ear cleaners, systemic oral ketoconazole or itraconizole is useful for refractory yeast otitis cases or for yeast otitis cases where there is also stenosis. These systemic compounds may reduce the pruritus associated with the yeasts, but they have not been shown to reduce otic yeast numbers.

In mild cases of Malassezia otitis externa, the external canal can be cleaned by the owner at home to facilitate removal of excessive exudate accumulation associated with otitis externa. Acidic ear cleaners with a pH of less than 5.5 inhibit yeast growth. The ear cleaner or flush is used daily for 7 to 10 days by filling the ear canal to overflowing, massaging the base of the ear, and allowing the solution to remain in the ear canal for 5 minutes. The loosened debris is wiped off of the concave pinnal surface with a dry cotton ball. This procedure is repeated once daily. When the ear canal is clean, the cotton ball will remain fairly white when the solution is wiped away. At that time, home ear cleaning is reduced to once weekly.

Malassezia otitis is secondary to a primary skin disease, so during the maintenance phase of treatment, the underlying skin condition needs to be identified and treated. Failure to resolve the primary cause of the otitis results in chronic Malassezia ear infections.

EAR CLEANING TECHNIQUES

Louis N. Gotthelf, DVM
Animal Hospital of Montgomery
Montgomery, AL

When exudates and excessive cerumen accumulate in the ear, removal of these secretions is an essential part of good ear therapy. Many veterinarians skip this important step. Ear cleaning techniques can be very profitable in addition to just being good medicine.

Ear cleaning by itself can contribute to healing and reduction of inflammation by removing many of the chemicals and organisms that contribute to the disease process. Enzymes such as collagenase and lysozyme cause problems in the ear and their removal decreases the cytopathic effect on the ear canal epidermis. Cytokines found in the exudates recruit inflammatory mediators. Volatile fatty acids in ceruminous ears directly increase inflammation. Once these compounds are removed, resolution of the ear disease may result. Sometimes ear cleaning will help dislodge a foreign body, like plant awns, from the ear canal.

After the primary cause of the ear disease and the type of infection present, if any, are determined, the next step is to anesthetize the patient so that a thorough cleaning of the ear canal can be done. The depth of anesthesia should be deep, since the ear canal is highly innervated. A light plane of anesthesia will result in the patient shaking the head during the procedure. An endotracheal tube is placed so that if the eardrum is ruptured, material will not be aspirated from drainage through the auditory tube into the retropharynx. If the procedure is long, gas anesthetics can easily be connected.

Good visualization of the ear canal after flushing helps to ensure that the vertical and horizontal canals are clean and free of debris. Irregularities of the ear canal can be seen after cleaning. Ulcers, fissures, folds, tumors, hyperplastic glands and polyps may be uncovered after cleaning. The efficacy of otic medications is enhanced when they are applied directly onto the cleaned epithelial surface.

When the ear(s) are so filled with wax and debris that there is occlusion of the canal, the exudates and wax must be removed prior to treatment. Vertical ear cleaning is very easily accomplished, but it is a challenge to make sure that the horizontal canal is clean and that the eardrum is intact. There are two types of cleaning that need to be done in the ear. When the eardrum cannot be visualized, mechanical cleaning should be done first to physically remove the debris. After the eardrum has been seen and it determined to be normal, then chemicals can be used in the ear canal to hasten the cleaning process.

MECHANICAL CLEANING

Cotton swabs or Q-tips should not be used in the ear canal for cleaning. The abrasive cotton swab can ulcerate a friable ear canal if used in an in/out or rotating manner. Due to the funnel shape of the ear canal, debris will be pushed forward as the swab is advanced into the small diameter of the horizontal canal and can result in packing the debris into the horizontal canal or pushing it through a ruptured eardrum into the bulla. There are some uses for cotton-tipped applicators. The absorbent cotton material may help remove liquid in the ear canal. The swab is laid onto the canal and removed when saturated. The abrasive action may be useful for laser procedures in the ear canal to help remove the char, a byproduct of laser dessication. Ear swabs are also used to get cytological samples from the ear canal.

Buck ear curettes are useful for scraping the ear canal to dislodge large pieces of wax and epithelial shreds. These atraumatic, blunt curettes are available in various loop sizes and angles and some have a circular cutting surface (Dermal Curette), which helps cut or remove a piece of a tumor for histopathology. Ear loops consisting of a loop of wire at the end of a handle are also available. Curettes are useful for harvesting cells for cytology when a tumor mass is suspected. Some curettes have a handle on them for blind curetting in the ear canal, but with the use of the video-otoscope, curettes are designed with long, narrow shafts to back load into the 2-mm channel of the otoscope probe (Ear Curette Set, C-Med Surgical). That way, the curetting is done under video visualization.

Many instruments are used in the ear canal, such as alligator forceps and hemostats, but because they are used blindly, extra caution should be taken to prevent excessive trauma and eardrum rupture. Endoscopic instruments are used through the video-otoscope. Grasping forceps are the most useful to remove foreign material or hairs. Instrumentation used in this manner is very precise, atraumatic, and is viewed on the video monitor.

Warm water or saline solution under pressure is used frequently to remove material in the ear canal. Bulb syringes and syringe/catheter combinations are fine for flushing large pieces of debris. Water picks have also been employed for this purpose. A new instrument has been designed to provide independent flushing and suctioning pressures (Ear-I-Gator, MedRx) for "pressure washing" the ear canal. Using a two channel hose, trumpet valves for suction and flush are connected to a common port. This port accommodates the flanged end of a catheter so that the catheter can be introduced into the ear canal. This is usually done with a 5-French polypropylene urethral catheter with the closed end cut off that is threaded through the 2-mm working channel of the video-otoscope. Precise flushing and suctioning of debris can be accomplished with the open ended urethral catheter. In addition, a constant high flush pressure dilates the ear canal making examination of the deeper structures easier.

CHEMICAL CLEANING

Care must be taken in the selection of a flushing agent, since so many ear cleaners contain materials that are potentially ototoxic when the eardrum is not intact. Prior to using an ear cleaner, read the label to see if it can be used if the eardrum is damaged. Many manufacturers are now placing a warning on their labels that says "Caution: Do Not Use if the Eardrum Is Ruptured."

With so many products available to veterinarians for ear care, it is important to understand that these products often fall into one of three categories. *Cerumenolytics* are detergents that emulsify ear wax for easy removal. *Ear flushes* are liquids that aid in removing pus, mucus, and serum from the ears. *Drying agents* decrease moisture in the ears and desiccate the surface keratinocytes. Moisture is a predisposing factor allowing growth of organisms in the ear canal. Many ear products also contain steroids, antibacterials, and antifungals. Prior to using these products, understanding the activity of each of the components of these compounds aids the veterinarian in determining which situations are appropriate for different products.

Until a determination of the integrity of the eardrum is made, the choice of flushing solutions should be limited to non-detergent, non-alcoholic type of flushing solutions. Physiologic saline and dilute povidone iodine are safe flushing materials to use if the eardrum is not intact or its integrity is suspect. When used as warm solutions (98°F) these solutions act to soften wax and loosen other debris.

When using a cerumenolytic compound, like dioctyl sodium sulfosuccinate (DSS)(KlearWax, DermaPet), which is almost universally used as an otic detergent, water must be used with it. It is helpful to put the cerumenolytic in the ear canal, add some water, massage the ears, and let the detergent work for a minimum of 5 minutes. Then the emulsified material can be easily washed out of the ear. All of the detergent should be flushed out with a large volume of water including that in the horizontal canal. Based on otic examination, this process may need repeating if there is still debris in the ear canal. DSS ear flushes should not be dispensed to owners because they cannot remove all of the detergent properly. They should not be used if the eardrum is ruptured because of ototoxicity. In the event an ear cleaner is required with a ruptured eardrum, a product containing squalene (Cerumene, Evsco) can be safely used.

After the flushing procedure, all liquid should be removed by suction from the ear canal. This will allow re-examination of the ear canal and will allow topical medication to be put on the surface epithelium.

HOME EAR CLEANING

Numerous products are available for maintenance ear cleaning by the owners at home. Because exudates and waxes will continue to accumulate in the ear canal during therapy of ear disease, some home care is required. During the course of therapy, which may be 2 to 3 weeks, home products are used two or three times daily, followed by antimicrobial ear medications, but after this time, their frequent use will contribute to maceration of the ear canal. Keeping ear cleaning chemicals in the ear prevents normal cerumen from coating the ear canal epithelium. Cerumen provides a protective moisture barrier to prevent excessive moisture from damaging the ear canal cells. Re-examination and cytology after 2 weeks will give information as to continued frequent use of a home ear product. If the ear canal is healing and is quiet, once or twice weekly ear cleaning may be needed.

MANAGING DIFFICULT EAR INFECTIONS

James O. Noxon, DVM. Diplomate ACVIM
College of Veterinary Medicine
Iowa State University, Ames, IA

Bacterial infections of the ear are considered perpetuating factors. In other words, they are secondary to some condition or event that initiates inflammation. Bacterial ear infections are common problems in dogs, and although present in cats, are much less common. The bacteria isolated most often from inflamed ears of the dog are *Staphylococcus intermedius* and *Pseudomonas aeruginosa*. Other bacteria that may be isolated include: *Escherichia coli*, *Proteus* spp, other staphylococcal species, *Klebsiella* spp, *Enterococcus* spp, *Corynebacterium* spp, streptococci, *Clostridium* spp, and other bacteria on occasion.

GENERAL RULES OF ENGAGEMENT

The successful management of any ear disease requires the following:

1. **Cleaning the ear canal.** At some point in the management of otitis externa or media, the canal should be thoroughly cleaned. This will allow better evaluation of the extent of the problem and remove debris (eg, wax, hair) that will interfere with distribution, and possibly activation, of medications instilled into the ear. Some ear cleansers, such as those containing lactic acid and salicylic acid (EpiOtic, Virbac), have some antibacterial properties, which may also help resolve some bacterial ear infections.

2. **Clear identification of the organism(s) involved.** In some cases, such as when cocci are the only organisms involved and for first time otitis cases, cytology may be sufficient to identify the types of organisms involved.

   Bacterial culture is indicated when 1) cytology reveals only rod-shaped bacteria, 2) the condition is a recurring infection and organisms of any type are seen on cytology, 3) the infection has failed to respond to appropriate medications (and owner compliance has been good), and 4) when otitis media is present.

3. Glucocorticoids are usually helpful. Glucocorticoids have anti-inflammatory effects, and therefore reduce inflammation, reduce edema and swelling to allow topical medications better access in the canal, and reduce pain and pruritus associated with inflammation (allowing better patient compliance with application of medications). Glucocorticoids may be applied topically and/or systemically depending on the severity of the hyperplastic changes, pain, and owners' abilities to apply medications.

4. **Hyperplastic changes should be addressed immediately.** Severe hyperplastic changes interfere with application of topical medications and trap exudate and debris in the ear canal.

Patients with hyperplastic changes are treated with oral prednisone (at 1–2 mg/kg, PO daily for 7–10 days, then every other day for 5–7 doses), topical glucocorticoids (eg, flucinolone plus DMSO), and/or intralesional glucocorticoids (eg, triamcinolone) if the changes result in complete closure of the ear canal.

PHARMACOLOGIC CONSIDERATIONS

Antimicrobial therapy may be delivered systemically or topically. The advantage clinicians have in the management of ear infections is the option to deliver the medication by the topical route. This allows us to: 1) deliver the medication directly to the area affected, and 2) to deliver the antimicrobial agent in concentrations that greatly exceed concentrations that can be achieved by systemic routes. This is especially of interest when considering the use of concentration-dependent antibiotics, such as fluoroquinolones or aminoglycosides.

Because of the topical option available to manage otitis externa and media, bacterial culture and susceptibility data often misrepresent the effectiveness of an antimicrobial agent for ear infections. Minimum inhibitory concentrations are of the greatest value since they may indicate that an antibiotic cannot achieve inhibitory concentrations, even at the highest concentrations reached by instilling concentrated antibiotics directly into the ear. In contrast, Kirby-Bauer results will provide information on the resistance or susceptibility of an organism based on known or extrapolated breakpoint concentrations, which may be greatly exceeded by the direct instillation of drug into the ear.

Important Concept: an antibiotic may still be effective in treating a bacterial skin infection, even though a culture and susceptibility test (using Kirby-Bauer methods) indicates that the organism is resistant to that drug.

In addition, the location of the infection within the ear plays an important role in management of the infection. Middle ear infections (ie, otitis media) generally require thorough cleaning of that ear cavity to facilitate treatment. Certainly, infections within the middle ear are more difficult to reach with topical medications, though that also depends on the integrity of the tympanic membrane. Topical medications may reach the middle ear if the ear drum is ruptured; however, it is appropriate to employ systemic therapy in those cases, as well as any topical treatment that might be indicated.

VETERINARY FORMULATIONS

There are a limited number of veterinary otic products for use in dogs and cats (Table 1). The antibacterial agents found in products available in the United States include antibiotics (gentamicin, enrofloxacin, neomycin, thiostrepton) and antiseptics (aluminum acetate, acetic acid). Antimicrobials found in commercial otic preparations outside the US include polymyxin B sulfates, norfloxacin, marbofloxacin, and fusidic acid. In addition, there are several veterinary products that are used in the ear canal, even though they are not labeled for use in the ear. These products have not undergone the requirements for labeling and are generally labeled as "lotions" or "flushes." Since there are so few commercial otic products for veterinarians to use in bacterial ear infections, a large number of "homemade" formulations have been promoted at continuing education seminars and are spread by word of mouth throughout the veterinary community. Certainly, many of these work very well; however, the majority have not been tested for safety or to ensure that the active ingredients have remained active when mixed with other products.

BASIC THERAPEUTICS

Overall success of antibacterial therapy depends upon the following factors:

- The efficacy of the active ingredients
- Route of administration of anti-bacterial medications
- Removal of obstructions (eg, wax, hair) from the ear canal (topical)
- The technique used to instill topical medications (topical)
- The formulation of the medication (topical)
- The volume of medication instilled (topical)
- The integrity of the tympanic membrane (topical)
- Treatment duration

In all cases when topical therapy is used, the owners MUST be educated about application of medications. This should include having the owner instill medication, IN THE PRESENCE of the veterinarian or technician. Owners should massage ears for 15 to 30 seconds after instilling medication and to use proper amounts of medications.

Ear medications are most often in the form of an ointment (emulsions of lipid in water) or as a solution (aqueous or other carriers). Emulsions containing lipids will enhance penetration of the active ingredient into the skin of the ear, however, most of these ointment formulations are so viscous, that they fail to penetrate down deep into the ear canal. They are especially ineffective in the presence of a heavy growth of hair in the canal. Less viscous medications are more likely to allow medication to distribute deeper into the canal, especially when there is significant hair in the ear canal or when the canal is hyperplastic.

Once-daily treatment is generally sufficient for most cases of otitis, though severe infections *may* benefit from twice daily treatment. Treatment should be continued until there is no clinical or cytologic evidence of active disease. The minimum recommended treatment time (with topical therapy) is 30 days.

Volume of medication: The volume of medication applied into the ear during treatment appears to be *critical*. Enough medication should be applied to ensure delivery to the deepest part of the ear canal (by the tympanum). Failure to apply sufficient quantities to penetrate to these areas seems to be a major cause of treatment failure.

Recommended volumes:

< 10 kg	0.4–0.5 mL
10–20 kg	0.5–0.7 mL
> 20 kg	0.7–1.0 mL

The integrity of the tympanic membrane is critical in determining the best treatment   medication is instilled directly into the middle ear. To the author's knowledge, no commercial ear medications have been evaluated for the potential to cause ototoxicosis if the medication is instilled into the middle ear. The best practice is to avoid topical therapy, if the tympanic membrane is torn or absent. However, there are some clinical indications, based entirely on anecdotal evidence, that vinegar: water (1:2), dilute ticarcillin (3%) in saline, dilute enrofloxacin, and enrofloxacin (parenteral formulation) are anecdotally considered safe in dogs.

SYSTEMIC THERAPY

Topical therapy is considered sufficient to manage most bacterial infections of the external ear canal, if the above recommendations are followed. Systemic therapy is indicated when:

- The infections are recurring and severe
- There are concurrent infections elsewhere, such as the skin, that are caused by the same organism
- When owners are incapable of instilling topical medications (eg, elderly, arthritis)
- When the patient is uncooperative due to pain or temperament
- When there are severe hyperplastic changes in the ear canal that preclude the ability of topical medications to distribute deep into the canal
- When inflammatory cells are abundant on cytology
- When otitis media is present

In general, the choice of antimicrobial for systemic therapy may be based on historical evidence of efficacy for staphylococci, though these organisms can develop resistance to the commonly used antibiotics. Culture and sensitivity data should be used to help select the best antimicrobial for systemic therapy against *Pseudomonas* bacteria.

Pseudomonas Otitis

Pseudomonas ear infections are often considered the most difficult of ear infections to clear. Unfortunately, there are very few studies of topical and/or systemic therapies that provide sufficient evidence of the efficacy of the many options for treatment of *Pseudomonas* ear infections that are discussed in the literature. However, several therapeutic options are considered clinically effective for these infections, despite the lack of good studies to support that clinical impression. Some treatment options include:

- Topicals containing polymyxin B (Ak-Trol®, Akorn: neomycin, polymyxin B sulfates & 0.1% dexamethasone ophthalmic solution) or (Neomycin and polymyxin B sulfates and 1% hydrocortisone Otic Solution, Bausch & Lomb). May be useful to pre-treat with Tris-EDTA. Most *Pseudomonas* isolates are very sensitive to this antibiotic; however, polymyxin is not active in suppurative environments, so it is important to clean the ear thoroughly before using this antibiotic.

- Topical tobramycin (available as generic ophthalmic drops). Other aminogylcosides, including gentamicin and amikacin, are often effective for *Pseudomonas* infections. Ototoxicity is a potential problem with aminogylcosides. These agents should not be used if the ear drum is ruptured.

- Topical fluoroquinolone antibiotics, such as Baytril Otic (Bayer) (containing enrofloxacin and silver sulfadiazine). Enrofloxacin remains a very effective antibiotic for the treatment of *Pseudomonas* infections. Remember, susceptibility data may be misleading because the concentrations of enrofloxacin achieved in the ear can greatly exceed the serum concentrations.

- Silver sulfadiazine (SSD) has been demonstrated in vitro to be highly effective against resistant strains of *Pseudomonas*. SSD is commercially available as a 1% cream, which may be diluted 1:9 in water, and as a 1% solution in Baytril.

- Topical ticarcillin-clavulinic acid (Timentin®-SmithKlineGlaxo) or ticarcillin (Ticar®-SKG. This antibiotic retains activity for 24 to 36 hours at room temperature or when refrigerated.

> AT ISU, we will take one 3.1 g vial of Timentin and dilute it with 100 mL of sterile saline. 1.0 mL aliquots of the 3% suspension are drawn into individual syringes (with about 0.5 mL of air) and the syringes are frozen. The content of one syringe is instilled into each infected ear twice daily (thus....four syringes daily for bilateral disease). Each vial of Timentin will make enough medication to treat a dog with bilateral disease for 25 days. Frozen ticarcillin will remain active for approximately 30 days.

- Tris-EDTA solution: Two commercial products (TrizEDTA™, DermaPet, T8™-DVM) contain this solution. There is good evidence that the T8 solution is more appropriate for staphylococcal infections, while both the T8 Solution and Triz-EDTA are highly effective for *Pseudomonas* infections. These products are usually administering into the infected ear 15 to 30 minutes prior to an antibiotic. They are well-documented to enhance the activity of some antibiotics, especially aminoglycosides and fluoroquinolones.

Systemic antibiotic therapy (eg, marbofloxacin) is indicated for otitis media when the tympanic membrane is intact. Systemic medications are generally not highly effective if used without concurrent topical antimicrobial therapy. If it is completely absent, thorough middle ear flushing is recommended. Antibiotics, such as ticarcillin and enrofloxacin, may be infused directly into the middle ear. (There are not studies to confirm their safety when used in this manner, but there is abundant anecdotal evidence to suggest these drugs are safe when infused directly into the middle ear.)

One very important key to successful treatment of *Pseudomonas* otitis is the concurrent use of glucocorticoids, preferably systemically. Glucocorticoids reduce the pain that is associated with this condition- and thus will make application of topical medications easier and more effective. In addition, glucocorticoids reduce the inflammation, which also reduces the discomfort ant swelling that accompanies this condition. Naturally, any allergy testing should be done *prior* to initiation of glucocorticoid therapy.

> KEY Point: Glucocorticoid therapy is an important and necessary component of the treatment of *Pseudomonas* infections of the external ear canal!

Of course, proper cleansing of the ear, systemic therapy with an appropriate antimicrobial agent, and management of the primary factor are also part of managing *Pseudomonas* infections of the ear!

> KEY Point: Patients with *Pseudomonas* infections tend to get other secondary infections, most often yeast infections, immediately after the *Pseudomonas* is cleared. This is probably because application of topical medications to clear the bacterial infection tends to leave the inflamed ear moist, and thus more susceptible to yeast infections. Therefore, we recommend prophylactic anti-yeast therapy be initiated as soon as the bacterial component of the otitis is controlled.

SUMMARY

Bacterial infections of the ear may be successfully managed if the above principles are followed. The keys include: thorough cleaning of the ear canal and middle ear (if necessary), identification of the causative organism through cytology and/or culture, selection of an appropriate antimicrobial agent and delivery system, proper application of medicine into the ear, identification and control of the primary and other perpetuating factors, and good follow-up otic care.

Table 1. Veterinary Products Used to Treat Otitis Externa *

Name	Antibacterial Agent(s)	Other Ingredients	Drops / mL	Recommended Dosing	Maximum Duration
Animax	Neomycin Thiostrepton	Nystatin Triamcinolone	49	3–5 drops Variable frequency	Variable
Baytril Otic	Enrofloxacin Silver sulfadiazine		30	< 35 lbs: 5-10 d. bid > 35 lbs: 10-15 d. bid	14 days
Bur-Otic HC	Aluminum acetate	Hydrocortisone Propylene glycol	38	5 – 10 drops daily	5 days
Conofite *	Miconazole		44	"light covering"	NG
MalAcetic HC	Acetic acid Boric acid	Hydrocortisone	41	"apply liberally"	NG
Mometamax	Gentamicin	Clotrimazole Mometasone	40	< 30 lbs: 4 drops daily > 30 lbs: 8 drops daily	7 days
Otomax †	Gentamicin	Clotrimazole Betamethasone	37	< 30 lbs: 4 drops daily > 30 lbs: 8 drops daily	7 days
SynOtic		Flucinolone Dimethyl sulfoxide Propylene glycol	39	4–6 drops bid	14 days
T8 Keto*		Tris EDTA Ketoconazole	24	"flush liberally"	NG
Tresaderm	Neomycin	Thiabendazole Dexamethasone Propylene glycol	40	5–15 drops bid	7 days
Triz EDTA Ultra+Keto*		Tris EDTA Ketoconazole	23	"apply liberally"	NG

Products with asterisks are NOT labeled for use in ears, but are often recommended for use in otitis.
† = Similar products are available from various companies, but were not evaluated.
NG = not given.

REFERENCES
1. Morris DO. Medical therapy of otitis externa and otitis media Vet Clin North Am. 2004;34:541-555.
2. Hariharan H, Coles M, Poole D, et al. Update on antimicrobial susceptibilities of bacterial isolates from canine and feline otitis externa. Can Vet J. 2006;47:253-255.
3. Cole LK, Kwochka KW, Kowalski JJ, et al. Microbial flora and antimicrobial susceptibility patterns of isolated pathogens from the horizontal ear canal and middle ear in dogs with otitis media. J Am Vet Med Assoc. 1998;212:534-538.
4. Cole LK, Kwochka KW, Kowalski JJ, et al. Evaluation of an ear cleaner for the treatment of infectious otitis externa in dogs. Vet Therap. 2003;4:12-23.
5. Nuttall T, Cole LK. Evidence-based veterinary dermatology: a systematic review of interventions for treatment of Pseudomonas otitis in dogs. Vet Dermatol. 2007;18:69-142.
6. Barrasa JLM, Gómez PL, Lama PG, et al. Antibacterial susceptibility patterns of Pseudomonas strains isolated from chronic canine otitis externa. J Vet Med. 2000; 17:191-196.
7. Noxon JO, Kinyon JM, Murphy DP. Minimal inhibitory Concentrations of Silver Sulfadiazine on Pseudomonas aeruginsa and Staphylococcus intermedius Isolates from the Ears of Dogs with Otitis Externa. 13th Proceedings Annual Members' Meeting of the ACVD/AAVD, Nashville, TN, April 18, 1997, pp 72-73.
8. Nuttell TJ. Use of ticarcillin in the management of canine otitis externa complicated by Pseudomonas aeruginosa. J Small Anim Pract. 1998;39:165-168.
9. Farca AM, Piromalli G, Maffei F et al. Potentiating effect of EDTA-Tris on the activity of antibiotics against resistant bacteria associated with otitis, dermatitis, and cystitis. J Small Anim Pract. 1997;38:243-245.
10. Carlotti DN, Guaguère E, Koch HJ, et al. Marbofloxacin for the systemic treatment of Pseudomonas spp. suppurative otitis externa in the dog. In: von Tscharner C, Kwochka KW, Wilemse T (eds.): Advances in Veterinary Dermatology 3. Oxford: Butterworth Heinemann, 1998, pp 463-464.

HOW TO APPROACH A CASE OF CHRONIC OTITIS

Rod A.W. Rosychuk DVM, Diplomate ACVIM
College of Veterinary Medicine and Biomedical Sciences
Colorado State University, Ft. Collins, CO

When working towards diagnosing and treating a case of chronic otitis externa, it becomes imperative to recall the factors that are responsible for the generation of otitis externa. Primary factors are those which are responsible for initiating inflammation in ears. Atopy is the most common primary factor encountered in the dog and the most common cause of chronicity with respect to otitis. Less commonly encountered, but still important canine primary factors include food sensitivity, foreign body, hypothyroidism (causing ceruminous otitis), primary idiopathic seborrhea (causing ceruminous otitis), ceruminous cysts, and neoplasia. Although other primary factors, such as zinc-responsive dermatosis and autoimmune diseases (eg, pemphigus), may also cause otitis, they are usually a relatively minor part of a more generalized skin disease. The list of primary factors in the cat includes ear mites, atopy, food sensitivity, foreign body, idiopathic ceruminous otitis, aural polyps, ceruminous cysts, neoplasia. Perpetuating factors are those that keep inflammation active within ears, even if the primary factor has been removed /resolved. These factors are definite contributors to chronicity and may indeed be the factors responsible for making an otitis case chronic. They include secondary infections (*Malasssezia*, bacteria), proliferative changes, debris within ears (eg, ceruminoliths) and medication issues (overtreatment, undertreatment and reactions to medications). The accumulation of significant amounts of debris within ears perpetuates otitis in that debris can be a source of irritation, can serve as a nidus for infection and can prevent medications from getting to where they should in the ear. Proliferative changes produce a microenvironment that can harbor debris and micro-organisms. The presence of a concurrent otitis media will potentially "re-seed" the canals with organisms, even if the canals have been well managed with topical therapy. Over-treatment may macerate the epithelial lining of the ear, producing chronic, low-grade inflammation. Reactions to medications (eg, propylene glycol) may also perpetuate inflammation within ears.

PATHOPHYSIOLOGY OF OTITIS EXTERNA

The pathologic changes associated with otitis externa in some ways tend to be relatively similar, regardless of the underlying primary cause. However, the degree of change (eg, ceruminous gland hyperplasia, ectasia, and fibrosis) may vary with the breed.

With more acute otitis, there is edema and inflammatory cell infiltrate within the dermis. With chronicity, the epidermis becomes hyperplastic and potentially thrown in to folds (ie, papillary hyperplasia). With chronicity, sebaceous glands may increase in numbers, remain the same or decrease in numbers. Chronic inflammation may result in ceruminous glands becoming widely dilated. This contributes to dermal thickening and narrowing of the lumen. Dilated ceruminous glands may appear as small "bumps" on the surface of the canals (giving the lining of the ear a "cobblestone" or "chicken skin" like appearance). Dermal inflammation around apocrine glands, combined with epidermal hyperplasia may result in occlusion of ductal openings and predispose to gland rupture. This appears to contribute significantly to inflammation, fibrosis and pain.

Folliculitis may proceed to a furunculosis and its attendant dermal inflammation. With chronicity, the dermis may develop significant fibrosis, which contributes to the tissue thickening seen with chronic otitis.

In some individuals, canal thickening is diffuse and results in stenosis of the horizontal and/or vertical canals. In others, the ear will throw up proliferative nodules that occlude the horizontal canal (eg, Cocker spaniel).

With severe, chronic, deep-seated inflammation, there is a tendency to have the soft tissues of the ear calcify. This calcification is considered to be a permanent change and contributes to permanent stenosis within the ear.

It would appear that the cocker spaniel is more likely to develop ceruminous gland hyperplasia and dilatation (ectasia) with chronic inflammation and have relatively less firbrosis. In other breeds, dermal fibrosis tends to predominate. The cocker spaniel tends to develop soft tissue calcification more rapidly and frequently than other breeds.

APPROACH
Find and Resolve or Control Primary Factors

When diagnosing and managing a case of chronic otitis, major emphasis must be placed on defining an underlying primary factor, if possible. Emphasis is placed on:

1. **History**
   a. **Seasonality** – If otitis is seasonal, suggests atopy
   b. **Unilateral vs. bilateral** – Unilateral problems suggest foreign bodies, chronic infections that have not been adequately dealt with, ceruminous cysts, polyps, or neoplasia. Bilateral problems are more likely to be associated with atopy, food sensitivity, hypothyroidism, idiopathic seborrhea in the dog and ear mites, atopy or food sensitivity in the cat. However, it is important to note that allergic disease (atopy and food sensitivity) in both the dog and cat can be predominantly unilateral in some individuals.
   c. **Owners observation of more generalized skin disease.** In the dog, more generalized pruritus (foot, flank or perineum) suggests atopy or food sensitivity. Many atopic dogs will have recurrent or chronic otitis as the first sign of their atopic otitis externa, but, usually within months, they will develop more generalized signs of pruritus. Food sensitive individuals may also follow this pattern. However, up to 20% of the patients that are

diagnosed with food sensitivities will have otitis externa as the only sign of their allergy – ie, with no more generalized signs of pruritus noted. If the problem is restricted to the ears over long periods of time (eg, 1–2 years), food sensitivity would therefore become a more likely diagnosis than usual. Atopic or food sensitive cats may have otitis as the only manifestation of their allergies. They may also have any of the myriad of clinical signs associated with allergic disease (eg, excessive grooming, alopecia and dermatitis due to self trauma, miliary dermatitis, indolent ulcers, eosinophilic plaques, eosinophilic granuloma, pruritius restricted to the head or face or chin dermatitis.

  d. **Previous therapies:**
    i. Response to therapy – ie, parenteral steroid responsiveness might suggest underlying allergic disease.
    ii. An individual who has had multiple previous topical antibiotic therapies is more likely to have a more resistant population of bacteria

2. **Dermatologic Examination**
   The physical examination must include a thorough dermatologic examination because of the common association of otitis with dermatologic diseases (allergy, hypothyroidism, primary idiopathic seborrhea in the dog; allergy in the cat). Auricular cartilages should be palpated for lack of compressibility (suggesting severity and extent of proliferative changes) or calcification. Severe calcification generally is associated with a very poor prognosis for medical management. A brief neurologic examination of the facial region is also indicated, looking for evidence of middle ear disease (Horner's syndrome, xeromycteria or dry nose, facial paresis or paralysis) or otitis interna (nystagmus, head tilt). The bulla area can be palpated for a pain response, which might suggest an otitis media.

3. **Diagnostics for Primary Factors**
   a. Restrictive diet trial – Started early in the management of the otitis. If the problem is indeed due to a food sensitivity, the restrictive diet will make resolution of the otitis more rapid and topical and systemic therapies will be more effective. Diet trials are usually longer than those used for atopy. Initially, one has to work at resolving secondary infections and inflammation, then slowly discontinue anti-inflammatory medications until the patient is only on an ear flush and the restrictive diet. In this way, it is possible to see what the diet alone is capable of doing for the problem. It may take 3 to 4 months on a restrictive diet to make this assessment. To prove the presence of a food sensitivity, the patient can be challenged with the patient's previous diet.
   b. **Intradermal testing or in vitro serologic testing.** Consideration should be given to doing

these early in the workup, prior to steroid therapy.
   c. Screening for hypothyroidism
   d. If it is unclear as to whether lesions within ears are proliferative (a product of chronicity) or neoplastic, then affected tissues should be biopsied.

Document Perpetuating Factors
(ideal to keep good records of these findings to compare progress from examination to examination).
1. **Cytology** – looking for *Malassezia*, bacteria, inflammatory cells. The finding of neutrophils and bacteria suggests a deeper seated infection and warrants systemic antibiotic therapy.
2. Otoscopic or video otoscopic examination- note the integrity of the tympanum, nature and amount of ceruminous debris, proliferative changes (and severity).
3. **Culture** – if bacteria are persisting in the face of therapy; if "rods" noted on cytologic examination and the patient has been on various topical antibiotics in the past (suggesting a greater chance for multiple drug resistance).
4. **Radiographs or CT or MRI** – to evaluate for the presence of calcification of the auricular cartilages and to assess for the presence of otitis media. The finding of fluid/debris within the middle ear warrants sampling from the middle ear for cytology and culture and sensitivity testing (e.g. myringotomy if tympanum intact). Middle ear disease also warrants systemic therapy. Radiographs/CT also provide prognostic information. If there is significant bulla wall disease (moderate to severe sclerosis, thickening, any lysis), the prognosis for the medical management of the problem is poor. It has been shown that CT is more sensitive and specific for defining middle ear disease than are radiographs. CT has been used as the "gold standard" for defining middle ear disease.
5. **Myringotomy** – It has been suggested by some that a myringotomy be performed on all chronic cases of otitis externa wherein the tympanum is intact, because of the high incidence of middle ear disease noted in these patients. Myringotomy is especially indicated if the tympanum is discolored (whitish, brown, vascularized). This higher incidence of concurrent otitis media has not been the experience of the author and others. Discoloration of the tympanum is a common finding in any case of otitis externa wherein debris has been sitting on the surface of the tympanum for some time. A myringotomy is more readily rationalized if the tympanum is intact and there are neurological signs of otitis media or interna or radiographic or CT/MRI evidence of fluid or debris within the middle ear. However, it is also important to note that performing a myringotomy is a relatively easily performed and safe procedure and should be considered if the clinician has a higher degree of concern for the presence of otitis media.

Manage Primary Factors, Where Possible

For example, foreign body removal, restrictive diet trial, oral glucocorticoids or cyclosporine for allergies, etc.

Manage Perpetuating Factors

The most common perpetuating factors encountered in cases of chronic otitis externa are secondary infections, ceruminous debris within the canals and proliferative changes.

Ceruminous Debris Removal

It is imperative that a clean ear be achieved in the workup of any case of otitis externa. In the author's experience, one of the more common perpetuators of otitis are ceruminoliths that fill the horizontal canal, just in front of the tympanum. These are commonly encountered in both dogs and cats. Adequate removal usually requires anesthesia and thorough deep ear cleaning. It would appear that the induction of inner ear dysfunction (head tilt, nystagmus, ataxia, deafness) appears to occur more commonly in cats than in dogs following these "deep ear cleaning" procedures. In the author's experience, these side effects can be minimized by flushing (through open-ended tomcat catheter) and suctioning (suction unit attached to a 14-gauge teflon catheter; utilizing a suction unit which allows for the control of variable degrees of suction; alternative would be a hand held flush/suction unit (such as the Storz Vetpump II). The use of grasping forceps through a video-otoscope can greatly facilitate the removal of such debris. The use of ear curettes, alligator forceps and blind "feeding tube" flushing and suctioning is to be discouraged. Flushing is usually done with just saline. If concretions are dry, the heavy oil product. Cerumene (EVSCO/Vetoquinol) can be worked in to the debris to both soften and lubricate and facilitate its removal. This product does not appear to be ototoxic. Other ceruminolytics can be used, but if the tympanum is found to be perforated, they should be thoroughly flushed out of the middle ear.

PROLIFERATIVE CHANGES

The reduction of proliferative changes usually requires both topical and systemic therapy. The major question to be asked when selecting topical therapies is whether the tympanum is intact. In most cases of proliferative otitis, the tympanum cannot be visualized. If so, consideration should be given to using products that do not contain potentially ototoxic ingredients. When proliferative changes are severe, the major initial goal of therapy is to "open up" the canals. If this cannot be achieved, then the prognosis for medical management of the otitis is poor and the ear or ears are likely candidates for surgery (total ear canal ablation and lateral bulla osteotomy).

Systemic Therapy

1. **Systemic glucocorticoid** (eg, starting at 1–2 mg/kg/day prednisolone/prednisone for 2 weeks, then 0.05–1 mg/kg for 2 weeks, then 1 mg/kg every other day for 2 weeks, then 0.5 mg/kg every other day for 2 weeks). The decision as to where in this dosage range one should start therapy is dictated by the severity of the disease. Systemic glucocorticoid therapy is generally maintained until proliferative changes have been significantly reduced.
2. **Oral cyclosporine** – As a steroid alternative for longer-term reduction of proliferative changes associated with allergic disease, especially when the patient is intolerant of steroids (although we often still do aggressive glucocorticoid therapy early in the cyclosporine regimen – ie, for the first 2 weeks).
3. **Systemic antibiotic** (if bacteria present cytologically) - chosen on the basis of cytology initially – cephalexin for cocci, ciprofloxacin or marbofloxacin for rods; +/- culture and sensitivity testing
4. **Systemic anti-*Malalssezia* therapy** (if *Malassezia* present on cytology) – for dogs – ketoconazole at 5–10 mg/kg BID, fluconazole at 2.5–5 mg/kg q 24 hours or itraconazole at 5 mg/kg q 24 hours and for cats – itraconazole at 5 mg/kg q 24 hours.

Topical Therapy if Tympanum is Intact

1. **Topical glucocorticoid/antibiotic/antifungal preparations:** if the tympanum is intact, all options are acceptable. For proliferative changes, the author tends to favor ointments over solutions for improved contact time. All products are used BID. Medications are "scripted out" with a syringe and multiple dose vial to assure adequate volumes of medication are applied (eg, cocker spaniel will be treated with 0. 4 mL per treatment.
2. **Ear flush** - Routine cleanser/dryer (eg, EpiOtic Advanced, Virbac) or a TrisEDTA product, if warranted (eg, T8 Keto by DVM pharmaceuticals, if "rods" seen on cytologic examination).

Topical Antibiotic and/or Anti-Malassezia Therapy if The Integrity of the Tympanum is Unknown or the Tympanum is Known to be Perforated

1. For bacteria, injectable enrofloxacin (22.7 mg/mL): dexamethasone sodium phosphate (4 mg/mL) at a ratio of 1:2
2. For *Malassezia* consider dexamethasone sodium phosphate: 1% miconazole (1:1)
3. For bacteria and *Malassezia* consider a mix of enrofloxacin: dexamethasone sodium phosphate: 1% miconazole (1:1:2).

Topical Potent Glucocorticoid – Appears to be Safe if Tympanum not Intact

1. Synotic (fluocinolone and DMSO) +/- enrofloxacin (22.7 mg/mL) – 2:1 mix (should be tolerated well in middle ear).

Ear Flush if Integrity of Tympanum Unknown

1. Dilute vinegar and water (1:2)
2. TrisEDTA (TrizEDTA, DermaPet)
3. Cerumene (Vetquinol)

Intralesional Glucocorticoids

Intralesional glucocorticoids are used at the time of deep ear cleaning (when patient anesthetized) to hasten the resolution of proliferative changes and to lessen the amount of systemic glucocorticoid necessary to reduce proliferative changes. We utilize triamcinolone acetonide (2 mg/mL); spinal needle (3.5", 22-gauge); injected following cleaning; 0.1 mL injections into proliferative lesions or if 360 degree proliferation, administer in a "ring" of 3 points around wall, with each "ring" 1–2 cm apart. The maximum triamcinolone dosage that this author usually uses in a 30- to 40-pound dog is 6 mg. Repeat administration may be considered in 3 to 4 weeks. When intralesional therapy is used, dosages of systemic therapy are usually reduced There is usually a lesser need for very aggressive oral glucocorticoid dosages, ie, instead of starting at 1–2 mg/kg/day, start at 0.5–1 mg/kg/day of prednisone/prednisolone.

Ear "Wicks"

Ear wicks are "sponges" that are supplied compressed for ready placement. Upon exposure to tissue fluid and topical medications within the ear, the sponge expands putting gentle pressure on proliferative changes within the ear and allows for rapid dispersion of topical medications throughout the canal. The wick is placed while the patient is under general anesthesia and usually removed in 5 to 7 days (again, under a short general anesthesia). This therapeutic attack has the potential for more rapidly resolving proliferative changes and more effectively dispersing both topical antibiotics and steroids.

Laser Therapy

It is possible to laser some proliferative lesions (hyperplastic ceruminous glands) with either CO_2 or diode lasers. This may facilitate an increase in the diameter of the ear canal and reduce secretions.

Followup

It is very important that patients be rechecked every 2 to 4 weeks while on these more aggressive regimens to resolve infections and reduce/resolve proliferative changes. Once maximal benefit has been noted, a decision must be made regarding topical maintenance therapy (eg, for allergies).

CHRONIC MANAGEMENT OF ALLERGIC OTITIS EXTERNA

Consider long-term maintenance therapy with a topical glucocorticoid product devoid of an antibiotic.

- Less severely inflamed ears – eg, MalAcetic HC (DermaPet, acetic acid, boric acid, surfactant, hydrocortisone), Bur-Otic HC (Virbac; propylene glycol, water, Burrow's solution, acetic acid, benzalkonium chloride); once every 48 to 72 hours long term.
- Less severely inflamed ears – Some success in managing chronic allergic otitis has been associated with the chronic use of Zymox Otic or Zymox Otic with 1% hydrocortisone (Pet King Brands) or Maxi/Guard Zn Otic (Addison Biologic Laboratory) on an every other day to twice weekly basis
- Many allergic patients are prone to recurrent *Malassezia* colonization/infections. Topical hydrocortisone is often not potent enough in these individuals to reduce their "flares" of allergic otitis. Improved control may be achieved with a mix of 1:2 or 1:1 dexamethasone sodium phosphate and 1% miconazole (Confite, Mallinckrodt)). The ratios are changed in accordance with the primary problem being managed within the ear (inflammation vs *Malassezia*). A common application protocol for this mix in a Golden retriever sized dog would be 0.5 mL twice weekly, as a long term maintenance regime

Combine these long-term topical glucocorticoids with routine flushes using a combination cleanser/dryer.

REFERENCES

1. Angus JC, Lichtensteiger C, Campbell KL, Schaeffer DJ. Breed variations in histopathologic features of chronic severe otitis externa in dogs: 80 cases (1995-2001). J Am Vet Med Assoc. 2002;221(7);10000-1006.
2. Rohleder JJ, Jones CJ, Duncan RB, Larson MM, Waldron DL, Tromblee T. Comparative performance of radiography and computed tomography in the diagnosis of middle ear disease in 31 dogs. Vet Radiol Ultrasound. 2006; 47; 5-52.
3. Doust R, King A, Hammond G, Cave T, Weinrauch S, Mellor D, Sullivan M. Assessment of middle ear disease in the dog: a comparison of diagnostic imaging modalities. J Small Anim Pract. 2007; 48:188-192.
4. Moll FR, Eeg PH, Berger N. Laser ear surgery. In: Gotthelf LN (ed.): Small Animal Ear Diseases: An Illustrated Guide, 2nd ed. St. Louis, MO: Elsevier Saunders, 2005, pp 361-364.

PSEUDOMONAS OTITIS

Rod A.W. Rosychuk, DVM, Diplomate ACVIM
College of Veterinary Medicine and Biomedical Sciences
Colorado State University, Ft. Collins, CO

GENERAL COMMENTS

Pseudomonas aeruginosa is a gram-negative "rod-shaped" bacteria that is ubiquitous in the environment. It is one of the more commonly encountered secondary infections associated with canine otitis externa, especially chronic otitis. It is one of the most common organisms associated with otitis media in the dog. Although other gram-negative "rod-shaped" bacteria are also associated with otitis externa and media (*Proteus, E. coli, Klebsiella, Enterobacter* sp), *Pseudomonas* is the most commonly encountered. *Pseudomonas* and other gram-negative "rods" are not found in the cytology of normal ears.

Pseudomonas is intrinsically resistant to many antibiotics and rapidly develops multi-drug resistance.

Pseudomonas infections are usually secondary to a primary factor that has initiated inflammation within the ear (eg, in the dog - atopy, food sensitivity, foreign body, primary idiopathic seborrhea, hypothyroidism, autoimmune disease such as pemphigus foliaceus, etc.) Predisposing factors (increased environmental humidity, swimming, hair in ears, stenotic horizontal canals) essentially amplify the deleterious effects of these primary factors. Perpetuating factors, such as proliferative changes, debris within the ears and otitis media support the persistence of disease in the ear, even if the primary factor is no longer active. Therapy for *Pseudomonas* infections is very importantly not only directed at resolving the infection, but also at resolving / controlling primary and perpetuating factors involved. The control of primary and perpetuating factors is also very important in preventing recurrences of infection.

CLINICAL SIGNS

The presence of a *Pseudomonas* infection is usually heralded by the presence of purulent exudate within the ear. Affected ears are often very inflamed, swollen and painful and may be eroded or ulcerated. *Pseudomonas* is also a relatively common secondary infection in chronic, proliferative cases of otitis externa.

EFFECTS ON TYMPANUM

Pseudomonas infections are more likely to be associated with breakdown of the tympanum and the concurrent presence of otitis media. This likely has to do with the proteases produced by this organism. Otitis media is even more common if the canals are hyperplastic and stenotic. When a *Pseudomonas* infection is known or suspected (based on cytology or culture) and the tympanum is not visible, consideration should be given to the use of topical antibiotics/products with less potential for ototoxicity, working on the premise that the tympanum may be perforated. The presence of a *Pseudomonas* infection may also provide the rationale for the performance of a deep ear cleaning, early in the course of the therapy. This would allow for the removal of organisms and potentially irritating debris and would also allow for the assessment of the integrity of the tympanum.

CYTOLOGIC FINDINGS

Cytologic examination will reveal "rods" and usually neutrophils on cytologic examination. *Pseudomonas* is usually the only organism associated with the infection, but can occasionally be found with other bacteria or *Malassezia*.

CULTURE

Acute *Pseudomonas* infections that have not received significant topical antibiotic therapy in the past are often treated with antibiotics chosen empirically, based on our knowledge of efficacy. These include gentamicin, polymixin B, and enrofloxacin. With the advent of concurrent TrisEDTA therapy, many *Pseudomonas* infections may be successfully treated, even when they show resistance to the antibiotic being used (eg, enrofloxacin or gentamicin). Culture is indicated when there is a history of unsuccessful topical therapy using these antibiotic regimens. These are usually chronic cases. Culture and sensitivity testing data is of particular importance in choosing systemic therapy. Samples for cultures should be taken from both the canals and, if involved, the middle ear. These can be combined for purposes of culture (to lessen cost). It has been shown that the strains and sensitivity patterns of *Pseudomonas* organisms cultured from the horizontal canal may differ from those cultured from the middle ear.

When submitting cultures from cases with suspected *Pseudomonas* infections, it is important to request sensitivities for antibiotics that are known to have good efficacy for treating this organism. While several of these are usually present on routine antibiograms (eg, gentamicin, amikacin, enrofloxacin), several are not (ticarcillin, polymixin B, ciprofloxacin, marbofloxacin). These should be requested at the time of submission. It is important to note that the susceptibility or resistance to one fluoroquinolone does not imply susceptibility or resistance to all (or any) other fluoroquinolones.

THERAPY
General Comments

- The overall quality and quantity of studies reporting the efficacy of various treatments for *Pseudomonas* infections of the ear are low.
- Many of the drugs listed below have the potential to be ototoxic if they pass through a perforated tympanum into the middle ear and subsequently into the inner ear. Although the incidence of ototoxicity is low in the dog, the author does tend to choose drugs that are considered less likely to cause ototoxicity when the tympanum is perforated or if the integrity of the tympanum is unknown and there is a high index of suspicion for perforation.
- The author prefers to dispense most topical antibiotics in "multi-dose" vials that allow the owner to draw up the medication in a graduated syringe.

This facilitates more accurate dosing. Most "Golden retriever" sized dogs receive 0.5 mL; small dogs and cats 0.3–0.4 mL, and large-breed dogs such as St. Bernards, 0.8 mL per treatment. If the inner aspect of the pinna is involved in the pathologic process, it is imperative that the owner be instructed to topically treat these areas.

- Tris-EDTA has been a very beneficial addition to our armamentarium of treatments for *Pseudomonas* otitis. Tris-EDTA has been shown to increase the susceptibility of various bacteria (*Pseudomonas aeruginosa*, *Staphylococcus aureus*, *E. coli,* and *Proteus mirablis*) to several antibiotics (enrofloxacin, cephaloridine, or kanamycin).[5] It has also been shown that Tris-EDTA has some inherent antibacterial activity. There are currently three Veterinary Tris-EDTA products on the market. T8 solution (DVM Pharmaceuticals) also contains benzoyl alcohol, which enhances its antibacterial effects. It contains surfactants which provide some cleansing activity. There is some question about its increased potential for ototoxicity because of these additives. T8 Keto (DVM Pharmaceuticals) has an ingredient profile as for T8 but also contains ketoconazole, which provides anti-*Malassezia* effects. TrizEDTA (DermaPet) contains Tris-EDTA , but none of the additives noted above for the T8 and T8 Keto products and for this reason, has been suggested to be safe in the middle ear (not ototoxic). The Tris-EDTA products are used to flush the ear 10 minutes prior to instilling topical antibiotics such as enrofloxacin (see below).

Topical Therapies for Acute, First-Time or Infrequently Recurrent *Pseudomonas* Infections (Tympanum Intact or Thought to be Intact)

- The empiric antibiotics we tend to reach for when "rods" predominate on cytologic examination are:
  o Gentamicin (ie, Otomax or Mometamax; Schering-Plough Animal Health). Gentamicin is effective against a significant number of *Pseudomonas* strains (50–60%). It is potentially ototoxic.
  o Polymixin B - Polymixin B is effective against as many as 95–100% of the *Pseudomonas* organisms seen in association with otitis in the US, where polymxin B is not used in routine ear preparations. Example: Cortisporin Otic solution (Glaxo Wellcome; polymyxin B, neomycin, 1% hydrocortisone). This is a human product. Polymixin B is potentially ototoxic.
  o Baytril Otic (Bayer; 5 mg/mL enrofloxacin, 10 mg/mL sliver sulfadiazine). Silver sulfadiazine is effective against a broad spectrum of gram-positive and gram-negative bacteria, including *Pseudomonas*. It is, at best, only a mildly effective therapy for *Malassezia*. The product appears to be well tolerated within the middle ear. It does not contain a steroid. If a steroid influence is necessary (and it often is), then a steroid drop or systemic steroid therapy would be used in addition to the Baytril Otic.
  o These products are used BID initially.
  o These antibiotics also work well against other gram-negative organisms.
- Choices of flushes are extensive in this scenario and include:
  o Tris-EDTA-containing product (eg, T8 solution, T8 Keto, or TrizEDTA). These products are used to flush the ear twice daily (about 10 minutes prior to application of topical antibiotic-containing product).
  o Acetic acid containing products (e.g. 2% acetic acid, 2% boric acid; MalAcetic Otic (DermaPet) or dilute 5% white vinegar and water – 1:2). Acetic acid is noted to have unique anti-*Pseudomonal* effects. Used once or twice daily (author usually uses it once daily).
  o Cleanser/dryers - EpiOtic Advanced (Virbac; contains monosaccharides reported to reduce *Pseudomonas* adherence to epithelial cell surfaces) . EpiOtic (Virbac) alone, without monosaccharides was shown in one study to have efficacy against *Pseudomonas* when used as the only therapy for *Pseudomonas* otitis (ears flushed twice daily for 2 weeks). The salicylic acid and lactic acid along with PCMX (parachlometaxylenol) likely contributed the antibacterial effect associated with this product. These cleanser/dryer flushes are most routinely used once daily.

Topical Therapies to Consider with More Chronic, Persistent or very Recurrent Infections or Based on Culture and Sensitivity Testing (Potential for Ototoxicity is Noted for Each)

Flushes:
- Tris-EDTA-containing product (see above). There is some debate as to whether the benzoyl alcohol containing products are safe within the middle ear. For this reason, the author favors the use of TrizEDTA (DermaPet) in these scenarios. However, others have used the T8 Keto product in ears with perforations and are not aware of encountering problems.
- Acetic acid containing product (see above). Dilute vinegar and water (1: 2) appears to be well tolerated in the middle ear.

Topical Antibiotics:
- Enrofloxacin mixes utilizing injectable (22.7 mg/ml) enrofloxacin; these formulations should be "safe" in the middle ear; ears pre-treated with TrisEDTA .
  o 1:2 enrofloxacin:dexamethasone sodium phosphate (for moderate steroid effect). Used BID.
  o 1 part enrofloxacin to 1 part dexamethasone phosphate to 2 parts 1% miconazole (Conofite; Schering-Plough Animal Health) (for concurrent anti-*Malassezia* effect). Used BID.

- o Saline and enrofloxacin 1:1 to 1:2. Used BID.
- o 3–4 mL enrofloxacin to 8 mL Synotic BID (for potent steroid effect; eg, proliferative ear disease)
- o Enrofloxacin mixed with a Tris-EDTA solution: when using these products in combination, the author tries to achieve a final concentration of 10 mg/mL of enrofloxacin (ie, 13 mL of 100 mg/mL injectable enrofloxacin per 118-mL bottle of T8 solution). Others have claimed similar success with concentrations of 4–5 mg/mL of enrofloxacin. The combination product is used BID to initiate therapy (ear is filled with the combination and massaged in). The author has used a combination of enrofloxacin and TrizEDTA in middle ears, without apparent ototoxicity. Due to the lack of an anti-fungal component to this product (TrizEDTA), a flare of *Malassezia* otitis may occasionally be seen during therapy. However, if the T8 Keto product is used, this should not be a problem.

- Ticarcillin or ticarcillin and clavulonic acid (Timentin; GlaxoSmithKline). Ticarcillin has proven to be a very beneficial therapy for resistant *Pseudomonas*. The reconstituted product is suggested to have a shelf life of only 2 to 3 days. The shelf life is prolonged to one month with freezing of the reconstituted product. The author uses Timentin; 3.1-g vial; reconstitute with 26 mL (100 mg/mL); freeze in 4-mL aliquots; thaw and use each 4-mL aliquot over 2 days; 1/2 mL in each ear BID. Others have suggested: reconstitute a 6-g vial of ticarcillin with 12 mL of sterile water. Divide equally into 2-mL portions in syringes and freeze (will remain stable for 3 months); this is the "stock solution." To make up the ear treatment solution, thaw and mix a 2-mL aliquot of concentrate with 40 mL of normal saline. Divide this into four 10-mL aliquots and freeze. Clients should keep these frozen; one aliquot should be thawed at a time, keeping it refrigerated, and used for no longer than 1 week. Anything remaining after 1 week should be discarded and another aliquot thawed. Ticarcillin appears to be well tolerated in the middle ear.
- Silver sulfadiazine 1% cream. Very efficacious therapy (although the author has seen resistant cases) – eg, Kendall Thermazene (Kendall Co.; diluted 1:9 with water) or powder (Spectrum Pharmacy; www.spectrumRx.com; make up 1% solution). Ear should be cleaned prior to application to enhance efficacy. May promote re-epithelialization in ulcerated ears. Silver sulfadiazine appears to be well tolerated within the middle ear.
- Amikacin injectable (dilute 250 mg/mL to 50 mg/mL) 4 to 8 drops of 50 mg/mL BID or tobramycin (human ophthalmologic preparation). Both aminoglycosides are potentially ototoxic and should not be used in ears with a perforated tympanum.

Complications of Antibiotic Therapy

When antibiotic or antibiotic/steroid combination products are used in the ear for treating bacterial infections, it is not uncommon to see opportunistic, secondary *Malassezia* infections develop. These are diagnosed based on cytology and are usually readily resolved with topical +/- systemic anti-malassezia therapy. They may be prevented with the use of a product such as T8 Keto, which contains ketoconazole.

Systemic Antibiotics

There is some evidence supporting the efficacy of systemic antibiotic therapy alone in treating bacterial otitis (improving 43% or resolving 28% of cases in one study). Systemic antibiotic is indicated when the canals are hyperplastic or proliferative, erosive or ulcerated and/or there is otitis media or it is difficult for the owners to topically treat the ears. However, it is important to note that the author has treated many cases of *Pseudomonas* otitis externa +/- media with just a topical antibiotic alone (eg, combination of Tris-EDTA and enrofloxacin or combination of ticarcillin and acetic acid flushes). The author's antibiotics of choice are ciprofloxacin (15–20 mg/kg BID) and marbofloxacin (4–5.5 mg/kg/day). This is based on some in vitro data that has shown these antibiotics to be superior to other fluoroquinolones for treating *Pseudomonas*. Enrofloxacin would be used at a dose of 10–20 mg/kg/day. The fluoroquinolones are concentration-dependent antibiotics. On an antibiogram, if the bacteria is reported as sensitive (S), the lower dosage range is used; if intermediate (I), then the higher range is used. If the bacteria are resistant (R), then the antibiotic should not be used. Appropriate antibiotics for systemic use are best chosen on the basis of culture and sensitivity testing. Alternative injectable systemic antibiotic considerations for very resistant *Pseudomonas* would include ticarcillin or ceftazidime (ticarcillin, 60–75 mg/kg BID SQ or ceftazidime 30–50 mg/kg SQ BID) for 2 to 3 weeks. These injections can be given at home by the owner.

Systemic Glucocorticoids

Systemic glucocorticoids are not contraindicated in the treatment of *Pseudomonas* infections. An exception may exist in the presence of an osteomyelitis of the bulla or petrous temporal bone, wherein there is the potential for extension of infection in to the calvarium.

Glucocorticoids will rapidly reduce inflammation and pain and facilitate the owner's ability to topically treat the ears. In general, anti-inflammatory dosages of prednisone/prednisolone are used (starting at 0.5–1.0 mg/kg/day). With chronic, proliferative otitis, it becomes important to "open up" the canals. This allows topical antibiotic to come in contact with the lining of the length of the canals. Depending on the degree of proliferation and stenosis, more aggressive glucocorticoid dosages may be required (eg, moderate to severe proliferative changes – starting at 1–2 mg/kg/day prednisone for the first 1 to 2 weeks, then gradually taper).

Management of Concurrent Primary and Perpetuating Factors

As noted previously, the successful management of *Pseudomonas* infections also emphasizes the need to resolve/control primary and perpetuating factors that are key to the pathogenesis of otitis. This may mean initiating a restrictive diet trial to rule out or control a food sensitivity; treating with glucocorticoids for underlying allergies; emphasizing the need to have all debris removed from the ears at some time in the management of every case of otitis; resolving proliferative changes, etc.

FOLLOW-UP

Patients with *Pseudomonas* otitis externa and/or media should be rechecked every 2 to 3 weeks until the organism is no longer present on cytologic examination. The finding of even rare "rods" on cytologic examination warrants continued therapy. Treatment for at least 1 to 2 weeks beyond apparent resolution of infection is warranted for proliferative otitis and otitis media. The duration of topical and systemic therapy for otitis media is usually at least 4 to 6 weeks.

REFERENCES

1. Cole LK, Kwochka KW, Kowalski JJ, Hillier A. Microbial flora and antimicrobial susceptibility patterns of isolated pathogens from the horizontal ear canal and middle ear in dogs with otitis media. J Am Vet Med Assoc. 1998;212;534-538.
2. Martin Barrasa JL, Lupiola Gomez P, Gonzallez Lama Z, Tejedor Junco MT. Antibacterial susceptibility patterns of *Pseudomonas* strains isolated from chronic canine otitis externa. J Vet Med B Infect Dis Vet Public Health. 2000; 47;191-196.
3. Cole LK, Kwachka KW, Hillier A, et al, Ciprofloxacin as a representative of disc diffusion susceptibility of enrofloxacin for bacterial organisms from the middle ear tissue of dogs with end stage otitis externa. Vet Dermatol. 2006;17(2);128-133.
4. Nuttall T, Cole Lynette C. Evidence-based veterinary dermatology : a systematic review of interventions for treatment of *Pseudomonas* otitis in dogs. Vet Dermatol. 2007;18;69-77.
5. Farca AM, Piromalli G, Maffei F, et al. Potentiating effect of EDTA-Tris on the activity of antibiotics against resistant bacteria associated with otitis, dermatitis and cystitis. J Small Anim Pract. 1997; 38;243-45.
6. Cole LK, Luu DH, Rajala-Schultz PJ et al. In vitro activity of an ear rinse containing trimethamine, EDTA and benzoyl alcohol on bacterial pathogens. Am J Vet Res. 2006; 67;1040 – 1044.
7. Cole LK, Kwochka RW, Kowalski JJ, et a.: Evaluation of an ear cleanser for the treatment of infectious otitis externa in dogs, Vet Therap. 2003; 4;12-23.
8. Palmeiro BS, Morris DO, Wiemelt SP, et al. Evaluation of outcome of otitis media after lavage of the tympanic bulla and long-term antimicrobial drug treatment in dogs: 44 cases (1998-2002). J Am Vet Med Assoc. 2004;225;548-553.
9. Carlotti DN, Guaguere E, Koch HJ, et al. Marbofloxacin for the systemic treatment of *Pseudomonas* spp. suppurative otitis externa in the dog. In: von Tscharner C, Kwochka KW, Willemse T (eds.): Advances in Veterinary Dermatology 3. Oxford: Butterworth Heinemann, 1998. pp 463-464.

FELINE EAR DISEASE: SO MUCH MORE THAN "EAR MITES"

Rod A.W. Rosychuk, DVM, Diplomate ACVIM
College of Veterinary Medicine and Biomedical Sciences
Colorado State University, Ft. Collins, CO

ETIOPATHOGENESIS OF FELINE OTITIS EXTERNA

The etiopathogenesis of otitis externa in the cat can generally be divided into various factors. **Primary factors** are those that are noted to cause inflammation in ears. The most common primary factors are ear mites (*Otodectes cynotis*), suggested to be responsible for about 50% of the cases of otitis externa seen in the cat. The next most commonly encountered primary factors are hypersensitivities (atopy, food sensitivity). Other primary factors tend to be much less common and include foreign bodies, other ectoparasites (Demodex, ticks), keratinization/lipid disorders (idiopathic ceruminous otitis), and autoimmune diseases (eg, pemphigus foliaceus).

Predisposing factors are those that produce an environment conducive to the development of otitis externa. They include increased environmental temperature and humidity and systemic diseases, including immunocompromising viral infections such as feline leukemia virus (FeLV) or feline immunodeficiency virus (FIV). Obstructive lesions, such as aural polyps, ceruminous cysts/adenometous hyperplasia, and neoplasias, often function as predispositions to otitis initially. They do so by producing accumulations of ceruminous debris. Once the masses become large and fill the ear canal, they become a primary source of irritation within the ear and can be thought of as primary factors.

Perpetuating factors are those that are capable of perpetuating the otitis even if the primary factor has been removed/resolved. In the cat, these include bacterial infections, fungal infections (eg, *Malassezia pachydermatis*), ceruminous debris (eg, ceruminoliths), proliferative changes (marked thickening of epidermis/dermis), otitis media, and treatment errors (eg, overtreatment, undertreatment, inappropriate treatment).

DEMODEX

Cats with generalized *Demodex cati* infestations may have mites within the ears and a concurrent, usually mild otitis externa. Cats with generalized demodicosis are usually suffering from some underlying immunocompromising disease. Mites are usually easily found by swabbing the ears and doing a microscopic examination of debris that has been placed in mineral oil on a slide.

A focal form of demodicosis may occur in the cat wherein the mite problem is restricted to the ears. The otitis is usually bilateral and characterized by the accumulation of large amounts of brown, waxy debris. Pruritus and signs of discomfort are variable. Diagnosis is by swabbing (as noted above). In the author's experience, most cats with this problem have not been noted to have significant intercurrent immunocompromising disease. Therapies have included:

1. Topical ivermectin – 1 part injectable ivermectin (10 mg/mL) to 9 parts propylene glycol – treat once every other day
2. Systemic ivermectin per os – 0.3 mg/kg once daily or once every other day
3. Amitraz (Mitaban, Pharmacia and Upjohn; 19.9%) – 1 mL in 30 mL of mineral oil or propylene glycol. Treat once every other day. Make up new solution once every 2 weeks
4. Topical Tresaderm – every 24 hours or BID

ATOPY

Atopy tends to be under-diagnosed as a cause of otitis externa in the cat. The incidence of otitis seen in atopic cats appears to be less than that seen in the atopic dog. Otic involvement may be concurrent with more generalized skin disease, but may also be the only sign of atopy (ie, ears are the only area affected). Atopic otitis externa is usually bilateral, but may be predominantly or entirely unilateral. The most common secondary infection appears to be with *Malassezia pachydermatis*, although secondary bacterial infections (eg, *Staphylococcus intermedius*; much less commonly gram-negative organisms including *Pseudomonas*) are also seen. Progression to otitis media via perforation of the tympanum is not uncommon. In the author's practice, atopic otitis externa is the most common cause of aural hematoma seen in the cat.

Diagnostics routinely employed include otoscopic or video-otoscopic examination and cytologic examination. Cultures are only done when resistant bacteria are suspected (ie, bacteria persisting in the face of an apparently appropriate antibiotic; large numbers of "rods" on cytologic examination, suggesting the possibility of a more resistant gram-negative infection). Radiographs or CT to look for the presence of otitis media are done when proliferative changes or severe debris accumulation prevent observation of the tympanum (in chronic cases) or neurologic signs suggest the possibility of otitis media/interna. If middle ear disease is present, it should be seen radiographically (unlike in the dog, where it may be missed in as many as 25% of cases). The finding of a peripheral eosinophilia and basophilia in a complete blood count (CBC) is common in atopic cats. Biopsies from affected areas commonly show increased numbers of mast cells and eosionphils (suggesting a hypersensitivity disorder but not defining the type of hypersensitivity disorder). The above diagnostic aids are considered supportive. The diagnosis of atopy is largely based on history and rule out (eg, seasonality; rule out food sensitivity).

Therapy

Therapy for a "flare" of atopic otitis is directed at resolving secondary infections, reducing inflammation and removing debris from the ears. Some controversy exists within the veterinary community about preferred treatments for otitis externa in the cat (topical versus systemic). Because of the increased propensity of the cat to develop ototoxicity related to the use of some topical medications, some clinicians only use systemic therapies in managing otitis externa in the cat. These include oral glucocorticoids to reduce inflammation, oral antibiotics to resolve secondary infections and oral antifungals to resolve secondary *Malassezia* infections. The author generally uses topical and/or a combination of topical and systemic treatments, depending on the severity of the problem and the integrity of the tympanum. Therapies to consider when the tympanum is intact include:

- Combination products such as Tresaderm (neomycin, thiabendazole, dexamethasone) or Otomax (Schering-Plough Animal Health; contains gentamicin, clotrimazole, betamethasone) are used in the ears BID to initiate therapy. Mometamax (Schering-Plough Animal Health; contains gentamicin, clotrimazole, mometasin) is used once daily.
- Because the ear canals of the cat are relatively much shorter than in the dog, much debris from the ears can be shaken out, without the need for otic flushes. If necessary, the otic flushes used most commonly by the author in cats include EpiOtic Advanced (Virbac), MalAcetic Otic (DermaPet), and, for drier concretions, Cerumene (EVSCO/Vetquinol). T8 and T8 Keto (both from DVM Pharmaceuticals) and TrizEDTA (DermaPet) are used as both a cleanser and enhancer of antibiotic activity. Flushing regimens are often less aggressive than in the dog – ie, beginning once every other day. They are often not started for 2 to 4 days after anti-inflammatory medications are started to facilitate greater tolerance to the flushing procedure. An exception might be with TrisEDTA containing products if they are being used prior to the instillation of a topical antibiotic–containing product. This is often done twice daily to initiate therapy.
- Oral glucocorticoids can be used if the ears are severely inflamed, if very painful, or if very proliferative. Start at anti-inflammatory dosages (prednisolone, beginning at 1–2 mg/kg/day).
- Oral antibiotics – Based on cytologic examinations: Clavamox, clindamycin, azithromycin, cephalexin, marbofloxacin, enrofloxacin for cocci; marbofloxacin, Clavamox for rods (rods are usually gram-negative bacteria).
- Oral antifungal – Primarily used if there are significant proliferative changes within the ears – itraconazole (5 mg/kg every 24 hours).

Therapies to consider when the tympanum is perforated or integrity of tympanum unknown:

- Flush
  - Dilute white vinegar and water (1:2 or 1:3 dilution) – used daily or every other day

- TrizEDTA (DermaPet) – Usually used to flush the ear about 10 minutes before placing appropriate antibiotic-containing product in ear.
- Cerumene (EVSCO/Vetoquinol; potentially very messy) – Usually used once every other day; ear filled, massaged in, then several hours later, flushed out with dilute vinegar and water (1:2). Usually used for softening/lubricating drier concretions.
- Topical Antibacterial/Antifungal Therapies
  - For bacteria (cocci) – Mix of dexamethasone sodium phosphate (2 parts) and enrofloxacin (injectable, 22.7 mg/mL) (1 part); use BID.
  - For bacteria (rods, suggesting gram-negative bacteria) – Mix of enrofloxacin (22.7 mg/mL) and TrizEDTA (Dermapet) – enrofloxacin concentration of 10 mg/mL. Fill ear BID. If a steroid influence is necessary, consider systemic treatment.
  - For *Malassezia* – Mix of 1 part dexamethasone sodium phosphate and 1 part 1% miconazole (Conofite; Schering-Plough Animal Health); BID therapy; Note: True safety of 1% miconazole product (with respect to ototoxicity) is unknown; the author, however, has found it to be well tolerated. Alternative would be to consider systemic anti-yeast therapy.
  - For *Malassezia* and bacteria – Combination of 1 part dexamethasone sodium phosphate, 1 part enrofloxacin, 2 parts 1% miconazole. BID

CERUMINOLITHS – COMMON PERPETUATOR OF PROBLEMS IN ALLERGIC EARS

It is common to see concretions of material that have accumulated within the horizontal canals (covering the tympanum) in allergic cats. This debris serves as a nidus for infection, is a source of irritation, prevents medication from reaching the deeper aspects of the ear canal, and may perforate the tympanum. This debris is often difficult to remove with "at home" flushing. It is best flushed from the ears under general anesthesia. It would appear that the induction of inner ear dysfunction (head tilt, nystagmus, ataxia, deafness) appears to occur more commonly in cats than in dogs following these "deep ear cleaning" procedures. In the author's experience, these side effects can be minimized by flushing (through open ended tomcat catheter) and suctioning (suction unit attached to a 14-gauge Teflon catheter; utilizing a suction unit which allows for the control of variable degrees of suction; alternative would be a hand held flush/suction unit such as the Storz Vetpump II). The use of grasping forceps through a video-otoscope can greatly facilitate the removal of such debris. The use of ear curettes, alligator forceps and blind "feeding tube" flushing and suctioning is to be discouraged. Flushing is usually done with just saline. If concretions are dry, the heavier oil product Cerumene (EVSCO/Vetoquinol) can be worked in to the debris to both soften and lubricate and facilitate its removal. This product does not appear to be ototoxic. Other ceruminolytics can be used, but if the tympanum is found to be perforated, they should be thoroughly flushed out of the middle ear.

Proliferative Changes

The author most commonly encounters proliferative changes in ears (thickening of epithelium, dermis) is association with chronic allergic disease in cats. Proliferative changes are usually diffuse in nature and target the entrance to the vertical canal. The more rapid reduction of proliferative changes is most commonly associated with the use of both systemic and topical glucocorticoids. The author has also used intradermal injections of triamcinolone (2 mg/mL; maximum of approx. 4 mg per cat) following deep ear cleaning to hasten the resolution of these lesions and reduce the need for more aggressive oral glucocorticoid regimens.

Management for Chronic Atopic Otitis Externa

- Overall, major emphasis should be placed on managing the underlying allergy. The two most successful alternatives that have been used by the author are testing and hyposensitization (benefiting 60–70% of patients) and oral cyclosporine (5–10 mg/kg/day), benefiting 70% of patients. Other alternatives for managing allergic otitis externa have been much less successful in the authors hands (antihistamines such as chlorpheniramine, amitriptylline), and omega 3 fatty acids.
- As an alternative to systemic management of atopy or as an adjunctive therapy in those individuals who are not adequately controlled by systemic therapy, consideration can be given to chronic topical maintenance management: 1:1 mix of 1% miconazole and dexamethasone sodium phosphate (4 mg/mL) twice weekly.

FOOD SENSITIVITY

Otitis may be concurrent with more generalized dermatologic signs but disease may also be restricted to just the ears. Although the otitis is usually bilateral, it may be predominantly unilateral. The most common secondary infections are with *Malassezia*. Affected individuals may have circulating peripheral eosinophilias and basophilias. Skin biopsies from the ear are often characterized by significant increases in mast cells and eosinophils, suggesting the presence of a hypersensitivity disorder. Diagnosis is by history, rule out and by assessing response to a restrictive diet (home prepared, novel protein; commercial novel protein or hydrolysate). During the early phases of the diet trial, every effort must be made to normalize the ear (resolve infections, remove debris, resolve proliferative changes). Medications are then slowly withdrawn to see if the problem remains controlled with just the diet alone. Duration of the diet trial is often 8 to 12 weeks or longer to meet the guidelines given above. The diagnosis of food sensitivity is usually confirmed by challenge. Exacerbation of otitis is often prompt (frequently 3 to 7 days) if food sensitivity is ultimately proven to be the source of problem.

IDIOPATHIC CERUMINOUS OTITIS EXTERNA

Some normal cats produce a very fine layer of a light oily secretion that lines the canals of the ear. This is often seen on the end of the otoscope cone after otoscopic examination. The author considers this to be "normal" finding in these cats. However, there is a subset of cats who have what is referred to as a "ceruminous" otitis wherein excessive amounts of cerumen are produced within the ears. These accumulations may be associated with mild inflammation. This problem may predispose to secondary Malassezia and/or bacterial infections. The controversy regarding this syndrome centers around whether this is a primary ceruminous otitis externa (i.e. primary seborrheic otitis externa) or the manifestation of low-grade allergy. At present, the author has come to support the latter suggestion. Most successful therapies have involved the chronic use of a topical, steroid containing product. We most commonly use a formulation mde up of dexamethasone sodium phosphate 4 mg/ml and 1% miconazole mix (1:1). 0.3 mls is place in each ear twice weekly.

FELINE CERUMINOUS CYSTS/CERUMINOUS CYSTOMATOSIS

Ceruminous cystomatosis is a non-neoplastic disorder that is relatively commonly seen in cats. Ceruminous glands become dilated with a brownish secretory material. Although the secretions are brownish in color, grossly the lesions are a very dark blue. Lesions may be solitary or grouped and may originate anywhere from the tympanum, throughout the canals and over the proximal and medial aspects of the medial pinnae and base of the ear. The reason for cyst formation is not known. It has been suggested that the lesions may be a sequel to otitis externa. In the author's experience, it does appear that the concurrent presence of otitis externa does tend to worsen the clinical manifestations of this syndrome (more lesions, lesions larger), but otitis does not actually cause the lesions.

When ceruminous cysts are small, even in the ear canals, they are usually not symptomatic. As they become larger within the horizontal canal, they may become a predisposition to otitis by partially occluding the canal and resulting in the accumulation of debris. This produces a favorable microenvironment for yeast and bacterial proliferation. The ear becomes symptomatic with the development of these infections or if the lesion or lesions occlude the ear canal. With canal occlusion, debris accumulating behind the lesions may eventually perforate the tympanum and accumulate within the middle ear. Unless the lesions are occluding the canals, they are often tolerated and do not require therapy. In the presence of a concurrent, allergic otitis, control of the allergic and secondary infection components (eg, chronic topical steroid /antibiotic/anti-fungal product) may reduce the numbers and size of lesions. The most effective options for management include surgical resection, cryosurgery or laser removal. Surgical resection involves the removal of as much of the cystic tissue as possible utilizing biopsy or grasping forceps. The removal of remnant material is facilitated by the use of biopsy forceps through a video otoscope. The ears are treated with a steroid containing product for 3 to 4 weeks following the procedure. The incidence of regrowth is variable. Laser removal of especially the base of the cysts is very effective for removing tissue and reducing the incidence of regrowth. Difficult to remove lesions or recurrent lesions may require ear canal ablation.

AURAL POLYPS

Polyps are most commonly noted in young cats (variably reported with a mean age of about 1 year; range of 2.5 months to 18 years). Although most are unilateral, polyps can be bilateral. Most polyps appear to grow from the epithelial lining of the epitympanic cavity/tympanic cavity, then extend either through the tympanum in to the horizontal canal or down through the auditory canal in to the posterior pharynx. Although uncommon, it is possible to have polyps grow in both directions (about 10% of cases). It has also been hypothesized that polyps may grow from the epithelial lining of the auditory canal or nasopharynx, although this would appear to be uncommon. Histologically, polyps consist of a core of loosely arranged fibrovascular tissue with variable numbers and types of inflammatory cells throughout (lymphoplasmacytic; lymphoid aggregates/follicles; pleocellular inflammation). This core is covered by a stratified squamous to ciliated columnar epithelial layer that thickens, producing a capsular effect.

Clinical signs associated with aural polyps include signs of otitis externa (head shaking, scratching ears, otic exudate), and/or the development of neurologic signs (Horner's syndrome, head tilt, nystagmus, ataxia). Growth in to the posterior pharynx is suggested by nasal discharge, sneezing, sterterous respiration, dyspnea, and dysphagia.

The etiology of polyps remains unknown. The young age of involvement and the notation that polyps may affect littermates suggests the potential for a genetic predisposition. It would be more attractive, however, to assume that an inflammatory process, perhaps initiated by an infectious agent that has ascended through the auditory canal, may play a role. Recently, attempts have failed to document the presence of viruses (calicivirus and herpesvirus) in polyp tissue. Attempts to retrieve the DNA of various infectious agents (Bartonella, Mycoplasma, and feline herpesvirus 1 (FHV-1) from 14 polyps and the middle ears of normal cats revealed only FHV-1 DNA from 2 of 14 normal bulla and Mycoplasma DNA from 4 of 13 polyps. The significance of this (i.e. possible association with Mycoplasma) requires further study. Although secondary bacterial infections are reasonably common, no particular bacterium appears to be over represented and systemic antibiotic therapy alone fails to significantly benefit the problem.

Current therapies of choice include removal by traction/avulsion or removal by ventral bulla osteotomy. Traction alone (through the ear or through the posterior pharynx) results in an overall cure in about 60% of cases. A significant reduction in the incidence of recurrence following traction has been noted in cats treated with oral prednisolone following traction removal. Glucocorticoids were used at anti-inflammatory dosages (1–2 mg/kg/day to initiate therapy) over several weeks. It would appear that traction/avulsion alone is more effective for nasopharyngeal polyps. Patients with nasopharyngeal polyps are less likely to have radiographic evidence of polypoid tissue within the middle ear, suggesting that they may grow from the auditory tube and are more completely removed with traction. A higher incidence of recurrence, following traction alone, has been associated with aural polyps. In another study, an increased incidence of recurrence appeared to be associated with the presence of radiographic evidence of tissue density within the middle ear and in individuals with both otic and respiratory signs. Ventral bulla osteotomy is noted to cure the vast majority of cases.

The author primarily deals with cats with aural polyps. Essentially all have had radiographic or CT evidence of soft tissue density within the middle ear. The authors therapy of choice for aural polyps is to remove as much of the polyp as possible from the ear via traction/avulsion. Deeper tissue removal is facilitated by utilizing biopsy forceps directed through a video otoscope. Cytologic examination dictates the need for systemic and topical antibiotic therapy. Post avulsion, the ear is flushed with dilute vinegar and water (1:2 to 1:3). Post avulsion, the cat is treated with oral prednisolone, beginning at 2–3 mg/kg/day for 2 weeks, then 1–1.5 mg/kg/day for 2 weeks, then 0.5–0.75 mg/kg/day for 2 weeks, then 0.5–0.75 mg/kg once every other day for 2 weeks (6–8 weeks of therapy). This therapeutic attack has resulted in regression of remaining inflammatory tissue within the middle ear and healing of the tympanum (as documented by video otoscopy). The author is not aware of recurrences utilizing this protocol.

REFERENCES

1. Faulkner JE, Budsberg SC. Results of ventral bulla osteotomy for the treatment of middle ear polyps in cats. J Am Anim Hosp Assoc. 1990; 26:496-499.
2. Donnelly KE, Tillson MD. Feline inflammatory polyps and ventral bula osteotomy. Compend ContinEduc Pract Vet. 2004; 446–453.
3. Anderson DM, Robinson RK, White RA, Management of inflammatory polyps in 37 cats. Vet Rec. 2000; 147; 684.
4. Veir JK, Lappin MR, Foley JE, Getzy DM. Feline inflammatory polyps:historical, clinical and PCR findings for feline calici virus and feline herpes virus-1 in 28 cases. J Feline Med Surg. 2002; 4:195.
5. Klose TC, Rosychuk RA, MacPhail CM, Hawley JR, Veir J, Schultheiss P, Lappin MR. Association between upper respiratory tract infections and inflammatory aural and nasopharyngeal polyps in cats (Abstract), J Vet Intern Med. 2007; 21: 628.

PAIN MANAGEMENT METHODS FOR TREATING OSTEOARTHRITIS

Mike Conzemius, DVM, PhD, Diplomate ACVS
University of Minnesota, St. Paul, MN

Degenerative joint disease (DJD) or osteoarthritis (OA) is typically a progressive disorder that affects diarthrodial joints. It is characterized by the destruction of cartilage and subchondral bone and changes in the synovial fluid and periarticular tissues. Osteoarthritis can develop from instability, chronic inflammation, incongruity, and disease processes that create cellular pathology. Approximately 20% of all dogs in North America have OA and associated pain and lameness. Prior to instituting treatment, a definitive diagnosis must be made, beginning with the patient signalment. Osteoarthritis can affect dogs of any age but as age increases the probability of OA developing and causing clinical signs increases. Owners might report that their dog tires easy during a walk, no longer can go up the stairs or jump, has a lameness or pain in the morning or after exercise, or has a change in behavior. The clinical signs will likely wax and wan over a period of days or weeks. On physical exam, the diagnosis can be made by finding muscle atrophy, localizing pain to a joint(s), determining that a joint has a decreased range of motion, or finding an increase in joint size from periarticular fibrosis. Plain or stress radiographs and arthrocentesis can confirm impressions from the clinical exam. It is critical to make a diagnosis of joint pain during the clinical exam and to confirm that OA is present and related to the pain with the assistance of radiographs. Most would agree that the radiographic presence of OA increases the probability that a dog will have associated joint pain. However, as stated before, it is important to understand that the radiographic presence of OA, by itself, does not necessarily imply that a patient will have clinical signs of disease. Radiographs are an excellent way to diagnose the presence of osteophytes but are a poor indicator of the health status of the cartilage and/or joint capsule. In addition, it has been demonstrated that there is no correlation between the presence of radiographic OA and clinical function in dogs with OA after surgery for a torn cranial cruciate ligament, hip dysplasia, and OA after repair of a lateral humeral condylar fracture. The simple explanation is that inflammation, not osteophytes, cause pain and lameness.

The treatment of idiopathic OA is either nonsurgical or surgical. Nonsurgical treatment should almost always be tried first and in many cases will be successful. While OA is a slowly progressive disease, there are undoubtedly inflammatory flares that can be managed medically. Nonsurgical management should focus on treatments where science provides evidence of efficacy. Many owners have limited financial resources so advice should be made to optimize those resources. If the dog is overweight, weight loss can be effective. Several publications have demonstrated that weight loss alone as a treatment can provide significant relief and improve limb function in dogs with joint pain from OA. In addition, in dogs that have had an orthopedic disease(s) that are predisposed to OA (eg, rupture of the cranial cruciate ligament, fragmented coronoid process, hip dysplasia) patients should be maintained at a body condition score of 4 to 5. Food intake restriction has been demonstrated to slow the onset and progression of OA in dogs with hip dysplasia. Daily activities like leash walks should be encouraged. Consistent, low-load use of the limbs will not only provide joint range of motion which is needed to improve cartilage and synovial lining health but it will also assist in the management of the patient's body weight and begin the reversal of any disuse muscle atrophy that had developed. Swimming can also be very helpful. Specifically, aquatic therapy provides buoyancy (which eliminates ground reaction forces), multiplanar resistance to the muscles and when dogs swim they use their joints with more flexion than during land based activities. Although it is important for the patient to have exercise restriction this should only be done when the joint is very painful during the early phases of treatment. In general, exercise restriction should also be limited to only a few days to a week and when the patient is "having a bad day."

Since treatment of inflammation is one of the primary ways to improve patient function, we should have a better understanding of the principal inflammatory pathways. Most clinicians first think of the arachidonic acid pathway when thinking of inflammation. This pathway can be further broken down into the cyclooxygenases (COX) and lipoxygenases (LOX), which can act as mediators of inflammation but also have other important and necessary roles in the body. Steroids work towards inhibition of the entire arachidonic acid pathway and most nonsteroidal anti-inflammatory drugs (NSAIDs) work to completely or selectively inhibit the cyclooxygenase pathway. It is my opinion that when choosing a NSAID one can look at many things but the drug's ability to focus the effect on the COX-II isoenzyme should have a major role choosing a NSAID. The use of NSAIDs is a large component to the long-term management of patient's suffering from OA. While many NSAIDs are available over the counter, there are several that have gained approval by the US Food and Drug Administration (FDA) for OA in dogs. In most circumstances, using an approved drug makes more sense than having a patient begin with an over the counter medication. Finally, while most NSAIDs can be used safely it is important to understand their risks and contraindications. While this will be discussed in detail, understanding that most complications are related to the gastrointestinal tract in required. I recommend that each NSAID prescription include a message to stop the use of the drug and contact a veterinarian if vomiting, diarrhea, or loss of appetite develops. A second important note is to avoid using FDA-approved NSAIDs with aspirin or steroids.

Additional aspects of nonsurgical management of canine OA that have scientific evidence of efficacy are prescription diets that are high in omega-3 fatty acids. While the details are beyond the scope of this article, I would suggest that the scientific method has been followed when demonstrating that at least some of these prescription arthritis diets are beneficial. Specifically, when used they reduce inflammatory mediators in the serum, active agent can be found to be increased in the synovial fluid and, perhaps most importantly, dogs with lameness from OA improved when dogs treated with a control study diet did not.

Tramadol is an analgesic and antitussive agent that has shown efficacy in humans and has gained in popularity in veterinary medicine. Tramadol and its active metabolites exert their mode of action through opiate, adrenergic, and serotonin receptors. While it seems to have many potential advantages, the pharmacokinetics of the oral drug in dogs differs markedly from that in people, with a much faster elimination half-life and systemic clearance and a variable maximal plasma concentration. The drug can apparently be safely given but to the best of my knowledge strong evidence of a consistent analgesic effect in the dog is lacking with the available oral formulation.

Matrix metalloproteases (MMPs) are a large family of enzymes that degrade the extracellular matrix. The expanding MMP family of structurally related enzymes contains members with the capacity to degrade almost all of the components of the extracellular matrix (ECM). These enzymes are divided into three groups on the basis of their substrate preference: 1) Collagenases degrade connective tissue collagen: MMP-1, MMP-8, MMP-13; 2) Gelatinases degrade basement membrane collagens: MMP-2, MMP-9; and 3) Stromelysins degrade ECM proteoglycans, laminin, fibronectin and gelatin: MMP-3, MMP-10, MMP-11. Production of MMP-1, MMP-3, and MMP-9 is greatly enhanced by pro-inflammatory cytokines such as interleukin-1 (IL-1) and tumor necrosis factor alpha. Serine proteinases are also linked to IL-1 and mediate degradation of cartilage proteoglycans and collagen. Monitoring of serum and synovial MMP levels may prove a useful means of monitoring response to treatment in diseases in which these cytokines are central.

Prevention of further cartilage destruction is another approach for the treatment of OA. These agents, which historically have been called *chondroprotective agents*, are now more commonly referred to as *disease-modifying osteoarthritis drugs* (DMOADs). DMOADs are products that claim to prevent, reduce, or reverse cartilaginous abnormalities (principally by enhancing chondrocyte and synoviocyte metabolism). In addition, many products claim to have an anti-inflammatory effect by reducing mediators of inflammation in the joint. I believe it is important to separate injectable polysulfated glycosaminoglycan (PSGAG) which is a DMOAD that has been approved by the FDA for use in dogs, and oral DMOADs, which have essentially no regulation and should be referred to as nutraceuticals or nutritional supplements. PSGAG is a mixture of highly sulfated glycosaminoglycans, the major component of which is chondroitin sulfate (CS), which is extracted from the bovine trachea and lungs.

Over the years, a sufficient number of studies have demonstrated the efficacy of the injectable formulation of PSGAG for consistent clinical use. (Unfortunately, the exact mechanism of their action remains unknown.) In vitro, PSGAGs have been shown to significantly inhibit serine proteinases, prostaglandin E2, and several catabolic enzymes including elastase, stromelysin, metalloproteases, and hyaluronidases.[5,6] Additional in vitro work has demonstrated that PSGAGs have an anabolic effect with the ability to stimulate the synthesis of protein, collagen, proteoglycans and hyaluronic acid. Finally, cultured rabbit and human chondrocytes have shown increased synthesis of proteoglycan and hyaluronic acid in the presence of PSGAG.

In vivo, work evaluating PSGAG has been performed in several species. Perhaps the most important information is that following an intramuscular injection the drug is widely distributed to the tissues including the cartilage, meniscus and synovial fluid. In humans, an increase in the concentration of hyaluronan (a major constituent of synovial fluid and the boundary lubricant for the synovial lining) has been reported as a result of treatment with PSGAG.[9] Evaluation of the PSGAG has been performed in dogs. In dogs that had their cranial cruciate ligament surgically transected, it was reported that PSGAG-treated dogs had lower collagenase concentrations.[2] However, it is important that there is evidence that the use of intra-articular PSGAGs immediately following joint surgery is contraindicated[8] and they should not be should in dogs with suspected bleeding disorders.[3] In a group of very young dogs with canine hip dysplasia that were treated with PSGAG and studied until skeletal maturity, dogs treated with PSGAG had significantly better hip conformation and fewer pathologic and biochemical abnormalities on the femoral head when compared with dogs in the control group, evidence of a disease-modifying effect.[7] In addition, in dogs with radiographically confirmed traumatic or degenerative OA, dogs that received Adequan Canine at a dose of 2 mg/lb IM twice weekly for 4 weeks had a significant improvement in lameness scores when compared with dogs treated with saline. This type of blinded, placebo-controlled study is critical when making a decision if a medication should be widely instituted in the clinical arena or not. However, not all the evidence is supportive. In one blinded, prospective clinical study, the efficacy of a nutraceutical in dogs with OA was evaluated. Three different doses of the nutraceutical were studied and, although dogs in each group improved, no group showed a significant improvement when compared to the dogs that were treated with placebo.[4] This data would suggest that patients might benefit the most from parentally administered PSGAGs if treatment begins early in the degenerative process.

Orally administered PSGAGs (eg, Cosequin) are frequently touted as providing a similar therapeutic effect as the injectable formulations. They, however, are not regulated by the FDA, are considered nutritional supplements or nutraceuticals, and do not have an overwhelming amount of supportive evidence that they are effective in many clinical situations. However, they continue to be commonly prescribed by veterinarians and used by pet owners because they are exceptionally safe (GI problems in about 1% of cases) and have the potential to help. It is advertised that oral nutraceuticals provide the patient with a supraphysiologic concentrations of the precursors necessary for the synthesis of hyaline cartilage. Although most contain glucosamine and chondroitin sulfate, scientific evidence supporting that these precursors reach the joint and help to form new hyaline cartilage is scarce. Recent information would suggest that Cosequin, when administered orally to Beagle dogs at a dose of 1500 mg of glucosamine and 1600 mg of chondroitin, is bioavailable.[1] It was reported that after a single dose 12% of glucosamine and 5.0% of chondroitin was available. The bioavailability of chondroitin increased dramatically with longer-term use. However, it is important to note that this study reported blood concentration, not concentration in the target tissues. Another potential problem with nutraceuticals is that since there is no regulation, the quality of the medication in the bottle is left up to the manufacturer. Some speakers have suggested that the actual concentration of glucosamine and chondroitin in these over-the-counter supplements varies widely. All of these concerns are also true for nutritional supplements that have been added to dog food.

Hyaluronan (HA) is a nonsulfated glycosaminoglycan and is considered a *symptomatic slow-acting drug for osteoarthritis* or SYSADOA. Intra-articular (IA) injections of hyaluronan-related medications have increased in popularity as the formulations have improved. Empirical evidence from colleagues and from my own experience would suggest that many patients will improve for 3 to 12 months from a single or series of injections. Following aseptic preparation of the joint to be treated, I remove as much synovial fluid as I can and then inject 1 to 3 mL of HA. Light sedation of the patient is generally necessary. The only concern with the use of IA medications is the increased risk for iatrogenic infection or with latent infection that might cause a problem during joint replacement surgery. I do not recommend the use of IA steroids.

Alternative treatments for OA are a plenty and include magnets, nutrients, collagens, shark fin, herbs and spices, chiropractic, acupuncture, vitamins and minerals, fish oils, and the list goes on and on. How can one determine whether these are effective treatments for OA? The answer lies in the scientific method: Either there is scientific evidence generated from a neutral party of efficacy when compared with a control group, or there is not.

REFERENCES

1. Adebowale A, Du J, Liang Z, Leslie JL, Eddington ND. The bioavailability and pharmacokinetics of glucosamine hydrochloride and low molecular weight chondroitin sulfate after single and multiple doses to beagle dogs. Biopharm Drug Dispos. 2002;23:217.
2. Altman RD, Dean DD, Muniz OE, et al. Prophylactic treatment of canine osteoarthritis with glycosaminoglycan polysulfuric acid ester. Arthritis Rheum. 1989;32:759.
3. Beale BS, Goring RL, Clemmons RM, et al. The effect of semi-synthetic polysulfated glycosaminoglycan on the hemostatic mechanism in the dog. Vet Surg. 1990;19:57.
4. DeHann JJ, Goring RL, Beale BS. Evaluation of polysulfated glycosaminoglycan for the treatment of hip dysplasia in dogs. Vet Surg. 1994;23:177.
5. Ghosh P, Smith M, Wells C. Second-line agents in osteoarthritis. In: Dixon JS, Furst DE (eds): Second-line Agents in the Treatment of Rheumatic Diseases. New York: Mercel Dekker, 1993, pp 363-427.
6. Howell DS, Carreno MR, Pelletier JP, et al. Articular cartilage breakdown in an alpine model of osteoarthritis: Action of glycosaminoglycan polysulfate ester (GAGPS) on proteoglycan enzyme activity, hexuronate, and cell counts. Clin Orthop Rel Res. 1986;213:69.
7. Lust G, Williams AJ, Burton-Wurster N, et al. Effects of intramuscular injections of glycosaminoglycan polysulfates on signs of incipient hip dysplasia in growing dogs. Am J Vet Res. 1992;53:1836.
8. Todhunter RJ, Minor RR, Wootton JAM, et al. Effects of exercise and polysulfated glycosaminoglycan on the repair of articular cartilage defects in the equine carpus. J Orthop Res. 1993;11:782.
9. Verbruggen G, Veys EM. Influence of an oversulphated heparinoid upon hyaluronate metabolism of the human synovial cell in vivo. J Rheumatol. 1979;6:554.
10. KuKanich B, Papich MG. Pharmacokinetics of tramadol and the metabolite O-desmethyltramadol in dogs. J Vet Pharmacol Ther. 2004; Aug;27(4):239-46.

AN INTEGRATED APPROACH TO CANCER PAIN CONTROL

James S. Gaynor, DVM, MS, Diplomate ACVA & AAPM
Animal Anesthesia and Pain Management Center
Colorado Springs, CO

The treatment of cancer has become more commonplace in veterinary practice as knowledge, drugs, and therapeutic techniques evolve. While some cancers still are not very effectively treated, many owners will attempt various measures at prolonging their pet's lives. Regardless of the prognosis, it is vitally important to attempt to alleviate the pet's pain. It is estimated that cancer pain can be effectively managed in 90% of humans with currently available drugs and techniques. There is no reason to believe that the same success could not be achieved in small animals.

There are four main steps in assuring that pain management is optimized in veterinary patients.

- Assure that veterinarians have the appropriate education and training about the importance of alleviating pain, assessment of pain, available drugs and potential complications, and interventional techniques.
- Educate the client about realistic expectations surrounding pain control and conveying the idea that most patients' pain can be managed. This involves letting the client know that owner involvement in evaluating the pet and providing feedback on therapy is crucial to success. The veterinarian and owner should all participate in developing effective strategies to alleviate pain. Client involvement also helps decrease the potential feeling of helplessness.
- Thoroughly assess the pet's pain at the start and throughout the course of therapy, not just when it gets severe.
- Have good support from the veterinary practice or institution for the use of opioids and other controlled substances.

DRUGS AND TECHNIQUES FOR ALLEVIATION OF PAIN

Drug treatment is the cornerstone of cancer pain management. It is effective and affordable for most patients and owners. The general approach to pain management should follow the World Health Organization ladder which is a three step hierarchy (Figure 1). Within the same category of drugs, there can be different side effects for individuals. Therefore, if possible it may be best to substitute drugs within a category before switching therapies. It is always best to try to keep dosage scheduling as simple as possible. The more complicated the regimen the more likely that non-compliance will occur. Mild to moderate pain should be treated with a non-opioid such as a non-steroidal anti-inflammatory drug (NSAID) or acetaminophen. As pain increases some type of opioid should be added to the regimen. As pain becomes more severe, increase the dose of the opioid. Drugs should be dosed on a regular basis, not just as needed, as pain becomes moderate to severe. Continuous analgesia will facilitate maintaining patient comfort. Additional doses of analgesics can then be administered as pain is intermittently more severe. Adjuvant drugs can be administered to help with specific types of pain and anxiety.

Nonopioids

Nonopioid analgesics include drugs such as acetaminophen, carprofen, deracoxib, firocoxib,

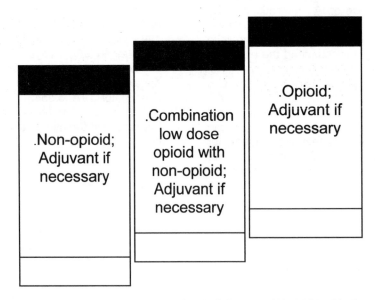

Figure 1. The general approach to pain management should follow the World Health Organization ladder, which is a three step hierarchy.

meloxicam, piroxicam and tepoxalin (Table 1). All except acetaminophen are considered nonsteroidal anti-inflammatory drugs (NSAIDs). Despite the low anti-inflammatory activity of acetaminophen, it possesses beneficial effects of analgesia, minimal risk of bleeding in thrombocytopenic patients, decreased gastrointestinal effects, and synergism with opioid analgesics, such as codeine. Acetaminophen should be avoided in cats due to their inadequate cytochrome P-450 dependent hydroxylation.

Mild to moderate pain, especially that arising from intrathoracic masses, intra-abdominal masses, and bone metastases, can be relieved with NSAIDs. When pain increases, NSAIDs have an opioid-sparing effect so that better analgesia than be achieved with lower doses of opioids. Nonsteroidal anti-inflammatory drugs have central analgesic and peripheral anti-inflammatory effects mediated via inhibition of cyclo-oxygenase. The choice of NSAID ultimately depends upon available species information, clinical response, and tolerance of side effects. Most NSAIDs have been formally investigated only in dogs, leaving anecdotal information for use in cats. The most common side effect of NSAID administration in dogs is gastric irritation and bleeding due to loss of gastric acid inhibition and of cytoprotective mucous production normally promoted by prostaglandins. Other side effects include renal failure and hepatic dysfunction that may lead to failure. Nonsteroidal anti-inflammatory drugs which are more selective for inhibition of cyclo-oxygenase-2 (COX-2) seem to have fewer gastrointestinal effects and potentially fewer renal effects. Therefore, more selective COX-2 inhibitors, such as carprofen, deracoxib, firocoxib, and meloxicam should be considered priority NSAIDs in cancer patients. A blood chemistry panel should be performed prior to initiating NSAID therapy. If there is evidence of liver or renal disease, dehydration or hypotension, another approach to therapy should be considered. The combination of NSAIDs with certain other drugs, such as cisplatin and methoxyflurane, may induce renal toxicity. Therapy with NSAIDs may also inhibit platelet function leading to bleeding and oozing. Therapy with NSAIDs should be stopped if this occurs. If clinical effectiveness is not achieved with one NSAID, it should be discontinued and another started 7 days later to avoid additive or synergistic cyclo-oxygenase inhibition effects. Aspirin should be avoided in dogs due to the increased possibility of gastrointestinal bleeding, even with buffered formulations. Administering misoprostol can help provide gastrointestinal protection during the switchover period. All cancer patients should be closely monitored for gastrointestinal bleeding if receiving NSAID therapy during chemotherapy that may induce thrombocytopenia.

Opioids

Opioids are the major class of analgesics used in the management of moderate to severe cancer pain. They are most effective, predictable, and have low risk associated with them. The most common parenteral opioids used in small animals are morphine, oxymorphone, hydromorphone, fentanyl, codeine, meperidine, buprenorphine, and butorphanol. Parenteral opioids should be used in the perioperative period and should be discontinued when a patient can be switched to oral medication. Common oral opioids (Table 2) include morphine, oxycodone, and codeine with or without acetaminophen.

As a patient's pain increases, the required dose of opioid also increases. Veterinarians may be reluctant to administer high doses of opioids for fear of adverse side effects. It is important to remember that veterinarians have an ethical obligation to benefit the patient by alleviating pain. Opioids can be administered while managing side effects to maximally help the patient. Side effects of opioid administration include diarrhea and vomiting initially, constipation with long-term use, sedation, and dysphoria. The initial gastrointestinal effects occur most frequently with the first injection in the perioperative period and usually do not occur with subsequent dosing. These effects usually do not occur with oral dosing. When sending a patient home with oral medications, it is important to discuss with the owner that dosing is very individual. It is possible that a given dose is perfect, does not provide enough analgesia, induces sedation, or induces dysphoria or excitement. Adjusting of the dose requires excellent doctor-client interaction. Bradycardia is also possible after opioid administration, but is most common when opioids are administered parenterally. If bradycardia occurs, an anticholinergic, such as atropine or glycopyrrolate, should be administered, rather than discontinuing the opioid.

Tricyclic Antidepressants

Tricyclic antidepressants, such as amitriptyline and imipramine block the re-uptake of serotonin and norpeinephrine in the central nervous system (Table 2). They also have antihistimine effects. These drugs have been used in humans for the treatment of chronic and neuuropathic pain at doses considerably lower than those used to treat depression. Veterinarians have not used tricyclic antidepressants in this manner. Presumably, they have similar analgesic properties and enhance opioid analgesia as they do in humans.

OTHER PAIN RELIEVING MODALITIES

Local or whole body radiation can enhance analgesic drug effectiveness by reducing metastatic or primary tumor bulk. Radiation dose should be balanced between the amount necessary to kill tumor cells and that which would affect normal cells. Mucositis of the oral cavity and pharynx can develop after radiation to the neck, head or oral cavities, resulting in impaired ability to eat and drink. Mucositis therapies include analgesics, sucralfate, 2% viscous lidocaine, and green tea rinses.

Bony metastases are one of the most common causes of pain in advanced cancer. Some tumors cause osteoblastic metastsases, but most can cause oseolytic lesions. Administration of biophospanates, such as pamidronate, reduces pain and pathologic fractures in humans. Biophosphanates accumulate on bone surfaces and inhibit osteoclast-induced resorption, favoring bone formation. This therapy is expensive but has been used clinically in dogs and cats. Intravenous administration of strontium-89 has also been shown to provide analgesia related to bony metastases in approximately 50% of humans, but is also uncommon in veterinary patients.

Acupuncture can be used as a pain-relieving modality, often when conventional therapy does not work. It is also useful in conjunction with other therapy to allow lower doses of drugs that may have significant side effects. While some practitioners have difficulty accepting acupuncture because of Traditional Chinese Medical explanations which may be scientifically untenable, it is important to remember that there exists well-documented physiologic theory and evidence for its clinical effects. Details about acupuncture are discussed elsewhere. In general acupuncture analgesia is extremely useful for pelvic, radius/ulna, and femoral bone pain as well as cutaneous discomfort secondary to radiation therapy. Acupuncture also helps alleviate nausea associated with chemotherapy and some analgesics, as well as promoting general well being.

SUMMARY

Control of cancer pain is within the capabilities of most veterinarians and is achievable in most animal cancer patients with techniques that are currently available. Once veterinarians and technicians gain a good knowledge base about pain and its therapy, pain control should be achievable by following these simple ABCs:

- Assess the pain. Ask for the owner's perceptions.
- Believe the owner. The owner sees the pet every day in its own environment.
- Choose appropriate therapy following the WHO ladder and other more specific paradigms.
- Deliver therapy in a logical coordinated manner.
- Empower the clients to actively participate in their pet's well being.

Table 1. Non-opioid Analgesics

Drug	Dog Dose	Cat Dose
Acetaminophen (Tylenol®)	5–10 mg/kg PO q 8 hrs	CI
Carprofen (Rimadyl®)	2.2 mg/kg PO q 12 hrs	UK
Carprofen (Rimadyl®)	4.0 mg/kg IV, SC ONCE	1–3 mg/kg SC ONCE
Deracoxib (Deramaxx®)	1–4 mg/kg PO q 24 hr	UK
Firocoxib (Previcox®)	5.0 mg/kg PO q 24hr	UK
Meloxicam (Metacam®)	0.2 mg/kg SC ONCE	0.1–0.3 mg/kg SC ONCE
Meloxicam (Metacam®)	0.1 mg/kg PO q 24 hr	0.1 mg/kg PO q 24 hr for days then tapering
Tepoxalin (Zubrin®)	10 mg/kg PO q 24 hr	UK
Piroxicam (Feldene®)	0.3 mg/kg q 24 hrs for 2 days then 0.3 mg/kg q 48 hrs	0.3 mg/kg q 48 hrs
Misoprostal (Cytotec®))	2–5 µg/kg PO q 8 hrs	UK

CI = Contraindicated for use in cats; UK = unknown dose
*Carprofen dosing, efficacy, and side effects have not been well established in cats. The oral dose is empirical based on pharmacokinetics in cats
*Synthetic prostaglandin E used to increase the protective effects of endogenous prostaglandins ($PGE_{2\square}$) and prevent GI ulceration.

Table 2. Oral Opioids and Adjunct Drugs to Management of Pain for Dogs and Cats*

Drug	Dose
Morphine	0.5–1.0 mg/kg PO q 6–12 hrs
Sustained release morphine	0.5–1.0 mg/kg PO q 12–24 hrs
Oxycodone	0.2–0.3 mg/kg PO q 6-12 hrs
Codeine	1 mg/kg Po Q6–12 hrs
Codeine (30 mg) with acetaminophen (300 mg)	1 mg/kg codeine = 10 mg/kg acetaminophen q 12 hrs
Clomipramine (Clomicalm®)	2–4 mg/kg q 24 hrs
Amitriptyline (dog) (Elavil®)	1–2 mg/kg q 12–24 hrs
Amitriptyline (cat) (Elavil®)	2.5–12.5 mg /cat q 24 hrs
Imipramine (dog) (Tofranil®)	0.5–1.0 mg/kg q 8 hrs
Imipramine (cat) (Tofranil®)	2.5–5 mg/kg q 12 hrs

* Doses are the same for dogs and cats unless otherwise described.

FRINGE THERAPIES: FRINGE RESULTS?

James S. Gaynor, DVM, MS, Diplomate ACVA & AAPM
Animal Anesthesia and Pain Management Center
Colorado Springs, CO

Clients tend to come into our exam rooms with many different ideas on how to treat their pet's arthritis, both the pain and as a disease. Virtually all of the products are not drugs, and therefore have not undergone the scrutiny of the FDA approval process. In addition, most products have undergone very little to no research. As a result, there is likely no scientific basis for their use. We know that any product can induce a placebo effect and that any company can choose to just report good testimonials and anecdotal information. A number of products have apparent efficacy and varying degrees of research to support their use. These include glucosamine/chondroitin products, oral hyaluronic acid formulations, Microlactin®, and elk antler velvet.

GLUCOSAMINE-CONTAINING SUPPLEMENTS

There is ongoing controversy surrounding glucosamine-containing products for the treatment of osteoarthritis. The first important concept with these products is to recognize that not all products are created equally. A study from the University of Maryland in 2000 indicated that 80% of glucosamine-containing products do not contain the amounts of glucosamine as indicated on the label. One way to help assure quality of ingredients is to find products that follow US Pharmacopaeia (USP) standards. The next important aspect is to recognize that not all glucosamine formulations have the same in vivo effects. For example, glucosamine sulfate is not nearly as efficacious as glucosamine HCl. After getting past the glucosamine, it is important to look at the other ingredients in the formulation.

Like glucosamine, chondroitin sulfate efficacy can vary depending on its particular formulation. Most products have high-molecular-weight chondroitin, which is absorbed very little from the gastrointestinal (GI) tract of humans, dogs, and horses. Low-molecular-weight chondroitin, a small molecule, is a proprietary formulation found in Cosequin® and Dasuquin® and has associated data showing its absorption from the GI tract.

While glucosamine HCl and low-molecular-weight chondroitin have been documented to have significant bioactivity in cartilage, their combination with manganese has a greater effect. Manganese has a catalyst effect, increasing bioactivity a significant amount.

Perna canaliculus, green-lipped muscle, can be found in some products such as Glycoflex III®. While the data is old, it has been shown to be effective at pain relief, at least in the laboratory setting.

A number of published papers have shown that Cosequin® (glucosamine HCl, low-molecular-weight chondroitin, and manganese) has many beneficial effects on cartilage in dogs and other species. This combination has also been shown to be a preventative effect. Patients receiving Cosequin® prior to an acute joint injury heal more quickly than those who start to receive it afterwards.

Glycoflex III® has Perna canaliculus, glucosamine HCl, manganese, methylsulfonylmethane (MSM), DMG, vitamins E&C, grape seed extract, glutathione, and selenium. Only the first three components have known efficacy associated with them. However, there is emerging data that Glycoflex III® may reduce the severity of cartilage breakdown and synovitis and appears to have an anti-inflammatory effect. Data is still pending on its effect in clinically affected patients.

When evaluating data for any glucosamine-containing product, be sure the material being presented by a company representative actually pertains to the particular product and not that of another manufacturer. This can happen quite frequently. Beware!

HYALURONIC ACID

Hyaluronic acid (HA) exists naturally in all living organisms. It is found in greatest concentrations in the synovial fluid of joints for lubrication, the vitreous humor (fluid) of the eye, and in the skin. Hyaluronic acid plays an important role in tissue hydration, lubrication and cellular function, and is able to hold more water than any other natural substance. Hyaluronic acid is a special mucopolysacharide. Its concentration decreases with osteoarthritis. (Figure 1). When present in a joint, even a joint with minimal or no cartilage, it can provide a cushion effect. High-molecular-weight HA has been shown to provide better joint lubrication than low-molecular-weight HA.

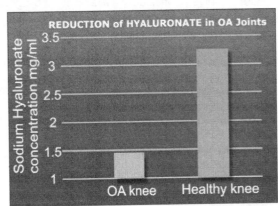

In a healthy knee, sodium hyaluronate has a concentration between 2.5-4 mg/ml. This concentration is reduced two to three times in osteoarthritic (OA) joints.

Figure 1. Graphical representation of the quantity of hyaluronic acid in normal and knees and those with osteoarthritis.

Injectable hyaluronic acid is available as an FDA-approved drug for use in horses (Legend®). There are no FDA-approved oral versions of HA. However, there is good evidence that high-molecular-weight HA is absorbed through the GI tract and provides good knee lubrication in humans. There are no comparable animal studies, but clinical impressions of many veterinarians are that oral HA can act as a good adjunct to increasing pain control in dogs and cats with osteoarthritis.

MICROLACTIN

Duralactin® contains MicroLactin®, a patented special dried milk protein from the milk of hyperimmunized cows. Partially purified preparations inhibit inflammation in many laboratory animal models. The anti-inflammatory activity is bioavailable both orally and systemically, is effective regardless of the etiology of the inflammation, and appears to function with no evidence of gastrointestinal tract irritation.

Unlike steroids and nonsteroidal anti-inflammatory drugs (NSAIDs), Duralactin® has no demonstrable cyclo-oxygenase (COX) inhibiting activity or short- or long-term toxic effects in any species studied thus far. This is especially important for dogs in which long-term management of musculoskeletal disorders is indicated and the extended use of steroids or NSAIDs is contraindicated.

In a recent placebo-controlled study in dogs showing signs of osteoarthritis, Duralactin® induced a significant improvement in standardized and patient-specific questionnaire scores and in owner global assessments (Figure 2).

ELK ANTLER VELVET

Elk antler velvet is harvested from the male elk during the velvet stage of growth, when the antler contains the most nutritional value. The inner cartilaginous matrix, not the outside velvet covering is used as the supplement. The bioactive components of the antler velvet include type II collagen, glycosaminoglycans (chondroitin sulfate),

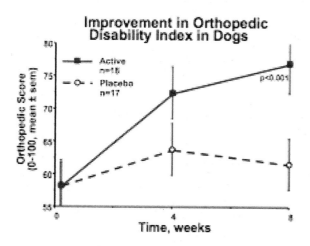

Figure 2. Duralactin® (active) induced improvement in dogs versus placebo.

polysaccharides, growth hormone, and various prostaglandins.

Elk antler velvet has been shown to aid in the performance of human athletes and may help with osteoporosis in women. In a double-blinded, placebo-controlled study, CanEVA–K9® (Canadian Elk Velvet Antler of Dogs) was effective in alleviating the clinical signs of arthritis in dogs and improved ground reaction forces. In addition, investigators observed that the dogs receiving CanEVA® had a significant reduction of muscle atrophy, suggesting a myotrophic effect.

HOW TO TREAT THE ARTHRITIC CAT: MANAGING CHRONIC PAIN

B. Duncan X. Lascelles, BSc, BVSC, PhD, MRCVS, CertVA, DSAS(ST), Diplomate ECVS and ACVS
Director, Comparative Pain Research Laboratory
Director, Integrated Pain Management Service
College of Veterinary Medicine
North Carolina State, University Raleigh, NC

Suggested doses of analgesics that may be used for the alleviation of chronic pain in the cat are listed in Table 1. **Only one of these drugs is approved for use in chronic pain, and only in the EU.** Some drugs are approved for inflammatory or painful conditions in the cat in certain countries, and doses for the control of chronic pain are extrapolated from these.

The doses given come from the authors' experience, and the experience of others working in the area of clinical cancer pain control. Sources of information are given. Where sources of information are not given, there is no information on this drug as an analgesic in the cat.

Table 1. Analgesics for Alleviation of Chronic Pain in Cats*

Drug	Cat Dose (mg/kg)	Notes	Published Source of Information/ Reference on Analgesic Efficacy in Cats
Paracetamol (acetaminophen)	Contraindicated	Contraindicated—small doses rapidly cause death in cats.	—
Amantadine	3.0–5.0 mg/kg PO q 24 hrs	This drug has not been evaluated for toxicity but is well tolerated in dogs and humans, with occasional side effects of agitation and GI irritation. May be a useful addition to NSAIDs in the treatment of chronic cancer pain conditions. The 100-mg capsules need to be re-compounded for cats.	†
Amitriptyline	0.5–2.0 mg/kg PO q 24 hrs	Appears to be well tolerated for up to 12 months of daily administration. Has been used for interstitial cystitis, and somnolence (<10%), weight gain, decreased grooming, and transient cystic calculi were observed during treatment in some cats (see ref). May be a useful addition to NSAIDs for treatment of chronic pain conditions.	1
Aspirin	10 mg/kg PO q 48 hrs	Can cause significant gastro-intestinal ulceration	2-4
Buprenorphine	0.02 mg/kg sublingual q 6–7 hrs	The sublingual route is not resented by cats and may be a good way to provide postoperative analgesia at home. Feedback from owners indicates that after 2–3 days dosing at this dose, anorexia develops. Smaller doses (5–10 mcg/kg) may be more appropriate for "long-term" administration, especially in combination with other drugs.	5
Butorphanol	0.2–1.0 mg/kg PO q 6 hrs	One study suggests using oral butorphanol after surgery may be beneficial. Generally considered to be a poor analgesic in cats except for visceral pain, however the author has found it to be useful as part of a multimodal approach to cancer pain therapy	6

Table 1. Continued.

Carprofen	Not enough data to enable recommendations for long term administration	—	—
Etodolac	Not recommended	—	—
Flunixin meglumine	1 mg/kg PO daily for 7 days	Daily dosing for 7 days results in increased rate of metabolism of the drug, but a rise in liver enzymes, suggesting liver toxicity may be a problem with prolonged dosing.	7
Gabapentin	5–10 mg/kg q 12 hours	Appears to be particularly effective in chronic pain in cats where an increase in sensitivity has occurred, or where the pain appears to be excessive in comparison to the lesion present.	
Glucosamine/ chondroitin sulfate combinations	Approx 15 mg/kg chondroitin sulfate PO q 12 to 24 hrs	This combination appears to produce mild anti-inflammatory and analgesic effects in cats more predictably than in dogs. Can be used in conjunction with NSAIDs, opioids and amantadine.	
Glucosamine/ chondroitin sulfate combination with avocado/soya extracts	Labeled dose	This preparation has only just become available, but the addition of ASU (Dasuquin®) appears to boost the analgesic effects of Glu/Cho4. Can be used in conjunction with NSAIDs, opioids and amantadine.	
Ketoprofen[§]	1 mg/kg PO q 24 hrs; maximum 5 days	Probably well tolerated as pulse therapy for chronic pain, with a few days "rest" between treatments. Has also been used by some at 1mg/kg every 3 days long term. Another approach has been to use 0.5mg/kg daily for 5 days (weekdays) followed by no drug over the weekend, and this is repeated.	8
Meloxicam §	mg/kg PO on day 1, followed by 0.05mg/kg PO daily for 4 days, then 0.05 mg/kg every other day thereafter, OR 0.025 mg/kg daily. Approval has recently (June 2007) been gained in Europe (EMEA – the equivalent of the FDA) for long-term (unlimited) use of meloxicam in the cat at 0.1 mg/kg on day 1, followed by 0.05 mg/kg daily	This drug is particularly well received by cats due to its formulation as a honey syrup. Also, the drop formulation makes it very easy to gradually and accurately decrease the dose. The suggested dosing regimen has not been evaluated for clinical toxicity	8,9, 10
Morphine (oral liquid)	0.2–0.5 mg/kg PO t.i.d. –q.i.d.	Best compounded into a palatable flavored syrup; however, cats usually strongly resent this medication. Morphine may not be as effective in cats as it is in dogs.	

Table 1. Continued.

Morphine (oral sustained release)	Tablets too large for dosing cats	—	—
Piroxicam	1 mg/cat PO daily for a maximum of 7 days. If longer term medication is considered, suggest every other day dosing, but see note at right.	Daily dosing for 7 days results in a slight increase in the half-life. The active drug decreases significantly over a 10-day period after compounding in an aqueous solution. In the author's experience, significant drops in PCV (presumably due to GI hemorrhage) occur in up to 30% of cats after 2–3 weeks of drug therapy.	11
Prednisolone	0.5–1.0 mg/kg PO q 24 hrs	Can be particularly effective in cancers associated with significant inflammation (such as squamous cell carcinoma of the oral cavity in cats). **NOT to be combined with concurrent NSAID administration**	†
Tolfenamic acid [§]	4 mg/kg PO q 24 hrs for 3 days maximum	—	—
Tramadol	1–2 mg/kg once to twice daily	Not yet been used extensively by the author for the treatment of chronic pain in cats. However, early results are encouraging, but neurological side effects are more readily seen in the cat compared to the dog, and dosing should be started at the low end.	†
Transdermal fentanyl patch	2–5 μg/kg/hrs	A 25μg/hr patch can be applied to an "average" cat (7.7–11 lb; 3.5–5.0 kg). In smaller cats, other methods of providing analgesia should be sought as it is not recommended to cut patches in half and covering half of the patch gives unpredictable results. The patches may provide 5–7 days of analgesia in some cases. Following removal at 3 days, the decay in plasma levels following patch removal is slow.	12,13
Vedaprofen	0.5 mg/kg q 24 hrs for 3 days	Has not been evaluated for chronic pain, but was evaluated for controlling pyrexia in upper respiratory infection, and for controlling post-operative pain following ovariohysterectomy	14

* Adapted from Lascelles BDX. Drug therapy for acute and chronic pain in the cat. Int J Pharm Compounding. 2002;6:338-343.
† From author's and colleagues' experience.
§ Drug indicated is licensed and approved for use at the stated dose (for an indication other than cancer) in one of the following countries: United States, United Kingdom, Australia, New Zealand.

REFERENCES

1. Chew DJ, Buffington CA, Kendall MS, et al. Amitriptyline treatment for severe recurrent idiopathic cystitis in cats. J Am Vet Med Assoc. 1998; 213:1282-1286.

2. Lau AT, Graham GG, Day RO, et al. Effect of aspirin on ulcer site blood flow in cat stomachs. Am J Physiol. 1992; 263:G155-160.

3. Villar D, Buck WB, Gonzalez JM. Ibuprofen, aspirin and acetaminophen toxicosis and treatment in dogs and cats. Vet Hum Toxicol. 1998; 40:156-162.

4. Whittle BJ, Hansen D, Salmon JA. Gastric ulcer formation and cyclo-oxygenase inhibition in cat antrum follows parenteral administration of aspirin but not salicylate. Eur J Pharmacol. 1985; 116:153-157.

5. Robertson SA, Lascelles BD, Taylor PM, et al. PK-PD modeling of buprenorphine in cats: intravenous and oral transmucosal administration. J Vet Pharmacol Ther. 2005; 28:453-460.

6. Carroll GL, Howe LB, Slater MR, et al. Evaluation of analgesia provided by postoperative administration of butorphanol to cats undergoing onychectomy. J Am Vet Med Assoc. 1998; 213:246-250.

7. Taylor PM, Winnard JG, Jefferies R, et al. Flunixin in the cat: a pharmacodynamic, pharmacokinetic and toxicological study. Br Vet J. 1994; 150:253-262.

8. Lascelles BD, Henderson AJ, Hackett IJ. Evaluation of the clinical efficacy of meloxicam in cats with painful locomotor disorders. J Small Anim Pract. 2001; 42:587-593.

9. Lascelles BDX, Hansen BD, Roe SC, et al. Evaluation of client-specific outcome measures and activity monitoring to measure pain relief in cats with osteoarthritis. J Vet Intern Med. 2007; 21:410-416.

10. Clarke SP, Bennett D. Feline osteoarthritis: a prospective study of 28 cases. J Small Anim Pract. 2006; 47:439-445.

11. Heeb HL, Chun R, Koch DE, et al. Multiple dose pharmacokinetics and acute safety of piroxicam and cimetidine in the cat. J Vet Pharmacol Ther. 2005; 28:447-452.

12. Franks JN, Boothe HW, Taylor L, et al. Evaluation of transdermal fentanyl patches for analgesia in cats undergoing onychectomy. J Am Vet Med Assoc. 2000; 217:1013-1020.

13. Glerum LE, Egger CM, Allen SW, et al. Analgesic effect of the transdermal fentanyl patch during and after feline ovariohysterectomy. Vet Surg. 2001; 30:351-358.

14. Lopez S, Pertuy S, Horspool L, et al. Vedaprofen therapy in cats with upper respiratory tract infection or following ovariohysterectomy. J Small Anim Pract. 2007; 48:70-75.

ADJUNCTIVE DRUG THERAPY FOR CANINE OSTEOARTHRITIS PAIN

B. Duncan X. Lascelles, BSc, BVSC, PhD, MRCVS, CertVA, DSAS(ST), Diplomate ECVS and ACVS
Director, Comparative Pain Research Laboratory
Director, Integrated Pain Management Service
College of Veterinary Medicine
North Carolina State University. Raleigh, NC

Osteoarthritic disease is the most common cause of chronic pain in dogs, involving about 20% of the US canine population, or up to 12 million dogs. Clinical experience and a review of experimental studies reveal that nonsteroidal anti-inflammatory drugs (NSAIDs) may not provide complete pain relief in all cases of canine osteoarthritis. In human medicine, a multimodal pharmacologic approach is used frequently for chronic pain associated with osteoarthritis. A multimodal approach has also been suggested for the alleviation of chronic pain in veterinary species.

This suggestion stems from the recent understanding of central nervous system changes that result from the constant input of noxious signals from the periphery. Pain transmission involves multiple pathways, mechanisms, and transmitter systems. Therefore, it is unlikely that a single class of analgesic, whatever the dose, will provide complete pain relief. Clinical experience confirms this. The combination of two or more classes of analgesics (eg, concurrent use of opioids, NSAIDs, and local anesthetics) is more effective for perioperative pain control. A similar multimodal approach is recommended for chronic pain management, such as that associated with cancer or osteoarthritis. The analgesic effect from these drugs is often synergistic. Therefore, smaller doses of the individual drugs can be used, thus decreasing the likelihood of side effects from any one drug.

However, there is no published scientific evidence that multimodal drug therapy is of benefit over monomodal therapy in veterinary patients suffering from osteoarthritis. Any suggestions and recommendations are based on information extrapolated from the human literature own clinical experience. The effectiveness and toxicity of multimodal therapy is an area of active research in veterinary medicine, and recommendations may change as data are generated.

INTEGRATING NSAID, ADJUNCTIVE DRUG, AND NON-DRUG THERAPIES

The benefit of nondrug therapies in osteoarthritis pain management is also relatively undefined in the veterinary literature. Clinically, the analgesic therapeutic effects of acupuncture, electroacupuncture, acupressure, and transcutaneous electrical nerve stimulation have not been fully investigated, nor has the analgesic effect of physical therapy (cold and heat therapy, massage therapy, passive physiotherapy, hydrotherapy, and active controlled exercise, including swimming). However, despite the lack of experimental evidence for their efficacy, clinical experience supports the use of such modalities in conjunction with NSAID and adjunctive drug therapy as appropriate. The desired clinical outcome is better control of patient discomfort and an overall decrease in the amount of drugs needed.

In 2002, the American Pain Society published the first evidence-based, multidisciplinary arthritis pain management guideline. This document outlines the detrimental effects of untreated chronic pain, the need for comprehensive pain assessment, and the evidence-based medicine recommendations for multimodal drug therapy and concurrent multimodal nondrug therapy. The use of multiple classes of drugs and the integration of drug and nondrug therapies can be called *integrated multimodal pain therapy*.

RATIONALE FOR ADJUNCTIVE DRUG USE

Adjunctive drugs are drugs used together with NSAIDs to provide greater osteoarthritic pain relief. Adjunctive drug classes include opioids, N-methyl-D-aspartate (NMDA) receptor antagonists, tricyclic antidepressants, anticonvulsants and calcium channel blockers, sodium channel blockers, and polysulfated glycosaminoglycans. The most commonly used individual drugs are amantadine, tramadol, gabapentin, amitriptyline, and Adequan (Luitpold Pharmaceuticals) (see Table 1).

Opioids

Opioids act at all levels of the pain pathway—peripherally and centrally at the spinal cord and at higher centers. Four opioid receptors have been cloned: mu, delta, kappa, and ORL-1. Little progress has been made on the development of synthetic opioid drugs that will produce analgesia without the classic opioid side effects in dogs, such as sedation and gastrointestinal ileus leading to constipation. In the next few years, most progress with opioids will probably be made by defining their interactions with other systems. For example, there appears to be an interaction between the NMDA receptor and the opioid receptor in the dorsal horn of the spinal cord and a positive interaction between the alpha-2-receptor and opioid receptor. Harnessing these interactions by using a multimodal analgesic approach should provide greater therapeutic effects in the future. Recently, there has been interest in redefining the role of opioids and opioid derivatives in chronic pain states in people, and both the American and Canadian pain societies have endorsed the use of opioids for osteoarthritis as part of a multimodal approach.

Transdermal fentanyl can be used but is expensive for long-term use, and recent concerns about its safety in people may lead manufacturers to pull fentanyl patches from the market in the future. The recent advent of buprenorphine patches in human medicine hold promise for providing longer-term pain relief than with fentanyl patches. The buprenorphine patch has not been evaluated in dogs, but work has been performed in cats.

Oral opioid medications, such as codeine, codeine-combination drugs (such as acetaminophen with codeine), morphine, methadone, and butorphanol, can be administered to dogs, although very little is known about their efficacy in dogs. Oral opioids are subject to a high first-pass effect in the liver, and recent work has demonstrated that oral morphine and oral methadone are not well absorbed in dogs, casting doubt on their efficacy as canine analgesics. This area needs further work—both to define the potential overall usefulness of oral opioids in dogs and to evaluate other specific oral opioids, such as codeine and butorphanol.

Oral tramadol, however, was found to be absorbed sufficiently. Tramadol is an opioid derivative that also has actions on the serotoninergic and alpha-adrenergic systems. Tramadol's analgesic efficacy is a result of complex interactions between opiate, adrenergic, and serotonin receptor systems. It has been used successfully in osteoarthritis pain management in people and is now recommended as part of a multimodal drug therapy for osteoarthritis pain control. One report in dogs is encouraging. Animals with chronic osteoarthritis were treated with a low dose of ketoprofen (0.25 mg/kg orally once daily) or low dose ketoprofen plus tramadol (5 mg/kg of prolonged release form orally once daily) for 28 days. Dogs receiving both drugs had a significant improvement in pain scores, and even after treatment was discontinued, they continued to improve. The dogs in the ketoprofen-only group remained static and had more incidences of acute flare-ups than the other dogs after the end of treatment.

NMDA Antagonists

The NMDA receptor plays a key role in inducing and maintaining central sensitization, a change that appears to be present in chronic pain states. The use of NMDA receptor antagonists appears to be of benefit in arthritis models where central sensitization is present. Given that even a brief noxious input to the spinal cord can induce central changes, NMDA antagonists have been studied in the treatment for most types of pain. NMDA receptors have also been found on unmyelinated axons in the peripheral nervous system, suggesting that they play a role in primary nociception. Memantine, amantadine, ketamine, and dextromethorphan are uncompetitive NMDA antagonists that have been used clinically in people with neuropathic pain. However, there are no reports of NMDA antagonists being used to treat osteoarthritis pain in people. Research indicates that dogs probably do not make the active metabolite from dextromethorphan necessary for NMDA blockade.

I have been evaluating the NMDA antagonist amantadine (3 to 5 mg/kg orally once daily) as an adjunct to NSAID use in canine osteoarthritis and consider it to augment pain relief with a low incidence of side effects (agitation and diarrhea). The dose of amantadine was decided upon on the basis of known kinetics, clinical observations, and pilot data. Although I have not performed toxicity studies on amantadine, others have. In repeated studies conducted over a two-year period, a dose of 40 to 80 mg/kg resulted in deaths after 30 weeks of administration, a dose of 40 mg/kg resulted in one death (out of eight dogs) after 47 weeks of administration, and a dose of 8 mg/kg was not associated with any adverse signs. The deaths were

attributed to vomiting and seizures. In my experience and based on the results of a recently completed clinical trial in my laboratory, the oral NMDA antagonist amantadine appears to be effective in treating canine osteoarthritis when combined with an NSAID. The development of more specific NMDA antagonists is an exciting area being pursued by several manufacturers. However, the development of clinically useful and targeted NMDA antagonists is hampered because the NMDA receptor exists in numerous forms, the form changes rapidly after nociceptive input, and the form and quantity may differ significantly from one type of painful stimulus to another.

Tricyclic Antidepressants

Tricyclic antidepressants have been used for many years for the treatment of chronic pain syndromes in people and are becoming widely used for the modulation of behavioral disorders in animals. Given that many behavioral disorders are due to chronic pain, tricyclic antidepressants may not directly affect behavior but rather the pain itself, which results in behavior modification. Antidepressants, such as amitriptyline, clomipramine, imipramine, maprotiline, fluoxetine, and paroxetine primarily inhibit the reuptake of various monoamines (such as serotonin and norepinephrine). Many of these drugs have mixed actions, which may be an added benefit (eg, amitriptyline has some effect on the norepinephrine system and on histidine and cholinergic receptors). These drugs have been used in people for the treatment of chronic and neuropathic pain at doses considerably lower than those used to treat depression. Amitriptyline has been used successfully for feline interstitial cystitis, a syndrome associated with chronic pain, but as of yet, the use of these drugs in animals has not been systematically evaluated. Tricyclic antidepressants should probably not be used concurrently with drugs that modify the serotonergic system, such as tramadol.

Anticonvulsants and Calcium Channel Blockers

Many anticonvulsants, such as carbamazepine, phenytoin, baclofen, and gabapentin, have been used for chronic pain, including neuropathic pain, in people. Gabapentin, a structural analogue of gamma-aminobutyric acid, and the more recently introduced pregabalin, appear to be the most effective of the anticonvulsants for neuropathic pain. Their mechanism of action appears to be binding to the alpha-2-delta subunit of calcium channels, thereby modulating the activity of calcium channels. Calcium channels participate in the process of nociceptive transmission at the level of the neuronal synapse in the central nervous system. Calcium channel modulators have been demonstrated to reduce pain, allodynia, and hyperalgesia. The indications for their use are unclear for veterinary patients, but they may be useful as an adjunct to other analgesics, especially for neurogenic pain, neuropathic pain, and pain from certain cancers, such as bone tumors. Although there is considerable information on gabapentin as an anticonvulsant in dogs, there is no peer-reviewed information on its use for osteoarthritis pain, although recent studies in rats suggest it may play a role in the management of osteoarthritis pain. I use gabapentin for neuropathic, neurogenic, and osteoarthritic pain at relatively low doses of 5 to 10 mg/kg twice daily.

Sodium Channel Blockers

Alterations in the level of expression, cellular localization, and distribution of sodium channels are strongly associated with neuropathic pain. Although not convenient for most patients, intravenous lidocaine has proven effective for neuropathic pain in people. I have used it as part of an intravenous cocktail for the treatment of neurogenic pain, such as nerve root entrapment pain, lumbosacral pain, and severe osteoarthritis pain. There is increasing interest in transdermal lidocaine patches for osteoarthritis in people. Currently no information exists on how to use these agents safely and effectively in animals, although one study has evaluated the kinetics of lidocaine absorbed from patches applied to dogs. Mexiletine, phenytoin, carbamazepine, oxcarbazepine, and lamotrigine have all demonstrated sodium channel blocking properties, but their use in people has been limited by inconsistent efficacy, drug-drug interactions, and side effects.

Polysulfated Glycosaminoglycans

In the United States, one polysulfated glycosaminoglycan is approved by the Food and Drug Administration for dogs—Adequan. It is used for the potential modification (decrease) of osteoarthritis progression. Theoretically, it modifies the disease cycle by reducing proteoglycan degradation and inhibiting cytokine synthesis and activity. Adequan also stimulates glycosaminoglycan synthesis and results in an increased concentration of hyaluronan. Adequan is a semisynthetic heparinoid, the major component of which is chondroitin sulfate. The extra sulfate groups that are synthetically added to chondroitin sulfate to produce polysulfated glycosaminoglycan appear to increase the efficacy of this molecule to inhibit enzyme activity. Presumably the extra sulfate groups increase the available charge area for interaction of polysulfated glycosaminoglycan with active enzymes.

A number of studies have evaluated Adequan in a variety of scenarios. One study has shown a beneficial effect in reducing the progression of hip dysplasia in puppies. Other studies have shown positive effects on the metabolism of cartilage explants. A study evaluating the effects of Adequan on pain and lameness in adult dogs with hip osteoarthritis found a benefit (although not statistically significant) to the administration of Adequan. The drug was administered intramuscularly to 84 dogs every 3 to 5 days for a total of eight injections. Treatment response was analyzed based on changes in lameness, range of motion, and pain on manipulation of the hip joints. Dogs that were given 4.4 mg/kg of Adequan showed the greatest improvement in orthopedic scores, whereas dogs in the placebo group showed the smallest

improvement. However, the differences in clinical improvement among the four treatment groups were not statistically significant.[51] Overall, it appears that Adequan can have a mild analgesic effect, it is compatible with other therapies mentioned, and it is devoid of side effects.

NEUROBIOLOGICAL SIGNATURE OF OSTEOARTHRITIS

In recent years, researchers have noted that chronic pain results in a unique set of changes in the peripheral and central nervous system, and these changes vary depending on the disease. These changes have been referred to as the *neurobiological signature* of the disease. Understanding the neurobiological signatures for different disease processes should lead to the development of novel, targeted, and more effective treatments.[52] Currently, details of pain neurobiology associated with naturally occurring osteoarthritis are scant. Further research should allow for more informed choices regarding efficacy of the currently available drugs.

MULTIMODAL USE OF ADJUNCTIVE DRUGS

Despite the scarcity of clinical evidence to guide practitioners, the following points summarize a currently suitable approach to multimodal osteoarthritis pain management:

- NSAIDs, acetaminophen, or steroids usually form the analgesic base when treating osteoarthritis pain, and all of the above-mentioned drugs can be administered safely with these.
- Generally, the above-mentioned drugs are most effective when used with NSAIDs; however, in dogs that are intolerant of NSAIDs, steroids, or acetaminophen (or where these are contraindicated), they can be used alone or in combination with each other.
- It appears that NSAIDs and the above-mentioned drugs can be used in combination for many months. Amitriptyline and tramadol should probably not be used concurrently.
- A suitable order in which to add adjunctive drugs to NSAID therapy would be Adequan, tramadol, amantadine, and then gabapentin. Tramadol will probably provide the fastest analgesic result; the others take a variable amount of time to have a measurable effect.
- The drugs should probably be added one by one, allowing five to seven days to assess the potential for drug intolerance (sedation, vomiting, or agitation) and the need for dosage adjustments before adding the next one.

REFERENCES

1. Hedhammar A, Olsson SE, Andersson SA, et al. Canine hip dysplasia: study of heritability in 401 litters of German Shepherd dogs. J Am Vet Med Assoc. 1979;174:1012-1016.

2. Johnson JA, Austin C, Breur GJ. Incidence of canine appendicular musculoskeletal disorders in 16 veterinary teaching hospitals from 1980 to 1989. Vet Comp Orthop Traum. 1994;7:56-69.

3. Moore GE, Burkman KD, Carter MN, et al. Causes of death or reasons for euthanasia in military working dogs: 927 cases (1993-1996). J Am Vet Med Assoc. 2001;219:209-214.

4. Lascelles BD, Main DC. Surgical trauma and chronically painful conditions—within our comfort level but beyond theirs? J Am Vet Med Assoc. 2002;221:215-222.

5. Budsberg SC, Johnston SA, Schwarz PD, et al. Efficacy of etodolac for the treatment of osteoarthritis of the hip joints in dogs. J Am Vet Med Assoc. 1999;214:206-210.

6. Holtsinger RH, Parker RB, Beale BS, et al. The therapeutic efficacy of carprofen (Rimadyl-V) in 209 clinical cases of canine degenerative joint disease. Vet Comp Orthop Traum. 1992;5:140-144.

7. Vasseur PB, Johnson AL, Budsberg SC, et al. Randomized, controlled trial of the efficacy of carprofen, a nonsteroidal anti-inflammatory drug, in the treatment of osteoarthritis in dogs. J Am Vet Med Assoc. 1995;206:807-811.

8. Freedman GM. Chronic pain. Clinical management of common causes of geriatric pain. Geriatrics. 2002;57:36-41; quiz 42.

9. Manek NJ, Lane NE. Osteoarthritis: current concepts in diagnosis and management. Am Fam Physician. 2000;61:1795-1804.

10. Mullican WS, Lacy JR. Tramadol/acetaminophen combination tablets and codeine/acetaminophen combination capsules for the management of chronic pain: a comparative trial. Clin Ther. 2001;23:1429-1445.

Additional references are available from the author upon request.

Table 1. Adjunctive drugs used in canine osteoarthritis pain management*

Drug	Dose for Dogs	Comments
Amantadine	3–5 mg/kg orally once daily	• May take up to 2 weeks to see positive effects • Side effects appear to be mild agitation in some dogs • Marketed as 100-mg capsules. Suggest one capsule for dogs weighing 20–37 kg, and two capsules for dogs weighing 37–65 kg.
Amitriptyline	0.5–2 mg/kg orally once daily	• Bitter taste • Should not be used concurrently with tramadol
Gabapentin	5–10 mg/kg orally twice daily (up to 10 mg/kg three times daily)	• Most common side effect appears to be sedation
Polysulfated glycosaminoglycan (Adequan)	5 mg/kg intramuscularly twice weekly for 4 weeks, then once a month	• No noted side effects
Tramadol	4–5 mg/kg orally twice or three times daily	• Side effects appear to be sedation and vomiting (likely opioidergic effects) • Should not be used concurrently with amitriptyline

* This table outlines the doses for some of the adjunctive oral drugs used by the author to help alleviate chronic osteoarthritis pain in dogs. Although all of these drugs are available in the United States, not all are approved for use in dogs. Most of the drugs have not had comprehensive efficacy, kinetic, or toxicity studies carried out in dogs and are being used empirically based on extrapolation from human medicine and clinical experience. There has been no comprehensive evaluation of the toxicity when these drugs are administered simultaneously. Evaluation of these drugs is being undertaken by a number of investigators, and new information may result in changes in the recommended doses. These drugs are for use in combination with NSAIDs, steroids, or acetaminophen; however, they can also be used on their own to provide pain relief in canine osteoarthritis.

SHOULD WE BE RECOGNIZING AND TREATING NEUROPATHIC PAIN?

B. Duncan X. Lascelles, BSc, BVSC, PhD, MRCVS, CertVA, DSAS(ST), Diplomate ECVS, Diplomate ACVS
Director, Comparative Pain Research Laboratory
Director, Integrated Pain Management Service
College of Veterinary Medicine
North Carolina State University, Raleigh, NC

Dealing with pain is a significant challenge for owners of companion animals and the provider of their medical care. Pain can be difficult to assess, and the veterinarian must work closely with the owner in assessing level of pain, and response to treatment. Neuropathic or neurogenic pain can be particularly frustrating, as the drugs used most frequently for chronic pain control, NSAIDs, often do not provide sufficient relief.

This article discusses drugs that may be useful for the treatment of neuropathic or neurogenic pain. Drug options include NSAIDs (COX-1 sparing, coxibs and dual inhibitors), acetaminophen, N-methyl-d-asparate (NMDA) antagonists (amantadine), ion channel modulators (gabapentin; sodium channel blockers), and mixed analgesics (tramadol). There is currently no information to guide the clinician on which drugs or combinations to use in particular circumstances, but it is generally recognized that a multimodal approach (concurrent use of more than one type of drug) is necessary, and treatment may need to extend for considerable periods of time. It must be remembered though that managing pain goes far beyond the administration of medications. It includes optimizing body weight, optimizing nutrition and nutritional supplementation, implementing a home exercise program, making appropriate use of safe and effective ambulation assistance devices, and optimizing the home environment. This therapy must be tailored to the individual animal, should be multimodal, and needs constant re-evaluation for efficacy and toxicity.

WHAT IS NEUROPATHIC PAIN?

Neuropathic pain is most often described as a malfunction in the nervous system that usually follows direct injury to the nerve or to certain regions of the spinal cord or brain. As such, neurogenic pain (pain from the injury or compression of the nervous system) likely has considerable overlap with neuropathic pain, with neurogenic pain often leading to neuropathic pain. For the purposes of this article, the two will be considered together. Indeed, they both share common hallmarks: allodynia, hyperalgesia, and hyperpathia (Table 1).

DEFINING NEUROPATHIC PAIN IN THE CLINIC

Neuropathic pain is usually described as pain that originates from a damaged nerve or nervous system (www.painconnection.org/MyTreatment/MayoClinic_glossary.asp), but there are many other definitions found if one performs an Internet search:

- Abnormal pain that outlasts the injury and is associated with nerve and/or central nervous system changes (www.nationalpainfoundation.org/MyTreatment/articles/CRPS_PainDefinitions.asp)
- Pain that results from pathologic change in nerves (www.health.qld.gov.au/diabetes_chd_resource/resources/glossary/glossary_n.html)
- Pain due to nerve damage, often severe and often described as burning (www.conquerchiari.org/Glossary.htm)
- Pain initiated or caused by a primary lesion or dysfunction in the nervous system (shsskip.swan.ac.uk/Information/Pain%20Terms.htm)
- Pain originating from the malfunctioning of the nervous system. (www.uhn.ca/programs/spine/glossary.asp)
- Pain which is transmitted by a damaged nervous system and which is usually only partially opioid responsive (www.portfolio.mvm.ed.ac.uk/studentwebs/session6/54/pain_definitions.html)
- Prolonged and intractable neurogenic pain. (www.qvhs.com.au/Dict-Ref/dict/pain.htm)
- Pain initiated or caused by a primary lesion, dysfunction, or transitory perturbation in the peripheral or central nervous system. (shsskip.swan.ac.uk/Information/Pain%20Terms.htm)
- Arising from damage, trauma, inflammation or degeneration of the afferent nerves (nerves passing messages from the periphery towards the central nervous system). (www.qvhs.com.au/Dict-Ref/dict/pain.htm)

The fact that there are so many definitions indicates that neuropathic pain is not easily defined. In human beings that can communicate, neuropathic pain is often defined as being present by the experiences perceived by the patient, such as:

- Shooting, burning, stabbing, radiating; often spontaneous (dysesthesias)

Table 1. Characteristics of Neuropathic and Neurogenic Pain

Allodynia:	Pain following a normal innocuous stimulation
Hyperalgesia:	Pain disproportionate to a noxious stimulation
Hyperpathia:	Increasing pain with repetitive stimulation:
	o After response (continued pain after stimulation)
	o Radiation of pain to adjacent areas after stimulation

- Pain is associated with stimuli which do not normally evoke pain (allodynia)
- Response to a pain stimuli is exaggerated (hyperalgesia)

There is no definition of neuropathic pain that has been proposed in veterinary medicine, but a good working definition would be: **"Persistent intractable pain, disproportionate to any physical disease process".**

WHAT CAUSES NEUROPAHTIC PAIN?

In humans, neuropathic pain has been divided into peripheral and central. Some causes of neuropathic pain are:

- Peripheral neuropathic:
  - Postherpetic neuralgia, HIV infections, trigeminal neuralgia, diabetic neuropathy, compression by tumor, sciatica, post-surgery, post-dental surgery, radiation, vincristine chemotherapy
- Central neuropathic:
  - Post-amputation stump, post-stroke pain, multiple sclerosis

Some common causes of nerve injury are listed in Table 2. Again, there is no information on possible causes of neuropathic pain in animals, but some likely causes are:

- Nerve root entrapment
- Osteosarcoma
- Post neurological surgery
- Interstitial cystitis
- Following multiple surgeries where perioperative pain was not well controlled multi-surgery
- post amputation
- post de-claw

Clearly, neuropathic pain does not occur every time the above conditions occur, for example, neuropathic pain does not occur every time an amputation is performed. It is not possible to predict when neuropathic pain will occur, but the above list is a list of conditions the author considers can be associated with neuropathic pain in animals.

Table 2. Causes of Nerve Damage and Possible Neuropathic Pain

Damage to Nerve:	Cause of Damage:
Section	Trauma
Stretch	Trauma
Compression	Tumor / mechanical
Chemical	Chemotherapy / other
Radiation	Cancer treatment
Metabolic	Diabetes
Viral	HIV
Immune	Paraneoploastic

DRUG THERAPY FOR NEUROPATHIC/ NEUROGENIC PAIN

Neuropathic pain is not a single entity, but rather includes a range of poorly understood heterogenous conditions that differ in etiology, location and initiatingcause. Because of this, and our poor understanding of the neurobiology of neuropathic pain, it is currently impossible to define which drugs work best in certain situations. The following groups of drugs should be considered, and the approach of the clinician should be to use a multimodal drug approach; that is, to use more than one class of drug concurrently. For severe pain such as associated with nerve root entrapment, the author will hospitalise the patients, and use continuous intravenous therapy with drugs from the following classes.

NONSTEROIDAL ANTI-INFLAMMATORY DRUGS.

NSAIDs often form the basis of treatment of chronic pain. The fact that they are generally fairly effective in a variety of chronic pain conditions is due to their multiple mechanisms of action. In general, they interact with the cyclo-oxygenase enzymes (COX-1 or COX-2 or both), or cyclo-oxygenase and lipoxygenase (LOX) enzymes (dual inhibitors), inhibiting the production of many prostanoids (and leukotrienes [dual inhibitors]) involved in facilitating pain transmission. However, NSAIDs also act on other COX- or LOX-independent systems to help inhibit the transmission of pain. Although they are generally considered poorly effective for neuropathic pain, they should probably still be considered, but used in conjunction with other drugs.

OPIOIDS

Like NSAIDs, opioids are considered poorly effective for the treatment of neuropathic pain in human medicine. However, given the difficulty we have in accurately defining neuropathic pain, and understanding the mechanisms in animals, they are worth trying. Oral opioid medications, such as codeine, codeine-combination drugs (such as acetaminophen-codeine), morphine, methadone, or butorphanol can be administered. Very little is known about the efficacy of oral opioids in dogs. Oral opioids are subject to a high 'first pass' effect in the liver, and recent work at NCSU Pharmacology and Comparative Pain Research Laboratories suggests it is very difficult to provide any analgesia in dogs using oral morphine (immediate or extended release) or oral methadone. Transdermal fentanyl can also be used but is expensive for long-term use, and recent concerns about their safety in humans (http://www.fda.gov/medwatch/SAFETY/2005/safety05.htm#Fentanyl) may lead to fentanyl patches not being available in the future. The recent advent of buprenorphine patches in human medicine holds promise for providing longer term pain relief than with fentanyl patches. Side effects of opioids include sedation and gastrointestinal ileus, leading to constipation.

TRICYCLIC ANTIDEPRESSANTS

From the medulla oblongata and mesencephalon, there are descending inhibitory serotoninergic and noradrenergic pathways that reduce pain transmission in the spinal cord. Many drugs act on these descending inhibitory systems; however, the development of specific analgesics acting on serotonin (5HT) receptors has been confounded by the many different types and subtypes of serotonin receptors.

The tricyclic antidepressants (TCAs) have been used for many years for the treatment of chronic pain syndromes in people. Tricyclic antidepressants, such as amitriptyline, clomipramine, fluoxetine, imipramine, maprotiline, and paroxetine primarily inhibit the reuptake of various monoamines (serotonin for clomipramine, fluoxetine, and paroxetine; noradrenaline for imipramine, amitriptyline, and maprotiline). Tricyclic antidepressants can also interact with 5HT receptors, and thus work by augmenting the body's descending analgesic systems. These drugs have been used in humans for the treatment of chronic and neuropathic pain at doses considerably lower than those used to treat depression. Amitryptiline has been used successfully for interstitial cystitis in cats, a chronic pain syndrome, but as yet, these drugs have been systematically evaluated in animals. The TCAs should probably not be used concurrently with drugs that modify the serotinergic system, such as tramadol.

ANTICONVULSANTS

Many anticonvulsants such as carbamazepine, phenytoin, baclofen, and more recently gabapentin, have been used for chronic pain, including neuropathic pain, in people. Gabapentin, and the more recently introduced pregablin, appear to be the most effective for neuropathic pain. Gabapentin is a structural analogue of GABA (gamma-aminobutyric acid) and was originally introduced as an anti-epileptic drug. There is now considerable interest in gabapentin and pregablin as treatments for neuropathic pain. The mechanism of action appears to be binding to the alpha-2-delta subunit of calcium channels (see below). The indications for gabapentin are unclear for veterinary patients, but it may be useful as an adjunct to other analgesics, especially for neurogenic pain, neuropathic pain and pain from certain cancers such as bone tumors. Recent basic science studies in rats suggest it may have a role to play in the management of pain from osteoarthritis.[4] There is no peer-reviewed published information on its use in dogs.

NMDA ANTAGONISTS

Preclinical evidence indicates that hyperalgesia and allodynia following peripheral tissue or nerve injury depends on NMDA receptor-mediated central changes in synaptic excitability. Memantine, amantadine, ketamine and dextromethorphan are uncompetitive NMDA antagonists that have been used clinically in humans for neuropathic pain. Work at NCSU indicated that dogs probably do not make the active metabolite from dextromethorphan necessary for NMDA blockade.

The author has been evaluating the NMDA antagonist amantadine (3–5 mg/kg orally once daily) as an adjunct to NSAID use in osteoarthritis and considers it to augment pain relief with a low incidence of side effects (mainly agitation and diarrhea). The dose of amantadine was decided upon on the basis of known kinetics,[6] clinical observations and pilot data. Although we have not performed toxicity studies on amantadine, toxicity studies have been performed. In repeated dose toxicity studies conducted over a 2-year period, a dose of 40 to 80 mg/kg resulted in deaths after 30 weeks of administration; a dose of 40 mg/kg resulted in one death (out of 8 dogs) after 47 weeks of administration; a dose of 8 mg/kg was not associated with any adverse signs.

MIXED ANALGESICS

Although not classified as a true opioid, tramadol has weak binding affinity at mu-receptors and is thought to activate monoaminergic spinal inhibition of pain although this may not apply to non-primate species. It can be administered by multiple routes and is effective for chronic pain in humans and seems remarkably devoid of the usual undesirable side effects of opioids such as respiratory depression, nausea and constipation. Its kinetics have been studied in beagles. One unpublished report in dogs is encouraging. Animals with chronic OA were treated with a low dose of ketoprofen (0.25 mg/kg PO daily) or low dose ketoprofen plus tramadol (5 mg/kg of prolonged release form PO daily) for 28 days. Dogs receiving both drugs had a greater improvement in pain scores, and even after treatment was discontinued they continued to improve while the dogs in the ketoprofen-only group remained static and had more incidences of acute flare ups after the end of treatment that the ketoprofen-tramadol animals. There is no information on its efficacy in canine or feline neurogenic or neuropathic pain.

SODIUM CHANNEL BLOCKADE

Alterations in the level of expression, cellular localization, and distribution of sodium channels are strongly associated with neuropathic pain. Although not a convenient mode of delivery for most patients with neuropathic pain, intravenous lidocaine has proven effective for neuropathic pain in humans. The author has used it as part of an intravenous cocktail for the treatment of neurogenic pain, such as nerve root entrapment pain and lumbosacral pain. There is increasing interest in transdermal lidocaine patches, although there is currently no information in animals on how to use these safely and effectively. Mexiletine, phenytoin, carbamazepine, oxcarbazepine, and lamotrigine have all demonstrated sodium channel blocking properties, but their use in humans has been limited by inconsistent efficacy, drug-drug interactions and side effects.

CALCIUM CHANNEL BLOCKADE

Calcium channels modulate nociceptive transmission at the level of the neuronal synapse in the central nervous system. The role of L, N and P/Q type voltage gated calcium channels, varies with the nature of the neural injury. Calcium channel antagonists have been demonstrated to reduce pain, allodynia and hyperalgesia. A growing body of evidence points to a distinct pattern of calcium channel expression in animal models of neuropathic pain, suggesting that understanding the neurobiology of individual diseases may allow targeting of the ionic channel remodeling. Gabapentin and pregablin interact with the alpha-2-delta subunit of the voltage gated calcium channel, and have both been shown to be effective in various neuropathic pain states in humans. Although there is considerable information on gabapentin as an anticonvulsant in dogs, there is, as yet, no information on its use for neuropathic or neurogenic pain. However, the author finds this particularly useful drug for neuropathic or neurogenic pain, at relatively low doses of 5 to 10 mg/kg twice daily.

CONCLUSION

We have a suspicion that neuropathic pain occurs in our veterinary patients. We do not know what drugs are effective against this type of pain, but the drug classes reviewed are appropriate choices based on what we know about the mechanisms of neuropathic pain in animal (rodent) models.

We have much to learn about both the efficacy and toxicity of certain individual and various combinations of drugs. Although much information can be successfully transferred from human medicine, veterinary patients are significantly different from humans in terms of drug metabolism and efficacy, and also probably in aspects of pain neurobiology. It is important that we obtain evidence-based medicine on the management of veterinary patients, and that we keep in mind which recommendations are based on opinion, and which on scientific evidence. Suggestions given in this review may well change in the future as more information becomes available about what drugs are effective in treating neuropathic pain. In the light of little scientific information in this area, the successful use of multimodal drug and non-drug therapy for suspected neuropathic pain can be greatly increased if veterinarians counsel clients on potential adverse effects and proactively ask for feedback on safety and efficacy, documenting this accurately. This will only occur successfully if the animal is re-evaluated, and the owner interviewed regarding progress, on a regular basis.

REFERENCES

1. Kukanich B, Lascelles BD, Papich MG. Pharmacokinetics of morphine and plasma concentrations of morphine-6-glucuronide following morphine administration to dogs. J Vet Pharmacol Ther. 2005; 28:371-376.
2. Kukanich B, Lascelles BD, Aman AM, et al. The effects of inhibiting cytochrome P450 3A, p-glycoprotein, and gastric acid secretion on the oral bioavailability of methadone in dogs. J Vet Pharmacol Ther. 2005; 28:461-466.
3. Chew DJ, Buffington CA, Kendall MS, et al. Amitriptyline treatment for severe recurrent idiopathic cystitis in cats. J Am Vet Med Assoc. 1998; 213:1282-1286.
4. Fernihough J, Gentry C, Malcangio M, et al. Pain related behaviour in two models of osteoarthritis in the rat knee. Pain. 2004;112:83-93.
5. Kukanich B, Papich MG. Plasma profile and pharmacokinetics of dextromethorphan after intravenous and oral administration in healthy dogs. J Vet Pharmacol Ther. 2004;27:337-341.
6. Bleidner WE, Harmon JB, Hewes WE, et al. Absorption, distribution and excretion of amantadine hydrochloride. J Pharmacol Exp Ther. 1965; 150:484-490.
7. Vernier VG, Harmon JB, Stump JM, et al. The toxicologic and pharmacologic properties of amantadine hydrochloride. Toxicol Appl Pharmacol. 1969;15:642-665.
8. KuKanich B, Papich MG. Pharmacokinetics of tramadol and the metabolite O-desmethyltramadol in dogs. J Vet Pharmacol Ther. 2004;27:239-246.
9. Devor M, Govrin-Lippmann R, Angelides K. Na+ channel immunolocalization in peripheral mammalian axons and changes following nerve injury and neuroma formation. J Neurosci. 1993; 13:1976-1992.

EPIDURAL ANALGESIA: QUICK AND EFFECTIVE!

Ross H. Palmer, DVM, MS, Diplomate ACVS
James L. Voss Veterinary Teaching Hospital
Colorado State University, Fort Collins, CO

Relief of pain and suffering is at the very core of our professional oath. There may be no other service that we provide for which pet owners are more willing to pay us. Our mission is to relieve pain and our clients want pain relief for their pets—that's a really good fit! Pain management does not have to be difficult and it certainly does not have to be expensive to be effective. In fact, some of the very most effective pain management tools for the orthopedic patient are the least expensive. With a little effort and forethought we have the ability to make pain management one of our greatest profit centers and sources of professional pride!

There are two key strategies to highly effective pain management in the orthopedic surgical patients:

1. **Pre-emptive pain relief** – Pre-emptive pain management refers to the treatment of pain *prior* to the onset of noxious stimuli (such as surgical manipulations). This decreases the intensity and duration of postsurgical pain and minimizes the likelihood of establishing a chronic pain state. This may include the preoperative use of opioids, nonsteroidal anti-inflammatory drugs (NSAIDs), alpha$_2$ agonists, or epidural analgesia.
2. **Multimodal analgesia** – Multimodal analgesia is achieved by the simultaneous administration of two or more analgesics or analgesic techniques. Since various classes of analgesics have additive or synergistic actions when administered near the same time, the dosages can often be reduced while the analgesic effects are amplified. When employed preemptively, multimodal analgesia helps to inhibit surgery-induced peripheral nociceptor sensitization and "wind up" changes at the spinal level.

TECHNIQUE FOR EPIDURAL INJECTIONS

Pre-emptive epidural pain relief has been one very effective component of our multimodal approach to analgesia for pelvic limb orthopedic surgery. Intravenous fluid therapy and monitoring of blood pressure, electrocardiogram, and respiration are assumed with these more advanced surgical procedures being performed on the pelvic limbs. The routine use of epidural marcaine and/or opioids in our patients has dramatically reduced the concentration of inspired isoflurane that we administer, but it is very dependent upon proper technique. When properly performed, epidural pain management oftentimes allows our patients to inspire 1.25% to 1.5% isoflurane with no elevation of heart rate or respiratory rate during even the most aggressive osteotomies or periosteal elevation procedures. The skill is relatively easy to learn. I prefer to position the anesthetized dog in sternal recumbency (unless pelvic or spinal fractures contraindicate this position). Clip hair from between the space of ilial wings. A line connecting the cranial edge of the wings of the ilia overlies the roof of L7. Just caudal to this line, there is typically a palpable depression between the L7 and sacral dorsal spinous processes. After palpating my landmarks, a standard presurgical scrub preparation is performed. Sterile gloves are donned for placement of the spinal needle (includes a stylet). In large dogs I typically use a 20-gauge, 3.5-inch spinal needle. In smaller dogs, I typically use a 22-gauge, 2.5-inch spinal needle. The needle and stylet are advanced toward the palpable lumbosacral depression. The needle is advanced until a distinct pop is felt as the ligamentum flavum is penetrated. If the needle first contacts bone, it is withdrawn slightly and redirected until the ligamenum flavum is punctured. Next the stylet is removed and the needle is observed for flow of cerebrospinal fluid (CSF) or blood. If blood or CSF flows from the needle, I typically withdraw the needle and reconfirm my landmarks (CSF flow is more common with inadvertent puncture at L5-L6 or L6-L7). Once properly positioned, the syringe is attached to the spinal needle. If properly positioned, there is no resistance to injection. If resistance is encountered, the needle is withdrawn, the stylet replaced, and the needle is repositioned. With concentration and a little practice, accurate and reliable epidural injection can be made in 5 minutes or less including the time to prepare the patient. While I do not advocate relying on any single method of analgesia, epidural pain management has been the most effective addition to our armamentarium in recent years.

SUMMARY

With a little dedicated effort, epidural pain management can allow a veterinary clinic the opportunity to earn the distinction of "excellence in pain management" while simultaneously developing a new profit center! Our patients benefit, our clients are happier with our services, and our profitability is enhanced. Everybody wins!

CHRONIC PAIN IN DOGS AND CATS

Lysa Pam Posner, DVM, Diplomate ACVA
College of Veterinary Medicine
North Carolina State University, Raleigh, NC

One of the most challenging and often frustrating parts of veterinary practice is the management of chronic pain. Advancement in veterinary science as well as changing cultural attitudes toward pet ownership has increased the number of patients requiring management of chronic and terminal conditions. The goal for this article to review the pain pathways and discuss treatment options for chronic pain syndromes.

REVIEW OF THE PAIN PATHWAY

Definition of pain from the IASP (International Association for the Study of Pain): "An unpleasant sensory and emotional experience associated with actual or potential tissue damage, or described in terms of such damage" and "The inability to communicate verbally does not negate the possibility that an individual is experiencing pain and is in need of appropriate pain-relieving treatment."

Nociception is the detection of a noxious stimulus (that in humans results in "pain"). Some authors argue that animals have nociception and not pain because they do not have the emotional experience that is part of the pain definition. In this author's opinion, there is no reason to believe that animals do not experience pain very similarly to humans.

Nociceptors are free (naked) nerve endings that encode mechanical, chemical, thermal energy into electrical impulses. Fibers of primary sensory neurons include:

- Aβ fibers: large myelinated low threshold fibers that transduce pressure and innocuous sensations.
- Aδ fibers: small myelinated, high threshold fibers that transduce sharp well localized pain.
- C fibers: small unmyelinated (slow), high threshold fibers that transmit slow, burning, diffuse pain.

Aδ and C fibers have a variable distribution and density.

Somatic nociceptors are both deep and superficial in the skin, subcutaneous tissues, muscles, tendons, joint capsules, periosteum, subchondral bone, and fascia.

Visceral nociceptors are located in the peritoneum, pleura, internal organs, and blood vessels. They are mostly silent nociceptors (c-fiber) and respond to distention, spasm, ischemia, and inflammation. Thus they respond little to cutting, burning, or crushing. Interestingly, visceral nociceptors (vs. somatic nociceptors) are not always activated in life threatening disease not always painful (ie, perforation).

Classic Pain Pathway is Divided into Four Parts

Transduction: Stimuli from periphery to neural pathway, 1st order neurons, are naked nerve endings in periphery with cell bodies in dorsal horn ganglia. They encode mechanical, chemical, thermal or electrical stimulus that is "transduced" to afferent action potentials on Aδ or C fibers. The action potentials are propagated by Na$^+$ channels. First-order neurons synapse with neurons in dorsal horn (second-order neurons). *Peripheral sensitization* occurs when damaged cells produce chemical mediators, which act synergistically to promote vasodilation, increase permeability and recruit inflammatory cells which results in lowers threshold for Aδ and C fiber activation.

Transmission: rostral movement of action potentials within pain pathway. Transmission of action potential occurs via ascending spinal tracts within the spinal cord. The spinothalamic tract (STT) is most prominent nociceptive pathway although many alternative routes are present. The transmission of second-order neurons terminates in the thalamus.

Modulation: Inhibition or enhancement of signal Inhibition of nociceptive signal can occur peripherally via local effects at the nociceptor: local anesthetics, opioids, and (nonsteroidal anti-inflammatory drugs NSAIDs) can act those peripheral sites. More centrally inhibition can occur at the dorsal horn of the spinal cord; opioids, serotonin, α-2 agonists, and N-methyl-d-aspartate (NMDA) antagonists can decrease pain transmission.

Enhancement of nociceptive signal can occur peripherally due to primary hyperalgesia from allogens (pain producing substances) from the tissues (eg, histamine). Central enhancement can occur due to secondary hyperalgesia and windup.

Perception: Conscious perception of noxious stimuli is generally considered pain. Third-order neurons transmit information from the thalamus to higher (cortical) brain centers. The cerebral cortex is considered the target for noxious stimuli. If a patient is anesthetized with a general anesthetic and a toe is clamped, the entire pain pathway is activated up to the cerebral cortex (which is asleep). Without the conscious perception the patient does not "feel" pain. However, if the general anesthetic is turned off, the entire pathway is activated and the patient will feel the pain. By decreasing the activation of the pain pathway during anesthesia the veterinarian can limit the pain felt by the patient upon awakening.

ACUTE VERSUS CHRONIC PAIN

Acute Pain

Acute pain generally occurs in proportion to the stimulus, is relatively short lived, and is well modulated by drugs like opioids or NSAIDs.

Chronic/Neuropathic Pain

Chronic pain is long lasting (in humans, it is considered to be longer than 6 months in duration) and often is not proportional to the stimulus. Chronic pain can be quite frustrating to treat, as it often responds poorly to classic analgesics (eg, opioids, NSAIDs). Chronic pain can occur due to progression of disease that does not resolve (eg, osteoarthritis) or can be progressive (eg, neoplasia), or due to wind-up of the central nervous system.

Wind-up/Central Sensitization

Central sensitization occurs due to changes in dorsal horn neuron excitability. Briefly, there is a summation of potentials, which causes seconds of nociceptive activation to produce minutes of post-synaptic depolarization ("wind-up"). The wind-up phenomenon is mediated by NMDA receptors which bind glutamate and tachykinin receptors that bind substance P (SubP) and neurokinin A. Activation of NMDA receptors (where ketamine binds) increases sensitivity to glutamate. Furthermore, there is a decrease in threshold, so that lower threshold stimuli can be perceived as pain (e.g. Aβ fibers). Thus, wind-up can result in an increased responsiveness and a zone of secondary hyperalgesia (increased sensitivity in neighboring areas).

Breaking Cycle of Wind-up

Treating central sensitization/ wind-up often requires a multimodal approach. Better results are seen by choosing to attack more than one part of the pain pathway at a time.

DRUG OPTIONS
Opioids

Opioids have been the mainstay of analgesia in both humans and animals, however, they are often are less effective when treating chronic pain, and the side effects (drowsiness, parenteral administration, GI stasis) can preclude their use long-term. There are some opioid based drugs that are useful in chronic pain treatment.

Tramadol is by classification a mu-opioid agonist, but much of the analgesia is reported to come from its inhibition of the reuptake of norepinephrine and serotonin. Tramadol is gaining favor in the veterinary community because of it efficacy and ability to be administered orally. However, tramadol should be used with caution in patients taking monoamine oxidase inhibitors or tricyclic antidepressants, which also increase circulating serotonin levels. Elevated serotonin levels can lead to "serotonin syndrome," which can be expressed as drowsiness, restlessness, altered mentation, muscle twitching, high body temperature, shivering, diarrhea, unconsciousness, and death. Tramadol dose: Dogs: 1–5 mg/kg. BID-QID. Cats: 1.0–5.0 mg/kg every 12 hours (suspension available). High doses may cause anorexia.

Fentanyl patches have become quite popular for treating pain in a variety species. The ability to provide fairly steady state analgesia for days and while at home is advantageous. At the high end of the dose animals may become sedated, but usually do not. Cats in particular can have a positive behavior change while the patch is being used. After placement, therapeutic levels are reached in the cat in ~6 hours and ~12 hours in the dog. Patches are designed to last ~3 days, but differences can occur with differences in uptake; warm skin facilitates uptake whereas cold skin decreases uptake. The success of the patch is often based on good skin contact. Patches should NOT be cut. Fentanyl has a large human abuse risk.

Buprenorphine is a partial mu agonist, which means it has a ceiling effect (ie, after a certain dose, giving more does not result in more analgesia). Due to the pH of the cat's mouth (~9.0), buprenorphine can be administered transmucosally (not orally) at 0.02 mg/kg (20 µg/kg). Research has shown that transmucosal administration is as effective and intravenous (IV) administration in cats. It is unclear and unlikely that the same is true for dogs.

NMDA (N-methyl d-aspartic acid) Antagonists

NMDA antagonists (ketamine, amantadine) have been shown to interrupt wind-up. NMDA antagonists can also potentiate the effects of opioids. Interrupting wind-up can be accomplished at sub-anesthetic doses with minimal risks for behavior changes, but needs to be given intravenously. Ketamine is a commonly used dissociative injectable anesthetic and amantadine is an oral formulation that can be administered once daily. Amantadine dose: dog and cats 3–5 mg/kg PO SID. Amantadine is available in 100-mg capsule or a foul tasting 10 mg/mL liquid. Amantadine can be given with other drugs and may take days to weeks to reach full effect. Ketamine is generally administered as constant rate infusion (CRI) for at least 12 hours and usually 24 hours at 5–10 µg/kg/min. The ketamine dose is sub-anesthetic and should not produce any behavioral changes.

Nonsteroidal Anti-inflammatory Drugs (NSAIDs)

NSAIDs have become a common analgesic used in humans and animals alike. They are potent analgesics and work by interfering with prostaglandin synthesis in the arachidonic acid inflammatory pathway. NSAIDs are popular because they are available in many oral preparations that owners can administer at home. Although inhibiting prostaglandins results in analgesia, the inhibition of homeostatic prostaglandins can be detrimental. NSAIDs can interfere with stomach lining protection, renal blood flow, and coagulation. Patients with a vomiting or diarrhea history or who have been administered corticosteroids should also not receive NSAIDs. Interestingly there is great individual variation in patient response, ie, some patients will respond more favorably to carprofen than to meloxicam or vice versa. Remember also that there are species differences to metabolism, dosing (both amount and frequency) as well a licensing. It is beyond the scope of this talk to review all the NSAIDs available.

Local Anesthetics

These drugs work by interrupting neural transmission of pain via blocking sodium channels. They are effective at producing analgesia. Limitation of use of local anesthetics include, short duration of action (2–6 hours) and the need for parenteral application (injection perineurally). In treating chronic pain, multiple injections are not practical, but the placement of "soaker-catheters" may have its place. Additionally the introduction of Lidoderm® patches provides another option. Lidoderm patches can be cut to appropriate sizes.

Gabapentin

Gabapentin has been used in humans to treat many pain states including; inflammatory pain, diabetic neuropathy, malignant pain, central pain, complex regional pain syndrome, and trigeminal neuralgia. Gabapentin was designed as a structural analog of GABA, an inhibitory neurotransmitter, however the analgesic effects appears to be mediated via voltage-dependent calcium ion channels (VDCC). Many of these channels in the dorsal root ganglia and spinal cord are upregulated after peripheral nerve injury. Gabapentin has been successfully used by the author in both dogs and cats. Dogs: 2.5–10 mg/kg PO SID–TID. Cats: 50 mg PO BID–TID. If gabapentin is discontinued in a patient, they should be weaned off over 2 to 3 weeks to prevent seizures (reported in humans) and a rebound pain phenomenon.

Bisphosphonates

Bisphosphonates are drugs that restrict the action of the osteoclasts (the cells that destroy bone). They reduce the breakdown of the bone, and can be used to reduce the risk of fracture and reduce discomfort of skeletal neoplasia. They have a wide safety margin (approved for use for 20 years in humans); however, side effects can include hypocalcemia and renal toxicity. Pamidronate is an IV bisphosphonate that has been shown to provide pain relief in ~50% of dogs with skeletal neoplasia. Dose: pamidronate IV, at 1–2 mg/kg over 2 hours every 21 to 28 days.

Alpha-2 Agonists

Alpha-2 agonists (xylazine, medetomidine) are profound sedatives and analgesics. In human medicine, alpha-2 agonists are used for rescue analgesia when opioids have failed. Although they produce reliable analgesia (SQ, IM, IV, epidurally) they also provide significant sedation (and cardiovascular effects). The sedative properties may be appropriate for hospice care, but often prevents their use in day-to-day management.

Resiniferatoxin

Resiniferatoxin (RTX) is an ultra-potent capsaicin analog (active ingredient in hot chili pepper). RTX binds at the vanilloid (VR1) receptor which is a ligand-gated sodium/calcium cation channel that is expressed by small sensory neurons (unmyelinated C-fibers). C-fibers transmit noxious, inflammatory, thermal information. Binding of RTX to VR1 receptor causes prolonged increase in the free intracellular calcium concentration which results in calcium toxicity of the neuron and subsequent neuronal desensitization. The advantage of targeting C-fiber information is that RTX can stop inflammatory/hyperalgesic/cancer/osteoarthritis pain while maintaining normal proprioception and mechano-sensation. Furthermore, since the effect is via toxicity of the neuron, the effects can last weeks to months. A limitation for its use is that the drug activates the pain pathway before it desensitizes it! RTX is still experimental although capsicin cream is available in alternative medicine stores.

Palliative Radiation

Palliative radiation is a useful adjunct for non-treatable neoplasia.

SAMPLE PROTOCOLS
Osteoarthritis

Mild osteoarthritis is usually controlled with NSAIDs. For patients that do not respond to NSAIDs or for whom the effect is insufficient, the addition of amantadine is often helpful. Severe osteoarthritis may respond to the addition of gabapentin or tramadol to the above combination.

Skeletal Neoplasia

Skeletal neoplasia often responds well to gabapentin with and without tramadol. Bisphosphonates used every 3 weeks can increase comfort and decrease the incidence of pathologic fracture. Palliative radiation can also increase comfort.

Neurologic Pain

Pain associated with neurologic disease (eg, intravertebral disease), neuritis, and amputation often respond well to gabapentin +/- amantadine. If the disease can be corrected (eg, IVD), then patients can often be successfully weaned from the drugs

Terminal Care

End-stage disease is often accompanied with anything ranging from discomfort to extreme pain. Treatment choices need to balance quality of life issues. Tramadol and fentanyl patches are good choices for home care. Depending on the cause of pain, amantadine and gabapentin can be used too.

REFERENCES

1. Robertson SA, Johnston S, Beemsterboer J. Cardiopulmonary, anesthetic, and postanesthetic effects of intravenous infusions of propofol in greyhounds and non-greyhounds. Am J Vet Res, 1992; 53(6): 1027-32.
2. Eisenberg E, Pud D. Can patients with chronic neuropathic pain be cured by acute administration of the NMDA receptor antagonist amantadine? Pain. 1998; 74(2-3):337-9.
3. Fan TM, et al. Evaluation of intravenous pamidronate administration in 33 cancer-bearing dogs with primary or secondary bone involvement. J Vet Intern Med. 2005;19(1): 74-80.
4. Karai, L., et al. Deletion of vanilloid receptor 1-expressing primary afferent neurons for pain control. J Clin Invest. 2004;113(9):1344-52.

POSTOPERATIVE PAIN ASSESSMENT IN CATS – HOW DO I KNOW MY TREATMENT IS WORKING?

Sheilah A. Robertson, BVMS (Hons), PhD,
Diplomate ACVA and ECVA, MRCVS
College of Veterinary Medicine
University of Florida, Gainesville, FL

Pet cats outnumber dogs in the US yet our understanding and treatment of pain in this species has lagged behind that for dogs. Veterinarians consider surgical procedures in dogs and cats to be equally painful, but treat cats less often.[4] This under-treatment of pain results from the *difficulty in recognizing and assessing pain*, lack of species-specific data on analgesic agents, fear of side effects, and the lack of licensed products for cats.

PAIN ASSESSMENT

To treat pain we must recognize it and quantify it in some way so we can assess the efficacy of our interventions. Pain is a complex multidimensional experience with both sensory and affective (emotional) components. Because animals, and some sub-populations of humans are nonverbal, the International Association for the Study of Pain (IASP) added the following important caveat to its definition of pain: "The inability to communicate in no way negates the possibility that an individual is experiencing pain and is in need of appropriate pain relieving treatment".

Pain is subjective and no one can "feel" another person's pain. Even after the same surgical procedure, humans do not experience the same quality and intensity of pain so how can we determine with any degree of certainty what an animal feels? Put simply, in humans, pain is what the patient says it is and in animals it is what we say it is.

There is no gold standard for assessing pain in animals at this time. Many different scoring methods that include physiologic and behavioral variables have been published, but few are validated. Assessment systems must take into account different types and sources of pain, for example, abdominal versus musculoskeletal pain. As more studies focus on species-specific pain behaviors our ability to recognize and treat pain in animals will improve but at present the assessment of pain in animals is subjective and inaccurate. However, ignoring pain simply because we have difficulty measuring it condemns our patients to undue suffering.

Acute Pain Assessment Tools

Several studies have focused on assessing acute postoperative pain in cats, but no system has been validated or rigorously tested. In cats, the correlation between easily measured physiologic (objective) variables such as heart rate, respiratory rate, and blood pressure,[1,12] has been disappointing. No study found a consistently reliable objective measure, which is not surprising since these parameters can be affected by many factors other than pain; for example fear. Plasma cortisol and β-endorphins are components of the "stress response" to anaesthesia and surgery and much effort has been expended trying to correlate these hormones with pain in laboratory and clinical trials. Plasma cortisol is unreliable in cats as a direct indicator of pain.[1,6,8,12] Pressure platform gait analysis can be successfully used in cats[9] and this may provide an objective method of assessing pain after procedures such as onychectomy, at least in research settings.

Mechanical nociceptive threshold testing with devices such as palpometers has proved a useful technique for evaluating both primary (wound) and secondary (remote areas) hyperalgesia in cats. Changes in wound sensitivity have correlated with visual analogue scoring in cats,[11] suggesting that wound tenderness should be incorporated into an overall assessment protocol.

Scoring Systems

All scoring systems that depend on human observers must by definition be subjective to some degree and leave room for error, which could be either under-, or over-assessment of the animal's pain. Any system that is used must be valid, reliable and sensitive. Without strictly defined criteria and use of well-trained and experienced observers, many scoring systems are highly variable; one scoring system may show an analgesic agent to be effective yet another will show that same analgesic to be ineffective. These differences are inevitable if a system is insensitive and results in large interobserver variability.

The most basic pain scales are the simple descriptive scales. These usually have four or five descriptors to choose from such as no pain, mild, moderate, severe or very severe pain. Although simple to use these scales are extremely subjective and do not detect small changes in pain. Numerical rating scales are similar to simple descriptive scales but with numbers assigned for ease of tabulation and analyses; for example no pain would be assigned the number 0, and very severe pain the number 5. This system implies equal difference or weighting between each category, which is not the case. A further development of these systems is a categorized numerical rating system where certain behaviours are chosen and assigned a value.[1]

In an attempt to improve on discontinuous scales, the visual analogue scale (VAS) has been widely used in veterinary medicine. This tool consists of a continuous line, anchored at either end with a description of the limits of the scale, for example **no pain** at one end and **severe pain** at the other end. The observer places a mark on the line that they think correlates to the animal under observation and this is later translated into a number by measuring the distance of that mark from zero. These scales can be improved by adding a descriptor that says "worst possible pain for *this* procedure," because the worst pain associated with a castration is likely to be different from the worst pain after a thoracotomy. Holton and others[3] compared the use of a simple descriptive, numerical rating and visual analogue scales for assessing pain in dogs following surgery. They showed significant observer variability, which could be as high as 36%, with all three scales.

The use of a dynamic and interactive visual analogue scale (DIVAS) as an extension of the classic VAS system. With this system, the animals are first observed undisturbed and from a distance and then approached, handled and encouraged to walk or move around. Finally the surgical incision and surrounding area is palpated and a final overall assessment of pain is made. This approach overcomes some of the deficiencies of purely observational systems; for example a cat may lie very still and quiet *because* a wound is painful and this would go undetected without interaction with the animal. The DIVAS system has been used to assess postoperative pain in cats[5,11] and when performed by one individual unaware of treatments it detected differences between analgesics and between treated and untreated cats.[5]

In humans, multidimensional systems such as the McGill pain questionnaire that account for intensity but also sensory and affective (emotional) qualities of pain have provided a more comprehensive assessment of the patient's pain. Multidimensional systems are particularly important when self-reporting is not possible but must incorporate components that are proven to be sensitive and specific to pain (for example, facial expressions in infants) in the species being studied.

It is now accepted that quantitative measurements of behavior are the most reliable methods for assessing pain in animals and that if the methodology used to develop and validate these systems is rigorous they can be objective with minimal observer bias.[2] Knowledge of the normal behaviour for the individual being evaluated is essential and deviations from normal behaviour suggest pain, anxiety, or some combination of stressors. Currently there is no published "library" of validated pain behaviors in cats.

Suggestions for Creating an Acute Pain Scoring System

Each practice should choose a scoring system that fits their specific needs, and this may require some trial and error. Whichever one is chosen should be user friendly and readily used by all caretakers and should be an integral part of the animal's postoperative evaluation. After temperature, pulse and respiration are checked, pain, which has been coined the "fourth vital sign," should also be assessed. A scale should include both noninteractive and interactive components and rely heavily on changes in behavior.

How Often Should Animals be Assessed?

The health status of the animal, extent of surgery/injuries, and anticipated duration of analgesic drugs determine the frequency and interval of evaluations. In general, evaluations should be made hourly for the first 4 to 6 hours after surgery provided the animal has recovered from anesthesia, has stable vital signs, and is resting comfortably.

Patient response to analgesic therapy, and expected duration of analgesic drug(s) administered, will help to determine frequency of evaluations. For example, if a cat

is resting comfortably following the postoperative administration of buprenorphine, it may not need to be re-assessed for two to four hours. Animals should be allowed to sleep following analgesic therapy. Vital signs can often be checked without unduly disturbing a sleeping animal. In general, animals are not woken up to check their pain status; however this does not mean they should not receive their scheduled analgesics.

Continuous, undisturbed observations, coupled with periodic interactive observations (open the cage, palpate wound, etc) are likely to provide more information than occasionally observing the animal through the cage door. Unfortunately, continuous observations are not practical for most clinical situations. In general, the more frequent the observations, the more likely that subtle signs of pain will be detected.

Behaviors Suggestive of Acute Pain in Cats

Cats that adopt a hunched posture, sit quietly and seek no attention, or resent being handled are likely experiencing pain. A cat sitting quietly in the back of the cage after surgery may be painful; however, pain would not be recognized if the caregiver expects to see more active signs of pain such as pacing, agitation, or vocalizing. In one of the few studies where detailed behavioral ethograms have been constructed, a hunched or tucked up posture appears to be correlated with acute pain in cats following abdominal surgery.[13] This has been corroborated by preliminary work at Glasgow University (Robertson, unpublished data). In addition a head down posture, with eye-lids half closed and eyes held in a slanted position may correlate with pain. One of the many commonly reported problems following onychectomy is excessive licking and chewing of the feet.[7]

An important component of pain assessment is palpation of the wound. Cats will often shake their paws and try to bite at their feet if bandages after declaw surgery. In general many cats dislike (shake, bite, "freak out") any restrictive dressings including the tape used to secure intravenous catheters. These behaviors could indicate pain or dislike of the bandage so it is important to differentiate between these two.

REFERENCES

1. Cambridge A, Tobias K, Newberry R, et al. Subjective and objective measurements of postoperative pain in cats. J Am Vet Med Assoc. 2000;217:685-690.
2. Holton L, Reid J, Scott EM, et al. Development of a behaviour-based scale to measure acute pain in dogs. Vet Rec. 2001;148: 525-531.
3. Holton LL, Scott EM, Nolan AM et al. Comparison of three methods used for assessment of pain in dogs. J Am Vet Med Assoc 1998;212:61-66.
4. Lascelles B, Capner C, Waterman-Pearson AE. A survey of current British Veterinary attitudes to peri-operative analgesia for cats and small mammals. Vet Rec. 1999;145:601-604.
5. Lascelles B, Cripps P, Mirchandani S, et al. Carprofen as an analgesic for postoperative pain in

cats: dose titration and assessment of efficacy in comparison to pethidine hydrochloride. J Small Anim Pract 1995;36: 535-541.

6. Levy J, Lapham B, Hardie E, et al. Evaluation of laser onychectomy in the cat. 19th Annual Meeting of the American Society of Laser Medicine and Surgery. Lake Buena Vista, FL, 1999.

7. Patronek GJ. Assessment of claims of short- and long-term complications associated with onychectomy in cats. J Am Vet Med Assoc. 2001; 219:932-937.

8. Robertson SA, M. Richter, Martinez S. Comparison of two injectable anesthetic regimens for onychectomy in cats. Am Coll Vet Anesthesiologists Annual Meeting. Atlanta, GA, 1995.

9. Romans CW, Conzemius MG, Horstman CL, et al. Use of pressure platform gait analysis in cats with and without bilateral onychectomy. Am J Vet Res 2004;65:1276-1278.

10. Slingsby L, Jones A, Waterman-Pearson AE. Use of a new finger-mounted device to compare mechanical nociceptive thresholds in cats given pethidine or no medication after castration. Res Vet Sci. 2001;70:243-246.

11. Slingsby L, Waterman-Pearson A. Comparison of pethidine, buprenorphine and ketoprofen for postoperative analgesia after ovariohysterectomy in the cat. Vet Rec. 1998;143: 185-189.

12. Smith JD, Allen SW, Quandt JE. Changes in cortisol concentration in response to stress and postoperative pain in client-owned cats and correlation with objective clinical variables. Am J Vet Res. 1999;60: 432-436.

13. Waran N, Best L, Williams VM, et al. A preliminary study of behaviour-based indicators of pain in cats. Animal Welfare. 2007;16(S):105-108.

THE IMPORTANCE OF INTEGRATED FLEA CONTROL

Sharron Barnett, BS, MS
Novartis Animal Health US, Inc
Greensboro, NC

The history of the farmer's fight against insects in the production of food and fiber is replete with examples of the development of insecticide resistance and its impact on the cost and effectiveness of insect control programs. Successful growers must stay well versed in the nuances of insect control and the use of multifaceted Integrated Pest Management (IPM) programs that are the hallmark of insect management in today's agriculture. Many important lessons can be learned from the management—or sometimes lack of management—of insects of economic importance in crop protection. The experience of the producer of food and fiber in insect control techniques has relevant applications in veterinary medicine and should be considered in control strategies against fleas on dogs and cats. History clearly shows us the sustainable insect control is not best left to chance, but instead should be carefully planned and executed.

CASE HISTORY FROM AGRICULTURE

In Enterprise, Alabama stands a statue to the boll weevil. Placed in the center of this cotton farming town in 1919, its inscription praises the contribution of the insect to the prosperity of the citizens of Enterprise.[8] How did the boll weevil, which was the most destructive insect pest of cotton until recent history, improve the prosperity of farmers in Enterprise, Alabama?

The boll weevil was introduced into the US from Mexico in 1892 and by the early 1900s had made the production of cotton unprofitable in many places in the Deep South. Over the next 80 years, insecticide application onto cotton to combat the boll weevil and another insect pest, the boll worm, comprised 25% of the total insecticide usage on agricultural crops.[1] In spite of heavy reliance on insecticides, cotton pests continued to plague growers by building resistance to the pesticides used to control them. The combined cost of insecticides and crop losses due to insects caused many farmers to transition from the production of cotton to alternate crops. This transition resulted in great prosperity to the farmers in Enterprise, Alabama; hence the statue. However for others, failure to control insect pests with the chemical means available resulted in financial disaster and the decline of cotton production in the US.[9]

Today, the boll weevil is almost eradicated in the US and application of insecticides for the control of the bollworm have declined significantly. The control of insects on cotton (and most other agricultural crops) is achieved through Integrated Pest Management (IPM) Programs that includes not only the judicious use of insecticides but a variety of other control techniques. These complex programs include cultural practices, use of attractants, the insect-resistant plant varieties, biological controls and other techniques. One of the main goals of IPM is to reduce exposure of insects to chemicals with the same mode of action to delay or avoid the onset of resistance. Due, in part, to the adoption of IPM programs, cotton has once again become a profitable crop.

RELEVANCE TO VETERINARY MEDICINE

What relevance does the experience of the cotton farmer have in our control efforts against fleas on dogs and cats? Simply put—the principles are the same. Fleas, like all insects, have the ability to develop resistance to many of the chemicals we use to control them, if those chemicals are used unwisely. What steps can we in veterinary medicine take to ensure the sustainable control of fleas now and in the future?

THE IMPORTANCE OF INTEGRATED PEST MANAGEMENT

The foundation of a successful IPM program is an understanding of the insect pest and the basic tenants of resistance management. We all know that the cat flea is a formable enemy. Both sexes are obligate parasites on their host. Females lay up to 28 eggs per day and a total of up to 2000 in her lifetime.[2] What we may not consider is that this constant exposure of fleas to any insecticide placed on the pet, combined with the reproductive capacity of the flea can contribute to its ability to develop resistance to insecticides. Resistance is defined as "The selection of a heritable characteristic in an insect population that results in the repeated failure of an insecticide product to provide the intended level of control when used as recommended."[5] Simply put, it is the inherited ability to survive treatments that have previously been used successfully. Resistance occurs when naturally occurring genetic mutations allow a small proportion of the population to survive treatment. If this advantage is maintained by continual exposure to the same chemical, these genetic changes are passed to offspring so that eventually resistant individuals become numerous in the population.[5] Several factors contribute to the development of resistance in insects, including the persistence and frequency of application of the chemical used, the rate of reproduction of the pest species and the genetic isolation of the pest population. A history documenting the ability of a given species to develop resistance is a good indicator that the pest can develop resistance to compounds in the future.

There are several mechanisms observed in insects that can result in resistance to insecticides including metabolic, altered target-site, penetration, and behavioral resistance.

Metabolic resistance is the most common mechanism seen in insects and involves the detoxification of insecticides by enzyme systems. Commonly, elevated levels or activities of esterases confer metabolic resistance although there are additional types of enzymes that may play a role.[3] Metabolic resistance in insects has been identified to major classes of insecticides including organophosphates, carbamates, organochlorines, and pyrethroids.

Target site resistance is the second most common mechanism of resistance in insects and is caused by changes at the site where the toxin is active. Changes, such as the *kdr* mutation, in the amino acid sequence in the sodium channels of nerve cell membranes leads to a reduction in sensitivity of the binding of DDT and pyrethroids thus conveying resistance. Likewise, changes in acetylcholinesterase have been shown to cause insect resistance to organophosphates.[4]

Reduced penetration resistance occurs when the integument of the insect or the digestive tract lining becomes more imperious to insecticides thus reducing the amount of toxin actually absorbed.[7] Reduced penetration is often a contributing factor and not a sole mechanism of resistance in insects.

Behavioral resistance occurs when changes in behavior helps insects to avoid the lethal effect of insecticides.[6] As with reduced penetration resistance, behavioral resistance is usually a contributing factor and not a sole mechanism in resistant insects.

Since continual exposure to insecticides with the same mode of action can provide the selection pressure responsible for the development of insecticide resistance, several factors should be kept in mind when flea control recommendations are made.

- Use an integrated approach
  o The inclusion of several different control strategies including both chemical and non-chemical methods should be considered.
- Select chemical controls wisely.
  o Chemical controls with different modes of action should be rotated or used concurrently. This includes the use of both adulticides to remove the adults and IGRs or IDIs to kill the immature stages. This will reduce the selection pressure on any single chemical class.
- Educate your clients regarding the proper timing and application methods for the products recommended.
  o Products should always be used as directed, keeping in mind that improper dosing can speed the onset of insecticide resistance. Increased frequency of application (in excess of label recommendations) or use of a product at a dose higher than recommended on the label, in response to resistance development should be avoided.
- Educate your clients on flea life cycle and stress non-chemical controls.

  o Vacuuming, removal, and washing of pet bedding and other non-chemical techniques that were historically part of flea control recommendations should be included in flea control programs of today. Non-chemical control techniques can kill resistant insects and keep them from passing their genes to the next generation.

Although there are many products approved for flea control today, they belong to relatively few chemical classes. Care should be taken, through judicious use of these products, to ensure they provide the level of control needed today and in the future.

REFERENCES

1. Allen Woodburn Associates Ltd/Managing Resources Ltd. Cotton: The Crop and its Agrochemicals Market, 1995.
2. Dryden MW. Host association, on-host longevity and egg production of *Ctenocephalides felis*. Vet Parasitol. 1989;34:117-122.
3. ffrench-Constant RH, Park Y, Feyereisen R. Molecular biology of insecticide resistance. In: Puga A, Wallace KB (eds.): Molecular Biology of the Toxic Response. Philadelphia: Taylor & Francis, 1999, pp. 533-551.
4. Hinkle NC, Wadleigh RW, Koehler PG, Patterson RS, et al. Mechanisms of insecticide resistance in a strain of cat fleas (Siphonaptera: Pulicidae). J Entomol Sci. 1995;30:43-48.
5. IRAC. Prevention and Management of Insecticide Resistance in Vectors and Pests of Public Health Importance. Insect Resistance Action Committee (IRAC), 2006, 50 pages.
6. Kunz SE, Estrada MO, Sanchez HF. Status of *Haematobia irritans* (Diptera: Muscidae) insecticide resistance in northeastern Mexico. J Med Entomol. 1995;32, 726-725.
7. Scott JG. Investigating mechanisms of insecticide resistance; methods, strategies and pitfalls. In: Roush RT, Tabashnik BE (eds.): Pesticide Resistance in Arthropods. New York/London: Chapman Hall, 1990, pp 39-57.
8. Shoffner R. Pest of Honor, The Story of the World's Most Unusual Monument, The Enterprise Ledger, Enterprise, Alabama. 1988, 46 pages.
9. Strickland AE. The strange affair of the boll weevil: The pest as liberator. Agricult Hist. 1994;68(2):157-168.

GIARDIA? NOW YOU SEE IT, NOW YOU DON'T? OOPS, NOW YOU SEE IT AGAIN!

Dwight D. Bowman, MS, PhD
College of Veterinary Medicine
Cornell University, Ithaca, NY

Nothing parasitic seems to be causing more consternation amongst practitioners right now than *Giardia*. No matter when or what the topic of parasitology discussed, if there are practitioners in the room and someone mentions the word "*Giardia*," the discussion will be dominated by this topic. It can go on for hours. The reality is that nothing has changed, except that now it can be diagnosed. The development of an in-house test for patient-side testing has created a situation where this little creature that lives in the intestines of dogs and cats with, AND without, causing clinical signs is co-opting a great deal of clinical time from other conversations.

There are several questions that are the major points of discussion. Does it cause disease? Do you treat animals without signs? How long after treatment do you recheck? (and do you?) What do you do if it does not clear? Is it a zoonotic agent? Are dogs and cats infected with the same thing? What about the vaccine?

The first consideration is whether or not *Giardia* causes disease. Well, we know based on the same test that has caused all the consternation, the IDEXX Snap® *Giardia* Test, that there are an awful lot of positive dogs and cats. This was not really a surprise to parasitologists, because we were good at running zinc sulfate flotations and had been seeing *Giardia* cysts in the feces of animals without signs regularly. Thus, we were not really all that surprised when the IDEXX test showed that the United States was populated by a lot of positive dogs and cats. So, it obviously does not always cause disease. The problem is that it sometimes causes disease. Sometimes dogs and cats develop intractable diarrhea, and they have large amounts of these organisms in their feces. It seems that what is going on in dogs and cats is probably similar to what occurs in people. *Giardia* is the most commonly diagnosed flagellate of the human intestinal tract. Surveys throughout the world in people have demonstrated a background prevalence of between 2% and 25% with higher prevalences in toddler aged children and lowest levels in adults. In people, a survey of fecal samples collected as floaters in public swimming pools in the United States revealed a background prevalence of 4.4% of the formed fecal samples that were collected. It seems that the infection is relatively endemic in the human population, but as Dr. Beaver et al stated in 1984 in *Clinical Parasitology*, 9th edition: "In the United States, the epidemiologic pattern has changed from the typical picture, possibly because of a decrease of immunity acquired in childhood within the population as a consequence of improved sanitation and standard of living. Today epidemics of giardiasis are being observed among adults, presumably due to fecal contamination of food and drink. More commonly, giardiasis is seen as a cause of travelers' diarrhea in adults, especially among visitors to certain centers, notably Leningrad." The thing is, dogs and cats are living the same lifestyles now as their owners, and they may not be being exposed as young animals any longer, and this might make them susceptible to infection as adults with concomitant signs.

Does one treat dogs and cats that are shedding cysts or are antigen positive if they do not have clinical signs? Well, the answer just a few years ago would have most likely been "Nope, don't bother." However, we are no longer thinking along the same lines any more; we may be wading towards the wrong shore, but we are moving in the direction of treatment. The thing is, if dogs and cats get sick now because they get infected, then there is reason to think that they should be stopped from shedding the agent if they are positive. The easiest way to think about this is to pretend (if you are not one) that you are a parent or grandparent. Then, ask the question: If my child (or grandchild) was in daycare and one of the other children was found infected with *Giardia*, would I want that child treated? Or, if my child or grandchild was diagnosed with *Giardia*, would I want them treated? See, this is anthropomorphizing, but the reality is that this is how people think, and well, you will probably treat.

So, if you treat, when do you check to see if the treatment has been successful? We used say, back in the days when we were looking for cysts or trophozoites, check before 7 days. The reason was that the prepatent period is right around 7 days. Thus, if you wait more than 7 days, you are liable to be dealing with reinfection. However, with the antigen detection tests, it appears that the recommendation that is being made is 2 weeks. So, we have a prepatent period and a recommendation to wait 2 weeks after the prepatent period in order to allow the antigen to clear. So, you're stuck. Some people say not to recheck. This is fine if you are treating a dog or cat with signs that gets better, but is problematic in treating for the clearance of cysts or antigens from the feces of a dog or cat without signs of disease.

So, how often do you continue the treatments if the infection does not clear? This becomes hard to determine in the case of the animal without clinical signs from the infection. The question is do you treat until there are no more cysts or antigen present in the feces? Sometimes, this can involve three or more treatments with metronidazole and fenbendazole. Sometimes, the infection will not appear to clear even after three treatments.

Currently dogs and cats are considered to mainly be host to their own form of *Giardia* that is currently called an Assemblage by the molecular biologists. Dogs are hosts to Assemblages C and D, cats to Assemblage F, and people to Assemblages A and B. It seems that for the most part there is not significant sharing of the two pathogens between pets and people, and this is borne out in part from the fact that we do not routinely have outbreaks of giardiasis among veterinary students like we do with the *Cryptosporidium* species, *Cryptosporidium parvum*, that is highly zoonotic and infects young dairy calves. Also, according to a personal communication form Dr. Xiao at CDC, Assemblages C and D have yet to be found in fecal samples that are submitted to the Centers for genotyping. Unfortunately, it is not yet 100% clear that dogs and cats may not pose some risk. Dogs have been reported in Germany to be host on rare occasions with Assemblage A, and cats from Mississippi and Alabama have been found to be hosts also on occasion with Assemblage A. The problem is that we are unclear what this means in the way of zoonotic transmission. There may be some risk, and more importantly, if owners are concerned about *Giardia*, you will never be able to convince them that there is not any real risk anyway.

Finally, the question arises as to how good is the vaccine that is available for *Giardia* prevention? The vaccine has its supporters and detractors. The papers presenting the work supporting the claims seem to indicate that it was efficacious in preventing infections in beagles and kittens. However, there has been work showing that the treatment of dogs with existing *Giardia* infections has had little to no effect on the standing infections. Overall, the jury still seems to have not reached a verdict on the vaccine. However, it has the advantage that if a dog is vaccinated, there is no reason to look for the infection unless it has signs of disease. Also, there are some puppy and kitten boarding and day-care facilities that require the vaccine for admittance to the facility.

REFERENCES

1. US Department of Health and Human Services. Prevalence of parasites from fecal material from chlorinated swimming pools – United States, 1999. Morbid Mortal Weekly Rep. 2001; 50(20): 4110-4122.
2. Beaver PC, Jung RC, Cupp EW. Clinical Parasitology, 9th edition. Philadelphia: Lea & Febiger, 1984, 825 p.
3. Barutzki D, Thompson RCA, Wielinga C, Parka U, Schaper R. Observation on *Giardia* infection in dogs from veterinary clinics in Germany. Parasitol Res. 2007; 101: S153-S156.
4. Vasilopulos RJ, Rickard LG, Mackin AJ, Pharr GT, Huston CL. Genotypic analysis of *Giardia duodenalis* in domestic cats. J Vet Intern Med. 2007; 21:352-355.
5. Olson ME, Morck DW, Cen H, Preliminary data on the efficacy of a *Giardia* vaccine in puppies. Can Vet J. 1997; 38:777-779.
6. Olson ME, Morck DW, Cen H, The efficacy of a *Giardia* vaccine in kittens. Can J Vet Res. 1996; 60:249-256.
7. Anderson KA, Brooks AS, Morrison AL, Reid-Smith RJ, Martin SW, Benn DM, Peregrine AS. Impact of *Giardia* vaccination on asymptomatic *Giardia* infections in dogs at a research facility. Can Vet J. 2004; 45:924-930.
8. Payne PA, Ridley RK, Dryden MW, Bathgate C, Milliken GA, Steart PW. Efficacy of a combination febantel-praziquantel-pyrantel product, with or without vaccination with a commercial *Giardia* vaccine, for treatment of dogs with naturally occurring giardiasis. J Am Vet Med Assoc. 2002; 220:330-333.

HEARTWORM DISEASE – NEW INFORMATION AND IMPLICATIONS FOR THE NORTHERN US

Dwight D. Bowman, MS, PhD
College of Veterinary Medicine
Cornell University, Ithaca, NY

We are currently in the process of examining data collected by the IDEXX corporation for information gleaned from their surveys using in-house tests and laboratory data for the pathogens *Dirofilaria immitis*, *Borrelia burgdorferi*, *Ehrlichia canis*, and *Anaplasma phagocytophilum*. The analysis is not yet complete, but it is giving us the opportunity of examining a very large data set for the presence of heartworm antigen as detected by the tests that they have been selling and running in house. This article will examine the data only dealing with heartworm, and will concentrate on the northern states of the United States, basically with those states north of the 37th parallel, eg, north of Norfolk, VA, the union of the Ohio and Mississippi Rivers, and Fresno, California.

The SNAP® 3Dx® test (IDEXX Laboratories, Westbrook, ME) is an in-clinic ELISA that will detect *D. immitis* antigen, in canine serum, plasma, or whole blood. In 2001 the test became available for commercial use as a replacement option for in-clinic "heartworm only" screening protocols. Starting in 2001, IDEXX began offering practice rebates toward the cost of the SNAP 3Dx assay in exchange for practices keeping a log of all test results performed. The offer was extended to veterinary practices across the United States; therefore, the clinic geographic distribution was randomly selected. These practices agreed to use the SNAP 3Dx assay exclusively for all regular canine heartworm screenings, and submitted the results on an IDEXX-provided data sheet. Heartworm data was not collected for the years 2002 to 2003. Clinic enrollments began in September of each year and typically continued through spring. In September of 2006, IDEXX introduced the SNAP® 4Dx® Test, which added the ability to detect *A. phagocytophilum* antibody. Thus, for 2006 and 2007, the data was collected using SNAP 4Dx assay.

To increase the distribution and number of data points for the *D. immitis* database, data were retrospectively mined for the years 2001 to 2006 from the IDEXX Reference Laboratories network and added to the data set generated by clinics on the SNAP assays. The reference laboratory evaluations were performed on the IDEXX PetChek® microtiter plate. The laboratories' heartworm results were analyzed for duplicate test results in a given year, and subsequent results for an individual dog within the year were excluded from the analysis.

The number of practices that submitted samples totaled 2,573, consisting of 5,626,926 data points from over 3 million dogs from all 48 contiguous states. Evidence of at least one agent was found in dogs from every state considered. For the animals, there is no data on their travel history, so it is not known whether or not the dogs that tested positive had traveled outside their state or not.

The southeastern states (AL, AR, FL, GA, KY, LA, MS, NC, OK, SC, TN, TX, VA, WV), the Northeast (CT, DE, MA, MD, ME, NH, NJ, NY, PA, RI, VT), and the Midwest (IA, IL, IN, KS, MI, MN, MO, ND, NE, OH, SD, WI) tended to use mainly in-house tests, while in the West (AK, AZ, CA, CO, HI, ID, MY, NM, NV, OR, UT, WA, WY), with the exception of California, it appeared as though most of the tests were done within the centralized facilities. However, the two sets of data points give fairly good coverage for the nation in general. The overall prevalence for the Northeast was 0.6% of samples tested, for the Midwest was 0.8 %, and for the West was 1.2% (interestingly, higher than the Northeast or Midwest). South Dakota was the only state in which no infected dogs were detected. There were counties with fairly high percentages of positive dogs in North Dakota, Montana, Wyoming, and coastal Washington and Oregon. As would be expected, the map of prevalences demonstrated the highest percent positive rates within individual counties occurring mostly in the Southeast, but there were two clusters in California, where more than 6% of dogs tested were positive [Shasta County, Yuba and Sutter Counties]. There were a number of counties in northeastern Colorado with high percentages of cases, but basically most of the northern counties had a fairly high percentage of positive dogs. There were cases in northern Utah, western Idaho, and even in Montana and North Dakota.

During the presentation, we will discuss the individual counties within states in more depth, and will consider the specifics of infection by state. We will also examine the number of tests performed per state and the relationship of number of tests run to the percentage of positive dogs detected. We also hope to look at the general elevation of the different counties in an effort to determine if we can detect any impact this factor may have on the level of infection.

HEARTWORM DISEASE – NEW INFORMATION AND IMPLICATIONS FOR THE SOUTHERN US

Dwight D. Bowman, MS, PhD
College of Veterinary Medicine
Cornell University, Ithaca, NY

We are currently in the process of examining data collected by the IDEXX corporation for information gleaned from their surveys using in-house tests and laboratory data for the pathogens *Dirofilaria immitis*, *Borrelia burgdorferi*, *Ehrlichia canis*, and *Anaplasma phagocytophilum*. The analysis is not yet complete, but it is giving us the opportunity of examining a very large data set for the presence of heartworm antigen as detected by the tests that they have been selling and running in house. This article will examine the data only dealing with heartworm, and will concentrate on the northern states of the United States, basically with those states south of the 37th parallel, eg, south of Norfolk, VA, the union of the Ohio and Mississippi Rivers, and Fresno, California.

The SNAP® 3Dx® test (IDEXX Laboratories, Westbrook, ME) is an in-clinic ELISA that will detect *D. immitis* antigen, in canine serum, plasma, or whole blood. In 2001 the test became available for commercial use as a replacement option for in-clinic "heartworm only" screening protocols. Starting in 2001, IDEXX began offering practice rebates toward the cost of the SNAP 3Dx assay in exchange for practices keeping a log of all test results performed. The offer was extended to veterinary practices across the United States; therefore, the clinic geographic distribution was randomly selected. These practices agreed to use the SNAP 3Dx assay exclusively for all regular canine heartworm screenings, and submitted the results on an IDEXX-provided data sheet. Heartworm data was not collected for the years 2002 to 2003. Clinic enrollments began in September of each year and typically continued through spring. In September of 2006, IDEXX introduced the SNAP® 4Dx® Test, which added the ability to detect *A. phagocytophilum* antibody. Thus, for 2006 and 2007, the data was collected using SNAP 4Dx assay.

To increase the distribution and number of data points for the *D. immitis* database, data were retrospectively mined for the years 2001 to 2006 from the IDEXX Reference Laboratories network and added to the data set generated by clinics on the SNAP assays. The reference laboratory evaluations were performed on the IDEXX PetChek® microtiter plate. The laboratories'

heartworm results were analyzed for duplicate test results in a given year, and subsequent results for an individual dog within the year were excluded from the analysis.

The number of practices that submitted samples totaled 2,573, consisting of 5,626,926 data points from over 3 million dogs from all 48 contiguous states. Evidence of at least one agent was found in dogs from every state considered. For the animals, there is no data on their travel history, so it is not known whether or not the dogs that tested positive had traveled outside their state or not.

The southeastern states (AL, AR, FL, GA, KY, LA, MS, NC, OK, SC, TN, TX, VA, WV), the Northeast (CT, DE, MA, MD, ME, NH, NJ, NY, PA, RI, VT), and the Midwest (IA, IL, IN, KS, MI, MN, MO, ND, NE, OH, SD, WI) tended to use mainly in-house tests, while in the West (AK, AZ, CA, CO, HI, ID, MY, NM, NV, OR, UT, WA, WY), with the exception of California, it appeared as though most of the tests were done within the centralized facilities. However, the two sets of data points give fairly good coverage for the nation in general. The overall prevalence for the Southeast, as expected, was higher than that for the other regions of the country; the number for the southeast was 3.9%. As would be expected, the highest levels of prevalence detected by the testing were in the coastal regions and along the Mississippi River. There also seems to be an increase, perhaps due to increased testing in urban centers such as Dallas, Austin, San Antonio, Birmingham, and Atlanta. One of the most striking features were the high prevalence levels of infection detected in the western states of southern California, Arizona, and New Mexico. This may be a bit skewed by the larger size of counties in the western US, but there were definite pockets of infection detected around Santa Fe, NM, and in many of the eastern and central counties in Arizona. There were cases throughout southern California and but the increases in prevalence seemed to begin north of Santa Barbara. There were also a fairly high percentage of cases reported from the southern corner of Nevada.

During the presentation, we will discuss the individual counties within states in more depth, and will consider the specifics of infection by state. We will also examine the number of tests performed per state and the relationship of number of tests run to the percentage of positive dogs detected. We also hope to look at the general elevation of the different counties in an effort to determine if we can detect any impact this factor may have on the level of infection.

DIAGNOSTICS AND PREVENTION FOR HEARTWORM DISEASE IN DOGS: CHANGES IN HOSPITAL POLICY

Ray Dillon, DVM, MS, MBA, Diplomate ACVIM
College of Veterinary Medicine
Auburn University, Auburn, AL

DIAGNOSTICS

With the development of improved immunodiagnostic testing for heartworm disease of dogs, the use of these tests have often been relegated to the sole determination of heartworm status in dogs. Knowing the use of macrolides in dogs, even when adult heartworms are present, will typically decrease microfilaria numbers and decrease the "usefulness" of microfilarial detection. The current working application of antigen testing in practice is to consider these tests to be either positive or negative for heartworms; as an absolute, this has created problems. From a practical point of view, most all antigen tests will be positive if there are 3 to 5 adult female heartworms. However, because these assays only detect glycoprotein from gravid female heartworms, false-negative tests will result from all-male infections, low worm burdens, and immature worms. A study by the author of spontaneous heartworm infections in dogs in the Southeastern United States demonstrated that one third of all infections were unisex infections. A negative antigen test should not be equated with "a dog with no heartworms" to the client.

Because there is a rough relationship between the number of mature adult female heartworms and the amount of antigen present, some methodologies allow of a semi-quantitation of worm burden based on antigen load. However, many of the in-house techniques have been optimized to assure that borderline test results have a definite color change. Therefore, the most consistent means of equating antigen load is using micro well techniques where the intensity of the color change is determined by an instrument and threshold positive benchmarks has been established. In these technologies, the high intensity of the color has been correlated with antigen load, and high worm burdens can be anticipated. In these cases, death of a large number of heartworms can be anticipated to be associated with severe acute lung injury, regardless of clinical signs or radiographic disease.

THREE-MONTH DISEASE CYCLE OF HEARTWORMS

By common definition, Dirofilaria immitis is discussed as having a 6-month life cycle (infection of host through development and sexual maturity). The assumption that clinical disease does not develop until the parasite is a 6-month-old adult is incorrect.

The initial arrival of immature L5 in the small pulmonary vessels of the lungs is associated with an intense eosinophilic pulmonary reaction and clinical and radiographic signs may be present in this 3- to 6-month post-infection period. This 3-month disease cycle precedes the production of microfilaria and circulating antigen by 2 to 3 months. Because of the difference in the host immune reaction, and mortality of the immature L5 worms, the clinical signs, diagnosis, and effects of prophylaxis are different in the dog vs the cat with heartworm infection.

LIFE CYCLE FROM THE HOST'S VIEW POINT

Adult females (27 cm long) and males (17 cm long) normally reside in the pulmonary arteries and right ventricles without causing major occlusion of blood supply. Microfilariae (315 µm long and 6–7 µm wide) are discharged into the blood stream and survive 1 to 3 years. The number of circulating microfilaria in dogs is increased in warm ambient temperature, after eating, and late at night. The microfilariae are ingested by a mosquito during feeding. The infective larvae (L1) migrate to the stomach and then the mouthparts (L3) during development. The rate of development can be as short as 8 days at 30°C or as long as 28 days at 18°C. After a mosquito acquires the microfilaria (L1), adequate exposure to warm temperatures must occur during the relatively short lifespan (1 month) of many of the mosquito vectors. The infective larvae are deposited on the skin of an animal when the mosquito feeds again and the L3 enters through the bite wound. A maximum of 10 to 12 L3 can be transmitted by a single mosquito.

The L3 stages molt to L4 and L5 (adults) and migrate to the pulmonary arteries arriving as L5 (1–2 cm in length) approximately 75 to 90 days after infection. These small L5 are distributed mainly to the caudal distal pulmonary arteries, and over the next 2 to 3 months, develop to sexually mature adults and migrate back toward the right ventricle. If both sexes are present, microfilaria are produced 6 to 7 months after L3 exposure and can be detected in the blood in the dog, rarely in the cat. The common detection methods for adult antigen are positive typically about 6 to 7 months after infection. High enough quantities of the glycoprotein to be detected are only associated with fully mature adult female heartworms.

INITIATION OF DISEASE-3 MONTHS AFTER INITIAL INFECTION

With the arrival of L5 as 1.5-cm worms in the right and left caudal arteries, small vessel disease and lung parenchymal pathology are initial insults. As would be expected of any foreign body of this size, the parasite is ejected out the pulmonary outflow tract and most are deposited in the right and left caudal pulmonary arteries. Consequently, initial damage associated with the 3- to 6-month post-infection period is most noted in these arteries and caudal lung lobes. The host response to the infection during this initial insult is inflammatory and eosinophils can be detected in the alveolar space and interstitium.

In dogs, the majority of L5 which arrive in the lungs will survive and develop into adult heartworms. In cats, there is a high mortality rate of the initial L5 worms. Some cats will have all of the L5 will die during the next months and have no adults at 6 to 7 months post infection but have lung pathology.

As the worms increase in size and grow up the pulmonary arteries towards the heart, the surface arterial lesions become more evident. The periarteritis allows additional leakage and inflammation will extend into the lung parenchyma. At the distal capillary bed level, even the alveolar septa will develop edema and injury of the capillary beds. These lesions are significantly worse associated with dead and dying worms. High flow at critical times of early lesions will promote fibrosis rather than normal repair. Demonstration of heartworm antigen in interstitial areas distal to the physical presence of heartworms emphasize that the inflammatory response is throughout the pulmonary parenchyma. The microvascular lesions are severe when worms are alive, but become exaggerated associated with worm death. Type 1 pneumocytes are disrupted from the endothelial cells, leaving many of the alveolar sacs as denuded airways. Although more severe in lobes where heartworms are dying, similar lesions can be demonstrated in other lobes. The author has produced similar histologic lesions with cell free extracts of adult heartworms. The resultant lung injury is typical of Adult Respiratory Distress Syndrome (ARDS). During these critical times of natural or induced worm death, the lung develops severe periarteritis, interstitial edema, and acute inflammatory interstitial disease. The ciliated bronchial columnar epithelium can also be damaged and undergoes necrosis.

HOSPITAL POLICY

With the above information, the hospital policy should make the owner aware of the reliability of positive testing for heartworms, but should also be made aware of the possibility of heartworm disease in the face of a "negative antigen test." The possibility should be discussed with owners that in heartworm endemic areas, dogs with immature heartworms may be presented when they are 4, 5, or 6 months old (ages when hospitals will not test young dogs.) If these dogs are not tested until one year later, a dog with immature worms may be a "positive heartworm" dog next year, even when the owners have administered the macrolide monthly during the year. At this point, the veterinarian suspects lack of owner compliance, the owner suspects the veterinarian, the veterinarian then suspects the products efficacy, and yet it often is simply lack of hospital policy to warn the owner that immature heartworm infections are not detected by any antigen testing method.

The mechanism by which a hospital can avoid such issues is to recommend antigen testing 4 months after initiation of heartworm preventative to determine if an immature infection was present at the initial time of presentation. In heartworm endemic areas where mosquito seasons are concurrent with the age of a puppy, this would include dogs 4 to 6 months of age.

PREVENTION OF PRIOR INFECTION

In administration of monthly macrolides, owners are frequently told that this will prevent any infection over the previous month. The term "reach back effect" has been more recently been changed to "safely net" to define the fact that monthly macrolides used for over 12 months consecutively has the ability to kill some of the immature heartworms. However, there is not a 3- or 4-month preventative effect from any macrolides because by 3 or 4 months after the infection, the immature adult heartworms are already in the distal pulmonary arteries and lung disease has been initiated. However, the death of these immature adult heartworms over the next months is still more clinically advantageous that having fully mature adult heartworms develop. No doubt there are differences in efficacy of the various macrolides in their ability to kill immature heartworms, yet the ability of heartworms, during administration of macrolides, to become adults and produce antigen still confuses the issue for veterinarians and clients.

PRACTICAL APPLICATION

Because of the difficulty in educating clients and staff, the redefinition of heartworm disease to a "three month disease cycle" will assist veterinary medicine. Because of the new information about the disease caused by immature (3- to 6-month old) adult heartworms in cats, redefining heartworm disease to a 3-month disease fits both species. Dogs and cats both get immature adult heartworms arriving in the pulmonary arteries as 2-to 4-cm worms by 3 months after initiation infection. Neither can be diagnosed by antigen testing or echocardiography. Typically, the immature L5 develops to become an adult in dogs and can be only diagnosed 3 months later if antigen or microfilaria are produced. Typically in cats, many of the immature L5 die in the pulmonary artery of cats and cause bronchial disease and may never develop adults, thus no antigen or echocardiographic image develop. Some cats may also have L5 develop into adult heartworms which may or may not be antigen positive.

This description of heartworm disease as a 3-month disease can be used with owner who have both cats and dogs; and can be used to explain why retesting of dogs after initial presentation is needed because immature heartworms cannot be detected, and why in cats with bronchial disease the antigen test is often negative, and why antigen testing before initiating prevention in cats has limited application. The 3-month heartworm disease cycle can be used to educate both dog and cat owners.

HEARTWORM DISEASE OF CATS: IMPLICATIONS OF LUNG DISEASE

Ray Dillon, DVM, MS, MBA, Diplomate ACVIM
College of Veterinary Medicine
Auburn University, Auburn, AL

The last 30 years have increased the basic understanding of heartworm disease in the cat and emphasized the clinical importance of this disease. Several basic concepts have been confirmed by research in clinical practices, shelter cat populations, and experimental studies:

- Cats develop bronchial disease as a consequence of immature heartworms which never become adult heartworms
- Cats get immature heartworms as early as 75 to 90 days after infection and immature heartworms die creating lung and arterial disease which persist for up to 8 months
- Cats which develop lung disease from immature heartworms which die may be antibody positive for only a few months
- Cats with immature heartworms will be antigen negative and echocardiographically worm cannot be visualized
- Some cats do develop adult heartworms which may live for over 3 to 4 years in client cats
- After adult heartworm develop, the inflammatory reaction of the lung is reduced in cats and symptoms may be limited for long periods of time
- The death of immature as well as adult heartworms may be associated with acute lung injury
- Some cats which develop adult heartworms develop minimal clinical signs prior to acute death
- Most cats which develop adult heartworms survive the infection as the worms die over the next 2 to 4 years

The weight of the evidence has defined that wherever there is heartworm disease of dogs, there is heartworm disease of cats; it just does not present the same way as heartworm disease of dogs.

RESPONSE OF THE CAT LUNG TO ADULT HEARTWORM

If the course of a *D. immitis* infection is evaluated chronologically, the changing nature of the disease is evident. As the parasite first arrives in the lungs as early as 75 days after being infected by a mosquito, the lung responds with intense inflammation and "asthma-like" symptoms may develop. The cat has specialized macrophages (pulmonary intravascular macrophages, PIMs) in the capillary beds of the lung that are not present in the dog. If the mature parasite develops, the clinical signs may be intermittent or absent.

The adult parasite seems to be able to suppress the macrophage function in the lung. The cat will have classic radiographic and histologic findings of feline heartworms, but may not show clinical signs. After the adult parasite develops, the pulmonary parenchymal changes and even enlarged caudal pulmonary arteries on VD radiographs may decrease. However, at the time of worm death, the suppression of macrophage function is decreased and the lungs become extremely inflamed and the specialized macrophages may become important in the intense reaction. The result is a non-functioning lung and an acute respiratory distress syndrome. Although this reaction can occur as the result of even a single worm burden, spontaneous death of cats from heartworm infection is uncommon compared to clinical disease associated with the early 3- to 6-month disease.

Usually severe dyspnea is associated with heartworm disease and especially that which results in death as the consequence of an adult heartworm dying. After the removal of dead heartworms, there may be continued inflammatory lung disease in some cats. Following a clinical group of cats in Italy, client cats were positive on antigen tests and echocardiographically for over 3 years.

RESPONSE OF THE CAT TO THE EARLY INFECTION

The disease associated with feline heartworm infection is a moving target, with the pathology, and resulting clinical signs, dependent on the stage of the life cycle involved. Early arrival of L5 results in classic asthma-like radiographic and clinical signs. In cats during this early part of the infection, coughing and dyspnea can be intermittent. A peripheral eosinophilia may or may not be present. Typically, the cytology of bronchoalveolar lavage (BAL) reveals an eosinophilic reaction which continues even if all the immature heartworms die. The radiographic pattern can be dynamic and right-sided cardiac changes are not present. The inflammatory pattern in the lung parenchyma is peribronchial but may be severe enough to be a diffuse alveolar pattern. Pulmonary arterial patterns may be normal although if the periarterial inflammation is severe, the right and/or caudal pulmonary arteries may appear enlarged. Often, the inflammatory lung pattern is severe enough that the pulmonary arteries cannot be visualized. The arrival of immature L5s in the 75- to 90-day post-infection period probably represent a time frame where many immature heartworms are dying, causing inflammatory lung disease, even in cats which develop adult heartworms. Even in experimental cats with adult heartworms, the finding of heartworm fragments 6 and 8 months after infection with L3 would confirm that immature heartworms have a higher mortality rate than in dogs, where almost all become mature adult heartworms.

THREE-MONTH DISEASE CYCLE – DIAGNOSTIC CONSIDERATIONS

With the initiation of pulmonary disease at 3 months after the infection, pathology and clinical signs may be present 3 months before antigen or microfilaria would be present in the blood and 3 months before heartworms could be visualized echocardiographically. Thus, dogs and cats with lesions during this early phase are "heartworm negative" by the typically applied screening tests used in practice. Although the radiographic and histopathologic lesions are present during the early phases (months 3 to 6 post L3 infection) in the dog, rarely are dogs presented for clinical signs during this time frame. However, because of the intense reaction of the cat lung to the arrival of these 2- to 3-cm L5 at 3 months and/or the reaction of the lung to the higher mortality of these early young adults, clinical signs are frequently noted during this stage of the infection.

Some cats will develop these early lesions and become antibody positive, but over time (3 to 6 months) the young adult parasites in the distal pulmonary arteries all die. Although this form of heartworm infection could be considered as "self-curing," lesions were induced, clinical signs may have developed, and long-term consequences of this infection are unknown. The alveolar and bronchial changes associated with this early form of the disease will clinically and radiographically mimic "feline asthma." Cats will develop an eosinophilic BAL cytology, radiographic bronchial lesions without pulmonary arterial changes, and clinical signs of coughing and/or dyspnea will respond to typical corticosteroid therapies. Cats that are heartworm antibody positive have been successfully infected with the L3 which have molted to the L4 and L5, typically (depending on the test methods) lived 2 ½ to 3 months, and may or may not have gone on to arrive in the distal pulmonary arteries as L5.

In a study of cats presented to practicing veterinarians with a history of coughing and/or dyspnea, 42% were initially heartworm antibody positive. When cats with radiographic lesions and/or positive serology were examined over a 3-month time frame, the changes demonstrated that this infection is dynamic and a diagnostic challenge. Discordant serologic results between test methods can occur because each identifies a different antibody during the initial phases of the infection. Over the course of the 3-month observation period of client cats, 60% of cats presented for the first time for coughing were heartworm antibody positive at least on one test and had radiographic disease consistent with heartworm disease.

HEARTWORM-ASSOCIATED LUNG DISEASE (HARDs)

The *HARDs* term has been coined to describe the lesions associated with the arrival and death of immature heartworms (2–3 cm) as early as 75 to 90 days after infection. It is important to point out that this pathology develops also in cats which then develop adult heartworm infections as well. The radiographic lesions are identical in cats which have only immature adult heartworms and those which develop adult heartworms. Thus, the HARDs term can be used in cats which develop adult heartworms as well.

With the new understanding of the effects of immature heartworms on cat bronchial disease, the most likely time to identify this syndrome would be 3 to 6 months after the peak mosquito season in heartworm areas. Testing of chronic bronchial cats would prove to be unlikely to identify cause and affect relationships because even if the lung disease were induced by immature heartworms, the antibody test would most likely be negative 3 to 4 months after the initial insult.

The clinical and experimental evidence continues to support the basic fact that immature heartworms often infect cats, cause bronchial and lung disease, and no physical evidence (worm fragments) or antibody to heartworms can be identified as early as 2 to 3 months after worm death. The author used this phrase to describe heartworm disease in cats to clients: "The juvenile delinquent form of heartworms is a hit and run driver in cats. The immature forms come in, create disease, and any evidence that they were the cause is often gone by the time we arrive on the scene."

THREE-MONTH DISEASE CYCLE – PREVENTATIVE CONSIDERATIONS

The obvious position for veterinary medicine is to prevent disease. The profession has been timid in recommending heartworm prevention to cat owners. The supporting evidence of the clinical studies of coughing client cats, shelter cat studies, and experimental studies have all confirmed that bronchial disease of cats can be caused by heartworms, even if adult heartworms never develop. Prevention of heartworm disease should be recommended to both dogs and cats where heartworm disease is present.

TREATMENT AND COMPLICATIONS OF HEARTWORM DISEASE IN DOGS

Ray Dillon, DVM, MS, MBA, Diplomate ACVIM
College of Veterinary Medicine
Auburn University, AL

Although the clinical signs of heartworm disease have been documented, the exact pathogenesis of the disease is multi-factorial. As complicated as the disease process is when heartworms are alive, the dramatic changes associated with the death of heartworms, either spontaneously or induced, are clear indications of the dramatic host versus parasite reaction.

REACTION OF HOST TO HEARTWORM DEATH

Based on experimental transplantation of dead heartworms or administration of extracts of homogenated worms, the death of heartworms is associated with severe pulmonary edema and loss of alveolar Type I cells and even ciliated epithelium lining the bronchi. The acute necrosis was noted to be more severe in dogs than in cats. Pulmonary capillaries were often obstructed by plugs of platelets and eosinophils. No increase in pulmonary intravascular macrophage (PIM) phagocytosis was noted in cats with dead heartworms. Type II cell hyperplasia, showing evidence of the repair of lung injury, was more common in cats than in dogs. Based on lung scans and histopathology, infarction of the lung associated with dead heartworms was occasionally observed in dogs but was rare in cats. The death of heartworms results in severe capillary bed fragility, loss blood into the alveolar space, and causes the type of lung injury associated with adult respiratory distress syndrome (ARDS) in humans. The acute lung injury from dying heartworms is not a direct toxic effect of the worm byproducts, occurs in dogs and cats with no prior exposure to *D. immitis*, and is related to the worm mass and rate of worm death.

Typically heartworms die and fragment over a period of weeks. After the death of mature adult heartworms, even those which have just died and have been surgically implanted in normal Beagles, the adult worms slowly collapse, lose the rigid appearance, fold over, and lodge in the most distal pulmonary artery. However, embolization and infarction of pulmonary parenchyma rarely occur as collateral circulation provides adequate oxygenation. Even in dogs with no prior adaptation via ancillary arterial supplies, normal dogs which had 14 dead heartworms surgically implanted did not develop areas of infarction based on radioisotope lung scans, although blunting of pulmonary arteriograms suggest occlusion of distal flow. In addition, contrary to popular assumption, significant increases in pulmonary hypertension and decreases in cardiac output are not associated with this death and gradual fragmentation of whole heartworms in the pulmonary arteries.

However, critical to the dog and cat with dying heartworms is the intense pulmonary parenchymal change associated with heartworm death. The intensity of the pulmonary parenchymal changes would appear to be directly related to mass of heartworms and somewhat related to rapidity of the breakdown of the physical structure of the worm itself. Increased pulmonary blood flow associated with increased cardiac output causes alveolar flooding and in the dog, pulmonary consolidation and capillary bed fibrosis.

ADULTICIDAL THERAPY – COMPLICATIONS

The most serous complication of heartworm adulticidal therapy is 2 to 3 weeks after heartworm death. Acute lung injury is compounded by endothelial sloughing, pulmonary vascular obstruction, and intense platelet activation. Dyspnea after adulticide therapy in dogs should be considered an emergency and nasal oxygen and glucocorticoid therapy are required to stabilize damaged lung parenchymal damage. Although the dogs may appear in shock, the cardiac output is usually maintained. Large volumes of intravascular colloids should not be administered and central venous pressure carefully monitored. If significant pulmonary embolization with vascular occlusion has occurred, large volumes of fluids will increase end-diastolic right ventricular pressure resulting in poor perfusion of the right ventricular free-wall and myocardial failure.

Some dogs with severe thromboembolism of major pulmonary arteries may present with significant dyspnea and what appears to be relatively "clear" lung fields, which are hypoperfused caudal lung lobes. Most dogs with dying heartworms have significant activation of platelets that cannot be blocked even with extremely high doses of aspirin. Thrombocytopenia (<100,000/µL) is common 2 to 3 weeks after adulticide administration even in asymptomatic heartworm dogs. If platelet counts below 100,000/µL are noted, dogs should be screened for disseminated intravascular coagulation (DIC). In the absence of DIC, many dogs will respond to oxygen and glucocorticoid therapy within 24 hours. Because of the fragile nature of the capillary beds of the lungs, complete rest should be maintained. After 24 hours of supplemental oxygen, arterial partial pressures of oxygen below 70 mmHg reflect severe diffuse lung injury and often a poor prognosis. Heparin therapy, administration of warfarin derivatives, and clot lysing agents have not been demonstrated to be clinically effective during the crisis.

Early aggressive intervention with glucocorticoid administration continues to provide the best clinical approach during the post-adulticidal period. Because the initial studies demonstrated that daily administration corticosteroids protected adult worms to thiacetarsamide, increased the myointimal proliferation, and increased the incidence of severe embolism, corticosteroids have been advocated only at the time of thromboembolism. Low dosing of alternate-day corticosteroid administration has been advocated to treat the periarteritis in heartworm dogs, and has definite indications in dogs with severe eosinophil pneumonitis.

Although the first 3 weeks are critical after adulticide therapy, residual worm fragments in small pulmonary arteries can be demonstrated for up to 6 weeks. Strict exercise restriction and maintaining a low cardiac output is important to facilitate lung repair rather than encourage fibrosis. The reversibility of pathology cannot be predicted based on initial radiographic pattern. Dogs with significant elevations in pulmonary vascular resistance at presentation have irreversible morphologic changes in the pulmonary beds. In addition, an intense response of the dog to worm death may alter the initial clinical impression that the disease state was mild. Because some of the cardiovascular response to heartworm disease is vasoactive, not mechanical, and removal of the heartworms encourages repair, not fibrosis, most owners report clinical improvement after the successful removal of heartworms.

RAPID ADULTICIDAL APPROACH

The use of melarsomine has provided an effective method of killing adult and immature adult heartworms. Compared with thiacetarsamide, which did not affect immature worms and had poor efficacy on young mature female heartworms, the increased efficacy of melarsomine also increases the risk associated with heartworm death. Because the clinical signs are often not related to heartworm burden, the number of heartworms that are going to insult the lungs cannot be accurately predicted based on the classification system provided with melarsomine. Thus, although an active dog could be classified as severe grade 3, there could be a low worm burden. The alternative is that a class 1 dog with no clinical or radiographic signs that is primarily a sedentary dog could have a large worm burden. The death of a large number of worms regardless of the clinical condition of the dog can result in severe complications.

Based on an unknown heartworm burden in client dogs, where monies are not a major concern to the owners, the safest approach to a dog with heartworms is a staged heartworm kill. One injection of melarsomine and then a 1-month rest, followed by two injections over 24 hours can result in elimination of approximately 30% of the worm burden initially. After 1 month to resolve the pulmonary insult, two injections would eliminate the rest of the worm burden. However, this approach also requires the prolonged restriction of activities during this 2-month period of staged heartworm death. In areas where large heartworm burdens are common, this three-dose approach is the standard recommended therapy for all heartworm-positive dogs.

SLOW ADULTICIDAL APPROACH

Based on a series of studies by several investigators, there is a consensus, but not agreement on the efficacy, that administration of the monthly preventative medications over a 1-year to 18-month treatment will result in a reduction in the number of adult heartworms. With some differences in the experimentations where variables of age of worms, dosing duration, and worm numbers varied, there is evidence to demonstrate that there are long-term adulticidal effects associated with dosing of monthly preventatives. The adulticidal effects of monthly preventatives demonstrate efficacy in this descending order: ivermectin with pyrantel pamoate,

milbemycin, and selamectin. (Moxidectin Sustained Release administered as a single dose or 3 doses separated by 6 months does not appear to demonstrate a significant adulticidal effect.) Although many of the studies demonstrate a decrease in total worm burdens related to controls, the complete clearance of all the worms in individual dogs (important to clinical medicine) is less defined.

Based on results of studies with ivermectin with pyrantel pamoate, in which use for 16 months was 56% effective on 8-month-old worms and use for 29 months was 95% effective for 7-month-old worms in experimental Beagles, it has been suggested that administration of monthly preventatives is an alternative method of treating clinical heartworm infection. In regards to the adulticidal activity of monthly preventatives, the key question to clinical medicine - **"Is this a good thing or a bad thing?"**

Understanding that the dogs in the various studies did not demonstrate significant clinical signs associated with the "gradual" worm death, the immediate response would be encouraging even though the total worm mass was not removed in many of these studies. However, experimental studies using purpose breed dogs in confined space for the duration of the experiment would reflect a similar clinical scenario of cage resting a client dog for the 1½ to 2 years of worm death and lung injury. Experimental dogs with similar worm burdens, as in these studies, have been administered two doses melarsomine per 24 hours with 99% efficacy over 3 to 4 weeks and have not demonstrated significant clinical signs; but once again the dogs were cage confined.

Acute lung injury is associated with the death of heartworms, regardless of the cause. Increased flow though the disease pulmonary capillary beds can result in fibrosis and extend to hemoptysis and in the extreme, ARDS and death. In the clinical practice of heartworm disease management, it is vital to know when the heartworms die and thus when the lung injury is induced and limited exercise is necessary. In a dog which has no physical activity, this may be a moot question. However, of concern is an active dog in which it is known that even with live worms, the increased cardiac output is associated with increased pulmonary fibrosis and increases in pulmonary vascular resistance. The **unanswered question** is whether an active dog with worms dying over a gradual period of time will have a greater tendency to develop these lesions as a consequence of the prolonged lung insult. Lung injury is more severe in studies where monthly preventatives were more "effective" at killing 4-month-old L5 adults. Acute consequences of "slow adulticidal" therapy with monthly preventative medications have been anecdontal reports. Clinical trials using unconfined dogs to determine the real risk of adulticidal activity of monthly preventatives have not been reported.

In active dogs, the use of monthly preventative medications as an adulticide should be used with caution. Owners of dogs receiving such therapy should be advised that any respiratory difficulty should be considered an emergency. Owners should also be advised that this therapy is not as efficacious as the current recommended adulticide melarsomine and a negative antigen test does not equate with successful elimination of all adult heartworms.

THE WOLBACHIA QUESTION

The last 10 years has produced extreme scientific interest in *Wolbachia pipiens,* an intracellular bacterium that is present in all stages of the heartworm lifecycle and is an endosymbiont necessary for microfilaria production. Recently, the entire *Wolbachia* genome has been identified in the DNA sequences of several species of flies. That the associated antigen can be identified in many organs of dogs and cats infected with heartworms is unquestioned. Differences in immune responses to dogs and cats with and without *Wolbachia*-infected heartworms have also been identified. The total elimination of *Wolbachia* in heartworm-infected dogs even with long-term and high doses of doxycycline has been difficult. The concentration of *Wolbachia* in spontaneous heartworm infection would appear to be very diverse, and Wolbachia were still present in heartworms even in dogs treated with doxycycline for 8 months,

Trying to eliminate *Wolbachia* prior to adulticidal therapy has not been associated with improved clinical outcome or decreased histopathologic scoring of lesions. Long-term use of ivermectin plus doxycycline for 24 weeks prior to and during a staged (three dose) use of melarsomine was associated with less gross pathology than melarsomine alone. Given the problems associated with owner compliance, a regimen of long-term daily medications for 8 months has inherent clinical limitations. The decrease in worm burden with long-term ivermectin prior to melarsomine would have experimental support, but prior studies where exercise was not limited during long-term ivermectin-only therapy in clinical studies would continue to suggest limited application of this treatment to sedentary dogs only. The use of doxycycline alone was not associated with significant decrease in worm burdens or improvement in pathology. Extremely high doses of doxycycline also decrease inflammatory responses in their role as metalloproteinase inhibitors, also confusing the *Wolbachia* issue.

The use of doxycycline alone as an adjuvant to standard melarsomine treatment does not at this time have significant clinical data to support the practice. Given the minimal side effects of tetracycline, other than induction of antibody-resistant bacteria, the use of tetracyclines has become routine in some hospitals. Although the evidence to support this practice is clinically supported, there would appear to be minimal risk. The impact of this intracellular bacterial continues to be of interest to clinical veterinary medicine.

FELINE PARASITE PREVENTION STRATEGIES

Christian Epe, Dr. med. vet., Diplomate EVPC
Institute for Parasitology
Department of Infectious Diseases
University of Veterinary Medicine Foundation
Hannover, Germany

The feline parasite spectrum comprises a range of endoparasites as well as ectoparasites. Among the most important endoparasites are protozoans such as *Giardia, Isospora, Sarcocystis, Toxoplasma, Neospora,* and *Babesia.* A wide range of helminths such as roundworms and hookworms, whipworm, tapeworms (*Taenia, Echinococcus*), lungworm (*Crenosoma, Angiostrongylus*), and heartworm also play an important role in cats. Finally, ectoparasites including fleas (*Ctenocephalides felis* and others), ticks, and mites/mange, as well as more rarely occurring genera such as lice, mosquitoes, midges, and sandflies, are found on cats. For some specific parasites, treatment and control is just one aspect of the problem; the ability to of some parasites to transmit other diseases can cause the major veterinary problem, whether the cat is the vector (ie, necessarily included in the transmitted agent's biology and development as host, eg, *Leishmania,* heartworm) or just a mechanical transmitter (eg, flies for many bacteria),

As far as focusing on a prevention strategy, the species that are most important vary from continent to continent or even country to country. Nevertheless, the availability of information or expertise with specific existing control programs can help in certain cases to develop a strategy. This article focuses on the applied clinical aspects and comments on current control and prevention programs.

ENDOPARASITES

For many of the **protozoan endoparasites**, preventive strategies such as improving hygiene and interrupting or avoiding infection and transmission cycles are the core tools for controlling the diseases. In many cases, therapy is able to cure the disease, but is not able to eliminate the parasite from the host's body. For protozoans like *Toxoplasma gondii,* this is even more important because of the risk of zoonotic infection and the epizootic infection risk to livestock and – for instance, abortus risk – than as a severe disease for the final host cat itself. For *Toxoplasma,* prevention strategies focus on meat control and increased hygienic measures for pregnant seronegative women, rather than treating the patently infected final host which is simply not practical due to the biology of *Toxoplasma.*

Isospora felis is another protozoan enteroparasite, that is found worldwide. Although drugs for curative treatment are available within the class of sulfonamides and quinacrine, there is no persistent efficacy. This leads helps to cure the disease, but only on a short-term basis, which is unsatisfying in heavy reinfection scenarios. Here again, stringent hygiene to reduce the population of coccidia is the only way to control the cause, which to be honest is easier to recommend and to describe than to do in many cases. Individual factors, such as specific conditions, surface material, outdoor access and many others can make control a difficult task.

Hemoparasitic protozoans such as *Babesia* are found in the cat, but only rarely. *Babesia felis* is the most common *Babesia*-like species worldwide, and its prevention is related to therapeutic attempts with primaquine phosphate. However, this drug is not without side effects and the therapeutic dosage of 0.5 mg/kg IM is close to lethal dosage for the cat (1.0 mg/kg).

In the southern and southwestern US, another piroplasm, *Cytauxzoon felis,* is of great importance. Described in the 1970s (Kier, 1979), this parasite leads to severe illness in cast, with anemia, depression, icterus, and spleno- and hepatomegaly. Since it is very similar to the biology of *Theileria* spp, it has this synonym, too. As a therapeutic treatment, imidocarb (5 mg/kg IM, twice 2 weeks apart) or diminizine (2 mg/kg) is recommended. Prevention strategies recommend tick control for cats sharing an environment with bobcats (*Lynx rufus*) as natural reservoir. Vaccination as done for some *Babesia* species is still under investigation and might be a possible tool in future.

Leishmania spp is reported in cats from across the world, but cats do not seem to be a major host and, therefore, do not play an epidemiological role. Despite some case reports, a common recommendation for therapy has not yet been published. Prevention is the same as canine *Leishmania* prevention efforts, focusing on sandfly control and prevention.

Among the parasitic **helminths**, a wide range of **trematodes** is present in cats. As predators, cats can be infected by even more trematode species as a result of their fish-eating behavior. So many trematode cycles include fish species as intermediate hosts; however, for many of the trematodes described in cats, the full cycle has not been described completely, making it difficult to assess the risks and or draw any epidemiological conclusions. For most of these trematodes, no therapy has been described. The use of praziquantel has been suggested anecdotally, but this is off-label use and there has been no case report-based documentation. For more details, see the excellent work of Bowman et al.[2]

Among the **cestodes**, the most important species in cats are *Spirometra mansonoides* (treatment with praziquantel and bunamidine), *Dipylidium caninum* (praziquantel, epsiprantel, flea control), *Taenia taeniaeformis* (praziquantel, mebendazole, nitroscanate), and *Echinococcus multilocularis* (praziquantel). But many more tapeworms have been described in felids,[2] in different parts of the world and sometimes have local importance. Although serving as a potential definitive host for *E. multilocularis,* cats do not seem to play a major role in its epizootiology. Even in highly endemic areas like Switzerland, the new recommendations do not favor chemoprophylaxis of cats, since hardly any cases are described and the risk for further environmental contamination through cats or infection of humans seems to be negligible (ESSCAP recommendation, see www.esccap.org). Therefore, no prevention strategy can be stated. *Spirometra mansonoides*, however, at least in the US, is of public health importance because it causes the human sparganosis, mainly in southeastern part of the country. The recommendation is to prevent cats from preying on the intermediate hosts like frogs, water snakes, or rodents, and not allowing them to roam freely. In some cases this may be against the natural behavior of cat and owner, so it hardly seems to be a reliable prevention strategy. A regular treatment (ie, at least monthly, since the development is described to vary between 10 and 30 days in the cat) with elevated doses of praziquantel (30–35 mg/kg) is reported to be effective.[2]

Among the **nematodes**, *Toxocara cati* is one of the most common gastrointestinal helminths in domestic felids.[7] It has veterinary and zoonotic relevance. The documented infection rates in Western Europe range between 8% and 76% for *T. cati* in cats; the rates in the US range from 10% to 85%.[1,3,5,6] In contrast to its canine representative, *T. canis,* studies have shown that the parasite does not develop arrested somatic larvae that are responsible for lactogenic infections of subsequent litters (Epe & Kraemer, 2006). A vertical infection via the queen's milk could only be recorded in animals having an acute infection during late pregnancy. Nevertheless, all other biological features of roundworms, particularly the longevity of infectious eggs in the environment, still cause major risks for spreading roundworm in catteries and shelters or in other cat-holding conditions. Consequences of an infection with the cat hookworm *Ancylostoma tubaeforme* are similar, leading to regenerative anemia and weight loss after either oral infection with L3 through eating of paratenic hosts like rodents or larvae from environment, or percutaneous infection with L3. Other nematode species like *Strongyloides* spp, filaroidea like *Brugia* spp or *Dirofilaria* spp, *Physaloptera* spp, *Trichuris felis*, metastrongylids like *Aelurostrongylus abstrusus*, or *Thelazia* spp occur in different parts of the world with direct or, sometime indirect cycle involving intermediate hosts, usually either prey of cats or arthropods. Therefore, prevention strategy includes preventing cats from hunting (impossible for all feral cats and wild felids, often difficult for most of free-ranging cats), or from contact with arthropods. Persistent efficacy of the anthelmintic compounds used to control nematodes in cats is of advantage in the prevention scenario, but for curative treatment all broad spectrum anthelmintics are useful. The widely used benzimidazoles (fenbendazole, febantel/pyrantel) as well as pyrantel, as a representative of the tetrahydropyrimidines, are highly effective therapeutic anthelmintics. Benzimidazoles eliminate the existing worm burden; however, they do not have a persistent efficacy. Macrocyclic lactones on the other hand proved to be persistent, and data from studies on dog roundworm showed them to be highly efficacious. So far for companion animals and especially

cats, selamectin (Stronghold®/, Revolution®, Pfizer Animal Health), milbemycin oxime (Milbemax®/ Sentinel®/Interceptor®, Novartis Animal Health) and moxidectin (Moxidectin/Imidacloprid, Advocate®, Advantage Multi®, BayerHealthCare AG Germany) are marketed as registered products for cats. In addition, a new product with emodepside, belonging to the class of cyclo-octadepsipeptides has been registered for cats for a few years in Germany (Profender®, BayerHealthCare AG, Germany).

ECTOPARASITES

The arthropod parasite spectrum of cats comprises mites (*Demodex cati* and *D. gatoi*, *Cheyletiella blakei*, *Otodectes cynotis*, *Notoedres cati*, *Sarcoptes scabiei*), ticks (*Ornithodoros* spp, *Otobius* spp, *Ixodes* spp, *Dermacentor* spp, *Amblyomma* spp, *Haemaphysalis* spp), insects (*Felicola subrostratus*, Culicidae, Ceratopogonidae, Simuliidae) with fleas (*Ctenocephalides felis*) and other facultative myiasis-causing insects.

A prevention of the latter and all blood-feeding mosquitoes, midges, muscoids, and sandflies follows the regular use of insecticides and, if possible with good repellent efficacy in a more or less monthly application evolved in the last decades due to the abilities of new marketed insecticides, mainly but not only applied as spot-ons. The predominant groups are ticks and fleas. Table 1 summarizes the characteristics of the ectoparasiticides currently available.

For **acaricides** ("tickicides") a clear trend can be noticed in the last decades towards a spot-on application, and almost all compounds registered claim a 4-week efficacy (or persistence) for a monthly interval between applications. Besides spot-ons, collars with longer duration of efficacy as prevention of tick and other insect infestation are marketed as well. Still, older products for wash or bathing application are on the market, but often with shorter duration of efficacy. Therefore, those drugs have the risk of owner noncompliance because of the need for repeated application at shorter intervals. In our observation, the market share for these products has decreased in the last few decades for that reason. It is important to keep in mind that sometimes the dose- limiting species are different for the different compound classes, which sometimes leads to insufficient prevention, especially towards the end of the monthly interval, if in certain regions these species occur in high numbers causing a high infestation pressure. In most cases, an increase of applications with reduced intervals (ie, from 4-week to 2-week interval) can compensate for this problem. Resistance is hard to monitor, since no identical standardized laboratory techniques are used and are difficult to implement. However, case reports show the presence of resistance in certain parts of the world. The registered products for cats in Germany are listed in Table 2.

Table 1. Different Currently Available Ectoparasiticide Compound Classes

Product Chemistry:	Mode of Action
• Organophospates (OPs) (Cythioat, Diazinon, Dichlorvos, Fenthion,	Cholinesterase Inhibitor
• Hexachlorcyclohexan)	
• Carbamates (Propoxur)	Cholinesterase Inhibitor
• Pyrethroids/Pyrethrins (Cypermethrin, Flumethrin, Permethrin)/	Neurotoxic
• (Pyrethrum-Derivative, Acarine)	
• Phenylpyrazole (Fipronil, Pyriprol)	Block of GABA Cl-Channels
• Macrocyclic Lactones (Selamectin, Moxidectin, Milbemycin)	Opening of GABA Cl-Channels
• Chloronicotinoide (Imidacloprid, Nitenpyram)	Agonists of postsyn. cholinerg Nicot. Recep.
• Semicarbazone (Metaflumizon)	Na-Channel-Antagonist

Table 2. Acaricides Registered in Germany for Treatment of Ticks on Cats

Substance	Brand Name	Manufacturer	Application	Dosage mg/ kg KGW	Duration max.	Compound Class
Dimpylat	Varia	Varia	Collar		Ab 10d, Mon.	OP
Fipronil	Frontline	Merial	Spot-on, Spray	6-15	1-3 Months	Phenylpyrazole
Fipr., Methopren	Frontl. Combo	Merial	Spray	7.5 - 15	1-3 Months	Phenylp., IGR
Propoxur	Bolfo	Bayer	Collar		5 Months	Carbamate
Pro+Flumethrin	Kiltix	Bayer	Collar		7 Months	Carb., Pyr

Registrations in Germany; Source: Vetidata.de; Status: July2007; no responsibility can be taken for the correctness and completeness of this information.

Control and Prevention of fleas using **insecticides** is distinguished between the curative therapy of an existing flea infestation and the prophylaxis/prevention of an infestation. The first is performed using adulticides with an as quick as possible knock-down effect. The existing residual efficacy of modern insecticides helps in also treating reinfesting adults from environment. Spot-ons need to be applied on the skin (and not the hairs), sprays should reach he complete body surface for complete efficacy. For flea prevention, the reinfestation from the animals nest and environment has to be reached by the application as well. Either with modern persistent adulticides, newly reinfesting adult fleas will be killed within the duration of efficacy, or insect growth regulators (IGRs) are combined with adulticides. These IGRs (lufenuron, pyriproxifen, fenoxycarb) act as hormone analogues on different developmental stages of the flea population. As an example, the registered products for cats in Germany are listed in Table 3. For heavy (re-)infestation scenarios a single use of either adulticides or IGRs will not be effective, a combination of them of the so called integrated flea control, including measures as treatment of environment with insecticides, but also vacuuming, cleaning of animals nest and clothes etc. helps to increase the effect of the control measures. But the correct use, ie, correct dosage, correct application and correct intervals are crucial for success. Also, other animals in the unit or household can act as a reservoir and need to be included in the control.

CONCLUSION

North America has proved in the past and Europe seems to be proving now that so-called "travel parasitosis" is increasing in formerly non-endemic regions. This happens due to either i) travelling pets which join the owners on vacation – classical example are pets in Europe importing diseases from the Mediterranean basin to Central Europe – or ii) imported pets which are transferred from endemic to non-endemic regions. European examples are mainly animal welfare organizations that import pets from Greece, Spain, and other Mediterranean destinations to Germany or UK. This is challenging the European veterinarians in diagnosing and controlling these diseases, as well as the pet population in these countries, facing formerly unknown new diseases as (parasite) naïve animals. The same anecdotes are reported in connection with the spread of heartworm disease, for example, through US, partly connected with movement of people (army) together with their pets, which took the parasites with them to new regions. Thus, it is even more important, that suitable prevention schemes in place. These have to be tailored to the individual case and need the be selected from the available broad range (anthelmintics) or the less-broad range (acaricides for cats) of drugs.

Table 3. Insecticides Registered in Germany for Treatment of Fleas on Cats

Substance	Brand Name	Manufacturer	Application	Dosage (mg/kg)	Duration (max)	Compound Class
Dimpylat	Varia	Varia	Collar		months	OP
Fipronil	Frontline	Merial	Spot-on, spray	6-15	1-3 months	Phenylpyrazole
Fipronil, methopren	Frontline Combo	Merial	Spray	7.5-15	1-3 months	Phenylpyrazole, IGR
Lufenuron	Program Tablets	Novartis	Oral	10	4 weeks	IGR
Imidacloprid	Advantage	Bayer	Spot-on	10	4 weeks	Neonicotinoide
Imidacloprid/ Moxidection	Advocate	Bayer	Spot-on	10	4 weeks	Nicot., ML
Nitenpyram	Capstar	Novartis	Spot-on	1	1 day	Neonicotinoide
Propoxur	Bolfo	Bayer	Collar		5 months	Carbamate
Pyriproxifen	Cyclio	Virbac	Spot-on	2	3 months	IGR
Selamectin	Stronghold	Pfizer	Spot-on	6	4 weeks	ML
Metaflumizon	ProMeris	Fort Dodge	Spot-on	12.5	1 month	Semicarbazone

Registrations in Germany; Source: Vetidata.de; Status: July2007; no responsibility can be taken for the correctness and completeness of this information.

REFERENCES

1. Al-Jabr, OA, Storey, DM, Akrigg, A, et al.: Prevalence of *Toxocara* ova in dog faeces. *Vet Rec*:211-212, 1997.
2. Bowman DD, Hendrix CM, Lindsay DS, Barr SC: Feline Clinical Parasitology. Iowa State University Press. ISBN 0-8138-0333-0. 2002
3. Erhard, T, Kernbaum, S: *Toxocara canis* et toxocarose humaine. *Bull Inst Pasteur* 77:225-287, 1979.
4. ESSCAP 2006. ESCCAP Guideline 1: ESCCAP Guideline No. 1: Worm Control in Dogs and Cats. www.esccap.org
5. Franc, M, Cadiergues, MC, Marchand, A, et al.: Intestinal parasitism in dogs and cats. Results of an epidemiological survey in France. *Rev Méd Vét* 148:147-150, 1997.
6. Overgaauw, PAM: Prevalence of intestinal nematodes of dogs and cats in the Netherlands. *Vet Quart* 19:14-17, 1997.
7. Parsons, JC: Ascarid infections of cats and dogs. *Vet Clin N Am* 17:1307-1313, 1987.

INTEGRATED MANAGEMENT OF TICK-BORNE DISEASES: A PRACTITONER'S APPROACH TO TICK BIOLOGY, CANINE LYME DISEASE, AND ANAPLASMOSIS

Steven A. Levy, VMD
Durham Veterinary Hospital
Durham, CT

TICK BIOLOGY

Ticks are second only to mosquitoes as vectors of pathogens. The microbial pathogens transmitted include protozoa, bacteria, and viruses. Ticks may also cause toxicosis, hypersensitivity, and paralysis as well as blood loss anemia. They infest birds, mammals, reptiles and amphibians. Lyme disease, the most important vector-borne disease in the United States and Europe, is transmitted by the bite of a tick infected with *Borrelia burgdorferi*. Traditional approaches to managing tick-borne diseases have focused on the etiologic organisms and their clinical presentations in the companion animal patient. However, a vector-based approach can use the common link in all cases to generate an integrated management of tick-borne diseases (IMTBD) that can work for each organism or even coinfections with multiple agents (Table I). The common link in IMTBD is tick biology. Understand the tick vector is a key first step to understanding the complex events occurring at the vector–pathogen–host interface.

TAXONOMY AND PHYLOGONY OF TICKS

Ticks are members of the phylum arthropoda and have a general body shape similar to the parasitic mites.

There are two large families and one small family of ticks in the order Acarina and suborder Ixodida. The large families are the hard ticks, Ixodidae and the soft ticks, Argasidae. The family Nuttalliellidae is unique and contains only 1 species, *Nuttalliella*. There are 19 tick genera and nearly 850 species. The family Ixodidae (hard ticks) is further divided into two phyletic lines: Prostriata contains all of the ticks in the genus *Ixodes* (about 250 species) and Metastriata contains 12 Genera and about 425 species. The familiar genera *Amblyomma*, *Dermacentor* and *Rhipicephalus* are all metastriate ticks. There are major anatomic, physiologic, and behavioral differences between the Ixodid and Argasid ticks.

LIFE CYCLES OF TICKS

The life cycles of the hard ticks all involve 4 stages: egg, larva, nymph and adult. Ixodid ticks may use 1-, 2-, or 3-host life cycles and in all cases the parasitic stage must feed to repletion on a host prior to molting or egg laying. Three-host ticks are the most common vectors for canines. In 3-host life cycles each parasitic stage feeds to repletion on a separate host and leaves that host to molt in the environment or, in the case of fed females, to lay eggs. In some cases of multi-host life cycles the hosts may be individuals of the same species (eg, *Rhipicephalus sanguineous* which will parasitize dogs in all three stages) and in other cases the hosts may be from a variety of species (eg, *Ixodes scapularis* which may parasitize nearly 100 different mammal, bird, and reptile species). Adult female Ixodid ticks feed for many days, take a large blood meal, leave their host and lay thousands of eggs in a single large mass in the environment.

Table I. Integrated Management of Tick-borne Diseases

Integrated Management Component	Tick, Pathogen, or Host Related
1) What tick species are active in your area? 　a) When are they active?	Tick Biology Related
2) What organisms can these tick species transmit?	Tick Biology and Pathogen Related
3) What are the signs of disease caused by these organisms? 4) What diagnostic tests are appropriate? 　a) Tests for exposure and infection. 　b) Tests for infection associated pathology.	Pathogen and Host Related
5) Has effective tick control been employed?	Tick Biology Related
6) Is there a vaccination available?	Host Related

Most Argasid ticks are nidicolous, inhabiting a nest, burrow, or other specific habitat centered around a single host species. After eggs hatch Argasid larvae take a rapid blood meal in minutes (or rarely, in hours). Fed larvae leave the host but remain in the nest or burrow where they molt to nymphs which will feed in from 2 to 8 nymphal instars. In each case the nymph takes a small, rapid meal, leaves the host and remains in the nidicole. Subsequent feedings may be on the same host or on another host of the same species that inhabits the same burrow or nest. Over the course of many years and at intervals of from 1 to 3 years, adult female Argasids take many rapid (hours), small meals and after each feeding lay hundreds of eggs in the nidicole where they hatch and larvae begin the life cycle again.

TRANSMISSION OF MICRO-ORGANISMS BY TICKS

Reservoir hosts are essential in the life cycles of tick-borne pathogens. Reservoirs maintain pathogens in the environment and ticks become infected when they take a blood meal from these infected reservoirs. Persistence of pathogens in ticks from stage-to-stage constitutes transstaadial transmission and is essential for disease transmission to new hosts. When infection spreads to the ovaries of gravid female ticks and organisms are present in newly hatched larvae transovarial transmission has occurred. Parasitism of individual hosts by multiple ticks may lead to co-infection of the host by multiple organisms.

TICK ADAPTATIONS THAT GIVE THEM A HIGH POTENTIAL TO BE VECTOTRS

Ixodids live up to several years, Argasids up to several decades. Long life perpetuates both tick species and pathogens within the tick. Various stages may survive over winter. Ticks may have multi-year life cycles and long starvation tolerance.

Slow, intracellular digestion of blood allows pathogens to escape digestive process in the tick's gut and protects pathogens in an intracellular location.

Ixodids produce large egg masses (up to 22,000 eggs in one oviposition). Argasids lay hundreds of eggs in each of many egg-laying cycles.

Ability to suppress host immune response to tick feeding allows for repeat feedings on the same host by many ticks without host rejection of ticks. Tick saliva contains pharmacologically active compounds (anticoagulants, immune modulators, antihistamine and others) that mediate the host response.

Elaborate physiologic mechanisms exist for water conservation and excretion. Ticks are able to tolerate low humidity and water starvation when they are off-host and to excrete large amounts of water during the blood meal on the host. Ticks utilize various mechanisms to survive and feed such as: diapause, strategically timed feeding and drop-off rhythms, and elaborate pheromonal and hormonal control of functions like host and mate seeking

CO-INFECTION OF TICKS AND DOGS

Ticks may become infected with more than one organism when they feed on reservoir hosts that have multiple infections or when successive tick stages feed on reservoir hosts with single or multiple infections. *Ixodes scapularis* larvae and nymphs may be infected with *Borrelia burgdorferi* and/or *Anaplasma phagocytophilum* and carry these infections transstaadially to either nymph or adult stages after molting occurs. The result is a tick that has co-infection and the potential to transmit multiple organisms to the next host it parasitizes. Dogs may become co-infected when they are parasitized by individual ticks with multiple infections or more than one tick with single or multiple infections. In the northeast and Midwest, the coexistence of adult *Dermacentor variabilis* ticks with nymph and adult *Ixodes scapularis* ticks in the spring and summer months creates the possibility of dogs becoming infected with not only *Borrelia burgdorferi* and *Anaplasma phagocytophilum* but also the agent of Rock Mountain Spotted Fever, *Rickettsia rickettsii*. When the presence of the brown dog tick, *Rhipicephalus sanguineus* is factored in during warm months, *Ehrlichia canis* infection also becomes a possibility.

CO-INFECTION IS INCREASING

Magnarelli et al determined that in the mid-1980s 15.6% (10/64) of *B. burgdorferi* infected dogs and 0% (0/42) of *B. burgdorferi* negative dogs were infected with *E. equi* (now *A. phagocytophilum*). In an abstract accepted for presentation at the IXth International Congress on Lyme Borreliosis (NYC 2002) I tested dogs from my practice in Durham, CT in a study examining coinfection rates with the 2 organisms. C_6 ELISA was used to identify 15 *B. burgdorferi* positive and 15 negative dogs. Each dog was then tested for antibodies to *A. phagocytophilum*. Forty percent (6/15) of the Lyme infected dogs were coinfected while 6.6% (1/15) of the Lyme negative dogs were positive for *Anaplasma*.

The emergence of coinfection has continued to increase. In 2002, 2003 and 2004 I collected and froze serum or plasma from 621 dogs in my practice tested for *B. burgdorferi* infection using the C_6 ELISA (Table 2). In 2005 these samples were tested for antibodies to *A. phagocytophilum* allowing the incidence of single and coinfections to be determined. Single infection with *A phagocytophilum* was found in 23.8% (148/621), single infection with *B. burgdorferi* was found in 13.8% (86/621) and of a total of 159 dogs infected with *B. burgdorferi*, 45.9% (73/159) were co-infected with *A. phagocytophilum*.

The data in Table 2 reflect the trend towards increasing in co-infection of dogs with these two organisms vectored by the same tick species: *Ixodes scapularis* and *Ixodes pacificus*. This increase is due to the expanding range of the tick vectors, increased travel by pet owners with their dogs, and a tendency for families to move into tick environments.

Table 2. Co-infection with *Anaplasma phagocytophilum* (Ap) in Dogs Testing Negative Versus Positive for Lyme Disease (LD) in Durham, CT

Sample Collection	% Ap in LD Negative (Single infection Ap)	% Ap in LD Positive Co-infection Ap & LD
1985 + 1986	0	15.6
2002	6.6	40
2002-2004	23.8	45.9

IMPACT OF CO-INFECTION

The models used to characterize canine Lyme disease have employed field-caught *Ixodes scapularis* ticks from the northeast states. These ticks were likely to have been co-infected. Thus, the Lyme disease models may be, to some extent, models of coinfection induced disease. Further, when field-caught ticks were used to challenge dogs immunized with various Lyme disease vaccines, these dogs were often, unknowingly challenged with multiple tick-borne organisms. Early reports of dogs immunized against Lyme disease and displaying signs of the illness in the absence of western blot evidence of infection with *B. burgdorferi* may well have been describing canine anaplasmosis in naturally exposed dogs.

CANINE LYME DISEASE AND ANAPLASMOSIS

Both *Borrelia burgdorferi* and *Anaplasma phagocytophilum* are vectored by the same tick species, *Ixodes scapularis* in the Eastern and Midwestern states and *Ixodes pacificus* on the west coast (Figures 1 and 2). Dogs are infected after a tick feeds for from 24 hours (*Anaplasma*) to 48 to 72 hours (*Borrelia*). Signs of canine Lyme disease are most commonly associated with limb/joint disorder (Lyme arthritis) but severe and generally fatal nephritis and a rare syndrome involving heart block have been reported. Vaccination of dogs with a whole cell bacterin has been demonstrated to be safe and highly effective, especially when dogs are immunized prior to exposure to infected ticks. Anaplasmosis is a newly emerging disease of dogs and has been associated with Lyme-like signs including fever, lameness, lethargy and also uveitis. Both infections may be treated with doxycycline at a dose of 5 mg per pound twice a day for 28 days. Doxycycline may cause nausea and vomiting and it must be given with meals. Dogs infected only with *Borrelia burgdorferi* may be treated with amoxicillin at a dose of 10 mg per pound twice a day for 28 days. Other constitutional signs associated with affected organ systems should be treated appropriately.

INTEGRATED MANAGEMENT OF TICK-BORNE DISEASES

Tick control for the prevention of transmission of tick-borne organisms is accomplished only with rapidly acting acaracides that kill ticks before they have fed on canine hosts. Permethrin and amitraz affect gating kinetics of sodium channels and inhibit monoamine oxidase, respectively and can kill tick before they bite dogs, thus preventing disease transmission. Control of tick-borne diseases in dogs by immunization is limited only to Lyme disease. Dogs exposed to *Borrelia burgdorferi* are also often exposed to *Anaplasma phagocytophilum* by the same vector tick. Further, dogs living in Lyme endemic areas are also at risk for exposure to other tick species infected with other organisms. This highlights the need for an integrated management approach to address risk through all avenues and use of overlapping control strategies to produce a higher level of tick and disease awareness, effective surveillance testing, acaracidal prevention of feeding and organism transmission and finally, effective vaccination for dogs at risk of Lyme disease.

SELECTED REFERENCES

1. Barthold SW, Levy SA, Fikrig E, et al. Serologic responses of dogs naturally exposed to or vaccinated against *Borrelia burgdorferi* infection. J Am Vet Med Assoc. 1995; 207:1435-1439.
2. Elfassy OJ, Goodman FW, Levy SA, et al. Efficacy of an amitraz-impregnated collar in preventing transmission of *Borrelia burgdorferi* by adult *Ixodes scapularis* to dogs. J Am Vet Med Assoc. 2001; 219:185-189.
3. Levy SA, Lissman BA, and Ficke CM. Performance of a *Borrelia burgdorferi* bacterin in borreliosis-endemic areas. J Am Vet Med Assoc. 1993; 202:1834-1838.
4. Levy SA, Barthold SW, Dombach DM, et al. Canine Borreliosis. Compend Contin Educ Pract Vet. 1993; 15:833-848.
5. Levy SA, Magnarelli LM. Relationship between development of antibodies to *Borrelia burgdorferi* in dogs and the subsequent development of limb/joint borreliosis. J Am Vet Med Assoc. 1992;200:344-347.
6. Levy SA, Duray PH. Complete heart block in a dog seropositive for *Borrelia burgdorferi*: Similarity to human Lyme carditis. J Vet Intern Med, 1988; 2:138-144.
7. Levy SA, O'Connor, et al. Utility of an In-office C_6 ELISA test kit for determination of infection status of dogs naturally exposed to *Borrelia burgdorferi*. J Vet Therap, 2002; 3:308-315.
8. Levy SA. Use of a C_6 ELISA to evaluate the efficacy of a whole-cell bacterin for the prevention of naturally transmitted canine *Borrelia burgdorferi* infection. J Vet Therap, in press.

9. Levy SA, Clark KC, Glickman LT. Infection rates in dogs vaccinated and not vaccinated with an OspA *Borrelia burgdorferi* vaccine in a Lyme disease-endemic area of Connecticut. Int J Appl Res Vet Med, 2005; 3:1-5.

10. Sonenshine DE. Biology of Ticks, Volumes I and II, Oxford University Press, New York, 1991 and 1992.

WHERE ARE THEY? INCIDENCE AND GEOGRAPHIC DISTRIBUTION OF INTESTINAL PARASITES IN PET DOGS

Susan E. Little, DVM, PhD, Diplomate EVPC
Center for Veterinary Health Sciences
Oklahoma State University, Stillwater, OK

Despite the advent of highly effective, easily administered broad-spectrum parasite control products for dogs, infection with intestinal parasites remains a common finding in most veterinary practices. Many of the common intestinal parasites of pets, including ascarids, hookworms, whipworms, and *Giardia*, not only induce disease in dogs, they may also pose a risk of infection to people. Correct performance of fecal flotation using centrifugation and examination of the slide by a trained technician skilled at identifying parasites is essential to detecting the presence of intestinal parasites in our patients. However, understanding how common these parasites are in pets in a given area of the country is also critically important. Obviously, parasitic infections can only be diagnosed if a sample is submitted or obtained and a fecal flotation actually performed. Awareness of the threat of infection is often that first step needed to motivate both clinic staff and clients to collaborate in seeing that routine fecal flotations using centrifugation are conducted on every pet.

Previously published surveys have shown that over one third of all dogs in animal shelters are shedding eggs of at least one of the three major intestinal nematodes in their feces at any point in time (Blagburn et al., 1996). In the southern U. S., where a warm, humid climate facilitates survival of infectious stages of parasites such as hookworms in the environment, over half of dogs in shelters are shedding nematode ova.[1] However, the population of dogs in animal shelters is distinct from that of many pet dogs in both the level of veterinary care they have received and their overall quality of life prior to arriving at a managed facility. This previous lack of care likely contributes to higher-than-average rates of infection, including those with intestinal parasites. Nonetheless, surveys of shelter dogs clearly show that massive environmental contamination with canine parasites is occurring, and that the threat to pet dogs is a constant and ongoing reality.

Although the literature does contain some surveys of intestinal parasites in pet dogs, they often are somewhat dated, conducted in limited geographic areas or using sub-standard diagnostic techniques, or focused on only a single parasite species. This article reviews the common and important intestinal parasites of dogs and then provides a preview of data generated through analysis of a comprehensive database compiled by veterinary diagnostic specialists at Antech Laboratories to reveal the geographic distribution and relative prevalence of the major intestinal parasites of pet dogs. Wellness programs should include measures to actively seek to identify these infections when they occur through routine fecal examination, as well as proactively manage dogs to prevent infection with common intestinal parasites.

COMMON AND IMPORTANT INTESTINAL PARASITES IN PET DOGS

The most common and important intestinal parasites of dogs that fecal flotation is effective for diagnosing are listed in Table 1. Cestodes are also common in dogs throughout the US, but fecal flotation by any means is an insensitive method for identification of tapeworm infections. Infection rates with each of these parasites vary widely among individual dogs according to age, lifestyle, and a variety of other factors that influence both immune status and exposure rate. Recent national surveys of dogs in animal shelters or symptomatic dogs presenting with diarrhea have shown that infections with these parasites commonly occur (Table 1).

Table 1. Common and Important Intestinal Parasites of Dogs in the United States.

Parasite	Scientific name(s)	Disease Caused	Zoonotic Agent?	Reported Prevalence
Ascarids	*Toxocara canis*	Mucoid diarrhea, vomiting, malnutrition, ill-thrift	yes	14.5%[1]
	Toxascaris leonina	Considered minor	no	0.7%[1]
	Baylisascaris spp	Neurologic disease (larvae)	yes	ND
Hookworms	*Ancylostoma caninum*	Anemia, diarrhea, pruritus	yes	19.2%[1]
	Ancylstoma braziliense	Pruritus	yes	ND
	Uncinaria stenocephala	Considered minor	yes	1.0%[1]
Whipworms	*Trichuris vulpis*	Diarrhea, mucoid or bloody	no*	14.3%[1]
Giardia	*Giardia* sp	Mucoid diarrhea	**	15.6%[2]
Coccidia	*Isospora* spp	Diarrhea, may be watery, granular, or blood-flecked	no	4.8%[1]

*Despite occasional reports in the medical literature of human infections with *T. vulpis*, the consensus opinion is that *T. vulpis* should not be considered a zoonotic parasite at this time (CAPC Guidelines, 2007).[4]

**Human infection of *Giardia* from a dog or cat source has not been conclusively demonstrated in North America (CAPC Guidelines, 2007).[4]

[1]Shelter dogs determined to be positive by sugar centrifugation as summarized in Blagburn et al., 1996.[1]

[2]Symptomatic pet dogs determined to be positive by IDEXX SNAP *Giardia* Test as summarized in Carlin et al., 2006.[2]

ND = not done (national prevalence not previously reported)

Ascarids

Ascarids known to infect dogs in North America include *Toxocara canis*, *Toxascaris leonina*, and *Baylisascaris* spp. Infection with each of these parasites follows ingestion of a larvated egg from a fecal contaminated environment or, in the case of *T. canis* and *Baylisascaris* spp, ingestion of larvae in the muscle tissues of transport hosts. Ascarid eggs are long-lived in the environment and can persist to cause infections in animals for years. In the case of *T. canis*, infections commonly occur in pups in utero when larvae in the tissues of the dam are activated late in pregnancy to cross the placenta and begin migrating in the fetal pups. In this way, entire litters are born already harboring larval ascarids on their way to the small intestine of the puppies.

Pups with heavy *T. canis* infections may develop malnutrition, a pot-bellied appearance, and overall ill-thrift. Neonatal pups infected with massive numbers of larvae in utero may die acutely at 2 to 3 days of age due to the damage caused by migration of the larvae through the lungs as they make their way to the small intestine. Infections with *T. canis*, by far the most common of the three, are most commonly seen in dogs less than 6 months of age although prevalence rates greater than 10% have been reported for dogs 6 months to 7 years of age, and infections occur in older dogs as well.[1] In addition to causing disease in dogs, *T. canis* is an important zoonotic pathogen. Upon consumption of larvated ascarid eggs from the environment, people, particularly children, may develop visceral or ocular larva migrans. A particularly severe form of visceral larva migrans is caused by *Baylisascaris* spp, the larvae of which are neurotropic and tend to migrate in the CNS, causing damage and inciting inflammation.[6]

Hookworms

Hookworms reported from dogs in North America include *Ancylostoma caninum*, the common hookworm of dogs; *A. braziliense*, which is associated with sandy environs; and *Uncinaria stenocephala*, a relatively apathogenic hookworm occasionally reported from dogs and cats. Infection with hookworms occurs following ingestion of larvae from a contaminated environment or, in the case of neonatal pups, in the milk of the dam. Skin penetration, with subsequent dermal migration of larvae and pruritus, can also occur upon direct contact with active, motile larvae in the environment. Whether infection occurs by ingestion or skin penetration, the larvae make their way to the small intestine, where they begin developing to adults. Immature and adult hookworms in the small intestine feed on blood from bite wounds they create on the intestinal mucosa, and anemia due to blood loss can result when infection levels are high. *Ancylostoma caninum* is a voracious and wasteful blood feeder; anemia is commonly seen in pups heavily infected with this species although not with the less common *A. braziliense* or *U. stenocephala*.

Unlike with *T. canis*, where infection rates decrease somewhat but do not disappear entirely in adult dogs, the likelihood of infection with hookworms appears to remain relatively constant throughout the life of a dog.[1] The presence of an infection is most likely dependent on acquisition of larvae from a contaminated environment. Dogs with hookworm infections shed eggs into the environment. Under proper environmental conditions of warmth and humidity, larvae hatch and develop to the infectious third-stage. Larvae of *A. caninum* and *A. braziliense* readily penetrate the skin of hosts other than dogs, including people, migrate in the skin, and induce inflammation and the resultant sinuous erythematous track lesions known as cutaneous larva migrans. Adults of *A. caninum* also have been recovered via endoscopy from the intestine of human patients with eosinophilic enteritis and severe abdominal pain.[3]

Whipworms

Trichuris vulpis, the canine whipworm, infects dogs upon ingestion of larvated eggs from a fecal contaminated environment. Like those of ascarids, the eggs of *T. vulpis* are long-lived; once deposited in the environment, a source of infection is all but assured for many years. Although many *T. vulpis* infections are asymptomatic in otherwise healthy dogs, a large burden of whipworms in the large intestine of a dog can result in bloody diarrhea. *Trichuris vulpis* has a long prepatent period and perinatal infections from the dam to the pups are not known to occur. Although *T. vulpis* infections do occur in dogs less than 6 months of age, the rate of both infection and clinical disease is much higher in older dogs. As stated in the current CAPC Guidelines (2007),[4] "reports in the medical literature of human infections with *T. vulpis* … lack sufficient validation to consider *T. vulpis* a zoonotic parasite at this time."

Giardia spp

Giardia is a common, important parasite of dogs throughout North America with prevalence rates in symptomatic dogs (those with diarrhea and/or vomiting) exceeding 15% nationwide.[2] Although many canine infections with *Giardia* sp appear asymptomatic, this parasite can induce moderate to severe diarrhea in dogs. Infection is acquired by ingestion of cysts from a contaminated environment; fecal-contaminated water often serves as a source of the cysts. Both dogs and people develop disease from *Giardia* sp, and *Giardia* infections in dogs must be handled as though they present a zoonotic threat. However, infections in people in North America have consistently been shown to be *Giarida* strains of human origin. Disease in people in North America has not yet been linked to a canine source, and the role of canine infections in creating a risk of human infection, if any, has not been clearly established (CAPC Guidelines, 2007).[4]

Coccidia

Coccidia (*Isospora canis* and the *Isospora ohioensis*-complex) are also common findings on fecal flotation of dogs. In otherwise healthy dogs, infections with *Isospora* spp. are usually well controlled. However, diarrhea, which can be severe, may be associated with *Isospora* spp infection, particularly in young dogs that have not yet developed mucosal immunity. Dogs acquire infection with *Isospora* spp primarily upon ingestion of sporulated oocysts from a contaminated environment. Infection is common, with overall prevalence rates greater than 4%; oocysts are more commonly found in fecal samples from younger dogs, presumably due to naive immune status in the absence of prior exposure. Many enteric coccidia (eg, *Isospora*, *Eimeria*) are species-specific by nature; the *Isospora* spp of dogs are not known to infect or cause disease in people or other animals.

PREVIEW OF NEW DATA ON GEOGRAPHIC DISTRIBUTION OF INTESTINAL PARASITES IN PET DOGS

The Companion Animal Parasite Council is dedicated to providing education and information to veterinarians to assist them in their efforts to control parasites in pets. In collaboration with veterinary diagnostic specialists at Antech Laboratories, we have reviewed results of centrifugal flotation generated from testing fecal samples submitted by veterinarians from more than 1 million pet dogs in 2006 with a goal of determining where these infections occur geographically and which dogs are most likely to be infected. Those results are summarized here (Table 2). Although definite regional and age-related patterns of infection emerged, infection with each of these five common intestinal parasites of dogs was present in every region and age group of dog considered.

In this review of fecal flotation results from almost 1.2 million dogs in the US, 12.5% of all dogs examined were found to be shedding at least one species of parasite. On average, protozoa (*Giardia* and coccidia) were more commonly found than nematodes, a finding which differs from previously published surveys and may reflect both the success of practicing veterinarians at controlling intestinal nematodes in dogs under their care and the sensitivity of the technique used in analyzing these fecal samples. The high level of detection of both *Giardia* and coccidia by centrifugal fecal floation also resulted in a higher overall rate of detected intestinal parasitism in dogs in the West, a result that is in stark contrast to commonly held beliefs about the geographic distribution of parasites in pets in the US.

Giardia infections were more commonly reported from dogs from the West, with as many as 6.27% of dogs from this region found to be shedding cysts at the time of examination. Infections were least commonly detected in the Southeast, where infection with this parasite is known to be less common.[2] There was also a striking, albeit expected, age-related pattern to the presence of *Giardia* cysts in feces, with more than 12% of dogs less than 6 months of age actively shedding cysts at the time of examination; by 3 years of age the prevalence had dropped to 1% or less. Although any age dog in any area of the country is at risk for infection with *Giardia*, control programs for this parasite should take into consideration the marked regional and age-related distribution of this parasite.

Coccidia (*Isospora* spp) were also more commonly seen in the West and Midwest, with infection rates in Midwestern states approaching 6% of all dogs examined. As expected, *Isospora* spp were much more commonly found in dogs less than 12 months of age, and the highest prevalence (>11%) was seen in dogs less than 6 months of age. Acquisition of mucosal immunity likely limited, but did not eliminate, these parasites from fecal samples of adult dogs. Infection rates with *Isospora* spp in dogs from the South were significantly lower than that in dogs from the West and Midwest. This finding was surprising because a survey of shelter dogs showed slightly higher rates of *Isospora* infection in southern dogs. Nonetheless, the overall rate of infection was roughly similar in pet dogs in this data set (4.43%) and shelter dogs previously reported (4.82%[1]).

As expected, ascarids (predominantly *T. canis*) were found in dogs from every state and region considered, although infection was most common in the midwestern and western states and comparatively less common in the southeast. This regional prevalence, particularly the lower than anticipated infection rates in dogs in the South, may reflect greater use of year-round heartworm control products in dogs in the southeastern US as compared with other regions; all the commonly available heartworm control products also effectively control ascarids. *Toxocara canis* was present in all age groups of dogs examined although infection was much more common in dogs less than 1 year of age.

Table 2. Prevalence of Intestinal Parasites in Dogs in Different Regions of the United States

Region	Ascarids	Hookworms	Whipworms	*Giardia*	Coccidia
Northeast	2.18%	1.71%	1.48%	3.71%	4.23%
Midwest	2.60%	3.35%	1.50%	3.95%	5.95%
Southeast	1.56%	3.99%	1.45%	2.25%	3.00%
West	2.75%	1.37%	0.52%	6.27%	5.20%
Total	**2.23%**	**2.46%**	**1.23%**	**4.03%**	**4.43%**

Hookworms (predominantly *A. caninum*) were also found commonly in dogs in each region, although as expected, infections with hookworms were more than twice as frequently seen in dogs in the South and Midwest than in dogs in the Northeast or West. An age related protection from hookworm infection was not observed; dogs of all age groups were found to be shedding hookworm eggs at roughly equivalent levels. As with ascarids, frequent year-round use of heartworm control products with efficacy against intestinal parasites in pet dogs in the southeastern US may suppress hookworm infections somewhat, albeit not absolutely; the reported prevalence in shelter dogs from this region was more than 38%, compared to less than 3% in the West.[1]

Eggs of canine whipworms (*Trichuris vulpis*) were identified in 1.23% of all dogs in this study, with the highest rates of infection in dogs in the Northeast, Midwest, and Southeast. As in previous studies, the rate of infection in dogs in the West was lower than that in the rest of the country.[1] Infection with *T. vulpis* was most commonly seen in young adult dogs (6 months to 3 years of age) with rates of infection lower in young (<6 months) and aged (>7 years) dogs.

SUMMARY

Intestinal parasites remain a common finding even in well-cared-for dogs seen by veterinarians. In the data reviewed here, 12.5% of pet dogs were shedding eggs of at least one parasite, and many of these dogs were infected with multiple parasites. As with many infections, intestinal parasites are more common in young dogs, particularly those less than 6 months of age. However, for some of the parasites, such as *T. vulpis* and *A. caninum*, prevalence of infection increases slightly with age and remains high for most of the life of the pet. Routine testing of fecal samples for intestinal parasites using the appropriately sensitive approach of centrifugation with zinc sulfate or sugar solution is necessary if these infections are to be identified and treated. The Companion Animal Parasite Council recommends performing a fecal examination on all dogs, including those on year-round parasite control programs, one to two times each year. None of the available comprehensive parasite control products are efficacious against all the major intestinal parasites of dogs; routine testing is the only means of identifying and then eliminating these infections in pets.

In addition to routine testing for parasitic infections through fecal centrifugation, these data support continued vigilance on the part of veterinarians in recommending year-round intestinal parasite control products for dogs. This approach to parasite control is important and may explain, in part, the fact that pet dogs appear to harbor intestinal nematodes at a rate that is 10% to 15% that seen in shelter dogs. This remarkable level of control is no doubt augmented by the higher standard of living that pet dogs enjoy, and perhaps also reflects a shift to older overall age distribution among pet dogs. However, a similar decrease was not seen in rates of infection with *Isospora* spp between shelter dogs and pet dogs, suggesting that veterinary intervention may indeed lead to decreased levels of parasitism. The importance of veterinary intervention by recommending year-round comprehensive parasite control programs cannot be overemphasized; due to the frequency of infection in un-owned dogs and the resultant massive environmental contamination with infectious stages, in the absence of veterinary care and the use of broad spectrum parasiticides, intestinal parasitism could easily return to the pre-control levels in pet dogs which are now seen primarily in un-owned dogs.

Acknowledgements

Access to this comprehensive database was graciously provided by Antech Diagnostic Laboratories and was analyzed at Oklahoma State University in collaboration with Drs. E. Johnson and M. Payton; valuable support with database management was provided by R. Jacklitsch. Drs. M. Paul and B. Blagburn provided insightful comments on the analysis.

SELECTED REFERENCES

1. Blagburn BL, Lindsay DS, Vaughan JL, et al. Prevalence of canine parasites based on fecal floatation. Compend Cont Ed Pract Vet. 1996;18:483-509.
2. Carlin EP, Bowman DD, Scarlett JM, et al. Prevalence of *Giardia* in symptomatic dogs and cats throughout the United States as determined by the IDEXX SNAP Giardia test. Vet Ther. 2005;7(3):199-206.
3. Croese J, Loukas A, Opdebeeck J, Fairley S, Prociv P. Human enteric infection with canine hookworms. Ann Intern Med. 1994;120(5):369-74.
4. Companion Animal Parasite Council Guidelines, Ascarids, Hookworms, Whipworms, Giardia, Coccida. http://www.capcvet.org. Accessed October 1, 2007.
5. Dunn JJ, Columbus ST, Aldeen WE, Davis M, Carroll KC. *Trichuris vulpis* recovered from a patient with chronic diarrhea and five dogs. J Clin Microbiol. 2002;40(7):2703-4.
6. Gavin PJ, Kazacos KR, Shulman ST. 2005. Baylisascariasis. *Clin Microbiol Rev* 18(4):703-18.

Additional detailed references are available from the author upon request.

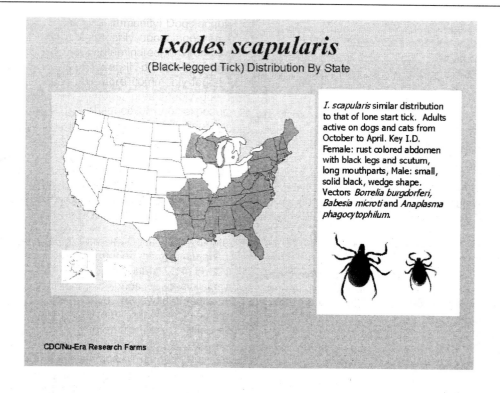

Figure 1. *Ixodes scapularis* and its range. Courtesy of Dr. J. Hair Nu-era Research Farms.

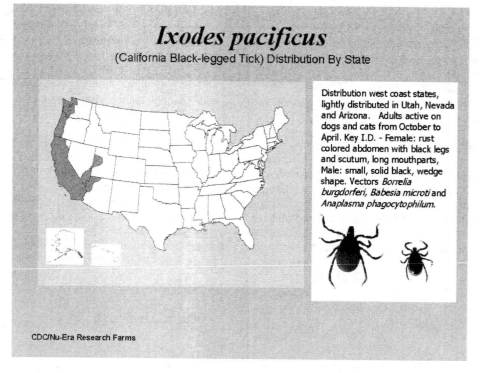

Figure 2. *Ixodes pacificus* and its range. Courtesy of Dr. J. Hair Nu-Era Research Farms.

TICK-BORNE DISEASE: INCIDENCE AND IMPLICATIONS FOR UNDERSTANDING LYME DISEASE, EHRLICHIOSIS, AND ANAPLASMOSIS IN DOGS IN THE EASTERN US

Susan E. Little, DVM, PhD, Diplomate EVPC
Center for Veterinary Health Sciences
Oklahoma State University, Stillwater, OK

Tick-borne diseases are increasingly recognized as critically important in both veterinary medicine and public health. In recent years, new disease agents have been identified in both animals and people, tick populations have increased in number and extent of geographic distribution, and the potential for transmission of disease agents to people and dogs appears to be increasing. Ticks play a critical role in creating and maintaining a source of these infections in pets as well as allowing transmission to pets and people. Throughout much of the United States, as many as six major tick species may be commonly found on dogs, and at least one stage or species of tick is active in any given month, creating a risk for year-round transmission of tick-borne disease agents (Table 1). Accurate interpretation of clinical evidence of disease and diagnostic test results is greatly aided by familiarity with the disease agents most common in a given geographic area. This presentation reviews the clinical presentation, natural history, and geographic distribution of the three most commonly recognized tick-borne diseases in dogs, incorporating data generated through a national voluntary veterinary reporting system developed and maintained by scientists at IDEXX.

Common, Important Canine Tick-borne Diseases

A large and diverse group of tick-borne disease agents infect dogs in the United States. Due to their common occurrence, the severity of illness induced in dogs, and the zoonotic nature of each causative agent, three diseases of particular importance will be discussed in these presentations: Lyme disease, anaplasmosis, and ehrlichiosis.

Lyme Disease

Lyme disease is commonly recognized in both people and dogs in hyperendemic areas of the United States, which includes northeastern, upper midwestern, and West Coast states. Dogs with Lyme borreliosis most commonly present with fever, anorexia, polyarthritis, and lymphadenopathy; although uncommon, protein-losing nephropathy associated with infection may result in edema, weight loss, vomiting, and diarrhea. In people,

Table 1. Common Ticks of Dogs in North America and the Disease Agents They Transmit

Tick Species	Common Name	Pathogen(s) Vectored
Amblyomma americanum	Lone star tick	*Ehrlichia ewingii*[1] *Ehrlichia chaffeensis*[1] *Borrelia lonestari*[1] *Rickettsia rickettsii*[*2]
Amblyomma maculatum	Gulf coast tick	*Hepatozoon americanum*[1]
Dermacentor andersoni	Rocky Mountain wood tick	*Rickettsia rickettsii*[1]
Dermacentor variabilis	American dog tick	*Babesia canis*[2] *Rickettsia rickettsii*[1] *Ehrlichia canis*[2] *Ehrlichia chaffeensis*[2]
Ixodes pacificus	Western black-legged tick ("deer tick")	*Borrelia burgdorferi*[1] *Anaplasma phagocytophilum*[1]
Ixodes scapularis	Eastern black-legged tick ("deer tick")	*Borrelia burgdorferi*[1] *Anaplasma phagocytophilum*[1]
Rhipicephalus sanguineus	Brown dog tick	*Ehrlichia canis*[1] *Anaplasma platys*[*1] *Babesia canis*[1] *Babesia gibsoni*[*1]

[1]Considered primary or main vector
[2]Considered secondary vector
*Vector-pathogen relationship in North America suspected but not confirmed

acute Lyme borreliosis is characterized by headache, fever, muscle and joint pain, and, in approximately 70% of patients, an expanding circular rash (> 5 cm diameter), termed *erythema migrans*, which develops at the primary tick bite or as a secondary lesion; erythema migrans is not recognized in dogs. If not treated in the acute phase, people may experience chronic, disseminated disease, which can result in arthritis, carditis, or neurologic disease; it is not clear if cardiac and neurologic disease is associated with *B. burgdorferi* infection in dogs (CAPC Guidelines, 2007).[1]

Borrelia burgdorferi is the only etiologic agent of Lyme borreliosis identified in people or dogs in North America to date. The organism is maintained in nature through a cycle involving rodents, primarily white-footed mice, as reservoir host and *Ixodes* spp. ticks as vector. Infection is transmitted to people or dogs via the bite of nymphal or adult *Ixodes* spp ticks that acquired the spirochetes when feeding on rodents as larvae or nymphs. Although *Ixodes scapularis*, the primary vector of Lyme disease in the eastern half of the US, is common in southern states, confirmed cases of Lyme disease in people or dogs are considered rare or non-existent in this region. The relative dearth of laboratory confirmed Lyme disease in the South is thought due to the fact that immature *I. scapularis* in this region prefer to feed on lizards rather than rodents, dramatically suppressing prevalence of infection in the ticks. Rodents infected with *B. burgdorferi* have been described from the southern US, but there appears to be no readily available bridge vector to carry infection from these infected rodents to people or pets. There has not been a report of a laboratory-confirmed case of *B. burgdorferi* infection acquired in a human patient south of Maryland or Virginia[6]); the veterinary literature available to date appears to support this regional distribution.[2]

Anaplasmosis

Granulocytic anaplasmosis is a relatively recently recognized disease of both dogs and people in the United States caused by infection with *Anaplasma phagocytophilum*. Dogs with anaplasmosis develop a mild to severe febrile illness characterized by lethargy, depression, and anorexia. Most clinically affected dogs also have moderate to severe myalgia; inflammatory arthritis and associated joint pain, although rare, has been reported in canine anaplasmosis patients. However, when arthritis does occur, co-infection with *B. burgdorferi* should be considered. Complete blood count reveals thrombocytopenia and lymphopenia in the majority of cases. In people, clinical signs of anaplasmosis include fever, malaise, headache, and myalgia. Disease may be severe, particularly in the elderly, and fatalities due to infection have been reported. Disease is more severe in both people and dogs when co-infections with other agents, such as *B. burgdorferi*, *Anaplasma* spp, or *Ehrlichia* spp occur (CAPC Guidelines, 2007).[1]

Infection of dogs with *A. phagocytophilum* is common in areas where dogs are frequently parasitized by black-legged ticks (*Ixodes* spp), such as the northeastern, midwestern, and West Coast states. Indeed, distribution of infection closely resembles that of Lyme disease as the two causative agents share a common maintenance cycle in nature; as with *B. burgdorferi*, rodents are considered the primary reservoir host for *A. phagocytophilum* and *I. scapularis/I. pacificus* ticks the major vector. However, *A. phagocytophilum* can infect a large variety of mammalian species, and other reservoir hosts may well be involved in creating a source of infection for ticks in nature. The geographic distribution of human anaplasmosis largely overlaps that of Lyme borreliosis, and most cases in the US are reported from the Northeast, upper Midwest, and West Coast states.

Ehrlichiosis

In the US, canine ehrlichiosis is most frequently caused by *Ehrlichia canis*, *E. ewingii*, and *E. chaffeensis*. Of the three, *E. canis* is the best known and causes both an acute and a recrudescing chronic febrile disease in infected dogs that is associated with thrombocytopenia, leukopenia, depression, and bleeding diatheses (CAPC Guidelines, 2007).[1] The organism is transmitted from infected to naïve dogs via *Rhipicephalus sanguineus* ticks, although *Dermacentor variabilis* may also serve as a vector for *E. canis*. *Ehrlichia ewingii* is a granulocytic ehrlichiosis agent which, in recent years, has been found to be more common in dogs than *E. canis* in some surveys, a predominance that is likely explained by the high exposure rates of dogs to the vector lone star ticks in many areas.[3]

Despite the common nature of *E. ewingii* infection in dogs, specific diagnostic assays for this pathogen are not widely available; identification of morulae in granulocytes on stained blood smears is possible in acute infections and remains the best patient-side method of confirming infection. Serologic cross-reactivity occurs among *Ehrlichia* spp., and IFA assays for *E. canis* or *E. chaffeensis* may cross-react with antibodies raised against *E. ewingii*. However, the widely available patient-side assays for *E. canis* and *A. phagocytophilum* do not result in false positives in *E. ewingii* infected dogs. While the majority of *E. ewingii* infections in dogs appear to be asymptomatic, clinical signs, including fever, polyarthritis, neurologic disease, and general malaise, have been associated with this agent. *Ehrlichia chaffeensis*, the causative agent of human monocytic ehrlichiosis, also infects dogs although the resultant disease is relatively mild. Co-infections with *E. chaffeensis* and other *Ehrlichia/Anaplasma* spp may result in more severe disease.

All three canine ehrlichiosis organisms have also been described as agents of human disease, with infections confirmed in people, although the majority of cases of human ehrlichiosis in the US are due to infection with *E. chaffeensis*. As in dogs, infected people develop a non-specific febrile illness characterized by headache, malaise, myalgia, and, occasionally, vomiting, diarrhea, or a rash. Human cases of ehrlichosis are largely limited to the hyperendemic areas in the southeastern and southcentral US, where *Amblyomma americanum* ticks are frequently encountered. Infections in this region are very common; in one pediatric study, 13% of children in endemic areas harbored antibodies reactive to *E. chaffeensis*.[4] While dogs serve as reservoir for both *E. canis* and *E. ewingii*, white-tailed deer are considered the primary reservoir host for *E. chaffeensis*.

NEW DATA ON DISTRIBUTION OF TICK-BORNE DISEASES

Commonly used and widely available veterinary patient-side assays (IDEXX 3Dx/4Dx SNAP) allow immediate detection of antibodies to *Borrelia burgdorferi*, *Ehrlichia*, and *Anaplasma*. As explained in the product insert material and on the IDEXX web site, the analyte for *B. burgdorferi* used in the 3Dx/4Dx SNAP assay is extremely specific for antibodies to this organism and cross reactions are not known to occur. A follow-up laboratory assay (quantitative C6) provides more information about the level of antibodies present, and thus indicates whether there is an ongoing, active infection in that dog that warrants antibiotic therapy or if the initial result is more consistent with prior exposure and a resolved infection. The *Ehrlichia* analyte in the 3Dx/4Dx SNAP assays is designed to detect *E. canis*, but will also produce positive results when antibodies to *E. chaffeensis*, but not *E. ewingii*, are present. Similarly, the *Anaplasma* analyte will also react with antibodies to *A. platys*. In collaboration with scientists at IDEXX, the results of serologic testing of dogs from across the US have been compiled (Table 2); an overview of this distribution and the significance these findings have for practicing veterinarians are described here.

Lyme Borreliosis

Antibodies to *Borrelia burgdorferi* were much more commonly reported from dogs in the northeastern and upper Midwestern states, where Lyme disease is considered endemic, than from dogs in the southern U. S. When considered on a regional basis, the rate of positive tests reported was 11.6% in the northeast and 1% in the Southeast (Table 2). However, when Virginia, where endemic Lyme borreliosis is well documented in the northernmost counties, was removed from the analysis, the rate of positive tests in the Southeast fell to 0.36%. Indeed, rates of positive dogs in Connecticut, where 18% of the dogs were reported to test positive to *B. burgdorferi*, are 50- to more than 200-fold greater

than those in the southeastern border states of Texas, Louisiana, Mississippi, Alabama, and Florida. A higher proportion of dogs were also reported positive from counties in northern California where Lyme disease is known to be endemic (2.9% to 5.0%) than from the state or the region as a whole (1.7% and 1.4%, respectively).

This pattern of high endemicity of Lyme disease in the northeastern states and relatively low endemicity in the South was expected and correlates well with documented human case reports for Lyme borreliosis. Nonetheless, occasionally dogs were reported from the southeastern US with antibodies to *B. burgdorferi*. These positive dogs may have acquired infections in endemic areas and then traveled to a non-endemic area. Alternatively, the results in these dogs may represent a low level of local transmission occurring in areas traditionally considered to be non-endemic for Lyme borreliosis. Veterinarians in Florida, Texas, and other areas of the South considered non-endemic for Lyme borreliosis occasionally report observing seroconversion to *Borrelia burgdorferi* with and without concomitant clinical disease in dogs with no history of travel out of the region.

Anaplasmosis

As with *Borrelia burgdorferi*, antibodies to *Anaplasma phagocytophilum* were more commonly reported in dogs in the Northeast, Midwest, and West Coast (Table 2). Prevalence rates in the northeastern states were more than 10-fold greater than those in the South, where infection with *A. phagocytophilum* is considered relatively uncommon. *Anaplasma phagocytophilum* is maintained in nature in a cycle similar to that of *B. burgdorferi*, with black-legged ticks (aka deer ticks) serving as vector and rodents as primary reservoir host. Thus, it is not surprising that the two share a common geographic distribution. This shared transmission cycle also means that co-infection with *A. phagocytophilum* and *B. burgdorferi* is frequently seen. Indeed, 2.0% of all dogs from the Midwest, and 1.4% of dogs from the Northeast were reported to harbor antibodies to both *A. phagocytophilum* and *B. burgdorferi*. In some focal areas, co-infection rates with these two organisms were as high as 10.9%. However, in the southern US, where both Lyme disease and granulocytic anaplasmosis are comparatively rare, co-infection rates were very low (0.1%; Table 2).

Table 2. Percent positive test results reported for *Borrelia burgdorferi*, *Anaplasma*, and *Ehrlichia* in domestic dogs in the United States

Region	B. burgdorferi	Anaplasma	Ehrlichia	Bb/Anaplasma co-infection
Northeast	11.6%	5.5%	0.3%	1.4%
Southeast	1.0%	0.5%	1.3%	0.1%
Midwest	4.0%	6.7%	0.4%	2.0%
West	1.4%	4.5%	0.6%	0.8%
National	**5.1%**	**4.8%**	**0.6%**	**1.3%**

Occasionally, dogs in areas where granulocytic anaplasmosis is considered low to non-endemic are found to harbor antibodies to *A. phagocytophilum*. As with *B. burgdorferi*, travel to and from endemic and hyperendemic foci of infection or a low level of local transmission may account for some of these positive dogs. However, in some cases, particularly in dogs without a travel history or in areas where a high proportion of the dogs test positive, the antibodies present are more likely generated to infection with *A. platys*, a platelet-dwelling *Anaplasma* sp of dogs thought to be transmitted between dogs by *Rhipicephalus sanguineus*, the brown dog tick. Unlike the analyte used to detect antibodies to *B. burgdorferi*, which is very specific, the *A. phagocytophilum* analyte will also react with antibodies generated against *A. platys*. This cross-reactivity is well explained in the 4Dx package insert and is most important to understand in areas where *A. phagocytophilum* is not thought to occur, which in North America is largely the same areas where *B. burgdorferi* is largely absent. *Anaplasma platys* can cause clinical disease in dogs, particularly when present in co-infections. Therefore, even when *A. platys* and not *A. phagocytophilum* is suspected to be responsible for the positive result, follow-up complete blood counts with enumeration of platelets is warranted; thrombocytopenia is an indication for doxycycline therapy in *A. phagocytophilum*/*A. platys* antibody-positive dogs.

Ehrlichiosis

Fewer dogs were reported as testing positive for antibodies to *Ehrlichia* than for *B. burgdorferi* or *Anaplasma*. Nonetheless, 0.6% of dogs had antibodies to *Ehrlichia* nationwide. In the South, the rate of positive dogs was more than twice the national average (Table 2). Cases of ehrlichiosis due to *E. canis* are considered more common in the southern US, where infestations of *R. sanguineus* are also more commonly seen, although this tick, in the absence of effective control programs, can survive indoors in kennels and homes virtually anywhere there are dogs. As with Lyme disease and anaplasmosis, a number of foci of infection were identified where prevalence rates were much higher than the average for the respective state or region considered. For example, in some areas in Missouri and Arkansas, the rate of positive dogs was 6% to 7%, more than 10-fold higher than the national average. Detection of antibodies generated to *E. chaffeensis*, as is known to occur with the analyte used in the 3Dx/4Dx SNAP assays, may explain some of these findings, as these areas of Missouri and Arkansas are well known as hyperendemic for human ehrlichiosis.[7] Alternatively, the analyte could be detecting antibodies to novel *Ehrlichia* spp. that have not yet been described. This assay does not detect antibodies to *E. ewingii*, but dogs may be exposed to other novel *Ehrlichia* spp. cycling in nature.[5]

CONCLUSIONS

Current data indicate that both *Borrelia burgdorferi* and *Anaplasma phagocytophilum* are cycling in hyperendemic areas of the northeastern, upper Midwestern, and West Coast states, whereas *Ehrlichia canis* is more widely distributed in the US, albeit at an apparent lower overall prevalence. However, there is evidence of exposure to at least one of each of these three tick-borne disease agents in every state and region considered. The presence of specific antibodies to *B. burgdorferi* in southern states is of particular interest. Should future work document endemic transmission in these areas, changes in vaccination protocols may be indicated, with vaccination of dogs considered in areas traditionally thought to be relatively free of Lyme disease. Vaccines are not currently available to prevent anaplasmosis or ehrlichiosis in dogs, and thus stringent adherence to tick control through routine administration of acaricides is necessary to block transmission of these and other tick-borne diseases. Routine screening for exposure to these organisms with appropriate subsequent laboratory tests to evaluate for presence of subclinical disease is also warranted. The wider than expected geographic distribution, which includes evidence of each infection in areas considered to be non- or low-endemic, supports continued vigilance by veterinarians in testing for tick-borne disease agents and indicates the need for increased research efforts to understand the transmission patterns of these important pathogens.

SELECTED REFERENCES

1. Companion Animal Parasite Council Guidelines, Vector-borne Diseases. http://www.capcvet.org.
2. Duncan AW, Correa MT, Levine JF, et al. The dog as a sentinel for human infection: prevalence of *Borrelia burgdorferi* C6 antibodies in dogs from southeastern and mid-Atlantic states. Vector Borne Zoonotic Dis. 2004;4:221–229.
3. Liddell AM, Stockham SL, Scott MA, et al. Predominance of *Ehrlichia ewingii* in Missouri dogs. J Clin Microbiol. 2003;41(10):4617-22.
4. Marshall GS, Jacobs RF, Schutze GE, et al. *Ehrlichia chaffeensis* seroprevalence among children in the southeast and south-central regions of the United States. Arch Pediatr Adolesc Med. 2002;156(2):166-70.
5. Seaman RL, Kania SA, Hegarty BC, et al. Comparison of results for serologic testing and a polymerase chain reaction assay to determine the prevalence of stray dogs in eastern Tennessee seropositive to *Ehrlichia canis*. Am J Vet Res. 2004;65(9):1200-3.
6. Wormser GP, Dattwyler RJ, Shapiro ED, et al. The clinical assessment, treatment, and prevention of Lyme disease, human granulocytic anaplasmosis, and babesiosis: clinical practice guidelines by the Infectious Diseases Society of America. *Clin Infect Dis.* 2006;43(9):1089-134.
7. Yabsley MJ, Wimberly MC, Stallknecht DE, et al. Spatial analysis of the distribution of *Ehrlichia chaffeensis*, causative agent of human monocytotropic ehrlichiosis, across a multi-state region. Am J Trop Med Hyg. 2005;72, 840-50.

Additional detailed references are available from the author upon request.

LAWS AFFECTING DRUG USE BY VETERINARIANS

Alistair I. Webb, BVSc, PhD, FRCVS, Diplomate ACVA
College of Veterinary Medicine
University of Florida, Gainesville, FL

A "**valid veterinarian–client–patient relationship**" is the core of legal and ethical use of drugs—both legend and controlled. When dispensing or prescribing any drug, a veterinarian should ensure he/she is acting within the elements of a valid relationship. This was initially defined by the AVMA but has more lately been codified in the Federal Regulations. A valid veterinarian–client–patient relationship exists when:

- The Veterinarian is responsible for medical judgments on the health and treatment of the animal(s) and the client (owner/agent) agrees to follow the veterinarian's instructions
- Through physical examination of the animal(s) and/or medically appropriate and timely visits to the premises where the animals(s) are kept, the Veterinarian is sufficiently knowledgeable of the animal(s) to make a general or preliminary diagnosis of the medical problem
- The veterinarian is readily available for follow-up in case of adverse reactions or failure of the regimen of therapy

Such a relationship can exist only when the veterinarian has recently seen and is personally acquainted with the keeping and care of the animal(s) by virtue of examination of the animal(s), and/or by medically appropriate and timely visits to the premises where the animal(s) are kept.

There are a number of laws that control how veterinarians use drugs in the practice of their profession. These originate from both Federal and State legislatures with the state laws often mirroring the federal laws. However, where there are differences, you must follow the law with the higher standard. The laws encompass (a) Drug abuse prevention and control, (b) Regulation of food, drugs and cosmetics, and (c) Conduct of veterinary practice. The latter is a State of Florida law only.

CONTROLLED SUBSTANCES

Although supported by almost identical Florida laws, the Drug Enforcement Administration (DEA) is the primary federal law enforcement agency charged with the responsibility of supervising the Controlled Substances Act through a system of classification and licensing.

Classification

Drugs and chemicals with abuse potential are classified into five schedules based on potential for abuse and their use in medical practice in the US.

SCHEDULE I – These have a high potential for abuse and no currently accepted medical use in treatment in the US. Examples include opium derivatives such as heroin and codeine methylbromide, as well as hallucinogenic substances (marijuana, LSD, THC, peyote, mescaline), and stimulants/depressants such as methaqualone and methylamphetamine. These drugs are not available to clinicians.

SCHEDULE II – This includes drugs available for medical use in the US but which have a high potential for abuse that may lead to severe psychological or physical dependence. Included in this category are opium itself, morphine, codeine, fentanyl, hydromorphone, methadone, meperidine, oxycodone, and oxymorphone. Etorphine hydrochloride and carfentanil are included but are in a subclass restricted to use in the restraint of wild and zoo animals. Also included are stimulants such as cocaine, phencyclidine, amphetamine, and methamphetamine as well as methylphenidate. The short-acting barbiturates amobarbital, pentobarbital, and secobarbital are included here also.

SCHEDULES III–V – These schedules do not differ in either storage or documentation requirements but rather in the severity of penalties assessed for legal infractions. Drugs in these schedules do not require any special form to place orders but rather can be done quite informally over the phone or by e-mail to a distributor who has copies of your current state and DEA registration. You are still required to keep invoices/packing slips annotated as the delivery data and confirmation that contents and packing list match. These together with details of the drug disposition have to be kept for 2 years and be readily available upon request by authorized regulatory inspectors (DEA, FDA, and DPR). They can be kept as a computer log but data losses by hardware failure is not an acceptable excuse – backups are therefore essential. Drugs in these schedules include thiopental, ketamine and Telazol, buprenorphine, narcotic-acetaminophen mixtures and anabolic steroids [C-III]; phenobarbital, chloral hydrate, and benzodiazepines.

Registration

The prime requirement of the controlled drug laws is that anyone who manufactures, distributes, or dispenses a controlled substance must register with the DEA. Although the DEA's clinically relevant regulations have been written primarily to cover physicians, pharmacists, and human hospitals, veterinarians are treated no differently than professionals from other medical fields Registration is for 3 years at a time. The fee was increased by 40% last November and the current fee $551. The certificate of registration is issued for that particular place of business and must be kept at that site. Any additional places of business where controlled drugs are stored require separate registration.

Practitioners must be licensed in the states where they are practicing and have a valid DEA registration to order controlled substances from distributors. No special form is needed for orders of drugs in Schedules III, IV, and V; however, in Schedule II, drugs must be ordered with the DEA's own form (Form DEA-222) which is pre-printed with the registrant's name and address.

Suppliers of any controlled drugs will require proof of your State and DEA registration.

Record Keeping

Schedule II Drugs: All records for Schedule II drugs must be kept separate from all other data. These records, required to be kept for 2 years, consist of records of receipt of all shipments and details of the disposition of those drugs. MINIMALLY - annotated as received carbons of the DEA's order form (DEA-222A), and the details of individual dispensings (client's name, date, species, dose administered). It is important that the administration of ALL scheduled drugs is included in the patient's medical record as it may act as proof of administration in the event of an inquiry.

Schedules III–V: A log must be kept of all deliveries (best to keep packing slip endorsed to show verified receipt and date). Individual details of drug disposition must be kept separately as for Schedule II or be "readily retrievable from ordinary business records". These data must be kept 2 years as well. The basic difference through schedules III through V is of decreasing penalties for criminal offenses with no difference in record keeping or storage requirements.

Inventory: Starting on the date DEA registration is received, a complete and accurate inventory of all controlled drugs on hand must be taken and repeated every two years. The inventory should have Schedule II items listed separately from other controlled drugs. The list must include your name, DEA number, the address where the inventory was performed, and is signed. It should be kept for at least 2 years and must be produced to a DEA officer on demand.

Dispensing: When dispensing for clients to administer at home, you must ensure that the drug is adequately labeled with your name, address, and phone number, plus the name of the owner and species of patient; dispensing and expiry dates; directions for use; and a warning that the drug must not be transferred to another patient. You should also use a childproof container unless specifically requested otherwise. Finally, when the drug is dispensed, do not forget to subtract it from inventory/records. The transfer of any controlled substance requires formal record keeping; an individual practitioner can deliver or transfer a controlled drug to another registrant as long as records are kept of the transaction. Since most veterinary practitioners do not administer or dispense large quantities of controlled substances, their activities generally are under less close governmental scrutiny although in recent years they have become a target beak-ins. If a theft or break-in occurs, it must be reported to both the police and the DEA. One rule in Florida that many practitioners seem unaware about is that once drugs are dispensed and leave your premises they cannot be returned and re-dispensed. This applies even if the packaging seems unopened.

Disposal: Despite the Act, the regulations are not clear here but do give individual DEA Offices power to establish local practices. To dispose of controlled substances you need DEA permission—Form DEA-41 in triplicate is prescribed for occasional disposals. Several years ago, the DEA contracted with a number of companies to act as it is agent in controlled drug collection and disposal—to find your nearest/economic contractor contact your local DEA diversion office. Today it seems that the DEA's position has softened somewhat and they regard drugs once dispensed/withdrawn to be of low interest to them, and these can be destroyed under controlled and witnessed conditions. You must keep records of such disposals.

Prescriptions: Requirements for prescriptions for controlled drugs do not vary from standard prescription format. It is mandated by Federal regulations that prescriptions for controlled drugs have the same basic elements as when you are labeling dispensed drugs. The script must be signed, dated, and have the prescriber's DEA number. It is recommended that the DEA number be written and not preprinted. Pharmacists who fill your prescriptions must retain them for 2 years. Controlled drug prescriptions only have a life of 6 months and repeats are not allowed for Schedule II drugs but up to five repeats are allowed for Schedules III–V.

Security: Veterinary practitioners who store controlled drugs and substances within their offices, hospitals, or clinics must keep these drugs in securely locked, substantially constructed cabinets or safes. Drug stocks should be kept to a minimum. Access to the storage area should be restricted to an absolute minimum number of authorized employees.

FLORIDA'S VETERINARY MEDICINE PRACTICE ACT

Florida's practice act has some specific restrictions on veterinarians administering, dispensing or prescribing drugs that can result in disciplinary action if not followed. These include:

- Prescribing unnecessary treatment
- Failing to keep contemporaneous written medical records
- Prescribing or dispensing legend drugs inappropriately or in excessive quantities
- Pre-signing blank prescription forms
- Failing to give owners of a patient, before dispensing any drug, a written prescription when requested
- Not obtaining an owner's informed consent when prescribing or dispensing drugs extra-label and the intend use is novel, unproven or experimental

FOOD, DRUG & COSMETICS ACT

The Food and Drug Administration's Center for Veterinary Medicine (FDA CVM) has been given the authority to govern the manufacture, distribution, and use of veterinary drugs. The Federal Regulations set requirements for drugs to be approved, which include demonstrating both efficacy and safety of the drug (to both the patient and humans who come in contact with the drug directly or by eating treated animals). Once a new animal drug clears this process, the FDA approval identifies the specific conditions for which the drug has been shown to be safe and effective as well as any restrictions for use. This information is part of the label or insert provided with each drug container. Although the same drug may be effective and safe for other uses or perhaps other species, the economics of a limited marketplace often prohibit a pharmaceutical company from performing sufficient additional research to seek wider approval. This fact and others often result in "extra-label" uses of drugs. This is when the drug is administered in a manor not covered by the conditions of the FDA approval; this can mean different doses, routes of administration, indications, and species. Such use used to be illegal but is now permitted for treatment of disease and/or pain but only to veterinarians acting within the confines of a valid veterinarian–client–patient relationship. Such use by laypersons or in mediated feed is prohibited. When companion animals are treated, the only restrictions are that the drug must be approved by the FDA in humans or animals and that the veterinarian is using good clinical judgment. In food-producing animals there are a series of requirement that must be met as well as correct record keeping of the decision and the identity of the animals involved. Of course, all drug use, label or off-label in any species can be curtailed by FDA if that use is "against the public interest".

EXTRA-LABEL DRUG USE IN FOOD-PRODUCING ANIMALS

Veterinarians are now given considerable latitude in the therapeutic use of animal drugs off-label as long as they inform livestock producers of the appropriate drug withdrawal times for food-producing animals and follow the following steps in deciding what drug and dose to use:

1. A careful medical diagnosis is made by an attending veterinarian within the context of a valid veterinarian–client–patient relationship;
2. A determination is made that there is no marketed drug (a) specifically labeled to treat the condition diagnosed, or (b) clinically ineffective in the animals to be treated;
3. Procedures are instituted to assure that identity of the treated animals is carefully maintained;
4. A significantly extended time period, supported by appropriate scientific information, is assigned for drug withdrawal prior to marketing meat, milk, or eggs and steps are taken to assure that the assigned time frames are met, and no illegal residues occur;
5. A drug approved for animals should always be used where possible before considering use of a human-labeled drug;
6. Records are to be maintained by the veterinarian for a minimum of 2 years documenting that the above steps were observed.

Despite this ability to use drugs off label there are drugs where extra-label use in food-producing animals is prohibited. The FDA considers this area to be of major regulatory priority and has demonstrated both the will and desire to prosecute offenders. The drugs currently in that list are chloramphenicol, clenbuterol, diethylstilbestrol, nitroimidazoles, nitrofurans, sulfonamides, fluoroquinolones, and glycopeptides. The FDA has reserved the power to add to that list and has recently done so in the addition of the last two antibiotic groups. The concern at protection of children exposed to drug residues is demonstrated by higher residue limits (tolerances) in milk and prohibition of a drug like phenylbutazone from use in lactating cows.

Two areas of FDA responsibility attracting attention are antibiotic resistance and compounding. The concern about *resistance* stems from the extent of antibiotic use by both the medical and veterinary professions as well as the use of antibiotics as growth promotants. Veterinarians need to be aware of the latest guidelines about prudent usage as well as exercising restraint in using newer drugs that have potential of significant application in humans.

The second concern is *compounding*. To be legal, compounding can only be done by a compounding pharmacist acting under a veterinarian's prescription issued within a valid veterinarian–client–patient relationship. Compounding can only be performed for a single client/patient and must not be a duplication of an already approved drug formulation. Compounding, by definition, is an extra-label use of dugs and therefore all of AMDUCA requirements have to be met. Remember, the onus for any toxicity of a compounded product is shared by the veterinarian who wrote the script and by the pharmacist for the accuracy of the compounding. Compounding pharmacists regard compounding as an art and guarantee neither absorption nor stability. Sterility of compounded parenteral medications is the responsibility of the pharmacist so veterinarians should make sure they know the training and facilities of pharmacists who compound for their clients. FDAs stand on banning use of bulk chemicals in compounding has been challenged in court and the latest implications will be discussed at the meeting.

WEB SOURCES
[Please note: this web is spelled with only one B]

DEA's diversion page
http://www.deadiversion.usdoj.gov/

FDA Center for Veterinary Medicine home page
http://www.fda.gov/cvm/

Veterinary Adverse Drug Experience Reports
http://www.fda.gov/cvm/adetoc.htm

Florida law On-Line [Veterinary Medical Practice]
http://www.leg.state.fl.us/Statutes/index.cfm?App_mode=Display_Statute&URL=Ch0474/ch0474.htm

Current drug shortage list
http://www.ashp.org/s_ashp/resolved_shortages.asp?CID=1500&DID=1544&sort=0

Verified Internet Pharmacy Practice Sites
http://vipps.nabp.net/verify.asp

FARAD home page
http://www.farad.org

NRSP-7 web site [minor species]
http://www.nrsp-7.org/

Veterinary PDA Programs
http://www.anmldr.com

Above URLs are valid as of August 2007

Footnotes
Potential for abuse is defined in the regulations as having properties of CNS stimulation, depression, or hallucination that creates a substantial likelihood of its being:

a) used in amounts that create a hazard in the user's health or the safety of the community

b) diverted from legal channels and distributed through illegal channels

c) taken on the user's own initiative rather than on the basis of professional advice

The Florida statutes specifically enable veterinarians to dispense controlled drugs and to supervise their administration by un-licensed personnel [term = direct supervision, which equates with responsible supervision rather than "immediate supervision" where the veterinarian's physical presence is mandated].

DON'T GET LEFT BEHIND: THREE CRITICAL WAYS TO KEEP YOUR VETERINARY PRACTICE COMPETITIVE, AND PROFITABLE

Jim Baum
Regional Sales Manager, Matsco
Emeryville, CA

Today's rapid advancements in veterinary technology and medical information have spurred an increase in specialized services and practices, with doctors delivering better care than ever for their patients. At the same time, this explosion in technology and species-specific information has produced intense, continuous pressure on veterinarians to remain current with new trends in order to stay competitive. The basic principle of business management that applies across industries holds true in the veterinary field—update, or stagnate.

Practices that are not continually updating their technology, facility, and even their practice style are destined to realize only incremental growth through price increases or a limited expansion of services. But with upgraded information technology and medical equipment, an expanded facility, or even a new approach to practice partnership, practices can increase productivity, customer loyalty, quality of care, range of services, and ultimately, their profits.

There are three fundamental ways to keep your practice competitive and profitable, and avoid getting left behind amidst the growing diversification in veterinary care.

UPGRADE TECHNOLOGIES TO INCREASE EFFICIENCY

Practices that are highly efficient can command higher fees while serving a larger number of patients. Today's advanced communications and equipment technologies have been shown to improve the efficiencies of the average veterinary practice, providing systematic and easy coordination and tracking of in-hospital referrals, procedures, medications, and client communications for every patient.

For example, integrated computer systems that link to your pharmaceutical companies, allow immediate access to patient charts and billing data, connect exam rooms with the front desk, provide client education, and deliver client emails, have been shown to significantly increase in-hospital productivity. In addition, comprehensive practice management software can assist you in managing the day-to-day details of running your practice, such as marketing, billing, scheduling staff meetings and processing new hires. Conversely, the wrong practice management software can be a big hindrance to efficiency and a productive practice.

In addition to integrated computer technologies, advances in medical equipment and procedures can improve the effectiveness of your practice with better diagnostic tools and solutions for your patients. Digital radiography, for instance, is becoming increasingly popular in veterinary medicine because it allows faster image processing time, eliminates the costs and hazards of film and processing chemicals, helps communicate diagnoses and treatment options to clients, and assists doctors and technicians in reviewing cases before and during treatment. It also facilitates remote consultations with specialists.

With new technologies that support increased productivity and efficiency, your practice can deliver higher quality services in less time, resulting in greater customer satisfaction and loyalty.

Of course, there's no "rule of thumb" for exactly how much your productivity will increase when you integrate new communications or equipment technology, as each practice is unique. But you can get a good sense of potential improvements in practice efficiencies by speaking with colleagues who have migrated to advanced technology about their experience.

You can also set meaningful goals for productivity improvements to offset your technology investment. For instance, track how long it currently takes to manage each patient visit—from scheduling and sending out appointment reminders, to billing and collections, updating charts and files, and referring patients to specialists. If you are able to attain a 10% to 20% increase in productivity through the integration of new computer technology and equipment, how much extra time will that leave your practice for additional appointments, procedures or marketing activities? You can also do a cost analysis to assess return on investment (ROI) taking into account expected income, equipment costs, labor costs, supply costs, DVM compensation, and maintenance costs.

Knowing When to Upgrade

One of the more difficult decisions you will make in upgrading or buying new systems and equipment is, "Should I make the leap into advanced technology now, or wait for the next generation of upgrades?" The answer is make the leap **now,** if at all possible, and keep upgrading as your practice grows.

Veterinary technology is advancing at a tremendous rate, with new equipment and computer software being introduced continually. So purchasing advanced technology is not an occasional investment. To stay at the forefront of the industry, you will want to develop a technology upgrade program that allows for investment in a new technology purchase every year or so. This should be a line item in every hospital's yearly budget.

The amount you invest will depend on the type of veterinary service you provide—specialists will obviously require a greater investment in equipment and materials than general practices. Your CPA and practice management consultant can help you outline a comfortable technology investment program that keeps your practice current and competitive. To help ensure a smooth implementation of your program, you might consider working with a lender that specializes in veterinary practice financing and understands your particular business needs.

EXPAND YOUR FACILITY TO ACCOMMODATE MORE PATIENTS AND SERVICES

Expanding your practice can help provide a more functional workspace, improving staff morale as well as quality of service for your clients and patients. In addition, a modern, expanded hospital communicates to your clients that you offer a high level of care for their animals, and allows you to offer new services such as animal training, boarding, day care and educational seminars, potentially leading to increased revenue and profits.

Many older facilities are not outfitted to accommodate the high-density scheduling or in-house client service training and staff meetings that are becoming more prevalent in veterinary practices. Expanding or building a new facility can also help increase work flow efficiency by providing a more functional workspace, and can serve to attract new clients as well as high caliber staff members.

How do you know when it's time to consider an expansion? When the size and quality of your facility hamper your potential for production and your ability to practice in an efficient manner. Most doctors know when they are "maxed out," with not enough hours in the day to meet the demands of their practice. In addition, when clients are waiting too long for appointments, it takes your staff too long to find or complete files, you have to turn away patients for lack of adequate cages and runs, or keep patients longer than should be necessary because of a shortage of technicians, then it's time to consider a hospital and staff expansion. The important factors to consider are:

- The cost to expand (including additional personnel and equipment costs), versus potential increased revenue from a larger clientele and range of services;
- The impact moving to a new location will have on your existing clientele and staff;
- The increased savings from greater efficiencies achieved through workspace design, technology and shared services;
- The costs of effectively promoting your new facility.

However, don't focus on costs alone. Consider also the potential for growth that an updated, expanded facility provides, not only in additional patients and higher priced services, but in client satisfaction and loyalty as well. Also, consider the professional satisfaction you will get from having a modern state-of-the-art facility.

CONSOLIDATE TO OFFER GREATER CLIENT CONVENIENCE

As veterinary medicine has become increasingly diverse with many practitioners specializing in a particular species or procedure, the tactic of combining several solo practices into a larger central hospital that serves an entire community has become a significant trend. This approach provides a range of services under one roof, delivering greater convenience and comfort for clients and ultimately better continuity of care for their animals.

The group practice is especially advantageous for clients when general animal diagnostics and care are combined with a range of specialties and surgical services that are typically outsourced, allowing for quicker response times, more efficient client communications and greater convenience by treating the patient in one facility. In addition, because of shared costs and specialties among participants, a group practice provides an opportunity to incorporate new technology that offers improved patient care and comfort, such as ultrasound, minimally invasive surgeries (laparoscopy, thoracoscopy, arthroscopy), joint replacement surgeries, stifle reconstruction, closed fracture repair with fluoroscopy, various scoping procedures, advanced imaging (CT, MRI, nuclear scintigraphy), and radiation therapy.

Ultimately, the group hospital can offer better continuity of care with veterinarians able to directly oversee the full health and recovery process for a patient and thereby gain a more comprehensive picture of the patient's overall well being. And because there are more participants to provide input to cases, oversee animal care and conduct client transactions, the group practice may generate greater efficiency as well. These are benefits your clients will recognize and gladly support through higher fees as appropriate.

You may also want to consider including critical onsite services in your facility that can add significant value for your clients without substantial overhead costs for you. For example:

- An effective pharmacy that provides more flexibility in meeting specifications for the exact medicine, strength, capsule size, dosage and flavor for each patient can be a valuable addition to your service offering, generating increased loyalty from your customers for this personalized service.
- Incorporating lab work in your hospital, such as blood and urine tests, allows greater control over the patient diagnostic process while providing higher quality care for patients and convenience for their owners. In addition, an onsite laboratory provides another revenue stream for the hospital.

By offering greater convenience, comfort and continuity of care, group practices can compete more effectively in their communities while simultaneously earning higher fees for premium services. In addition, by sharing investment costs with a number of participants, group practices can more readily stay current with trends in veterinary medicine with updated technology, services and equipment.

And finally, the group practice is better positioned to offer a range of opportunities for practice participants. For example, younger veterinarians can grow towards partnership status, while current owners may realize expanded retirement options through sale of their ownership to a member who is already familiar with the practice style and clientele.

ENSURING A POSITIVE RETURN ON INVESTMENT

Of course, providing higher quality of care, improving practice efficiencies and increasing customer convenience are all very worthy outcomes of your investment that will ultimately produce increased cash flow. But keep in mind that there is a cost associated with these new benefits. To ensure a quicker return on your investment, you will need to reassess your fee schedule and determine how much to increase client fees for advanced procedures.

Unfortunately, there is no simple formula for determining how much to charge for advanced procedures and their added benefits. Your management consultant and CPA can help you determine the appropriate fees for your practice. But clients understand the value of these services and appreciate the need to pay for them. In fact, if given a choice, most clients will happily pay extra for a shorter, more comfortable experience for their pet!

The key is that your customers will respect and appreciate the fact that you have kept up with advancements in veterinary medicine. In general, veterinary hospitals that have invested in upgrading or expanding their practice have not only recouped their costs in the short term, but recognized a significant profit as well. This is also a good way to add equity to the practice.

STAYING COMPETITIVE BY SATISFYING YOUR CUSTOMER

The veterinary field will continue to diversify as new technologies and procedures are developed, offering the promise of longer, healthier lives for a variety of animal species. Staying competitive and growing profits in this exciting, expanding career requires continually upgrading your practice with the latest advancements in order to give your clients and their animals the best service possible.

Whether you're adding technology, expanding your facility, or incorporating into a group practice, it's important to remember that staying competitive ultimately comes back to satisfying your customer. An excellent administration and customer service team, combined with leadership provided by the owners and a positive practice culture, create the foundation for a successful business that's well positioned to grow. And when your clients experience less waiting time, quicker results, thorough communications and healthier pets, they will return to your practice again and again, providing the continuity and resources for your practice to compete, and thrive.

By Keith Richter, DVM & Sina Afredi, Matsco. © 2007 Matsco. Reprinted with permission from Matsco for the 2008 NAVC Proceedings. For more information, contact Matsco at 866.4MY.PAWS (866.469.7297).

OPEN BOOK MANAGEMENT – MATRICES

Ross Clark, DVM
Kansas State University
Manhattan, KS

Louise Dunn
Snowgoose Veterinary Management Consulting
Greensboro, NC

Elise M. Lacher, CPA
Lacher McDonald & Co., CPAs
Seminole, FL

Charging for what we do is a problem in many veterinary practices. Services somehow don't get onto travel sheets/circle sheets or into charts. Discounts are given to team members, former team members, multiple pet owners, cat owners, dog owners, snake owners, what have you. Any excuse that can be thought of is frequently given as to why fees are too high or why clients can't or won't pay our fees. The team may be uncomfortable with charging large amounts for services that are provided. How can Open Book Management help with these issues?

Fees do communicate a practice's value to its clients. If clients won't pay for the services we provide, maybe the problem isn't with the amount charged, but the service provided. We consistently find that practices whose owners and team members truly believe that they offer the best client service and who truly do practice high quality medicine, fee issues are not a problem, either with the setting or collecting. That said; remember that high fees must be supported with excellent service. Increases to your fee schedule equalize the largest possible increase in profit. Most, if not all of a fee increase, falls immediately to the bottom-line.

There are many areas and influences that play a part in setting your prices. Pricing objectives, price flexibility, discounts, the legal environment, competition, costs involved in purchasing the items or providing the service, demand – you as an owner know that – does your team? Helping your team understand the costs of doing business and how they relate to the fees you charge for the services you perform all make for good team meetings.

The Mega study back in 1999 stated that there is an inelastic nature to the demand for veterinary services – clients will pay for value. This finding continues to be true. In looking for help in reviewing your fee schedule, remember that your accountant can be of tremendous help to you in this area. In reviewing the price/quality matrix, you will find that it is generally easier to look at your services and their related price along a continuum of quality from low to high and related pricing from how to high. Vaccinations may fall in the low quality, low price range, and surgery using the latest laser technique may be in a high quality, high price end of the scale. One thing we consistently find is that you can't have a price schedule that reflects low cost, high service and high quality medicine. Two out of the three is about the best you can do.

With Open Book Management as a centerpiece of your management program, team members are constantly reminded that there is a cost to the services they provide. As they become more aware that the light bill, and the rent, and the telephone company all need to be paid, the understanding will develop that the payments that they receive for the services that they perform all are part of the circle of doing business. If the service is poor and clients are unhappy, the money isn't received and the utility company turns off the lights. If the clients are happy, the pet leaves better off than when he came it, but we think the bill is too high so we don't charge what we should, the landlord evicts us because the landlord wants to be paid. All of this seems so obvious to us as practice owners, but it is not to many team members. They are used to handling their own expenses at home, generally, but making the transition to the practice, needs some training.

Once the team is trained in how Open Book Management works, tracking outcomes becomes the next logical place to be. This is where scorecards come into play. If we believe the statement that what gets measured gets changed, and if we believe that a well trained team will perform at the highest possible level, then using scorecards to help us achieve our goals will necessarily follow suit.

The purpose of scorecards is not to measure everything and understand nothing. We want to be setting goals in the practice and then developing scorecards to help us reach those goals. So many times, practice owners come back from great seminars with all of these new ideas. They implement them in their practices, hopefully, but then get bogged down with the day to day life issues. While the scorecards may continue to be tracked, it is easy to forget what the purpose of these cards was in the first place. We then find that practices have Excel spreadsheets tracking things that were meaningful ten years ago, but have no bearing on what the practice is trying to achieve today.

In this article we will be giving examples of scorecards that we have all used in practices to help the full team achieve the goals they want. The scorecards that we are using are examples of things that have worked in other practices. They may not all be relevant to your practice. It is important that the scorecards become part of the Open Book Management team training meetings, that they are discussed, modified as appropriate and actions taken based on what the scorecards are saying. If they are just more numbers that are looked at and then moved on without action being taken, scorecards are just one more management tool that isn't of any real value. We will be talking about and giving examples of productivity measures, such staff costs per transaction, veterinarian costs per transaction, revenue generated per square foot of the building, staff hours/transaction. Not only will the scorecards be given, but the meaning behind the scorecards. What are we trying to track and why? If we can cut the wait time to see a veterinarian, what affect should this have on the ATCs of the doctors?

The goal in keeping scorecards and tracking Key Performance Indicators is not just to make everyone Excel proficient. However, we do frequently find that having a working knowledge of Excel is almost a necessity when it comes to monitoring these results. We have started to require being proficient in Excel or at least to be willing to get the training, part of the job description and requirements for the position of Practice Manager. Getting back on track, the reason why measurements are taken is not just to keep schedules. We track the scorecards to measure how close we are actually coming to achieving the goals that we have set for the practices. Magic does happen when everyone is on the same page, with their sights set on the same goal.

What are some of the scorecards that might be important to you? Some of the basic things that should be tracked in any practice relate to production. A very basic Key Performance Indicator schedule would track revenue per doctor per month, number of transactions and the Average Transaction Charge for the month. We keep the production related to just the work that is done by the doctor in the room, plus dentals and radiographs. Why don't we put prescription refills and over the counter goods into these numbers? Because it brings down and distorts what the veterinarians are actually doing in their patient encounters. With information like this at your fingertips, you are able to see at a glance how your practice measures up to some of the external published benchmarks dealing with well run companion animal basic wellness practices. If you know that your doctors are averaging 300 to 350 transactions per month that they are seeing the appropriate number of clients for a practice that is performing up to par. If there are variances in the transactions, this information gives you concrete data with which to talk with your veterinarians. This is much more beneficial than "I just don't think you are doing your job."

Tracking non-doctor-related production also can give you key information that you can use in managing your practice. There are published benchmarks on ranges for what this range should be. If your practice falls outside this range, this can be a topic for meaningful team meetings. Putting in scorecards to track this number – macro scorecards for you to review as the Chief Financial Officer for your practice, but also micro scorecards for various departments in your practice to use to plug holes and improve on delivery of service to bring the overall number up to where it should be. Achieving the goal of performing at the level you want should be cause for a well deserved celebration.

Most practices want to track number of new clients seen each month. Instead of having to leaf through pages of your practice management software reports, capturing this data on your production report will let you know at a glance if you are within the recommended number of 30 to 40 new clients per month for a well established companion animal practice. If you are falling short, you can work on various ideas to raise the number. Having the information available to team members each month on a report that they have access to will help you stay on track of seeing the number of new clients that is realistic for your practice. We are all interested in new clients. However, most of us are aware that it costs a lot of money to attract and service new clients. Are you tracking retention of existing clients? Are you tracking new services for existing clients? Are you tracking referral sources? (And rewarding not only clients who spend a lot of money with you, your top 20% of revenue generating clients, but also rewarding those clients are referring their friends to you?)

The limit to the number of scorecards that you can have is only how creative you can be. Just remember, you don't want to fall into the trap of Measuring everything, and Understanding Nothing.

OPEN BOOK MANAGEMENT – LIGHTNING IN A BOTTLE, FINALLY PERFECTED

Ross Clark, DVM
Kansas State University,
Manhattan, KS

There are many new ideas that come down the pike each year promising to solve all of our management problems. However, according to the Harvard School of Business, Open Book Management is the greatest new management tool we have had in the last 75 years.

At the center of Open Book Management is training. The staff needs to be trained in what running a business is all about. While a veterinary practice is all about taking care of the animals, it is still a business that needs to be appropriately managed. While we frequently complain that employees don't think like us (the owners), if we look at it, most of them have never been involved with running a business so of course, they can't think like owners.

Opening the company books, to whatever extent you are comfortable with, is not going to be of much benefit to the staff if they don't know what they are looking at. So with Open Book Management, it is important that you train your staff in those things over which they have some control, so they can start to "think like owners."

With Open Book Management, accountability takes a front row seat. Since your staff now learns what things they should be looking at and how their performance fits into the running of the practice, they can start to be held accountable for the things that they have control over. Compensation plans can be used to help people perform to the level that you expect. In Open Book Management, team members start to see that all the money coming in the front door doesn't get to stay in the doctor's pocket. So sharing the good times with the bad times helps the team understand some of these issues.

Since team members have a better understanding of how the business side of the practice functions, we can actually seek and value input that they have into making their job and perhaps the overall management of the practice even more efficient and productive. Asking questions and suggesting new ways of implementing procedures is expected. They can also learn that they will have the freedom to try new things and if they fail, at least, hopefully, everyone learned from the experience.

Open Book Management meetings are held on a very regular basis to address the concerns of the four stakeholders of any veterinary practice:

- **The Pets** – Team's job is to make the patient as comfortable as possible and relieve pain whenever needed;
- **The Client** – Superior Client Service is expected and required;
- **The Team** – Working as a team, feeling you have done a good job, and all team members have the ability to progress and grow;
- **The Investors** – Profitability grows a veterinary hospital.

From our staff's perspective, the important issue to them in evaluating many of the ideas that we bring back from NAVC each year, is "What's in it for me?" Jim Harris wrote a book a number of years ago titled *Getting Employees to Fall in Love with Your Company*. He outlined five principles to make this happen. Each of these principles is embodied in the Open Book Management style of management. Let's review these principles.

Our job as practice owners is to capture the hearts of our team members. We need to set the example, become a true leader, and our team will follow us. So first and foremost we need to model the behaviors we want our team members to embody. If we believe that balancing work and family is important, we need to make sure that our team understands that work does fit into that equation, it is not "all about me." Most importantly, we need to have fun at what we do. If our practices are not fun places to work, it is going to be drudgery for all of us, not just our team members.

There needs to be open lines of communication in our practices. We talk about communicating, but communication between team members is just as important as communicating with our clients. With Open Book Management we actually have meaningful data with which to communicate. Instead of saying "you are not doing a good job," we can actually present data that we have taught team members to understand, and can show concrete examples of where we would like to see improvement. Veterinarians hate to confront people. We remove the confrontational aspect and are simply looking at results and asking for accountability.

Instead of relying on titles, we want to create partnerships with our team members. Each and every team member is important. We say this, but with Open Book Management we can show team members how exactly what they do contributes to the carrying out of the practice's mission. We reward team members for the performance they do to contribute to the overall success of the practice. While it is impossible to remove all subjectivity from this issue, how salaries are arrived at becomes much more transparent when using Open Book Management techniques.

Good team members always want to better themselves. They want to learn more. They want to be able to provide better services to their clients. With Open Book Management we are always seeking input from out team. Attending outside seminars and learning sessions is always viewed as an opportunity to share new skills with the other team members.

We are encouraging them to try new ideas and we don't criticize when these ideas don't always play out like they envision. It truly takes learning from our mistakes to a new level. Many times the first time a new idea is tried does not give us the results we are looking for. In Open Book Management the results are analyzed, the team makes recommendations, the idea is tweaked and generally everyone benefits from the process.

Peter Drucker, who is widely believed to be the Father of Contemporary Business Management, has stated that "As we advance deeper into the information and knowledge economy, the basic assumptions taught and practiced in the name of management are hopelessly out of date….Get the assumptions wrong and everything that follows is wrong." As the entire team is brought into the management environment, we spread the wealth of having to know everything about running our practices. Not only do we not have to "know it all," we don't even have to "do it all." When we have our team members understanding what it means to really be an owner, they will start thinking like owners. We will start to see decisions being made that do represent "thinking like owners." As doctors get freed up from all of the burdens of running the financial side of their practices, the practices become more fun places to work. The stress level of being a practice owner should start to decrease which should bode well for being able to bring associate veterinarians along the path to practice ownership. In the September issue of Veterinary Economics, it was stated that one of the main reasons that associates don't want to be a practice owner is because of the stress involved. If the duties of practice ownership are shared with a knowledgeable team, this should relieve the stress and hence make practice ownership a much more viable option to the next wave of potential practice owners.

Table 1. Comparison of Assumptions

Traditional Model	Open Book Management Model
Control	Order
Management	Leadership
Employees	Team
Creativity is at the top	Creativity at all levels
Knowledge is at the top	Knowledge at all levels
Specialization and division of labor	Generalization/owner mentality
Information is guarded	Information is distributed
People must be supervised	Teams become self policing
Ultimate goal is profit	Profit supports the mission

MARKETING YOUR PRACTICE IN YOUR COMMUNITY — "HIGH TECH–HIGH TOUCH" TACTICS THAT WORK

Pamela Cole, CEO, Owner,
Irvine Veterinary Services, Irvine, CA

Kate Knutson, DVM, Owner, Pet Crossing Animal Hospital, Bloomington, MN

MARKETING IS EVERYTHING!

Before beginning a discussion on marketing your practice in your community, it is important to begin with some general statements about marketing in general. Marketing in a veterinary practice setting is essentially delivering and promoting something of value to clients by providing services or products that meet client's needs.

Marketing includes virtually everything—from how your practice looks on the outside to the 'first impressions' made by staff that greet them—to how the lobby looks and smells. The experiences following those first impressions can either enhance a client's point of view or subtract from it.

Clients' "impressions" count heavily in providing veterinary services. Clients judge us by 'intangibles' such as perceived reliability and competence, empathy for them and their pets, and responsiveness to them in the form of personal care and attention.

Two key objectives of a marketing program are:

- Increase number of client visits
  - New clients
  - Increasing existing client visits
- Increase $ spent per visit

Both objectives are designed to increase fee income.

ARE YOU READY TO MARKET YOUR PRACTICE?

Most practice leaders think of marketing as advertising and promotion that focuses on reaching new clients outside the practice and using traditional advertising and promotional vehicles such as newspaper, display ads in telephone directories, or direct mail companies.

In reality one of the first places to begin marketing is 'inside' the practice. Important questions to consider before marketing 'outside' the practice:

- Have you developed a mission statement?
- Do you know "who you are" as a practice group?
- What are you and your team focused on delivering for your clients and patients?
- Why are you different than other practices?
- Does your practice team understand "who they are" and do they reflect this in both appearance and action "consistently"?
- Is your practice operationally prepared to 'welcome new clients'?
- Are you able to manage additional transactions upfront and in treatment?

ENGAGE YOUR STAFF IN THE INTERNAL MARKETING PROCESS

Developing a marketing program from the 'inside out' can be a great team experience:

- Involve the entire staff in developing a practice mission statement. If you already have one, re-visit it and ensure that it is still relevant.
- Solicit staff ideas on "what should be marketed" and what community programs that should be considered.
- Ask staff about what areas of "client compliance" need work.
- Develop practice protocols that mirror AAHA practice standards and assign sections to staff. Protocol development clarifies standards of care as an "internal compass" for all staff and encourages staff to "speak with one voice."

Are You A Client-Oriented Practice?
- Do you know who your clients are?
- How often do your clients visit and what age and kind of pets do they own?
- What are your clients' needs?
- Do you use client surveys to find out what you do well and what needs work?
- Are you able to operationally meet client's needs and exceed their expectations each time they visit?
- Where are your weak points and what could your team do to strengthen client service?

IMPORTANCE OF CONSISTENTLY DELIVERING QUALITY SERVICE

Remember that:

- It costs 5 to 6 times more to acquire a new client than it does to do business with a current client.
- Happy clients will tell 3 to 5 people about a good experience; a dissatisfied client will tell up to 20 people about a problem.
- 45% of pet owners cited a "friend or acquaintance's recommendation" as the reason for choice of veterinarian. Client referrals are the most important source of new clients!

WHAT DO CLIENTS WANT?
- I expect my Vet to be good with my pet!
- I want my Vet to treat me with respect!
- I want a Vet who answers all my questions, someone I can trust with my pet!

INTERNAL/EXTERNAL MARKETING TACTICS
I Expect my Vet to be Good with my Pet!
Internal
- Warm greeting at admittance that includes physical contact with pet and client.
- Relationship building in the exam room/special attention to pet.
- Special attention at release that focuses's on questions following exam and follow-up 'promise' with client.

External

- 'High touch' Web site photos that feature 'pets and people' in the practice
- Local tie-in with animal shelter volunteer work, fundraising, free shelter exams, shelter Web site presence
- Involvement with community activities and organizations that permit practice and vets to show care and concern (eg, Delta Society, senior centers, hospital visits with therapy dogs, rescue groups, and city animal care services)
- Pet loss donations to local pet welfare groups following euthanasia
- Puppy on-site preschool classes/obedience classes
- Annual "open house" for pets fundraiser using AAHA's open house kit and press materials
- Post your practice's "good deeds" on your Web site!

I Want my Vet to Treat me With Respect!

Internal

- Create a varied and unending supply of client handouts and use them!
- Use a file audit system that prepares staff prior to visits. Re-visit previous recommendations and follow up.
- Develop and audit telephone protocols at reception desk and throughout the hospital to assure that client conversations and requests are being met consistently.
- Develop and audit an appointment management system that consistently assures timely admittance and release. Post arrival times on files and measure "time spent" by clients in the practice service delivery system.
- Audit client call backs and follow ups. Audit files in then "re-file" section on a regular basis.
- Audit the quality and success of e-mail or postcard reminder systems.

External

- Honor clients' "need to know" by using "Pet Portals" Health Care Access Program.
- Be available more days and hours and let clients know.
- Change and update Web site content often and feature "news and views." Keep clients informed and position your practice as the "source for pet care information."

- Market your knowledge by using seasonal direct mail or e-mail that focuses on AAHA recommendations, such as:
  - AAHA Dental Care Guidelines
  - AAHA Senior Care Guidelines
  - AAHA Pain Management Guidelines

I Want a Vet Who Answers All my Questions, Someone I Can Trust with my Pet!

Internal

- Teach staff to offer options when your practice cannot meet a need. Show you care about the client's need even though you cannot meet it. Develop referrals that clients can trust.
- Create an imperative in your staff to research client questions. Be the source of pet care information for your practice and your community.
- Track client compliance in key areas of fee income and share with your staff regularly. Establish an imperative for quality care through compliance results.

External

- Contact local community newspapers, radio stations, community website editors to offer your services in answering questions about pet care.
- Volunteer for "career days" at schools.
- Invite community groups in for tours.

DEVELOP A MARKETING CALENDAR AND BUDGET

- What a marketing plan "is":
  - A plan of action that is "ongoing"
  - An ongoing activity that requires lots of work by the entire practice team
  - A journey and not a destination
- What it "isn't":
  - A silver bullet
  - A quick fix
  - A "one time" activity
- Budget
  - Plan to spend from 1% to 2% of fee income annually.
- Calendar:
  - Plan major programs or campaigns during slower times of the year.
  - Allow plenty of time—from 30 to 60 days prior to complete details and make contacts.

PRACTICE PARTNERING

Henry M. (Trey) Cutler III, JD
The Cutler Law Firm
Fort Collins, CO

The material provided in this article is intended for informational and educational purposes only and is not legal advice. Readers should consult with a licensed attorney for legal advice and to address specific concerns.

OVERVIEW

Welcoming a new partner into the ownership of a veterinary practice is one of the most significant developments that can occur in the life-cycle of a typical veterinary practice. Because the introduction of a new partner usually involves one or more veterinarian owners and one or more associate veterinarians who are buying in, all of the parties tend to be preoccupied with their existing full-time commitments to the practice. As a result, planning considerations can take a backseat, sometimes with disastrous results.

This article is designed to introduce some of the key issues that commonly arise in the context of veterinary practice partnering relationships, for the benefit of anyone considering such a relationship. This article particularly focuses on the terms of the "buy-sell" agreement among the original owner(s), the new partner(s) and the practice entity, as opposed to the terms of the original buy-in arrangement.

Prospective partners should be aware that there is no single partnering structure that is ideal for every situation. Factors such as the form of practice entity, and the relative ages, roles, financial strength, and health of the prospective partners can lead to significantly different partnering relationship structures. The discussion of the issues below is therefore intended as an overview only.

While the titles and formatting of the documents can vary, partnering relationships typically involve agreement by the parties to certain terms and conditions that are commonly referred to as a "buy-sell agreement." The main purpose of this agreement is to establish at the outset of the partnering relationship how the parties will deal with various contingencies or changes in circumstances that could arise in the future, such as the death, disability, divorce, loss of license, or termination of employment of one of the partners. These events are typically referred to as "triggering events." Buy-sell agreements also may address other terms, such as non-compete covenants and certain governance matters.

Practices can be owned through a variety of entities. For simplicity's sake, this article will generally refer to each co-owner of the practice as a "partner" or "shareholder" and will refer to the practice as being owned by a corporation. Thus, each partner or shareholder will hold shares in the entity that owns the practice.

REDEMPTION VERSUS CROSS-PURCHASE

One threshold issue for any buy-sell agreement is whether the prospective purchase of a partner's shares following a triggering event is to be made by the practice entity (a redemption) or by the other partner(s) (a cross-purchase). While redemption arrangements are simpler to draft and to administer, cross-purchase arrangements have the significant advantage of providing the buying partner(s) a step-up in basis for the shares purchased from the selling partner.

Hypothetical: Dr. Lisa Longview and Dr. Samuel Shortimer are co-owners of Quality Pet Care, P.C., a professional corporation (the "PC"), which has made an S election with the IRS and which owns and operates a veterinary practice known as Main Street Animal Hospital. Dr. Longview and Dr. Shortimer each hold 1,000 shares of the PC and currently each has a $1,000 tax basis in those shares. The practice is now worth $1,000,000.

Table 1 demonstrates the potential impact of the step-up in basis in a cross-purchase arrangement, assuming that Dr. Shortimer retires from the practice and his shares are purchased for $500,000, and assuming that Dr. Longview later sells all of her shares to one or more new buyers for a total of $1,000,000 (ie, the practice did not increase further in value).

The example below demonstrates the effect of a cross-purchase versus a redemption following the retirement of a partner, but the effect of the step-up in basis for the benefit of Dr. Longview, the remaining partner, would be the same, regardless the nature of the trigger event that gave rise to the purchase of Dr. Shortimer's shares.

Table 1. The Potential Impact of the Step-up in Basis in a Cross-Purchase Arrangement

Buy-Back Structure	No. of Shares Held by Dr. Longview After Buy-Back	Tax Basis in Shares Held by Dr. Longview After Buy-Back	Capital Gains for Dr. Longview upon Subsequent Sale of Her Shares for $1,000,000
Redemption	1,000	$1,000	$999,000
Cross-Purchase	2,000	$501,000	$499,000

If the capital gains of Dr. Longview are taxed at 15%, then she would pay an additional $75,000 [($999,000–$499,000) X .15 = $75,000] in capital gains taxes under the redemption structure, as compared to the cross-purchase structure.

TRANSFER RESTRICTIONS

As suggested above, the main purpose of a buy-sell agreement is to avoid later disagreement and possible litigation over the disposition of the partners' interests in the practice entity. So, partners must be careful to draft transfer restrictions that will be enforceable, or else they run the risk of undermining the time and effort that they put into creating the buy-sell agreement in the first place.

In the past, state courts have tended to not enforce a prohibition on transfer that required the consent of the other shareholder(s), although that result may seem misguided in situations where veterinarian partners rely extensively on each other's practice style and quality. While some recent court decisions reflect a more accepting view of this type of restriction if it is exercised reasonably and in good faith, the safer course is to draft transfer restrictions that provide some reasonable means for a partner to ultimately dispose of his or her shares (even if those shares are subject to options to purchase and/or rights of first refusal), in lieu of a flat prohibition on transfer.

TRIGGERING EVENTS: MANDATORY VERSUS OPTIONAL REDEMPTION

Typical triggering events for veterinary buy-sell agreements include death, disability, divorce, bankruptcy, loss of license, and termination of employment of a partner. Disagreements on certain major decisions, often referred to as impasse events, also may give rise to a trigger event, especially in 50/50 partnerships.

In the event of the death of a partner, buy-sell agreements typically provide for the automatic purchase of the deceased partner's shares, either by the corporation, or by the surviving partner(s). Life insurance policies are often obtained to provide the funding source for this mandatory purchase. Unfortunately, life insurance premiums are not deductible, whether they are paid by the shareholders, or the corporation. So partners will often obtain insurance on each other so that the surviving shareholder(s) can get the benefit of the step up in tax basis through a cross-purchase, as described above. In practices that have three or more partners, the partners have to either obtain multiple life insurance policies or provide for a trust that will receive the life insurance proceeds and use those proceeds to purchase the deceased partner's shares, if they wish to structure the purchase as a cross-redemption.

The disability, bankruptcy, loss of license, or termination of employment of a partner may give rise to either automatic or optional share purchase. As a general rule, the remaining partners typically do not want to remain partners indefinitely with someone who can't or won't continue working in the practice, or worse, with a bankruptcy trustee. Nonetheless, a mandatory purchase in these circumstances can sometimes create a significant financial hardship for the remaining partner(s), at a time when the practice may already be stressed by the departure of one of the partners. As a result, it is often beneficial to structure the buy-sell agreement so that it gives the surviving partner(s) or

corporation, or both, the option to purchase the shares of the other partner upon any of those triggering events, instead of obligating the remaining partner(s) to make the purchase at that time.

With disability and even termination of employment, the partners will need to carefully define what circumstances will actually constitute a trigger event. How long must someone be unable to work to be deemed "disabled," for example? Is a doctor's determination of disability required? If so, how is the doctor selected? If a partner near the end of his career is working only one shift per month, will the other partner(s) still be comfortable "pulling the load"? As is often the case with contracts, the devil can be in the details.

In two-veterinarian partnerships, especially those where the shares are split equally, or close to equally, the partners may ultimately desire to part ways due to significant disagreement over one or more key issues relating to the practice. If one partner wishes to leave much of the profit in the practice to fund capital expenditures and future growth, for example, while the other partner wants to take as much profit out as possible, the partners ultimately will have to either decide which direction the practice is going to take, or they will need to part ways.

If the buy-sell agreement provides a mechanism for handling those "impasse" situations, then the partners can potentially avoid months and years of legal wrangling and countless dollars spent on attorneys' fees. One such mechanism is sometimes referred to as a "shotgun" buy-sell.

Our friends from the hypothetical situation above, Dr. Longview and Dr. Shortimer, can help demonstrate how a shotgun buy-sell provision operates. If Dr. Longview and Dr. Shortimer have been unable to agree on a material issue, and that disagreement gives rise to the right to set a shotgun buy-sell in motion, then either of the partners may do so. Here, we'll assume that Dr. Shortimer initiates the shotgun buy-sell by providing the required notice to Dr. Longview, which indicates the price per share that Dr. Shortimer believes the Quality Pet Care, P.C. stock is worth. Dr. Longview will then have the right to elect to either buy Dr. Shortimer's shares or sell her own shares at the price per share determined by Dr. Shortimer. Since Dr. Shortimer will not know whether he is going to be buying or selling at the time that he determines the offered price, he should be highly motivated to establish a fair price.

If both partners have ready access to capital, then shotgun buy-sell provisions tend to produce a fair result. While it can be difficult to find acceptable third party financing for a buy-in, there are many sources of funds in the current lending market for a remaining partner who will own the entire practice upon the consummation of a buy-out. The buy-out can also be accomplished through a seller note, as discussed further below.

VALUATION

One of the benefits of the shotgun buy-sell mechanism is that it results in a share valuation. For other trigger events, the buy-sell agreement must establish either a price or a method for determining a price for the shares to be sold.

One method for determining the share price is by annual agreement of the partners. At least theoretically, this approach has the benefit of working somewhat like the shotgun buy-sell, in that the partners do not know whether they would be receiving the share price or paying it at the time of determination. The share price determination also would be made periodically, so that it does not get too "stale." Unfortunately, these arrangements do not tend to work well in actual practice, because the partners are busy with other matters and often fail to make the annual price determination, as originally contemplated. Unfortunately, the failure to make the price determination is the same as having no agreement on price at all, so this approach does not tend to be favored.

A second possible approach for determining the price of the practice shares is to establish a formula. Again, this approach has the benefit of establishing a method for determining the price when none of the partners know whether they will be buying or selling at the time that the formula is later applied. However, veterinarians should be wary of formulas that are based on "book value" or otherwise are not designed specifically for veterinary practices of their type. And even if a formula is designed for a particular type of veterinary practice, a formula that would result in a very fair price at the outset of a partnering relationship may yield a very unfair price many years later, due to changing conditions in the veterinary practice market.

A third approach is to provide that the share price will be determined by appraisal. If the appraisal approach is used, then the buy-sell agreement should clearly outline how the appraiser(s) will be selected and how their costs will be paid. Ideally, it should also indicate whether the appraiser shall consider factors such as minority discounts. If an appraisal has been used to determine the value of the practice's stock at the time of the buy-in, it can be helpful to provide that any subsequent appraisal shall be determined using the same methodology. Even if a buy-sell agreement provides for the shares to be valued by appraisal, the agreement should expressly provide that the appraisal (and its related expense) should only be necessary if the parties are unable to agree upon a value of the shares within a reasonable period of time.

In some cases, such as where a junior partner is buying in to the practice at a particularly attractive price, the senior partner may wish to provide for a discounted purchase price if the associate were to voluntarily leave the practice before a certain period of time. In this type of situation, the buy-in is being offered as a strong incentive for the junior partner to remain with the practice and to enhance its continued growth over an extended period of time. By either using some form of vesting or discounting the purchase price of the junior partner's shares (or both), senior partners can structure arrangements that best suit their particular practice transition goals.

FUNDING OF STOCK PURCHASES

As noted above, life insurance is commonly used as a funding source for stock purchases in the case of the death of a partner. Disability insurance is also available, although it tends to be expensive and thus not an ideal funding source. For all situations for which insurance does not provide a practical funding source, the buy-sell agreement can either require payment in cash or provide for the possibility of payment over a period of time. If the departing partner must be paid out in cash, then the remaining partner(s) or corporation, as applicable, may be challenged to find reasonable financing for the buy-back in a short period of time. As a result, many buy-sell agreements provide for the payment of the stock through a promissory note with a reasonable rate of interest. If the corporation is buying back the shares, the buy-sell agreement will often require the remaining shareholders to guarantee the promissory note for the shares.

The terms of buy-back promissory notes vary significantly. Sometimes they mirror the terms of the promissory note that was in effect when an associate bought into a practice. In other cases, the buy-sell agreement may provide for a promissory note with a shorter term, because the parties want to ensure that the payment does not stretch out over many years.

OTHER TERMS

Buy-sell agreements may also address other key matters between the partners. They often include mutual confidentiality and non-competition covenants, for example. In fact, in some states, a non-compete covenant that would not be enforceable with an employee would be enforceable when it runs between partners, and this may provide an existing owner with a strong incentive to offer the buy-in opportunity in the first place. Buy-sell agreements also can include governance provisions, to make it clear that unanimous or supermajority approval is required for certain key decisions, such as the admission of a new partner or the incurrence of significant capital expenditures or indebtedness.

Finally, partners who enter into buy-sell agreements for their practice entities should be sure to consider how they intend to handle any shared ownership interests in an entity that owns the affiliated real estate, if applicable. Is the real estate intended to be treated as a free-standing investment? Or should the partners be able to continue to participate in the ownership of the real estate only if they continue to own part of the practice? Again, results can vary depending upon the circumstances, but the parties would be wise to consider these issues at the outset of their partnering relationship.

CONCLUSION

The problems that can arise under buy-sell agreements tend to fall into one of two categories: the agreements either fail to plan for how key issues will be handled, or they handle key issues in a manner that later proves impractical. By taking the time to carefully focus on the types of issues discussed above, prospective partners in a veterinary practice can spare themselves significant stress and expense by developing a well-crafted buy-sell agreement that fits their particular circumstances.

Recognizing that relationships evolve, partners should keep in mind that buy-sell agreements can and should evolve as well, especially as new partners join as co-owners of the practice, for example. Partners should also recognize their own power to vary from the terms of a buy-sell agreement by mutual agreement if they wish. In other words, if they can agree to a different approach to a situation that later arises, they are always free to follow that different approach. If they cannot agree, however, then the buy-sell agreement should provide all parties with the peace of mind that there will be certainty as to how the matter will be addressed.

CHOOSING THE RIGHT FORM OF ENTITY (AND WHY IT MATTERS)

Henry M. (Trey) Cutler III, JD
The Cutler Law Firm
Fort Collins, CO

The material provided in this article is intended for informational and educational purposes only and is not legal advice. Readers should consult with a licensed attorney for legal advice and to address specific concerns.

OVERVIEW

Veterinary practices in the United States operate as sole proprietorships, partnerships, limited partnerships, limited liability companies, corporations, professional associations, and other forms of entities. Given the wide variety of entities available, it can sometimes seem a daunting task to pick the form of entity that is best suited for a particular veterinary practice.

This article explores some of the common options for the form of entity for a veterinary practice. It assumes that all of the operating assets, other than real estate, are held by the practice entity, and it highlights some of the implications of choosing one form of entity over another.

Except with respect to elections made with the Internal Revenue Service (for S corporations or limited liability companies, for example), the types of entity that can own and operate a veterinary practice are dictated by state law, and can vary significantly from state to state. As a result, any veterinarian who plans to establish an entity to own veterinary practice assets should consult with an attorney who is experienced in choice of entity matters in the state where the practice is located.

DO I NEED AN ENTITY AT ALL?

In the past, many veterinary practices have been operated as sole proprietorships and some continue to operate in that manner today. Generally, a sole proprietorship is a business that is directly owned and operated by an individual, not an entity. Since there is no separate entity with a sole proprietorship, there are no formation documents, ongoing entity records, or separate tax returns to prepare or maintain. Unfortunately, there also is no shield from liability for the owner's personal assets (including assets completely unrelated to the business) from the reach of the practice's creditors.

Given that today's society is unfortunately far more litigious than in years past, many veterinary practice owners elect to hold their practice assets in a separate entity, even though there may only be a single owner of that entity. For practices with multiple owners the decision is usually easier, as the owners need some means of collectively owning the practice assets, in addition to wanting protection of their personal assets from the liabilities of the practice.

So, practice owners who elect to operate as sole proprietorships (and multiple owners who elect to operate in the form of a general partnership) are taking the risk that they may lose more than the practice assets if the practice becomes insolvent or a significant liability event were to occur. Fortunately, significant liability events are rare, but they can occur when a person is seriously injured at the practice or in the case of intentional torts, such as harassment or discrimination claims, for example.

C CORPORATION, S CORPORATION, DOES IT REALLY MAKE A DIFFERENCE?

In a word, yes! Many practices are formed either as corporations or professional corporations through filings with the applicable Secretary of State's office, which results in the creation of a C corporation, from the IRS's perspective. Practice owners sometimes neglect to make an S election filing with the IRS, or decide not to do so, so that their practice entity remains a C corporation going forward. C corporations are taxed as separate entities and their dividends or distributions are taxed a second time when paid out to the corporation's shareholders. Generally speaking, S corporations do not pay taxes on the profits of the practice, because the practice's profits and losses are "passed through" to the shareholders and the shareholders will pay income taxes based on those profits and losses.

Practice owners are sometimes advised that they can "zero out" their profits in a C corporation by paying themselves bonuses at the end of the year, or through other means, and this is a common practice among veterinary practice C corporations. Those same advisors often neglect to explain the tax impact of being in a C corporation upon the sale of the practice when the owner or owners are ready to move on, however.

The potential tax impact of a sale of practice assets by a C corporation as compared with an S corporation is shown in Table 1. In both cases, the practice is being sold as an asset sale, because most buyers are unwilling to buy a practice through a stock sale due to the negative tax and liability consequences of a stock sale for a buyer. The table assumes that the selling corporation has $50,000 of remaining tax basis in the practice's assets, that the practice is selling for $1,000,000, and that the sale will result in long-term capital gains. The table does not address the additional impact of possible state taxes.

Since the shareholders of the C corporation will have to bear the burden of the corporate capital gains tax (at 35%) and the subsequent dividend/distribution tax (at 15%), their net proceeds are dramatically less than the S corporation shareholder's net proceeds, which are only subject to the individual 15% capital gains tax in the example above.

Given the magnitude of this potential "tax hit" upon the sale of the practice, practice owners who own practice assets through a C corporation may benefit from the conversion of their C corporations to S corporations. While the "built in gains" rules will limit the benefit of such a conversion for a period of 10 years, there still can

Table 1. The Potential Tax Impact of a Sale of Practice Assets by a C Corporation as Compared with an S Corporation

	C Corporation	Tax Rate	S Corporation	Tax Rate
Sales Price (Practice Assets)	$1,000,000		$1,000,000	
Tax Basis in Practice Assets	$50,000		$50,000	
Capital Gains*	$950,000		$950,000	
Less Corporate Capital Gains Tax*	−$332,500	35%	N/A	
Net Proceeds from Corporation	$617,500		$950,000	
Tax Paid by Shareholders*	−$92,625	15%	−$142,500	15%
Net Proceeds to Shareholders	$524,875		$807,500	

* The sale of the assets by the corporation will trigger capital gains taxes, and possibly income taxes as well, depending on factors including the allocation of the purchase price and possible depreciation recapture. In the example above, the entire $950,000 above the $50,000 tax basis in the corporation's assets has been assumed to be capital gains for illustration purposes.

be a significant benefit to converting, especially if the practice continues to increase in value and/or the owner(s) do not intend to sell the practice for at least 10 years. Although a full discussion of the built-in gains rules and other relevant factors is beyond the scope of this article, owners of C corporations are encouraged to consult with their attorneys and accountants to make sure that they understand the immediate effects of converting to an S corporation, as well as the effect of the built-in gains rules going forward.

IS AN LLC OR PLLC RIGHT FOR ME?

An limited liability company (LLC) or professional limited liability company (PLLC) could be a beneficial form of entity, depending on the specific circumstances. Usually, practice owners do not need the tremendous flexibility provided by LLCs in the structuring of the respective owners' interests in the profits, losses and tax benefits of the entity. As a result, S corporations are often favored over LLCs and PLLCs, especially since S corporations can also provide an opportunity for some payroll tax savings in certain situations.

WHAT OTHER FACTORS SHOULD I BE CONCERNED ABOUT?

In some states, veterinary practices must be owned in the form of a professional entity, such as a professional association, professional corporation or professional limited liability company, so practice owners and their advisors must be careful to review the applicable statutes and rules (and determine whether the relevant state authorities have adopted any formal or informal interpretations of those statutes and rules). Practice owners and advisors should also be aware that the form of entity can have a direct impact on how much the practice may have to pay in state franchise taxes, so they should confirm those tax effects as well.

CONCLUSION

Because the choice of entity considerations vary so much from state to state, it is critical to get the guidance of an experienced advisor in the state where the practice is located before making a choice of entity decision. As noted above with respect to C corporations, the original decision regarding the form of a practice's entity can have lasting consequences, so it is worth the time and effort at the outset to determine the best form of entity for you.

LETTERS OF INTENT FOR PRACTICE PURCHASES

Henry M. (Trey) Cutler III, JD
The Cutler Law Firm
Fort Collins, CO

The material provided in this article is intended for informational and educational purposes only and is not legal advice. Readers should consult with a licensed attorney for legal advice and to address specific concerns.

OVERVIEW

Although letters of intent are common tools in veterinary practice acquisitions, they vary to a surprising degree. This article explores the basic terms of letters of intent for the benefit of both prospective buyers and sellers.

WHY HAVE A LETTER OF INTENT?

Practices that are listed with brokers always have a listing price, so if a buyer is willing to pay that price, or the buyer and seller are able to agree on a different price, some may ask why the parties even need a letter of intent (LOI).

The short answer to that question is that an LOI ensures that the parties have agreed to all of the basic terms of the transaction before they commit significant additional resources (ie, time and expense) to move the transaction through to closing. As an example, if the parties have agreed on price, but not on the terms of the seller financing that will be required in order for the buyer to be able to pay that price, then the parties could unintentionally waste a significant amount of time and money on less important matters when they were actually at an impasse on a key issue.

WHAT TERMS SHOULD BE INCLUDED IN THE LETTER OF INTENT?

So, what are the key terms that should be addressed in a letter of intent? Assuming that there are no particularly unusual circumstances, a comprehensive LOI would address the following terms and conditions in no more than two to three pages:

- Sales price
- Categories of assets included and excluded from the sale
- Clarification regarding the treatment of seller's liabilities, including prorations
- Whether there will be any holdback, and if so, the amount and duration of that holdback
- If there will be seller financing, then the length, interest rate, and other terms of that financing
- Subordination of the seller financing to the primary financing, if applicable
- Lease terms, if the practice seller is retaining the practice real estate

- Key elements of the post-closing restrictive covenants with the seller
- Buyer's conditions to closing, including as applicable:
  - Obtaining financing on satisfactory terms
  - Completion of due diligence
  - Acceptable agreements with key practice members who will be staying at the practice
  - Acceptable lease agreement with a third party landlord
- Anticipated timeframes for negotiation of definitive purchase documents and the closing
- No shop provisions (see below)

And, for transactions that also involve the purchase of the practice's real estate:

- Appraisal of the real estate at an amount at least equal to the purchase price
- Clarification regarding how costs will be borne for title policies, surveys, appraisals, environmental site assessments, and closing costs

BINDING VERSUS NON-BINDING?

The great majority of LOIs are expressly non-binding. While this might seem to run counter to the general purpose of LOIs, it actually makes sense in most situations, since the buyer typically has not completed his or her due diligence on the practice at the time of execution of the LOI, and thus does not know all of the information that would be relevant in agreeing to purchase the practice.

While neither party is obligated to close the transaction on the terms outlined in the LOI, parties would be unwise to outline terms that they do not intend to fulfill. If either party were to do so, it would just be wasting its own time, as the other party will have a predictable negative reaction to a perceived "bait and switch" tactic. As a result, changes to the terms of a non-binding LOI are typically justified by a change in the underlying circumstances or the buyer's awareness of new material information relating to the practice.

NO SHOP PROVISIONS

One term that is usually made binding, if it is included in an LOI, is the no-shop provision. A no-shop provision is an agreement from the seller to work exclusively with the buyer for a limited period of time prior to the execution of the definitive purchase documents. The no-shop provision typically obligates the seller to not pursue any negotiations or discussions with other prospective buyers for a brief period of time, ranging from 30 to 60 days, after the signing of the LOI.

The no-shop provision is obviously beneficial to the buyer, who wants to make sure that his or her offer will be taken seriously and not used merely as a "stalking horse" to encourage another prospective buyer to offer better terms for the practice. For a seller who has identified a buyer prospect that looks promising, the no-shop provision is usually an easy concession to make, as the seller wants to encourage the buyer to move forward diligently in any reasonable way that the seller can.

CONCLUSION

To be most beneficial, a letter of intent will cover the key transaction terms, such as those listed above. If the LOI has been negotiated with input from both parties' respective legal counsel, then it usually saves substantial time and expense in the subsequent negotiation and drafting of the definitive purchase documents. Most of all, an appropriate LOI helps the parties focus on "first things first"—for the benefit of all involved.

STRATEGIES TO ENHANCE COMMUNICATION AND COLLABORATION BETWEEN SPECIALISTS AND GENERAL PRACTITIONERS – PART 1

Amanda L. Donnelly, DVM, MBA
ALD Veterinary Consulting
Rockledge, FL

As veterinary medicine has become more specialized in the last decade, concerns regarding the working relationship between specialists and referring veterinarians have been the focus of discussion for multiple organizations and associations in the profession. Discordant issues and communication challenges between specialists and general practitioners have been identified as both groups have expressed opinions about what constitutes a positive referral relationship.

ISSUES AND CHALLENGES FOR SPECIALISTS AND REFERRING VETERINARIANS

The number of specialists increases every year with approximately 60 individuals gaining certification by the American College of Veterinary Surgeons and 80 gaining certification by the American College of Veterinary Internal Medicine. The number of specialists in other disciplines such as dentistry, behavior, and dermatology is increasing as well. As more general practitioners interact with specialists on a regular basis, some areas of concern regarding the working relationship have become more evident for these two groups.

Economic Issues

General practitioners today are faced with a variety of economic concerns such as the loss of income associated with alternate-year vaccine protocols, a decrease in sterilization procedures due to pediatric spays and neuters being performed at shelters, income lost to over-the-counter medications and internet pharmacies, lack of business skills by veterinarians, downturns in the economy, and increasing veterinary student debt loads. Some veterinarians regard referral of cases to specialists as another area of potential lost revenue. Increasingly, general practitioners think twice before sending patients to specialists and are more likely to perform procedures such as ultrasound at their practice rather than referring these cases. Additional economic concerns of general practitioners include:

- Specialty hospitals that do not send cases back as soon as possible for follow-up at the general practice
- Emergency services affiliated with specialty hospitals that do not check with the referring veterinarian to see if they want a patient transferred back to the general practice but instead just refer the pet internally to a specialist for continued care
- Internal referrals between specialists. For example, an internist that refers a pet to the dermatologist or ophthalmologist for a consult rather than back to the general practitioner first to work-up the case
- Specialty hospitals that accept clients without a referral.
- Specialists that perform procedures or diagnostics that could have been done at the general practice

One of the most significant economic challenges for specialists is maintaining a profitable caseload. This can be a significant issue given the high overhead of specialty hospitals due to their physical plant size, sophisticated equipment, expensive inventory, and large number of employees. In some communities this financial challenge is magnified when specialists are in competition with other specialty practices in the area to retain referring veterinarians as clients and to attract pet owners. With the increase in the number of specialty hospitals, these practices are also now having facing competition when recruiting additional specialists. Other common economic frustrations reported by specialists include:

- **Timeliness of referrals.** Referring veterinarians not sending cases soon enough. Although the primary issue for specialists is one of patient advocacy, this becomes an economic issue if the specialist does not have the opportunity to see a case that should have been referred or if the client has run out of money by the time they are referred.
- **Receiving appropriate compensation for their expertise and consultation time.** This is increasingly becoming an issue for those specialists such as internists who spend a considerable amount of time doing phone consultations. The need to consider charging for their consultation time comes into play when specialists receive requests for phone consults from general practitioners that only want to discuss cases but do not refer patients or when specialists are asked to interpret laboratory tests that are performed by the referring practice.
- **Referring veterinarians misjudging clients' willingness to pay for specialty care.** Specialists often report that clients say they would have come much sooner if they had only known about the availability of the specialist. Specialists also report that pet owners often are willing to pay for specialty care even when the referring veterinarian indicated that they would likely not be able to afford care.
- **Limited awareness of pet owners about the availability of specialists.** Despite the increase in specialists and specialty hospitals, there are still a significant number of pet owners that have very limited knowledge regarding the scope of services offered by specialists.

Communication Challenges

General practitioners often cite a lack of effective communication by specialty practices as one of their biggest frustrations. Their concerns include:

- **Timely return of phone calls.** This is particularly disconcerting if referring veterinarians are waiting on a specialist to call them back regarding hospitalized referral patients or to discuss whether a case should be referred.
- **Lack of availability and accessibility of specialists.** This is an issue when general practitioners feel that specialists are not interested in routinely discussing cases, have limited hours, are always overworked and too busy to come to the phone, etc.
- **Referral reports that are not sent promptly or are never received.** This leads to breakdowns in communication with pet owners who expect the referring veterinarian to be informed and also requires staff time to track down the missing report.
- **Inadequate follow-up communication regarding referral cases.** This includes a lack of updates on hospitalized referral patients and a lack of follow-up information on patients that are being seen on an on-going basis at the specialty hospital.
- **Specialists that communicate in a condescending or disrespectful manner.** General practitioners have expressed that some specialists seem overly judgmental and critical of them when discussing cases.
- **Reports by clients that the specialist indicated the case was not worked up properly**
- **Poor client service to pet owners.** This includes reports from clients that the staff was unfriendly, the specialist had a poor bedside manner, or the specialist was not timely with updates about their pet.

Likewise, specialists have communication challenges at times with general practices. Specialists have voiced the following concerns:

- **Time to return phone calls.** One of the biggest challenges is finding enough time in a day to return calls to both groups of clients—the pet owners and the referring veterinarians. As specialists become busier they are increasingly finding it difficult to return a large number of phone calls and still provide excellent patient care and client service.
- **General practitioners that request phone consultations but never refer cases.** Due to their extremely busy schedules, specialists often return phone calls to these practitioners after first calling veterinarians who refer patients regularly.
- **Unavailability of practitioners when calls are returned.** Knowing that the referring veterinarian is anticipating a phone call, it is particularly frustrating to be told by a receptionist that "Dr. Smith is in an exam room and cannot come to the phone." In addition, specialists often return phone calls during lunch hours or after 5:00 or 6:00 PM when referring veterinarians are unavailable unless they have left alternate phone numbers with the specialty hospital.

- **Illegible medical records.** In many instances, the specialist cannot read the handwriting of the referring veterinarian on the medical records that are sent.
- **Incomplete medical records.** This occurs when problems occur with fax transmissions or when referring veterinarians fail to send copies of laboratory findings.
- **Inappropriate medical records and lack of a medical summary.** Many specialists are frustrated when general practices send pages and pages of medical records that are not relevant to the condition for which the patient was referred. Instead the specialist would like a written medical summary of the case.
- **Unrealistic or erroneous expectations given to pet owners by the referring practice.**
- **Referring veterinarians that are defensive when feedback is offered regarding cases.**
- **Keeping track of what type of follow-up is desired by all referring veterinarians.** Some practitioners want their cases sent back right away as soon as they are stable and some only want cases back once the condition is resolved.
- **Liability issues.** Given the litigious nature of our society, specialists must be careful when offering medical advice to general practitioners about patients that they have never seen or not seen recently. Specialists are also concerned about giving information that may not be in the pet's best interest- it is difficult to provide accurate information for a pet that the specialist has not examined.

Timeliness of Referrals

Many specialists have expressed concerns regarding the timeliness of referrals by general practitioners. It is disheartening to see patients that should have been referred sooner, especially if an earlier referral would have resulted in a quicker recovery or a positive outcome instead of death. Sometimes general practitioners recommend referrals but the client does not agree until the pet's condition has deteriorated. Specialists understand these circumstances occur and are not critical of referring veterinarians in these instances. They are, however, frustrated when general practitioners treat cases for multiple days in their hospital and then refer the patient on Friday afternoon or when it is too late to help the pet.

Another concern of specialists related to timeliness of referrals occurs when patients are not referred because general practitioners are not aware of the benefits of a referral: for example, a pet that would have an improved prognosis or longevity with chemotherapy.

SUMMARY

To address the above issues concerning communication and collaboration between specialists and referring veterinarians, a number of strategies and tools can be utilized which will promote a positive referral experience and integrate a team approach to patient care. These are discussed in Part 2 of this article.

STRATEGIES TO ENHANCE COMMUNICATION AND COLLABORATION BETWEEN SPECIALISTS AND GENERAL PRACTITIONERS – PART 2

Amanda L. Donnelly, DVM, MBA
ALD Veterinary Consulting
Rockledge, FL

In Part 1 of this article, we examined some of the relevant issues and challenges facing specialists and general practitioners today. To improve the working relationship between these two groups, efforts should be undertaken to enhance communication and collaboration. The following strategies and tools are presented as a means to achieve this goal.

IMPROVING COMMUNICATION BETWEEN GENERAL PRACTITIONERS AND SPECIALISTS

Enhanced communication is the biggest key to improving relationships between specialists and general practitioners. Both groups should strive to establish effective dialogue and maintain open lines of communication.

Verbal Communication

The best communication between two individuals occurs when both parties engage in a dialogue and commit to active listening. Dialogue is characterized by a desire to build mutual understanding and implies that a conversation is occurring. Referring veterinarians can facilitate dialogue with specialists by scheduling face to face meetings with area specialists and by visiting their facilities. It is much easier to talk on the phone with someone that you have met and have established rapport with. These meetings are beneficial in a number of ways. General practitioners can utilize these visits to become familiar with particular areas of interest or expertise for each specialist and to understand the full scope of services offered by the specialty hospital. When referring veterinarians know area specialists, they can offer assurances to clients that their pet will be seen by a specialist that they know personally and have confidence in their expertise. In addition, referring veterinarians should take the opportunity when meeting with specialists to emphasize the importance of receiving timely follow-up on referral cases and to convey what level of involvement they desire for cases that they have referred.

Likewise, specialty hospitals should establish a schedule of routine hospital visitations to referring practices to facilitate improved communication. These meetings afford specialists the opportunity to get to know referring veterinarians better, to educate them about their services, and to address any concerns about client service.

When general practitioners and specialists know each other, a foundation exists to facilitate improved communication. We tend to be less critical of those individuals we have established a relationship with and more likely to give them the benefit of the doubt when misunderstandings or breakdowns in communication occur.

Written Communication by Referring Veterinarians

Specialists often complain that referring veterinarians send medical records that are illegible, incomplete, not relevant to the referred condition, not sent ahead of time, and do not include a summary of the problem. Since it is highly unlikely that general practitioners are purposefully trying to aggravate specialists, specialty hospitals need to communicate with referring practices and let them know what they want in terms of medical records. This can be accomplished by sending a letter to all referring veterinarians advising them of the preferred protocols regarding submission of medical records. The letter would likely look something like this:

"In an effort to provide the best patient care possible for your clients' pets and to enhance our communication and collaboration with you as referring veterinarians, we are asking you to submit medical records using the following protocol:"

- Please fill out our referral forms whenever possible and submit prior to referral. We will provide your hospital with as many blank forms as you need.
- Please provide a written medical summary for the case you are referring. This can be included on our referral form, in the medical record or attached separately. This is particularly important if we cannot read the attending veterinarian's handwriting.
- We would like to receive medical records 24 hours prior to the pet's appointment. Our office will call to remind you to send records. It is also helpful if the client has a copy of the medical records in case there is a problem with fax transmittal.
- Medical records we desire include: only those pages of the pet's chart that are pertinent to the condition for which they are being referred-it is not necessary to send the entire record and copies of all laboratory tests.

Specialty practices can reinforce the desire for pertinent medical records by communicating this information during clinic visitations, continuing education events held by the hospital and when consulting with area veterinarians on the phone.

Referring veterinarians who are aware to the above information should take efforts to comply even if they are not contacted by specialty practices. It is helpful to check with area specialists to determine their preferences regarding submission of medical records or general practices may choose to simply establish a consistent protocol that best meets the needs of all parties.

Written Communication by Specialists

Specialty hospitals must adopt and follow consistent protocols to ensure that timely follow-up reports about referred cases are sent to referring veterinarians by mail or fax. The best way to achieve this is to assign a staff member to oversee written communications with referring practices. In general, referral reports should be sent within 24 hours of the time the patient is discharged from the hospital. Specialty practices should also enhance their communication with referring hospitals by faxing daily progress reports on hospitalized cases or patients receiving ongoing care.

Utilize Staff to Assist with Communication

A team approach involving the entire staff will enhance efforts to improve communication between specialists and referring veterinarians. All too often, healthcare team members at general practices are left out of the loop when a referral occurs. This can lead to frustration and a break down in communication. Client relations personnel need to be informed when patients are referred and should be familiar with the doctors at the specialty hospital so they can better field incoming calls from clients or specialists.

A white board or a notebook is helpful as a means to keep track of all referral cases. The following information should be logged: date of referral, which specialist the case was referred to, all status updates from the specialty hospital, all communications with the client, diagnosis, dates rechecks are due, etc. For general practices that hold rounds, status updates on referral cases should be included in discussions. It is best to designate a staff coordinator for referrals to oversee communication efforts. This may be the nursing supervisor, head technician, or office manager. Referring veterinarians should establish with the specialty practice if they want daily updates on referred cases. If they are unavailable to take phone calls, a technician should be designated to talk to the specialist to receive updates about cases.

Likewise, staff at specialty hospitals can be utilized to take the burden of some phone calls from referring veterinarians. Appropriate staff should be able to answer basic questions regarding fees, scheduling of appointments, which specialist should receive a case and even some technical questions. Specialty hospitals can enhance ongoing communication with area practitioners by designating an employee as a referring veterinarian liaison. This individual is the point person to handle all phone calls from referring veterinarians that cannot be quickly addressed by the front office staff.

ESTABLISH APPROPRIATE CLIENT EXPECTATIONS ABOUT THE REFERRAL PROCESS

Another important component to improving the working relationship between specialists and referring veterinarians is to effectively communicate appropriate expectations to pet owners regarding referrals. This helps to avoid misunderstandings and breakdowns in communication. Referring practices should give clients an idea of what to expect financially but should not quote fees. Referred clients should have some idea of what to expect when they walk into a specialty hospital. They should feel comfortable knowing that the referring veterinarian will communicate with the specialist and send all pertinent medical records. Clients should be advised that the specialist may not be able to quickly

provide an exact diagnosis, may not be able to provide a simple treatment and certain tests may need to be repeated. It is also wise for general practitioners to tell pet owners that they have made a tentative assessment but the specialist may have a different assessment or determine a different diagnosis.

To ensure that appropriate expectations are communicated to pet owners, specialists and referring veterinarians need to discuss the above issues when possible. For example, with respect to costs, a specialist such as a surgeon may be comfortable giving some fee estimates over the phone while other specialists may only want the client to be informed of the cost of the consult.

DEFINE ROLES FOR CASE MANAGEMENT

Since referring veterinarians within a community or even within a practice express variable degrees of desired involvement in follow-up case management, this issue must be discussed on a regular basis. When specialists and general practitioners know one another, it becomes much easier to keep track of the level of involvement that is desired. Specialty hospitals should try to document referring veterinarian's preferences regarding case management whenever possible. Some specialty practices do this with their computer software while others may need to generate a written reference document that contains this information. The type of information that is recorded would include information on whether a referring veterinarian does orthopedic surgeries, whether they tend to manage cases such as ketoacidotic diabetics, whether they have ultrasound capabilities, and so on.

When patients discharged from specialty hospitals require follow-up monitoring or treatment, the roles of the specialist and the general practitioner should be defined regarding who will provide these services. This avoids misunderstandings and confusion for the specialist, the referring veterinarian, and the pet owner.

IMPROVING TIMELINESS OF REFERRALS

One of the best ways to improve timeliness of referrals is for specialists to initiate efforts to increase the knowledge of referring veterinarians and inform them about the availability and scope of services they offer. To do this, specialists should execute targeted marketing objectives that encompass these goals. Tactics to achieve these types of objectives could include:

- Continuing education seminars on topics that afford specialists the opportunity to educate referring veterinarians about specific disease processes as well as highlight their expertise and services available to treat these type of cases
- Rounds at the specialty hospital for small groups of practitioners to discuss case management of diseases
- Lunch n' Learn seminars at area practices
- Newsletters for area veterinarians with articles targeted to raise the level of awareness about

specific case management or services offered by the referral hospital

CONCLUSION

To build positive relationships between specialists and referring veterinarians, efforts should focus on promoting a collaborative, team approach to veterinary care for pets and enhancing communication. When general practitioners and specialists work together effectively, opportunities exist to improve the quality of patient care, to enhance pet owner satisfaction and to improve the profitability for all practices.

TO REFER OR NOT TO REFER: IMPORTANT CONSIDERATIONS

Amanda L. Donnelly, DVM, MBA
ALD Veterinary Consulting
Rockledge, FL

In the last ten years the number of veterinary specialists in private practice has grown tremendously. Most medium-size cities have specialty hospitals and new practices are opening on a regular basis. Many major metropolitan areas now have multiple specialty hospitals. With this increase in availability of specialists, general practitioners now have the opportunity to refer pets locally for advanced diagnostics and treatments that were previously unavailable.

The increased specialization of veterinary medicine is viewed by some in the profession with mixed emotions. While access to the highest quality medical care for pets is desirable, referring veterinarians are grappling with the need to redefine which cases can and should be treated at general practices vs. which should be referred to specialists.

WHY GENERAL PRACTITIONERS MAY BE RELUCTANT TO REFER

Some general practitioners have indicated a reluctance to refer cases to specialists for several reasons. One of the biggest reasons cited is due to problems with communication. Referring veterinarians have expressed the following concerns with respect to communication with specialists:

- Critical or condescending attitudes conveyed by specialists when discussing cases
- Referral reports that are not received in a timely manner
- Phone calls not returned
- Specialists that have poor bedside manners with clients
- Specialists that are not interested in or too busy to discuss cases
- Lack of progress reports or follow-up communication about cases
- Not being informed if patients die or are euthanized at the specialty hospital

These communication issues are particularly troublesome for referring veterinarians if they result in pet owner dissatisfaction regarding the referral experience or they prevent timely referral of cases.

A second reason that some general practitioners may be reluctant to refer case to specialists is due to the perceived loss of income. Referring veterinarians already face a variety of economic concerns related to the loss of income associated with alternate-year vaccines, a decrease in sterilization procedures, over-the-counter medications, internet pharmacies, lack of business skills by veterinarians, downturns in the economy, and increasing student debt. Consequently, some regard referral of cases to specialists as another area of potential lost revenue. Increasingly, general practitioners think twice before sending patients to specialists and are more likely to perform procedures such as ultrasound at their practice rather than referring these cases.

In addition, referring veterinarians may be reluctant to refer cases if they fear they may lose the client. Some clients decide after visiting a specialty hospital that they want the specialist to provide all medical services for the pet whenever possible. In some cities there are specialty hospitals that are willing to see pet owners that have not been referred by a primary care veterinarian. This scenario is typically viewed negatively by general practitioners who increasingly are concerned that pet owners don't understand the referral process and will bypass visits to the family veterinarian.

Surveys have reported the following additional reasons cited by general practitioners for why they do not refer more cases: distance to nearest specialty hospital is too great, clients' inability to afford specialty care, and that the general practice could provide all the necessary services for clients.

DEVELOPING AN EFFECTIVE REFERRAL PROCESS

When deciding whether to refer clients to specialists, referring veterinarians should focus on what is in the best interest of the pet and the owner. Additionally, efforts to improve communication with veterinary specialists will help facilitate appropriate referrals and improve the referral experience for all parties.

Ethics and Standards of Care

Professional ethics should always be adhered to when deciding whether a referral to a specialty hospital is appropriate. Ethically, we as veterinarians must give clients honest assessments regarding their pet's condition and advise them of all their alternatives for medical care. If a pet requires 24-hour care and your hospital is closed at night, clients need to be advised that no one is present overnight to monitor their pet.

Likewise, medical standards of care should dictate whether referrals are appropriate. Unfortunately, standards of care can sometimes be debated. For example, most veterinarians would agree that a completely torn cruciate in a large dog should be surgically repaired. Whether the surgery should be performed by a general practitioner or a board-certified surgeon may be debatable. General practitioners that feel comfortable performing this surgery do not need to refer this case to a surgeon. Other less experienced veterinarians need to be honest with themselves and clients about their level of surgical expertise. It is always appropriate to inform clients about the availability of a boarded surgeon even when the referring veterinarian is confident about their surgical skills.

Deciding Where to Refer Your Patients

For those veterinarians practicing in cities with multiple specialty hospitals and/or veterinary teaching hospitals in close proximity, there may be several options when considering where to send referrals. General practitioners should first consider which specialist in the area has the most experience or qualifications seeing the type of case that is being referred. For example, a puppy with a congenital heart defect should ideally see a cardiologist if one is available. Many specialists have areas of interest or expertise within their specialty. It may be in the patient's best interest to send a pet with severe gastrointestinal disease to the internist who focuses on these types of cases rather than another internist whose primary area of focus is endocrinology.

A second consideration for referring veterinarians in deciding where to send cases is the availability of specific diagnostic equipment such as MRI or medical treatments such as radiation therapy.

Aside from the availability of specific services or the expertise of individual specialists, the most important factor when deciding where to send referrals is the presence of a positive working relationship with specialists. A positive referral experience is more likely to occur when general practitioners and specialists have developed a personal relationship and established effective lines of communication.

Treat All Clients Equally

General practitioners need to be careful not to pre-judge a client's willingness to pay or ability to afford specialty care. Referral to a specialist should be discussed with pet owners whenever appropriate regardless of whether the general practitioner thinks the client might have financial constraints or be reluctant to agree to advanced diagnostics or treatment. Surveys of pet owners have found that they are willing to spend a considerable amount of money on their pets. Specialists often report that pet owners indicate to them that they would have sought specialty care sooner if they had known about their services. The use of third party payment plans has also helped to increase the affordability of specialized care for many clients.

Consult with Specialists

Given the time constraints of busy practitioners and specialists, it is not always necessary or practical for both parties to discuss cases prior to referral. Most specialists feel that a written summary of the case and a copy of current laboratory findings is sufficient information to review prior to seeing cases. However, in some instances a phone conversation between specialists and referring veterinarians prior to referral is invaluable to enhance communication and improve continuity of care. These include:

- **Emergency referrals.** A phone call to the specialty hospital is necessary to confirm the availability of the specialist to receive the case, to determine which service will receive the case, and to inquire about any additional costs involved. These phone calls also helpful clarify expectations that should be communicated to the pet owner. A dialogue about the pet's medical condition helps the specialty hospital prepare for a critical case.
- **When the referring veterinarian is unsure of the diagnosis or prognosis for a pet.** Often a phone consult with the specialist helps facilitate timely and appropriate referrals. The specialist may suggest that further testing or treatment be done at the general practice prior to referral or they may advise the practitioner that there is nothing medically to be gained with a referral. On the other hand, specialists may confirm that a referral is in the best interest of the pet or they may educate referring veterinarians regarding treatment options they were not aware of.

Economic Considerations

When deciding whether to refer pets to specialists, referring veterinarians may need to consider the economics of managing the case at the general practice. Given the level of patient care that is necessary to successfully treat some pets, it may be more appropriate to send a pet to a specialty hospital that has more resources than a general practice.

SUMMARY

To answer the question of "To refer or not to refer," general practitioners should first consider the answer to the following questions:

- Have I adhered to my code of ethics and recommended the best possible medical care available for this patient including the option of a referral when appropriate?
- Have I withheld judgment on my client's willingness or ability to pay for specialty care?
- Am I aware of the specialty treatment options available and the expertise of the specialists in my area?
- Have I consulted with area specialists regarding any questions I have about whether it is medically beneficial to refer this patient?

By focusing on these questions, the answer of whether to refer a patient to a specialist should become clear.

IMPROVE PATIENT CARE AND INCREASE REVENUES BY WORKING WITH SPECIALISTS

Amanda L. Donnelly, DVM, MBA
ALD Veterinary Consulting
Rockledge, FL

Pet owners in many communities today have access to specialized, high-quality medical care that previously was only available at a university veterinary teaching hospital. In part, this is due to the migration of veterinary specialists from the academic setting into private practice. As the profession has become more specialized, some general practitioners have expressed concern about losing income to specialists and may think twice before referring cases that could be treated at their hospital. In some instances, the roles of the primary care veterinarian and the veterinary specialist are not clearly delineated. This can be confusing for pet owners and may negatively impact patient care. Instead of viewing the increase in veterinary specialists as a threat to the current status of general practice, referring veterinarians should see developing effective relationships with specialists as an opportunity to improve patient advocacy and actually increase hospital revenues.

IMPROVING PATIENT CARE

With the increasing specialization of veterinary medicine, it has become even more important to develop a team approach to patient care. By adopting a team approach, patient advocacy is enhanced and continuity of care can be maintained. As primary care-givers, general practitioners play a central, vital role in coordinating patient care for pet owners. When pets may are monitored and treated for specific medical conditions on a regular basis at a specialty hospital, the care provided by specialists should be an extension of the overall care provided by general practices. The family veterinarian should continue to assume responsibility for all preventative and wellness medical care. Referring practitioners play the important role of patient care coordinators for pets and in many instances are responsible for follow-up medical care recommended by specialists. It is not unusual for general practitioners to provide ongoing treatment and monitoring for patients with several medical conditions on multiple medications prescribed by specialists.

Referring veterinarians should maintain complete and thorough medical records for their client's pets. Aside from avoiding problems with liability, maintaining detailed medical records facilitates improved communication with specialists who may later being reviewing the pet's chart. Referring veterinarians should also collate referral reports from specialty hospitals and maintain them in the patient's medical file. Many pets today see multiple specialists during their lifetime or during the course of a disease. General practitioners need to communicate with specialists about the pet's entire medical history and condition. For example, if a patient is referred for orthopedic surgery, the surgeon should be informed if the pet has been seen by an internist for other conditions such as heart or endocrine disease. The referring veterinarian should not assume that the surgeon has access to the internist's records or that the client will relay this pertinent information to the surgeon.

For a team approach to patient care to be successful, general practitioners and specialists need to develop and maintain effective communication and collaboration. Given the demands of busy schedules and time constraints, veterinary staff members should be utilized to assist with communication between hospitals. Many specialty hospitals now have dedicated referring veterinarian liaisons or similarly titled employees whose main job function is to promote and maintain open lines of communication between referring veterinarians and the specialty hospital. For their part, general practices should designate "patient care coordinators" or "specialty practice liaisons" to assist with communication efforts with referral hospitals as well as with clients whose pets have been referred to a specialist.

NCREASING REVENUES

Most referring veterinarians enjoy having access to specialists within their community to answer questions, perform advanced diagnostics, and to accept referrals for difficult cases or those needing 24-hour care. Another less commonly discussed benefit of working with specialists is the increase in practice revenues that results when referring veterinarians develop an effective relationship with specialists.

Enhanced Client Satisfaction

One of the most obvious yet often overlooked aspects of enhanced financial success that results from specialty referrals is related to increased client satisfaction and retention. Today's pet owners are very bonded to their pets and trust general practitioners to provide excellent medical care including recommending referral to specialists when appropriate. Even if clients have cost constraints or decline a referral for other reasons, they appreciate that their family veterinarian cared enough about their pet to recommend the highest quality medical care. To maximize client's satisfaction it is imperative that general practitioners give them appropriate expectations regarding the referral process. Clients should be given some idea of what to expect financially and informed that specialists may need to repeat tests, cannot guarantee a definitive diagnosis, and may make a different assessment of the case. In addition, general practices should maintain some level of continued communication with clients who have been referred to a specialty hospital. This communication provides an opportunity to answer their questions and demonstrate compassion for them and their pet. These efforts help keep clients bonded to the general practice even when they may be visiting a specialty hospital on a regular basis.

Improved Profitability

When deciding to treat and manage sick patients at their hospital, referring veterinarians should consider the level of care that is needed and whether it is practical or profitable to keep the case. Patients needing constant monitoring and advanced patient care may require attention that cannot reasonably be provided by the technical team at a general practice. Dedicating one or more technicians to a patient requiring constant attention may not be a productive use of resources and general practices are often reluctant to charge appropriately for this level of care. Profitability can also be negatively affected if complications arise with a medical or surgical case. This may result from reluctance by general practitioners to charge for additional care, the cost associated with the loss of a client who finds out that specialized options were available or even liability issues. Referring veterinarians that focus on profit centers in their practice such as dentistry, senior care, pain management, diagnostic testing, feline medicine, and client service programs are more likely to improve revenues and attain greater profitability than those managing complicated cases best handled by a specialist.

Increased Patient Care and Longevity

As discussed above, patient care is often improved with referral to specialists. This enhanced patient care translates to increased life spans for many pets. When pets live longer, referring veterinarians are rewarded emotionally and financially by having the opportunity to provide continued care for the pet. To enhance the human–animal bond and promote longevity for pets, general practitioners should consult with specialists regularly to ensure that clients are afforded the highest level of medical care and have the opportunity to consider all treatment options.

Increased Knowledge and Revenue Associated with Case Follow-up

Referring veterinarians can generate additional service revenue in several ways by developing an effective relationship with area specialists. Specialists routinely comment that referring veterinarians miss opportunities to perform procedures and diagnostics prior to the referral that would have been helpful to expedite the case assessment. Those general practitioners that establish positive working relationships with specialists are more likely to gain this valuable feedback. In addition, service revenues increase as a result of recommendations by specialists for rechecks and follow-up diagnostics to be done at the general practice. Referring veterinarians that maintain effective, regular communication with specialists also enhance their medical knowledge and learn about diagnostics or procedures that they may be able to do at their practice in lieu of referring a case.

It is important to clearly establish the roles of the specialist and the general practitioner regarding case follow-up to promote continuity of care, avoid client confusion and to ensure fair compensation for both veterinarians. For example, in the case of an autoimmune hemolytic anemia patient, the general practice may perform follow-up CBCs on the pet once it is discharged from the specialty practice. This situation allows the client to return to their primary care veterinarian and affords the general practice the opportunity to gain revenue for follow-up diagnostic testing. However, if the referring veterinarian does not feel comfortable interpreting the laboratory results and needs to consult with the internist for treatment recommendations, then it is reasonable for the specialist to be compensated for their time and expertise. A number of specialty practices have instituted protocols to address this type of scenario. Most clients are happy to be able to take their pet back to their regular veterinarian and pay the specialist a reasonable laboratory interpretation fee when necessary.

To facilitate effective relationships and communication with specialists, referring veterinarians should take the following steps:

- Get to know area specialists personally. It is much easier to communicate with someone you know and have established a relationship with.
- Visit all specialty hospitals in your area to gain a better understanding of what services they offer and to meet with specialists.
- Participate in any rounds, journal clubs or continuing education seminars provided by specialists. These events are educational and provide an opportunity for relationship building.
- Give specialists feedback about their marketing efforts such as newsletters. If these materials provide new and useful information, this is important for specialty hospitals to know so they continue this investment.
- Become a welcomed face at your local specialty hospital. Referring veterinarians that regularly refer cases and develop friendly rapport with specialists and their staff gain a number of perks such as free review of radiographs and valuable in-the-halls advice on case management

SUMMARY

Changes in the veterinary profession in the last decade are viewed both negatively and positively depending on your perspective. Changes related to the increased specialization of veterinary medicine should be embraced as an opportunity to create a win–win scenario for general practitioners, specialists, and pet owners. The benefits of effective communication and collaboration between specialists and referring veterinarians include improved patient care and outcomes, improved financial success that results from a team approach to veterinary care and strengthening of the human–animal bond for pet owners.

TRAIN YOUR TECHNICAL STAFF TO A HIGHER LEVEL OF COMPETENCY

Amanda L. Donnelly, DVM, MBA
ALD Veterinary Consulting
Rockledge, FL

Veterinary practices often struggle with the goal of recruiting and retaining a top-notch, highly trained technical staff. In part, this is due to a veterinary technician shortage. Another contributing factor is the relatively high employee turnover rate within the veterinary industry due to poor wages or inadequate job satisfaction. An even more prevalent reason that practices do not always have a highly competent healthcare team is that management has not devoted the necessary resources to developing and instituting effective training programs for the hospital. The following steps will assist in efforts to improve training for your technical staff.

DEFINE IMPORTANT AREAS OF COMPETENCY

To develop effective training programs, managers should first define the desired areas of competency for the technical staff. The primary focus for evaluating the proficiency of veterinary assistants and technicians is usually directed at assessing their technical skills such as their ability to set intravenous catheters and perform laboratory tests. Although technical skills are critically important, they are only one area that should be defined as an area of desired competency for the technical staff. Technicians should be proficient in all of the following areas.

Technical Skills

When evaluating an employee's technical skills, managers should consider the individual's roles and responsibilities as well as their level of education. For example, registered or certified technicians are typically held to a higher standard than those technicians who do not have a degree. Of course, some technicians that are not certified but have been trained in-house also have outstanding technical skills. The technical proficiency of veterinary assistants and technicians may be related to their years of experience, the quality of care provided by the practice and whether management has empowered the staff to utilize their skills. To help facilitate assessments of technical proficiency, managers should develop a written list of technical skills required for each job position in the practice. The required technical skills are different for veterinary assistants, level 1 technicians, level 2 technicians, ICU technicians, and credentialed veterinary technician specialists.

Client Communication Skills

Veterinary technicians should be utilized extensively to assist with client education. This includes discussing preventative heath care with clients, presenting treatment plans, giving discharge instructions, nutrition counseling, and discussing the value of medical services. To communicate effectively with clients, the technical staff must be confident, skilled at interacting with emotional clients and committed to providing exceptional client service.

Time Management

The technical staff should have the ability to multi-task and prioritize job responsibilities. Technicians are often faced with juggling the demands of a busy workday that includes multiple anesthetic procedures, performing laboratory tests, overseeing patient care, and interacting with numerous clients. It is imperative that they are organized to facilitate smooth operations and enhanced productivity for the practice.

Teamwork

Another important area of competency for the technical staff is the ability to function as a team. A highly skilled technician is less valuable to the practice if they only want to work independently or have a poor attitude. Managers should assess each employee's willingness and desire to work collaboratively with the rest of the healthcare team.

ASSESS STAFF PROFICIENCY AND TRAINING NEEDS

Next, management should assess the proficiency of the technical staff in the above four categories. To successfully implement training that results in increased competency, managers should thoroughly assess individual strengths and weaknesses of healthcare team members. It is important to note levels of specific competency particularly when evaluating technical skills. For example, a technician may be proficient placing intravenous catheters in most dogs but not have developed the expertise of placing them in cats or puppies. When assessing the skills and knowledge of the technical staff, managers should consult with the veterinarians and supervisors in the practice for their feedback. In addition, employees being evaluated should be asked to fill out a self-evaluation.

Another means to evaluate the skill level of the team is to look for problems with staff accountability and lapses in client service. Oftentimes, the underlying cause of lack of accountability or inconsistent service is a lack of training.

ESTABLISH AND UTILIZE HOSPITAL TOOLS TO IMPROVE TRAINING

To implement a successful training program for the hospital, the management team should adopt an organized approach and think of staff training as an operating system within the practice. This operating system needs to be supported by hospital tools. To facilitate effective training and bring your staff to a higher level of competency, make sure your practice is utilizing the following tools:

Job Descriptions

Detailed, written job descriptions should be part of your hospital employee manual. Job descriptions help to define roles and responsibilities for each job position in the hospital. They are also useful as a tool to assist with new hire training. Job descriptions should have sufficient detail to clarify all the job duties for team members and they should be updated regularly.

Job Expectations

Staff should also be given job expectations, which outline how an individual is supposed to do their job and how they are to act while at work. Job expectations might include being clocked-in and ready to work promptly at the start of a shift, working with a positive attitude, a no gossip rule, and always treating clients with kindness. Specific job expectations for a technician might include items such as strict adherence to aseptic techniques when placing intravenous catheters and lubricating endotracheal tubes before they are passed for anesthesia.

Written Training Manual

The hospital training manual is used primarily as a reference for certain hospital policies regarding medical services and to assist with new hire training. A hospital training manual should include:

- Hospital policy information such as drop-off policies, how to handle wildlife and strays, vaccine protocols, prescription refill procedures, etc
- Medical terminology and abbreviations used in medical records
- Client service standards
- Check-off lists for skills training for each job position
- Protocols for running quality control tests for laboratory equipment
- Radiation safety information and standards
- OSHA information and policies
- Inventory protocols
- Information on hospital preventative health care programs–ie, senior care programs

UTILIZE MULTIPLE RESOURCES FOR TRAINING

To provide basic training, opportunities for career advancement and on-going continuing education, practices should take advantage of a variety of training resources for the technical staff.

In-House Training

When implementing in-house training, it is important to first outline who will provide training on specific topics. One of the most overlooked aspects of staff training is to make sure that the person providing the training understands the expectations of management, is willing to provide the training, and has the skill set to provide the training. It is very frustrating for new hires to receive training from someone who has a negative attitude or cannot adequately assist them by answering their questions or demonstrating superior skills.

In addition to the written tools mentioned above, in-house training for the technical staff can be provided by senior technicians and veterinarians. Most hands-on skills such as animal restraint, placement of catheters, and performing laboratory tests are taught in this

manner. To ensure proficiency in these technical areas, supervisors should provide oversight until the employee being trained has mastered the skill consistently.

In-house training is enhanced by assigning mentors to new employees and by offering timely feedback about job performance. A coaching management style is especially helpful when providing training to improve communication skills, time management and teamwork.

Staff Meetings

Staff meetings serve as an excellent means to provide training to multiple team members at once. Time during staff meetings should regularly be devoted to training, which can be facilitated, by associate veterinarians or senior technicians. Industry representatives are another resource available to provide staff training on a variety of topics and new products.

Online Courses or Rounds

Multiple organizations and associations now offer many online courses for technical staff on a variety of topics. If employees participate in online courses, they should be compensated for their time and be expected to share with the rest of the staff the highlights of their training. Staff should also be encouraged to access online discussion boards for networking and to exchange ideas.

Maintain a Resource Library

Books on technical topics, practice management, OSHA, client service, grief and nutrition are all excellent additions to your library. DVDs and CDs are another means of providing in-house staff training. Multiple team members can listen to an audio CD or watch a training DVD as part of their new hire training or to gain on-going education. To ensure learning retention, supervisors need to be responsible for quizzing employees regarding the content of these training tools. The exhibit hall at major veterinary conventions is a good place to look for a variety of training resources for your library.

Seminars and Conventions

The leadership team should encourage and expect the technical staff to participate in ongoing continuing education by attending seminars at local or state veterinary medical association meetings and national veterinary conferences. The veterinarians and managers of the practice should review the seminar information ahead of time with employees to make sure they attend sessions that will be the most valuable. Employees should report highlights of their key learning's at the next staff meeting after the conference.

CONCLUSION

To train the technical staff to a higher level of competency, practices need to devote sufficient resources to this operating system. These resources include time and money. Owners must allocate a portion of the budget for staff training. Managers must take the time to develop an organized training plan that includes written hospital tools and incorporates multiple training resources. And finally, management must provide ongoing mentoring and make continuing education training part of all employees' developmental plans. This commitment to training will result in a more efficient veterinary healthcare team that will enjoy greater job satisfaction. This in turn will lead to enhanced patient care, improved client service and greater productivity for the hospital.

TALKING TO CLIENTS ABOUT TREATMENT PLANS AND FEES

Amanda L. Donnelly, DVM, MBA
ALD Veterinary Consulting
Rockledge, FL

Discussing fees can be one of the most uncomfortable and frustrating interactions the veterinary healthcare team has with pet owners. Often veterinarians or staff are afraid that clients will not agree to treatment or that they will become angry about the associated cost. One of the biggest reasons veterinary practices approach talking to clients about treatment plans and fees with so much trepidation is that employees have not been adequately trained to present plans in an effective manner.

EFFECTIVE PRESENTATION OF TREATMENT PLANS

Veterinary hospitals should have an organized, standardized approach to presenting treatment plans to pet owners. Take the following steps to establish an effective protocol for discussing treatment plans with clients.

1. After examining patients, the veterinarian should make appropriate recommendations for medical care to the client and discuss the details of treatment such as the benefits of medical services, anticipated course of therapy, and prognosis. The veterinarian should then tell the client that a veterinary healthcare team member will be in shortly to review the itemized treatment plan with them. If the client asks about fees, the veterinarian should explain that the technician can also review the associated costs of services.
2. Veterinarians should advise clients whenever there is a need for long-term care or the possibility of referral to a specialist. Clients also need to understand the scope of care and time period that is included in the treatment plan.
3. For most medical treatments or surgeries, it is best if the treatment plan is presented to clients by a trained veterinary assistant or technician. The technical staff is typically more capable of answering questions about medical treatment than front office personnel.
4. Discussion of treatment plans and fees should take place in an exam room or consultation room. This gives clients privacy and will help make them more comfortable asking questions.
5. If the client has questions that the technician cannot answer or has financial constraints and cannot authorize all treatment recommendations, then the technician must inform the attending veterinarian who may need to talk to the client again.
6. The pet should be admitted to the hospital from the exam room and the client should be told when to expect an update about their pet.
7. Staff should be prepared to take deposits from clients while they are still in the exam room especially if there is congestion in the waiting room or if the client is emotional.
8. The exception to the above protocol is when presenting pet owners treatment plans and associated fees for routine preventative healthcare. These types of plans are often reviewed at the front desk by the client relations staff so that clients are aware of the expense involved with routine services.

INCREASING COMPLIANCE WITH TREATMENT PLAN RECOMMENDATIONS

Owner compliance with treatment recommendations has been evaluated by the veterinary industry in recent years and there appears to be a consensus that pet owners do not always understand the value of our services. To better communicate the value of veterinary services, the healthcare team must first understand the client's perspective regarding how they evaluate their need for veterinary medical services.

Understanding Client's Product Knowledge and Involvement

When deciding whether to purchase a veterinary product or agree to a veterinary service recommendation, clients base their decision on what is referred to as "product knowledge" and "product involvement." Product knowledge is the amount of information a client has acquired about a particular product or service. The extent of product knowledge influences the client's evaluation of a veterinary service and their willingness to purchase the service. A client that is familiar with heartworm preventative because they have used it for years is likely to quickly agree to purchase this product. On the other hand, a client making a decision about hospitalizing their critically ill pet for intravenous fluids may never have faced this situation. They may be reluctant to agree to care and need time to understand their options or alternatives. Product involvement refers to the perceived importance or value of a service for a client. Factors that can influence a pet owner's product or service involvement include their attachment to their pet, their product knowledge, the age of the pet, marketing influences, social interactions and whether the recommendation is for a wellness or an emergency service.

By appreciating that variable degrees of product knowledge and involvement exist for clients, the veterinary healthcare team is more likely to focus on effectively communicating the value of veterinary services. When veterinarians and staff adequately convey the value of services, they heighten a client's product knowledge and involvement which helps to increase treatment compliance.

Communicating the Value of Veterinary Services

The next step to communicating value to clients is to make sure that all staff members understand and agree with the value of the hospital's services. A veterinary technician that does not believe in premium nutrition is not likely to convey the value of feeding a pet a senior diet. Likewise, a newly hired technician that is unfamiliar with laser surgery may not be comfortable discussing the benefits of this procedure with clients. Staff meetings are an excellent time to discuss the value of veterinary services. Both the client relations staff and the technical staff should be trained to convey the value of routine preventative healthcare services to pet owners. In addition, the technical staff should be able to provide clients with details about medical services and the associated benefits in language that clients can easily understand. If gaps in training are identified or employees demonstrate discomfort associated with certain client interactions, discussion during staff meetings should focus on these areas.

Once employees understand the value of veterinary services, they are much more likely to communicate this value to clients. However, it is important to emphasize the need to give clients consistent messages regarding the benefits of veterinary services. Staff members should be trained to always highlight the benefits of services to clients even when the client has purchased similar services in the past.

Overcoming Resistance

Inevitably pet owners demonstrate resistance when presented with treatment plan recommendations. When this occurs, the veterinary team should be trained to identify possible underlying causes for an owner's reluctance to agree to services and how to overcome objections. Aside from concerns regarding fees, clients may experience several emotions that influence their willingness to agree to our services. These include the following:

- Fear that their pet will experience pain or discomfort associated with procedures or hospitalization
- Fear that testing will reveal serious or terminal disease. This fear can be especially heightened if the pet may have a condition or disease that is similar to another family member such as diabetes or cancer
- Sadness associated with being away from a hospitalized pet
- Fear that the pet may die while hospitalized
- Anger at the pet or another family member. For example, the client may be angry at their teenage son who left open the gate resulting in the pet leaving the yard and being hit by a car.
- Skepticism about the value of services since their neighbor had a similar situation and the pet died
- Fear of what family, friends, or co-workers will think about their willingness to pay for certain services
- Concerns about who will be available to give the pet follow-up care at home

The best means to identify the cause of an owner's reluctance to agree to services is by asking open-ended questions such as "What concerns do you have about the treatment plan I have presented for Tigger?" Staff members should endeavor to engage clients in a dialogue about their concerns and encourage them time to voice specific objections. Clients may need some time alone to consider their treatment options or they may need to call other family members. Never rush clients when they are making important medical decisions regarding their pet's care unless it is a life-threatening emergency.

Once team members identify the cause of an owner's reluctance to comply with treatment recommendations, the best approach is to demonstrate genuine empathy towards the client regarding their objections and to focus on patient advocacy and the human–animal bond. Pet owners should be treated with compassion and gently reminded that the medical services recommended are in the best interest of their pet. The benefits and value of medical services often need to be reiterated to clients. It is also useful to ask clients "How can I help you make this decision?" This question may uncover further questions the client has or may lead the client to treatment acceptance. Clients often state at this point comments such as "I know I need to have this done for Tigger, I just needed to talk about it."

DISCUSSING FEES WITH CLIENTS

Unfortunately, staff and veterinarians alike tend to let their concern for the client's ability to pay interfere with their discussions regarding medical services. Sometimes veterinarians are conservative in their recommendations, eliminate services from the treatment plan, or even discount services if they are concerned about an owner's financial constraints. The entire veterinary healthcare team should not feel the need to apologize for the cost of services but instead should remain committed to providing the best care possible to pets and focus on communicating the value of this care to pet owners.

Understanding Client Emotions

Although pet owners today are typically very bonded to their pets, it is not unreasonable to expect them to react negatively to the high cost of medical care. This is especially true when clients are confronted with expenses associated with unexpected medical illnesses or traumas. The veterinary team should be prepared to handle clients' reactions to fees by following these steps:

1. Let clients vent their emotions. The most frequent emotion is one of anger. The staff needs to understand that clients are not necessarily angry at them but just upset about the situation.
2. Validate the client's emotion. Use compassionate phrases such as "I understand that this is a difficult time for you and you have every right to be upset about being faced with these unexpected expenses."
3. Reinforce the value of the services. The staff should attempt to keep the client focused on the benefits of medical care, not just on associated fees.
4. Offer assistance as deemed appropriate. This may involve giving the client time to make a decision, answering questions, or offering payment options.

Determine Ability to Pay Versus Willingness to Pay

Since many pet owners express concern about the cost of veterinary services, it is important to differentiate an individual's ability to pay versus willingness to pay. Often clients are open about their financial constraints and in these instances, discussion of treatment plans and fees is dictated by the client's financial limitations. To increase the affordability of care for clients, practices can offer third party payment plans. Often these plans allow clients that cannot afford to pay for services upfront to spread the cost of treatment over multiple months.

For a majority of clients that have the ability to pay for veterinary services, their willingness to pay is the key to treatment acceptance. A client's willingness to pay for treatment recommendations is determined by their recognition of the need for the services offered. The higher the perceived need, the more likely the client is to agree to treatment recommendations.

SUMMARY

When the healthcare team is sufficiently trained to present treatment plans and associated fees to pet owners, hospital compliance rates and client satisfaction will increase. Efforts to train staff should focus on understanding the client's perspective regarding medical services, effectively presenting the value of services to clients and being prepared to respond to clients' emotions and resistance to recommendations.

MANAGING BY CORE VALUES

Amanda L. Donnelly, DVM, MBA
ALD Veterinary Consulting
Rockledge, FL

Most veterinary businesses, regardless of size, are started by individuals who have a vision of how they would like the business to operate and some idea of their desired long-term goals. Unfortunately, business owners do not always fully develop and define their vision for employees. This lack of planning and communication on the part of the business owner often results in problems with the successful execution of daily operations and achievement of short- and long-term goals.

Veterinary practice owners should consider whether they have clearly defined and articulated the vision and mission of the business to all employees. In addition, the leadership team should take the additional step of developing core values for the practice which serve as an important foundation for effective management.

DEFINITIONS

Developing a vision, mission statement, core values, and business strategy are all part of the strategic planning process for any business. The terms *vision* and *mission* are often used interchangeably. These statements refer to the purpose and goals of the business. When a company has both a written vision and mission statement, the vision usually refers to a long-term goal. Mission statements can be one sentence or several paragraphs. The mission or vision statement defines the focus of a business and highlights the most important operational goals.

Core values are words or statements that define how a business will conduct business. Core values usually encompass values with respect to how all employees of the business will interact with each other and customers. Companies may refer to their core values as "our beliefs," "our promise," "our commitments," or "standards." Examples of core values for a veterinary practice might include:

- Treating all pets with compassion and respect
- Making all clients feel welcome and special
- Honesty
- Communicating value to clients
- Treating co-workers with respect
- Providing high quality patient care

WHY CORE VALUES ARE SO IMPORTANT

Core values serve as a foundation for effective management for two primary reasons. First, they serve to define how the veterinary practice will conduct business and clarify the expected behavior for all employees in the workplace. For example, when employees understand that "providing high quality pet care" and a "commitment to client education" are core values of a practice, they know that their actions need to support and enhance these efforts. Core values help to focus the veterinary healthcare team on achieving hospital goals in a manner that is consistent with the vision of the practice owner.

Second, core values serve as a foundation for talking to staff about accountability. When lack of accountability is a problem, managers can point out that the team member's behavior does not adhere to the core value for the hospital. For example, if tardiness is a problem, managers should discuss that "respect" is a core value of the practice. When an employee is tardy, they are showing a lack of respect for their co-workers. If "providing exceptional client service" is a core value for the practice then this should be emphasized when discussing lack of accountability with respect to meeting client service standards. Employees are much more receptive to dialogue that is focused on core values. A discussion about inconsistent job performance no longer sounds like nagging but instead focuses on how adherence to core values is necessary to fulfill the mission of the practice.

HOW TO MANAGE BY CORE VALUES

To effectively manage a veterinary practice by core values takes time and patience. This is particularly true if the leadership team is transitioning to this type of management for the first time. Follow these steps to manage by core values:

Develop written core values. If your practice does not have written core values, these need to be developed. To be effective, limit the number of core values to the range of 4 to 10. If you have a long list of values, they start to be come less meaningful. Core values can be established with or without input from key staff members. Ideally, they should be developed in a planning session that includes the leadership team, all ...managers, and key employees. This session can be facilitated by the owner, the practice manager, or a practice management consultant. One of the advantages of staff participation is that employees are more likely to buy-in to future discussions about core values if they were part of the development process.

Disseminate and discuss core values with staff. Once you have established written core values, they must be distributed to the entire staff. To avoid having your core values just be words on paper, they need to be discussed with the healthcare team. Owners and managers need to engage the staff in dialogue about what the core values really mean and what specific types of behavior are consistent with the values.

Use core values as a foundation for human resource management. Core values should be incorporated into communication between managers and employees. If managers do not consistently reference core values when discussing staff behavior and job performance, they remain words on paper.

Discuss core values during new hire training. A discussion of the hospital's core values should be part of the training program for all newly hire employees. This serves to reinforce the practice culture and keeps new team members focused on how to act to help achieve the practice's mission.

IS EMPLOYEE BURNOUT AFFECTING YOUR SUCCESS?

Amanda L. Donnelly, DVM, MBA
ALD Veterinary Consulting
Rockledge, FL

Burnout has long been identified as a problem in high-stress professions such as veterinary medicine. For those working in veterinary practices, burnout may be related to an individual's inability to adequately deal with stress associated with a busy schedule, lower wages, demanding clients, life and death decisions, and high morbidity or mortality rates.

Although, consciously or unconsciously, practice owners realize that burnout can be a problem for employees, many owners and managers do not give enough consideration to whether employees with burnout are negatively affecting the success of the practice.

CLINICAL SYMPTOMS OF BURNOUT

Burnout is typically defined as a gradual progression of mental, emotional, and physical exhaustion related to a person's work environment. Employees with burnout tend to feel that their work efforts do not correlate with rewards, recognition, and job satisfaction. Symptoms of burnout may include feelings of hopelessness, powerlessness, resentment, and cynicism. Left untreated, burnout can lead to depression and feelings of unhappiness that negatively affect an individual's personal life and health.

Burnout also can include symptoms associated with stress such as irritability, depression, lack of concentration, fatigue, headaches, gastrointestinal disorders and high blood pressure.

Compassion fatigue is a particular type of burnout often identified in individuals in the medical profession. It occurs when people care significantly for others without taking care of themselves. Compassion fatigue can be the result for veterinary employees who become so invested in helping pets and owners that they eventually reach a point where they have nothing left to give. Veterinarians and staff that work in emergency hospitals or specialty hospitals are at increased risk due to the high morbidity and mortality rate and the high-stress environment associated with these types of practices. Symptoms of compassion fatigue are similar to those associated with burnout. People suffering from compassion fatigue may also experience decreased feelings of joy and personal accomplishment, low self-esteem, diminished ability to balance empathy and objectivity, and obsessive worry about not being able to do enough for clients and pets.

HOW BURNOUT AFFECTS YOUR PRACTICE SUCCESS

Although employees with burnout may have a history of superior job performance, they can negatively affect your practice in a number of ways. First, individuals with burnout develop a pessimistic outlook regarding their work environment. They often adopt poor attitudes which can result in conflict with co-workers and management. Employees with negative attitudes lower morale on the team and enhance stress in the work place. Not all employees with poor attitudes are experiencing burnout but it should be considered as a possible cause especially when an employee slowly acquires a negative attitude over a period of employment.

Second, employees with burnout are not good providers of exceptional client service. They may have good intentions but simply do not have the energy or enthusiasm required to meet and exceed client expectations. Management teams that notice lapses in client service should identify whether the underlying cause is related to a lack of training, poor attitudes, poor job fit, or perhaps burnout.

One of the worst ways burnout can affect your practice is decreased productivity. Employees experiencing burnout are less productive in large part due to a variety of negative emotions and fatigue. Employees with burnout also may experience more illness, be chronically tardy or have excessive absenteeism all of which can lower productivity for the practice.

MINIMIZING STRESS AND BURNOUT

Although stress doesn't directly lead to burnout, it may be a contributing factor. Those employees that become stressed and do not possess healthy coping skills are predisposed to burnout. Efforts to decrease stress for veterinary employees should be undertaken to make the workplace more enjoyable and to minimize the likelihood of burnout. Even if employees do not demonstrate all the clinical signs listed above, if they say "I feel burned out," this should be a strong clue that management needs to take action to offer assistance to this individual.

RECRUITING THE RIGHT PEOPLE EVERY TIME

Tracy Dowdy, CVPM
Management Resource Group
Grapevine, TX

Finding and keeping good employees has arguably been the most difficult task facing the veterinary profession for some years. Without these employees, veterinarians will not be able to offer the high levels of medical and surgical care that they wish to, nor will they be able to provide the kind of client service that keeps clients returning to a practice and allows the business to prosper financially.

Why specifically is employee retention important?

- Direct, tangible costs of attrition are high
- Intangible productivity loss costs are high
- Loosening of client loyalty when bonded with departing employees
- Disruption to operations
- Client loss due to poor service
- Emotional toll

The important points to remember are:

- Good employee morale = client satisfaction
- Good employee morale = competitiveness in the market
- Good employee morale = higher individual earnings

According to consultants at People Solutions, Inc. employees rarely leave for more money or better opportunities. Instead, they leave because they do not like feeling stupid and it is easier to leave than stay.

Why do employees feel stupid on the job?
- Some really are
  o Poor hiring
  o Little to no training
  o Poor management

Why is it easier to leave than stay?

- Low unemployment
- Attitude of employers
  What does it take to retain employees?
- Leadership
- Treat people as individuals
- Effective hiring
- Competitive salaries and benefits
- Outstanding training programs
- Good management
- Flexibility (tasks, work schedules, etc.)
- Personal fulfillment

The most critical step in retaining good employees is to know what they want. The days are gone when all that mattered to employees was having a job (any kind of a job) and getting a regular paycheck. The employee-employer relationship is now an equal one and employers must offer more than money to keep the kind of staff they need to effectively run the practice.

Unfortunately, employers frequently do not know what employees want. Kenneth Blanchard (author of *The One-Minute Manager*) surveyed 10,000 employees about what made them satisfied with their jobs. He also surveyed managers and supervisors as to what they thought made employees satisfied with their jobs. Interestingly enough, the answers were very different.

Employees listed the top five components of job satisfaction as being:

- Appreciation of work done
- Feeling of being "in on things"
- Help with personal problems
- Job security
- High salary or wages

Employers thought the things that made employees satisfied were as follows:

- High salary or wages
- Job security
- Promotion in the company
- Good working conditions
- Interesting work

The truly remarkable finding from this study is that the top three items on the employees' list were the last three items on the employers' list. Therefore, employers need to remember:

- What you want is not what everyone wants
- Don't assume you or your managers know what employees want
- Employees have a wide variety of motivators
- The best way to find out what employees want is to ask them

HIRING AND INTERVIEWING

The first step in retaining employees is effective hiring. Interviewing and hiring employees is not an easy task. Mike Best, President and CEO of MJDesign, recently said about their holiday hiring program, "If the person came in and filled out the application, we basically hired them unless they were followed by a policeman." While veterinarians often feel this same level of desperation when looking for employees, it is not the way to get the ones who will truly be an asset to your practice.

Why do interviews fail?

- You don't know the job
- You don't know the culture
- You don't get enough information about the applicant
- You don't probe
- You focus only on skills
- You don't remember information after the interview

The key components of a job include the organization chart, job description (ie, duties) candidate requirements, and organizational culture. Components of effective job descriptions include:

- Position title
- Reporting responsibility
- Basic purpose or mission of the job
- Principal job duties and responsibilities
- Minimum education, experience, and skill and personal characteristic requirements
- ADA requirements

Take the time to do the job descriptions correctly and put them in writing. Involve the people who do the job now; managers often find that what employees are actually doing is different from what they thought they were doing! Do not just focus on specific skills; also look at the personality attributes that are important to the position. And once you've taken the time to write the job descriptions, use them. Make sure employees understand these are only guidelines of general duties (ie, they may be asked to do something not on the list) and be sure and update the descriptions as the jobs change.

It is also important to understand your practice culture and whether or not a potential employee will fit in well. Your practice culture is the personality of your business and includes multiple components. Some are superficial (such as the dress code); others run deeper and include the goals, philosophies, and core values of the business. Practice cultures can be flexible versus rigid, stable versus innovative, or filled with outgoing people versus more reserved individuals.

Obtaining information about the candidate is the next step and this usually comes from the job application, resume, interview and references.

Everyone should fill out a job application (even if they submit a resume) because it contains information not usually seen in resumes and supports the practice's efforts at non-discrimination.

The application should be completed in pen and should include a section that the candidate signs attesting to the truth of the information.

What should a manager look for in the resume and job application?

- Typos, grammar, spelling, handwriting
- Gaps in employment
- Frequent moves
- Lack of career progression
- Job objectives
- Skills match to job requirements
- Lack of accomplishments
- Grades
- Avocations
- Professional affiliations

The next information-gathering step is the interview. Current interviewing theory states that past behavior is the best predictor of future behavior. Therefore, your goal is to identify situations in the candidates past that are similar to circumstances they will encounter in your clinic and see how they reacted to them. You then want to determine if those reactions are what you need in the position you are hiring for. Interview components include:

- Introduction
- Questions
- Company information
- Candidate questions
- Selling
- Next step

Listening skills are critical to the interviewing process and include the following:

- 80/20 rule
- Utilize silence
- Judge content, not delivery
- Restate responses
- Resist distractions
- Retain an open mind

Ask the same questions of all candidates and tailor them to the job. For example, you won't ask a potential 16-year old kennel worker "What is your philosophy of management?" but this would be an acceptable question for a potential practice manager.

Because the employee market is so tight, plan on giving a "sales pitch" to the potential employee. Tell them what is unique about your practice and why they should want to work there. Be positive, but also be honest and realistic. Key interviewing techniques include:

- Plan the interview process
- Take the time to do it properly
- Be friendly and interested
- Have multiple people interview the candidate
- Train everyone on how to interview effectively
- Ensure privacy
- Eliminate interruptions
- Take notes

Evaluating candidates after the interviews is the next step. Compare the skills and knowledge of the candidates to the requirements of the job, but don't place excessive emphasis on technical skills. These can be taught—attitude cannot. Assess the candidate's personal qualities to see if they match what you need and remember that employees usually fail due to personal characteristics, not skills, abilities, or knowledge. When evaluating candidates:

- Look at your notes
- Use same requirements to judge everyone
- Remember that the ideal candidate doesn't exist
- Determine if they fit the corporate culture
- Consider punctuality, pleasing manner and voice, appropriate dress
- Consider patterns of behavior

- Consider likes and dislikes
- Gather feedback from others in your clinic
- Be specific in your reasoning
- Avoid reactionary hiring!

Always check references—not only can they give you valuable information about a potential employee, but the very act of having checked may help you avoid potential legal complications should a problem develop.

EMPLOYEE ORIENTATION...DO YOU DO IT?

Tracy Dowdy, CVPM
Management Resource Group
Grapevine, TX

In most veterinary practices, new employees are thrown into their position with virtually no formal orientation or training. Employee's perceptions of their job and role in the practice are determined by first impressions. Keeping in mind that you never get a second chance to make a first impression, your practice should make absolutely sure that new hires feel welcomed, valued, and prepared for what lies ahead during their new employee orientation. If the manager of the practice is not prepared for the employee on the first day of employment, most times it communicates to the employee their position is not important and "it's just a job and not a career." However if done correctly, your new employee orientation can solidify the new employee's relationship with your practice.

New employee orientation is the process you use for welcoming a new employee into your practice. New employee orientation needs to be spearheaded with a meeting with the practice manager. The practice manager needs to have an employee handbook prepared that should contain the following information:

- A welcome letter
- The job description
- A phase training guide with timelines and a checklist
- Employee policies
- Standards handbook
- A copy of the employee's first performance appraisal

During the initial meeting with the new employee, the practice manager should give the new employee information about safety, the work environment, the practice culture, company history, the organization chart and anything else relevant to working in the practice. It also often includes an introduction to all the team members in each department and training on-the-job.

Let's look at each item listed above in more detail. The welcome letter should be customized to the new employee and signed by the practice owner and/or the practice manager. Below is an example of a welcome letter:

Dear Julie,

We are pleased you have joined our team at Advanced Animal Care Centre. With genuine concern for our clients and their pets, we are committed to provide them with the highest veterinary care possible. We strive to use the latest technology and techniques available for our clients and patients. As a veterinary health care team, the staff of the Advanced Animal Care Centre works together to promote public education, to prevent disease and to alleviate the suffering of animals.

The principles of cooperation and openness, combined with the personal characteristics of honesty, integrity, and willingness to help each other, are the foundation of our practice.

Our employees are second only to the quality of veterinary medicine that we practice. We believe that our staff members are the clinic's most valued assets. We will do everything within our power to help you become an integral part of our team as quickly as we can.

We always welcome any suggestions or ideas that you feel would benefit the practice. We encourage employees to share their concerns, seek information, provide input, and consult with the veterinarians at any time to discuss and work toward the resolution of any problems or issues that may arise.

Job descriptions should be included in the orientation. Employers need to maintain a balance between too much and too little information in job descriptions yet should include as many job duties and expectations as possible. Employers should be particularly careful to include any physical requirements for the job such as lifting, standing, walking, working frequent overtime, working weekends, rotating shifts, and exposure to particular conditions such as weather and chemicals. The performance standards for a position will reflect the content of job description. Start with the essential duties and have standards for those. The job description should also include unexpected job duties and should state that the employee may be asked to perform other duties as required. Overall, job descriptions should reflect the reality of the employee's job as closely as possible. Needs may also change on a daily basis, so job descriptions should specifically provide for this flexibility in a properly drafted description.

A phase training guide is necessary for the new employee. It gives the employee a road map to how they are going to learn all of the duties, roles and responsibilities in their position. In addition, assign a mentor to the new employee who can be responsible for making sure the training is accomplished. The mentor should be someone who has longevity in their position in the practice as well as a desire to teach others. It would be advantageous to compensate the mentor for taking on the additional responsibility of training the new employee.

Provide the new employee with the practice's employee manual and standards handbook. Employee benefits play an increasingly important role in the lives of employees and their families and have a significant financial and administrative impact on the practice. It would be highly recommended to have an attorney review and/or draft your employee policies to protect the practice from liability. Implement and draft a standards handbook that defines the practices standards based on the core values and vision of the practice. Utilize the standards handbook as a training tool as well as a way to hold the employee accountable for how to service and communicate with clients and conduct themselves in the practice with other team members.

Give the new employee a copy of their first performance appraisal form. Explain to the employee their will be receiving a performance review in 30 days and they need to fill out the form and evaluate themselves. Now the employee has a clear understanding of the expectations of their performance by reviewing the form's contents.

Lastly, follow up with the new employee. Ask the right questions.

- How is it going?
- How can I help you fine tune this job over time?
- What do you find most challenging about your job? What is not challenging enough about it?
- What have you learned about our practice that surprises you (either good, or not so good)?
- How can I help you get more of what you want from this practice? We want you to be happy here!

ARE YOU LOSING THEM AS FAST AS YOU ARE HIRING THEM?

Tracy Dowdy, CVPM
Management Resource Group
Grapevine, TX

You recruit. You hire. You train. Within a year, they leave. Many employees in veterinary practices consider their work a job versus a career. A 2005 survey by Career Systems International reports that almost half—48.4%—of the 7,600-plus respondents claim that "exciting work and challenge" top the list of reasons for staying at a job. Second on the list, at 42.6%, is "career growth, learning, and development." And "working with great people" is number three at 41.8%.

You can prevent new employee "disconnects" and hold on to good people by taking a few preventive steps. According to Abraham Maslow in his book, *Maslow on Management,* humans have particular needs. The foundational need humans have is physiological: food, water, and shelter. Then we have the need to feel safe, socialize with other humans, and build our self-esteem. Once all of those needs are met, we have the need for self-actualization, which means we want to be part of something bigger than ourselves. We have the need to serve society and community. When your practice has a vision towards serving clients and patients and the healthcare team plays an integral part in that vision, they will be more loyal to the practice.

It is very important for the healthcare team to buy into a clear defined vision beyond their normal job description. People are more motivated to devote energy to organizations with a service goal. Spiritual sustenance can be obtained from a job because employees will be proud to do a job that is congruent with their personal principles and values. Do you have a vision and core values that your employees share? Below is an example of core values and a vision for a veterinary practice.

Core Values:
- Equality
- CompassionLoyalty
- Respect
- Commitment
- Fun
- Honesty
- Teamwork
- Personal Responsibility

Vision:
1. Our practice shares knowledge with the entire healthcare team to fully meet the needs of our clients and patients.
2. We set and maintain high service standards and holds individuals accountable to those standards.
3. We foster an environment of loyalty, respect and equality. We recognize and celebrate the diversity among our clients and our staff.
4. We are committed to providing excellent care to our patients, our clients and each other 24 hours a day
5. We are committed to open and honest communication.
6. Every team member is committed to a clear, shared vision of our future.
7. We are compassionate to all clients and their pets.
8. We strive to be a national leader in veterinary healthcare.
9. We value training to promote education and growth

People want to do work that they love, that allows them to play to their strengths, and that they feel makes a difference. Are they doing it? Staff empowerment is the key to developing a loyal team. Training and empowerment allows team members to feel happy and confident about their contribution to the practice. Utilizing the healthcare team in practice is a win-win scenario. Their roles and responsibilities contribute to production and profits of the practice and in return, they are able to earn more money due to their increased contributions.

Developing a positive culture in your practice is critical to keeping good employees. What is the climate in the practice?

Negative:
- Controlling
- Oppressive
- Secretive
- Suspicious
- Disrespectful
- Divisive
- Political

Positive:
- Empowering
- Supportive
- Open
- Trusting
- Respectful
- Unifying
- Professional

What is a positive work environment? It is not a fun-filled place with a lot of warm fuzzy stuff or for relaxation. It is a positive supportive climate which is conducive to creative work; it is cooperative and civil workplace that is relatively free from bad mouthing, backstabbing or petty bickering. Every Chick-Fil-A store has a plaque engraved with this principle: "Associate yourselves only with those people you can be proud of—whether they work for you or you work for them." Can you say that about your team?

The leadership needs to set the tone. The leaders of the practice have to communicate and anchor the vision with the entire healthcare team. Leadership must have a well-defined, easily understood vision for the entire practice. There needs to be total agreement on the vision across all levels, functions, and divisions in the practice. All leaders must be committed to the transformation effort and are committed to seeing it through.

According to RHI Management Resources, these are the top two mistakes companies make in managing their employees: 61% say there is not enough communication and 19% say they do not feel appreciated for the work they perform. Conduct weekly meetings with the entire healthcare team. It creates a forum to keep the vision at the forefront of everyone's mind, it opens the lines of communication with leadership and the healthcare team, it gives the opportunity to show appreciation, and it holds everyone accountable to the standards and policies set in the practice.

CREATING RAVING FANS WITH YOUR CLIENTS

Tracy Dowdy, CVPM
Management Resource Group
Grapevine, TX

Adopting a successful strategy from corporate America, savvy veterinary practices are catching on that a commitment to exceptional client service is arguably the most significant, sustainable distinguishing factor in today's crowded and fickle marketplace. Increasingly, veterinarians and their teams are being trained in the essentials of client service, client satisfaction is assessed in qualitative and quantitative ways, and a service environment in the professional ranks is becoming standard operating procedure. But the truly exceptional practices are taking this to the next necessary level—they are developing a service culture throughout the entire organization, involving the support staff, too.

Practices who engage in satisfaction assessments with their clients hear it regularly—clients will praise the receptionist who went out of his or her way to get an answer to a question and praise a technician who always recognizes the client's pet. Likewise, these assessments uncover the dissatisfaction of clients who have had less than pleasant experiences—complaints about the lack of "going the extra mile," comments on sloppy correspondence, irritation with employees who go by the book without considering the client's special needs or circumstances. Individually, any of these examples may not cause a client to change practices, but collectively, the overall impression of the service they receive could send them packing.

The trends of the veterinary profession today are creating a tough and challenging practice climate, so it is a perfect time to turn to successful initiatives from outside the veterinary community to see what lessons can be learned. For example, those who have ever been a guest at a Ritz Carlton hotel are not surprised that this hotel has won the coveted and prestigious Malcolm Baldridge National Quality Award two times. Exceptional service, known as "The Ritz Carlton Mystique," is their standard, and it's what keeps their customers coming back repeatedly. A look at some of the twenty points in their "Credo" shows the factors that distinguish them and offers valuable lessons for forward-thinking practices, too:

- "The Credo is the principal belief of our Company. It must be known, owned and energized by all."
- "The Three Steps of Service are the foundation of Ritz-Carlton hospitality. These steps must be used in every interaction to ensure satisfaction, retention and loyalty."
- "It is the responsibility of each employee to create a work environment of teamwork and lateral service so that the needs of our guests and each other are met."

- "Each employee is empowered. For example, when a guest has a problem or needs something special you should break away from your regular duties, address and resolve the issue." (Source: Ritz Carlton web site, http://www.ritzcarlton.com)

How can veterinary practices ensure that they are developing a service culture that will keep their clients happy and well served? By institutionalizing the process, many practices have some measures in place, but few practices have a well-defined, formally structured, ongoing program. Veterinary practices that are successful at the process of institutionalizing a service culture engage in many similar activities, including the following: they develop written guidelines and protocols; they brand the service program (eg, give it a name and an identity); they communicate the fundamentals and importance of the program at every level and every opportunity; they find quantifiable ways to measure results; they conduct ongoing assessments; and they continuously seek to develop program enhancements.

There are many factors that could be included in a staff service program, several of which are explained here.

Employee Involvement: One of the hallmarks of the Ritz Carlton program is the expectation that all employees be involved in enhancing service, finding new ways to deliver exceptional service, and participating in the ongoing improvement of the program. This type of involvement is an accepted part of the culture—a norm. For veterinary practices that are not quite at this level, consider other, more tangible ways to foster employee involvement such as a contest, incentives, awards, etc.

Client Service Standards: To help employees understand what level of service excellence the practice is striving towards, develop written client service standards. These standards could include things such as acceptable procedures for returning phone calls, protocols for replying to requests, frequency of communications with clients, billing procedures, etc. Many practices have standards in place, but they are not regularly shared with staff or clients. To make them a normal part of the practice's culture, communicate them far and wide—post them on bulletin boards, include them in employee manuals, and post them on the web site or Intranet.

Training: Training is a critical component of implementing a successful staff initiative. Just developing a service mentality is not enough. Practices must help employees understand how these concepts translate into action on the job. There is a multitude of ways to accomplish this type of training. Here are a few examples: during orientation, through an ongoing series of "Lunch and Learn" sessions, in booklets and pamphlets, by bringing in guest speakers from companies who have successful programs, during retreats, etc. The possibilities are endless, and practices should hold the variety of training forums frequently. When conducting training, some of the methods that have proved to work best include imparting success stories, role-playing various scenarios, using visioning techniques, and listening to actual clients.

Rewards and Recognition: Reinforce the culture and service concept often by using rewards and recognition. An interesting feature of the Ritz Carlton's program is that monetary or other tangible awards are not offered to employees who go the extra mile, because they are just doing what is expected of them as employees of the chain. However, regular recognition and "atta boys" are given, particularly during weekly "lineups," a process in which everyone in a specific hotel gathers for information and updates.

Empowerment: Empower employees to take responsibility for client service. Don't make someone ask permission first before going the extra mile. If something is handled poorly, investigate the motive first—if what was done was the only or best way to handle a situation to keep a client happy, then deal with the consequences and don't reprimand the staff member. Reinforce the intentions and successful results. Engage in behaviors that will cause staff to want to take responsibility and initiative.

Quantify and Evaluate: Find ways to quantify the impact of staff participation in service—measure things such as the number of times a particular employee had a positive experience with a client or note how few complaints were received. Evaluate the success of efforts by asking clients for their feedback. This can be done through written surveys or face-to-face interviews. Ask specific questions that will allow an assessment of success or areas for improvement.

Become a Student: The best way to help staff do a better job at client service is to learn lessons from other practices and industries that are successful in this area and then impart that knowledge to them. Advise all to keep their eyes and ears open, and when something makes sense, think about how to translate that to the veterinary practice environment. For example, the Ritz Carlton includes "Guest Preference Tabs" as a part of each employee's uniform. It provides an easy mechanism for the employee to note and record guest preferences in their computer system, which is then used to enhance service on the guest's next visit. A recent guest requested an "egg crate" to soften her mattress, and on a next visit to a different Ritz Carlton,

had an egg crate ready and waiting without having to repeat the request. How could this translate to a veterinary practice? Give each employee a pre-printed pad on which they could note client's preferences, and then have these entered into the practice's practice management software. Then, whoever works with this client in the future can receive a briefing on preferences such as whether the client would rather leave the exam during the vaccinating their pet or stay during the procedures. Other companies noted for providing innovative and excellent client service include Arthur Andersen, Saturn Corporation, Microsoft and amazon.com, to name a few. These companies are not shy about blowing their own horns, and one can learn a lot about their customer service programs by simple visits to their web sites.

Don't forget the internal clients either. Veterinary practice staff supports the efforts of the owners—the veterinarians—so developing institutionalized internal programs and standards has great benefit as well. It always helps when people have clear expectations and ground rules for working together. Applying the fundamentals of an external client-focused program to an internally focused service initiative will strengthen the practice at a very critical and fundamental level.

The benefits of an institutionalized client service program are far-reaching and impact clients, staff, and veterinarians—everyone involved in the process of delivering or receiving veterinary healthcare. Besides the obvious, staff who are asked to do more than just "show up" at work every day achieve greater job satisfaction and stability, as well as personal growth and satisfaction.

Sounds simple, doesn't it? But then, so does losing ten pounds—we're told to just eat right and exercise. However, just knowing the right things to do doesn't mean we put them into practice. In this busy world, there is competition for our time, resources and creative energy. Client service programs must compete with skills training, a technology onslaught, skyrocketing salaries and the myriad other things keeping the days full and management meetings lively. But remember, without clients and their pets veterinary practices wouldn't exist. So, doesn't it make sense to put client service initiatives at the top of the priority list? It will surely keep those practices that do ahead of the rest.

OPEN BOOK MANAGEMENT – THE NUTS & BOLTS OF FILE PREP FOR BETTER PATIENT CARE, CLIENT EXPERIENCE, AND INCREASED PROFITS

Louise Dunn
Snowgoose Veterinary Management Consulting
Greensboro, NC

Working smarter, not harder, should be the mantra of every business today. It seems there's too much to do in too little time. Everybody is clamoring for your attention. Your clients want more face time to discuss their pets' health. Your hospital team members want more of your attention and constant input to make sure that they're succeeding in their respective roles. And your business demands are increasing as you continually look for new ways to boost your bottom line, draw clients in and deliver top-notch care— all while growing your business.

With all this demand, how are you to succeed in business and still practice the best veterinary medicine?

Start with your hospital team. Remember, you can't lead the band and play all the instruments. Creating a well-balanced, highly talented team is essential to working smarter and delivering the quality of care that will bond clients to your practice for the long haul. As the practice leader, it's up to you to give them the tools they need to perform their jobs and work as efficiently as possible.

BE PREPARED FOR CLIENT VISITS

At Snowgoose Veterinary Management Consulting, we believe that utilizing "tools from the trenches" is just smart business. Take file preparation, for example. If your team isn't already mastering this process, rally your team members for a training session today.

All too often when I visit hospitals in my consulting business, I see team members making a critical mistake: pulling patient records the day of that patient's visit. If your team is doing this, you're missing out on an important opportunity to enhance patient care, improve the overall client experience and increase your revenue.

All hospital records should be pulled well in advance of any client visit instead of being pulled the minute the client walks in the door. This allows you and your team time to review the pet's medical history and flag any necessary preventive care procedures that the pet may need. Thus, you can give the client a heads-up on the necessary procedure and educate him or her on the importance of preventive health care. Starting the client education process early will help boost your compliance rate and give you an opportunity to talk with clients about future care options. It also increases clients' expectations on the level of care they can expect from you and your team.

To ensure your hospital team is on board with this important process, consider creating a handy checklist of key steps that need to be completed to prepare for every client visit. This simple reminder will help your hospital team members get into the habit of file preparation so that it becomes second nature to them.

As an aside, another benefit of pulling clients in advance, especially for practices that capture the pet's picture in their practice management software, it gives the client service representatives (the receptionists) the opportunity to refamiliarize themselves with the pets. Imagine the "wow" factor when you great the pet by name as they walk up to the front desk!

TRY OPEN BOOK MANAGEMENT

Being a veterinarian involves more than just practicing good medicine and celebrating the human-animal bond. Veterinarians must know viable business practices to be successful.

Making smart business decisions, focusing on client compliance and building a winning team is all part of the Circle of Care. In a nutshell, patient care + the client experience + your business = the Circle of Care.

In order for you to complete this circle, you must:

- Develop or cultivate a team that treats your clients just as well as you treat them
- Create an environment that energizes staff
- Give your team the tools they need to be successful

One business practice that can help you be successful is Open Book Management. It enables team members to understand how their job performance affects the practice's bottom line. According to the Harvard Business School, Open Book Management has had the greatest impact of any business idea in the last 75 years.

The Open Book Management process shares a broad array of data with team members, including key performance indicators, and gives practice owners and the management team a step-by-step way to measure performance at every level of the business.

Team members are positively impacted by the Open Book Management process as well. The skills they learn will help them in their professional and personal lives. They will begin to feel more a part of the practice when they directly share in its successes and failures. Open Book Management empowers and encourages team members to share information to build a happy, dynamic, successful team and business. And that's what will set you apart from your competitors.

Using Open Book Management skills will help to develop the skills team members need to better interact with clients. Team meetings are not just run by the veterinarian or the practice manager. Team members are given assignments to do or investigate and then they must report on their findings at subsequent meetings. Accountability is taken to a whole new level using well run Open Book Management meetings. As team members work on developing their presentations and getting findings across to other team members, a spill over benefit to the practice is them learning how to interact with clients on helping to reinforce the need to follow through on recommendations made by the veterinarians.

Accountability is a term that is bantered about freely in management circles today. We struggle with trying to get our arms around this concept when dealing with our team members. Again, using Open Book Management ideas, each meeting ends with a list of ideas that team members will work on for the next meeting. The entire staff is aware of the assignments and the target date for their completion. Now, instead of the practice manager or the veterinarian having to always be the "bad guy" because team members are not doing their job, it is the team member who has to report to the entire rest of the team that they did not follow through and complete what was asked of them. This places accountability squarely where it should be – in the collective lap of the entire team.

Having a mission statement for our practice and a vision of how we are going to get there is another topic that is heard a lot about. However, what does this mean for our practice? Many times this is brushed off as one of those "touchy, feeling" things that really isn't important. However, if we want to have our team really take ownership of their jobs, they need to know what their job really is and what role their job place in the overall achievement of the practice's mission. Having the mission statement being very much a part of the team meetings is important. At various meetings throughout the year it is important to reinforce with team members how their particular jobs contribute to the overall mission statement. Seeing on the various scorecards the improvement that is made by implementing various things that are discussed helps reinforce in a positive way what we are trying to achieve. It takes training to a whole new level. It not only trains staff in what we want done, but actually shows them the "why" of what they are doing. When we talk generational issues, "why" is very important to many of our younger team members. Open Book Management shows the "why."

Profit is to many team members a four letter word. We aren't out to make money, we are here to love animals and make them better. As stated in the companion article article by Elise Lacher in this proceedings on understanding the practice's financial statements, profits are essential if the practice is to carry out its mission of providing the best in medical care to the patients who walk through the front door. Making a profit is generally understood by most practice owners. Many times, veterinarians feel that they bear the entire weight of trying to make the money to cover the costs of running a practice today. With Open Book Management, we are able to spread the wealth. It is no longer just the practice owner who has to worry about covering the light bill, the animal care attendant understands that if the bag of dog food wanders out the back door, they do get feet, you know, that cost absolutely affects them getting the raise they think they deserve. Responsibility for the profitable running of the practice now is a team effort.

While Open Book Management is frequently thought of as sharing financial information with the staff, it is so much more than that. It starts with the numbers, but spills over into human resource leadership, team development, communication, client service – all those areas that we feel are so important in today's practice environment.

YOUR HOSPITAL IS ONLY AS GOOD AS YOUR WEAKEST STAFF MEMBER

Byron S. Farquer, DVM
Simmons Pacific
Oakdale, CA

Donald Erceg
VETMARK: The Veterinary Marketing Company
Portland, OR

Hire for attitude and train for skill, a motto coined by Southwest Airlines, is generally ignored in the medical profession. Why is it that we tend to define practice positions established basically upon a framework of duties that require certain skills and hire someone to fill that role, only to then be disappointed in the performance? Perhaps too often veterinary staff is hired for skill when what we should be doing is hiring for attitude first. A sign adorns one large corporation that says, "We don't train people to be nice, we simply hire nice people." You can train, and teach skill sets. You can improve and foster advanced application, but it is rare, at least at the adult level that we hire from, you will be able to instill positive work ethic and attitude.

SOUTHWEST AIRLINES MODEL

Southwest Airlines has been profitable every year in its 30+ years of history, even after 9/11. Why? Great management, service, quick routing? Interestingly a major component of that success relates to having an incredibly dedicated work force, founded upon positive attitude, empowering employees, and garnishing it with respect. As former CEO Herb Kelleher said, "We are not an airline company with great customer service. We are a great customer service organization that happens to be in the airline business." Now, substitute "veterinary" for "airline" into the last sentence. Hiring the right people has been a hallmark of Southwest.

They look for people with an attitude that is positive, creative, and people-oriented. Are you still looking for "5 years experience as a kennel assistant, Acme Vet Tech correspondent graduate, good MS Word skills and familiar with Cornerstone"? Southwest trains for the rest, the skill set, and it REALLY works. That's not to say possession of certification (registered technician) should be ignored. It's also a vital component to your staff. But hiring for attitude might really serve you better when it's placed at the top of the criteria list. Customers are NOT #1 at Southwest—employees are, period. If you treat your employees right, they will treat your clients right. And, at Southwest, "outrageous customer service" is commonplace. It takes getting the right people on the bus, then getting them in the right seats. Veterinarians continue to miss the first critical step: the right people. The seats are the skills required. So the second step is ensuring the person you have on the bus (your practice) is matched correctly with their skill set (the right seat), but that first requires gathering great attitudes (the right people).

Southwest Airlines created a great company personality by adhering to the following key points.

- Never give up
- Focus on people
- Be resourceful, willing and able
- Promote esprit de corps
- Know what you do best, and quit doing what you can't do best
- If push comes to shove choose humor over skill

So, how do you translate great customer service over to a veterinary practice? Answering the phone by the third ring, minimizing on-hold times, returning calls promptly, keeping waiting times short, fresh flowers, water and coffee and a snack, current magazines that are right for your clients (*Popular Mechanics* vs. *Oprah*), progress reports, beeper access for critical patients, carrying pet food to a client's car, umbrellas, using the pet's proper gender and the most overlooked of all, eye contact with a big smile.

HIRING INTERVIEWS

Do you hire individually or in a group setting? At Southwest, much of the hiring is "group interviewing" and although answers are important, more important is the way in which the other candidates interact. Do they pay attention while someone else is answering a question? Are they genuinely interested in the others? Here's a common "trick" employed by companies that share this same group interaction and behavior observation mentality. An interview candidate enters a room with a couple of casual dressed company personnel, and is required to wait a short time. In walks a suit or two, and the interview apparently starts, although it actually started earlier. Who's in causal clothing? Key management. And the suits? Anyone. The point of the exercise is to observe how the interviewee acts not knowing who the big cheese is, and how all are treated in the room. Adaptable to veterinary medicine? Sure. Have your key receptionist or practice manager put on typical kennel help attire, and adorn your junior employee with business attire. Tour the practice, observe interactions. Does your practice manager receive the same interaction and respect as your well-dressed posed manager? If not, consider how this interviewee will treat these people in a work setting. When you hire someone, do you have him or her come to the practice in person with a resume? If so, how did they treat your front office staff? Were they neat and clean and professional? We can tell a GREAT deal from that personal contact. Today you can actually purchase the "perfect" resume online, so watch how much you put into resumes. Ever heard the comment "I want to be a veterinarian rather than a physician because I'm not really a people person". Wow—did we all learn quickly that veterinary medicine is most certainly a people business! So we always hire "people oriented" employees right? Wrong! I've passed many a recluse during practice visits, toiling after their daily tasks, and certainly not elevating the perception of the practice as a friendly, caring environment when interacting with clients. You need to hire people-people that will accept empowerment, stay within the policy guidelines but welcome your given freedom to think and adjust to the moment. You need to let go a little. Let the employee color outside the lines. I didn't suggest you let them color on the table (significantly deviate from set policies). Let employees take ownership of their role in besting client service at your practice and you will have the makings of a team. That won't be enough, however, since all good teams are captained by great leaders. You must fill that role in order for your team to succeed and survive.

LEADERSHIP

Good leaders are made, not born. If you have the desire and willpower, you can become an effective leader. Good leaders develop through a never-ending process of self-study, education, training, and experience. This guide will help you through that process. To inspire your team into higher levels of teamwork, there are certain things you must be, know, and do. These do not come naturally, but are acquired through continual work and study. The best leaders are continually working and studying to improve their leadership skills.

Leadership is a complex process by which you influence others to accomplish a mission, task by the application of your beliefs, values, ethics, character, knowledge, and skills. Ownership gives you the power to accomplish certain tasks and objectives in the practice but this power does not make you a leader. It simply makes you the boss. Bosses tell staff what to do; leaders inspire a desire to do it. Leaders make people want to achieve high goals and objectives.

Your staff will evaluate your leadership skills not by what you say but by what you do. They will watch to see if you walk your talk. They can tell immediately if you are an honorable and trusted leader or a self-serving tyrant who misuses your authority of ownership. Self-serving leaders can force employees to obey but can't force them to follow.

What makes a person want to follow a leader? People want to be guided by those they respect and who have a clear sense of direction. To gain that respect, be ethical above all else. Then develop and communicate a clear vision for the future of the practice.

Here are a few important words that will help you become a better leader:

- The six most important words: "I admit I made a mistake."
- The five most important words: "You did a good job."
- The four most important words: "What is your opinion?"
- The three most important words: "If you please."
- The two most important words: "Thank you."
- The one most important word: "We"
- The least most important word: "I"

THE PRACTICE CULTURE

If you already own or have acquired a preexisting practice, you have inherited a practice culture—a set of attitudes, beliefs, and a way of working. Every practice has a culture that was formed to considerable degree by how the owner responded to problems and opportunities. If you are fortunate the former owner was a good leader who set high standards and goals across the entire spectrum of services offered by the practice.

Both employees and clients can quickly sniff out the culture of the practice. Values reflect the concern the organization has for its employees, customers, investors, vendors, and surrounding community. These values define the manner in how business will be conducted and what type of business the organization will engage in. Each practice has its own distinctive culture. It is a combination of the founders, past leadership, current leadership, crises, events, history, and size. This results in routines and rituals; "way we do things."

Culture represents the shared expectations and self-image of the organization. The mature values that create "tradition" or the "way we do things here." Things are done differently in every practice. The collective vision and common folklore that define the institution are a reflection of culture. Changing a preexisting culture is not easy but, everything you do as a leader will eventually affect the culture of your practice.

VISIONING

As owner and leader, it is up to you to set the direction for your organization: to provide vision, purpose, and define goals. Then, with the future clear in your mind's eye, it is up to you to recognize the need for change and to choose the time frame and means of implementation. As owner you must find what is broken and fix it. As leader you must take what is not broken and make it better. Treat every project as an opportunity for improvement, for getting closer to your vision of excellence. Good practices convey a strong vision of where they will be in the future.

When setting goals, keep these points in mind:

- Goals should be realistic and attainable.
- The goals should improve the organization (morale, monetary, etc.).
- Your employees should be involved in the goal-setting process.
- A program should be developed to achieve each goal.

TEAM BUILDING

Team building is so important that it should become a persistent passion in your business culture. You can google the internet for additional resources and regional seminars that will help you develop your team building skills. This is not a skill you were born with. It is something you will have to learn and practice. Along with your skills as a doctor, your abilities at team building and team leadership will have the greatest impact on the success of your practice.

Keep in mind that vision is the most important aspect of making a team successful. Teams perish when they don't clearly see the vision that describes why they are doing what they do and where they are going. Workers want to be successful and they know the only way to do that is by following and achieving great goals.

The team leader is the one person who understands the ultimate project objectives, each step of the way, and who guides the rest of the team down this path through clear vision setting and effective communication. As a small business owner, becoming a great leader is not a job you can shirk if you hope to succeed.

WHY DO YOU WANT TO BECOME AN OWNER?

Byron Farquer, DVM
Simmons Pacific
Oakdale, CA

Donald J. Erceg
VETMARK: The Veterinary Marketing Company
Portland, OR

OWNERSHIP: IS IT FOR YOU?

In addition to a successful professional career, practice ownership can be one of the most emotionally and financially rewarding things we can achieve. In order for this to occur, a practice must change hands. This seemingly daunting process can, when done correctly, be quite painless. When done poorly, the effects and financial damage resulting from a poorly designed plan can last for decades.

Before you decide to do a start-up or buy a practice you need to decide if ownership itself is right for you. A number of items need consideration. You'll be your own boss, but can you give directions and provide leadership for others? Do you have any management skill, and importantly an interest to learn more? Can you handle risk and failure emotionally? Have you assessed the impact on personal time, the restriction of geographic mobility (tied down), and can you juggle ownership with medical duties? Braake's study on higher incomes determined the following common characteristics in our profession. Those that earned more owned practices, had more years in practice, worked more hours, and had a higher financial acumen than others. You need to access your medical experience, and your financial health.

WHAT OPTIONS EXIST FOR YOU? START UP, BUY-IN, AND BUY-OUT

Start Up — One exciting path to becoming an owner is starting a practice "from scratch." Because of the high costs and the lack of income in the initial period, this option is becoming less common in recent years, at least done the traditional way. This is, in part, due to the financial pressures created by large student loans, which were not present twenty years ago. As a result, it has become hard for young practitioners to have little or no income for any extended period. The advantages are that the new owner can choose the exact location, floor plan, equipment, and immediately personalize the practice to suit his or her needs. The disadvantages are the initial cost with no income, and the more restrictive financing options available. There is notable risk in this strategy because of no previous practice history or income. Cost for a startup would likely range from a low of $150,000 up to $450,000 for a leasehold practice and even more if real estate is purchased, so this is often a limiting factor, considering there is no instant income stream.

Today more than ever, you should approach a practice start-up using the property tools and techniques. This includes choosing your location wisely (siting), studying the demographics and psycho-graphics, and NOT simply choosing your location out of convenience (I already live nearby). Too often we see yet one more small struggling practice that recently wedged its way into an already oversaturated market. Quit it. It doesn't make good business sense, the fun of building something new will wear off quickly, and the pain of frustration and struggle is going to haunt you. Plan well, do it right, in the right spot and you will be handsomely rewarded. What is needed to achieve success? A well thought-out plan.

Buy In — Buying into an existing practice, especially the practice in which the associate is already employed, is becoming more and more common as there are more and more multi-DVM practices. This is a lower risk strategy than a start-up because there is a current track record and following the buy-in, usually little, if anything, changes. It allows the buyer to obtain management experience, using the senior owner as a mentor. The financing is often done by the senior owner and at favorable terms, so that can be an additional benefit. The disadvantages are that the buyer usually has little power or ability to institute changes or to personalize the practice as long as he or she is a minority owner. It can take many years to become the controlling owner, depending upon the purchase structure.

It is important to seek professional assistance with a buy-in because of the many issues that need to be resolved. There are significant tax issues that can mean many thousands of dollars, depending upon the purchase structure. In one case, a buyer was able to realize a tax savings in excess of $200,000 by purchasing the practice assets rather than stocks in the corporation! There are a myriad of legal issues that need resolution as well. How will the non-compete agreements be worded? What happens if either owner wants out? How will the partners be compensated fairly? What if one of the partners develops a drug addiction problem, or worse, dies? In short, a comprehensive and thorough buy-sell agreement must be crafted by an attorney who is knowledgeable with contract law.

Finally, employing a veterinary consultant or a buyer's agent or a neutral facilitator is invaluable to help negotiate a purchase that is fair, to assist in obtaining financing, and to keep everyone focused on the final goal. The veterinarians' time is best spent doing what they do best, practicing veterinary medicine. In a busy practice (usually the case in practice seeking a partner to buy-in), there is little extra time left to deal with the many issues and decisions related to a buy-in. Without someone to push, prod, and shepherd the whole process to a successful completion, it is all too common to see it drag on and on for many months or even years and eventually completely stall.

Buy Out — This is still a common entrance strategy and offers some distinct advantages. It has many of the benefits seen in start-ups such as ability to quickly personalize the practice and be in complete control of management. It also has some of the advantages of a buy-in because there is an existing cash flow and client base which reduces risk (lenders LOVE reduced risk!) and provides immediate income to the buyer. Because there is no other owner, the lender can be in "first" lien position, which makes financing for this type of purchase the easiest to obtain (as opposed to a partial buy-in or a start-up). The disadvantages of buying out an existing practice involve, mainly, the psychology of "going it alone." Although sometimes the previous owner will continue to work in the practice and help, it is more common to see a relatively short transition period. Therefore, it is important that the new practice owner have the skills and confidence to step into the role of the sole owner. Not only does that require medical skill, but it also requires a desire to learn the management and a willingness to take risk. This is what we call an "owner mentality."

In the next decade, an increasing number of baby boomers will approach retirement age. As their practices are listed for sale, the number of buyers may not increase at the same rate as sellers resulting in a market situation that strongly favors the buyer. Of those who are buying, we would expect to see more shared ownership by two unrelated buyers as well as a great selection of really super practices available for purchase.

Is buying a small practice a good thing? Isn't it a lot cheaper? Often in purchase price but recall that small grossing practices have little or no excess profit beyond a basic salary for the owner. That's fine if you already own it and have it paid off. But how is a buyer supposed to make payments to the bank and make a salary? Can't you just grow it to overcome the short fall? I ask you, can you grow it? That's something you absolutely need to know. Is it an underutilized practice or is it in its terminal stages of death? Small practices are either diamonds in the rough, or just plain rough. They can be an exciting opportunity when there is a neighboring practice that can be acquired and merged, reducing community redundancy and improving profitability. By eliminating the duplication of fixed costs, facilities and equipment (and to some extent duplication of staff), the merger of two practices can result in a more efficient and sellable practice entity later.

If you are considering starting a mixed practice also consider purchase of an existing one. It's a buyer's market—hands down. You can often acquire great facilities and receive a very good transition from the owner which ensures your successful capture of pre-existing clients.

Further complicating the situation, are various external factors influencing the marketplace. These factors, largely beyond the control of our profession, include interest rates, lender's view of veterinary practice loan risk, the economic health of the US as well as national security threats (terrorism, war, etc.). All of these factors can influence practice ownership opportunities and behavior and their occurrence is unpredictable.

So why do this anyway? Why not just remain an associate? The holy grail of ownership is equity. At the end of 10 years you will have nothing to show for your 40 to 50 hours a week as an associate other than ten W-2's. You have nothing to sell, and have had to fund your entire life with post-tax, earned income. As an owner, however you will earn equal to or more than most associates, and at the end of the same 10 years have a practice paid off that has sellable value. Assume an associate works in a $500,000 practice and earns $750,000 in 10 years, places $20,000 in an IRA and diligently saves another $123,000 (assumes a 10% ROI). She has a comfortable lifestyle. Net worth from the effort? $143,000. Same doctor chooses ownership instead of associate position. Ten years expire, same savings and IRA, but the doctor also has a paid off practice available for sale. Net worth: $643,000. That's a half a million dollars difference in your financial future.

Finally, when considering your entrance to ownership, planning remains key. If existing practices do not match the profile that you seek, strategic planning and time (1–2 years) may be required to better position yourself. Depending on your current situation relocation may need to be addressed. A keen awareness of the current and future market conditions can guide your planning. If you are considering buying in the next 2 years, getting your team together followed by a valuation and/or feasibility analysis done on the practice (new or existing) now can go along way to prevent you from being unprepared.

In all ownership changes, it is beneficial to use the advice of professionals. The ownership path can be navigated alone, and many have done so. Failure, or delayed success, tends to be more common using this approach, but some obviously succeed. Statistically, buyers and sellers that chose to surround themselves with a proper team of advisors have much higher success rates, and higher levels of long-term success. Consider this process a team sport. The players include appraiser, transition specialist/broker, CPA–tax advisor, attorney, lender, escrow/title company, marketing consultant, and practice management consultant.

RECOMMENDED READING

1. Farquer B, Wiseman L. Your Veterinary Practice, Buying, Selling & Merging. Adagio Press, 2006.
2. Farquer B, Erceg D, Guenther J, Pinger S, Sammons K, McCormick D. SmartStart Practice – Success Kit. SSP Press, 2006, 2007.
3. Monheiser L. Starting Your Own Veterinary Practice. AHHA Press, 2006.
4. Monheiser L. Buying a Veterinary Practice. AHHA Press, 2006.
5. Kawasaki G. The Art of the Start. Penguin Group, 2004.

BUILD IT AND THEY WILL COME

Byron S. Farquer, DVM
Simmons Pacific
Oakdale, CA

Donald Erceg
VETMARK
Portland, OR

Gone are the days when the veterinarian would come to a town that had no doctor, buy an old two-story house, tack a shingle to the front of the house that read "Veterinarian," and set up shop of the main floor. There was the doctor and his wife. He did the medicine. She was receptionist, bookkeeper, animal handler, and practice manager—a perfect manifestation of the nineteenth century American Mom & Pop small business model. There was a lot to envy in this style of life for the "Doc" and his family. He could take a 2-hour lunch at home and hang out a "gone fishin'" sign when trout season hit.

COMPETITION DRIVES CHANGE

The day a second veterinarian moved into town, things changed. The needs of the clients would begin to become more important than those of the doctor. Now the pet owners could choose. What would they base their choice on? Both men were doctors—from the consumer's point of view both were qualified. Convenience became a big issue. Doctor "x" might be open during the lunch hour or after work. Doctor "y" might be closer to the house or easier for driving and parking (location, location, location). After issues of convenience, the consumer had to rely on her senses: which hospital "looked" the best? To the consumer, you are as good as you look.

YOUR BUILDING IS YOUR BEST BILLBOARD

As a small business, veterinary hospitals have limited funds for advertising. For the most part, advertising is restricted to the yellow pages, some direct mail, the internet, word of mouth, perhaps some occasional radio and newspaper and, rarely, television. The biggest, most important advertising is the practice building and sign. Location, architecture, and design can have a huge impact on the success of the practice. If you are as good as you look, it is very important to not only look your best, but to also look better than the competition.

OUR CHOICES ARE IRRATIONAL

What happens when a potential client drives by or walks into your hospital? The psychological effect of this experience can be tremendous. The client is a walking litmus test of sensory input. Unconsciously the hospital layout, design, colors, noises and odors make their mark. As humans, we decide whether we like something or someone in one fifth of a second! Many of the factors in this decision are invisible to the conscious mind. In other words, they are irrational. People should choose doctors and hospitals based on a careful examination of their success rates, medical protocols, pain management programs, diagnostic skills, an so on. Unfortunately, people are human and base their retail choices on their feelings.

Over the last 15 years we have heard countless veterinarians complain that they practice the best medicine in town and still are barely scraping by economically. As if proof were needed, this was a clear demonstration that a medical degree is no guarantee of business and financial success! Business administration is a different skill set. Success in the retail world depends on our ability to please and delight the consumer.

BUILD IT AND THEY WILL COME

There is evidence that a practice can increase its revenues 20% just by building a new facility. Building a new facility in the right location is the single biggest step you can take toward success. The question is what kind of facility should you build? In today's marketplace, there are usually many more than two doctors in town. The secret to prevail in today's crowded marketplace is to not only meet the client's needs, but to exceed them. The race is on to surprise and delight the client. This makes the jobs of architect, interior designer, and landscaper more important than ever. The top architects serving the veterinary marketplace have responded with impressive, award-winning designs that offer an exciting backdrop to quality medical care and high-touch service. It also has to be functional, not just pretty AND in the right location. A great facility starts with a great location, and that isn't as intuitive as one might believe. Gut feelings, wet finger placed windward, or reliance upon general data isn't going to be sufficient in many cases. You should reach for professionals to help you decide if your initial assumptions are correct.

YOUR POTENTIAL TRADE AREA

The first and most important factor is the potential trade area for each of the locations you are considering. By definition, a trade area is the area that contains the majority of your active clients (typically 80%) and it represents your key market. Because you do not have clients to use to establish the trade area boundary, you need to use a conservative estimate for the boundary of that potential area.

In most cases the best way to estimate your potential trade area is to establish a boundary based on drive time to (or from) the practice location. Drive times take into account factors that a basic radius ring does not such as the influence of lakes, roadways (or lack thereof), golf courses, mountains, etc. These factors can increase or decrease your potential trade area.

So what drive time should you use for each of your sites? This depends on several factors including the services that you are planning to provide, whether the area is urban, suburban or rural, and the level of traffic congestion. In general, consumers are typically more willing to drive further in rural and suburban areas than they will in urban areas. Trade area analyses done on actual client distributions (by address mapping) resulted in the following drive time ranges. It is important to note that these are reference points to help get you started. You may want to adjust these based on the characteristics of the location you are considering.

- 10–5 minutes for small animal practices
- 30–40 minutes for a kennel or emergency practice
- 45–50 minutes for a specialty practice
- 30–40 minutes for mobile and large animal practices although the limit tends to be your preference with respect to how far you are willing to drive from client to client.

DATA COLLECTION

Once you have delineated your potential trade area you need to collect the demographic data that will aid you in comparing the different locations. Naturally, there are a many different variables you can use and different variables for different types of services.

What information should you collect? There are two categories of information that you should collect. First, the information on the community that will help you decide whether you can live and become a member of that community. The second category focuses on the demographic variables that reveal information on the community's need for veterinary services. Some of the most important to find include the number of households, the average household income, the aggregate income for the area, and the percentage of pet ownership. You can also collect information on home ownership, income distributions, and consumer expenditure variables such as "Pets and Supplies" and "Veterinary Services."

As you collect information on your target locations, you will also need to identify and learn about the alternate service providers, ie, the competition, influencing your potential trade area. This includes developing an estimate of the total number of veterinarians that are influencing your trade area.

PRE-EXISTING PRACTICES

What if you are interested in a pre-existing practice? Think again about the steps laid out above. Each one still applies; however, the one denominator here is that location is already chosen. You should consider using this same criteria to evaluate the current and future potential of a pre-existing practice. For instance, if you map out the client data base (using zip codes and the practice's database details) you might find a pattern with a rather round shape or perhaps one that has a long neck stretching from a larger cluster of clients. Now super impose the pre-existing practices in the area. What if you determine two new practices have a virtual chokehold on the neck of the distribution? That could mean these clients will switch in the near future. It continues to amaze professional consultants just how many practices are opened up each year with nary a look at the community data in enough detail to determine the likelihood of success. For many, availability of an affordable leasehold and convenient proximity to home is the only criteria considered.

"Facility costs are the third-largest expense for most hospitals. Only staffing costs and drug and medical supply expenses rank higher. Of course, your facility also plays a major role in revenue generation. The building acts as a working asset," says Veterinary Economics Editorial Advisory Board member Gary Glassman, CPA.

"When you look at industry averages, two full-time, small animal practitioners should generate approximately $940,000 of gross revenue out of an average of 2,500 square feet," says Glassman. When you look at these numbers by profit center, about 35% of your building space will be allocated to overhead and is not direct income-production space. "You need these areas—including offices, bathrooms, an employee lounge, and most of your reception area—to manage the business functions of the practice," says Glassman, a partner with Burzenski & Co. PC in East Haven, Connecticut.

So you better do your math, twice. Breaking down areas of the facility into profit or revenue generating centers helps you plan for the got-to-haves and the nice-to-haves, and when budgets get tight you'll know which to keep. Even different areas can cost different amounts to operate. Areas can become more efficient over time with growth in the practice's revenue. Some areas like radiology remain underutilized early on, as a small practice grows from a few radiology appointments to many per month later on. Other areas will quickly become outpaced by growth. Where tripling the gross revenues the patient count has little effect on radiology room needs; however, exam room space will quickly be at a premium. In planning, be sure to account for exam rooms for the future. They don't have to be built out now, but it is one of the biggest limiting factors in practice facilities that stifles long-term growth and functionality next to treatment centers. You can create "double sized" exam rooms initially, populating the room only on one side with sink, and exam table to save costs, later adding a wall to divide it. Other options include using a large space for doctor's offices, then later when demand dictates it, convert the doctor offices that were physically preplanned to be next to existing exam rooms into additional exam rooms and move the doctor offices to a different area that originally started out as unfinished or minimally finished space. Growing into a building is often cost effective as construction costs are frozen in time for major foundation, roof and wall structures, and sometimes future zoning restrictions prevent expansions.

All this space doesn't come cheap. The 2005 Well-Managed Practice Study found that nearly 13% of respondents plan to remodel their current facility in the next 2 years, and expect to spend an average of $316,000. Another 14% plan to expand their current facility, spending an average of $841,667. And 8% plan to build a brand-new facility at an average cost of $1,324,556. This means paying close attention to doing the right things, right, at the right time.

And all of this needs to be addressed within the context of building a better facility. Meaning its not just the act of controlling sound and odor, and making floor plans that have logical placement of rooms and efficient people movement, but it speaks to designing a better facility consistent with the needs and expectations of a business that intends to provide excellence in customer service, appeal to the senses of the client, and leave them with an "oh wow" experience. This isn't to be confused with some of the facilities built recently that elicit an "oh wow" from an architectural view point alone, an "oh wow" from your checkbook. You are wanting one that really creates an "oh wow" from a business management, profitability, consumer appeal and marketing view point. A well-designed practice, albeit probably expensive, if done right will exponentially thrust a practice upward and onward far further than just a "pretty" facility. Anyone can spend $2,000,000 and create a Taj Mahal, but proper planning requires more. You have to embrace not only the materials choice and workmanship knowledge of good architects familiar with veterinary industry facilities and needs, but it's wise to elicit help from architects with high-end retail and entertainment industry experience. You are reaching for the sweet spot where functionality meets appeal. This rather obscure concept isn't explained by simply looking to high quality materials, vaulted ceilings, or sky lights. The magic occurs when the architects can create the intangible ambiance that the general public finds so appealing and comforting, and invokes positive actions, whether it be product sales or purchased services. Think about some of the great restaurants, stores, social gathering spots that had that great feel. Studies prove you'll spend more, and importantly be more satisfied about it when you are in these types of settings, but does that extra expense to build a showcase make sense economically?

Using a basic example lets assume the following:

Hard Costs

Land	$230,000
Building sq. ft.	3500
Cost/sq.ft.	$220
Total Building Costs	$770,000
Total Hard Costs	$1,000,000

Soft Costs

Architectural -Vet	$44,000
Consultant	$20,000
Engineering	
Civil	$7,000
Environmental	$2,000
Structural	$8,500
Mechanical	$4,500
Regulatory	
Tap/permit fees	$4,500
Financing	
Appraisal	$3,000
Construction Loan	
Origination Fees 1%	$7,700
Interest Rate 8.5%	$19,550
Closing Costs	$4,500
Contingency 3%	$30,000
Total Soft Costs	$155,250

Total Project Costs	$1,155,250

Financing

Equity 20%	$231,000
Long Term Loan	
Principal	$924,250
Period	20 yr
Interest	8.5%
Loan Payment/Year	$94,503

Operating Expenses (Annual)

Real Estate Taxes	$9,000
Insurance	$6,500
Utilities	$8,400
Maintenance	$4,100
Total Operating Expenses	$28,000

Required Cashflow	
(Rent paid by Practice)	$122,503
Per Month	$10,209

As you can see it really adds up fast, but here we must decide what it takes to crack that nut each month. In pre-existing practices, the calculation is somewhat easier. You have a known financial performance and you can determine how much of the cashflow can be allocated to cover the monthly payment. Start-ups have a much more difficult task of using estimations and assumptions to predict as closely as possible, the financial performance of the practice.

To avoid a lengthy discussion on pro-forma development, and start up predictive indices, we will assume a pre-existing practice in a leasehold will be relocating to this new facility. Breakdown the known. If the practice sees 24 patients a day at with an ATF of $134, working 5.5 days per week, we could expect $70,752 in revenue. Since the typical well-managed practice consumes 40% of revenue in wage costs and another 20% in drugs and supplies there would be a mere $28,301 to pull all other expenses from including this $10,209 payment. Some leasehold rent is available, but the budget remains tight. You should be concerned IF you designed this facility strictly from a function-only basis—that is, if it has been designed only from the premise of good surfaces that feces wash off of, and plenty of electrical outlets. On the other hand if you have designed a facility that appeals to those intangible qualities described above, creating a real "wow" experience, not just a "wow" look, AND you deliver on your promise of customer service, the nut to crack suddenly appears less formidable. Here's why. Painting, new signage, fresh sealed blacktop, cleanliness and organization have all been shown to be extremely influential on customer buying habits and satisfaction. Tests too numerous to site have shown this to be factual. Recent studies indicate customers that are happy, calm or comfortable spend more, rate higher satisfaction levels, and in medical or technical settings have shown to retain more information or instruction. In a veterinary setting this translates to better acceptance of your best workup, more extensive or deep invoices

1219

(all you want to do, not just minimal workups) and clients that retain and remember instructions both of which lead to better case success rates. You can expect better client compliance when they hear, understand, and feel good about your recommendations. You can cure or treat more patients successfully when you don't have one arm tied behind your back resulting from mistrust, financial or perception limitations of the client. In order to perform well clients have to be very satisfied with the entire experience and that includes the "building visit" experience. Does it really matter to the bottom line? Ask yourself this question. "Could you sell $4.05 cups of coffee at Denny's as effectively as you can at Starbucks? We know the answer is no, because people endure the cost in exchange for the benefits derived, including among many things, the ambiance of the store itself. If you want a new facility, then you better build one that you can sell $4.05 coffee in, and not one that should be selling 'cupppa joe for a buck.'

IF YOU BUILD IT, WILL THEY REALLY COME?

Why go to the trouble to give attention to anything but the floor plan and materials? Can I really build a facility that embraces all that the consumer wants, loves, and subconsciously responds to, and will it actually make my practice better than if I just do the utilitarian approach?

Dr. Tom Van Meter is a strong case in point, illustrating the progression from traditional functionality into state of the art embracement of consumer psychology.

His original practice, located in a 1600 square foot block construction building, typified the classic veterinary facility—basic, utilitarian, and unassuming. It was clean, but "cold" visually, and portrayed sterility and function. Revenue grew as the practice did until it began to peak. A professional marketing firm re-branded the practice, addressing many of the above issues including signage, and color, and created a boutique approach to image. Sales that were flat at $503K or declining once again grew 20% to 25% over the next 22 months, proving that how your building looks and its match to your practice's self-proclaimed image is critical for success. Valuation of the practice changed also, moving from $300K to $450K in the same period. Growth again occurred from a local merger, but soon they were busting at the seams, with carts parked in hall ways and elbows bumping against one another. A new facility was imminent; however, a divergent path existed. Either choose function only, stay with the traditional approach that the doctor will design the floor plan, chose easy to clean materials, and the spouse will pick the colors, or choose to do it right, embracing all that is described in this article. He chose the latter. Today there stands a facility that is beautiful, functional, and appealing. Where covered entry ways and courtesy umbrellas are available for rainy days, fresh brewed Starbucks coffee and fresh baked chocolate chip cookies replace the otherwise familiar odors of a practice waiting room, framed art and fresh cut flowers adorn the rooms, and small touches like heated exam tables for cats and small dogs, typed visit reports given to each departing client, exercise areas, and bar-less cage doors help round out the "wow" experience. And the "wow" shows up on the P&L too. This practice has consistently posted 20% growth rates, clients drive upwards of an hour past other veterinary providers, and new client numbers reach as high as 200 per month. That's 200 per month, not per year, and support staff and doctors routinely drop off resumes seeking employment. Revenues exceed $3MM and practice value is respectably >$2MM. This practice financially performs well, AND delivers on its customer service promises. It does it more effectively and efficiently than would be possible in the traditional designed practice, or the Taj Mahal that looks pretty but lacks true attention to the very rules that govern successful retail and entertainment architecture.

All of this makes sense only if we understand what business we are in. If we think we are in the business of being really good doctors in the most efficient and practical way possible, this makes no sense at all. If we are in the business of making clients feel good while providing great and compassionate medical care for their companion animals, then it makes a great deal of sense. Then we have to ask ourselves, what kind of facility built in what kind of location will make them feel the best? Every owner will be tempted to make her or himself the center of focus in the practice and will be tempted to accept architecture and design that pleases him or her. The wise owner will endorse the vision of a client-centered practice and will insist on an esthetic based on what the client wants. It is the client who is the key to the financial success of every veterinary hospital.

So yes, if you build it they WILL come. And if you do it right, they will come in droves.

HOW CAN YOU SUCCESSFULLY MARKET THAT BUSINESS?

Donald J. Erceg
VETMARK: The Veterinary Marketing Company
Portland, OR

Byron Farquer, DVM
Simmons Pacific
Oakdale, CA

LIFESTYLE MARKETING

Successful veterinary advertising targets the world of the woman who is the primary consumer of small animal veterinary services, paying particular attention to the issues of quality pet care, compassion, convenience and, most importantly, to "getting her" as a person. Health care for her "family" is a job she takes very seriously. She wants quality care and she will pay a premium to get it. Marketing is a way of reaching out to her and telling her that your hospital is the one for her. In deconstructing the success of marketers like Martha Stewart, Oprah Winfrey, Nike, and Starbucks, we can see that "lifestyle marketing" is the most powerful form of marketing. If you can reach out and touch her in the core of her lifestyle she will, indeed, beat a path to your door.

BUILDING YOUR BRAND

Brand names control market share in the retail world. Again think Nike and Starbucks. Do people prefer their products because of scientific proof of excellence? No. People prefer brand products because they trust them more. It makes them feel better to buy Nikes. Effective brand marketing for veterinary hospitals tells the family health care giver the woman, that you "get her"—that you understand that her pet is part of her lifestyle and your hospital is totally centered on her and her pet as the center of your universe. Your brand marketing is a promise to deliver to her a client-centered practice that stresses quality, compassionate pet care delivered with high-touch client service. The final part of good marketing is keeping your brand promises.

To develop a home in the public mind, you must first develop a compelling image for your hospital. Many doctors associate Image with the hospital logo. The logo is only the beginning. Your image is everything you look like, smell like, sound like. Everything about your practice that touches the senses of the consumer builds your image. Great care should be paid to your hospital name, logo, colors, choice of type faces, style of layout, use of photographs. Usually, the final choices are made by the doctor/owner. A strong argument could be made that the doctor/owner is the least qualified of all people to build a company image. "I like it" or "I don't like it" is a terrible way to make those decisions because he or she has no qualifications or experience to make good decisions regarding the development of corporate image. Just as graphic designers and marketers are not qualified to practice medicine, doctors are not qualified to develop corporate identities. That important job should be entrusted to a professional agency with a proven track history in image development. It is accepted truth that an attorney who chooses to represent himself has a fool for a client—even though the attorney is trained to practice law. How much more foolish is it for a practice owner to develop his own public image—a job for which he is totally untrained?

KEEPING YOUR BRAND PROMISES

Historically, veterinary hospitals have seen clients as passive recipients of services and products. As the experts, doctors and technical staff have thought of themselves as the top of the organization's hierarchy, while clients were at the bottom. Client-centered hospitals elevate clients and their pets to the top position.

It is not difficult to see what a well-run, client-centered company looks like. One only has to make a list of highly successful companies like Nike, Disney, Nordstrom, Starbucks. What makes them successful? They all place the client at the center of their universe.

Their advertising spends more energy talking about the client than about their companies. A visit to one of their stores leaves no doubt about what they are trying to do: they are trying to make me, the client, happy. An interviewer on National Public Radio visited a Starbucks outlet in Watts, a still depressed neighborhood in Los Angeles, and asked a young minority person drinking a fancy latte why he was here paying $3.50 when he could clearly save money by buying his cup of coffee elsewhere. His answer was revealing: "Where else could I go around here and feel this good for only $3.50?" It may be expensive coffee, but it is cheap happiness.

Nordstrom will assign you a personal consultant who will keep track of your sizes, favorite brands and colors, and will call you about new products and special deals. Most people are not wealthy enough to hire personal assistants. Nordstrom gives you one. Talk about relational marketing! Nordstrom makes you feel important because you are important—you are the most important person in that store!

Visitors to Disney World will have to look long and hard to find an impolite, disgruntled employee. Yet the starting wage is lower than the starting wage at most veterinary hospitals. If you don't know how to make people happy, you don't get hired by Disney. Disney World exists for one and only one reason—to make the visitor feel good.

Nike is not about Phil Knight. Oprah is not about Oprah Winfrey. Martha is not about Martha Stewart. They are all dedicated to making you feel good about yourself. Just Do It (Nike). Go For It (Oprah). Be True To Your Nature (Martha Stewart). Your hospital should not be about you, the doctor.

Customer loyalty, customer goodwill, is the most valuable asset a company possesses. Coca Cola could sell off all of its physical assets, all of its property and bottling plants, and it would still be worth billions of dollars. Why? Customer loyalty.

A PARADIGM SHIFT

Adopting a client-centered approach may require a shift in the attitudes of doctors and staff. Many doctors believe that technical proficiency is the measure of their worth and, therefore, is the most important thing in the hospital. This emphasis makes the doctors the central focus of the hospital. Every major decision regarding the hospital, location, operations, staffing, décor, etc is at the pleasure of the owner/doctor. As a result, staff members spend a lot of time and energy trying to keep the doctors and owners happy. That time and energy is best spend trying to make the client happy.

Even while trying to deliver high quality service, the doctors and technical staff have assumed that, as the experts, they know what is best for the clients. In client-centered hospitals, clients are considered first and foremost at every point in the planning, implementation and evaluation of service delivery. *Clients are the experts on their own needs and wants.*

How can we best serve the owner/pet bond? Creating a client-centered hospital has to become the mission of each and every member of the hospital team. This leads to a client-centered culture that always places the client first. A happy, delighted, well-served client is the cornerstone of good practice management and financial success.

CLIENT-CENTERED BENCHMARKS

High-touch Service. It is both profitable and socially responsible to provide client-centered, high-touch service. It is the right thing to do.

Happiness. Everyone wants to be happy. Focus your energy on the client's happiness and the rest will follow.

Relationships. While technical proficiency may be number one with the doctor, his or her relationship to the client is more important to the client. This makes bedside manner more important to the client's happiness than the doctor's medical skills.

Customer Satisfaction. Customer satisfaction is no longer the goal. Companies like Nike, Starbucks and Nordstrom have raised customer expectations far beyond "satisfaction." The new goals are "delight," "awe" and "surprise."

Committed to Excellence. Every hospital says that it is committed to excellence and has a tradition of quality. But is it committed to making the client feel good? For the client-centered practice, client happiness is the definition of excellence.

Feeling Good. Most of us equate "happiness" with "feeling good." Everything the client sees, hears, touches, and smells should have the single purpose of making that client "feel good." Remember, providing great care for the client's pet also makes the client feel good. What are some practical, simple steps that can be taken to create a client-centered practice?

A CLIENT-CENTERED CHECKLIST

- Write a mission statement that makes client happiness number one. Post that mission statement where the clients can read your commitment to them.
- Have staff create and commit to a list of ways to make clients feel good.
- When a client walks in the door, what words or actions will make it clear that the client is the most important person in the room?
- Is the bathroom easily accessible and pleasantly appointed?
- Are the magazines chosen to suit client taste or doctor and staff taste?
- Does your seating make clients comfortable?
- Is there music to listen to? Was it selected to please the client or the receptionist?
- Is the hospital meticulously, obsessively clean?
- Is the hospital well ordered: a place for everything and everything in its place?
- Have medical staff evaluate their own attitudes about who is number one.
- Does the medical staff religiously honor client appointment times?
- Do the doctors honor the client's need-to-know by taking time to explain their examination in detail to the client?
- How is their bedside manner? Do they look clients in the eye? Listen to them? Avoid talking down to them?
- Respect the value of the client's time.
- What is the longest time a person is kept on hold on the telephone?
- What is the average waiting time for a client in your lobby?
- Develop a relationship with the client.
- Address the client by name.
- Call the client after every procedure to see how the patient is doing.
- Keep good records of clients' preferences for appointment times, pet food brands, etc.

FROM TIRES TO PET CARE

All of us feel good when we walk into a store or business where the staff exudes a passion for their work and are upbeat and energetic. In the Western states there is an amazingly successful chain of tire stores called Les Schwab. Their brand is best represented by the high-energy staff that run to get your car, run to get the tires for the car, run your invoice back into the office. Their high, optimistic energy is contagious and spills over to the client. It makes the client feel good. Their bathrooms are meticulously clean. To seal the deal, they delight the client by providing free, theater-style popcorn while the client is waiting for the tire change. Finally, they want you to bring your car in for free periodic checkup and rotation of the tires! A fringe benefit to the Les Schwab Tire Company...people love working there. You can feel the pride they have. It is palpable. They are proud to offer you such good service. Your pet hospital should be even more concerned about developing a reputation for high-touch service than the Les Schwab Tire Company. Understandably the public has higher expectations for a medical facility than for a tire store. You should, too. As owner, your primary job is that of leader and the first and best way to lead is by setting the example for others. If you want to develop a culture of service in your hospital, you must yourself develop and perfect your own dedication to service.

Recommended Reading
1. Beckwith H. Selling the Invisible: A Field Guide to Modern Marketing. Time Warner, 1997.
2. Cialdini RB. William Morrow 1984. Influence: The Psychology of Persuasion. AAHA Press 1998.
3. Smith CA. Client Satisfaction Pays: Quality Service for Practice Success. The Path To High Quality Care: Practical Tips for Improving Compliance. American Animal Hospital Association, 2003.

WHAT BUSINESS ARE YOU IN?

Donald J. Erceg
VETMARK: The Veterinary Marketing Company
Portland, OR

Byron Farquer, DVM
Simmons Pacific
Oakdale, CA.

In this segment we are going to take a look at some companies and individuals who are super successful, like Nike, Starbucks, Martha Stewart, and Oprah Winfrey. If we can deconstruct their formulas for success, we can use the formulas to make your hospital successful. To follow their model we will need to answer two important questions: 1. What business are you in—what are you selling? 2. To whom are you selling it—which is your target audience?

WHAT BUSINESS ARE YOU IN?
This might sound like a dumb question. Conventional wisdom would say that you are in the business of providing medical care for animals. In the same manner, it might seem that Oprah is in the business of selling magazines and Nike is in the business of selling running shoes. Nothing could be further from the truth. Oprah is in the business of selling a way for women to feel good about themselves: We are all in this together. We can do it. We can reach our goals. "Go for it." Nike is not selling running shoes; they are selling a way for us to feel successful. Whether we are overweight and struggling to walk a mile, or a world-class runner in a marathon, we can do it: "Just do it." Martha Stewart is not selling magazines or towels. She is selling the belief that, as a woman, you can have that beautiful home with everything in its place. More than that—you owe it to yourself to "be true to your nature." The founder of Revlon cosmetics said "In the factories we make perfume. But in the stores, *we sell hope.*" All of these businesses are clearly focused on the consumer.

WHAT ARE YOU SELLING?
To see what business you are in, you have to look in from the outside, the way your client does. You may think that you are in the business of providing medical care to companion animals. Your clients, however, may think it is your business to support the human–animal bond by making them and their pet feel good. It's true that good medical care supports this bond, but so does healthy pet food, classes in pet behavior, quality grooming, community pet service, etc. The veterinarian may be tempted to focus on the delivery of quality medical services. The successful veterinary hospital is client-centered and focuses on the needs of the client.

WHO IS YOUR TARGET AUDIENCE?
All successful business is tightly focused on the end-user or consumer of product or services. To underscore the obvious, Medicare supplemental insurance is targeted at senior citizens, not high school students.

Who is the primary target for small-animal medical services? At first blush it might seem to be anyone who owns a pet. In an absolute sense, this is true. But from a marketing and positioning point of view, you need to be more precise. You can't be everything to everyone. You need to focus your business on the largest market segment of pet owners who actually use your veterinary services: Male or female, young or old, rich or poor, well educated or not, white collar or blue collar. After developing a good demographic picture of your client, you can develop a marketing message that speaks to his or her concerns and needs.

On a nationwide basis, most pets are owned by families with children. Within the family, the primary caregiver is the mother. She is the one responsible for choosing and taking the children to a pediatrician and, likewise, for choosing and taking the family pet to the veterinarian. In the words of the wonderful, old show on national public television, Rumpole of the Bailey, your target audience is "she who must be obeyed." She is both your target audience and the source of your financial success as a hospital.

If you want to be super-successful by all business and professional measures, place your client and her needs and wants and lifestyle solidly in the center of your practice. Measure your facility and landscaping and front-end staff and all service questions by her needs. Serving the bond between her and her pet is why your hospital exists. Remember, it is she who defines how that bond is best served, not you and your staff. To find out how she defines great service, you have to pay attention to her and you have to ask her. Developing a client-centered practice is your most important job as practice owner.

WHAT DO WE KNOW ABOUT HER AS A CONSUMER?
When it comes to medical care for her family, cost is not her primary concern. Surveys show that cost of treatments ranks no better than seventh in her list of concerns regarding veterinary care. The following list addresses the concerns that rank much higher on the priority of concerns:

- **Quality medical care.** She is the family caregiver and this is a job she takes very seriously. She wants to provide the very best care possible. An 82 year-old woman who lives below the poverty line on less than $900 a month manages to spend $30,000 on healthcare for her pet Boston Terrier. Providing good care was a very high priority and she scrimped everywhere else to make it possible.
- **Convenience.** She has to wear a lot of hats. She is probably employed, is a homemaker, soccer mom and maybe community volunteer. Time is very precious to her. How can you save her time? Provide a convenient location, easy parking, short waiting times, early morning drop-off and after-work pick-up, entertainment for her human children, one-stop-shopping for medical care (food, medicine, grooming, doggie daycare). Remember that she will

spend money to buy time to spend more time with her children, go to the gym to work out, or just have time to rest.

- **Community Service.** She places a very high value on public service and corporate good citizenship. Contribute to civic causes and let her know that you are doing so. You will score even higher position points if you become a conduit for her to contribute: organize an effort to establish a dog park in your community, become a resource for training her and the pet for therapy or other good work.
- **Compassionate Care.** She wants you to love her pet the way she does.
- **Bonding.** You cannot sell a woman on product or service alone. She wants to build a relationship with you and your staff. Get to know her and let her get to know you.
- **Feeling Good.** Like the rest of us, she likes to feel good. You can help her feel good by creating a hospital environment that is well ordered and pleasantly appointed, has soothing music, and offers comforting refreshments like coffee and chocolate.

GOING UPSCALE

A cursory examination of the retail world in the United States reveals a simple truth: society is moving from quantity of consumption to quality. Big box retailers like Target feature designer kitchen equipment and designer furniture. High thread count all cotton sheets are the rule, not the exception, at the on-line Overstock. High-end retailers like Crate & Barrel and Renovation Hardware are multiplying like rabbits. They are all marketing to your consumer. To see how you measure up as a retail service, don't compare yourself to other veterinary hospitals. Compare yourself to Martha Stewart, Oprah Winfrey, Nike, Starbucks, Crate & Barrel. They are the ones competing for her attention and setting the standards of serving her. If you understand that you are in a retail business as they do, you will do well.

BE THE FEEL GOOD HOSPITAL

While "feeling good" is a state of mind or personality, it has a chemical neurological underpinning. When people feel good, there is a rise of neurotransmitters like serotonin and oxytonin zipping around in the amygdala. There are things you can do to cause the level of these neurotransmitters to increase. For example, just the smell of chocolate can cause serotonin levels to increase in many women, or the sight of a puppy, or even something as simple as a smile or a compliment. Making people feel good is not manipulation, it is good manners and good business.

MEDICAL EXCELLENCE IS NOT ENOUGH

From the client's point of view, medical excellence is taken for granted. You are a doctor after all, so isn't your proficiency in medicine and surgery all that matter? Think again.

WHAT IS PRESUMED EXCELLENCE?

At one time being a highly qualified and medically competent doctor was all that was expected in practice. You hung a shingle, people brought their pets to you. At one time, there were many animals and very few veterinarians. People patronized practices because they needed pet medical service and the choices were few, often only one. Bestowed upon you, this degree of doctor comes with great public respect. Your clients consider you an expert already, commanding automatic trust and respect. In fact, studies show your doctor title caries some degree of automatic trust and general acceptance of your opinion, on any topic, regardless of your expertise. That means that before you open your mouth or pick up your scalpel and prove otherwise they believe you to be an expert. Look around your office. Very few people in their circle of friends have graduate degrees, certificates and licenses. BUT you are not unique. Your clients have that same feeling about **all** veterinarians. The suffix "DVM" will NOT attract clients. Where once being the veterinarian in town was all it took to collect new clients, today competition is keen. In many areas there are too many veterinarians. Thirteen practices in Tucson, AZ within 3 miles of each other, 9 in Santa Barbara, CA and whopping 23 in central Los Angeles. Simply having the title DVM is not enough today.

Do clients really care if you're a good doctor? Yes, of course your clients care that you are proficient and qualified. Today, things move very fast, and people rely on mental shortcuts to deal with the amazing amount of information and decisions required to navigate through life. Robert Cialdini describes this process in detail in his book *Influence: The Psychology of Persuasion*. For most of us we know the general principle as "first impression." Our minds use specific conditioned responses and shortcuts to quickly evaluate and instruct us how to act or react to any situation. This phenomenon is alive and well in your practice, each and every client is influenced by its principles. Society has also changed. Americans are embracing "trading up," a behavioral shift affecting the purchasing habits of buyers. This action refers to the willingness to pay a premium for goods and services that are perceived as higher in quality, performance, value AND remain emotionally significant to the buyer. This is well described by Michael Silverstien and Neil Fiske in the book *Trading Up, the New American Luxury*. Why does a shipping clerk earning $25,000 annually treat herself to silk sleepwear from Victoria's Secret, a young professional purchase a $100 specialty wine, and a middle class family purchase a $4000 Viking stainless-steel stove when a serviceable generic range was included from the builder? The answer lies in the willingness of consumers to pay a premium for desired products and services that are emotionally important to them. Make no mistake; these same consumers have no tolerance for over-priced, under-valued items or services. Don't be surprised to find the Jaguar driver shopping at Target for tableware, or the hourly retail worker shopping for a new $50,000 vehicle. Perception and emotion, not reality and logic, drive many purchase decisions.

Therefore, quite frankly, the consumer cares less about what you know than how you look, act, and how much you care about their pet. They already presume you are an expert, well educated, so immediately lend a critical eye to the rest of the picture. Interestingly, we also live in a unique time when the quality of service (been to the local restaurant lately?), cleanliness, and professionalism are at an all time low. Forty years ago the masses would have marched in the streets demanding a return to chivalry, high moral and ethical standards, and respect. Today, we barely whimper our dissatisfaction with yet one more lousy cold hamburger.

That presents an enormous opportunity for you to distinguish your practice in the market place. If you give your clients a fabulous experience in sight, sound, smell, and personal interaction, they not only will eat it up, they will pay a premium for it. Are you having trouble getting clients to accept the $1000 invoice? Is it too expensive for the BMW driving client or is it perceived as being overpriced or of low value? Look around your practice. Close your eyes and listen, and smell. Is it something else overcoming their acceptance of your expert skills?

Your hospital, staff, and everything about you must within seconds reach inside and grab their hearts, never letting go. By the time you have a chance to work on their minds the opportunity is gone. When we evaluate our own colleagues, we look at their levels of training, diagnostic capabilities, and the overall quality of medicine they practice in determining if they are "good" practitioners. Clients do not have the ability to make these judgments, so they make their decisions on what they do understand, such as how you present yourself, how you act, and, most importantly, **how much you care.** Most veterinary clients are women, age 25–45, educated, with kids, and make the family's health care decisions. Like it or not, your hospital screams in silence to your clients that you care (or that you don't). Remember, you have only one chance to make a first impression! The first thing clients see is your sign. This is hugely important and often the ONLY thing the public will ever see. Is it bright, clean, simple, easy to read, and does it tell WHO you are? Is your parking lot clean and well-striped with easy access for your elderly clients? As clients approach the front door, do you have planters with attractive, healthy plants, or are they dried up and dead? The new client may think, "Hmm, if they can't even keep PLANTS alive, I wonder what else dies here?" Are there spider webs dangling in the doorway? Are there children's chocolate-colored fingerprints all over the windows or are they spotless? They ask to themselves, "If you don't even care about keeping the bathroom clean, I wonder if you keep your surgery suite clean."

Most veterinarians are providing "task-driven service." Your client requests a service, vaccination, surgery, or presents the pet with a medical problem and requests you find a solution. You then provide a standard level of service and the client pays you.

Done. Your client is satisfied. Are you sure? He or she got what was expected perhaps but often nothing more. Picture the client receiving an incredible experience, way beyond what is expected? Not only will they pay you happily studies prove they will pay more.

Clients are usually not qualified to choose professionals with a critical eye. If you ask your neighbors for a recommendation for an attorney, they might say, "I just adore Janet Smith. She is so nice and I love her office and her staff. She always calls me right back and she also has a German Shepherd Dog just like mine. She is an excellent attorney. I highly recommend her!" Do any of these qualities really speak to her legal abilities? Not really, but she DOES have an enthusiastic referring client. Your clients will judge you on the things they CAN use to judge you, things that they understand and those that they are absolutely qualified to render an opinion on: cleanliness, odor, attitudes, promptness, creature comforts (coffee, e-mail access, free phone, refreshments, pleasing sounds, etc.) They are not equipped to judge your surgical ability, but they CAN look at the incision and see that it is neat, straight, and not blood soaked. They will notice instantly if Fluffy smells like urine or feces upon release, or if she has just been brushed, nails clipped, and a little bow in her collar.

Like it or not, veterinarians are in the service and retail business. You must adhere to the rules of the game. You must create an environment unlike all others in your industry, and emulate the star performers found in different industries your clients interact with daily. Then, after that important screening function is complied with, you really need to buckle down and provide excellence in medical care. This isn't an about face on the preceding information. Providing excellence in medical and surgical services is critical to your continued success as a veterinary service provider. When you practice good medicine, you increase your case success rates. When that occurs, patients improve and clients are satisfied. The details about understanding that you are first and foremost in a customer service business ensures that you set an environment and hospital culture that embraces that clients trust, and allows the client to "see" just how good a doctor you really are. With a strong positive emotional interaction between practice and client, communication pathways stay open. Instructions get relayed, home therapy and treatments are administered correctly, and pets win. It's only after you have ensured that you really understand AND buy into the fact that "you are not a veterinary hospital with great customer service. You are a great customer service organization that happens to be in a veterinary business" will you actually be able to achieve greatness on the medical side. In speaking to hundreds of veterinarians over the years, a significant number express dissatisfaction and frustration with the public not fully realizing how hard they work at being a good doctor and often how much better the quality of medicine is at their practice than their formidable competitor's practice nearby. One common theme we have witnessed in these situations is that many of these practices have significant deficiencies in the customer service area. Interestingly fate often brings us the ability to visit the very competing practice in question, and despite some of them having arguably deficiencies in medical standards, these practices often excel in customer service. It's not fair, but it's reality.

RECOMMENDED READING

1. Trout J. The New Positioning: The Latest on the World's #1 Business Strategy. McGraw Hill, 2006.
2. Beckwith H. Selling the Invisible: A Field Guide to Modern Marketing. Warner Books, 1997.
3. Levinson JC. Guerrilla Marketing: Secrets for Making Big Profits from your Small Company, 3rd edition. Houghton Mifflin Company, 1998.
4. Postrel V. The Substance of Style. HarperCollins Books, 2003.
5. Silverstien M, Fiske N. Trading Up, the New American Luxury. Penguin Group, 2003.
6. Cialdini,RB. William Morrow 1984. Influence: The Psychology of Persuasion. AAHA Press, 1998.

TRUE PRACTICE PROFITABILITY—HOW DOES YOURS COMPARE?

Karen E. Felsted, CPA, MS, DVM, CVPM
Gatto McFerson, CPA's
Santa Monica, CA

The Brakke Management and Behavior Study empirically demonstrated the importance to practice owners of understanding the finances of their practices and how few owners really do. Bottom line: The majority of practice owners don't understand financial terms and those that do, make more money. Only half of the group understood "pre-tax profits" and "cash flow." Only 10% to 20% of the respondents could choose the correct definition of the other terms in a multiple-choice format. And it makes a big difference in earnings—Male owners who answered three or more questions right had personal incomes of 7% greater than those who didn't and female owners who answered three or more questions right had incomes that were 19% higher than those who didn't.

In addition to the obvious impact on current cash flow, profitability also is a critical determinant of practice value. Historically, practice owners have assumed (and with good reason) that when they decided to sell their practices there would be buyers ready to purchase them and willing to pay a good price. In other words, they have assumed there was value in these businesses that could be transferred to someone else. Of course, there have always been a few practices for which this assumption didn't hold true. A buyer couldn't be found or what buyers wanted to pay wasn't remotely what the seller thought the practice was worth. Typically, these practices have been easy to identify and had several traits in common. They tended to be smaller practices with owners who had not focused much on the business side of things. Often the facility and equipment were old and the doctors hadn't kept up with the changes in medicine as much as perhaps they should have. These practices had little profit in them and, because the bulk of practice value is determined by profitability, the practices had little value. Fortunately, there weren't too many of these practices.

However, in the last few years, the number of practices with no or little value has been increasing—to the point where the Valuation Committee of the Association of Veterinary Practice Management Consultants and Advisors coined the term "No-Lo[SM] practice" to describe these practices. More and more practices, when appraised, did not have the value that would normally have been expected. And, in almost all cases, the owners of these practices were totally unaware of the problem. Some of these practices had traits in common with the practices that have historically had little or no value. They were small practices with a low level of profitability and couldn't keep up with changing client demands regarding service, quality of medicine, advanced technology, and improved facilities. The other practices with no or little value, however, were a surprising group. On the surface, these practices would appear to be doing very well. They are located in very attractive facilities, practice good medicine, have all the latest equipment and a large support staff, offer comparatively high compensation and benefits to their employees and, in the owners' eyes, cash flow is strong. However, practice value is largely based on profits and the very factors that make these practices look attractive on the surface are those that are reducing profitability.

Understanding the profitability of a practice is one of the most important concepts necessary to manage a veterinary hospital well. Calculating the true operating profitability of a practice is not a simple task. None of the standard financial or management reports a practice usually gets show this figure. Neither the taxable income from the tax return nor the net income from the profit and loss statement represents true profitability. This doesn't mean those reports are improperly prepared; it simply means the reports required by the IRS or accounting standards for small businesses weren't designed to determine profitability. No one report will give a practice all of the financial information it needs to make intelligent operating decisions; unfortunately, the report that seems to be prepared least often is the one that calculates true practice profitability. Because practice owners and managers aren't used to getting this kind of information, they generally don't know what the true profitability of their practice is. The first time many owners realize their true profitability is when their appraiser talks to them about it.

Operating profit is the difference between the operating revenues and expenses of a practice. Operating revenue and expenses include only items normally and necessarily seen in the day-to-day operations of the practice such as fees for professional services and drugs and medical supplies expense. These items should be stated at fair market value rates. For ease of comparison with other practices, the profit margin is generally stated as a percentage—this is calculated as practice profits divided by gross revenue. Some of the items that must be calculated differently to determine operating profit versus taxable income or net income include: practice owner payments, facility and equipment rent if these items are owned by the practice owner and leased to the practice, services provided by family members to the practice, depreciation, interest on debt and perks.

Owner compensation is one of the most significant adjustments and almost always has to be calculated differently in determining operating profits than would be done for the tax return or other reports. Owners often arbitrarily determine an amount they will be paid through their payroll system; this amount often has no correlation to the actual medical, surgical and management work the owner does in the practice and therefore the tax return or income statement looks as if the practice is more or less profitable than it really is. IRS regulations also dictate how some aspects of owner payments must be handled and these regulations vary by entity type. For example, owner compensation must be reported differently for a C corporation than for a partnership. A practice may appear to be more or less profitable than it really is simply because of these regulations.

So how do you calculate operating profit? Net income per the financial statements or tax return is the starting point. Various adjustments are made from there.

- Add back: depreciation, amortization, and interest on debt
- Deduct the estimated average amount spent on equipment per year—purchasing equipment is a true operating expense of the practice but depreciation as determined by tax law is not the best estimate
- Determine how much the owner was paid during the year and what it was comprised of (salary, rent, etc.)
- Adjust owner compensation to represent a fair compensation for medical/surgical work—20% of personal production is a good average in a small animal practice
- Adjust owner compensation for management work—management expense generally averages 3–4% of gross revenues—if you have a practice or office manager, the owner should get less than 3% of revenues as management compensation
- Adjust rent expense to fair market value if paid to owner at a rate greater or less than fair market value
- Adjust equipment lease expense to fair market value if paid to owner at a rate greater or less than fair market value
- Determine the $ amount of personal perks paid by the practice and remove this expense—perks would be items not necessary to the operation of the practice but paid by the practice generally to gain a tax advantage (examples include excess meals and entertainment, excess auto costs, swimming pool payments, personal furniture, trips to Tahiti, etc.)
- Deduct the cost associated with free services provided to the practice—family members may provide bookkeeping or other services to the practice at no charge—if the practice had to hire someone to do this work, there would be a cost involved and this should be included as an expense
- Remove any true non-recurring income or expenses such as one-time insurance proceeds or expenses related to a natural disaster
- Recalculate net income
- Divide the new net income by gross revenue

The resulting percentage is the true operating profit of the practice—how does it compare to other investments you have, and to other practices? Eighteen percent would be considered superior, 13% to 16% average, and less than 13% is below average.

If your profits aren't what you want them to be, what can you do about it? A lack of profitability either comes from revenues that are too low, expenses that are too high, or a combination of the two. Expense management is often the easiest to understand and is discussed first.

What practices don't do when making the decisions to invest in equipment, staff, or facilities is to make sure that the costs will lead to increased levels of revenue and thus profits. For example, how much space and what kind of building is really necessary to practice veterinary medicine? Operating out of the Taj Mahal can be very psychically rewarding but may not be good financially. For example, if a practice moves into a beautiful, new facility and the rent doubles, will there be a sufficient increase in revenue (and more importantly profits) to cover this rent increase?

The same goes for the addition of staff. A doctor's work life may be much easier and personally rewarding with three techs trailing behind him or her during the day, but does this doctor actually produce more revenue with this additional support staff? If not, the cost of the staff is eating into the profitability of the practice. Other staff problems seen in practices include the hiring of low-level, minimum wage staff that can't do the job properly, too many part-time employees and a lack of training and supervision. All of these lead to inefficiencies in getting the job done.

Declining revenue or a lack in growth of revenue is the other factor contributing to a lack of profitability. Practices often don't focus specifically on growing revenue because it's harder for them to determine what to do. In many cases, they've also been fortunate in that the revenue has just seemed to be there. If they don't have the 12% to 13% growth they did a few years ago, owners often assume that's just because the practice has matured or the demographics of their area are changing and that there is nothing they can do about it.

The reality is quite different, however, for many practices. Generally, there is much a practice can do to keep revenues strong even if located in a demographically challenged area. For example, are fees appropriate? It's not uncommon to see a practice that hasn't increased fees in 2 years or has only increased a few of them by a small percentage. Most expenses rise annually because the providers of those goods and services raise their prices—this is true of staff costs, drugs and medical supplies and the various other goods and services used by a typical practice. If the practice isn't raising its fees at least 5% per year, profitability will suffer even if nothing else changes in the practice.

Lack of attention to discounts and missed charges can also lead to declining revenue. Even a small amount of products or services given away by well-meaning doctors or other team members can significantly decrease revenue and profitability. Missed charges, those not deliberately given away, can also dramatically reduce the profit margin. Capturing charges is generally about having good systems in place and is essential to efficient operations. It is a rare practice who doesn't experience these problems on a fairly regular basis.

Understanding not only the profitability of the practice but the kinds of factors that lead to this state is critical. Until the practice has an idea of the root causes of the problem, it is difficult to determine what the correct solution is. Working with a financial advisor or practice consultant may help in not only gaining a greater understanding of the issues impacting profitability but in identifying and implementing solutions.

BUILDING AN EFFECTIVE ANNUAL REVENUE BUDGET

Karen E. Felsted, CPA, MS, DVM, VCPM
Gatto McFerson, CPA's
Santa Monica, CA

WHY BUDGET?

Budgeting, however dull or intimidating it may appear to be, is nonetheless an essential tool for just about anything you plan to do within your hospital.

- "If you don't know where you're going, how will you know when you get there?"
- "If you can't measure it, you can't manage it."

Budgeting is an essential planning tool for improving the medical and surgical services offered by a practice, increasing revenue, estimating cash flow, setting fees, analyzing expenses, monitoring cash flows and specifying operational changes.

Besides providing this very specific financial data, a budget forces planning which helps in the early identification of problems and in determining why circumstances might be expected to change in the future, and what could be done about it.

Budgeting is also an excellent way to communicate goals to the entire hospital staff, and to ensure that these goals are coordinated. Although the focus of this article is on the revenue side of the budget, expenses should still be included in the budget so that the impact on cash flow of all planned programs can be seen. This article includes information on budgeting for both areas.

STEPS TO CREATING A BUDGET

- Gather the basic information
- Input historical data into a spreadsheet program
- Identify the financial changes expected in the practice next year
- Identify the changes the practice would like to see in the practice next year
- Determine the budget for next year

Gather the Basic Information

Start the budgeting process for the next year three to four months before the end of the current year. First, collect the profit and loss statements (P&L) or tax returns from the past 2 full years as well as a year-to-date statement from the current year (Table 1).

Although the P&L statements from accounting software may provide more detail than the tax return, it is essential that the P&L figures are reconciled to those in the tax return, which is the most reliable source of financial data for the practice. This may require some work to determine how separate line items in the P&L were grouped together to produce the figures in the tax return, but it is essential that this happens.

The practice management information system (PMIS) has a report that shows revenue by category. Categories most frequently seen include vaccination income, surgery income, anesthesia revenue, dentistry income, laboratory income, hospitalization, food sales, pharmacy sales, and so on. In some PMISs, two reports must be printed—one for the service categories and one for the product sale categories.

Table 1. Year-to-Date Profit and Loss Statement

ID	SERVICE TYPE DESCRIPTION	YEAR TO DATE	
		FREQ	SALES
010	VACCINATIONS	499	$116,197.50
020	PROFESSIONAL SERVICES	653	$223,373.72
030	SURGERY	131	$86,982.18
040	ANESTHESIA	24	$21,583.92
050	LABORATORY	187	$108,126.22
055	RADIOLOGY	42	$30,967.75
060	HOSPITALIZATION	125	$31,972.17
065	BOARDING	681	$44,037.31
075	DENTAL	38	$36,828.48
080	MISCELLANEOUS	3	$0.00
085	GROOMING	10	$1,366.51
500	LABORATORY	3	$1,076.83
PH	ANTIBIOTICS	2,485	$150,299.41
FOO	FOOD & PRESCRIPTION DIETS	709	$44,520.76
SUP	OTC SUPPLIES	85	$3,901.99
		5,675	$901,234.75

Input Historical Data into a Spreadsheet Program

A spreadsheet program is superior to a paper and pencil budget because it is faster, more accurate and also allows for "what if" scenarios. To enter a budget it is only necessary to know spreadsheet basics: how to input data, how to sum data and do simple arithmetic calculations. More and more people already have these basic skills, but if training is necessary, the basics are easily obtained by courses on disk or from a book, from instructor-led courses at local community colleges or computer stores, or from a family member or friend. With these skills, it is easy to prepare the budget that is illustrated in Table 2.

- Input the data from the last two year's financial statements as well as the YTD information from the current year
- Annualize the partial year data
- List revenue and expense categories down the side, and the dollar amounts and percentage of gross revenues for each year across the top
- The net income or taxable income line should be a formula subtracting all the expenses from the revenue. This must match the net income on the tax return.

The percentage column is important because it shows variable costs versus fixed costs and allows for an analysis of the consistency of revenues and expenses even when dollar amounts change.

The percentage category calculation is the revenue or expense line item divided by the total gross revenues.

Revenue shown on the income statement will usually consist of just one line so use the revenue category report as mentioned above, to break this out. It is very likely that there will be difference between the total on the revenue by category report and the financial statements and tax return. To deal with this:

- Put it in a line item called "unidentified revenue"
- If its more than 1% of gross revenue and can't be explained by the growth in receivables, the difference needs to be investigated
- Data entered above results in practice profit or taxable income. The most useful budget is one that shows cash flow. To convert the exiting budget to cash flow:
- Add back depreciation
- Subtract principle payments on loans and capital leases

Identify Expected Practice Changes

The next step is to identify practices changes that are fairly certain to happen, such as fee increases, rent or utilities increases; new hires not fully represented in current year financials and raises.

Identify Desired Practice Changes (Generally Expense Items)

Goals can be those of the practice and owner, they can be personal and professional, they can be financial and non-financial. Sample goals are as follows:

- Purchase of new equipment
- Attend a particular CE conference
- Hire more staff
- Hire a new veterinarian
- Give the staff a raise and more benefits
- Provide more training for the staff

It is important to quantify the financial aspect of each goal. Most goals are about spending more money. To achieve these new goals, the practice needs to make more money or spend less money. This frequently involves changing the areas in which the practice is spending money and focusing more on revenue.

Table 2. Preparing a Budget

	Actual results		Actual results		Budget amounts	
	2005	%	2006	%	2007	%
Revenue						
Fees for services	$852,339	100.00%	$912,675	100.00%		
Total Revenues	852,339	100.00%	912,675	100.00%		
Cost of Professional Services						
Animal disposal	4,673	0.55%	5,788	0.63%		
Drugs and medical supplies	70,344	8.25%	75,222	8.24%		
Laboratory costs	27,466	3.22%	32,175	3.53%		

Determine the Budget for Next Year

The starting point for next year's budget is the information just entered above. For the expense items, enter fixed expenses as the dollars you expect them to be. The cost of medical services is best entered as a percent of the revenue, based on prior year percentages of revenue. Change all expenses to include all known changes as well as those brought about by your goals.

Revenue is generally much more difficult to estimate than expenses. There are several ways, however, to look at it and to make meaningful estimates.

- The prior year revenue figure can, of course, be increased by any known fee increases.
- Some amount can be added for growth in transactions based on history.
- The biggest revenue planning opportunity, however, is through the addition of new programs and services. Several examples are shown below.

Increasing the Frequency of Services Currently Offered

For example, perhaps the practice would like to focus on increasing the frequency with which preanesthetic blood profiles are performed.

First of all, what needs to happen logistically in the practice to insure the success of this type of program? First, the doctors must be consistent in making these recommendations for preanesthetic bloodwork. They may need to set standards among themselves as to when they will do so. At what age will blood work be recommended? At what age what will it be required? Specifically what tests will be done?

Staff people must be able to talk intelligently about the benefits of preanesthetic lab work to clients. If they cannot explain those benefits know, training needs to be done to help them learn to do so. Receptionists must have the time to talk with clients about this recommendation when clients drop their pets off. The practice may need to add another receptionist during the morning rush so that receptionists have the time to educate clients.

Also, there will need to be enough technicians to perform the additional lab tests before surgery starts. Technicians also need to feel comfortable reminding the doctors if they forget to mention preanesthetic bloodwork to clients.

How would you calculate the effect of this on the budget? (This thought process can be applied to any similar revenue item.)

- Calculate the number of preanesthetic profiles the practice did in the prior year
- Calculate what percent this was of total anesthetic procedures
- Decide by what amount the practice would like to increase this percent
- Calculate the increase in both revenue and expense from this increase

Offering New Services

One way to increase the profitability of a practice is through the offering of new services. Careful planning should go into this decision, however, in order to maximize the benefits. One service that can help with this goal is grooming. This service, however, must be implemented well in order to be profitable and not turn into a management nightmare.

Grooming, by itself, is not usually highly profitable. However, the medical services generated from grooming clients is where the additional revenue comes from. Do not leave this to chance—if you are going to offer grooming, do it right. The first step in making this a profitable service is to train your groomer.

- Include them in all hospital meetings and training
- Treat them as part of the team
- Teach them to recognize basic medical problems—eyes, ears, nose, teeth, skin, lumps and bumps
- Include client service training

Groomers obviously aren't doctors, but there is no reason they can't discuss basic medical issues with clients in the same way that receptionists and technicians do. When the groomer identifies a potential medical issue, they should discuss it with the client and offer to have a doctor look at the pet. Ideally, the groomer will call the client so the pet can be examined while it is still at the practice. Any findings noted by the groomer should be listed on the grooming report card.

As with most services, effective marketing makes a difference:

- Convenient hours for drop off and pick up of pet
- Convenient way for drop-off owners to talk to groomer
- Window between grooming room and reception area so people can watch the service
- Introduce groomer in hospital tours
- Frequent groomer cards
- Gifts for good pets
- Business cards
- Grooming seminars
- Before and after photos on reception area walls
- Before and after pictures to send with client
- Give hospital support staff a free groom for every 10 referrals

Budget revenue estimates can be made by calculating the medical revenue expected to be brought into the practice by offering grooming:

- No. of grooms/day X average fee charged for grooming
- No. of ears referred X average fee for treatment
- No. of skin problems referred X average fee for treatment
- No. of dentals referred X average fee for treatment
- etc.

The total should be decreased by an estimate of the revenue generated from clients who would have come to the practice even if grooming services were not offered

And, of course, estimates for the associated costs of the groomer and the medical treatment must also be included in the expense side of the budget.

New medical services may also be a source of increased revenue. Many new medical services will involve the purchase of new equipment and yet these purchases are often made without much thought. Effective planning will involve all aspects of the service expansion decision—client needs, doctor interest, staff expertise—as well as the financial aspect.

For example, a veterinary practice may want to purchase an ultrasound unit costing $30,000. This is an expensive piece of equipment and if this is the first such ultrasound to be owned by the practice, it may not be clear if there will be enough usage to justify the purchase. It is unlikely the payback on the machine will occur within the first year or two and other questions will also have to be addressed.

- What kinds of cases will benefit from an ultrasound exam?
- Are all the doctors in the practice committed to using the machine?
- How will the doctors be trained in its usage?
- Will outside interpretation of the images need to be made during the early months of usage? How much will this cost?
- Will additional support staff be needed if the ultrasound is used frequently?
- How will clients be educated as to the benefits of the new diagnostic tests?
- How will the machine be financed?

- Are there timing issues to consider in the acquisition?
- What fees will be charged for the exams?

There are a number of techniques that are extremely useful in analyzing the purchase of new equipment. These techniques can be used in contemplating the purchase of just one asset (for example, the ultrasound) or in comparing the benefits of two different assets (for example, an ultrasound versus a laser surgical unit.) Two of the more commonly used financial techniques are payback period analysis and net present value analysis. These figures can then be input into the overall budget to determine the impact of these potential programs on the cash flow of the practice.

Finalization of the Budget

Creating a viable budget is an iterative process; there will generally be multiple changes before deciding on a final choice of goals. Critical to the process is net cash flow desired next year and the importance and viability of individual goals

Hints for a Successful Budget
- Be liberal with expense estimates and conservative with revenue estimates
- Leave room for surprises
- Start with a simple budget and then use it to calculate the effect of more complicated plans
- Get help when you need it
- Give yourself the time needed for the process
- Be sure that you have accurate in-house accounting system
- Compare your revenue and expense ratios to industry revenue and expense ratios
- Be sure to get staff input

DEALING WITH WHINY, GOSSIPY, PROBLEM-CHILDREN EMPLOYEES IN YOUR PRACTICE

Karen E. Felsted, CPA, MS, DVM, CVPM
Gatto McFerson, CPA's
Santa Monica, CA

It doesn't matter if you have whiny, gossipy or any other kind of problem-children employees in your practice; the issues need to be managed in a similar way. Four things to remember:

- Communicate expectations
- Act like a leader
- Manage behavior, not personalities
- Fire the ones that need to be fired

COMMUNICATING EXPECTATIONS

One of the most essential aspects of leadership is the intangible quality of "vision." Leaders need to have a clear idea of where they want to go and the energy and enthusiasm to inspire followers to reach that goal. Consider the following nine steps you can take to communicate your goals to your employees and to inspire them in making progress toward your objectives:

- Expect the best from your people and you will usually get it.
- Praise employees in public.
- Give credit where credit is due.
- Show interest in and appreciation for your staff in many ways.
- State suggestions and requests clearly.
- Explain the reasons behind your suggestions.
- Give your people goals, a sense of direction, something to strive for.
- Give frequent constructive performance reviews with plans for betterment.
- Tell employees what your priorities are, particularly when they change.

ACT LIKE A LEADER

If you want your people to take responsibility for their work and to behave in a certain way, then you have to do the same. If you complain about clients, you have given the staff permission to do the same. If you come in late, you have effectively told the staff it is OK to do so. By setting a good example, you can establish standards for accountability that your employees will take seriously. When you're wrong or make a mistake, admit.

MANAGE BEHAVIOR, NOT PERSONALITIES

How criticism is presented is critical. The most important point to remember is: Evaluate the behavior, not the person.

Example: "John, you have no initiative."

When you say this to John, his first reaction will be to get defensive. He knows you are talking about a big character flaw and he is busy thinking up all the times he has demonstrated initiative. Plus he really doesn't know what you are talking about so doesn't know what to fix.

Example: "John, we need you to let the doctors know when a boarding animal is lethargic or not eating. This is the fourth dog this week we haven't been informed about."

John still knows there are areas he needs to improve in but he knows the specific behavior to fix. And he doesn't feel his character has been decimated.

FIRE THE ONES THAT NEED TO BE FIRED

At some time, a few of the problem children need to be fired. No one likes doing it but do it the right way.

- Define the problem clearly to the employee in behavioral terms
- Review communication of expectation
- Look for contributing causes
- Document, document, document
- If appropriate, prepare a performance improvement plan and give the employee a chance to improve
- Don't wait too long
- Be specific with the employee when their job is in jeopardy
- Make sure treatment is consistent among employees
- Consider talking to your attorney if the issue are sensitive
- Have a plan for replacement in mind
- Learn from your mistakes

EQUIPMENT PURCHASE FOR FUN AND PROFIT – PART I

Karen E. Felsted, CPA, MS, DVM, CVPM
Gatto McFerson, CPA's
Santa Monica, CA

Three factors are essential to the practice of quality medicine and surgery:

- A doctor with a high level of knowledge and skills in veterinary medicine
- An appropriate range of high-quality equipment for both diagnostics and treatment
- An appropriate range of safe and effective therapeutic agents

If any one of these factors is missing or of substandard quality, patient care will suffer.

In this article, the second factor, equipment, will be discussed. Unfortunately, equipment usually cannot be purchased JUST because it contributes to high-quality care. It must also pay for itself.

Most veterinarians make their most comprehensive purchase of equipment at the time they buy or start a practice. However, any successful hospital must be continually replacing and upgrading equipment as well as purchasing new technology if they are to continue offering the highest quality of care to their clients and their patients.

Whether a doctor is buying one piece of equipment or several, the principles are the same.

It must first be understood what the goal of the acquisition is. Will the new equipment improve patient care? For example, the purchase of a CT scanner may allow for more accurate diagnoses. Will the new equipment lower the operating costs related to the provision of services? A new blood chemistry unit may lower the direct costs incurred in running a blood profile because less maintenance is required for the unit. An automatic processor may improve staff efficiency and lower staff costs because the time needed to develop radiographs is less. Will the new equipment increase revenues? Use of a laser surgery unit may allow a practice to increase the surgical fees charged. Often, more than one of these goals is met with the acquisition of a single piece of equipment. For example, an IV fluid pump will often reduce staff costs related to monitoring fluid administration as well as improve patient care by more accurately ensuring patients receive the volume of fluids needed.

If a practice buys a piece of equipment that does not meet one of the above goals, the purchase usually falls into either the coat rack or toy category. The first category includes all the equipment purchased that is never used, sits in a corner, gathers dust, and is used to hang coats on. The second category includes all the equipment purchased and used occasionally, but never consistently or profitably. Coat rack equipment purchases are a failure in all regards. Toy equipment may provide much enjoyment and satisfaction to the purchaser and is not necessarily a bad decision, but the purchaser must understand that instead of making a wise, profit-generating business decision, he or she is instead using part of his or her profits to purchase a fun item, much in the same way as they might use those profits to purchase a lake house.

As noted earlier, the most significant purchase of equipment in dollar terms often comes when a veterinarian buys or starts a practice. However, this may not be the time during which the buyer can exercise total choice in type of equipment, brand, or features. The buyer of the practice does not usually have much choice in what equipment he or she will receive as part of the practice purchase. Generally the purchase is a package deal, although there may be some room for purchase price negotiation if certain equipment is seriously outdated or in need of repair.

Veterinarians starting their own practice from the ground up theoretically have total flexibility in purchasing equipment; however, most doctors cannot purchase everything they'd like to have at the outset due to lender restrictions and limited personal capital. In these cases, it is necessary to decide which equipment and of what quality is essential to the start-up of the practice and which items can remain on the wish list until further money is available. The purchase of used equipment from veterinary or human medical companies or on an internet auction site can help reduce the initial capital outlay. However, the quality of these may vary greatly and care should be taken in selecting your vendor, particularly with a high-dollar piece of equipment.

The decision to purchase an individual piece of equipment by a practice with a reasonable cash flow is often the time when the veterinarian can exercise the most choice in selection. "Selection" doesn't just mean picking the equipment one is most interested in learning to use with the features most desired. Selection also includes performing the financial analysis necessary to determine if the equipment purchase will likely increase the profits of the practice.

The term **capital budgeting** involves all of the financial planning and analysis tasks associated with buying capital assets. Capital assets are those with a life of greater than one year and expected returns over a period greater than one year. The one-year cut-off is somewhat arbitrary but conforms to the concept of current and long-term assets and liabilities that is standardly used in financial statement preparation. Almost all equipment purchased by a hospital is expected to have a life of greater than one year.

The process of capital budgeting can be loosely divided into two sections—analyzing the acquisition of certain assets for profitability and, assuming that a transaction appears to be a sound one, determining if the cash flow necessary to finance the transaction will be available from the business or must be obtained elsewhere.

There are many considerations, financial and managerial, associated with planning and implementing the purchase of assets of this kind. The decision to purchase some capital assets may be an easy one—for example, it may be clear that the practice needs a new anesthetic machine and even though this is a long-term asset, its cost is not too great and the practice already uses this type of equipment daily; therefore the decision is clear-cut.

The purchase of more expensive assets and those not previously used in the practice, however, requires more planning and forethought than does the purchase of equipment or supplies with a much shorter life. As with any asset, it is important to understand why the new equipment is necessary. Mentioned earlier were the most common reasons: to improve patient care, to lower operating costs (either direct costs or via increased staff efficiency), or to increase revenues.

However, because the cost of certain capital assets is high, the positive results may not be seen immediately and other aspects of a practice may also be impacted by the purchase, the risk associated with their purchase is much greater. Clearly, a $500 piece of equipment that sits in the corner and gathers dust is not nearly as much of a problem as a $15,000 such item. For example, a veterinary practice may want to purchase a CT scanner costing $110,000. This clearly is much more expensive than an anesthesia machine and if this is the first such scanner to be owned by the practice, it may not be clear if there will be enough usage to justify the purchase. Many questions need to be addressed.

- What kinds of cases will benefit from a scan?
- Are all the doctors in the practice committed to using the machine?
- How will the doctors be trained in its usage?
- Will outside interpretation of the images need to be made during the early months of usage? How much will this cost?
- Will additional support staff be needed if the scanner is used frequently?
- How will clients be educated as to the benefits of the new diagnostic tests?
- How will the machine be financed?
- Are there timing issues to consider in the acquisition?
- What fees will be charged for the imaging?

There are a number of capital budgeting techniques that are extremely useful in analyzing the purchase of new equipment. These techniques can be used in contemplating the purchase of just one asset (for example, the scanner) or in comparing the benefits of two different assets (for example, a CT scanner vs. MRI equipment).

As with any analysis, good data is critical to good results. A number of variables will be used in these calculations such as the cost of the equipment, the additional annual costs associated with the asset (such as a service contract or supplies), the expected cost savings to be obtained from usage or the anticipated increase in revenues. If these items are not accurately estimated, the results of the acquisition analysis may be erroneous. For example, cost of equipment does not just include the sticker price. Other components of cost

include tax, installation, training, and interest costs if the asset is financed.

Some of the more commonly used financial techniques are payback period analysis, net present value calculations, and breakeven analysis. Breakeven analysis will be covered in Part 2 of this article.

The **payback period** is the number of years necessary to breakeven on the purchase of the asset. After this point, the practice will start to realize a profit on the acquisition assuming the figures used in the analysis are accurate and reality conforms to the assumptions made in the analysis. The payback period is calculated as:

$$\frac{\text{Total purchase price}}{\text{Annual net income (ie, revenue minus operating costs for a year)}}$$

Example:

The Felsted Cat Clinic is planning to purchase a CT scanner with a total cost of $114,000. Dr. Felsted already has a large storage room in her clinic that can be converted to house the scanner. This conversion will cost about $4,000. The average fee charged to clients per procedure will be $655. On average the practice estimates it will perform 5 scans per week or 260 per year at a cost to the practice of $195.60 each. Costs to the practice include veterinarian compensation related to provision of the service, staff time, and supplies. Additional annual operating costs average $21,665 for maintenance, electricity and interest.

$$\text{Payback period} = \frac{\$114,000}{((\$655 - \$195.6) \times 260) - \$21,665}$$

$$= 1.17$$

In other words, it will take 1.17 years to pay for this machine before any profits will be made by the clinic on this service.

The payback period is not the only tool that should be used in analyzing an asset purchase. Acquisitions with the shortest payback period may not be the ones that are ultimately the most profitable to the practice. It is also important to remember that the time value of money has not been factored into this calculation.

Net present value (NPV) analysis estimates the total cash outflows involved with the purchase of an asset compared with the total inflows. A positive outcome equals a profitable purchase. NPV analysis also incorporates the time value of money into the calculations.

The difference in value depends on the interest rate used in the calculation. Differences get larger with higher interest rates and longer payback periods.

While this calculation gives more accurate information, it is also more difficult to do and many small business owners will enlist the aid of their accountant or financial advisor in performing this calculation.

Continuing the example used above, the NPV analysis for the first five years of the life of the scanner is as follows. The first chart calculates the cash flow related to the purchase as well as the income expected each year less operating costs and maintenance.

Year	Cash out	Cash in	Net flow
0	($114,000) (purchase)		($114,000)
1	($69,882)	$170,300	$100,418
2	($68,335)	$170,300	$101,965
3	($66,660)	$170,300	$103,640
4	($89,846)	$170,300	$ 80,454
5	($62,881)	$170,300	$107,419
			$379,896

The next chart calculates the discounted cash flow using present value factors.

Year	Net cash flow	8% PV factor	Discounted net cash flow
0	($114,000)	1	($114,000)
1	$100,418	.926	$92,987
2	$101,965	.857	$87,384
3	$103,640	.794	$82,290
4	$80,454	.735	$59,134
5	$107,419	.681	$73,153
			$280,947

After allowing for the time value of money, it is expected that use of the new scanner will generate profits of $280,947 during the first five years. If this analysis is done on a monthly basis instead of an annual basis, the payback period turns out to be 1.24 years instead of 1.17 years due to the time value of money.

This analysis could be performed over the full expected life of the equipment in order to estimate the total profitability. If this were done, any amounts expected to be realized from the sale of the equipment at the end of its life should be recognized as an inflow and any costs of disposal should be recognized as an outflow. This is a useful calculation when comparing the potential profitability of two or more pieces of equipment.

Tax effects and alternative financing can be included for even more precise analysis, but those calculations are beyond the scope of this document.

(Costs related to purchasing and operating a CT scanner were graciously made available by TW Medical Veterinary Supply.)

EQUIPMENT PURCHASE FOR FUN AND PROFIT– PART 2

Karen E. Felsted, CPA, MS, DVM, CVPM
Gatto McFerson, CPA's
Santa Monica, CA

Some of the more commonly used financial techniques used in analyzing the purchase of new equipment are payback period analysis, net present value calculations, and breakeven analysis. Payback period analysis and net present value calculations are discussed in Part 1 of this article.

Breakeven analysis is a very useful tool for studying the relationships between revenues, fixed costs, and variable costs. It is particularly helpful in analyzing the consequences of starting or expanding a business or when acquiring significant pieces of new equipment.

The breakeven point is the level of sales that will just cover all costs, both fixed and variable. Variable costs are those that fluctuate directly with revenue. For example, variable costs in a veterinary practice would include anesthesia, drugs, and supplies. If no patients are seen, none of these items are used and there is no associated cost.

Fixed costs are those that do not fluctuate with revenue over some range of this revenue. For example, the rent paid to lease the building a veterinary practice is located in is a fixed cost. Even if no clients come in the door and no revenue is generated by the practice, the business still has to pay rent. Very few fixed costs, however, are fixed forever over the life of the business. A two–exam room veterinary hospital may spend $1500/month in rent payments for the facility. This amount will be the same whether the practice generates $300,000 or $600,000 in revenue per year. There will come a point; however, at which the building is simply too small to accommodate any more clients or any more revenue growth. In order to continue growing the business, facility expansion will have to occur and this cost will increase. Rent is a fixed cost over a very wide range of revenue (in this case from $0 to perhaps $900,000) but at some point the cost will change. It is important recognize that if there were no fixed costs, there would be no breakeven point. A practice would have no costs if it had no revenue.

Some costs that don't fluctuate directly with revenue but must be increased over shorter ranges of revenue than an item like rent are often called semi-variable costs—staff salaries would be an example in a veterinary clinic. At the breakeven point:

Revenue = fixed costs plus variable costs

or

Revenue = total costs

Breakeven analysis can be used very effectively for new equipment decisions. For example, let's assume the Felsted Cat Clinic has been in existence for 5 years and has been doing very well. Dr. Felsted decides to buy a CT scanner and wants to know how many scans she will have to do in order to pay off this machine in 2 years. The machine costs $114,000 and the average fee charged to clients per view is $655.00. Costs to the practice for each scan are $196.00 and include veterinarian compensation related to provision of the service, staff time, and supplies. Annual maintenance, interest and electricity costs for the scanner average $21,665.

$$\text{Number of scans} = \frac{\text{Fixed costs } (\$114,000) + 2 \text{ years operating costs } (2*(\$21,665))}{\text{Profit per scan } (\$655–\$196)}$$

$$= 342$$

Dr. Felsted must do 342 scans in order to pay for this machine and start making a profit. Since she anticipates doing 5 scans a week (260 per year) she feels this machine can be paid for in a reasonable amount of time. It is important to note that this is a fairly simple example that excludes the time value of money.

While breakeven analysis is very useful in understanding the relationships between transaction volume, prices and costs, it does have some weaknesses. As with all analyses, reasonable estimates are essential. The linear assumptions made may not hold true in all cases; for example, as the volume of transactions increases, variable costs may increase or decrease on a per unit basis.

(Costs related to purchasing and operating a CT scanner were graciously made available by TW Medical Veterinary Supply.)

SUCCESSION PLANNING—WHAT DOES THIS MEAN AND WHAT DO YOU DO?

Karen E. Felsted, CPA, MS, DVM, CVPM
Gatto McFerson, CPA's
Santa Monica, CA

In formal terms, succession planning is the process to be followed in finding replacements for key individuals in an organization. In small businesses such as veterinary medicine, it often means, "who am I going to sell my practice to?" However, even in the smallest of practices, the process, if it is to be successful, isn't as simple as that.

Succession planning isn't just about choosing a successor; it's about choosing one who will be successful. To do that, the current owners of the practice need to have a good understanding of what has made the practice successful so far and what skills the new owners must have in order to keep the practice successful in the future. Identifying these skills and finding and mentoring this individual can be very time-consuming. Of course, if you're going to sell the practice in its entirety, will have no financial involvement in it after the sale and don't care if it fails once you're gone, you can ignore finding the right person and just sell to anyone. But most people aren't in this position financially or have more of an emotional interest in seeing what they've built continue to do well so they need to pick the right successor.

A successful exit strategy begins with understanding why you want to sell; common reasons are listed below:

- Ready to fully retire
- Want to decrease workload
- Desire to change careers
- Desire to practice more medicine
- Health issues
- Divorce
- Location/demographics of practice are poor
- Management frustrations
- Financial issues
- Want to bond associate to practice

Intertwined with the whys are the goals you want to achieve along with or through the sale; some common ones include:

- Financial security
- Leaving of a legacy
- Staff security
- Clients taken care of
- Transparent changing of the guard

These are the questions and issues that are most difficult to deal with and take the most time. Once they are answered rest of it is almost easy.

The most common options in transitioning a practice include a partial sale to an associate, a full sale of the practice either to an associate or an outside buyer, a sale of the practice to a corporate group, or a merger.

Selling part or all of the practice to an associate is the most common sale type and the easiest if you can manage it. It presents the greatest opportunity to know if the buyer is the right fit and has the right skills. If you are the owner of a C corporation, a partial sale of stock to an associate can be a great way of dealing with a thorny tax issue. Even though you may know the buyer well, the transaction should be handled as if this was an unknown individual and the usual due diligence and legal activities carried out.

Selling to an outside veterinarian is another option frequently seen. It is not as attractive as selling to an associate because it can be harder to locate the buyer and sales cost may be incurred that wouldn't be involved in an associate buy-in. And the seller may not have as much choice in selecting the specific person he or she wants to take over the practice and perpetuate the legacy. However, many practices are successfully transacted in this way.

Another option available to bigger practices (two to three doctors with $1,000,000 in revenues in desirable locations) is sale to a corporate buyer. This can be a very attractive option for many owners; however, the owner will likely be required to stay with the practice for several years and won't have the freedom and flexibility they had as owner.

A merger is a great idea if you can find the right partner. This can be a slow process but is still the fastest way to grow a practice and increase potential associate buyers. Finding the right partner, however, is difficult and it is critical to get one with the same values and philosophies as you. Hearing the same cliché over and over is very boring but clichés are clichés because they are true and this one certainly is. A merger is like a marriage and you need to want to be with your partner long-term. A corporate divorce is no prettier than a marital one.

No matter which of the options above you end up going with, many of the "logistics" regarding practice valuation, financing, legal work, etc will be similar. Planning is key and you must start early. If you need to do an S corp election, find the right partner, or need to significantly improve the practice value, 10 years is not too soon. Three to 5 years may be enough for fine-tuning value.

A core team of advisors is essential—practice appraiser, practice consultant, CPA, attorney and possibly a broker. Some of these roles can overlap but they will all need to be filled by someone. Your advisors can help you avoid some of the common pitfalls encountered in succession planning:

- Lack of business strategy
- Unrealistic value expectations
- Rationalizing of management and leadership qualities of buyer
- Lack of understanding of process

What can you do know to start the process?
- PLAN, PLAN, PLAN
- PONDER, PONDER, PONDER
- NAIL DOWN NEEDS AND WANTS

TRENDS IN PRACTICE VALUATION

Karen E. Felsted, CPA, MS, DVM, CVPM
Gatto McFerson, CPA's
Santa Monica, CA

Historically, practice owners have assumed (and with good reason) that when they decided to sell their practices there would be buyers ready to purchase them and willing to pay a good price. In other words, they have assumed there was value in these businesses that could be transferred to someone else. Of course, there have always been a few practices for which this assumption did not hold true. A buyer could not be found or what buyers wanted to pay was not remotely what the seller thought the practice was worth. Typically these practices have been easy to identify and had several traits in common. They tended to be smaller practices with owners who had not focused much on the business side of things. Often the facility and equipment were old and the doctors had not kept up with the changes in medicine as much as perhaps they should have. These practices had little profit in them and, because the bulk of practice value is determined by profitability, the practices had little value. Fortunately there were not too many of these practices.

In the last few years, however, the number of practices with no or little value has been increasing—to the point where the Valuation Committee of the Association of Veterinary Practice Management Consultants and Advisors coined the term "No-Lo[SM] practice" to describe these practices.

More and more practices, when appraised, did not have the value that would normally have been expected. And, in almost all cases, the owners of these practices were totally unaware of the problem. Some of these practices had traits in common with the practices that have historically had little or no value. They were small practices with a low level of profitability and could not keep up with changing client demands regarding service, quality of medicine, advanced technology, and improved facilities. The other practices with no or little value, however, were a surprising group. On the surface, these practices would appear to be doing very well. They are located in very attractive facilities, practice good medicine, have all the latest equipment and a large support staff, offer comparatively high compensation and benefits to their employees and, in the owners' eyes, cash flow is strong. However, practice value is largely based on profits and the very factors that make these practices look attractive on the surface are those that are reducing profitability. A lack of profitability either comes from revenues that are too low, expenses that are too high, or a combination of the two.

All of the above traits of the new No-Lo[SM] practice cost money—attractive new buildings, state of the art equipment, high levels of compensation and benefits, and large levels of support staff. What practices do not do when making the decisions to spend these amounts of money is make sure that the costs will lead to increased levels of revenue and thus profits.

For example, how much space and what kind of building are really necessary to practice veterinary medicine? Operating out of the Taj Mahal can be very psychically rewarding but may not be good financially. For example, if a practice moves into a beautiful, new facility and the rent doubles, will there be a sufficient increase in revenue (and more importantly profits) to cover this rent increase?

The same goes for the addition of staff. A doctor's work life may be much easier and personally rewarding with three techs trailing behind him or her during the day, but does this doctor actually produce more revenue with this additional support staff? If not, the cost of the staff is eating into the profitability of the practice. Other staff problems seen in practices include the hiring of low-level, minimum wage staff that cannot do the job properly, too many part-time employees, and a lack of training and supervision. All of these lead to inefficiencies in getting the job done.

Declining revenue or a lack in growth of revenue is the other factor contributing to a lack of profitability. Practices often do not focus specifically on growing revenue because it's harder for them to determine what to do. In many cases they've also been fortunate in that the revenue has just seemed to be there. If they don't have the 12% to 13% growth they did a few years ago, owners often assume that's just because the practice has matured or the demographics of their area are changing and that there is nothing they can do about it.

The reality is quite different, however, for many practices. Generally there is much a practice can do to keep revenues strong even if located in a demographically challenged area. For example, are fees appropriate? It's not uncommon to see a practice that hasn't increased fees in two years or has only increased a few of them by a small percentage. Most expenses in a practice rise annually because the providers of those goods and services raise their prices—this is true of staff costs, drugs and medical supplies and the various other goods and services used by a typical practice. If the practice isn't raising its fees at least 5% per year, profitability will suffer even if nothing else changes in the practice.

Lack of attention to discounts and missed charges can also lead to declining revenue. Even a small amount of products or services given away by well-meaning doctors or other team members can significantly decrease revenue and profitability. Missed charges, those not deliberately given away, can also dramatically reduce the profit margin. Capturing charges is generally about having good systems in place and is essential to efficient operations. It is a rare practice that doesn't experience these problems on a fairly regular basis.

Understanding not only the profitability of the practice but the kinds of factors that lead to this state is critical. Until the practice has an idea of the root causes of the problem, it is difficult to determine what the correct solution is. Working with a financial advisor or practice consultant may help in not only gaining a greater understanding of the issues impacting profitability but in identifying and implementing solutions.

WOW YOUR CLIENTS, WOW YOUR BOSS

David B. Gerber, DVM, BA
Simmons & Associates Northwest, Inc.
Coeur d'Alene, ID

David F. King, DVM, BS
Simmons & Associates Southcentral, Inc.
Scurry, TX

WHAT MATTERS TODAY

No longer is having highly qualified doctors and staff good enough. That is EXPECTED and taken for granted and does not make you unique. It's what your clients can actually see and understand, on their terms, that allows them to make decisions about where to seek veterinary care.

When those of us in the profession evaluate other practices, we tend to look at the quality of medicine they practice n determining whether they are "good" practitioners. Clients do not have the ability to make these judgments, so they make their decisions on what they **do** understand, such as how you present yourself, how you act, and, most importantly, **how much you care**.

We can divide the "how you present yourself, how you act, and how much you care" into two areas. First is the facility itself, and second is how you treat clients on a personal level. First, let's look at the facility.

THE HOSPITAL

Like it or not, your hospital screams to your clients that you care (or that you don't). Remember, you have only one chance to make a first impression!

There are several outdoor items that deserve attention and are often overlooked because you likely enter from the back and don't ever see the clinic from the clients' view. Think like a new client and try to see what they see. Remember, on that first visit, they are looking VERY carefully for any clues that will tell them how much you care.

Sign. The first thing clients see is your sign. This is hugely important and often the ONLY thing the public will ever see. Granted, you have little control over this, but it is worth mentioning to your boss since it is so important. Is it bright, clean, simple, easy to read, and does it tell WHO you are?

Parking Lot. A tiny parking lot that is difficult to navigate can be a major deterrent, especially for your elderly clients who still drive the big "boats" and sit way low in the seat, barely able to see over the steering wheel. You may not be able to change that, but you might suggest to your boss to consider leasing spaces from a neighboring business for the staff parking. Is the lot clean and well-striped? Someone should have the duty EVERY morning to pick up any trash and, generally, police the lot.

Plantings. As clients approach the front door, do they find planters with attractive, healthy plants, or are they dried up and dead or full of weeds? The new client may think, "Hmm, if they can't even keep PLANTS alive,

I wonder what *else* dies here?" Are there spider webs dangling in the doorway? Are there children's chocolate-colored fingerprints all over the windows? They ask themselves, "If you don't even care about keeping the windows clean, I wonder if you keep your surgery suite clean." As they first enter the hospital, you want them to ALREADY be impressed. By the time you have a chance to say, "Hello," they have already begun to decide if they made the right or wrong choice.

The **waiting/reception area** is a biggie. Let's lose the term "waiting" because none of us wants or likes to wait. How about the "greeting" area? Isn't that what you are really doing? Or should be? We'll get to that in a bit. When we go to a physician's office the first we see is the cleanliness. This is obvious.

Magazines. Then I go right to the magazine rack. This can be very telling. I recently went to my physician's office (always a long wait, less than pleasant staff) and the NEWEST magazine was from 2005. Really. Hmmmm, I wonder if they are also three years behind reading medical journals. I commented on the old magazines to the receptionist. Her expected response was, "Oh, that's not my job." Geez. Interestingly, the very next day I went to my dentist's office. Clean reception area, bottled water and fresh coffee, and a good variety of magazines. The OLDEST magazine there was two months old. What a difference! So, keep the magazines up to date and have a nice variety. They don't all need to be old *Field & Stream* or *Guns and Ammo*. Remember, 70% to 80% of your clients are women, 25 to 45 years old. How about *Newsweek, National Geographic,* or *Cooking*? It's not that hard!

Odors. A most important "detail" is the odor or lack thereof. Several years ago, Veterinary Economics surveyed a large group of clients, asking them why they changed veterinarians. The number one reason was bad odor. Either it smelled like a kennel or it smelled like a hospital. There really is no substitute for cleaning. Masking odors just doesn't work. It must be clean to not smell—and the best smell is no smell at all.

Fresh flowers. This is one of those details that really shows you care. I recently visited a practice with a nice vase of yellow roses. Next to it was a small stack of business cards from a local florist. The local florist made a "deal" with the practice manager. They would bring in and leave a fresh vase of flowers once a week in return for being allowed to leave their cards on the counter. What a great idea! Clients loved it.

Cookies. The smell of freshly baked chocolate chip cookies is pretty hard to resist. It says, "You are welcome here. We are glad to see you. We care about you." With inexpensive convection countertop ovens and pre-made cookie dough that you simply slice and bake, this is another inexpensive and simple "perk" you can offer to your clients.

Coffee. Not just any old coffee. Having freshly brewed coffee available is always well received, but you can be a cut above if it is Starbucks or other premium coffee. Be sure to have the Starbucks label visible! For those who don't drink coffee, inexpensive bottled water can be kept available as well.

The reception area is a great place for a fish tank or a clinic bird. If there is a bit of a wait, they provide some entertainment that fits well in a veterinary hospital. We had a cockatiel for awhile and he was the source of much humor and enjoyment. Kind of a mess, but that can be cleaned up!

Courtesy phone and computer. As we have said, most clients are women and often busy moms. They are trying to accomplish the work of three people in one day. If they can turn any waiting time into productive time, the wait becomes an asset rather than a liability. (Of course, NO wait is always better.) Providing a private area with a phone that has long distance blocked is most appreciated. Also, providing a computer with internet access can allow clients to access email or do simple web searches while they wait. These services tell your clients that you care about them and that their time is valuable and the added cost is minimal.

Kids. Many moms have to bring their children along, which can be quite distracting. Attention to clients' *children* could be the most important marketing tool you have. Most moms love their kids more than life itself. Remember, who are your clients? If you also show them how important their children are, they will not soon forget. Surgical glove balloons, little dog treats, take-home magnets, or tiny stuffed toys are always a hit. Play areas with TV monitors showing cartoons not only show that you value children, it also gives Mom a break to relax a bit and concentrate on what the doctor is saying about Pookie. One high-tech practice even had a TV camera in this area with monitors in all the exam rooms so Mom could allow her kids to stay up front while she still was able to keep an eye on them while in the exam room with Pookie.

Ok, the very short wait is over and you escort your new client into the **exam room**. Although it is changing, the majority of hospitals are decorated by men. White, painted walls, plain everything, functional, but, boring. Who are your clients? They understand decorating, at least a lot better than most men. Usually clients have a few minutes alone in the exam room, giving them time to "examine" it closely. So, again, paying attention to details is important. Wallpaper on a wall or two, nice furniture that is not stained with cat urine, framed pictures, and some sample jars are all good. Drug company posters thumb tacked to the walls are NOT good. They deserve a frame if they are worthy of hanging up. Be sure the heating and cooling is comfortable.

Although we would like to think that the wait in the exam room is very short, indeed, it still is a good idea to have some reading material available, more of a medical nature. Maybe have a few pharmaceutical brochures on flea control or dentistry, or in-house hand-outs on different diseases or surgeries. A few toys might also be appropriate, but, rather than leaving the toys in the exam rooms, we have found it works better if the receptionist gives the moms a small basket of toys and books to take into the exam room and then return at the conclusion of the appointment. For those situations where Mom, two cats, a dog, and three children are all crammed into the exam room, how about assigning a staff person to take the kids on a clinic tour (to see all the cool gross stuff you keep in jars) or accompany them to the play area for a "mini" day care. Mom WILL love it and will likely comply a lot more readily with your recommendations.

Client education board. Another fun and inexpensive project you can do without any involvement from your boss is to install corkboard information boards. 12" square, decorative cork can be glued onto the wall to create a bulletin board in each exam room. A different staff member can be chosen each month to select a theme (dentistry, fleas, Lyme disease, parasites, hysterectomy, ACL surgery, ultrasound, etc.) and create a graphic informational display. The creativity can be fun and provide an excellent educational tool for doctors or technicians while they are talking with clients.

Restroom. One last area that is most often overlooked is the public restroom. It has been shown that women (remember they are most of your clients) will often subconsciously judge a business based on the appearance of the bathroom. It isn't necessary to remodel, but a couple hundred dollars will make a huge difference to most "plain Jane" bathrooms. You know, white walls, cheap toilet paper, paper towels, a bar of dirty soap, and open trash can. How about a nice wallpaper border along the ceiling, incandescent lights, cloth hand towel (yes, it needs to be checked often), "cushy" toilet paper on a nice free-standing stainless stand, liquid soap in a nice pottery dispenser, maybe a plant in the corner if there is natural light.....you get the picture. You will be surprised at how many clients, after they use this first-class restroom, will come back up front and comment on how nice a hospital this is, and not really be aware that it is because of their impression of the restroom.

Finally, regarding the hospital itself, paying constant attention to the details of how it looks makes a huge difference to clients. They DO notice. Pay attention to keeping the trash emptied and odor-free, full paper towel holders, no burnt-out light bulbs (that means NO burnt-out light bulbs), pet-waste free in front of the hospital (this may need to be checked several times/day), floor and counters free of excess pet hair, etc. It's the little things that make the difference.

OUTRAGEOUS CLIENT SERVICE

Again, it's not so much about what you know (you are EXPECTED to be knowledgeable and competent), but how much you care. We have addressed some of the issues specifically related to the hospital itself. However, even more important is how everyone in the practice treats clients.

You are the one who controls how you treat clients. They will know immediately whether you see them as valued and important, or as a bother and interruption to your day. One practice we visited had a "mood chart" on the wall in the back (Figure 1).

Each morning, the staff decided what mood the doctor was in that day. Good or bad, it set the whole "mood" for the practice. Although the practice owner is ultimately responsible for the culture of the practice, he

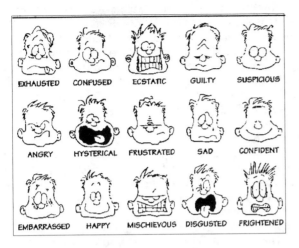

Figure 1. Mood chart.

or she will surely appreciate efforts that result in practice growth, increased revenues and, finally, more profit. This may require you to transcend a negative attitude, but YOU have control over yourself.

Following are a few ideas you can use to help you separate your hospital from the crowd; to create an experience for your clients that will "knock their socks off." You are not looking for "satisfied" clients, you are looking for clients who are wildly enthusiastic about you and go out of their way to tell their friends and neighbors that your hospital is THE ONLY place to take their pets. Period. You are looking to create "hospital groupies."

When your clients enter the hospital, do you always acknowledge them immediately? Even if things are hectic, a simple nod or eye contact shows the clients they have been recognized (that they are important). How many times have YOU entered your physician's office and waited for several minutes before anyone even acknowledged you? Did it make you feel important? I am a strong disciple or "groupie" of Southwest Airlines (more on that later), and, whenever I approach the ticket or check-in counter, someone at least nods, winks, waves a hand, OR SOMETHING. Last year I was forced to fly on another airline (which, in my opinion, is noted for customer *dis*-service). I approached the ticket counter and waited for over four minutes (yes, I timed it), listening to the agent complete a casual conversation with a friend while not so much as even glancing up. By the time she finally did acknowledge me, a paying customer, I was ready to strangle anyone with that airline's logo.

At this point, I should emphasize that you people who work in the front reception area "hot seats" are the heroes of your practices. Your job is rapid fire, you are the first (and last) to deal with disgruntled or stressed pet owners, you are expected to be able to diagnose and treat most diseases on the phone, and when you don't, be willing to absorb the wrath of the pet owner wanting the answer to "a quick question." Of course, most of the time you have two lines on hold while trying to locate the doctor who is on the phone with her stock broker, the other three lines are ringing, a HBC just walked through

the door in the arms of a hysterical client, and there is a rottweiler snarling and hoping for the split second he can tear the limbs off the cat next to him. Oh yes, I forgot the client who is checking out and her charge card has been denied and she indignantly is demanding to use the phone to call that "damn bank" again, since they do this to her all the time just because she is a few days late with her payments. Sound a little familiar? Yes, you are the heroes, and here I am telling you that you need to smile, be pleasant, and assure the next person you speak with that he or she is THE most important person in your day. It's not easy and most veterinarians couldn't do it. That's why we run to the safety of the treatment room as soon as we can.

It takes a special person to be able to pull off, with grace and style, the job of the "receptionist," "client care specialist," or whatever name you use. I had a receptionist, Sally, who was efficient, friendly, careful with details, and liked people. But, she was easily stressed, and showed it. One time, I saw a dog with some problem that really should have been seen the day before, and I mentioned that to the client. She told me that she DID call the previous day, but, hearing Sally's voice, she said to Sally, "I can tell you are really busy. I am sorry that I am bothering you today. I'll call back tomorrow." Fortunately, she did.

We have become accustomed to poor service in all arenas and have come to expect it, so it is actually quite easy to stand out in the crowd. How often have you ordered a hamburger, only to receive a cold, greasy, overcooked chunk of tasteless food? Part way through your meal the waitress comes and asks you how it is. More often than not, you will answer, "It's fine." But will be the last time you ever visit that restaurant, and, yet, they never know. Consumers vote with their dollars. We generally hate confrontation, so it is much easier to say, "It's fine" and then never go back. There is so much poor or mediocre service that offering better than the norm is just not that hard!

Most businesses provide "task-driven service." You provide a standard level of service and then your client pays for that service. Done. Your client is satisfied. He or she got what was expected. Not less, not more. Or, how about if you provide a drop dead incredible experience, way beyond what is expected? Not only will they pay you happily and pay more, but they will be anxious to tell their friends what a fantastic veterinarian you are. As Garrison Keillor said, "Be better than you need to be. Be unreasonably good."

Most of us are not qualified to choose professionals with a discriminating eye. We are not schooled in the intricacies of dentistry, law, accounting, stock brokerage, or insurance. If you ask your neighbors for a recommendation for an accountant, they might say, "I just adore Bob Smith. He is so nice and I love his office and staff. He always calls me right back and he also has a German Shepherd just like mine. He is an excellent accountant. I highly recommend him!" Do any of these qualities really speak to the accounting ability of Bob Smith? Not really, but he DOES have an enthusiastic client. Your clients will judge you on the things they CAN use to judge you. Things that they understand and are familiar to them. Cleanliness, smells, attitude, timeliness, amenities (coffee, email access, free phone, etc.) They are not equipped to judge your doctors' surgical abilities, but they CAN look at the incision and see that it is not blood soaked. And they will note if Pookie smells like urine or feces upon release after surgery, or if she has just been brushed, nails clipped, and has a little bow in her collar.

When you have captured their hearts, they will be yours forever, and with a passion. And, they will happily listen to and abide by your recommendations. They will spend much more for something that tugs at their hearts. Today's pets are no longer commodities, they are full-fledged family members.

"Price checkers" usually aren't! They are really pet owners attempting to choose a new veterinarian and price is the only piece of information they know to use for comparison. After all, if everything else were equal, price would be a valid means of comparison. Therefore, treat "price checkers" for what they usually are— conscientious pet owners trying to make the best choice for their pets. Engage the caller in a conversation about the pet and the procedure and offer the price LAST. This will show the callers that you are interested in them and their pets and that your clinic cares. If they are able to perceive more value at your clinic than at the other clinics they have called, price will quickly diminish in importance. Since these calls do take time, it may be wise to get a name and number and call back when you have a bit more time. That will also allow time to get an address to mail a small packet of information about the hospital. These people are worth the time. Many of these callers can be converted to clients instead of nuisances. Can you imagine a more highly targeted marketing program than to a pet owner who calls YOU and is in need of veterinary services now? It just doesn't get any better than that.

We have seen some practices that actually have a person who does nothing but answer the phone and is situated in a back office. The results can be remarkable.

Handwritten sympathy cards. Most clinics use some form of sympathy cards. However, a note, handwritten by the attending veterinarian, has infinitely more meaning than a card with only a signature. If possible, make every effort to send a personal note every time a pet dies. Clients will remember these notes for years into the future, long after they no longer have pets. Some clinics even send a small potted plant or cut flowers every time. Whatever you do, nothing will be more appreciated ever.

Clinic cat. Put those cats to work. Many clinics already have clinic cats, dogs, birds, etc. Consider creating special business cards for these "helpers" to use for recheck appointments, referral rewards, etc. Feature their pictures in brochures, newsletters, and newspaper columns. Our clinic cat, Pansy, had his own, pink business cards. He also ran a biweekly column in the local newspaper, *Pansy's Petpourri*, which cost us nothing more than the time to write the articles.

Reminders. It is inexpensive to have a bunch of reminder cards printed with YOUR message and a cute cartoon. Virtually every veterinary software program will print reminders for routine services, but they are highly impersonal and bland, even when printed on cute full-color stock cards. Few clients have any clue what a DA2PL/CPV or a FVRCP is. They do, however, understand, "It is time for us to see you and be sure you are healthy. Call us for your annual checkup and brag to your friends about the gold star on your perfect report card." It also adds an additional personal touch to send reminders to the pet instead of the owner, which some software programs allow. As practices rely less and less on vaccinations, doesn't it make sense to emphasize complete physical exams instead of vaccines on the reminders?

Target and personalize your mailings. When promoting a new service or product, it is not necessary to reach ALL of your clients, but only those who will benefit. For instance, if you have recently become skilled in doing cataract surgery, targeting dogs only and those over ten years of age would be the most productive. As your mail lists gets more and more refined, the chances of success become greater and greater. Because of the small numbers, it also allows you to send them HAND addressed and HAND stamped (first class, of course!), a refreshing change in our highly automated time. The chances of the mailing being read increase dramatically. As an example, one clinic sent a highly targeted mailing to 250 clients. 50% of them answered and 50% of those purchased the new service! Blanket mailings usually receive only a 1% to 3% response rate.

Healthy pet report cards. Dr. Gerald Snyder first published this idea many years ago. It forces the examining DVM to look at all the various organ systems and comment on each. It thus dictates performing a thorough physical exam. Because the report card provides a template, it encourages consistency among the different DVMs in a multi-DVM practice. It gives the client something to take home and review. It contributes to the perceived value of the visit, and, remember, it is not the cost, but the cost in relation to service that matters. The report cards are completed by the DVM and maybe in bright felt pen for emphasis. An added touch is to have the receptionist apply a stick-on gold star if everything is normal.

Pet ID card/cage tag. Simple, quick, and inexpensive, this wallet-sized ID card has all of the pet's vaccination details included along with the DVM's signature and a photo of the pet. On the reverse side is a clinic business card. It is all laminated together. Total cost is less than $2.00 and is a fantastic marketing tool. A similar process can produce a cage tag.

VALUE VS. PRICE

But there is a caveat. It is OK to have high fees, BUT the value must be there. Consumers are savvy and demand value. And they should. Raise your fees. That's not a problem as long as you raise your level of service *even more*. Value does not mean cheap; it means that the product or service was more than worth the cost, whatever that may be.

Let's assume for a moment that you have just landed on Earth, a seasoned space traveler. You are told that, to get around on this planet, you will need a means of transportation, a car. So you head down to Auto Row and decide to look at cars at two dealerships to be sure you are getting a good VALUE. The first is the Yugo dealership. The cars, although small, seem to have all the necessary requirements. They have doors, windshields, four wheels, two seats, a steering wheel, a heater, and even a thing called a radio. When turned on, they "go." They are a bit noisy and rattly, the trim doesn't line up too well, and the seats aren't so comfortable, but they do "go." You ask a few questions of the salesman, a young hip-hop sort of guy, with an earring, slick greasy hair, and an IPod hanging from his shirt pocket. He can't really answer any of your questions abut the car, but he assures you this Yugo is a great deal. And, the prices are in the $8,000 range. Is this a good value? You really don't have a clue. Your eyes keep noticing the hamburger wrappers and old French fries strewn on the cracked blacktop lot.

Now you go next door to the other dealership. They are selling cars called Mercedes Benz. On first glance, they look pretty similar to the Yugo. Doors, windshields, four wheels, two seats, steering wheel, a heater, and a radio. But a huge difference is the price, at around $90,000. Whoa. As you recover from your shock, an "automobile consultant" approaches you in her business suit. She offers you some fresh coffee or bottled water and invites you to look around at your leisure. She gives you space but mentions that she is available to answer any of your questions. As you walk through the lot, you can't help but notice the impeccable attention to detail. All the cars are spotless as is the lot itself. No trash, freshly striped. The paint on the cars is clearly superior to the Yugo. The doors close with a thud instead of a clank. Finally you ask the "consultant" to explain why this car's cost is so different from the Yugo's. She gladly shows the seats that are covered with luxurious leather. The "heater" is not simply a heater, but a "climate control system." The "radio" is actually a surround sound stereo system with high-end Bose speakers. Of course, everything is constantly monitored by the invisible computer. She points out the multifaceted safety features, again, not evident to the unschooled. In short, she is able to explain with specifics why this car commands a handsome price. She discusses the superior warranty, the no-cost "roadside assistance program," and free oil changes for 2 years. At no time does she downplay or compare to the Yugo, but she

simply points out why the Mercedes is such a good value.

The above example can easily be transferred to your practice. You don't need to tell potential clients how you are "better" than the other practices. You need to be sure they understand all of the things you do that provide a value far in excess of the cost. Will this approach convince everyone that you are a good fit for their needs? Of course not. Not everyone drives a Mercedes either.

THE MAGIC OF SOUTHWEST

Southwest Airlines has been profitable for every quarter in its 30+ years of history. It is the ONLY airline to continue that consistently even after 9/11. A major component of that success relates to having an incredible work force, and treating the employees with respect.

Hiring the right people has been a hallmark of Southwest. They look for people with an attitude that is positive, creative, and people-oriented. Then they train for the rest---and it REALLY works. *Customers are NOT #1 at Southwest---employees are.* If you treat your employees right, they will treat your clients right. And, at Southwest, "outrageous customer service" is everything. As former CEO Herb Kelleher said, "We are not an airline company with great customer service. We are a great customer service organization that happens to be in the airline business." Now, substitute "veterinary" for "airline" into the last sentence.

So, what is great customer service in a veterinary practice? Some of it we have addressed above. But it is also such things as answering by the 3rd ring and not allowing clients to be on hold, returning calls promptly, keeping waiting times short, fresh flowers, current reading material, hand-written sympathy cards, helping clients to their cars, lending an umbrella, using the pet's proper name and gender (always!), saying "thanks," having fun.

THE BOTTOM LINE

We are in the era of customer service, value, and convenience. Offering high quality medical care is a given, but will not be sufficient to grow your practice in the future. How you treat your clients and their pets will determine your level of success. It's not that hard, especially with poor service abounding everywhere. You can stand out from the crowd by implementing some of the ideas above and many more of your own. It will cost a little, but the increase in practice growth can be astonishing.

PURCHASING MEDICAL RECORDS—
DO THEY HAVE VALUE?

David B. Gerber, DVM, BA
Simmons & Associates Northwest, Inc.
Coeur d'Alene, ID

David F. King, DVM, BS
Simmons & Associates Southcentral, Inc.
Scurry, TX

WHY BUY MEDICAL RECORDS?

"Why should I buy them when I can get them for free?" is the routine question we hear. True, if a practice closes its door, you will get SOME of the records for free, but not all, unless you are the ONLY other practice in the area. Assume for the moment that a practice is in the center of four surrounding practices. On average, each practice will get 25% of the records for free. But what about the other 75%? Why should you care? Because the profit is so large.

The typical small animal practice has a profit margin of 12% to 18% after all expenses. With a records-only purchase, the profit on THAT new stream of income is at least twice as much or often 40% to 45%. Why? It is primarily due to the fact that the hard costs (rent, utilities, other facility costs) do not travel with the records. They are already paid by the acquiring practice.

So, what are the costs that WILL remain? Included would be the cost of additional DVM compensation, drugs and supplies, some additional administrative expenses, and some additional staffing and miscellaneous costs, which will look something like this:

DVM expense	25%
Drugs and supplies	18%
Administrative (additional)	5%
Extra support staff, misc.	12%
TOTAL costs	60%
PROFIT	40%*

*As compared to the normal 12% to 18% in a regular practice

But does this always work? Not by a long stretch. In short, "all the stars need to line up" just right. The questions that need to be asked are:

1. Does the acquiring practice have the excess capacity to absorb the new business without incurring major capital costs (additional space, etc.)?
2. Do the demographics work?
   a. Are the trade areas very similar?
   b. What are the drive times between the two locations? Are there any barriers such as a freeway?
   c. Are the practice cultures similar?
   d. Will the selling owner help with a transition and, preferably, work in the new location for a period of time?
   e. Can the phone number of the selling practice be transferred? This is CRITICAL!

If all of the above fits, this acquisition/merger strategy can be an excellent opportunity, and one that is largely overlooked by the veterinary profession.

PRACTICE VALUE, PRICE AND MARKETABILITY

David B. Gerber, DVM, BA
Simmons & Associates Northwest, Inc.
Coeur d'Alene, ID

David F. King, DVM, BS
Simmons & Associates Southcentral, Inc.
Scurry, TX

VALUE AND PRICE

Is there a difference between price and value? Price is an arbitrary number that someone puts on an item, a guess of what the market will bear. It can be based on formulas, comparisons, market experience, and so on, but it is still basically a guess. Some people confuse the terms and look at the results of some formula someone (hopefully with experience) used to come up with a number as the value. However, the actual definition of Fair Market Value is what a willing seller is willing to take and what a willing buyer is willing to give after the item has been exposed to the market for a fair amount of time. So the value is what it will sell for in the market. Only at one time does Price = Value, at closing. Is a Babe Ruth autographed baseball worth $10K? Not to most, but if someone is willing to pay that for it then it seems to be. The problem is that there are so many different factors that come into play that make valuing (or pricing) a practice so subjective. It often takes market experience and not just formulas to get it right.

VALUE AND MARKETABILITY

Just like value and price, value and marketability are not necessarily the same thing. Simply because a practice has a certain calculated "value" does not mean it will sell for that price. In the strict sense, value relates mostly to numbers, formulas, and objective data to arrive at what a practice is really "worth." Marketability also takes into account the intangible, subjective qualities of a practice to help establish a proper selling price. For instance, a highly profitable, well-run practice in Aspen, Colorado would have a very different "value" from that same practice in downtown Newark, New Jersey. Marketability has a huge effect on what a practice can actually sell for and needs to be considered during the valuation process. That is why is it is so important to hire a practice appraiser who specializes in veterinary practices and one who also is familiar with the geographic area.

WHAT DETERMINES PRACTICE VALUE?

Certainly gross income is necessary or there will be no available money to pay for expenses or for profit. More importantly, the impact of gross income level is mostly psychological because many people STILL try to correlate it with value. If a practice is priced above a year's gross revenue, there is artificial market resistance. Conversely, if it priced at a small fraction of a year's gross there may be a false perception that it is a "good deal."

Net income is far more important and actually determines how much money is available for profit—the money that will be available to buy the practice. Net income plays a huge role is determining practice value.

Practice growth contributes an intangible value. Wouldn't one rather purchase a practice that is growing robustly than one that is shrinking, even if the net income were equal?

Geographic location is of paramount importance when it comes time to sell. Most buyers have definite ideas about where they want to live.

Competition, whether it is stiff or non-existent, must be considered as an influential part of value.

Tangible asset value is the value of the equipment and the inventory. This has considerably less influence on value than most people think. It is income that buyers want, not "stuff." Of course certain equipment is necessary, but too much equipment does not increase value.

Other factors such as long-term, loyal, skilled employees add value, as does a reasonable transition period by the selling doctor. A small, "high touch, boutique" practice typically has more loyal clientele than does a high volume, "low cost" practice. A practice in a permanent location as opposed to a mobile practice will have more transferable goodwill because the clients will more easily remain with a fixed-location practice, hence, more value.

SUMMARY

When buying or selling a practice, it is important to understand the differences between value, price, and marketability. It is okay not to know why they are different (that should be left up to the folks with market experience) but just know that they are different. In a nutshell, understand that practice value, price and marketability are about more than just numbers.

DO YOU HAVE A LOW-VALUE PRACTICE— AND NOT EVEN KNOW IT?

David B. Gerber, DVM, BA
Simmons & Associates Northwest, Inc.
Coeur d'Alene, ID

David F. King, DVM, BS
Simmons & Associates Southcentral, Inc.
Scurry, TX

WHAT IS A NO-LO™ PRACTICE?

Over the past several years, practice appraisers and brokers have become aware of a growing and disturbing phenomenon in our profession. There has been an increase in the number of practices with values substantially lower than would be expected. Since practice value is closely tied to profit, the fact is that these practices have very low profitability. But what is even more disturbing than low profit is that *the vast majority of these practice owners are completely and totally unaware that a problem exists*. Since, traditionally, many veterinarians have relied on their practices and real estate as the bulk of their retirement funds, this is especially alarming.

The Valuation Committee of the Association of Practice Management Consultants and Advisors (AVPMCA) has decided to address this emerging trend of very low profit and, therefore, low valued practices and has dubbed them No-Lo™ practices.

There is no practice or type of practice that is immune. However, there are two common threads that run throughout every one of these practices. The first is that they have very little profit. The second, which is also almost universal, is a complete lack of awareness of the problem by the owners.

These are usually larger practices, generally in expensive stand-alone buildings owned by the practice owner, very well-equipped, offer high-touch superior care, are well (over) staffed, provide a great working environment, and the owner is a generous individual who wants to "share the wealth" with his/her staff. Result? Low profit.

To the commonly, these practices are superb practices in all ways and, clearly, should carry high values. In fact these are often award-winning practices.

So, what's going on? These practices gross in the upper areas, usually above $1M and they are in very expensive hospitals. Here's an example.

Gross	$1,000,000
Real estate value	$1,500,000
Owner takes home	$ 275,000

So what's wrong with this? Let's look closer. An owner should be paid four ways:

1. Pay for producing income,
2. Pay for management,
3. Rental income,
4. Profit simply for being an owner, and it is THIS piece that is the basis for practice value.

If there is nothing left for #4, the practice has little or no value because there is no money available for a buyer to use to pay for the practice loan. Let's continue with our example.

1. Owner produces $350K, so, at a 22% compensation rate, he gets $77,000.
2. Management compensation should total 3% to 4% of gross. He has a full-time manager, so he gets only 1% of the gross, or $10,000.
3. Rental income on $1,500,000 @ 10% of building value is $150,000.
4. So, the remainder (profit) is $38,000.
5. TOTAL OWNER COMPENSATION = $275,000
6. Practice value typically will be 3 to 6 times the profit. So, in our example, the value would be somewhere between $114K and $228K! (3 to 6 times $38K) YIKES!

WHY DO OWNERS ALLOW THIS TO HAPPEN?

- **Owner is "making enough."** The majority of veterinarians are highly compassionate and caring. They are not greedy. When they see that they are making more money than the others in their practices, they want to "share the wealth." Many feel guilty about making more than their staff members. They don't feel pressured to keep profits at an optimum level. Is that wrong? Of course not, but it needs to happen intentionally, not accidentally.

- **Employees are overly compensated and "over-benefited."** This is a direct result of the owner's need to share the wealth. It brings joy to owners to be able to pay top wages, provide top-quality health and dental insurance, send all staff to CE meetings, have a generous vacation policy, and to contribute liberally to employee retirement plans. But, again, there is a cost to the profit of the business.

- **NO expense is spared to provide the best possible customer and patient care.** When there seems to be enough money to go around, it becomes easy to add services and "extras" that don't add to the ultimate profit of the practice. Some of these probably do enhance the business, resulting in more enthusiastic clients and more repeat business, but some of these, frankly, make little difference to clients.

- **Not managed for profitability.** Many owners receive their monthly financial statements, look to see if there is a positive number at the end, and throw the statements in a drawer. Nobody ever showed us HOW to analyze for true profitability, so it becomes difficult to track if you don't know where to look. In essence, most owners have not been given the tools to properly read their financial statements so that they can be used a management tool.

ARE THERE SOLUTIONS?

Of course; the first is to diagnose the problem. Financial statements need to include a more accurate breakdown of what the owner is actually making for each of the four components listed above (production pay, management pay, rent, and finally, profit). If the remaining amount for profit is low, then the problem exists.

Two things are for sure. First, if the desire is to increase the value of the practice, the profit margin needs to increase. Period. That can be done by either increasing revenue without a parallel increase in expenses, OR reduce expenses while maintaining the level of revenue. Second, if the above is either not possible due to location, competition, demographics, or whatever, OR not desirable, then the status quo will continue and the owner needs to remain satisfied with the current situation.

In order to remedy the problem, it is often necessary to employ the expertise of an outside veterinary consultant who can examine both the revenue side (fees, missed charges, excessive discounting) AND the expense side (poor ordering, overstocking, employee compensation packages, and general "leakage"). Many of these No-Lo™ practices can be turned around, but it does require change and vigilance to the many everyday details. Remember, "If you keep doing what you have always done, you will keep getting what you have always gotten."

A FINANCIAL PHYSICAL FOR YOUR PRACTICE

Gary I. Glassman, CPA
Burzenski & Company, P.C.
East Haven, CT

Just like a yearly pet's physical, your practice should have a look under the hood at least yearly. Understanding the financial condition of your hospital enables you to make intelligent financial decisions, plan for capital expenditures (equipment purchases) and avoid cash flow issues that may arise through out the course of the year. What should you check on to make sure the practice is running smoothly? The hospital's finances are broken down into five categories: Assets, liabilities, equity, income, and expenses. Assets, liabilities, and equity are reported on a balance sheet and income and expenses are reported on an income statement. Assets and liabilities are broken down into categories know as current assets and current liabilities. These are defined as having a life cycle of one year or less. Anything beyond one year is defined as another asset or long term liability.

Begin your check-up with the assets of the practice.

CASH

How much is available on average at all times? Do you maintain an adequate cash balance? You can judge this by maintaining 30 days of obligations in the bank at all times. Thirty days of obligations will include vendor bills, credit card debt, and payroll for a month. Smaller practices may average $30,000 to $35,000 while larger practices may average $80,000 to $100,000. Does your practice have to much cash on hand? Excess cash makes it an unproductive asset and consideration should be given to a distribution to owners for personal investment or additional retirement contributions. If you are always running out of cash, it is a good sign that the practice is suffering from profitability issues or too much cash is being drawn for the owner's benefit and to the detriment of practice obligations. In these cases, cash flow projections or cash flow budgeting should be considered so a picture can be taken of what and when issues with bill payments will exist. Seasonal sales can also affect cash flow and should be planned for.

ACCOUNTS RECEIVABLE

How much are they and what's the percentage of gross revenue? An accounts receivable aging should be run each month. These can be printed from your veterinary software. This will tell you how much is owed by each client and how old their account balance is. Accounts receivable should not run more than 2.5% of gross revenue in a small animal practice and 11% in a large animal practice. Develop a good accounts receivable collection policy and keep activity up to date. Turn uncollected accounts over to a collection agency in a reasonable time period and follow through to small claims court or write them off. The IRS only recognizes bad debts if you report on an accrual basis of accounting and you have exhausted all means of collection; otherwise you have a sales allowance.

INVENTORY

What are the inventory issues? The first is do you know how much you have? Many practices do not take a physical inventory count and have no idea how much drug and supplies they have on hand. Seventy-five percent of practices do not use or only use limited portions of their veterinary software's inventory system. If you report on an accrual basis of accounting you must report the full inventory value of all drugs and supplies for tax purposes. If the inventory value or quantity on hand is an unknown, it is not possible to manage it effectively. Use the inventory module of your veterinary software completely. It is a significant tool in controlling quantity levels, reorder points, and pricing. Take a complete physical inventory of what's on your shelf at least once a year. Adjust inventory counts within the veterinary software.

Inventory is an essential asset of the hospital offering full service care, but the cost to maintain it can be expensive. A hospital should turn its inventory completely over four to five times a year or once every 90 days. The formula to compute this is as follows:

$$\frac{\text{Drug and supply costs}}{\text{Average Inventory}} = \text{Inventory turns}$$

Example:

All Pet Animal Hospital has $24,000 of inventory at the beginning of the year and $30,000 at the end of the year. During the year they have $130,000 of drug and supply purchases. Their inventory turns are 4.81 times or once every 76 days

$$\frac{\$130,000}{\$27,000 \text{ (A)}} = 4.81 \text{ times}$$

(A) Average inventory on hand = 24,000 + 30,000 = 54,000 ÷ 2 = 27,000

Days inventory = 365 days ÷ 4.81 times or 76 days

Many hospitals carry similar drugs for treatment of the same symptoms or ailments usually because of doctor preference. When doctors do not agree on the same drugs it increases inventory costs. Every $100 of inefficient inventory adds $8.00 in carrying costs. When doctors can agree on common drugs and supplies, it reduces inventory costs and adds to the bottom line.

Don't carry too much inventory. If too much exists, send back the excess. Most vendors will take it back, but beware of the restocking charges.

EQUIPMENT EXPENDITURES

Most practices reinvest in new equipment each year. Plan on reinvesting 1% to 2% of your gross revenue yearly. Make equipment purchases that will not only further the medicine of your practice but also be economically viable by providing a return on your investment (ROI) at 20% to 25% of the equipment's cost yearly.

LIABILITIES

Now let's look at liabilities of the practice. How much are they? What type of debt does the practice have and what is its cost? One way to measure the financial performance of the hospital is to look at its Current Ratio. This is found by dividing current assets by current liabilities. Many lenders look at this as sign of financial strength for the practice. Current assets would be found by adding cash, accounts receivable, and inventory. Current liabilities can be found by adding accounts payable, credit card payable, payroll taxes payable, sales tax payable, and current portion of long-term debt. The industry average is 2 to 1, which means that for every $1 dollar of current liability there is $2 of current asset. Divide current assets by current liabilities to get the result.

$$\text{Current ratio} = \frac{\text{Current assets}}{\text{Current liabilities}}$$

Common questions you need to ask concerning liabilities:

- Do I pay all my bills in 30 to 45 days, except for deferred billing items?
- Do I pay all credit card balances in full each month? If not, what is the interest rate on the cards?
- What type of bank debt do I have? Is the interest rate floating (variable) or is the rate fixed?
- What type of leases do I have and when are they due?
- Should I be refinancing or consolidating any debt?

Another common measurement tool for determining practice financial strength is commonly referred to as determining the debt to equity ratio. The calculation for this is as follows:

$$\text{Debt to equity ratio} = \frac{\text{Total debt}}{\text{Practice equity}}$$

The more debt the practice has, the weaker it is in financial strength. The industry average is .3 to 1.

EQUITY OF THE PRACTICE

How much is it? Most veterinary hospitals are service type businesses and do not build a significant amount of equity in the practice. Most veterinarians build their wealth outside of the practice individually.

INCOME OF THE PRACTICE

Where does the practice generate its income from? Use your veterinary software to tell you. Analyze it monthly and track it in your accounting software (Quickbooks). A hospital revenue analysis within the financial statement might look like example in Figure 1.

When hospital revenue areas look weak, look for issues within control systems to make sure all income is being earned. Here are items to consider in each area:

- Clinic Services
  - Are fees for exams and vaccines separated and charged appropriately?
  - Are sick pet visits charged when a medical issue arises but started as a wellness exam?

Do medical exams which are extended for eye, neurological, or orthopedic reasons become extended exams and charged as such?

XYZ Veterinary Hospital
Income Statement
For the years ended December 31, 2007 and 2006

	2007	%	2006	%
Sales				
Vaccinations	$ 67,541	12	$ 60,282	12
Professional services/examinations	118,196	21	105,493	21
Medicines	118,196	21	105,493	21
Laboratory/diagnostics	95,682	17	85,399	17
Surgery	39,999	7	35,164	7
Radiology	28,142	5	25,117	5
Anesthesia	22,514	4	20,094	4
Treatments	16,885	3	15,070	3
Hospitalizations	16,885	3	15,070	3
Dentistry	11,257	2	10,047	2
Prescription diets	22,514	4	20,094	4
Food	5,628	1	5,023	1
Retail	5,627	1	5,024	1
Discounts	(5,628)	(1)	(5,023)	(1)
Total Sales	$562,838	100	$502,347	100

Figure 1. A hospital revenue analysis.

- Pharmacy
  - Revisit mark-ups on drug and medical supplies
  - Revisit hospital dispensing fees. Does the hospital have:
    - A counted and label fee?
    - A separate label fee for items sold in full bottles or tubes?
  - Does the hospital have set minimum prescription prices?
- Diagnostics
  - Do x-ray prices include an interpretation fee?
  - Does the hospital charge for different size films and additional views?
  - Does the hospital add on clinic expenses when outside ultrasound specialists come in to do procedures?
- Hospital Services
  - Are surgeries and anesthesia procedures timed and billed accordingly?
  - Do hospitalization fees incorporate time spent by the nursing staff and the DVM?
  - Are hospitalization fees considered for day cases as well as overnight cases?
- Lab Services
  - Revisit markups on outside lab services. Are prices current with outside lab price schedule?
  - Do in-house lab prices reflect the cost of the test, equipment, and related payroll costs to run and interpret test results? Are invalid tests considered a part of the cost of service?
- Over the Counter Sales
  - Revisit markups on all items.

HOSPITAL FEES AND DISCOUNTING

Owners and associates should be reminded that they have a responsibility to adhere to their fee schedule. This point should be stressed to the associates, if not made a part of their contracts. If an associate has an issue with hospital fees, it should be either brought to a doctors' meeting for a resolution among all or brought to management's attention in a one-on-one session. The use of hospital estimates should be mandated. Clients need a clear understanding of expected charges. When clients receive unexpected bills, they get angry. This usually creates billing issues and eventually bad debts. Bad debts reduce the bottom line.

With most veterinary software, monthly accounts receivable reports can be created on a per-doctor basis. These should be printed for each doctor so they may review the status of unpaid balances related to their clients. This does not mean they need to have the responsibility to collect the account but certainly be made aware of it and to assist with collection when appropriate. Practice owners should also share with associates how much of their accounts receivable are written off each month. Hospital accounts receivable for small animal companion hospitals should never exceed 2.5% of the hospital's revenue and not more than 11% for large animal practices.

To further assist practice owners and associates, if the veterinary software allows, a daily fee exception report should be run by doctor to monitor fee overrides. This information should be shared with all doctors. Fee overrides should not be permitted.

Also, practices should monitor all manual discounts given. These should not be allowed. To alleviate any ill will regarding compassionate care, a doctor charity account can be set up for each associate for which they have the ability to use for free or reduced fee care. We recommend a $1,000 limit per doctor.

EXPENSES OF THE PRACTICE

You can not make money cutting expenses in a hospital. The best you can do is to control them. Budgeting is the best way to do that. Also, benchmarking your practice to the industry averages will let you know if you are in line with others. The industry averages for the most common expenses are shown in Table 1.

Table 1. Industry Averages for the Most Common Expenses	
Expenses	**Industry Average**
Drugs and supplies	15- 18%
Laboratory	3-3.2%
Utilities	1-1.2%
Office expense	1.5%
Insurance	0.8%
Advertising	1-1.2%
Continuing Education	0.6%
Postage	0.6%
Salaries and Wages	
Associate DVMs	11%
Receptionists	6-8%
Technicians	9-10%
Administrative Staff	3-4%
Rent Expense	6-8%
Payroll Taxes	2%
Repairs & Maintenance	1.2%
Advisors	1.5%

USE OF INTERNAL CONTROLS TO PREVENT FRAUD IN YOUR PRACTICE

Gary I. Glassman, CPA
Burzenski & Company, P.C.
East Haven, CT

ESTIMATES OF FRAUD IN THE UNITED STATES

Consider the following estimates of fraud in the United States:

- Health agencies estimate fraud represents 10% of the nation's health care bill at a cost of $75 to $130 billion a year.
- The tax gap, which is the difference between what people owe the government and what they pay, exceeds $200 billion a year.
- The IRS estimates that electronic tax filing fraud costs the government billions of dollars a year. For example, in one 10-month period, fraudulent electronic returns increased 105%.
- Thirteen percent of credit card sales resulted in loss due to fraud. For example, fraud losses at MasterCard exceed $300 million a year.
- Losses related to telephone fraud exceed $10 billion a year.
- Some 60% of Americans have shoplifted. An estimated 200 million shoplifting incidents a year cost US businesses almost $12 billion or about $150 per family per year.

THE PERVASIVENESS OF DISHONESTY

Not only are the losses to fraud very high, but the estimates of the number of people who commit or would commit a dishonest act are also very high. Consider the following:

- The director of fraud and security for a large consulting company stated that of every 10 workers, three look for a way to steal, three would steal if given an opportunity, and four would usually be honest.
- Two out of three college students admit to cheating on exams.
- An Institute of Management study found that 87% of managers were willing to commit fraud if it would make their organizations look better.
- A study of 400 people found that 47% of top executives, 41% of controllers, and 76% of graduate-level business students were willing to commit fraud by understating write-offs that cut into their company's profits.

WHAT IS THE DEFINITION OF FRAUD?

Fraud is defined as an intentional act of deceit for the purpose of gaining an unfair advantage that results in an injury to the rights or interests of another person. This can be accomplished through presentation of false or misleading information, suppressions of the truth, lies, tricks, and cunning. Fraud perpetrators are often referred to as white-collar criminals to distinguish them from criminals who commit violent crimes.

THREE STEPS TO FRAUD

To commit most frauds, a perpetrator must take three different steps: (i) the theft itself; (ii) converting the asset to personal use; and (iii) concealing the fraud.

Theft

Theft involves stealing something of value, such as cash, inventory, tools, supplies, equipment, or data. It can also be an intentional reporting of misleading financial information.

Conversion

The perpetrator converts the assets into a form that can be used personally. Conversion is usually required for all stolen assets except cash.

- Stolen checks must be deposited to an account from which the perpetrator can withdraw funds.
- Information (such as trade secrets or confidential company data) is often sold to someone such as a competitor.
- Industry experts estimate that computer companies annually lose up to $200 billion in computer chips due to armed robbery and employee theft. In some circles, computer chips are better than gold. Their theft is being referred to as the crime of the electronic age.

Employees who steal computer chips must convert them to cash. A sophisticated black market exists, and the chips often change hands as much as ten times in three days. When some companies run short, they often end up buying their stolen chips back.

The following example illustrates the conversion practices discussed above. On the advice of its trusted manager, a brand-name carpet manufacturer approved purchase orders replacing looms described by a subsidiary as deteriorated past reconditioning. Instead of being discarded or sold to a dealer, the used looms, which were in perfectly sound condition, found their way to another building in a town close by, along with skilled workers to man them. In a short time, a new low-priced carpet maker was bidding against the original brand.

Concealment

The perpetrator must conceal the crime in order to avoid detection and to continue the fraud. Concealing a fraud often takes more time and effort and leaves behind more evidence than the actual theft does. Where there are checks and balances in the system, the perpetrator often must "cook the books" to avoid detection.

- The theft of cash may require the employee to doctor the bank reconciliation and/or make false accounting entries to avoid detection.
- Taking cash takes only a few seconds, but altering records to hide the theft can be more challenging and time consuming. One effective way to hide an

employee theft is to charge the stolen item off to an expense account. For example, an employee could steal $10,000 and charge it off to miscellaneous expense. Or, a payroll clerk could add a fictitious name to the employee payroll records, intercept the paycheck, and cash it. The company would be missing funds, but the books would be in balance because there was a debit to wages expense and a credit to cash.

In the case of expense accounts, the perpetrator's principal exposure is limited to a year or less, because expense accounts are zeroed out at the end of the year.

If perpetrators chose to hide the theft by affecting another balance sheet account, they would have to continue to hide it. Hence, one of the most popular ways to cover up a fraud is to hide the theft in an income statement account.

One of the most effective ways to prevent the theft/conversion/concealment process is to have an effective system of internal controls. When such a system is in effect, fraud is made much more difficult. The internal control system must either be overridden or two or more perpetrators must collude with each other.

THE NATURE AND ELEMENTS OF FRAUD

A typical fraud has a number of important elements or characteristics.

- The perpetrator of the fraud must have gained the trust or confidence of the person or company being defrauded. This confidence makes it possible for the perpetrator to commit and conceal the fraud. For this reason, fraud schemes are often referred to as cons (from the word "CONfidence").
- In contrast to most other crimes, a perpetrator uses trickery or cunning to commit the fraud rather than force. Instead of using a gun, a knife, or physical force to commit a crime, perpetrators use false or misleading information. The intent is to get someone to give them money or assets. They hide their tracks by falsifying records or other information about the asset.
- Most frauds, once begun, are rarely terminated voluntarily by the perpetrator. The greed of the perpetrators is such that they continue to exploit the opportunity to obtain extra funds. The following factors can contribute to reasons why perpetrators may continue a fraudulent scheme:
  - o They begin to depend on the "extra" income and cannot afford to stop.
  - o When faced with the prospect of having additional money at their disposal, many move to a higher lifestyle that requires even greater amounts of money.
  - o Most perpetrators will take as much money as they think their particular scheme or method will allow them to take. The amount taken is usually limited only by the success, perpetrators have in concealing their actions or in the accidental or

contrived opportunities the perpetrator is able to discover and/or create.
  - o Some frauds are self-perpetuating. If perpetrators stop, their actions would be discovered, and they would get caught.
  - o Fraud perpetrators rarely save or invest what they embezzle. In all of the cases that one particular fraud expert has investigated or read about, he has only uncovered two perpetrators that saved the money embezzled. One perpetrator converted the money to gold bullion and stashed it in his basement. The other put the money into trust funds for her grandchildren.
  - o If the perpetrators are not caught shortly after they begin, they typically become more confident of their scheme. Many get greedy and take larger amounts of money. These larger amounts are more prone to be scrutinized, and a scheme that might have gone undetected for some time is uncovered because the amounts taken rise to unacceptable levels. Such perpetrators usually make a mistake that leads to their apprehension. In time, the sheer magnitude of the amount of the fraud leads to its detection.

    Example: At one auto repair shop, the accountant, a lifelong friend of the shop's owner, embezzled ever-increasing funds from the shop over a 7-year period. In the last year of the fraud, when the embezzler took over $100,000, the owner, facing bankruptcy, eventually had to fire the accountant and have his wife take over the bookkeeping. When the company began doing better, the wife began looking into the reasons for the recovery. She uncovered the fraud.
  - o The most significant contributing factor in most frauds is the failure to enforce existing internal controls.

WEAKNESSES IN CONTROLS

Some of the most commonly overlooked weaknesses that make embezzlement easier for the dishonest employee are as follows:

- Checks received in the mail go directly to the person who records, posts them, and prepares the deposits, with no independent record being made of the receipts.
- Bank statements go directly to the person who reconciles them.
- Checks and cash are allowed to accumulate before being deposited.
- Cash sales are loosely handled and sales slips are not accounted for by renumbering.
- There is no separate cashier to reconcile daily cash receipts with sales slips.
- Cash register amounts are not compared with bank deposits.
- Monthly statements are mailed by the very same person who works on accounts receivable without

- being checked by a superior and compared to the accounts receivable schedule.
- Customers report discrepancies on their statements, but no one in authority attempts to reconcile them.
- Accounts receivable are never confirmed with the customer.
- Uncollectible accounts are simply written off without being first turned over to an attorney or collection agency for collection.
- No one bothers to count and review petty cash because the fund is only a few hundred dollars.
- Petty cash slips are made out in pencil and are not canceled after use.
- No one cancels invoices, vouchers, supporting documents and checks to make sure they are not resubmitted for payment.
- Invoices are often paid without the initials of the person who is supposed to authorize their payment.
- The person authorizing payment of invoices does a perfunctory examination of the supporting documents: receiving reports, purchase requisitions, freight bills, etc.
- Physical inventories are not compared to book inventory figures and differences are not satisfactorily explained.
- Anyone with packages can walk out of the plant or other facility without question.
- Payroll checks are distributed by the same person who prepares the payroll or maintains the time records.
- The person signing payroll checks does not scrutinize the payroll, has little idea of its approximate total, or who the employees are.

Some businesses may not have sufficient personnel to provide the desired segregation of functions, but if the proper procedures are carefully followed, they can reduce the possibility of losses due to employee dishonesty.

SOME COMMON METHODS OF EMBEZZLEMENT
Misappropriation of Cash Receipts
1. Cash Sales
   - Covered by:
     - Not recording sales; destruction or omission of sales slips.
     - Tampering with cash register tapes; understating footings of cash sales reports.
     - Charging customers more than the duplicate slip shows.
     - Controversial charges collected, but reported as uncollectible.
2. Collections on Accounts and Notes Receivable
   - Covered by:
     - Lapping (both of bank balances and – with currency collections – petty cash)
     - Kiting, or inter-bank check transfers
     - Write-off of accounts as uncollectible
     - Improper credits for allowances or discounts

- Entry in customer's accounts only, concealed by:
  - Over-footing of cash receipts and tampering with adding machine tapes
  - Tampering with bank statements, passbooks and customers' statements
  - Insertion of fictitious ledger sheets at time of an audit
  - Reporting fake robberies of cash
3. Receipts of Miscellaneous Income and Credits
   - Covered by:
     - Not recording (including proceeds of illegitimate note executed to company bank)
     - Recording as an exchange item

Misappropriation of Disbursements
1. Cash on Hand
   - Covered by:
     - Cashing vouchers a second time
     - Payment of the same expense out of petty cash and also by check
     - Use of fictitious vouchers
     - Raising amounts on legitimate vouchers
     - Cashing worthless "exchange" checks
     - Unauthorized borrowing by employees
     - Unclaimed wages and dividends pocketed or check endorsements forged and cashed through the petty cash fund
     - Transfer of cash from one fund to another at time of an audit
2. Cash with Banks
   - Covered by:
     - Fictitious creditors' invoices (checks cashed through petty cash, secret or falsely named bank accounts, or forged endorsements)
     - Increasing amounts on creditor's invoices; refund of excess pocketed or split with the creditor
     - Paying creditor's invoices twice and appropriation of the second check
     - Failing to record purchase returns, allowances, and discounts, and appropriating check or cash payments
     - Payment of fictitious refunds or allowances
     - Increasing telephone and electric bills, etc. by employee's personal bills from the same utility
     - Making off with the check properly drawn to the creditor
     - Padding payroll rates, time, production or number of employees
     - Fictitious advances to employees, and neglecting to deduct them from subsequent payrolls
     - Duplicating payment for the same payroll or invoice by two checks signed by each of two authorized officers or partners
     - Appropriating checks made out to "cash" or the bank, supposedly for creditor's account, payment of note or expense
     - Buying improper disbursements in personal accounts of partners and officers

- o Altering the name of a payee or increasing the amount of a check after signature
- o Forging checks and destroying them on return by the bank, concealed by forced footings in the cash journal, or by raising amounts of legitimate checks
- o Mingling cashier's funds with company funds and withdrawing company's funds after cashier's are exhausted
- o Charging illegitimate withdrawals to fictitious customers' accounts

Merchandise
1. Illegitimate Removal of Merchandise
   - Covered by:

- o Overstatement of lists of physical inventory
- o Unauthorized requisitions
- o Entry only in stock records of fictitious purchase returns

2. Reporting as received, items not received (usually associated with collusion between the creditor and the receiving clerk)

Miscellaneous
1. Undercharging customers through reduction in unit prices, quantities or calculation
2. Allowing officer or employee free services or merchandise, or at reduced rate, when not entitled
3. Manipulating financial showing to secure excessive commissions, bonuses or dividends

THE MOST COMMON FINANCIAL MISTAKES VETERINARIANS MAKE

Gary I. Glassman, CPA
Burzenski & Company, P.C.
East Haven, CT

1. Many veterinarians pay their bills too quickly. When vendors provide you payment terms stick with them. If they offer discounts for early payment, make the payment early. However, if they do not, don't pay the bill until it is due. Normal credit terms provide you an ability to usually wait 20 to 30 days before payment is due. If there is not an incentive to pay early, don't. Use the "float" to work for you and invest the money through a sweep account at your bank which can earn interest. If you are fortunate enough to sell a product before you have to pay for it, you are using other's money to finance your practice operation. There is no better way to do business.

2. Many enter into leases for the purchase of equipment without considering other options. Leasing can be expensive and the imputed interest cost to a lease is not always easy to determine. Also don't be confused by the different types of leases that exist. Some generate better tax treatment than others. Consider other methods of payment besides leasing. Straight financing at the bank is usually less expensive than leasing and paying cash may be an option with no additional cost.

3. Many do not competitive price shop for products and services. Vendors will quote you a price for a product or a service but is it their best price? Many times you do not know unless you competitive price shop. Many times your best price is not your first. You may also not make price the final reason for doing business with a particular vendor, but it never hurts to get competitive prices before making a final decision. Price comparisons can be shopped for insurance, credit card services, telephone service, drugs and supplies, lab services, etc.

4. Owner veterinarians don't pay themselves on production. Owner veterinarians should pay themselves on production to hold themselves accountable to the practice for what they produce. The pay rate can be 21 to 22% of their professional collected production. Holding themselves accountable will remind owners of the way they practice and how it reflects in their earnings. They should also reward themselves a management pay. When you find out what is left over, you have a better idea of what the practice produces as excess earnings that will formulate the practice goodwill value. It also helps the practice determine available funds to pay the owner. Owners should pay themselves their pay for services and then their practice bills. Once what is leftover is known, it can be distributed to the owner(s) as a reward for the privilege of ownership.

5. Veterinarians don't plan their finances. They fail to budget. Use budgets to set the financial direction of the practice with an expected result. This way you have a better chance of meeting your goal. Once a budget is completed, input it into your accounting program and print monthly internal financial reports that can measure the budget against the actual result. If you are using QuickBooks, consider using the budget module already in the program. It works great and it's simple to use.

6. Many owners do not involve their associates in the finances of the practice. While I do not believe it necessary to share all information, I do believe it is important to share the individual doctor production information, even if they are not paid on production, and other hospital income information. As the owner of a hospital, you are the team coach. As part of your role as a coach, you have to share the playbook and let the team know how they are doing. You should also set an expectation for the results. Most will comply with your request as long as you set reasonable expectations. Monthly monitoring should also be completed so you stay the course. Develop a monthly statistical report you can share with your staff and associates.

7. Many practices have the wrong or no retirement programs for their practice. Many also start these programs late. A retirement program is easy to implement, but implementing the right one may not be as easy. SIMPLE plans, 401k plans, Profit Sharing Plans, Defined Benefit plans, SEP plans: All of these different plans can come at you at once. All have different parameters for savings levels and those levels between you as the employer and what you have to give to an employee. Choose the right one by looking at your own retirement need first. Then consider your affordability factor and how much you should put away to meet your own retirement objective. Always ask your pension specialist to provide you with an illustration of what a particular plan might look like for you so you can see the impact on your cash flow and determine what tax savings will be created. Simple plans have deferral limits for 2007 of $10,500 with an extra $2,500 available for those age 50 and over. 401k deferral limits for 2007 are $15,500 with an extra $5,000 for those age 50 and over. With profit sharing plans you can put away up to $45,000 based upon $225,000 of compensation. Plans can be combined to provide larger deductions. For associates, participate at least up to the employer match. You are missing out on free match money if you do not. Consider the use of IRA accounts on top of maximum employer plans for additional contributions. Roth IRA contributions can be made, if single, up to $99,000 before phase out and for married individuals up to $156,000 before phase out.

8. Most do not plan for the right amount of life insurance and disability insurance. Not having the right amount of coverage can be devastating to your practice and your family. Work with a qualified financial planner, accountant, and attorney who may guide you in advising you of the proper amount of coverage.

9. Many wait too long before considering an exit strategy and do not plan for the expected financial results that will drive their practice value. The type of tax entity may also impact the eventual sale. Discuss the importance of taxes related to a sale with your tax advisor 10 years before the sale especially if you are a "C" corporation. Exit strategies should be considered and started 5 years before an eventual sale. Who on your staff may be interested in purchasing your practice? How much is it worth? Will you sell your practice to a corporate owner of hospitals or through a practice broker? Have a practice valuation completed so you are aware of the practice value. Know what your practice return on investment (ROI) is and how it changes year to year so you can monitor the value of the practice. You can do this by computing the net income of the practice before the payment to owners. Then subtract payment to the owners for the performance of veterinary services and management fees. What is left is ROI. Have your accountant compute this for you each year. Based upon industry statistics in small animal practice, the ROI should approximate 11 to 13% of gross sales.

10. Many will not consider the purchase of a client list from a competing practice that may be closing. The attitude is to wait until they close and take what comes your way. Over and over again you will find it more financially rewarding to pay for a solidified client base stored in a computer system with reminders already set up and with medical records. Make sure you also take the practice phone number. If you feel uncertain about buying the whole client list at once, try to work out a purchase where you pay for only what you get and keep. It is a purchase made on a retainage basis.

WHAT DOES IT TAKE TO GET MY LOAN APPROVED?

Gary I. Glassman, CPA
Burzenski & Company, P.C.
East Haven, CT

WHAT TO CONSIDER WHEN FINANCING
1) Required down payment
2) Interest Rate – what is it related to?
- Prime Rate – Bank Internal Prime Rate/NY Wall Street Journal Prime Rate
- Treasury Index Rate – 5 year Treasury Bill
- LIBOR (London Inter-Bank Offering Rate)
- The Sale of Debentures (Bonds) – SBA CDC Loan Program
3) Costs related to routine financing
- Bank points – Equals a percentage of financing
- Legal fees – Your fee/bank's fee
- SBA fees
- Appraisal fees – Bank usually hires appraiser but you pay
- Other bank fees (ie, Inspection Fees)
4) Guarantees required – who will sign?
5) Loan Covenants
- Minimum or compensating cash balances
- Minimum working capital ratio
- Minimum equity level
- Dividend payout limitations
- Subordination of notes or advances due to stockholders or owners
- Limitations on salary increases
- Acquisition of fixed assets
- Acquisition of additional debt
- Practice sale, merger, or acquisition
- Acquisition of additional insurance on life of owner, key manager, or guarantor
- Periodic financial reporting and extent, if any, of CPA involvement, ie, compiled, reviewed, or audited financial statements.
6) Life and disability insurance requirements

TYPES OF FINANCING TO CONSIDER

Apply for:	Normal Amortization:
Building Loan	15 to 25 years
Equipment Financing	5 to 10 years
Line of Credit	Yearly renewal
Bridge Loan	Interest Only

An appraisal of the building plans is critical to proper financing since the appraisal will be the source for determining how much the bank will loan for your project. The appraisal will be based upon the finished architectural drawings. The bank loan will be based upon a percentage of the final valuation. As an example, if land were purchased for $180,000 and the building plans were appraised for $800,000, your total project appraisal would be $980,000. If bank financing were 80%, the bank loan will be $784,000. The bank will usually require a copy of the contractor's contract before final approval of financing. Veterinary buildings are special-use facilities. Find the right appraiser who is qualified to determine the project's fair market value.

When determining what costs banks will finance, consider both the "soft" and "hard" costs. Soft costs relate to architectural fees, engineering and service fees, and legal and accounting fees for your project. Hard costs relate to the actual costs of construction. Most banks under conventional financing terms will not finance soft costs, but the Small Business Association (SBA) will. Consider all of your costs which need to be financed before deciding what type of financing to apply for.

PREPARING A FINANCING PROPOSAL
Your financing proposal should include information that can be expected to help a potential lender assess whether the loan principal and interest will be paid when due. Lending institutions have identified the following factors in descending order of importance in making those assessments:

- Quality of management
- Risk of default
- Size of loan relative to size of business
- Debt-to-equity ratio
- Intended purpose of loan
- Practice's liquidity position
- Type of repayment plan
- Type of collateral available
- Past profit trend
- Future profit trend
- Stability of profits
- Ease of sale of the practice's assets in case of liquidation
- Possible future profitable relations with borrower
- Loan activity at other banks
- Loan term
- Availability of financial statements
- Length of lender's relationship with borrower
- Expected size of deposits with lender
- Rate of return borrower earns on assets

Thus, it is probably a good idea for the financing proposal to include information about these factors or information that can be expected to provide a basis for reaching a conclusion about these factors.

The typical contents of a loan proposal may be classified as follows:

- Proposal summary
- Management profiles
- Description of the practice
- Specific information about the loan requested
- Practice financial statements – current, historical, and prospective
- Personal financial statements of the practice owner

- Practice tax returns for 3 years
- Personal tax returns of the practice owner(s) for 3 years

If the practice has a business plan, it should accompany the proposal, or relevant information in the business plan (for example, the description of the business and management) may be incorporated into the proposal. Some lenders have standard loan request packages that applicants must complete. The standard packages may vary somewhat from the contents recommended above, but ordinarily they will be substantially similar.

With your loan proposal in hand, interview potential lenders. Do not only consider your present bank. You will get the best offer by interviewing a minimum of four lenders and comparing their commitment letters. If you wish to stay with your current bank but they did not make the best proposal, negotiate.

TYPES OF FINANCING AVAILABLE
Conventional Financing
- Usually through a bank
- Usually requires 20% down payment; will loan 80% of fair market value of project based upon appraisal
- Usually will not finance soft costs
- Will usually amortize on a 15- to 20-year schedule but on a 5- to 7-year term with a balloon payment or rate re-opener
- Rates can be fixed, then turn variable
- Rates can be variable
- Rates usually based upon common index such as prime rate, LIBOR or 5- year Treasury Bill rate

SBA Financing
The US Small Business Administration (SBA) is a federal agency created to encourage, assist, and protect the interests of small businesses. The SBA does not offer loans directly to borrowers, but guarantees loans made to borrowers by lenders. In the past, the SBA offered direct loans to certain groups of borrowers such as Vietnam and disabled veterans, handicapped and low-income persons, and owners of businesses in high unemployment areas. Now, these groups are eligible for loans under the SBA 7(a) Guaranty Loan Programs, and the SBA urges lenders to relax certain loan term and collateral criteria for these groups of borrowers.

Under the 7(a) Guaranty Loan Programs, a lender issues the loan, and the SBA guarantees up to 85% of aggregate loans up to $150,000. Loans greater than $150,000 up to $2 million are guaranteed up to 75%. The maximum SBA guarantee is generally $1,500.000.

Interest rates may not exceed SBA specified maximums, which are tied to *The Wall Street Journal's* New York prime rate. Depending on the loan's term, interest rates on loans over $50,000 are based on the New York prime plus 2.25% to 2.75%. The loans are secured by real estate and other practice assets (such as equipment, machinery, accounts receivable, and inventory), and personal assets (such as stocks and

bonds). Borrowers are generally required to provide 30% to 50% of the company's capitalization. For loans to corporations, the SBA requires personal guarantees of principals with 20% or more ownership. Those guarantees may be backed by mortgages of the owners, principals, or their spouses. Typically, the borrower's debt-to-equity ratio, including the SBA loan, should not exceed 3 to 1.

A prepayment charge referred to as a subsidy recoupment fee must be paid by the borrower to the SBA for any loans meeting the following criteria:

- Maturity of 15 years or more
- Prepayment amount exceeds 25% of the outstanding balance of the loan
- Prepayment is made within the first 3 years after the date of the first disbursement of the loan proceeds

The prepayment fee calculation is based on when the prepayment is made. Under the 7(a) Guaranty Loan Programs, the participating lender conducts the initial interview with the borrower, forwards the loan application to the SBA, answers any questions from the SBA about the proposed loan, and closes the loan. Guaranteed loans are disbursed by the lender and guaranteed by the SBA. If the borrower defaults on the guaranteed loan, the SBA will buy an agreed-upon percentage of the loan balance back from the lender. Even though the SBA is restricted to a maximum guarantee of $1,500,000, regulations do not preclude individual participating lenders from setting higher or lower loan limits.

By law, the SBA can consider loan applications only from small businesses that are unable to obtain reasonable financing from other sources. The lender certifies to the SBA that it will not make the loan without an SBA guarantee, and this certification is generally accepted by the SBA as sufficient proof that the requested financing is otherwise unavailable.

To offset the costs of the SBA's loan programs to the taxpayer, the Agency charges lenders a guaranty and a servicing fee for each loan approved. These fees can be passed on to the borrower once they have been paid by the lender. The amount of the fees is determined by the amount of the loan guaranty.

Effective December 8, 2004, when the loan amount is from $150,000 up to and including $700,000, a 3% guaranty fee will be charged. For loans greater than $700,000, a 3.5% guaranty fee will be charged and for loans greater than $1,000,000 there is an additional up-front guarantee fee equal to 0.25% of the amount by which the loans exceeds $1,000,000.

In addition, all loans will be subject to a 55 basis point (0.55%) annualized servicing fee, which is applied to the outstanding balance of SBA's guaranteed portion of the loan.

Processing fees, origination fees, application fees, points, brokerage fees, bonus points, and other fees that could be charged to an SBA loan applicant are prohibited. The only time a commitment fee may be charged is for a loan made under the Export Working

Capital Loan Program.

Practice owners should be aware of certain disadvantages to SBA program loans. The loan process can be cumbersome unless the client is dealing with a lender that has significant experience with SBA loans. Also, SBA loans can be very inflexible. For example, SBA loans are not easy to restructure; thus, changing payment streams can be very difficult after these loans have closed.

SBA 7(a) Guaranty Loan Programs

The Regular 7(a) Guaranty Loan Program. The Regular 7(a) Guaranty Loan is similar to other bank financing arrangements in most respects and is the most frequently used form of SBA financing. SBA guaranteed loans are primarily used to provide working capital, to assist in the acquisition of equipment and other assets, and to buy real property.

Terms are negotiated between the borrower and the participating lender, subject to the approval of the SBA. The following maximum maturities are available:

Use of Loan Proceeds	Loan Maturity
Working capital	7 to 10 years
Machinery and equipment	Up to a maximum of 25 years
Real estate purchase or construction	Up to a maximum of 25 years

However, in no instance can the maturity of the loan exceed the life of the assets being financed. SBA loans are fully amortizing, so there are no balloon payments.

Disbursement of the loan proceeds is handled by the lender. Depending on the use of proceeds (for example, for working capital or construction), it may be made in one payment or in a series of payments over a period that, in general, does not exceed 6 months.

504 Program

Under Section 504 of the Small Business Act, certified development companies (CDC) offer 10 and 20 year loans to small businesses for acquisition of land and buildings (including machinery and equipment, professional fees, and other "soft costs"). A bank or financial institution selected by the borrower provides 50% or more of the project cost secured by a first lien. The CDC provides up to 40% (usually up to $2,000,000) of the project cost secured by a second lien. The borrower must put in a minimum of 10% of the project. The borrower negotiates terms within these parameters with the financial institution. The CDC interest rate is fixed. Generally, the rate is a few basis points more than that of US Treasury bonds at the loan date for the maturity selected. In addition, the borrower must pay fees amounting to approximately 3% of the debenture amount. These fees may be financed through the loan.

CHOOSING A LENDER

After the practice has selected a type of financing, it may have to choose among lenders. Some practices automatically choose the lender with the lowest total cost. However, all of the relevant factors should be considered. Other criteria the practice might consider include:

- Lender's size and ability to meet future needs
- Lender's knowledge of the borrower's business
- Lender's speed of making credit decisions (especially when obtaining a line of credit or other financing that must be renewed)
- Loan officer's status in the organization and the frequency with which loan officers are changed
- Types of costs and commitments imposed. (For example, some practices prefer not to maintain a compensating balance)
- Lender's flexibility in responding to special requests (such as foreign letters of credit)

NEGOTIATING THE FINANCING

After the financing proposal has been prepared and the potential lender identified, you should make plans to negotiate with the lender. The objective involves negotiations because each party seeks its own most advantageous position and the terms can influence the lender's decision about whether to provide the funds.

Points to be negotiated:

- Amount
- Interest rate and fees
- Term of the loan
- Repayment schedule
- Amount and type of collateral
- Guarantees
- Restrictive covenants
- Acquisition of additional insurance on the life of the owner, key manager or guarantor
- Periodic financial reporting and the extent of CPA involvement

Refer to the SBA Website for more information: www.SBA.gov.

TAX TIPS: AN UPDATE

Gary I. Glassman, CPA
Burzenski & Company, P.C.
East Haven, CT

Tax laws are forever changing and this year is no exception. Since taxes can take a significant amount of our earnings, it pays to know and understand the tax laws that are important for you and your practice. This clear understanding can save you money and keep you out of tax trouble.

TAX LAW CHANGES FOR 2006 AND 2007:

The Tax Increase Prevention and Reconciliation Act (H.R. 4297) was signed into law by the President on May 17, 2006. The President also signed the Small Business and Work Opportunity Tax Act of 2007 (H.R. 2206) on May 25, 2007. This new law began life as a tax reconciliation bill designed primarily to retroactively extend a number of popular tax breaks that expired at the end of 2005, and extend a number of tax breaks due to expire in future years. The 2007 bill was coupled with an increase in the federal minimum wage.

1. **The Alternative Minimum Tax (AMT)** – More people are finding that they have to pay AMT in addition to their regular income tax. The AMT tax rates are 26% and 28%. You will want to gauge your AMT exposure when you do tax planning. Here is a list of items that can trigger the tax:

- Claiming many exemptions for dependents
- Claiming large itemized deductions for job and other miscellaneous expenses
- Claiming a large itemized deduction for state and local taxes, including property taxes
- Generating a large capital gain transaction

For 2006, the AMT exemption amount for married taxpayers increased to $62,550 and for unmarried individuals to $42,500 (instead of dropping to $45,000 and $33,700, respectively), and nonrefundable personal tax credits may be claimed to the full extent of an individual's regular tax and AMT (instead of being limited to the excess of regular tax liability over tentative minimum tax). Without a law change, the AMT amounts for 2007 will drop to $45,000 for joint filers and surviving spouses, $33,750 for unmarried individuals, and $22,500 for married individuals filing separately.

2. **Maximize depreciation deductions** with the use of IRS Code Section 179. For 2007, this allows the expense of up to $125,000 of new equipment purchases in the year of purchase. Trucks and SUVs also qualify if they are used more than 50% for business and are over 6,000 pounds gross loaded weight for trucks or over 6,000 pounds gross vehicle weight for SUVs, but are now limited to a $25,000 deduction. Leased property should be under a $1 buy-out lease to qualify. The extended favorable Section 179 limits now remain in effect through 2010.

3. **The current tax rate** on capital gains and dividends is 15%. These current laws' favorable tax rates for capital gains and qualified dividend income remain in place through 2010 (instead of sunsetting after 2008).

4. **The Kiddie Tax** – Investment income of a child under age 14 was generally taxed at the parents' top marginal rate if such income exceeds the sum of the $850 standard deduction and the greater of $850 or the itemized deductions directly connected to the production of that investment income. This rule applies to a child's investment income regardless of its source and requires a calculation of the parents' "allocable parental tax." For tax years beginning after 2005, the age at which the kiddie tax applies is changed from under 14 to under 18 years of age. For years beginning after 2007, the kiddie tax age has been raised to under 19 and students under the age of 24. This recent change will affect millions of families. College age students will no longer be able to sell off their appreciated investment accounts set up by their parents to cover current tuition. At a minimum, taking out student loans with interest until the year the student turns age 24 will be necessary now to carry forward such a plan. However, the maximum tax of capital gains imposed on any stock sale might rise from 15% to 20%, adding another price tag to postponing income recognition.

5. **A traditional IRA** can be converted to a Roth IRA by paying the tax on the conversion and in the year of the conversion. Currently this conversion can only be made if modified adjusted gross income is $100,000 or less. This modified AGI limit on conversions of traditional IRAs to Roth IRAs, is eliminated to tax years beginning after December 31, 2009.

6. **If you have been in tax trouble** with an outstanding tax balance that you could not pay, the IRS offers you an offer-in-compromise program to settle your tax bill for less than you owe. For offers-in-compromise submitted on and after July 16, 2006, taxpayers must make partial payments to IRS while their offer is being considered.

THE ENERGY TAX INCENTIVES ACT OF 2005:

7. **Purchase of a hybrid vehicle** - Are there any tax advantages to buying a hybrid passenger automobile (passenger automobile that is propelled by both a gasoline engine and an electric motor that is recharged as the motor vehicle operates)?

Beginning in 2006, a tax credit of up to $3,400 is available. For new hybrid vehicles purchased in 2007, you can obtain a tax credit from $400 to $3,400 depending on the model. A credit is usually more advantageous than a deduction because a tax credit is subtracted dollar-for-dollar off the bottom line of your federal tax bill, while a deduction simply reduces taxable income.

The amount of the credit depends on the fuel efficiency of the vehicle. The more gas it saves, the higher the credit. However, calculating the credit is a bit complicated, with the exact amount of your credit depending on three separate factors; the weight of the vehicle, its fuel economy, and its lifetime fuel savings. This information should be available from your dealer.

The credit is set to expire at the end of 2010, but for many hybrid models, the incentive will end much sooner. That is because the law limits the credits to 60,000 vehicles from each automaker. Once a manufacturer has sold 60,000 hybrid vehicles, the tax credit for that manufacturer's hybrids is slowly reduced over the next five consecutive quarters, eventually dripping to zero. For other manufacturers, their hybrid cars will have the full tax credit for a longer period. Check with the dealer you plan on making your purchase through to make sure the credit from the manufacturer is still available.

8. New 10% personal tax credit for energy efficient improvements to existing homes. The lifetime maximum credit per taxpayer is $500 and applies for property placed in service after December 31, 2005 and before January 1, 2008. The credit is still good for 2007 improvements.

9. New deduction for energy efficient commercial buildings meeting a 50% energy reduction standard. The deduction (generally $1.80 per square foot, but 60¢ per square foot in some cases) is effective for property placed in service after December 2005 and before January 1, 2008

OTHER TAX ISSUES YOU SHOULD BE AWARE OF:

10. Cost Segregation Studies - If you are depreciating your hospital building over 39 years, you may be missing out on accelerated depreciation of certain components.

It is true that business buildings generally have a 39-year depreciation period. However, some items of property that are, seemingly, "part of the building" can, nevertheless, be depreciated over a period for shorter than 39 years. Generally, the speedier depreciation is available for items that service the equipment used in a building, but is not available for items that service the operation and maintenance of a building. The concept in getting quicker deductions is through cost segregation. Make sure your builder or architect provides you the documentation that cost segregates your project. A tax court case involving the Hospital Corporation of America set the stage. The court case allows building costs, if segregated, to be written off over much faster lives. If certain items can be considered tangible personal property, you may even be able to expense them under IRS section 179 in the year of purchase.

What costs are we referring to? Well, as an example, electrical wiring directly related to a piece of medical equipment or to computers can be considered part of the cost of the equipment and can be expensed or written off over 5 or 7 years. This might include wiring for x-ray machines or surgical lights. How about plumbing for a wet table or automatic processor? They should qualify for accelerated write off as well as the cost of cabinetry. When it comes to flooring, the cost of tile must be written off over 39 years but the cost of vinyl floor covering or carpeting qualify for a 7-year write off. Landscaping and paving is covered under a 15-year write off.

If you finished a building project in a previous year, it isn't too late to get the benefit of speedier depreciation for any other items that were incorrectly assumed to be part of your building for depreciation purposes. You don't have to amend your past returns (or meet any deadline for claiming tax refunds) to claim the depreciation that you could have already claimed. Instead, you can claim that depreciation by following procedures, in connection with the next return that you file, that will result in "automatic" IRS consent to a change in your accounting for depreciation. Among the results of the process will be a one-time downward adjustment in your income, equal to the amount of the unclaimed depreciation. There are, however, some things to consider before beginning the process. One consideration is that you must do the work, probably with the help of your contractors or other construction experts, of identifying and substantiating the qualifying costs. Another consideration is that, before starting the work, you must judge whether the work will result in overall tax savings greater than the costs of the work itself.

11. Consider selling a practice vehicle before trading it in. It may provide a current tax loss not otherwise available.

12. Reduce your taxable income by recognizing credit card charges as an additional expense even when the credit card is not paid and you report on the cash basis. The IRS views credit card obligations as debt and not vendor accounts payable.

13. **Consider IRS Section 125 plans for health insurance** if your employees are asked to contribute towards their health insurance costs. These plans can also be used for group term life insurance and short-and long-term disability insurance. In a more complicated format, they can be used for reimbursement of medical expenses not covered by insurance and dependent-care reimbursement. Pet insurance provided to employees is not included and must be considered a taxable fringe benefit included in the income of the employee each year.

14. Consider long term care insurance as part of your overall financial plan. The premiums are deductible within limits.

15. Separate the practice real estate from the practice entity and pay a fair market value rent. The industry average for rent expense is 5% to 8% of gross revenue. Generally, fair market value rent can range between $12 and $18 a square foot on a triple net basis depending on geographic location. Another way to look at fair market value rent is to pay 10% of the fair market of the property yearly based upon a current real estate appraisal.

16. Choose a retirement program for yourself and employees that matches your goals:

- Pension plan/money purchase plan
- Profit sharing plan
- 401K plan
- SEP plan
- Simple plan

New contribution limits are in effect for 2007. Use non-deductible IRAs when over the phase-out ranges for traditional or Roth contributions.

17. Late 401K Deposits - Sometimes it just happens. The person responsible for payroll takes a vacation and forgets to send the 401(k) deposit in prior to leaving. At the end of the year, the accounts are reconciled and low and behold, the missing contribution is found.

The Department of Labor (DOL) takes a very harsh position on this occurrence. This is considered a prohibited transaction (PT) and is subject to all sorts of sanctions. The PT must be immediately corrected and an excise tax is due for as long as it is outstanding. Additionally, if the correction is made in another plan year because it crossed over, two Form 5330's must be filed with a doubling of the excise tax.

Interest is due from the date is should have been made to the date of the correction. The DOL has provided worksheets for a safe-harbor computation on their website. Even if all corrections are made, the DOL can still impose a 20% penalty tax on the fiduciaries for the breach of their responsibility.

Clearly, this is an overkill for a minor infraction. To avoid the 20% penalty tax on the breach, you can file under the Voluntary Fiduciary Correction Program and the DOL will issue a no penalty letter.

To be on the safe side, always deposit the 401(k) contributions and loan repayments on each pay date. Most vendors accept electronic submission of the payroll data in an ACH deposit.

18. Pay family members for legitimate jobs and duties. Wages to a spouse require the payment of FICA and FUTA taxes. It may only be an advantage to pay your spouse if additional pension contributions are considered.

19.   Health Savings Accounts (HSAs) - Health savings accounts are designed to allow individuals to save for current and post-retirement qualified medical expenses on a tax-free basis. Any eligible individual who is covered by a high deductible health plan (HDHP) can establish and contribute to an HSA. Contributions are tax-deductible if made by an individual, or excluded from income if paid by and employer. Earnings in HSAs are not taxable, and distributions are not included in income if used to pay qualified medical expenses. Unused amounts remain in the account available for use in later years. Amounts contributed to an HSA belong to the individual, so continue to be available to an individual that changes employers or leaves the work force.

Establishing an HSA – Health savings accounts are set up with a financial institution (such as a bank or an insurance company). No permission or authorization from the IRS is necessary to establish an HSA. The HSA can be established though a through a trustee that is different from the HDHP provider.

Eligible individuals – To qualify for an HSA, an individual must meet the following requirements.

- Must be covered under and HDHP
- May not be covered under any other non-HDHP health plan

- May not be entitled to Medicare benefits.
- Cannot be claimed as a dependent on another person's return

Note: Individuals who are eligible for Medicare but not yet enrolled continue to qualify until the month the individual is enrolled.

HSA contributions – Contributions for the tax year:

- Must be made in cash or through a cafeteria plan.
- Can be made in one or more payments, at the convenience of the individual or employer, but cannot be made before the beginning of the tax year.
- Must be made by the return due date (without extensions) for the tax year

HSA Established by an Employee – The employee, the employer or both may contribute to the HSA. Contributions made by the employee are deductible from AGI. Contributions made by the employer (including contributions made through a cafeteria plan) are excluded from income and are not subject to employment taxes.

HSA Established by an Individual (Self-Employed or Unemployed) – The eligible individual may contribute to the HSA or any person (such as a family member) may contribute to an HSA on behalf of an eligible individual. Contributions made by the individual (or by any other person) are deductible from the individual's AGI. Contributions to a self-employed individual's own HSA are not taken into account in determining net earnings from self-employment.

Catch-up contributions – To encourage saving for health expenses after retirement, individuals who are age 55 or older by the end of 2005 are allowed an additional contribution. The catch-up contribution limit areas follow:

The additional contribution amount for tax years beginning in:

2007	800
2008	900
2009 and later	1,000

20. Employee vs. Independent contribution.

EMPLOYEE vs. RELIEF VETERINARIAN

To determine whether a worker is an independent contractor or an employee, IRS examines the relationship between the worker and the business, and considers all evidence of control and independence. The facts that provide this evidence fall into the following three categories:

- Behavioral control covers facts that show whether the business has a right to direct and control how the work is done through instructions, training, or other means, Employees are generally given instructions on when and where to work, what tools to use, where to purchase supplies, what order to follow, etc. And employees are often trained to perform services in a particular manner.

- Financial control covers facts that show whether the business has a right to control the financial and business aspects of the worker's job. This includes the extent to which the worker has unreimbursed business expenses; the extent of his investment in the facilities being used; the extent to which he can realize a profit or incur a loss. For example, independent contractors are more likely to have unreimbursed expenses, be available to work for others in the relevant market, and make a profit or loss.
- Type of relationship includes written contracts describing the relationship the parties intended to create; the extent to which the worker is available to perform services for other, similar businesses; whether the business provides the worker with employee-type benefits, such as insurance, a pension plan, vacation pay, or sick pay; the permanency of the relationship; and the extent to which services performed by the worker are a key aspect of the company's regular business. For example, an employee's relationship is more likely to be permanent and an employee is more likely to provide services that are a key aspect of the business.

Taxpayers who would like IRS to determine employee status can file Form SS-8, which reflects the factors noted above. The previous 20-point test used by the IRS is no longer valid.

FINANCIAL TOOLS TO MAKE YOUR PRACTICE EXCEL

Gary I. Glassman, CPA
Burzenski & Company, P.C.
East Haven, CT

What kind of things will veterinary owners need to do for the development of the business owner's skill set? They will need to learn to develop and use good information from hospital data to make business decisions. They will have to stop running their practices based upon what's in the checking account and rely more on the financial data from, reports that can be printed from the veterinary software, financial statements and budgets. Reports from the veterinary software will tell you instances of services and what type of products and services are being sold. Not only that but they can tell you who made the sale. They report taxable vs. non taxable sales and what is being given away in discounts. Budgets will assist in setting the hospital's financial direction and achievement of desired goals including profitability. Financial statements will provide a sense of the past and report patterns of income and expenses as well as profitability. Most practices today are data rich and information poor. Today's practice needs less data and more information. Peter F. Drucker said, "The fewer the data needed, the better the information. And an overload of information, that is, anything much beyond what is truly needed, leads to information blackout. It does not enrich, but impoverishes." So what information should you develop for your practice? Owners and managers need key operating information. They are sometimes referred to as the practice pulse points.

For tracking income and income statistics develop a report to track monthly sales, new clients, number of invoices, and the average per invoice. Do the same for each of the doctors and provide them a copy of all reports each month. Also track the amount of accounts receivable each month to make sure credit and collection policies are in control.

Once you determine what your centers of revenue are, prepare financial reports in a manor that reflects these centers. For instance, if the hospital has strong retail, boarding and grooming activity as well as the practice of veterinary medicine, then report on a cost center basis to determine profitability in each of these centers. It will draw your attention to those areas of the practice that need or don't need work. Hopefully all activity areas of the hospital are profitable, but segmenting your operation may find that some areas are more profitable than others or some areas operate at a loss. Once you understand your reporting requirements, set up you accounting system chart of accounts in a way that will allow you to accumulate the information so it can be seen this way. Set up a schedule to receive monthly internal financial statements. Most should be able to close their books by the 15th day of the following month and have an internal financial statement prepared by the 20th. Prepare a budget and make the statements comparative to budget. Also, make them comparative to last year's data. Prepare a budget based upon the same chart of accounts used to accumulate actual financial data so they will be comparative. Check the line items each month to determine where you might be out of line. Know where you stand in terms of profitability every month and whether you hit your budgeted target for profitability. Have your accountant provide you monthly standard entries every month for reoccurring items that effect profitability such as depreciation expense. Make sure whatever accounting adjustments your accountants make to complete your books and records are given to you so your records can match theirs. This will keep your record complete.

Understand that all costs in your hospital are either fixed or variable. Fixed expenses are those that remain the same regardless of the change in sales for the facility. These types of expenses include rent, utilities, insurance, etc. Variable expenses are those that move in direct proportion to sales. These costs include drug and supplies, lab costs and animal disposal costs. Once you can define these costs in your hospital, understand the nature and relationship of these costs to changes in your hospital's revenue stream. How do they affect profitability? For instance, if you improve compliance with blood work and provide 100 additional pre-anesthetic blood tests, how will affect profitability? Once you are past the cost of the test and the labor to run it and interpret it, the remainder of the additional fee falls to the bottom line and the impact can be significant. The fixed costs of the hospital don't change. It is important to note that veterinary medicine is a fixed cost business and a majority of the costs to run the hospital are fixed.

With a good understanding of fixed and variable costs, know what it costs to open your door every day. This can be calculated by determining your fixed costs and dividing it by the number of days you are open. Also, calculate a break even point for the hospital. The formula is:

$$\text{Breakeven in sales} = \frac{\text{Fixed costs}}{\text{Contribution Margin}}$$

The contribution margin = 1 – variable costs. Share this information with your staff.

THE MONTHLY STATISTICAL ANALYSIS REPORT

Consider developing a monthly statistical analysis report for your practice. Take a pulse of your practice by understanding the monthly statistics that are important and track them in a comparative format; month to month, year by year. The information which should be tracked comes from your computer generated monthly reports. The most important statistics are as follows:

- Monthly gross sales
- New clients
- Number of invoices
- Average per invoice (ACT)
- Monthly accounts receivable balances
- Doctor production – share this information with your doctors

THE BUDGET

Budgets should an integral part of your overall financial plan. With budgets in place you are more likely to control the financial destiny of the practice. The question always is; are you controlling your financial affairs or is the practice controlling you? While preparing a budget may not fully answer the question, it can certainly play a part in determining its financial success. It is the tool that quantifies the practice's goals and serves as a yardstick for measuring its degree of success. It will also relieve your sense of frustration resulting from a lack of direction.

What else can a budget be used for? Well not only can it be used for predicting income; it can be used to assist in controlling expenses. It can be used in such a way, that once completed, the information can be given to department heads or others who are put in control of practice areas such as payroll, inventory control, and administrative supplies to assist in controlling their areas of responsibility. If you hold them accountable, it is also very important that you provide feedback of actual expenses to budget so that they can see and measure how they are doing.

How do you get started preparing your budget? Set the budget utilizing a spreadsheet program like excel where it is easy to set totals and other calculations by formula. Budgets are meant to be flexible and subject to change so when you do so you want to make it easy on yourself for all other results to change as well. "What if" situations can easily be handled in this way. An alternative to the excel spreadsheet would be the utilization of QuickBooks 2007. See the May, 2004 issue of *Veterinary Economics*, page 16, for setting up a budget in QuickBooks. If you are a QuickBooks user and are not utilizing one of these versions, consider it. The 2007 version has an easy to use budget preparation tools that allow you to format your information the same way the QuickBooks chart of accounts is set up. Setting up your budget tool in the same format as you report historical information is important so you can make easy comparisons to actual results.

Where do the numbers come from? The past is always a great predictor of the future and finding past financial results and having them in front of you is important.

The starting place for your budget is income. The easiest way to project it is to do so by utilizing your veterinary software to determine your past year's monthly income. Enter these amounts onto the spreadsheet. Note the number of invoices generated each month and the average invoice. Then project this year's variable by looking at each component and determining how it will increase. When projecting invoices, consider any new programs or marketing you be doing that will increase the number of invoices. For instance, you may be planning a big dental promotion next February so you should take this into consideration when projecting how many invoices will be generated in the month of February. At the same time look at changes in the average invoice and take into consideration new marketing of services to existing clients or maybe changes in vaccine protocols. Also, don't forget to also consider any changes in the pricing structure that may take place. Once the revenue budget is complete, also prepare a budget for each doctor based upon the same methodology. Income budgets as a component of the entire process should be shared with staff and doctors. Once the process is complete, also remember to benchmark the actual results with the budget and share that information. This way, doctors and staff will have an ability to measure their performance in terms of what was anticipated. Significant variance between the budget and actual should be explained.

Once the income is complete, it's time to move to expenses. Expenses should be looked at in terms of those that are variable and those that are fixed. Fixed should be put into the budget as set dollar amounts in the month the expense is actually incurred. For instance, if the rent is $6,000 per month, then this amount is put into the budget every month for the same amount. Insurance may be a fixed amount but only paid in January, April, and July.

If this is the case, then the amounts anticipated to be paid should be input only in those months. The following is a list of fixed expenses which should be input into the budget based upon a fixed dollar amount:

- Employee Benefit Programs
- Professional Dues and Subscriptions
- Laundry and Uniforms
- Continuing Education
- Rent on premises
- Rent on business equipment
- Maintenance and service contracts
- Housekeeping and janitorial supplies
- Repairs and maintenance
- Real estate taxes
- Personal property taxes
- Insurance
- Utilities
- Telephone
- Advertising and promotion
- Business gifts and flowers
- Business Meetings
- Printing expense
- Computer supplies
- Office supplies
- Postage expense
- Accounting fees
- Legal fees
- Payroll processing fees
- Charitable contributions
- Business consultation services
- Bank charges
- Miscellaneous
- Depreciation expense
- Amortization expense
- Interest expense

Expenses that are not fixed by dollars are considered variable and in theory move in direct proportion to fluctuations in income. These expenses should be budgeted as a percentage of gross income. The following is a list of variable expenses that should be budgeted based upon a percentage of gross income:

- Drugs and medical supplies
- Lab costs
- Radiology costs
- Dietary products
- Surgery costs
- Dentistry costs
- Anesthesia costs
- Animal disposal
- Salaries and wages
- Payroll taxes

The variable expense percentages that are used should be based upon the historical past or based upon an anticipated target. For instance, a look at the previous year financial statements indicate that that drug and supply costs for 2003 were 18% of gross revenue but the industry target is 16%. You can base the cost at the 18% or 16% depending upon the target you are looking to achieve.

THE HOSPITAL FINANCIAL STATEMENT
Revenue Analysis

Enhance your financial statement with a full revenue analysis. A hospital revenue analysis within the financial statement might look like the following:

XYZ Veterinary Hospital
Income Statement
For the years ended December 31, 2007 and 2006

Sales	2007	%	2006	%
Vaccinations	$ 67,541	12	$ 60,282	12
Professional services/examinations	118,196	21	105,493	21
Medicines	118,196	21	105,493	21
Laboratory/diagnostics	95,682	17	85,399	17
Surgery	39,999	7	35,164	7
Radiology	28,142	5	25,117	5
Anesthesia	22,514	4	20,094	4
Treatments	16,885	3	15,070	3
Hospitalizations	16,885	3	15,070	3
Dentistry	11,257	2	10,047	2
Prescription diets	22,514	4	20,094	4
Food	5,628	1	5,023	1
Retail	5,627	1	5,024	1
Discounts	(5,628)	(1)	(5,023)	(1)
Total Sales	$562,838	100	$502,347	100

YOU, ME, & THE 360 REVIEW

James E. Guenther, DVM, MBA, MHA, CVPM
Brakke Veterinary Practice Management Group
Asheville, NC

As an owner or manager of a veterinary practice, you have invested a lot of time, money, and a significant amount of energy to build a successful practice. It is nearly impossible to achieve the success you desire without the creative juices of positive, productive team members. These same people need to know they are appreciated on a regular basis so they continue to grow both as people and as team members in your organization.

Besides daily pats on the back for a job well done the performance review is the next best way to ensure that each employee is growing and meeting their job expectations. The performance review is not an easy task and is often neglected or more likely put off for years because someone feels uncomfortable conducting the review.

Most performance reviews have been done either by the practice manager or the owner. Most if not all of these have come down to negativity of performance dating back as much as 6 plus months. What good has that accomplished both for the person or the practice? Have you considered these thoughts in performing employee reviews?

- Start with all of the positives about the person. In essence, what you are doing is a personalized SWOT analysis (*Strengths*, *Weaknesses*, *Opportunities*, *Threats*) of the employee. In any good SWOT analysis, you always start with the strengths of the person. This aids in creating a positive environment for friendlier discussion of the person's weaknesses.
- Don't be confrontational. The point of any performance review is to review the job performance of the employee and not their personal traits. Yes, those traits may be the cause but it is wiser to have the employee realize that possibility and discuss it than for you to do it.
- Become a good listener. It is not about you doing all of the talking. It is about listening to what they have to say and not being the center of the review.
- Be consistent with your reviews. There are plenty of evaluation forms out there that will work in getting you started. Consistency of your reviews makes them easier to perform and eliminates the need to constantly re-invent the wheel. It starts with being prepared ahead of time for the review.
- Document the review in the employee's personal file. This is as much the legal aspect of human resources plus it makes it easier to review and prepare before the next review.
- Regular reviews are a must—at the very least yearly—but it might be wise to consider more frequently for all employees, especially the new hires.

One of the newer approaches for performance reviews are the 360 reviews. You may be wondering what is a 360 review? It is a technique where by people above, below, and beside you review your performance. Scary, isn't it? Businesses and veterinary practices that have used it see the good and bad aspects of the program but have learned to tweak it to their needs. What are some of the good aspects of the program?

- The obvious one is more voices appraising the person and not just the owner/manager. The people talking are seeing things that one person does not always see. These are the people working with this person daily and their perceptions are important if the practice is ever going to become a team.
- In a multi-rater system, it can elevate the concept of accountability of the person within the team. A well-orchestrated program can improve communication and trust which are the foundation of a strong team.
- In the case of veterinary medicine, client service is very important for the success of the practice. A 360 review can aid in evaluating the quality, consistency, and responsiveness of the employee when dealing with their peers or the external client.
- It can aid in finding the weaknesses of the employee and in some cases the practice. These findings can be earmarked to improve training for the practice.

With any new program, there are always concerns that need to be evaluated and the 360 review is no exception. By understanding some of the perceived downsides you, the practice owner/manager, can tweak the system to reduce the negativity of the program. Some of these points are as follows:

- The 360 review can be a disaster if it does not support the direction or goals of the practice. This program can solve problems and create the team you desire if you are willing to listen, have trust, and good communication amongst the team. The goal is to continually improve the quality of service provided by making sure the providers are in tune with the goals of the practice.
- Do not focus on the negatives. If as a good human resource person, you have hired the best minds available who have the ability to learn the skill. As the old saying goes: "hire for attitude and train for skills." This type person has the positives, which mean the negatives are few and far between.
- The buddy system can inflate the reviews. This is why trust and communication are so important for the growth of the practice. Create checks and balances to reduce the likelihood of cronies making each other look great.
- With multiple people reviewing there is that much more paper to keep track of in an employee's file. This is not a big deal if you plan on how to streamline the process. Consistency means developing a good repeatable system.

The goal of this article is to make sure you realize performance reviews are very important for the growth of the person and the practice. For years, veterinarians considered employees a necessary evil. Today the employees are assets to be invested in and monitored for success both for their personal as well as practice growth. Performance reviews are a way to measure the success of your team and to continually improve on the quality of service your practice provides.

THREE STEPS TO IMPROVING SELLING THE INVISIBLE

James E. Guenther, DVM, MBA, MHA, CVPM
Brakke Veterinary Practice Management Group
Asheville, NC

What the heck is selling the invisible anyway? The answer is simple, service. You are in the service business, not the animal business that you originally thought you were in. The product is the animals you daily work on but the real business is the ability to sell peace of mind to the clients that bring the pets into your office. Don't settle for having merely satisfied clients; keep them "wowed" with the entire experience at your office. To accomplish this task let's look at *three* steps for improving the art of selling the invisible.

ATMOSPHERICS

Call it atmospherics, visuals, or even packaging—what you or better yet your client sees can completely influence their entire impression of you, your team, and your practice. The saying: "perception is reality" is totally accurate. Your eyes see quality and transform it into an experience. It is the visual cues that can give us clues about what to expect. Yes, as consumers we have standards of what is expected and when they have been exceeded a new and improved standard appears.

One of the most common occurrences in veterinary medicine is when a practice moves into a bright, shiny new facility and their gross goes up. Has the quality of medicine been elevated to new levels? Maybe. Has the team transformed into unbelievably knowledgeable people? Sometimes. Is it because it is a brand new, well designed, clean smelling, well landscaped, and incredible beautiful facility? Yes! Most new facilities will demonstrate double-digit growth for a few years after the move. The answer may lie in the knowledge that you have improved the experience of the client by creating a new image.

Atmospherics can be extended beyond just what the facility looks like. It is looking like you want to succeed. Harry Beckwith in his book *The Invisible Touch* states: "What impression do you make, then, when you appear to have invested very little in your own business—in your brochure, offices, business cards, presentations, advertisements? You're saying you lack confidence in your own enterprise. You are not confident enough to invest in yourself." He sums it up with "if you believe in your business, show it." Do you believe in your practice? If so, then don't be a penny-pinching veterinarian.

BRANDING

There is probably a little bit of timidness in veterinarians to consider creating a brand identity. The fear is not fully understanding: you already have one. It is your reputation! Are you going to embrace that brand, manage it, and grow it to its fullest potential or allow it fall by the wayside? The importance is to realize that when you want to sell peace of mind a brand (reputation) creates the power of the service.

Your name or reputation is an asset to be nurtured, managed, and to be improved on. It has taken many long hard years to develop the reputation that your name or brand stands for. It is something to take pride in and to instill confidence in your employees as well as your clients. Your clients have learned that you are the right fit for them. When you have achieved this level, you have created the preference or habit by which clients will return. At the same time, you are presenting a consistent product to your users. You cannot and should not even try to be all things to all people. Focus on your core business and develop the brand reputation that will set you apart from other veterinary practices. The choice is yours.

PEOPLE

Now you may ask why are people in this short list of steps to improve selling the invisible? One of the first thoughts is differences in how veterinarians in the past and the present hire their team. In the past, it appeared that one of the first prerequisites for hiring was the person needed to be an animal lover followed by being a people hater. Think about for a second. Veterinary medicine is a service business which means dealing with public all day long. Why would someone want to hire a person who is not comfortable or willing to talk to people? Sounds like a recipe for a disaster.

For your clients, you want to create a connection, both for their pets as well as themselves. You have read the surveys regarding why clients leave a practice. The top few reasons are not about money; it is about the practice not doing what they said they would do or not feeling attached to the practice. It has been shown that a large number of clients will pass several other practices to get to yours. In some cases, it is because the veterinarians are good or special but in a lot of cases, it is because of the people working in the practice that the client has a connection with. They have been made to feel important by someone in the practice. Why not find out and replicate this feeling to improve selling the invisible?

Practice ownership is getting more challenging each year while the number of pets is staying about the same. The slice of pie is getting smaller because of more practices opening up. It is up to you and your team of dedicated professionals to figure out how you can keep your clients and attract more. Creating a nice brand, improving the atmospherics, and hiring and training the right people will help improve selling the invisible.

HIRE THE BEST EDUCATORS YOU CAN

James E. Guenther, DVM, MBA, MHA, CVPM
Brakke Veterinary Practice Management Group
Asheville, NC

If you have not reminded yourself recently, you are in the service business. For years, most veterinarians and their staff assumed they were in the animal business. The reality of the situation is they are in the people business. They are working with people to give these clients peace of mind about the real and perceived problems with their animals.

In her book, *Practice Made Perfect* Dr. Marsha Heinke states the following: "Like any service-based industry, veterinary medicine depends on satisfied clients who make decisions about expending money on a discretionary commodity. Client satisfaction depends on trained, customer-focused employees. Insightful veterinary staffers learn to work effectively with people so that the animal can get the care it deserves."

For years veterinarians felt it was an asset to hire animal lovers and people haters. A problem started when these animal lover/people haters were made into receptionists and/or veterinary assistants. These individuals were ill equipped to handle the demands of meeting, greeting, and satisfying clients. In fact, their attitudes and lack of people skills could easily harm the financial aspects of the practice. They were not qualified to work with people let alone give the client the positive feeling that the practice could solve their pet's problems.

Veterinary medicine is in the people business. The profession has learned that making good recommendations to clients is an important element in the success of the both the profession and the practice. Recommendations are nothing more than giving someone the information to make an informed decision. Successful businesses do not sell anything to clients; what they really do is give information for the purposes of having the client make the best decision for the care of their pet. To accomplish this task of disseminating information to clients, practices will need to hire the best educators available and then teach them about the best care for pets.

Mark Opperman has always stated that a practice needs to hire "10's." What he is alluding to is hiring people that like people, enjoy educating, enjoy communicating, and in turn want to make a difference in the pets and people they meet. Whether you like it or not you are an educator and you need to surround yourself with people that love to communicate and teach.

As the phrase, "hire for attitude and train for skill" implies you are in the service business and you want smiling, happy people who can satisfy the needs of your clients. Think for a moment about one of those "aha" moments when the service was fantastic. It seemed as though the wait staff, receptionist, or whoever was able to read your mind and have whatever you needed right there. As a surgeon you probably have had a surgical technician who knew before you did what you were going to need. They like the wait staff were hired with a fantastic attitude and trained to enhance that skill. The training did not stop there but continued and continued to constantly improve their skills and the level of client satisfaction. What does your program look like?

Where do you start? The answer is to have a management plan in place. It starts with the needs and trends of the practice. You need to know where the practice is headed to be able to know who and when you will need to hire. There is an old saying you need to make sure you have the right people on the bus doing the right things knowing where they are going for success to occur. Do you have the right people doing the right things in your practice?

Once you know what you are looking for now you need to be able to budget for their salary. One of the complaints heard regarding employment in veterinary practices has been low pay and no chance for advancement. That is the old model. The new model is advancement is always an option and the pay is greatly improved. The philosophy that you get what you paid for is very true. Paying for an attitude and training for skills is good business.

Training is the biggest element in this process. In the past veterinarians hired people and threw them to the lions. If they survived, great but most of them did not. The practice was upset that it did not work out and the employee was devastated. The loss of an employee usually costs the practice in lost production, training, etc., costing the practice financially and emotionally. Can this scenario be prevented? The answer is yes, by hiring the correct person and training them properly.

Training is the area most practices fall short on. This is where the ability to communicate and educate come together. Whether it is the initial training or the continuous improvement training, most practices do not have a plan in place that teaches staff members to be educators. At the very beginning most practices use the "poor me or lack of time" concept to train. The formal education process in most practices is more one of "here are the manuals, go for it". This laissez faire attitude is exactly what you get. These are the staff members who are clueless as to what to do or say to clients. Even McDonalds trains their new hires to at least say, "Can I super size it for you". What type of initial training do you offer new hires? Does it teach them about the culture of the practice, products, the computer, SOP, employee manuals, as well as this is your job description?

Training does not stop with the initial training. It continues with client service meetings, CE, visiting practices, computer software user meetings, and more. Each opportunity to educate your team improves the likelihood that they will be better able to serve the client. The more you can "wow" your clients with consistency and reliability the more you, your team, the pet, and the client will be rewarded for a job well done. Hire the people with the best attitudes, train them, and allow them to educate the clients, and your practice will meet your goals.

WARNING SIGNS OF EMBEZZLEMENT

James E. Guenther, DVM, MBA, MHA, CVPM
Brakke Veterinary Practice Management Group
Asheville, NC

Have you often wondered what an embezzler looks like? They look like ordinary people who are doing ordinary things. They can appear to be the most trusted person on your team or they could be the newbie who you hired for the summer. There is no particular mold they are made from. What these people have in common is their ability to game the system. In the beginning, it is a challenge but then it progresses and becomes an addiction. Whether you like it or not someone has embezzled money, product, or something else from you in the last twelve months.

In any practice, safeguards against theft need to be implemented in the hospital policy book. Most of the time we limit our thinking to theft of money from the cash box, but there are other assets that need to be monitored. What about drugs, medical supplies, and even equipment? These are just as much an asset to the hospital as the money in the cash box. Theft, fraud, embezzlement, and dishonesty in any form can cause the financial failure of a practice in a very short time. The staff needs to know that dishonesty will not be tolerated. Your hospital policy book should list examples of what can lead to dismissal and/or legal action if any staff member is found to be dishonest.

What kind of internal controls have you developed in your practice to prevent monetary theft? Each practice is special and may need additional controls, but there are some basic or common guidelines that need to be implemented. These include the following:

- Keep the cash box in a secure place away from the public during the hours of operation.
- Make sure the cash box is stored in a permanently attached (to the floor or wall) safe with only the practice manager and owner knowing the combination. If at all possible, have the combination changed whenever there is a change in the front office staff to keep the likelihood of theft reduced.
- When hiring staff to handle invoicing and collection of money, make sure references are checked carefully. In the interview process for receptionist/cashier; require each applicant to perform a simple math problem to aid in the evaluation process. Remember that if you ask one person to perform the test all applicants for the position must do the same test.
- Cross train employees so they can handle the different processes in case of an emergency and as a means of understanding the jobs of other employees.
- Establish the amount of cash and change necessary in the cash box for making change for each shift. Most cash boxes will contain $50 to $150 in cash and change.

- At the end of each shift have the cashier going off and the cashier coming on count and reconcile the cash box to the Cash Drawer Verification report generated by the computer. The verification report will break down the payments into the various types (cash, check, credit card). If discrepancies appear, the cashier tracks them down and makes the necessary corrections (ie, a cash transaction may have been entered as a credit card transaction). Once everything is verified, a deposit is made and the verification report is attached for proof of reconciliation.
- Daily bank deposits should be made. It is advisable that the person creating the deposit is not the same person going to the bank.
- Have a locked slotted drop box where bank deposits are kept until taken to the bank.
- Require that a receipt of payment be made each time a transaction happens. This will ensure that a paper trail is employed to reduce the risk of theft.
- Make sure all receipts are consecutively numbered. This will be another safeguard against theft from the cash box.
- Each morning have another individual reconcile medical records, invoices, and day sheets for accuracy, which will ensure that all charges and payments have been accounted for.
- Separate the responsibilities in handling the entire monetary process. Have someone responsible for reconciling the day sheets and creating the deposit, another to make the bank deposit, and a third individual to reconcile the checkbook (usually the bookkeeper). There is no perfect system to prevent fraud. It is your responsibility to monitor by creating adequate checks and balances to reduce the risk.
- Check with your insurance carrier about coverage against theft.
- Do not cash checks from the cash box.
- If a cash refund is made from the cash box make sure a receipt is made that includes the name of the person making it plus their signature, the time, the date, the signature of the recipient, and the signature of a member of management.
- Consider setting a limit for a cash refund to ensure adequate cash for daily operations. If it is above the limit, the bookkeeper will write the client a check.
- Most computer systems have audit reports for transactions that are changed—ie, cash payment changed to no payment or a fixed price lowered (a $100 charge lowered to $10). The practice manager should review this report daily and ask about the entries. The practice manager should also review the end of the day payment reconciliation. The physical presence of management goes a long way in discouraging theft.
- Watch for changes in lifestyle. An employee who was always broke or always complaining about money problems and who now can afford all sorts of new things is suspicious.

- Always have the bank statement sent to the owner's home and then review the statement before taking it to the bookkeeper.
- Be observant and do not take anything for granted
- Use your financial statements to assist you in monitoring your assets. Physical inspection or counting along with reviewing the Balance Sheet will aid in monitoring these assets.

The policy you create to reduce theft or embezzlement is important. Don't take it lightly, but don't make it so restrictive that the staff is smothered by all the policy requirements and unable to do their job. Theft will happen in your practice. As situations occur that are not completely covered in your present policy manual, make the necessary changes in the policy and move on. A policy or procedure is a constant work in progress. The policy manual will always grow and will evolve into a more thorough manual with time. It is your responsibility to monitor, evaluate, and make the needed changes as the situations occur. There will always be loopholes and you will correct them when they are discovered. That is the best you can do.

LIFE IS GOOD IF YOU REMEMBER THE LAKE WOBEGON EFFECT

James E. Guenther, DVM, MBA, MHA, CVPM
Brakke Veterinary Practice Management Group
Asheville, NC

What in the world is the Lake Wobegon Effect? The name is from Garrison Keillor's *Prairie Home Companion* closing comments: "all the women are strong, all the men are good-looking, and all the children are above average." The implication is most everyone feels they are above average. In veterinary medicine, every owner feels they are better than their colleagues. If every practice feels they are better than any other practice in the area than everyone is equal or AVERAGE.

This feeling or complex is so common that psychologists have actually named the syndrome "The Lake Wobegon Effect" (TLWE). So, let's assume just for a brief moment that just maybe you are a victim of TLWE. As mentioned earlier, most if not all veterinarians have an element of this effect because without it you likely will not succeed as a practice owner. With that in mind, I believe there are ways to make this effect (and people's awareness of it) work in your favor. The idea is this: *somehow credibly demonstrate how you are actually above average.* The key word here is "credibly."

So, let's say you are recruiting an exceptional veterinarian to join the practice. Now, assume this veterinarian has decided they want to work for you but they are considering several other offers. I bet this individual has heard the following message from all of the practices they have interviewed with: "we practice exceptional medicine, have the best clients, and our team is nothing short of fantastic". Sound familiar?

Now, the mistake here is not so much that the above statements aren't true (maybe they are), but you are assuming that you are the only practice owner making these kinds of statements. In reality you probably are exceptional in some way but not in all categories. Your goal is not just to demonstrate how great you are—but why *your* practice when compared to the other offers is "well above average" in specific areas of interest. How do you do this?

1. Devise some measures of success that can be demonstrated to the individual. These can be survey results from clients; listen in or better yet be the guest speaker at your weekly client service meeting. Be creative in devising methods to demonstrate you are above average.
2. Take your measuring tools and compare them to national benchmarks. By comparison, an individual can make his or her own decision whether you are full of hot air or telling the truth.

The "above average" mindset needs to be proven instead of being assumed. It should be of great inspiration on your part to prove that you and your practice are exceptional and not merely above average. As a practice owner it is not your place or right to market your services as outstanding. You need to earn the reputation for quality medicine/surgery, exceptional client service, the greatest place to work, and that everyone is an integral part of the success of the practice. Who better to decide this privilege but the clients you work for. They are the ones who can bestow this honor upon you and your team.

AAHA several years ago conducted a survey asking pet owners what was most important to them when choosing a veterinarian. The choices were Empathy, Reliability, Responsiveness, Assurance, and Atmospherics. The top two were Reliability and Responsiveness. Clients want you to do what you said you would do it when you said you would do it. If this is the basis for developing a client friendly practice where your service is second to none and you have lived up to the reputation set by your clients then you have developed credibility.

It is your job to ask the right questions and develop the recognition and reputation that will keep clients swinging the door and enhancing the practice. Maybe in the future you can say: "where the doctors are knowledgeable, the staff is friendly, and the service is exceptional."

Moral of the story: Figure out a way to find what "average" really means in your context and devise credible ways to show how you are "above average" in ways that the clients actually care about.

HIRING, FIRING, AND RETAINING STAFF

Edward J. Guiducci, JD
Guiducci & Guiducci, PC
Denver, CO

A basic understanding of employment law is critical for every practice owner, manager, and team interviewing member. In most cases a little preventative maintenance and an awareness of potential problem areas can eliminate or substantially reduce a practice's exposure to a costly claim or judgment. Conversely, failing to be alert for warning signs of trouble can be disastrous. It is important that practice owners and managers recognize the cost to the practice goes well beyond a potential money judgment against the practice. The cost of hiring a lawyer to defend a claim through the initial state labor department or the federal Equal Employment Opportunity Commission ("EEOC") and the potential for a subsequent lawsuit in state or federal court can cost tens of thousands of dollars. It is also very expensive and in some instances impossible to obtain insurance to cover some employment claims. Thus, it is important to have owners and managers obtain a basic understanding of employment law.

The purpose of this article is to focus on situations where a practice owner, manager, or team interviewing member asks questions during interviews or makes personnel decisions that intentionally or unintentionally stray into areas that could expose the veterinary practice to discrimination claims. I will identify a few situations where personnel decisions have caused EEOC/state labor board complaints and/or lawsuits. This article is designed to bring a sense of awareness to practice owners, managers, and team hiring members and is not intended to and cannot identify all areas and issues that practice owners and managers must be knowledgeable about. It is also a fact that the "case law" pertaining to these claims is minimal compared to the number of cases "settled out of court."

PERSONNEL DECISION MAKING APPROACH

It is important that practice owners/managers focus on six steps that if followed will substantially reduce a practice's exposure to employment discrimination related claims.

Review and Comply with Policies and Procedures

Written policies and procedures can help veterinary practices of all sizes create consistency in a wide variety of human resource issues. However, written policies and procedures can become a problem if a veterinary practice fails to follow its written policies. Doctor/owners should not make policy decisions in the hallway. They should refer human resource (HR) decisions to the manager or policy manual(s). This is a frequent source of litigation. Practices must review and evaluate all policies and procedures and update them, as necessary. It is important not to adopt a policy unless management is willing to comply with the policy in all circumstances. Before taking action against an employee for a violation of a policy, the practice should consult all applicable policies to ensure that the practice has fulfilled any promises that it has made.

Consider the Effect of Written Job Descriptions

Written job descriptions can assist the practice in hiring, conducting performance reviews, and in analyzing whether an employee is "qualified." Having a written job description can assist the practice in determining whether it can "reasonably accommodate" the disabilities of the applicant under the Americans with Disabilities Act. However, a written job description can create liability issues if it is inaccurate or outdated. If a practice decides to prepare job descriptions, it must commit to doing the job correctly.

Hire Legally

Veterinary practices must take the hiring process seriously. To ensure compliance with the Americans with Disabilities Act, the Age Discrimination in Employment Act, Title VII, and a variety of state laws, practices should review application forms and advertisements, train managers in interviewing skills, and review the policies of the hospital with respect to background checks, information verification, and other screening processes. Practices should establish a written policy prohibiting discrimination in the hiring process and promptly investigate and resolve allegations in the hiring process.

Give Accurate, Periodic Reviews

Periodic, accurate reviews are invaluable in both improving performance and documenting deficiencies. Inaccurate reviews that make an employee "feel good" do not serve the practice well and can expose the practice to liability if it needs to terminate the employee for poor performance at a later date. Practices should review forms and procedures to ensure objectivity and regularity.

Maintain Records

Most veterinary practices maintain personnel files, applicant data, and other records relating to the employees. To ensure compliance with federal, state and local civil rights and confidentiality laws, every practice should scrutinize its methods of collecting, handling, and storing such records.

Establish a Discharge Process.

Terminations of employment where the practice and employee agree to the termination and terminations where the employee is terminated on an involuntary basis must be handled properly to avoid claims. This is a high-risk area that can give rise to the following issues: a) whether the separation from employment alleges violation to applicable state and federal law; b) whether the practice's policies were followed; c) how and when the final paycheck is prepared and delivered; d) whether and how the employees must be paid for unused sick, vacation or personal leave time; e) how the employee is notified of his or her rights under COBRA or an applicable state law and other applicable laws; f) how the practice will handle requests for references. Every veterinary practice should develop and follow a procedure for handling these issues in order to limit legal exposure.

SCREENING AND INTERVIEWING PROBLEMS

A common problem area for veterinary practice owners and managers is the screening and interviewing process. Claims and lawsuits can arise from the words and conduct of a hiring veterinarian, manager, or hiring team member towards prospective employees. Employees or rejected applicants most often sue based on federal, state or local anti-discrimination laws, implied contracts allegedly created during the hiring process, or misrepresentations concerning the terms and conditions of employment. Given these risks, anyone who interviews applicants or otherwise participates in the hiring process should be trained to recognize what can and cannot properly be said to an applicant.

An example is where a veterinarian screens and interviews all job applicants for her veterinary practice. She has had a problem with former employees marrying and having children causing the employees to either quit or take excessive absences. As a result, she now screens applicants by asking probing questions during his/her interview about the applicants (especially associate doctors) plans to marry and have children.

This is a clear case of inappropriate questioning of applicants by the practice. It is illegal to base any hiring or employment decision on a person's: age; race; national origin; religion; gender; or handicap/disability. The practice is exposed to an EEOC or state labor board complaint and/or being sued for discrimination

There are a variety of questions that must be avoided when interviewing a prospective employee. The questions should focus on knowledge, skills, and abilities that relate to the job for which applicant is interviewing. Some of the questions to avoid are:

- Health issues: The ADA prohibits "fishing" for information about an applicant's physical or mental condition. A practice can only inquire about the person's ability to perform specific job-related functions.
- Age (except to ask if applicant is over the age of 18)
- Race/national origin
- Marital status
- Number and/or ages of children
- Maiden name
- Childbearing, pregnancy and family obligations
- Medical condition, state of health, or prior illnesses
- Physical or mental disability prior to offer for employment
- Height or weight
- Prior workers compensation claims

- Bankruptcies or garnishments
- Arrests

So what **can** the hiring team ask during an interview?

- **Work experience** – An interviewer can ask the applicant questions about the areas of responsibility of his or her previous job; what he or she likes best or least; what work is the easiest and most difficult; ask about a typical day; ask about his or her supervisory experience; ask how his or her work related to others; raises; promotions; awards; achievements; attendance; reason for leaving; career goals; veterinary specific experience; familiarity with certain equipment and instruments; and whether or not the associate doctor is subject to a non-competition agreement.
- **Training, skills and knowledge** – You can ask the applicant to describe a typical day in his or her job. You can ask the applicant what he or she considers the single most important idea or accomplishment s/he has contributed to in his/her present job. You can also pose a typical problem in the current job and inquire how the applicant would handle the situation.
- **Personal attitudes** – You can ask if the applicant prefers to work alone or with others or with minimal or direct supervision; career goals. You can ask the applicant to tell you about why he/she wants the job, his or her hobbies and interests.

Health-Related Employee Issues

Many owners/managers ask employees unnecessary health related questions. They may ask "How are you feeling today?" or "You don't act like you are feeling well, is something wrong?" These questions are normally asked out of a true concern for the welfare of their employees. Unfortunately, these types of health-related questions can come back to haunt the practice. If the employee is later terminated as a result of failure to perform his or her job duties, the employee can allege that he or she was terminated for discriminatory reasons because the practice became aware of a medical disability through the questioning by a supervisor.

These types of questions frequently arise when a supervisor is managing performance problems of an employee that may or may not stem from a health problem. If a manager has an employee that is frequently tardy or absent he or she must have unambiguous policies on personal leave or sick leave and must consistently apply the policy to all employees.

It is also important that the manager address the problem he or she is experiencing with the employee as opposed to speculating on a reason for the problem. The owner or manager should never inquire about whether or not the employee is having a medical issue thereby instigating a discussion on a medical condition of the employee. If the employee responds to a counseling, warning or termination by giving a medical reason for his or her failure to perform, the supervisor is advised to comply with the Americans with Disabilities Act by discussing what reasonable accommodations can be made, if any. A veterinarian or practice manager should not ignore the issue or make work for the employee because the practice could later be held by a court to having waived its right to argue that it could not reasonably accommodate the disability. It is important that an owner or manager handle an employee with medical problems in the same manner that s/he handles non-disabled employees.

It is important for veterinarians and practice managers to consider the legal effects of their questioning of employee and job applicants. Although there may be sincere motivations for the veterinarian or manager's actions, misguided personnel decisions or questions can be devastating to practices.

CREATING AND NEGOTIATING AN ASSOCIATE CONTRACT

Edward J. Guiducci, JD
Guiducci & Guiducci, PC
Denver, CO

Most practice owners believe that the process of hiring an associate veterinarian is completed upon their locating an associate that is willing to work for an agreed upon wage and that has the desired clinical and interpersonal skills to work with the client base and the staff. Many practice owners believe that the process is over at that point in time and that there is little benefit to have a written associate agreement. After all, what do they have to lose?

ALL ASSOCIATE AGREEMENTS SHOULD BE IN WRITING

It is a good business practice to reduce any important verbal agreement to writing. An associate agreement is no exception and should be written and signed by both parties. This is true whether the associate is classified as an employee or an independent contractor.

All too frequently, veterinarians believe that the associate they want to hire will honor his or her commitment to the practice. They claim that it is unnecessary to have a written agreement because they are both honest and honorable individuals and it over complicates a straightforward relationship. The flaw with this logic is that two people will frequently interpret and remember different details from a verbal conversation. If you take two perfectly honest individuals and ask them about the specific terms of an agreement that arose after a verbal conversation, each one will focus on certain details that will frequently conflict with the understanding or memory of the other individual.

This problem can become serious if it involves terms of a verbal associate agreement relating to compensation or other significant issues. When this happens, the party that feels that he or she has been mislead (normally the associate) may start questioning whether the hiring veterinarian is honest or is trying to take advantage of him or her. The effect of such a scenario is that the parties who once believed the other to be honest begin to question the character of the other. This is especially important if the doctors work well together otherwise and were looking for a long-term business relationship.

This problem can easily be avoided by having a well drafted associate agreement or independent contractor agreement. A poorly drafted agreement that fails to address important issues is frequently no better than a verbal agreement because there remains a misunderstanding or ambiguity on important issues. It is also important to understand that ambiguities in written agreements are construed against the drafters of the agreements. The effect of this is that the party that drafts the agreement, frequently the hiring veterinarian, will have any ambiguous or missing sections construed in a light most favorable to the associate and against their legal interest. The legal system has evolved over hundreds of years to protect the weak by construing the ambiguous contract provision against the drafter.

Some of the major terms relating to business issues that should be included in a written associate agreement are as follows:

Term - When does the associate's employment begin and when does it end? Most associate agreements provide that the agreement can be terminated by either party and for any reason upon either 30, 60, or 90 days notice to the other party. In addition, you need to address what happens upon the associate's death or disability, loss of license, or other circumstances.

Duties and Hours - Define the associate's work schedule and specify the associate's duties and responsibilities. It is important for the practice to have a very broad and flexible definition of duties to avoid an associate who desires to narrow the scope of his or her job duties. There needs to be language permitting the practice to alter the specific tasks that are being undertaken by the associate so long as it falls within the broad definition in the associate agreement. The associate agreement should generally permit a practice to alter the hours of work by the associate, ie, on call, etc. Does the associate have the right to work in other practices? The associate agreement needs to specifically indicate whether or not the associate is permitted to work in other practices.

Compensation - How will you compensate the associate? Associates are commonly compensated on a fixed salary, a percentage of personal production or a combination of both. It is important that a practice owner or manager understand what the market rate is for associate compensation.

If the term of the associate agreement expires after one year, the associate agreement will need to be renegotiated and amended to extend the term and reflect any changes to its terms rewritten with the new compensation terms. If the contract automatically renews then the associate agreement will need to be amended to reflect new compensation terms.

Benefits - In addition to the associate's compensation, will you provide any employee benefits such as health insurance, disability insurance, paid personal leave for vacations, paid professional leave for attending continuing education, and other business functions? Will you pay for the associate's malpractice insurance, continuing education, dues, and other business expenses? The number of benefits offered in the marketplace varies considerably from practice to practice. Usually those associate agreements that are part of an eventual buy-in will provide more benefits than just a straight associate relationship.

THE ASSOCIATE SHOULD BE AN EMPLOYEE

The associate should generally be hired as your employee and not as an independent contractor. Many veterinarians desire to treat their associates as independent contractors to avoid withholding employment taxes and unemployment taxes from the amounts paid to the associate. However, whether the associate is an employee or independent contractor is often based on a number of common law factors that may or may not be present in the relationship. These factors vary from state to state depending upon specific rulings by the appellate courts of each state. More importantly, the Internal Revenue Service has developed a list of twenty factors that it examines in making a determination of whether a worker is an employee or an independent contractor for tax purposes. In normal associate relationships, the vast majority of associates should be classified as employees. If you treat your associate as an independent contractor, you could be subjecting your practice to an IRS audit and potential penalties and interest charges.

Many veterinarians are unwilling to classify their associates as employees because of the problems that can develop if the associate does not work out and they are forced to terminate the relationship. The hiring veterinarian is frequently uncomfortable about claims for unemployment filed by the terminated associate. Veterinarians need to accept the fact that unemployment insurance fees are simply a cost of doing business. They also need to have their individual state laws examined to determine whether they are protected from payment on unemployment claims if they terminate the employee during an established "orientation" or "probationary period" to determine if the employee will work out with the practice. Assuming that your state law permits "trial periods" for purposes of unemployment benefits, you could terminate the relationship within the trial period without being exposed to additional fees for unemployment claims by the terminated employee.

Veterinarians also need to understand that they will not be able to avoid discrimination claims by having their associates classified as independent contractors versus employees. Most state and federal discrimination laws are not based on the worker being classified as an employee versus an independent contractor.

OWNERSHIP OF CLIENT AND PATIENT RECORDS

Almost all of the associate agreements we have reviewed or drafted have contained a clause stating that all client and patient records are owned by the employer veterinarian. While this appears to protect the employer from losing clients to the associate, this protection is illusory. We all know that any client, at any time, has the right to request copies of their veterinary records and can transfer their animal's treatment to another veterinarian. If the associate agreement does not contain an enforceable covenant not to compete prohibiting the associate from practicing within a reasonable area of your practice, this clause will offer little or no protection for the hiring veterinarian.

TRADE SECRET PROTECTION

Any associate working for your practice has access to certain business information that you want to protect. When your associate becomes a former associate you will want the right to prevent the associate from utilizing this business information. The business information may be protectable under most states laws if it can be classified and maintained as a trade secret. Associate agreements need to contain broad language prohibiting the associate from utilization of the hiring veterinarian's trade secrets. However, in much the same fashion as the contract term providing the hiring veterinarian with ownership interest in the client and patient records this protection is also illusory. In order for a hiring veterinarian to protect its trade secrets the records and information must meet the definition of a trade secret under the specific state's law and specific steps must be followed protecting the trade secret. If the business information is not a "trade secret" under the applicable state laws or if proper steps to protect the business information have not been taken then the ability to protect the business information is lost. Courts around the country focus on a variety of factors to consider whether or not a trade secret exists. Some of the more commons factors are:

- How widely the information is known outside of the particular practice;
- How widely the information is known by employees and others involved in the practice;
- Steps taken to guard the secrecy of the information;
- Value of the information;
- Cost or effort involved in the development of the information;
- Cost and effort that would be required to duplicate or acquired by a third party.

In practice, a trade secret can be any information that provides a business with a competitive edge in the marketplace. Some common examples of business information that may constitute a trade secret in a veterinary office include client and patient lists, patient charts, and marketing strategies.

ATTORNEYS' FEES

It is important that your associate agreement contain language permitting you to recover your attorneys' fees if you are forced to file a lawsuit to prevent a terminated associate from violating a covenant not to compete. Most states require an attorneys' fees provision in an associate agreement before the enforcing veterinarian is entitled to recover the sums that he or she paid to their attorneys. Further, having such language in your associate agreement may influence a former associate to comply with its terms if he or she would have to pay your attorneys' fees as well as his or her own.

LIQUIDATED DAMAGE PROVISION

The majority of states permit parties to negotiate into contracts the amount of damages that a party will be entitled to recover if a breach of the contract or covenant occurs. These contract terms are called "liquidated damage provisions" and can be an effective tool to prevent an associate from violating a covenant not to compete or a non-solicitation provision of an associate agreement.

ASSOCIATE AREEMENT MUST BE ASSIGNABLE BY EMPLOYER

The associate agreement should provide that the employing veterinarian is entitled to assign the agreement to a new purchaser or a new entity. This is very important to the employing veterinarian if he or she would decide or need to sell or restructure the business. The value of a veterinary practice is frequently dependent on preventing key employee veterinarians from competing with the business after the acquisitions.

EMPLOYING VETERINARIAN MUST GIVE "CONSIDERATION" WHEN EMPLOYEE VETERINARIAN ENTERS INTO COVENANT NOT TO COMPETE

All states require that both parties to a contract give "consideration" in order for the contract to be enforceable. The legal concept of consideration requires that each party either give some right, interest or benefit or give up a forbearance or detriment. This is also true for associate agreements and covenants not to compete. In order for the associate agreement and the covenant not to compete to be enforceable, the employing veterinarian and the associate veterinarian must have each given consideration. An associate veterinarian obviously meets the legal obligation by agreeing to the restrictive covenant not to compete. The same can be said for the employing veterinarian if the associate veterinarian enters into the associate agreement prior to becoming an employee. A problem develops when the employing veterinarian imposes terms upon the associate veterinarian after he or she has been working for the employing veterinarian. The employing veterinarian has arguably not given any consideration if the associate veterinarian has already been an employee. If a court rules that consideration has not been given as a result of prior employment, the contract containing the covenant not to compete cannot be enforced and the employing veterinarian is at risk of the associate taking a portion of the clients of the practice.

In certain states, it has been held that the employing veterinarian has given consideration by permitting the associate veterinarian to retain his or her job. However, courts in many states have ruled that the employing veterinarian has not met its obligation simply by permitting the associate veterinarian to retain his or her job. In light of the uncertainty of this issue around the country, it is advisable for all employing veterinarian to provide the existing associate veterinarian with a sum of money for his or her entering into the associate agreement. This is especially important for an employing veterinarian in the event he or she wants to sell the

veterinary practice because the buyer could reduce his offer or refuse to purchase a practice based upon his perception of the risk that an associate veterinarian would leave and legally compete with the practice. An employing veterinarian can choose to give an existing associate veterinarian with consideration of a benefit other than a cash payment. There is no specific requirement on what the benefit needs to be or the value of the benefit. One example of consideration other than cash is payment of professional liability insurance, if not already provided, or additional funds for continuing education.

TIPS TO CONDUCT NEGOTIATIONS WITH YOUR ASSOCIATE

How can the terms of an associate agreement be negotiated without damaging the relationship of the hiring veterinarian and the associate veterinarian? The inherent problem in these negotiations is that there are conflicting goals. The goal of the hiring veterinarian is to obtain contract terms to protect his or her practice in the event that the relationship is not successful. This is in sharp contrast to the goal of the associate veterinarian who is interested in contract terms that will permit him or her flexibility if the relationship fails. There is a point in the negotiation of an associate agreement when these equally compelling goals conflict with each other and hard feelings can develop. Frequently, these hard feelings that arise during these negotiations have long-term effects upon the relationship of the parties to the negotiations.

There are a number of steps that a hiring veterinarian can take to minimize the risk of hard feelings developing during the negotiations.

Negotiate in a Neutral Site - Conduct the negotiations in a neutral site where there is no perceived power position. This approach is intended to place the associate veterinarian at ease. If a hiring veterinarian conducts the negotiations in his or her office, he or she is more likely to be perceived by the associate veterinarian as being in the power position.

Describe Expectations - A technique that can be successful is for the hiring veterinarian to describe his or her expectations of the associate veterinarian and his or her goals at the beginning of the negotiations. If the intention of the hiring veterinarian is to have a non-solicitation provision and covenant not to compete, it is important that this issue be brought up at an early point in the negotiations with the associate. This is also an opportunity for the hiring veterinarian to explain why he or she feels strongly about having these provisions. A common explanation for a hiring veterinarian to give to an associate veterinarian is that the associate agreements are designed to protect the hiring veterinarian until the two veterinarians have decided that the veterinarian should stay with the practice and become an owner. The hiring veterinarian should communicate that at the point that the hiring veterinarian and the associate veterinarian have decided to stay together, the owner's employment agreement will be restructured to be more beneficial for the associate veterinarian.

Talk to the associate veterinarian about what his or her compensation will be early in the negotiations. There is no benefit to delaying communicating what the hiring veterinarian's expectations are for compensation.

Do Not Rush the Associate - It is important to give the associate veterinarian enough time to analyze and fully understand what is being proposed. The associate needs to have an opportunity to have his or her own attorney review the draft associate agreement. A hiring veterinarian needs to keep in mind that this may be the first time that the associate veterinarian has dealt with associate agreements and may be very uncomfortable about the entire process.

NON-VETERINARIAN OWNERSHIP OF A VETERINARY PRACTICE

Edward J. Guiducci, JD
Guiducci & Guiducci, PC
Denver, CO

Historically, state law in the United States prevented non-veterinarian ownership of veterinary practices. The article examines the original justifications and whether or not these justifications continue to apply. We will examine current trends in changes to state laws and veterinary practice acts in the United States relating to non-veterinary ownership of veterinary practices. This article also focuses on legal options for non-veterinarians to own veterinary practices and alternative options structures that are slowly being accepted by veterinary boards across the United States permitting non-licensed veterinarians to be owners of practice assets and operations even when the state's veterinary practice act has not been amended to permit non-veterinary ownership. Certain practical issues that go beyond the legalities for non-licensed veterinary ownership of a veterinary practice are also covered.

WHAT IS THE RATIONALE FOR THE HISTORICAL PROHIBITION OF NON-LICENSED VETERINARY OWNERSHIP?

The historical prohibition on non-licensed veterinary ownership of veterinary practices was primarily based upon the fact that veterinary medicine is a licensed and regulated business. As part of the regulation of the veterinary profession, as with other licensed professions, veterinary practice acts in the United States prohibited non-veterinary ownership of veterinary practices in order to maintain the quality of service and protect the professional's independent judgment. The primary rationale that was utilized by the states in adopting their statutes was that the non-licensed veterinarian owners would impact the professional judgment of the licensed veterinarians.

WHAT ARE MODERN DAY VIEWS OF THE PROHIBITION OF NON-VETERINARY OWNERSHIP AND ITS IMPACT UPON THE VETERINARY PROFESSION?

There remain differing views in the veterinary profession as to the appropriateness of non-licensed veterinarians owning veterinary practices. The following are common arguments in favor of non-veterinarians owning veterinary practices, followed by some of the arguments that are propounded opposing non-veterinary ownership:

Arguments Supporting Non-Veterinary Ownership:
1. Relaxing the rules will permit the introduction and development of innovative forms of professional practices with the input of non-veterinarian owners.
2. Relaxing the rules will permit widows/widowers and the heirs of the veterinarians from having a hardship placed upon them with a forced "fire sale" upon the death of the veterinarian. This is especially a hardship for spouses that manage the practice side-by-side with their veterinarian spouse.
3. Relaxing the rules will provide more opportunities for an exit strategy by expanding the market to sell existing practices.
4. Relaxing the rules will provide opportunities for key employees to become owners and remain in the profession.
5. Relaxing the rules could have a positive effect on competition and might afford consumers a wider selection of services and costs.

Arguments in Opposition to Permitting Non-Veterinary Ownership:
1. The corporate bottom-line would control over professional ethics and the Veterinary oath. This would create an unethical influence that would damage the public.
2. It is bad for the profession for cities and other public or quasi-public entities to own practices and compete with private practices.
3. "If it ain't broke, don't fix it!" This would prevent unforeseen problems caused by non-veterinary owners of veterinary practices.

HAVE VETERINARY PRACTICE ACTS BEEN AMENDED TO PERMIT NON-VETERINARY OWNERSHIP IN THE UNITED STATES?

There has not been one uniform change in the United States to this issue. There have been the following four basic approaches by the states:

1. Amendment to state veterinary practice act and/or corporation act permitting non-licensed veterinary ownership of 100% of veterinary practices;
2. Amendment of veterinary practice act and professional corporation act to permit up to 49% ownership of a veterinary practice by non-veterinarians;
3. Various amendments of state statutes that are inconsistent with each other permitting corporate ownership through certain legal entities but not others, ie, professional corporation acts prohibit non-veterinary ownership but for-profit corporation acts permit non-veterinarian ownership.
4. No amendment to act thereby continuing the prohibition on non-licensed veterinary ownership of veterinary practice.

HOW DO NON-VETERINARIANS OWN AN INTEREST IN VETERINARY PRACTICES IN STATES THAT CONTINUE TO PROHIBIT NON-VETERINARIAN OWNERSHIP?

Non-veterinarians are prohibited from individually owning a veterinary practice or forming a for-profit corporation to provide veterinary medical services and directly receive the fee for these services that reside in states that prohibit non-veterinary ownership or majority veterinary ownership. The individual or corporation would in these states be unlawfully engaged in the practice of veterinary medicine, while the licensed veterinarian employed by the corporation or individual would violate the prohibition against permitting or allowing another to use his or her license to practice medicine and would be subject to having his or her license canceled, revoked, or suspended by the states' board of veterinary medical examiners.

This would appear to prevent a non-veterinarian from obtaining ownership of a veterinary practice in the states that have not amended their veterinary practice acts. However, there is another option. In some states a non-veterinarian is permitted to enter into an administrative services structure to work in conjunction with a veterinary professional services corporation that provides veterinary medical care. The basic premise of this approach is that the administrative services legal entity provides any and all services and staff that the veterinary professional services corporation needs to operate the veterinary practice except for hiring veterinarians and in some states licensed technicians. This includes providing the veterinary professional services corporation with leased space, equipment, furniture, instruments, marketing services, accounting services, billing services, general administrative services, training, recruiting of professional staff, etc. The majority of the fees that are generated by the veterinary practice are received by the veterinary professional services corporation but are then disbursed as service fees or reimbursement except for the professional personnel expenses of the veterinary professional services entity. This structure has satisfied many states' concerns to protect the public because the separate structure insures that the professional judgment of the veterinarians is not being controlled by non-veterinarian owners.

WHAT IS A TYPICAL ADMINISTRATIVE SERVICES STRUCTURE?

A typical administrative services structure involves a for-profit corporation being formed to purchase practice assets from a selling veterinarian to serve the role of an administrative services entity. A separate professional veterinary corporation is formed to provide professional veterinary services and one veterinarian will be the sole stockholder of the corporation to comply with state law. If one of the owners of the for-profit legal entity were a veterinarian then typically this person would be the sole shareholder of the professional legal entity. If the purchaser doesn't have a licensed veterinarian as part of its ownership, then a veterinarian would need to be hired by the veterinary clinic to provide the veterinary services and to hold the share of stock while employed.

Typically the practice assets that are sold as part of a veterinary asset sale transaction consist of an assignment of the commercial lease on the land and buildings (or a purchase of the land and building), all the fixtures, furniture and equipment of the practice, trade name and drug and office supply inventory of the practice as well as the telephone numbers, email addresses, web sites, client and patient records and goodwill. The structure will vary depending upon the state that the practice is located in because certain states prohibit the for-profit administrative services corporation from owning the client/patient records and goodwill. In these cases the purchase of the client/patient records and good will assets will be assigned to the veterinary professional services entity.

The administrative services agreement is a formalized contract that clearly identifies the rights and responsibilities of each of the for-profit administrative services entity and the veterinary professional services corporation. It will outline the services that will be provided and the fees that will be paid the for-profit administrative services company.

DUE DILIGENCE OF A PRACTICE PURCHASE: MINIMIZING A BUYER'S RISK

Edward J. Guiducci, JD
Guiducci & Guiducci, PC
Denver, CO

The term *due diligence* refers to the investigation and review a prudent buyer should conduct before purchasing the assets or ownership interest of a veterinary practice. A buyer has to make decisions on what, if any, due diligence that he or she needs or wants to conduct before closing on the purchase. The scope of the due diligence will depend in part on the buyer's knowledge about the practice, concerns that arise during the negotiations and from preliminary due diligence and the buyer's budget for due diligence. The purchase of a veterinary practice is one of the most expensive and risky purchases of a buyer's life. It is important that a buyer conduct the necessary due diligence in order to ensure that the purchase is a good business decision.

WHEN SHOULD DUE DILIGENCE BE CONDUCTED?

A buyer must decide whether or not to conduct financial analysis of the practice prior to submitting an offer and obtaining a signed contract. This is a strategically difficult issue because a buyer doesn't want to spend money on evaluating a practice that he or she may not be able to purchase. On the other hand a buyer can run into problems it he or she submits an offer and obtains a signed contract before conducting financial due diligence in dealing with a seller who has the expectation of getting the full contract price. I have found that many deals fall apart when buyers attempt to renegotiate the purchase price after their due diligence uncovers problems because sellers have an expectation that they will receive the contract purchase price and are suspicious of buyers attempting to renegotiate the purchase price. A possible solution to this problem is to conduct a limited amount of financial due diligence before you have a submitted an offer and signed a purchase contract. A primary focus of this analysis would be to determine whether or not the buyer could afford the purchase by cash flowing the debt service. By having limited financial analysis conducted a buyer will have more information to work with before obtaining a signed contract and expanding the scope of the due diligence.

Another option is for a buyer to obtain a letter of intent from the seller that will provide an exclusive right to negotiate to purchase the veterinary practice assets or ownership interest until certain financial due diligence is conducted. This form of a letter of intent will require a seller to notify other buyers that he or she has entered into a letter of intent and to cease all negotiations with other buyers. This approach can prevent a seller from having unrealistic purchase price expectations while giving the buyer the assurance that the seller will not be negotiating to sell the practice to another buyer during the period of time that he or she is having the financial due diligence conducted. It is important to understand that this type of a letter of intent does not provide a buyer the same level of protection that a signed purchase contract would but it will prevent the seller from selling the practice out from underneath a buyer before the financial analysis is completed.

Once a buyer obtains a signed contract, a decision must be made as to the additional due diligence that needs to be conducted to create a comfort level before closing on the purchase. A buyer that has worked with the practice for an extended period of time should be able to limit the scope of the due diligence to areas of the practice that the buyer was not involved in. A buyer that learned of the practice from a listing in the local veterinary medical association publication or a practice broker should be much more thorough in conducting due diligence. A buyer must also consider the expense that will be incurred and decide how much of the due diligence that he or she can personally conduct as opposed to having lawyers and consultants perform.

THE IMPACT OF A PURCHASE AGREEMENT ON A BUYER'S DUE DILIGENCE

A properly drafted purchase agreement will require a seller to make specific representations and warranties regarding the practice assets or ownership interest that a buyer is entitled to rely upon in evaluating the purchase. These are generally very extensive and thorough. A few examples of common representations and warranties are: a) that there are no liens again the practice assets; b) that there have not been any material changes to the practice; and c) that the seller will be responsible for any and all pre-closing liabilities of the practice.

In addition to requiring a seller to make extensive representations and warranties about the assets being sold, it is a good practice for a buyer to require a seller to create lists of information and documents that it will represent are true and accurate and that a buyer is entitled to rely upon. A few examples of this are: a) previous 12 month's general ledgers, profit and loss statements, financial statements, bank statements and the previous 4 to 5 years of Schedule C tax returns if a sole proprietorship or corporate tax returns; b) a list of all furniture, equipment, examination and surgical instruments, trade fixtures, and other personal property owned by the seller located at the veterinary practice or used in connection with the veterinary practice; c) a list of all liabilities that the seller expects the buyer to assume and be responsible to pay, ie, commercial lease, postage meter lease, and so forth.

These warranties and representations, disclosures and attachments are very important to a buyer because properly drafted purchase agreements can create a valid claim for misrepresentation against a seller. Some buyers attempt to save money by relying upon the right to sue the seller for a misrepresentation instead of conducting independent due diligence to verify the information provided by a seller. It is important that a buyer conduct adequate due diligence to be comfortable that there is value in the practice and not simply rely upon being able to file a lawsuit because filing suit against a seller does not guaranty recovery of a buyer's damages.

A buyer needs to understand that it is very expensive to file suit to recover from a seller and that there is no guaranty that a buyer can recover the money that he or she is owed after obtaining a lawsuit judgment. Sellers that are sued can avoid paying on a judgment by filing for bankruptcy protection or spending the money that he or she was paid by the buyer before a buyer can recover the money that the seller was paid. It is also very expensive to hire a lawyer to sue a seller when the buyer is trying to focus his or her energy and resources on making the practice successful.

AREAS OF "DUE DILIGENCE" THAT A BUYER SHOULD CONSIDER CONDUCTING

This leads us into the areas of due diligence that a buyer should consider conducting. It is important to keep in mind that each practice is unique and due diligence must be tailored for the circumstances of each practice. Notwithstanding this fact, there are certain categories of due diligence that should always be considered by a buyer.

Financial Due Diligence

A buyer should always conduct financial due diligence to verify that the practice is worth the listed price. Financial due diligence is the process of verifying the financial information you are given from the seller and his or her representatives. It is important for a buyer to understand that practice valuations accept the financial information as being accurate as opposed to auditing the financial information that is provided. It is important to have an experienced practice appraiser that is a member of the Association of Veterinary Practice Management Consultants and Advisors (AVPMCA) to analyze the data and look for inconsistencies based upon the appraiser's knowledge of the industry.

Location Due Diligence

Location due diligence requires an analysis of the practice location and the demographics of the surrounding area to determine if there is a likelihood of continued growth of the practice. This category of due diligence also requires an analysis of the competitive situation within the practice's region and the availability of emergency and specialty services.

Building Due Diligence

Building due diligence is investigating the terms of the lease, the condition of the building and the legality of the use of the building. It is important that the lease be closely examined to determine whether or not the buyer can assign the lease. It is also important to determine the maintenance, repair and replacement obligations the buyer is responsible for under the lease. If the buyer will have significant replacement obligations (ie, HVAC, roof, parking lot, electrical, etc.) then the buyer should have an inspector examine and evaluate the current condition to avoid hidden expenses.

Furniture, Fixtures, and Equipment Due Diligence

Furniture, fixtures, and equipment due diligence is investigating the working condition of the furniture, equipment, examination and surgical instruments, and trade fixtures. It can require an examination of each item to determine whether or not the equipment is current and likely to continue to be operational with normal maintenance for an additional 5 years. This category also includes requiring the seller to identify all equipment that is leased and to provide copies of all equipment leases and maintenance contracts so that the buyer can make a decision to accept or reject the lease and maintenance contract obligations.

Human Resources Due Diligence

Human resources due diligence requires a buyer to investigate employee issues. This includes individual employees' positions, length of service, familiarity with clients, compensation and benefit packages and specific information regarding the employees' date of hire, date of last review, and date and amount of last raise. This area also includes investigating claims of discrimination or other labor law violations as well as determining which employees will not be staying with the practice.

Title and Lien Search Due Diligence

Title and lien search due diligence requires title searches to be conducted to be sure there are no liens against the assets a buyer is purchasing, including tax liens, uniform commercial code liens and lawsuits. Also, if there is a corporate seller there are other types of verifications of title and good standing.

SHOULD YOU USE A LETTER OF INTENT FOR YOUR PRACTICE SALE/PURCHASE?

Edward J. Guiducci, JD
Guiducci & Guiducci, PC
Denver, CO

Letters of intent are frequently used to list the basic terms upon which the parties have agreed to consider buying assets or ownership interest before the parties incur the expense of having attorneys prepare the formal transaction documents and begin due diligence investigations. In veterinary transactions, a letter of intent typically comes into play after a round of initial discussions about the proposed transaction.

REASONS TO USE LETTERS OF INTENT

There are many practical business and legal reasons to use of a Letter of Intent:

- **Financial Commitment to the Deal**: Signing a letter of intent, from a business perspective, indicates that each party is comfortable enough with the terms to spend the time and money that will be required to work towards negotiating binding purchase agreements.
- **Commitment to a Time Line**: A letter of intent will set forth a time line for negotiations to enter into purchase agreements, establish a deadline for completing due diligence investigation and establish a deadline for closing the transaction.
- **Nonbinding Terms**: Letters of intent for veterinary transaction purposes should be used to clarify the parties' agreement on basic terms and generally are drafted so that they are nonbinding. This means that either party can change his or her mind and walk away from the transaction for any reason. The only important exceptions to this are for confidentiality and no-shop terms, as follows:
  - **Confidentiality Terms**: Letters of intent should provide that all information that is disclosed to a buyer by a seller be kept confidential and returned to the seller.
  - **No-Shop Terms**: No-shop terms are exclusive negotiation terms of a letter of intent that require a seller to notify all interested parties that he or she has entered into a letter of intent and that he or she will not negotiate to sell to anyone else unless the letter of intent is terminated. This provision is designed to give a certain level of protection to a buyer who is incurring expenses in conducting financial due diligence prior to having a formal purchase agreement.
- **Due Diligence**: After signing a letter of intent and frequently before the finalization of formal purchase agreements, buyers will begin financial due diligence for the transaction. A buyer should be hesitant to spend too much money on negotiating formal purchase agreements until he or she is comfortable that the parties are close on the basic terms of the transaction. The financial due diligence should be started prior to entering into formal purchase agreements in order for the buyer to be comfortable that he or she is receiving value for the agreed upon purchase price. Sometimes buyers will start their financial due diligence investigation before a letter of intent is signed because they are uncomfortable agreeing to a purchase price until after they have had a consultant analyze the financials of the veterinary practice. This is a reasonable approach but a buyer needs to be cautious about spending too much money before the seller enters into a formal purchase agreement. Buyers need to understand that the formal purchase agreements will provide time for the buyer to complete due diligence to make sure that he or she is getting adequate value of the purchase price. If a buyer decides that he or she is not receiving value for the purchase price then he or she will be able to back out of the transaction.

CLOSING ADVICE

Letters of intent can save a veterinarian a lot of money by clarifying in writing the" basic" terms of an agreement before hiring a lawyer to prepare the purchase agreements. However, it is important to not sign a letter of intent until you have had discussions with your attorney and tax advisor and a review of the document by your attorney.

PRACTICE AFFILIATION: WILL IT WORK FOR ME?

Edward J. Guiducci, JD
Guiducci & Guiducci, PC
Denver, CO

WHAT IS PRACTICE AFFILIATION?

It has never been as expensive as it currently is to set up and operate a veterinary practice. It can cost hundreds of thousands of dollars to set up a veterinary practice with updated equipment.

A compounding factor in the current economics of veterinary medicine is the narrow profit margin in the industry. In most markets, veterinarians undercut their prices for core services in order to compete with large national chains. This undercutting of prices on core services has created an economic environment that is squeezing profit margins and making it more and more difficult to obtain the necessary profitability.

These economic realities have a bearing on any capital purchase by a veterinarian. Any veterinarian interested in opening a practice or updating his or her equipment or facilities must evaluate all of the options to avoid suffocating under the debt that would be incurred. The option that has historically been selected by veterinarians who cannot afford to acquire updated equipment or facilities is to enter into a partnership or co-ownership with one or more veterinarians. This would permit the veterinarian to purchase the equipment and update facilities with the combined resources and economy to scale to make it cost effective. Unfortunately, this approach also brings problems inherent in co-ownership of a veterinary practice. There are a multitude of issues that can and frequently do arise when a practice has multiple owners. Some of the more problematic areas for co-owners are: the sharing of profits and losses; this is especially evident when the veterinarians do not share similar work habits; as well as differences on division of new clients, spending habits, and staff management issues. Veterinarians frequently avoid co-ownership relationships because of these issues.

The concept of "practice affiliation" or "solo group practice" is a viable alternative to a traditional partnership or other form of co-ownership. The terms "practice affiliation" or "solo group practice" can be defined as an association of two or more veterinarians, each owning an undivided interest in the veterinary facility, for the sole purpose of sharing the veterinary facility and overhead expenses, while retaining separate, independent practices from one another. In its most simplistic form, it is a sharing of office space and equipment to minimize the expenses of operating the practice. In a more complex structure, it can be very similar to a partnership or joint ownership relationship.

Except in the most simplistic of structures, practice affiliations need to be structured as a separate legal entity with the individual veterinary practices or individual veterinarians being the owners of the new entity. This is very important if the practice affiliation markets the group under a name separate from the names of the individual veterinary practices. The marketing of a trade name is very expensive and the practice affiliation needs to take the necessary steps to reserve this name.

It is also important to have the practice affiliation operate as a separate legal entity for liability purposes. The goal needs to be to insulate the individual practices from lawsuits arising from actions of the other veterinarians. Certain legal entities provide the owners of an entity with insulation from liabilities of the entity. If the solo group is not formed as an entity that insulates the individual owners, the individual veterinarians could be named as parties to a lawsuit as a result of actions of one of the other veterinarians. Properly drafted legal documents created for the practice affiliation can create a defense to such a claim; however, the individual veterinarians would be forced to defend the litigation.

A creditor who chooses to name all of the individual veterinarians in a lawsuit will claim that the practice affiliation is a general partnership or a joint venture. This will provide the creditor with the legal authority to name the individual owners in the lawsuit because individual owners are personally liable for the entire debt of a general partnership or joint venture under the legal theory of joint and several liabilities. This could be avoided if the legal entity is a limited liability company, limited liability partnership, or a corporation where the individual owners have a shield from liability. Accordingly, it is important that the veterinarians protect themselves through the formation of a separate legal entity for the practice affiliation.

ALL PRACTICE AFFILIATIONS SHOULD HAVE A WRITTEN AGREEMENT

Although any important verbal agreement should be in writing, it is especially important in a practice affiliation. There are significant legal issues involving the legal relationship between the veterinarians that need to be addressed in a written practice affiliation agreement. These contract terms could ultimately save a veterinarian thousands of dollars in defense of a lawsuit that is focused on the actions of one of the other veterinary practices within the practice affiliation.

The form of the agreement will vary depending upon the type of legal entity that is created to operate the practice affiliation. If the practice affiliation is of a very simplistic form, the agreement between the parties will be of more significance because of the need for individual veterinarians to be protected from liabilities arising from actions of the other veterinarians. If the practice affiliation legal entity is of a form that will provide insulation from liability for the individual veterinarians, there are other issues between the individual veterinarians that remain very significant.

Some of the *major terms* that need to be included in a practice affiliation agreement are as follows:

- Statement as to separate ownership of veterinarians' practices
- Statement as to facility ownership

- Identification of practice affiliation assets and statement as to percentage of
- Term of agreement
- Name ownership
- Management structure
- Financial responsibilities of the veterinarians of the practice affiliation
- Rights to use of facilities of practice affiliation

- Sharing and compensation of staff
- Termination of practice affiliation
- Buy–sell terms
- Prohibition of solicitation of clients and covenants not to compete
- Allocation of new clients
- Ownership of telephone number
- Ownership of client and patient records

OPEN BOOK MANAGEMENT – UNDERSTANDING YOUR FINANCIAL STATEMENTS, THE LAB REPORT FOR YOUR PRACTICE

Elise M. Lacher, CPA
Lacher McDonald & Co., CPAs, PA
Seminole, FL

How many of you look at your financial statements each month? How many of you understand what your statements are telling you?

In this article, you are going to learn to use our financial statements as a tool to help you manage the business side of your practice. To begin, what are the basic financial statements? The Income Statement (or Profit and Loss Statement), the Balance Sheet, and the Statement of Cash Flows comprise the basic financial statements.

Most of the financial statements we encounter in working with veterinarians are prepared to reflect the fact that veterinarians are very poor business people so they should pay the least amount possible in taxes. And, judging from the statements we see, veterinarians have been very good at proving to the government that they don't make any money. While that may be a good idea from a tax perspective, it is not a good way to manage your practice. What is the alternative? Prepare the statements so that they help you manage the business side of your practice so you can achieve the goals that you want to achieve.

I have labeled this article, Understanding your Financial Statements, the Lab Report for Your Practice. How many laboratory tests do you use in your practices each week? I suspect more than one. Just like you use more than one lab test to practice medicine, we use more than one type of financial statement to manage the practices with which we work. We use one type to manage the practice; we use another kind to prepare the tax return. Perfectly legal! Perfectly necessary to have the information you need to achieve the results you want.

In this article, we are mainly going to be talking about the management use of financial statements. Open Book Management is more than simply posting your practice's financial statements on a screen and berating your staff for not achieving the numbers that you think are important. In this article, we are going to make sure that you, the owner, understand what your financial statements are saying and then we will look at what information you might want to share with your staff and some ideas as to how to share that information in a way that is meaningful for them.

The overriding consideration in sharing information is to give our team members the information they need in order for them to make good decisions in carrying out their duties in your practice. So often we berate our team because they are spending too much, but we never share with them what "too much" is. Part of the reason for this could very well be we don't know what "too much" is, so how can we expect our staff to know.

Let's discuss what a correctly prepared financial statement should look like, and what those statements are telling us. Our goal is not to turn you into CPAs. Our goal is to help you understand what the numbers are saying – much the way when you look at a lab report we don't want to turn you into a lab technicians – we just want you to understand if the patient is healthy or needs your help.

Most financial statements in veterinary hospitals today are prepared with one goal in mind – show the government that you aren't making any money and therefore you don't own any taxes. If we turn that around and use financial statements to help us manage our practices, we will have the information we need to see if we are managing our practices or our practices are running us. Again, let me say that it is perfectly legal to keep more than one set of books or financial statements for your business – one set for managing your practice, the other set for preparing the tax return. They are not the same. I am also not suggesting that by keeping multiple sets of books your accounting bill will become the largest single line item on your Income Statement. If you have a good accountant, he or she should be able to convert your management financial statements to your tax financial statements in about 15 minutes.

What is the difference between the two sets of statements? Basically, the difference is in presentation. The goal of management usage statements is to show you how well you are managing your practice to achieve the goals that you have for the practice. Those goals can be many, but they all basically center around one thing – to be as profitable as you can be in order to pay your staff appropriately, to buy the equipment you need to provide the very best medical care you want to provide, to give you an appropriate return for the risk you are taking in owning a business – whatever your goals are, the practice must be able to support those goals. The only way you know if you are on target or off target is to look at the financial statements and understand what they are telling you. Your financial statement should give you the information you need to manage your practice to achieve the goals that you want to achieve. From these statements you can pull the information you want to give to your staff to help them do their jobs better to achieve the practice's goals, especially as it relates to them. What's in it for me is still going to be the motivating force for many team members.

The financial statements that we recommend are formatted using the basic style that you will find in the AAHA Chart of Accounts. The overriding consideration we are going to be using is that the statements are set up to give you the information you need in order to make decisions. Too much information, you get drowned in the details. On the income statement, if every line item represents less than one percent of the total why bother? It won't do any good to make a change in this area because it is immaterial to the total outcome. Too little information and we don't have what we need to make a change. If Accounts Receivable aren't reflected on the Balance Sheet, if we have to go to another report to see what is owed to us by our clients, then we won't take the steps to give our team the tools they need to collect payment at time of service like the sign says at our front desk. But like Goldilocks and the Three Bears, if we have just the right amount of information, we will have what we need to make good decisions.

We will be talking about accrual vs. cash accounting, and about keeping multiple sets of books to meet the needs we have. Keeping multiple sets of books is perfectly legal – I don't want to go to jail, any more than I want you to go to jail. We want you to be able to get meaningful information from your financial records so that when you put together the various Key Performance Indicator schedules or scorecards referred to in the companion article in this proceedings by Louise Dunn, the scorecards reflect accurate and meaningful information. If you have bad information going into your scorecards, the decisions that your team members will be making will not be good decisions.

Let's consider the Balance Sheet first. The Balance Sheet is set up with three different categories, the Asset section (what the practice owns), the Liability section (what the practice owes), and the Equity section (what you own of the practice). The Balance Sheet is called a balance sheet because the Assets equal the Liabilities and Equity. If they don't, you have a problem and you need to get it fixed.

In the Asset section, it is again set up in a proscribed format: the Current Section lists the Cash, the Accounts Receivable, and the Inventory, and yes, for managing, we have Accounts Receivable and Inventory on the books. We want to have on your financial statements a one-stop place where you can go to find out all the information you need about how well your practice is performing. If you have to go to file cabinets to pull out information, no one has time to do that and "if you can't see it, you won't manage it." As your team gets better trained in being "owners," they will have the information and understanding of why accepting payment from clients at the time of service is important, why managing the inventory is important, and the financial statements should start to reflect the benefits of this increased knowledge.

The next section should be called Property, Plant and Equipment, or Fixed Assets. In this section we list all the big ticket items that the practice owns – the computers, the radiograph machines, and the reception room furniture. Your accountant generally keeps the backup schedules of all of the things that the practice has purchased over the years. On this list is the cost of the equipment, and how much it has depreciated, or declined in value over the years that you have owned it. Here is a major area in which management financial statements differ from the tax financial statements. Many of you have heard of Section 179 depreciation or Rapid Depreciation. This is a tax benefit to spur the economy in the direction that the government wants it to go. When people invest in big ticket items the government is happy and the economy improves. However, how many of you really believe that the

$100,000 digital radiograph machine that you purchased is only going to last one year? Hopefully, none of you! For tax purposes we show $100,000 of depreciation expense, but for management purposes, we really want to show that expense over the period of time that the DR machine is going to benefit our practice. A big difference in many cases!

In the other asset section, you will find things like security deposits and for those of you who have purchased a practice, it is here that you will find Goodwill listed. That represents the Blue Sky that you paid for when you purchased the practice. Again, for tax purposes, this gives you a major write-off; for managing your practice, hopefully your clients are going to stay with the practice, so writing off that investment is not meaningful.

Moving to the Liability section, we list what the practice owes in the next 12 months as current liabilities. These are items like payroll taxes, sales tax, credit card amounts due, and accounts payable. We want to know what immediate amounts are that we need to pay. We also want to know what we are going to owe over the long term – things like the remaining balance on the DR machine that we just purchased, the balance we owe on the practice purchase – a one-stop place to go that will tell us how much we owe.

The equity section is what it is – it shows us what we would walk away with if we sold all of the things the practice owns and paid off all of its debts. In theory, this is what is left over for us.

Turning to the income statement, here it should be set up in a very set pattern, based on the AAHA Chart of Accounts that can purchased from AAHA. You will note that the revenue section isn't one line item – Professional Fees. The revenue section is broken down into six to eight meaningful categories of revenue. You don't want to regurgitate your practice management software into your financial statements – you want to show the categories of revenue that you feel are important to you and which you will use to make decisions. If dentistry is important and it is running less than 1% of revenue, showing this on your income statement will help you and your staff focus your attention when dealing with clients.

Next we have the Cost of Goods sold section. This reflects the costs associated with the services you are providing. It shows the cost of the vaccines, the antibiotics, the lab charges for running those CBC reports, the food costs related to the prescription diets you sell. An inventory adjustment amount should be reflected. Part of our goal is to give your staff the training they need in order to manage your inventory, not spend all their time shopping for the lowest possible cost. We want this section of your income statement to reflect the cost associated with the revenue you took in that month.

Next we have the General and Administrative costs which are all the other costs that you incur in running your practice. Salaries should be broken out between support staff and doctors. This can be more or less detailed as you choose; the important point, however, is that you use your financial statements to reflect in a meaningful way the information you and your staff need to manage your practice and to think like owners. In addition to the raw numbers, your financial statement should include a percent column that shows a cost in relation to the revenue generated. If you don't know how to activate this on your accounting software, let me know and we will help you. The income statement should only be one page long; if it is much longer than this, your statement is too detailed, and it really isn't providing you the information you need.

If your financial statements are not prepared correctly, the Key Performance Indicators (KPI) schedules that you use to give data to your staff and that they will be using to make decisions will be incorrect. Bad information equals bad decisions, so make sure that the information you are providing your team is good information.

To begin sharing this information with your team, you are going to have to have some training sessions where you teach your team what this information means. It is basic to us that income coming in less all of the expenses we pay out equals what is left over. It is not always as apparent to your team.

One of the statements that very few accountants give to their clients is what I call the "Where Did the Cash Go" statement. If I were a real accountant, this would be called the Statement of Cash Flows. The problem with the presentation of a "real statement" is that it supposedly helps you if you are trying to analyze whether you want to invest in a Fortune 500 company. It doesn't help you much if what you really want to know is: If the bottom line of my financial statement says that I made $100,000 and I have $10,000 in the bank, "Where did all the cash go?"

Armed with an understanding of what the financial statements are telling you and having an accountant who will help you interpret what they are saying, you can begin to understand what these pieces of paper are telling you, just like you learned to read lab reports in Clinical Pathology in your second year of veterinary school.

PARTNERSHIPS – MORE THAN JUST SHARING TOOTHPASTE: PART 1

Charlotte Lacroix, DVM, JD
Veterinary Business Advisors, Inc.
Whitehouse Station, NJ

Elise M. Lacher, CPA
Lacher McDonald & Co., CPAs, PA
Seminole, FL

When we talk with veterinarians about their "perfect practice," we frequently receive mixed messages. Especially with companion animal practitioners, balancing personal and practice time is a high priority. They don't want to be spending all of their time at the office. That said, mention the word "partner" and many of them can tell one horror story after the other of people they knew who had partners in a business venture and what a nightmare it was.

When you take a look at the main reasons why business "marriages," ie, partnerships, break up, it all revolves around four main areas – Money, Power, Family, and Sex. Not very different from traditional marriages—the analogies can have far more similarities than differences.

The focus of this four-part article is to help individuals understand the process of becoming partners and then help them create partnerships that will help them realize their dreams, not their nightmares.

Today the word *partner* is in many ways over used. Our medical doctors want to partner with us in our medical care. Phone companies want to partner with us to take care of our communication needs. We are constantly told to partner with our clients, team members, vendors, and taken to extremes, even competitors. What does the word *partner* mean in the traditional sense? Basically a business partnership means that two or more people have joined together, pooling money and talents, and assuming a risk in order to create or build something together.

We are not talking about partnerships in the highly regulated Internal Revenue Service meaning of a partnership agreement and filing a form 1065 Partnership Tax Return and following IRS Code Section 721. We are talking about business partners without regard to their legal status as partners. They may be in a partnership, LLC, or corporation. What we mean is that these individuals own something together, generally a veterinary practice, and as such they have a duty to one another and the actions of one individual affect the other individual. Essentially, they sink or swim together.

Why do people want to take on a partner? Basically it is because you are much more likely to succeed in business with a partner than going it alone. Successful businesses are much more likely to be found where individuals pool their strengths and move forward towards a common goal than looking at the lone romantic individual who succeeds against all odds.

With the complexity of running a successful veterinary practice today, and the demands that we all have on our time and energy and skills, it is much more attractive to "share the wealth" than to try to do it all yourself. Having partners is often what makes ownership possible. Even the thought of providing extended hours in your practice becomes much more of a possibility if there are two or more owners available to provide coverage. With the high cost of opening and running a practice, sometimes the only way to have the financial strength is to share the burden.

Okay, we have set the stage. Before we go any further, however, we will digress for a moment with some warnings that are somewhat "touchy, feely" but can give you good advice as you start down this path:

- If you don't think you are a team player, don't even try
- Exercise extreme caution when selecting a partner
- If you don't need a partner, don't get one
- Legal documents, alone, are not going to keep you out of trouble
- If things don't feel right, work to fix it
- If you see potential problems, work to fix them while you are still "in love"

Some questions to ask before you start down the path: Why do you want to own a veterinary practice? I know it is to "provide high quality medicine for the animals and to create a good experience for all clients when they walk through the front door." But there is more to it than that. If you want it "your way or the highway," you might need to think about whether partnership is the route for you. Why do you want to have a partner? You get the cream of the work that way and can dump all the less desirable work onto your partner. Perhaps it's time to rethink your plans. Are there better alternatives available? Perhaps a strong practice manager would solve some of your needs and keeping the ownership entirely in your hands. And finally, are you choosing the best partner for you? While there are many people who could be good partners, just like choosing the spouse with whom you want to spend the rest of your life, your business partner is pretty much in the same category. Just like spouses, partners don't change after you tie the knot.

Now that we have covered some of the basics surrounding the partnership concepts, we are going to address some of the basics of putting together a successful partnership arrangement. As an aside, the documents do provide a good legal document that going forward will provide a measure of protection for the parties involved. Where I see the real benefit of the legal documents, however, is that if prepared properly, they provide an opportunity for the partners to really discuss issues and put out on the table viewpoints and concerns and approaches to issues that will be faced. For example, the structure of the transaction will influence the power distribution between the parties and this is generally an area that needs and should receive a great deal of thought and discussion up front.

In the discussions that are held about the various elements that should be covered in the contract, things will surface that should be dealt with before the knot is tied. Remember that definitions mean different things to different people. We all filter words through our life experiences. Fairness is simply in the eye of the beholder. Talking about what each person's expectations are concerning the business relationship will help to cut down on the distrust that tends to develop when things don't play out exactly as planned. Put money, time, and effort into the equation and this can be a recipe for disaster.

Some of the additional issues that need to be covered include an understanding of the personalities of all involved. Some of the questions that help to get an understanding of how the interaction between the parties will evolve include:

- Where do you prefer to focus your attention – inward or outward?
- How do you acquire information – sensing or intuition?
- How do you make decisions – thinking about it or how you feel about it?
- How do you view the outer world – by judgment or perception?
- How much time to you want to dedicate to the business versus personal life?
- What are your financial beliefs regarding debt, retirement, "fun" things?
- Management style – top down or collaboration of the team?
- Treatment of team members – hierarchy or equality?

PARTNERSHIPS – MORE THAN JUST SHARING TOOTHPASTE: PART 2

Charlotte Lacroix, DVM, JD
Veterinary Business Advisors
Whitehouse Station, NJ

Elise M. Lacher, CPA
Lacher McDonald & Co., CPAs, PA
Seminole, FL

In Part 1 of this four-part article, we began to consider the issues that need to be discussed before potential partners walk down the aisle to tie the proverbial business marriage knot. We are going to continue that discussion in this article because it is so critical that partners really know the person that they are marrying, in the financial sense. Partnership agreements are important, financial understanding is important, good advisors are important, but the most critical aspect of the relationship is that the person you are going to be spending the rest of your business life with is someone with whom you are very compatible. If it's not the right match, now is the time to back off. You can't change someone after the financial marriage any more than spouses change after a traditional marriage.

Every practice with whom we work talks about the high quality of medicine that they practice. That said, high quality medicine is very much in the eyes of the beholder. Now is the time for discussions about Standards of Care. What are your feelings about technology—is every "toy" a necessity? Continuing education—for the doctors, for the staff? Local or exotic places? Consistency of recommendations—does every doctor have the same script or is the care recommended dependent upon the doctor seen? Referrals—do we do everything possible in house or do we develop relationships with specialty hospitals? Other practitioners who may have an expertise in a given area?

What about ethical issues? What are our beliefs about convenience euthanasia, ear cropping, declawing cats, tail docking? Now is the time for these discussions. While the pet-related ethical issues are part of the beliefs that need to be ironed out, this is a business we are discussing. That opens up another whole area of ethical concerns. These issues can center around tax as well as general business matters.

In addition to these heavy ethical matters, there the practical concerns that revolves around the management of the hospital. Who is going to deal with Human Resource issues? How are prices going to be set and adjusted? A big marketing budget or are we going to rely on word of mouth and client referrals? How are we going to be spending our work-related time? Are we going to do emergencies or refer? Open weekends? Flex time during the work week? Is it okay if one of us runs for office with the local or state Veterinary Medical Association? If that takes time away from the office how is that going to be compensated? Are clients, clients of the hospital or are they individual doctor's clients?

Having control over your practice, where it is today and where it goes tomorrow is part of the thrill of owning your own practice. If there is only one of you, you can pretty much agree on these matters. When there is co-ownership of a company you can have tremendous control on these matters—if you all agree. If you can't agree, disaster can erupt.

The contract again, can provide that if you can't agree there are provisions for buy out or dissolution or forced mediation, or any number of ways to deal with the problem. Wouldn't it be better if some of the issues were addressed ahead of time to be sure that when disagreements arose, there were guiding structures built into the agreements to assist with a resolution where each could benefit rather than taking the path of dissolution?

One of the major areas of stress is most partnerships is the sharing of power. In veterinary practices, this can take a path very dissimilar from many businesses. With most traditional businesses, the issue is how to share power, or who is going to be "in control." In veterinary practices, we often see the opposite—who is going to be willing to assume the role of CEO? In any event, the issue of who is going to be the managing doctor, managing partner, operational chief, whatever you are going to name that role, but someone has to be the boss. Many times the solution to this issue, as proposed by veterinarians, simply doesn't work. We will share control—all decisions require a unanimous vote. Or, one will be the CEO and make the strategic long-term decisions, and one will be the manager and deal with the short-term decisions.

A better solution might be that before the knot is tied, the partners take a serious look at the practice needs and what each of the partners has to bring to the table. Practices need to differentiate roles to be efficient. Just like technicians should not primarily be doing receptionist's work, partners have different jobs to do. Once it is determined what each person's role is and the skills each brings to the table, it is then important to determine how they will coordinate their efforts. Once this is established, actually putting the conclusions onto paper, an organizational chart if you will, with job descriptions and responsibilities clearly outlined can be of major benefit. It is also important to understand that while it is important to separate roles and responsibilities, partners need to continually reconnect and share information. So in addition to the regular well-run staff meetings and doctor meetings, all successful practices need to have very well-run partner meetings.

Accountability in a partnership arrangement rises to a whole new level. The buzz word in practice management today is getting your team to be accountable for the things that they say they are going to do. Discussing ahead of time the level of accountability they want to maintain between themselves can prevent major problems down the road. If it is not spelled out ahead of time, then frequently the partner who most needs to be held accountability may resist all efforts to do so.

Accountability obviously means there is a consequence if performance is not up to some expected level. Tongue in cheek, it is much easier to hold team members accountable than fellow equals. Without real accountability, the alternative can be disastrous. They can truly cost the practice money rather than helping to generate the profits that all practices need to survive. Lack of accountability among partners can and does destroy good businesses. Nobody wants that to happen but avoiding performance problems among partners requires careful planning and generally lots of discussions. It rarely takes care of itself, so talking through these issues while everyone is still best friends is a good idea.

PARTNERSHIPS – MORE THAN JUST SHARING TOOTHPASTE: PART 3

Charlotte Lacroix, DVM, JD
Veterinary Business Advisors
Whitehouse Station, NJ

Elise M. Lacher, CPA
Lacher McDonald & Co., CPAs, PA
Seminole, FL

Let's explore in this article some of the details of the different entity choices. First, let's look at corporations. What we will be talking about here, for the most part, applies to C corporations, S Corporations as well as Professional Corporations and Professional Associations. Remember, the Personal Service Corporations are not a separate set of initials behind your name, they are a type of C corporation and the designation only applies to tax rate calculations.

When you decide that you want to be a corporation and receive the benefits of that type of entity, there are also certain responsibilities that you assume. You agree that you will have annual meetings of the shareholders and keep annual minutes of that meeting. Now many people are derelict in doing this, but if you are ever audited by IRS, or sued by a third party, one of the things that your lawyers and CPAs are going to insist upon is that the corporate minute book is brought up to date. It actually is much easier if once a year, at least, you sit down with your advisory team, and commit to writing what you have accomplished during the year and what you have agreed to do in certain areas. For example, if you have a retirement plan for your employees and you have decided upon a contribution to the plan, commit the amount to writing. If you have agreed to purchase an expensive piece of equipment, or decided to move the location of the practice, or open a satellite office, or made any major decisions affecting the practice, the shareholders, etc., these are the types of things that are put into the minutes. Talk to your advisors about what is appropriate for your practice.

In addition, upon forming the corporation, there should be stock certificates issued to the shareholders, and the money for those certificates paid to the corporation. Again, this is a step that is frequently overlooked. If the corporation has issued 100 shares of stock at a dollar value for each share, the shareholders need to write a check to the corporation for the amount of money represented by the number of shares that he or she owns. While this might seem silly, accomplishing each of these steps plays into the next topic.

One of the reasons why owners elect the corporate structure is for liability protection. Except for malpractice issues, being incorporated protects the shareholder's personal assets should a legal claim be won against the practice. That said, this protection exists if the "corporate veil" is intact. What this means is that if you have functioned as a corporation, kept your personal business separate from the business of the practice, played by the rules, and not intermingled personal and business assets, the corporate veil remains intact and the protection is there. Fail in any of the components and the corporate veil is pierced and one of the main reasons for incorporating disappears. Listen to your competent advisors in this area.

As mentioned an earlier article, C corporations require special planning and insight by you and your advisors to be sure that you are getting the benefit of the C corporation structure if it applies to you. If you are nearing retirement or thinking about transitioning 100% of your ownership of the practice to a third party, talk to your competent advisors very early in the process. The taxation of a sale of a C Corporation can be devastating if not prepared for properly.

S corporations present their own challenges. As mentioned previously also, C corporations pay taxes on their earnings, and S corporations are considered pass through entities. The profit an S corporation experiences flows through to the shareholders according to their ownership interest and is reported on the shareholders' individual income tax returns. It takes vigilant tax planning to be sure that there are no nasty surprises on April 15th because of this flow through of profits, not flow through of money from the corporation. This is something that shareholders frequently don't understand and if their advisors don't prepare them properly, there can be very nasty conversations when tax time roles around.

Using the corporate structure, "silent owners" or equity owners can play a role in helping veterinarians realize their dream of owning their own practice. In this scenario, individuals can purchase stock in the corporation—that is, they are capital investors versus sweat equity partners and play a minimal role in making management decisions, but can share in the increasing value of the practice over time. If you go this route, again, make sure you have competent legal and accounting advice and don't think that you can skip the whole discussion process of really getting to know the person you are taking on as an equity partner. Minority or equity shareholders are shareholders none the less and they have rights just like majority shareholders.

Co-owner agreements are sometimes what cause two people to wind up in a partnership even though they don't think this is what they are doing. As far as IRS is concerned, when two or more people enter into a business arrangement even without all the formalities of partnership agreements and the "paperwork," they are still in a partnership. "We'll cross that bridge when we come to it" doesn't work very well when issues arise in these types of arrangements. In a time of crisis, bridges are more likely to be burned than crossed.

Co-ownership arrangements can arise with no paperwork or employment agreements or other paperwork that wouldn't rise to the level of partnership agreements, but that puts you into the partnership arena none the less. If you are going to operate in the partnership arena, having formal partnership agreements at least puts you into an arena that provides for a spelling out governance policy, and hopefully provides for a predictable transfer of ownership interests.

Partnerships and S corporations and C corporations have very different provisions for distributions of profits and certain other allocations of profits, losses, and benefits. Again, this is not a course in taxation and accounting, but be aware that each of these is not created equal. You can inadvertently terminate your S election if you are not aware of or don't pay attention to the rules governing the distribution of profits. Distribution of profits in a partnership is generally governed by the partnership agreement. In the absence of a formal agreement anything goes. But this method of handling money can give rise to major dissention among the partners.

With Limited Liability Companies, many of the rules and regulations are still being hashed out in the court system and the IRS. That said, depending on whether you chose to be taxed as a corporation or a partnership generally determines if you follow corporate or partnership rules. Make sure you have an advisor who understands Limited Liability Companies if you chose to go down this path.

PARTNERSHIPS – MORE THAN JUST SHARING TOOTHPASTE: PART 4

Charlotte Lacroix, DVM, JD
Veterinary Business Advisors
Whitehouse Station, NJ

Elise M. Lacher, CPA
Lacher McDonald & Co., CPAs, PA
Seminole, FL

One of the key issues to be addressed in any arrangement with two or more people involved is transfer of ownership interests. Transfer of ownership interests can occur voluntarily—when one of the existing shareholders decides to retire, or the shareholders decide to admit a new person to the mix—or involuntarily. Involuntary transfer of ownership interests occur when someone is forced to sell their interest. This could occur from some triggering event, loss of a license to practice veterinary medicine, for example, or death or disability.

This is an area that you want to give a lot of thought to before forming the business arrangement, be it partnership, corporation or Limited Liability Company. Some areas that you want to be giving some thought include giving first right of refusal to existing shareholders/partners. This essentially means that before any of the ownership is given to someone new to the equation, the existing people have a right to purchase the shares or interest. Alternatively, the practice can have the right to purchase the shares as treasury stock. There should be some provision that shares can only be sold to qualified buyers.

Discussion needs to be given to how retirement of shareholders is handled. Also, what if a partner decides he or she is simply tired of the rat race and wants out? Handled the same?

Another area of concern that is frequently overlooked is what happens in the case of death or disability? Not all definitions of disability are the same. How do you want it defined in your agreement? This is an area that needs to be fully discussed before the pen is put to the paper. In the case of divorce or bankruptcy of one of the shareholders, how do you want that handled? I know, this will never happen in your practice, but the time to discuss the possibility is when the occurrence is remote that it will ever happen. Do you want to have a mandatory retirement age? If you or your partners can practice until they carry you out with your stethoscope on, are you entitled to the full privileges, including compensation and benefits that you were entitled to when you were a fully contributing member of the practice?

When the whole process of buy outs or transfer of interests is discussed, a key determining issue is "how much are the departing person's interests worth"? There are many ways to value a practice's worth: book value, fair market value, investment value. Spelling out in the paperwork, generally the shareholder agreement and/or the cross buy out agreement(s), how this is to be determined precludes problems developing at the time this is needed. This is an area that, again, you need competent advice from individuals who not only understand the veterinary profession, but understand the legal, accounting, tax, and valuation issues that are at stake.

Assuming that you can reach some kind of agreement on how the shares will be valued—a formula, or a full valuation by a competent appraiser, or something in between, how is the buy-out going to be funded? There are many variations to how this can be handled. Depending on the circumstances and the amount of money required, this can range from life insurance proceeds, to commercial financial, to promissory notes, to sophisticated deferred compensation plans. There is no "one size fits all" when it comes to this area of your discussions. You may have different funding patterns for voluntary withdrawals for the departing shareholder to move to Key West versus the sudden death of your key managing partner. Again, before the pen hits the paper is when you want to have these discussions.

Non-competition agreements are another area that is frequently overlooked in dealing with partnership issues. What can be equally troublesome are non-competition agreements that are pulled from articles that are read or agreements that other people are using. Non-competition agreements are generally a good thing. Their purpose is to prevent departing owners from directly or indirectly competing with the practice. They keep owners focused, preserve the goodwill of the practice, and reduce conflict of interests. They also have different enforceable components dependent on the state in which your practice, whether you are an owner or an employee, how they are worded, an so on. This is one more area where seeking competent advice is critically important.

What does it take to make your partnership work successfully? Throughout this four-part article, we have mentioned frequently that partners need to meet on a regular, meaningful time frame. To be meaningful to the attendees these meetings need to have as their agenda that communication is of the utmost importance. The attendees need to respect each other and to be open to agendas that might be setting stage for problems to develop. Sometimes it isn't what is necessarily said, but what is going on behind the scenes or in someone's head that needs to be addressed. Being in a partnership with other people requires a sense of humor. There is enough stress involved with running businesses today, without taking seriously the dictum that you have to have fun at what you are doing. Yes, it is possible to have fun and to be in partnership with other people. This is also a time when you don't want to sweat the small stuff. Keep your focus on what you are trying to accomplish—the mission statement for your practice. Put a good team in place, including outside advisors to help you on your journey. If you stick to doing the tasks that are appropriately yours and have a good team in place, you can have fun on your journey and actually achieve the goals that you set out to achieve.

SPECIALTY PARTNERSHIPS: WHAT TO CONSIDER BEFORE GETTING HITCHED

Charlotte A. Lacroix, DVM, JD
Veterinary Business Advisors, Inc.
Whitehouse Station, NJ

Co-ownership issues arise when a veterinarian becomes partners with other owners, or when two or more associates join to buy a veterinary practice. Becoming a co-owner of a veterinary practice is like getting married. It's important to agree on the principal terms governing the relationship *before* getting hitched.

CONSIDER THE FOLLOWING KEY CO-OWNERSHIP ISSUES

1. **Business Organization**. What basic form should the practice take? A "C" corporation, an S corporation, limited liability company (LLC), partnership (general or limited), or sole proprietorship? When buying less than all of a practice, the buyer usually must accept the existing structure. Even when buying 100% of already existing entity, adverse tax consequences often preclude transforming that entity. Those purchasing assets or starting from scratch have greater latitude. Selecting the right entity is a complex decision that should be thoroughly explored with the owners' accountant and attorney. Generally, tax considerations are determinative, but liability is also an important aspect. For example, while general partnerships often permit added flexibility, each partner is responsible for his share of the losses run up by the other partners (ie, joint and several liability). Thus, if a partner incurs malpractice losses exceeding the practice's insurance coverage, the other partners will be responsible for the shortfall.

2. **Compensation and Profits**.
   a. How will owners be paid for their efforts as veterinarians? Will their compensation be based on their individual gross revenues, on practice gross revenues, or will they be paid a flat salary? Or should it be a combination of the foregoing? Note that owners are almost always also employees of the practice to take advantage of various tax advantaged employee benefit plans.
   b. How will the practice's profits be shared? Should each owner's "take" be based on his ownership interest in the practice, his relative contribution to the practice's gross revenues, his ability to bring in new clients (ie, "rainmaking") or other factors? Some business entities, such as partnerships, allow more flexibility than others in distributing profits. Beware of the double taxation consequences of distributing dividends from a "C" corporation. "S" corporations are less flexible because the profits are distributed in proportion to ownership interest.

3. **Governance and Management.**
   a. Governance of the selected practice entity are addressed in its constituent documents or more frequently in an a shareholders' agreement (partnership agreements for partnerships, operating agreements for LLCs). When two equal co-owners join, typically all decisions will require unanimity, subject to perhaps dividing the day-to-day management duties among themselves. Three or more owners, particularly if they don't have equal shares in the practice usually require more complicated schemes. For example, majority vote needed for all decisions, other than certain enumerated strategic matters such as the acceptance of a new partner, or approving capital expenditures over a certain threshold, which require a super majority vote (eg, 66.66%) or even unanimity.
   b. Will the owners do the day-to-day managing themselves or hire a practice manager? Co-owners should consider their respective roles in this area and how their efforts should be compensated since they may be foregoing income generated from practicing veterinary medicine if their compensation is based on revenues. Compensation for management duties usually ranges between 2% and 4% of the annual gross revenues of the practice.

4. **Transfers, Withdrawals and Buy-Outs**.
   a. Because it is unthinkable to let strangers into the practice without the approval of all the owners, the shareholders' or operating agreement usually prohibits an owner from selling his interest to a third party...without at least first offering it to his partners.
   b. What happens when an owner dies, is disabled, goes bankrupt, gets his license revoked or just wants to retire? Or what happens to an owner who divorces and the divorce settlement awards an interest in the practice to the spouse? In all of these cases, the owners typically have either the option or obligation to buy-out the affected owner at a price based on the practice's appraised value. (In many agreements, the practice entity instead of the owners may purchase the affected owner's interest.) In the case of death and/or disability, some owners subscribe to life and/or "buy-out" disability insurance policies, the proceeds of which are used to fund the purchase.
   c. Owners selling a portion of their interest in the practice in anticipation of retirement sometimes wish to penalize the junior partners for withdrawing from the business before they have sold their remaining interest in the practice (ie, "you should not get out before I do"). These penalties usually reduce the price the junior partner can get for selling his interest.

5. **Non-Competition.** A clause prohibiting the owners from directly or indirectly competing with the practice, keeps the owners focused, preserves the goodwill of the practice, and reduces conflicts of interests.

Veterinarians seldom have time to do anything else than practice their profession. Nevertheless, it is far preferable to resolve co-ownership issues at an early stage rather than to wait until a dispute arises. Denial and misunderstanding are the handmaidens of messy divorces.

14 ISSUES YOUR VETERINARY PRACTICE PARTNERSHIP DOCUMENTS SHOULD (HAVE) ADDRESS(ED)

While we consider a two-partner practice; the basic issues are the same no matter how many partners there are. Their resolution just gets more complicated.

1. What happens when you die? Will your heirs receive a fair price, or *any* price for your investment in the practice? Will they remain locked into that investment forever? Will your heirs collect profits from the practice? What if the other partner (who is getting paid under his practice employment contract) has voting control and decides *not* to distribute profits?

If your heirs are to be bought out, who sets the purchase price? How and by whom is it paid? If part of the purchase price is paid with a promissory note, is same secured? How? What if the practice is not profitable enough to pay the note?

2. What happens when your partner dies? Your deceased partner's heirs are now *your* new partners.

Barring a fluke, your new partners will not be veterinarians. Does your State permit non-veterinarian practice owners? Will they want to be bought out or stay and collect profits from the practice (without contributing to profit generation, of course)? If the deceased partner was a large shareholder, or the majority interest holder, the heirs will also inherit your deceased partner's voting rights. Do you want to share practice management with, or *be managed by,* such persons? What if the heirs squabble among themselves, leading to management paralysis and/or litigation? Do you fancy having the practice run by a court-appointed receiver?

If the heirs are to be bought out, who determines the purchase price? How and by whom is it paid? If there's a note, is it secured? How?

3. What if you are permanently disabled? Will you receive a fair price, or *any* price for your investment in the practice? Will you remain locked into your investment forever? Will you collect profits from the practice? What if the remaining partner decides not to distribute profits?

If you are to be bought out, who sets the purchase price? By whom and how is it paid? If there's a note, is it secured? How?

4. What if your partner is permanently disabled? Will your disabled partner want to be bought out or stay and collect practice profits (without generating any of same)? A disabled partner's interests will be different then yours, so if he was the managing and/or majority partner, how will he run the practice? Will he *be able* to run the practice? What if the disabled partner is mentally disabled?

If your disabled partner is to be bought out, who determines the purchase price? How and by whom is it paid? If there's a note, is it secured? How?

5. What if your partner becomes mentally unstable? You don't want a mentally unstable person practicing veterinary medicine. But if such partner is the majority partner you can't fire him, because he, not you, controls the practice entity. The same problem arises for equal partners. Sure your mentally disabled partner could voluntarily remove himself, but can you rely on that? What if the majority partner has a guardian? How will the guardian run the practice? What if the majority partner or guardian fires *you*?

6. What if your partner should be fired as veterinarian-employee? Suppose your partner becomes lazy or his child becomes ill and decides to work significantly less hours or stop working altogether. Suppose your partner becomes a substance abuser and consequently unfit to practice veterinary medicine. Or he steals from the practice. Or he harasses employees and/or abuses clients and/or patients. The foregoing would be grounds for terminating a veterinarian employee. But if your partner is the majority or an equal partner you can't fire him (as explained in the preceding paragraph).

7. What if you no longer get along? Should the practice be dissolved? If not, who should leave? At what price should the departing partner be bought out? How and by whom is it paid? If there's a note, is it secured? How?

8. In a 50/50 practice how are disagreements handled? What happens when each party has equal voting/management rights and a serious disagreement arises? How will the resulting deadlock be resolved?

9. What if your partner wants to drop out, buy a boat, and sail around the world? Should your partner be permitted to withdraw? If not, how do you keep your partner from just resigning as an employee (in light of the constitutional prohibition of involuntary servitude)? If so, should withdrawal be subject to your partner reaching a certain age (eg, 55 or 60)?

What if your ex-partner discovers he's chronically seasick and comes back to set up a veterinary practice next store (using the client list he kept when he left)?

If a partner is permitted to withdraw, who determines the purchase price? By whom and how is it paid? If there's a note, is it secured? How?

10. What if your partner divorces? If the divorced spouse has, or is awarded, a portion of your partner's practice equity interest, the divorced spouse becomes a partner. *Ménages à trois* make great literature and film themes but ALWAYS end badly.

11. What if your partner goes bankrupt? Do you fancy your partner's creditor as your new partner? It won't be fun to have a bank running, or having a say in running, the practice. Worse, the bank likely will want to sell your partner's share to a competitor.

12. Who's got the land? The small animal practice's most valuable asset is its location, because most clients won't travel far for pet treatment. As zoning restrictions get ever tighter, good practice locations become ever rarer (and more expensive). If, as is frequently the case, one partner owns the practice premises, what happens when he dies, is disabled, withdraws, resigns, divorces and/or goes bankrupt?

13. What if another veterinarian wants to buy your partner's interest in the practice? Should your partner be allowed to sell without your approval? Should you have a right of first offer? A right of first refusal?

14. If your partner is not your retirement plan, then who is? If you don't have a firm agreement with your partner to sell your practice interest to him (or someone else) upon your retirement, then how are you going to retire using your investment in the practice as your nest egg? What if both partners want to retire at the same time?

Dr. Charlotte Lacroix owns a boutique law firm based in Whitehouse Station, New Jersey (908) 534-2065. Dr. Lacroix assists veterinarians and their attorneys nationwide with their business-related legal matters, including employment contracts, purchase and sale of veterinary practices, specialty practice issues, mediation and start-ups.

PEDIGREE DRUGS....WILL THE REAL DRUG STAND UP!

Charlotte Lacroix, DVM, JD
Veterinary Business Advisors, Inc.
Whitehouse Station, NJ

PEDIGREE PAPERS: FREQUENTLY ASKED QUESTIONS

Florida's Prescription Drug Pedigree law was recently amended by House Bill 371 during the 2006 Regular Session. This bill created an additional form of pedigree for direct purchase transactions and exempted drop shipment transactions from the pedigree requirements.

To assist the industry with the implementation of this law, the following Frequently Asked Questions are offered to provide direction for implementation. It is important to note that the recent changes to the pedigree law did not repeal or delay its implementation.

Rule promulgation will be required to implement the new requirements. It is the intent of the Department of Health to seek rules for the following issues:

- Wholesale distribution of prescription drugs for emergencies;
- Wholesale distribution of existing prescription drug inventories without pedigree papers;
- Returns of prescription drugs;
- Drop shipments of prescription drugs; and
- Definition of terms.

FREQUENTLY ASKED QUESTIONS
- General Pedigree Questions
- Direct Purchase Pedigree Questions
- Drop Shipment Questions
- Miscellaneous Questions

GENERAL PEDIGREE QUESTIONS
Which prescription drugs are subject to the pedigree requirements?

Prescription drugs subject to pedigree requirements include all prescription drugs labeled for human use, including brand-name prescription drugs, generic prescription drugs, and some medical devices that contain a prescription drug. An example of a medical device is a convenience kit; the US Food and Drug Administration (FDA) has treated any prescription drug component in such a kit as a drug, and Florida is, therefore, following the FDA's direction.

The only exceptions are for medical gases, veterinary prescription drugs, and any drug distributed under a limited veterinary prescription drug wholesale permit labeled for human use but sold to a veterinarian for animal use.

Who must provide a pedigree?

Anyone, including a repackager, who is engaged in the wholesale distribution of a prescription drug from, within, or into the state of Florida, must provide a pedigree, with two exceptions:

- The manufacturer of a prescription drug. A "manufacturer" includes the actual manufacturer; the NDA/ANDA holder, even though a contract manufacturer is used; and the distribution point for the manufacturer, whether the distribution point is owned by the manufacturer or is a contracted third party logistics provider for the manufacturer. If a manufacturer also engages in the wholesale distribution of any prescription drug that it did not manufacture, then a pedigree must be provided to the recipient of the drug; or
- A member of an affiliated group that distributes a prescription drug to a member warehouse or retail pharmacy. The affiliated group must be composed of at least 50 retail pharmacies, warehouses, or repackagers.

To whom must the pedigree be provided?

A pedigree must be provided to every person who receives a prescription drug from a wholesale distributor or repackager, including: a manufacturer; a repackager; a pharmacy; a medical practitioner authorized to purchase or possess the prescription drug; a person in Florida holding an exemption for authorized research, teaching, or testing; a hospital pharmacy; or anyone other than the patient.

Are end users required to pass a pedigree for prescription drugs that are returned to the wholesale distributor?

A pedigree is not required upon the return of a prescription drug to the wholesale supplier, or when the drug is adulterated or otherwise unusable and is transferred to a licensed reverse distributor or destruction facility. Please see 64F-12.012(3)(f), Florida Administrative Code (F.A.C.), for complete details of the return requirements for prescription drugs.

May I wholesale distribute a prescription drug, if the prescription drug is received prior to the pedigree?

No. Except for drop shipment transactions, a pedigree must be received prior to or contemporaneously with the receipt of prescription drugs (see section 499.005(29), F.S.).

What does "authenticating" a pedigree mean and how do I do it?

"Authenticate" means to affirmatively verify, before the distribution of a legend drug, that each transaction listed on the pedigree has occurred (see section 499.003(4), F.S.). In addition, section 499.0121(4)(d), F.S. requires:

Upon receipt, a wholesaler must review records required under this section for the acquisition of prescription drugs for accuracy and completeness, considering the total facts and circumstances surrounding the transactions and the wholesale distributors involved. This includes authenticating each transaction listed on a pedigree, as defined in Section 499.001(31), F.S.

Rule 64F-12.013(5)(d), F.A.C., sets out the following methods for authentication. Please see the rule in its entirety for full documentation requirements.

- Receipt of an invoice (or shipping document) from the seller to the purchaser, which may have the prices redacted;
- Telephone call to the seller;
- Email communication with the seller;
- Verification of the transaction per a web-based system established by the seller or an independent person that is secure from intentional or unintentional tampering or manipulation to conceal an accurate and complete history of the prescription drug transaction(s);
- Receipt of a legible and unaltered copy of a previous transaction's pedigree that has been signed under oath at the time of the previous transaction to support the transaction to which the pedigree relates; or
- Receipt of a pedigree in an electronic form from an automated system that was successfully opened and decrypted by an automated system.

Who must authenticate a pedigree and did it change during the 2006 legislative session?

A wholesale distributor or repackager must authenticate the information on the pedigree; a pharmacy, practitioner, or hospital is not subject to this requirement. The authentication requirement was not changed during the 2006 legislative session.

What do I do if I cannot authenticate the pedigree?

At a minimum, a wholesale distributor should not accept the prescription drug for which an accurate and completed pedigree has not been received; this prescription drug is deemed adulterated by law. Although currently there is no requirement under the law to notify the department, we encourage you to notify us if the information on the pedigree cannot be authenticated and the "problem" does not appear to be a simple typographical or similar error.

What is the definition of "wholesale distribution"?

"Wholesale distribution" means the distribution of a prescription drug to a person, other than a consumer or patient, with certain limited exceptions enumerated in section 499.012(1), F.S., and Rule 64F-12.001(2)(cc), F.A.C. "Wholesale distribution" does not include the act of dispensing or administering a prescription drug to a patient.

"Distribution" is further defined in section 499.003(15), F.S. as "to sell; offer to sell; give away; transfer, whether by passage of title, physical movement, or other; deliver; or offer to deliver." This means that a wholesale distribution includes both the sales part of the transaction as well as the physical movement of the prescription drug.

Is a pedigree required for the distribution of an active pharmaceutical ingredient (API) by a wholesale distributor or repackager?

Yes. APIs are prescription drugs by definition. Both wholesale distributors and repackagers must provide a pedigree when distributing an API.

Are there any exceptions or special provisions if I am an authorized distributor of record?

No. As of July 1, 2006, the concept of authorized distributor of record is no longer applicable.

DIRECT PURCHASE PEDIGREE QUESTIONS
What is the new form of pedigree created by HB 371, and when may it be used?

- The additional form of pedigree created by HB 371 ("direct purchase") consists of the following items:
- The statement "This wholesale distributor purchased the specific unit of the prescription drug directly from the manufacturer";
- The manufacturers' national drug code identifier and the name and address of the wholesale distributor and the purchaser of the prescription drug;
- The name of the prescription drug as it appears on the label; and
- The quantity, dosage form and strength of the prescription drug

Please note that the wholesale distributor must also maintain and make available to the department, upon request, the point of origin of the prescription drugs, including intracompany transfers; the date of the shipment from the manufacturer to the wholesale distributor; the lot numbers of such drugs; and the invoice numbers from the manufacturer.

The direct purchase pedigree may only be used where a wholesale distributor purchases and receives a specific unit of a prescription drug directly from the manufacturer of the prescription drug and distributes the prescription drug directly, or through an intracompany transfer, to a chain pharmacy warehouse or an end user. "Chain pharmacy warehouse" means a wholesale distributor permitted pursuant to section 499.01, F.S., that maintains a physical location for prescription drugs that functions solely as a central warehouse to perform intracompany transfers of such drugs to a member of its affiliated group as described in section 499.0121(6)(h)1., F.S.

How does the Department define "intracompany" as used in Section 499.003(31)(b)2.?

The term "intracompany" will be defined by rule, but is currently interpreted by the department to mean the distribution of prescription drugs between two establishments wholly owned by the same business entity.

How does the Department define "point of origin" as used in Section 499.003(31)(b)2.b.?

The term "point of origin" will be defined by rule, but is currently interpreted by the department to mean the location or locations from which the manufacturer transferred title and possession of the specific unit of the prescription drug.

Who is an "End User"?

An "end user" is a person authorized by law to purchase and receive prescription drugs for the purpose of administering or dispensing the drug, as defined in section 465.003, F.S.

May a retail pharmacy wholesale distributor use the direct purchase pedigree to distribute a prescription drug to an end user?

A retail pharmacy wholesale distributor may use this statement only when the retail pharmacy wholesale distributor purchases the specific unit of the prescription drug directly from the manufacturer and distributes the prescription drug directly to an end user; otherwise, a full pedigree must be used.

May a drug repackager provide a direct purchase pedigree?

This will depend on the repackager's operation.

YES, if a drug repackager purchases finished and fully labeled prescription drugs directly from the prescription drug manufacturer for placement in a convenience kit, provided that the drug repackager does not change the immediate container or label of the specific unit of the finished and fully labeled prescription drug received from the manufacturer. The department treats as a drug repackager the maker of a combination medical device containing any prescription drug component, as long as the FDA requires that such component comply with federal prescription drug regulations.

NO, if a drug repackager changes the specific unit of a prescription drug purchased directly from the manufacturer must. Examples of operations required to provide a full pedigree are:

- Companies that repackage bulk prescription drugs (APIs); and
- Companies that alter a packaging component that may have direct contact with the prescription drug (eg, repackaging from bottles of 500 dosage units to bottles of 30 dosage units.).

How do I handle existing prescription drug inventory on July 1, 2006 that was not accompanied by a pedigree?

The Department is in the process of promulgating rules regarding this subject. However, under the department's current interpretation, all existing inventory in commerce prior to July 1, 2006 may be distributed under pre-July 1, 2006 laws and rules if the wholesale distributor provides the department a list of such inventory by July 17, 2006 by disk, hard copy, or e-mail with file attached. Please mark inventory information "Trade Secret."

Please mail, fax, or electronically mail inventory information to:

Rebecca Poston, Executive Director
Florida Board of Pharmacy, and
Drugs, Devices and Cosmetics Program
4052 Bald Cypress Way Bin C#04
Tallahassee, Fl 32399-3255

Fax: (850) 413-6982
E-Mail: Rebecca_Poston@doh.state.fl.us

DROP SHIPMENT QUESTIONS
How do we handle drops?

House Bill 371 specifically authorized the receipt of a prescription drug without first receiving a pedigree for "drop shipment" transactions. A drop shipment transaction is defined as the wholesale distributor taking title to, but not possession of, a prescription drug and the prescription drug's manufacturer shipping the prescription drug directly to an end user or to a member of an affiliated group, with the exception of a repackager. The prescription drug manufacturer, wholesale distributor, and the end user or member of an affiliated group each have specific obligations in a drop shipment transaction:

- The manufacturer must provide, and the end user or member of an affiliated group must acquire, a shipping document within 14 days after the receipt of the prescription drug. The shipping document must contain the following information:
  o The name and address of the manufacturer, including the point of origin of the shipment, and the names and addresses of the wholesale distributor and the purchaser;
  o The name of the prescription drug as it appears on the label; and
  o The quantity, dosage form, and strength of the prescription drug.
- The wholesale distributor must provide an invoice and a sworn statement to the recipient of the prescription drug within 14 days after receiving a shipment notification from the manufacturer. The sworn statement is: "This wholesale distributor purchased the specific unit of the prescription drug listed on the invoice directly from the manufacturer, and the specific unit of prescription drug was shipped by the manufacturer directly to a person authorized by law to administer or dispense the legend drug, as defined in s. 465.003, Florida Statutes, or a member of an affiliated group, as described in s. 499.0121(6)(h), Florida Statutes, with the exception of a repackager." The invoice must contain a unique cross-reference to the manufacturer's shipping document. In addition, the wholesale distributor must also maintain and make available to the department, upon request, the lot number if not contained in the shipping document acquired by the recipient.

What is the penalty for failure to provide the required documentation in a drop ship transaction?

It is a third degree felony for the failure of the manufacturer to provide the shipping document; the recipient to acquire the shipping document; or the wholesale distributor to provide the invoice and sworn statement.

MISCELLANEOUS QUESTIONS

Can we use a Web site to provide the pedigree to our pharmacy customers?

Yes. A wholesale distributor may serve as a repository of a customer's pedigree if the wholesale distributor specifies on the customer's invoice or other distribution document the method for immediately accessing all pedigrees associated with each prescription drug. Please refer to Rule 64F-12.012(3)(a)2., F.A.C. for the entire rule language.

Will there be additional information and/or rules to implement Florida's pedigree requirements? Yes. Please visit www.doh.state.fl.us/pharmacy/drugs for the latest information.

VETERINARIANS' LEGAL LIABILITY FOR ZOONOTIC DISEASES

Charlotte Lacroix, DVM, JD
Veterinary Business Advisors, Inc.
Whitehouse Station, NJ

Mary W. Clark
Student, School of Veterinary Medicine
University of Pennsylvania, Philadelphia, PA

There are primarily two areas of law that regulate the conduct of veterinarians and help ensure that veterinarians act prudently and reasonably in their dealings with clients and their pets. The first is the civil court system, which adjudicates claims made by clients who allege that their veterinarians have acted carelessly. The second is the state board of examiners, which is an administrative office charged with enforcing a state's veterinary practice act. The state veterinary practice act sets forth laws to which veterinarians must comply in order to obtain and retain their veterinary licenses. In performing their daily clinical duties, veterinarians should be cognizant of these two areas of law, as they represent the two principle avenues by which clients may direct complaints and file claims of malpractice.

Receiving letters from the state board of examiners or a disgruntled client's attorney can be very distressing, sometimes causing veterinarians to respond impulsively and not always in their best interest. This is primarily the case with veterinarians who have been practicing for only a few years, as they are not likely to have been previously named in a lawsuit nor reprimanded by a regulatory agency. It is important for veterinarians to realize that the manner in which they initially respond to such allegations can have a significant impact on the final outcome. For this reason, it behooves veterinarians to become knowledgeable about the processes by which state boards and the courts adjudicate such allegations. The following zoonotic disease case example illustrates how these procedures work in real life.

DR. WILLIAMS' CASE

On a brisk October day, Mrs. McDonnell and her two young children bring Hobbes, a recently adopted 2-month-old kitten, to their local animal hospital where Dr. Williams is currently on duty. Mrs. McDonnell is surprised to see a new face; she has always seen the practice owner, Dr. Haus, for their 5 year-old Labrador retriever's annual visits. Dr. Williams explains that she was hired a few months ago and Dr. Haus is on vacation for a couple of weeks, and she would be happy to take a look at their new kitten.

Dr. Williams takes a fecal sample and performs a physical examination, noticing some mild nasal and ocular discharge. She also notices a few fleas and some patchy areas of alopecia and crusting, especially at the base of the tail. Dr. Williams explains that Hobbes probably has an upper respiratory infection and flea allergy dermatitis. Just then, one of the veterinary technicians informs Dr. Williams that there are four appointments waiting and a frantic client has just called to say that their dog was hit by a car and is on her way. Being the only doctor on duty, Dr. Williams knows she must act quickly. She returns to the exam room where Mrs. McDonnell is impatiently looking at her watch. She quickly performs a Wood's lamp test on Hobbes to rule out dermatophytosis (ringworm). Seeing that it is negative and knowing that lesions at the base of the tail are most often indicative of flea allergy dermatitis, she de-worms Hobbes, applies some topical flea preventative, and sends Mrs. McDonnell home with some Clavamox for the upper respiratory infection. She takes a deep breath and hurries into the next exam room.

Dr. Williams's hurried medical notes for Hobbes read: S: Owner brought kitten in for first visit. Recently adopted from an animal shelter. O: QAR, T = 104.3, mild dehydration, bilateral green ocular and nasal d/c, HR/RR WNL, multifocal areas of crusting patchy alopecia, esp. at tail base. Fleas. Fecal neg. A: Mild to moderate URI, flea allergy dermatitis. P: 0.21 cc Clavamox PO BID 2 weeks. Topical flea tx.

One night, a few days later, Mrs. McDonnell sees her 4-year-old son, Eric, rubbing his elbow. She notices a red crusting spot where he had been rubbing. Concerned, she calls her daughter Eliza into the room and asks if she has any itchy red spots on her skin. Eliza says no. Mrs. McDonnell, a kindergarten teacher, suspects that Eric contracted ringworm from one of his classmates at school. She immediately takes both of the children to their family pediatrician, Dr. Smith. During Eric's physical exam, Dr. Smith asks Mrs. McDonnell if they have any pets. Mrs. McDonnell doesn't see what that would have to do with anything until he explains that ringworm is a zoonotic disease, one that can be spread from animals to humans. He explains that it is quite possible that Eric could have gotten ringworm from their new kitten. Noting that Mrs. McDonnell seems to have a similar lesion on her own arm, Dr. Smith recommends that she and her husband visit their own physician.

After a visit with her physician confirming that she also has developed ringworm, Mrs. McDonnell contacts the school principal to notify her of the situation. She is told that she cannot come to work until further notice, as she might spread the disease to her students and the school wants to avoid angry phone calls or even lawsuits from angry overprotective parents. At the mention of lawsuits, Mrs. McDonnell thinks of her upcoming recheck appointment with Dr. Williams and wonders why she was never told about the risk of Hobbes transmitting ringworm to her family. Had she only known, she could have taken some precautions to avoid this whole mess. Thinking more and more about the situation and becoming increasingly frustrated, Mrs. McDonnell picks up the phone and cancels Hobbes' appointment for next week. She then makes an appointment with a different veterinarian. Finally, she telephones her sister-in-law, who happens to be an attorney.

On a Monday morning, 3 months later, Dr. Williams receives two frightening letters—one from a local attorney stating that she had been named in a negligence lawsuit being brought forth by Mrs. McDonnell. The second letter was from the Veterinary State Board of Examiners, requesting her response to allegations that she had "carelessly and negligently failed to inform a client about the risks associated with zoonotic diseases, and failed to perform appropriate diagnostic testing." Knowing that her boss had been out of town for Mrs. McDonnell's appointment, Dr. Williams knew she would soon have some explaining to do. What should Dr. Williams do?

RESPONDING TO ALLEGATIONS OF PROFESSIONAL MALPRACTICE

How veterinarians address such accusations will in part depend on whether the allegations are in the form of a lawsuit, state board complaint, or both. Regardless of the form in which the allegation is made, the first step a veterinarian should take is to carefully read the complaint and determine what is being requested of them and in what time frame. Once this information has been assimilated, he or she should gather pertinent medical records and any other documentation relating to the services in question and delineate their recollection of the events in chronological order.

In this case, the complaints allege that Dr. Williams failed to warn Mrs. McDonnell about zoonotic risks associated with having a pet, failed to perform the adequate diagnostic procedures required to rule out dermatophytosis, and failed to treat the pet accordingly. The facts indicate that Dr. Williams examined Hobbes, made a diagnosis of upper respiratory and flea allergic dermatitis, and performed one diagnostic test to rule out dermatophytosis without informing the owner. Dr. Williams should carefully review the medical records to corroborate her recollection of the events. Unfortunately in this case, because the documentation is poor, it will be a scenario of Dr. Williams's word against Mrs. McDonnell's. For example, it will be difficult for Dr. Williams to claim that she informed Mrs. McDonnell of zoonotic risks, or that she even attempted to rule out dermatophytosis with any diagnostic testing, as there is no such notation in the records. Since Dr. Williams has a legal obligation to maintain medical records, the fact that she hasn't done so adequately will imply that she also was careless with her medicine. As she reviews the records, Dr. Williams should write down the events that led to Mrs. McDonnell's complaint. Most veterinarians will find this helpful since it will refresh their memories, help them develop a consistent "story" as to what happened, and provide a draft from which to develop a written response.

So as not to compromise her defense in the lawsuit, Dr. Williams should immediately upon receiving the complaint, contact her professional liability insurance carrier and ask for advice. However, if Dr. Williams suspected earlier that Mrs. McDonnell was likely to pursue legal action, she should have contacted her insurance carrier at that time. Insurance carriers may differ in how they handle negligence actions, but usually require the defendant to fill out a claims form in which the veterinarian describes the circumstances that led to the claim. A claims representative then reviews the facts, makes a recommendation as to a course of action, and may assign an attorney to the case if the complaint cannot be settled quickly. In this case, if Mrs. McDonnell is offered a settlement and rejects it, it is likely an attorney would be assigned to defend Dr. Williams since in this case failing to diagnose, treat, and warn the client of zoonotic risks of dermatophytosis is likely to be deemed negligent.

In dealing with the letter from the state board, Dr. Williams should be aware that she will most likely be defending her conduct at her own expense, since professional liability insurance carriers generally do not provide coverage for state board actions (exception: AVMA-PLIT and ABD Insurance and Financial Services now offer a limited policy insuring against state board actions). While Dr. Williams may respond on her own, it is usually advisable for her to obtain legal advice as to how she should respond to the allegation(s) and at the very least have an attorney review her letter. In drafting her response, Dr. Williams should not underestimate the time and effort it will take to address all the issues in the complaint, in an organized and articulate manner. Responses that are disorganized, incomplete and difficult to follow often lead to further investigation by the board, whereas a professional, organized, and complete response is more likely to warrant an early dismissal of the charges. Additionally, Dr. Williams may find it helpful to consult with other veterinarians to determine whether they routinely perform Wood's lamp tests and fungal cultures on all patients with tail-base alopecia and crusting; do they then inform their clients of the zoonotic risks of contracting dermatophytosis, even if they are convinced of a different diagnosis? This will assist Dr. Williams in determining whether she acted within the standard of care and provide an indication as to her liability.

NEGLIGENCE

The burning issues for Dr. Williams of course, are whether she was negligent in failing to (a) accurately diagnose and treat Hobbes, (b) warn Mrs. McDonnell of the zoonotic risk associated with dermatophytosis and, (c) maintain proper medical records. Our courts and juries decide negligence on a case by case basis in light of the specific facts and circumstances of each situation, but veterinarians should be aware of a few general principles. First and foremost, it is important to note that a veterinarian can be found negligent even if he or she did not intend to cause harm. Simply put, "I didn't mean to" is no defense to "you should have known better." A simple mistake, if deemed careless, can lead to liability.

Second, veterinarians can be found negligent even if the rest of their colleagues would have acted in the exact same way. Judges can determine that the entire industry is at fault if it is in the public's interest. Judge Leonard

Hand, a famous judge once wrote in his opinion "[c]ourts must in the end say what is required; there are precautions so imperative that even their universal disregard will not excuse their omission." Hence, it is a false security to rely on what the rest of your colleagues are doing.

To recover damages from a veterinarian based on negligence, a client must prove four elements by a preponderance of the evidence, meaning it is more likely than not that the veterinarian erred:

Duty of Care. Clients must show that their veterinarians "owed" them a duty of care to provide veterinary services of a certain standard. This element is easy to prove, because courts almost always find that once a veterinarian has agreed to provide veterinary services, the veterinarian also has assumed the legal duty to take reasonable care in providing such services. In our scenario, Dr. Williams clearly owed Mrs. McDonnell a duty to take reasonable care in providing veterinary services to Hobbes.

Breach of Standard of Care. A duty to provide services within the standard of care is breached when veterinarians fail to meet the standard of care as established by the veterinary profession, that is, when they fail to act with the level of skill and diligence commonly possessed by members of the profession in good standing. Mrs. McDonnell probably will be able to prove breach of duty if her attorney can show that veterinarians routinely perform fungal cultures in addition to a Wood's lamp test when multifocal alopecia and crusting is observed on physical examination. Conversely, Dr. Williams will attempt to establish that she did not breach her duty of care, by showing that most general practitioners do not perform fungal cultures or Wood's lamp examinations when they are convinced a different diagnosis due to characteristic lesions. It is at this stage that expert witnesses are hired to testify as to the standard in the case at hand.

Proximate Cause. Clients must then prove that the veterinarian's failure to provide services within the standard of care "proximately" or "closely" caused the harm suffered by the clients. If the harm suffered by the client is not a result of the veterinarian's actions or omissions, it would be unfair to hold the veterinarian responsible. In this case, it is not yet clear that Hobbes transmitted dermatophytosis to the McDonnell family. If a different veterinarian is able to prove that Hobbes was indeed infected with dermatophytosis and the isolated organism is the same as the one isolated from Mrs. McDonnell or her children, proximate cause will be relatively easy to prove. Suppose, however, that dermatophytes cannot be cultured from a trichogram performed on Hobbes. It would be more difficult to prove that the family's infection resulted from any failure on Dr. Williams' part.

Damages. Even after they have proved negligence, clients also must establish that they suffered harm resulting from such negligence. Since animals are considered as property under the law and most state courts do not recognize loss of companionship, this harm is usually in the form of an economic loss. As a result veterinary malpractice awards are usually much lower than in human malpractice cases and clients usually only recover the fair market value of the animal, costs incurred for veterinary care, and loss of income or profits in cases where the use of the animal is lost. However, we are seeing more and more states entertain the possibility of awarding non-economic damages and this is likely to increase the scrutiny with which standards of care are evaluated as well as the number of lawsuits filed against veterinarians. Since this case involves a zoonotic disease, as further described in the following section, Mrs. McDonnell may be able to prove that she and her family suffered harm resulting from Dr. Williams' negligence; she would then be awarded damages for medical expenses, lost wages, or emotional distress.

CASES

Dr. William's case is an actual case that has had some of its facts changed to accommodate the scope of this chapter. While there has not been an overly abundant number of published cases involving veterinarians and zoonotic liability, below are a few examples of cases which illustrate the reality of the risk and need for veterinarians to review their practice policies so as to minimize the risk of transmission of zoonotic diseases to their clients and their families.

Malicki v. Koci, 121 Ohio App.3d 723, 700 N.E2d 913 (1997) - Plaintiffs who received a parakeet as a gift and thereafter contracted psittacosis were allowed to maintain a negligence action against the pet store. Plaintiffs presented an affadavit from their expert witness that pet store owners knew that parakeets may carry chlamydia and yet exhibit no outward signs of illness or symptoms. Also, that psittacosis is a potentially deadly public health hazard; that purchasers of parakeets should be notified by the seller at the time they buy the bird that it may carry Chlamydia, and that sellers should recommend the buyers have the bird examined by an avian veterinarian especially for zoonotic diseases. *121 Ohio App.3d at 727, 700 N.E.2d at 915.*

Latham v. Wal-mart stores, Inc., 818 S.W.2d 673, 676 (Mo. App. E.D. 1991) - Store and store manager were *not* strictly liable under products liability law for injuries to purchaser's husband caused by contracting psittacosis from a bird purchased at the store where the evidence revealed the purchaser was an employee of the store who had the bird specially ordered, store was not in the business of selling birds, and the store had the bird for less than an hour before it was sold to the purchaser.

Steele v. United States, 463 F. Suppl.321 (D. Alaska 1978) - Optometrist found negligent in failing to refer a 4-year old child in a timely manner to an ophthalmologist. The court found the child lost his eye because of *Toxacara canis* and if the optometrist had promptly referred the child to an ophthalmologist, the child might not have lost his eye.

Baylis v. Wilmington Medical Center, Inc., 477 A.2d 1051 (Del. Super. 1984) aff'd 567 A.2d 418 (Del

1989) - Medical malpractice action for improper treatment of patient who was suspected of having toxocariasis probably contracted from her dog.

Placko v. Fawver, 55 Ill.App.3d 759, 13 Ill. Dec. 492, 371 N.E.2d 187 (1977) - Veterinarian who failed to take steps to assure the body of a suspected rabid cat was not disposed of, was found liable where, because no test could be performed to determine whether in fact the cat was rabid, child had to undergo series of painful rabies injections

SPECIAL CONSIDERATIONS REGARDING ZOONOTIC DISEASES AND NEGLIGENCE

The human–animal bond has evolved such that animals are often considered part of the family. The new strength of the human—animal bond has put our clients at greater risk of acquiring certain zoonotic diseases. Keeping our animal patients' best interests in mind will go a long way in maintaining client satisfaction and preventing most negligence complaints, but when it comes to zoonotic diseases, society demands that veterinarians also take into account preservation of client health as well as general public health. Zoonotic transmission of viruses, bacteria, and internal parasites poses a significant public health concern. Veterinarians have a responsibility to educate clients and staff about the risks of disease transmission as well as to adopt appropriate prophylaxis measures to prevent or limit such diseases. Because zoonotic diseases involve humans as well as animals, there are some special issues to consider beyond typical negligence cases only involving harm to animals. For more recommendations, see the table entitled *Practical Tips for Avoiding Complaints Regarding Zoonoses* at the end of this article, and *Sample Hospital Zoonosis Policy (companion animal), Selected Zoonoses of Importance*, and sample consent/release forms.

More Significant Damages. Negligence resulting in harm to the animal may not lead to significant damages awarded to the plaintiff. However, if the plaintiff himself is harmed, he can sue for medical expenses, lost wages, pain and suffering, etc. In addition, if anyone in contact with the plaintiff contracted the disease, each affected person can bring an individual case against the veterinarian. Greater sums of money are now involved, and it is easy to see how the amount demanded of the defendant could easily exceed the amount covered by his or her professional liability insurance. If this amount is exceeded, the veterinarian's personal assets will then be at stake. Thus, it is imperative that veterinarians be especially aware that simple omissions of tests or information can lead to serious consequences when it comes to zoonotic diseases and human injury.

Increased Animal Law Education. As a consequence of the interest in animal law and increased potential damages awarded to plaintiffs in malpractice suits, over 60 law schools now offer courses in animal law. In fact, several law schools are receiving million-dollar grants from game show host Bob Barker allowing them to offer these courses. In addition, lawyers are becoming wiser with developing methods to prove proximate cause in cases of veterinary negligence. The idea of using DNA markers as proof is no longer a futuristic notion—it is now a part of animal legal education.

Unpredictable Verdicts. Because veterinarians' duties with regard to zoonoses include providing information and advice to protect clients and their families against such diseases in addition to diagnosing and treating their pets, this adds an element of unpredictability to the outcome of these cases. It is much easier for veterinarians to concur as to the acceptable standard of care or "textbook method" for diagnosing and treating a specific disease than it is for them to agree on exactly how and when a client should be warned and advised about zoonotic diseases. One veterinarian may argue that verbal communication is sufficient, while another may insist upon supplemental written communication. Differences of opinion from veterinarians and jurors themselves about the standard of care when communicating zoonotic risks to clients ultimately lead to unpredictable verdicts from juries. It follows that instead of hoping that everyone else is of the same mind, veterinarians should err on the side of caution (ie, make stricter and more detailed written and verbal recommendations to their clients, documenting all communications in their medical records).

Client Requirements. Confounding matters even further, different clients will have different requirements when it comes to explaining the risks of zoonotic diseases. One client may have a significant level of medical knowledge and may require only a few comments on zoonotic disease. Another may need a more lengthy discussion on specific diseases, risks, and precautionary measures supplemented by take-home reading material and verbal repetitions. Each veterinarian must decide what his/her standard of communication will be to minimize legal risks and tailor this information for individual clients as necessary.

Reportable Diseases. Further, different jurisdictions may differ in which diseases they require veterinarians to report and the requirements may change over time. In consequence, it is important for veterinarians to be knowledgeable about these requirements. Once the veterinarian does report the disease, it then falls upon the government to warn the public. However, it remains the veterinarian's responsibility to warn the client of his or her risks.

Limits to the Veterinary License. Although veterinary practice acts and regulations authorize licensed veterinarians to practice veterinary medicine within a respective state, it is important to remember that these laws do not permit veterinarians to give medical advice to clients or practice human medicine in any form. This would include any sort of physical exam, suggesting a diagnosis, estimating exact risks of contracting zoonotic diseases, or even asking basic questions that could be construed as taking a medical history. While it is important to establish a relationship with a local physician to whom you can refer clients suspected of having a zoonotic disease or at risk of developing one, it is also important to limit the consultation only to discussing the disease itself, being careful not to offer any suggestions for human diagnosis or treatment.

RESPONDING TO CLIENT COMPLAINTS

Veterinarians often can avoid receiving letters from clients' attorneys and state boards by addressing client complaints long before client dissatisfaction leads to legal recourse. Clients often resort to litigation and or state board action when they believe their veterinarian either acted negligently or failed to respond appropriately to their concerns. When faced with a client complaint, veterinarians should consider the following:

Listen to the Client
- Clients who have complaints are often angry and need the opportunity to "vent."
- Veterinarians should show their clients that they are taking the matter seriously by listening carefully to what their clients have to say and taking notes of the conversation.
- Do not interrupt the clients since this will only anger them further and likely interfere with a clear understanding of the facts.

Remain Calm and Objective
- Avoid becoming defensive and emotional, since this may inadvertently reinforce the client's belief that the veterinarian acted inappropriately with respect to the care of the client's pet.
- A client's criticism of a veterinarian's actions, even when fully justified, does not necessarily mean that any negligence occurred. Veterinary medicine is an imperfect science and veterinarians are not omnipotent.

Communicate, Communicate, Communicate
- Many lawsuits are filed because veterinarians fail to adequately communicate with their clients. Often the client does not fully understand the diagnosis or proposed treatment and has unrealistic expectations as to the veterinarian's services and the respective outcome.
- Veterinarians can enhance communication and reduce potential misunderstandings by 1) obtaining informed consents, 2) providing fee estimates, 3) encouraging questions, and 4) providing handouts explaining the contemplated services.
- Veterinarians should use "plain English" when communicating to clients since medical jargon may not only confuse clients but also intimidate them, making them reluctant to ask important questions.

Show Sympathy and Concern
- Clients whose pets have died are often emotionally distraught and under certain circumstances may seek to blame someone, sometimes their

veterinarian, for their pet's death. Veterinarians who are compassionate and attempt to comfort their clients are more likely to diffuse their client's perception that the veterinarian should be held accountable for their pet's death.
- Veterinarians should not hesitate to recommend grief counseling for clients who appear to have difficulty coping with the loss of their pet. Several veterinary schools have such hotlines, including, the University of California at Davis, University of Florida, Colorado State University, Tufts University, Iowa State University, and Cornell University.

Coach the Staff
- Staff members can help diffuse client complaints and should be coached in what to do and say, if anything, when a client complains.
- The staff should remain professional at all times and avoid "offensive - defensive" discussions with clients who may be less intimidated by staff members and therefore more hostile to the staff as compared with the veterinarian.

EXERCISE CAUTION BEFORE ADMITTING FAULT OR OFFERING SETTLEMENT
- Veterinarians should avoid making apologetic statements that communicate an admission of fault, without seeking legal advice, since such admission may compromise their case in the event a lawsuit was later filed. Veterinarians with only a few years of experience are more likely to feel guilty and accountable for bad outcomes, even though there was no negligence. Remember that "feeling guilty" is NOT the same thing as "being guilty." Nor is a "bad outcome" the same thing as "negligence."
- Veterinarians should not offer to settle a malpractice charge or agree to any settlement offered by the client without first contacting their insurance carrier and/or attorney since it may be interpreted as an admission of fault, thereby prejudicing their case. Under certain circumstances, it may be appropriate to reduce the client's bill in an attempt to amicably and expeditiously resolve a dispute, but without admitting liability.

AVOIDING CLIENT COMPLAINTS

Just as "an ounce of prevention is worth a pound of cure," the best practice to avoid being dragged into a lawsuit or state board investigation is to take measures to avoid client complaints. Even if successful, Dr. Williams will spend a lot of time, effort and money defending herself in court and before the state board. In retrospect, it would have been far less costly and burdensome if Dr. Williams had informed Mrs. McDonnell of all the differential diagnoses concerning skin lesions and that there was a possibility that Hobbes did have a dermatophyte infection. At a minimum, Dr. Williams should have offered a fungal culture and recommended isolating Hobbes until a definitive diagnosis was made.

Veterinarians will save themselves a lot of grief if they periodically evaluate their practices to identify areas where preventive measures and procedures will help avoid complaints before they start. **In** addition, veterinarians should regularly consult with the staff, their colleagues and perhaps even their insurance carrier to ensure that they are aware of the latest preventive measures adopted by other practitioners. Keeping abreast of developments in the legal liability field should be an integral part of any veterinarian's continuing professional education. Because people are people, there is no way to prevent client complaints entirely. But in this area like many others, ignorance is dangerous and a preventive attitude is the best approach.

CONCLUSION

In the past few decades, there has been an apparent increase in the strength of the human–animal bond, changing society's expectations of veterinarians. Veterinarians are becoming increasingly viewed as protectors of general public health and with that responsibility has come increasing numbers of malpractice disputes. Being accused of malpractice can be a disconcerting experience for any veterinarian, but especially for associates who have been in practice for only a few years. These allegations can come in the form of a civil law suit or state board action and require a veterinarian's immediate attention so as not to compromise his or her defense. Preparing a defense against such allegations is facilitated by having knowledge of the law of negligence and an understanding of the adjudicatory process. Nonetheless, the best defense is to err on the side of caution by addressing client complaints when they first arise, using honed listening and communication skills, keeping abreast of the standard of care within the industry and adopting appropriate preventative measures.

REFERENCES

1. Allen CJ. Zoonosis: What are the legal risks? Are you protected from clients who will sue anyone for anything? DVM Newsmagazine. May, 2005.
2. Wilson JF. Understanding your legal liability and treatments for zoonotic disease. Zoonotic Diseases 102. http://www.vetmedteam.com.
3. Nolen SR. The human-animal bond: A legal liability for veterinarians? JAVMA 2002; 221(6): 762-763.
4. Beran GW. Legal Issues Affecting Veterinary Practice: Zoonoses in Practice. Vet Clin North Am: Small Anim Pract. 1993; 23 (5):1085-1107.
5. Tannenbaum J. Medical-Legal Aspects of Veterinary Public Health in Private Practice. Semin Vet Med Surg (Small Anim). 1996; 6 (3): 175-185.
6. Information Sheet: Zoonotic Diseases in Shelters. UC Davis Koret Shelter Medicine Program. 1997. http://www.sheltermedicine.com/portal/is_zoonotic_diseases.shtml.
7. CFSH: Animal Disease Information. The Center for Food Security and Public Health: Iowa State University. 2004-2006. http://www.cfsph.iastate.edu.
8. The T.J. Hooper [60 F.2d 737 (2d Cir. 1932)].
9. Wilson JF. Limiting legal liability in zoonotic cases. Consultant on Call: NAVC Clinician's Brief, May 2005.
10. New Claims Reveal Ever Present Danger of Human Injuries. Professional Liability. The AVMA Trust Report. June 1989; 8 (3).
11. Wilson JF. Legal Consents for Veterinary Practice. Priority Press: United States, 2006.

Dr. Charlotte Lacroix is CEO of Veterinary Business Advisors, Inc, a firm based in Whitehouse Station, New Jersey (908) 534-2065. Dr. Lacroix assists veterinarians and their attorneys nationwide with their business related legal matters, including employment contracts and the purchase and sale of veterinary practices.

Practical Tips for Avoiding Complaints Regarding Zoonoses

Obtain Liability Insurance
- Be sure to purchase professional liability insurance if it is not provided by your employer
- Contact your insurance carrier if a complaint is received or if a potential lawsuit is suspected.

Obtain Legal Counsel
- Be on the lookout for a good attorney who can provide future help with drafting complaint response letters

Educate Yourself
- Ignorance is not a defense against negligence!
- Remain knowledgeable about the latest information regarding ALL zoonoses observed in veterinary practice (new drugs, new case law, new technology, new guidelines)
- Maintain copies of statutes and regulations for your jurisdiction
- Maintain documents on how to diagnose and treat zoonoses
- Maintain a list of all reportable diseases
- Maintain contact information of government officials
- Establish and maintain relationships with local physicians to which you can refer clients at risk of developing zoonotic diseases. In turn, you should be available for physicians to consult regarding specific disease processes.

Educate Staff
- Develop a written policy on dealing with zoonotic diseases
- When new paraprofessionals are hired, familiarize them with the hospital's policy on zoonoses
- Use staff meetings to provide updates

Educate Clients
- Verbal communication
- Identify at-risk family members while still preserving client confidentiality
- Explain the risks of contracting zoonotic diseases from their pet and urge clients to see a physician (some hospitals may choose to have a consent form for this purpose)
- Advise clients of special instructions regarding pet care (isolation, hand-washing, treatment, etc.)Written communication
- Always supplement verbal communication with written communication. Have pamphlets regarding zoonoses readily available and give them to clients in the exam room. Also provide written discharge instructions clearly explaining any precautions that must be taken
- Veterinarians may choose to take a more active role by offering free educational programs to the public or becoming involved with the media
- Do not give medical advice to clients (no PE or dx)! Leave this to the physician

Perform Appropriate Diagnostics
- Brainstorm thoroughly, evaluating each disease category so that no possibly zoonotic diseases are missed
- Offer all appropriate diagnostic tests and explain the relative importance of each. Record any tests declined in the medical records

Keep Good Medical Records
- Record all diagnostics performed and all relevant communications with the client.
- Regardless of whether a client is agreeing to or refusing services, have them sign a well written consent/release form. Consent/release forms can help convince clients to comply with recommendations in addition to providing protection against lawsuits.

Sample Hospital Policy on Zoonoses

Our Hospital's Goals:
- Identify at-risk individuals (young, old, pregnant, and immunocompromised)
- Warn clients of zoonotic risks
- Accurately diagnose and treat zoonotic diseases in animals
- Educate clients on avoiding risks associated with zoonotic diseases

Zoonotic Diseases:

Dogs/Cats:	Birds:
Rabies	*Chlamydophila psittaci* (psittacosis)
Cryptosporidium	*Mycobacterium tuberculosis/avium*
Giardia	
Toxoplasma gondii (cats)	**Fish:**
Bordetella bronchiseptica (dogs)	*Mycobacterium*
Leptospirosis	Lymphocytic choriomeningitis
Campylobacter, E. coli, Salmonella	
Toxocara canis/cati (roundworms)	**Reptiles:**
Ancylostoma braziliense/caninum (hookworms)	*Salmonella*
Fleas (can transmit other diseases)	
Dermatophytosis (ringworm)	

Promoting Client Awareness:
- Pamphlets and posters regarding zoonoses must be clearly visible and available for client use
- If clients have any questions about a particular disease, please refer them to the veterinarian on duty and provide them with the appropriate pamphlet, making note of this in the medical record
- If the client desires additional information, refer them to the CDC website: http://www.cdc.gov/
- If a client suspects they have a zoonotic disease, advise them to visit their physician, and note this in the medical record
- For all new clients/clients with puppies and kittens/annual visits:
  o Verbally explain the different types of intestinal parasites found in cats and dogs. Explain the modes of transmission, emphasizing transplacental and transmammary transmission as important reasons why puppies and kittens are often born with GI parasites
  o Explain the importance of preventative deworming
  o Explain how humans can be infected with the same parasites and how it is important that proper hygiene and sanitation practices be used in order to decrease the risk of infection
  o Reiterate this information by distributing the appropriate pamphlets to these clients

Deworming Policy:
- Fecal exams are to be run at every wellness exam, followed by administration of deworming medication
- Puppies: deworm at 2, 4, 6 and 8 weeks old
- Kittens: deworm at 6, 8 and 10 weeks old
- Deworm all nursing females
- Adult pets: Deworm annually (3 times a year if owned by an at-risk owner), recommend monthly heartworm preventative which includes anti intestinal parasite activity, recommend monthly flea/tick control; don't forget to follow vaccination protocols

Non-Compliance:
- Any client refusing a fecal examination (or any other diagnostic test or veterinary service) must sign a consent/release form
- If the client refuses to sign, please alert your supervisor or the hospital owner

Client Refusal to Authorize and/or Pay for Recommended Diagnostic Testing and/or Treatment for Zoonotic Disease [11]

Client's name _____

I, the undersigned owner of the pet(s) identified below, decline _____ and/or treatment for my pet as recommended by this veterinary practice. I understand that this diagnostic test and treatment for _____ is aimed primarily at improving or maintaining the health of my pet. I have been informed that eliminating _____ from my pet is also important for the health of my family and the community.

According to the U.S. government's Center for Disease Control and Prevention, some animal diseases can be transmitted to humans, especially small children and immunosuppressed people. This disease can cause potentially serious health problems to humans, including

_____ .

In the event any person, including myself, contracts or develops a medical problem caused by this disease that could have been diagnosed and treated in my pet(s) by conducting this diagnostic test and/or prevented by administering the recommended treatment to my pet(s), I agree to hold the doctors and staff at this practice harmless for any of the fees related to the diagnosis or treatment of such symptoms or for any temporary or permanent injuries related to such an infection.

Name of Pet	Species	Sex	Age

_____   _____
Signature of Owner or Authorized Agent   Date

Authorization to Contact Client's Physician [5]

I _____ [owner], hereby request and authorize you, Dr. _____
[veterinarian] to write or telephone my physician, Dr. _____ [name and address of
physician] to inform Dr. _____ [name of physician] that my animal
_____ [name, species, and any further description of animal] has
_____ [name of disease].

I understand that this disease can be shared with or transmitted to humans. You have explained to me that I
should consult my physician to see whether or not I might have this disease and to discuss the risk to myself
and others who may have come in contact with this animal.

I further understand that it is my responsibility to make appointment to see Dr. _____ [name
of physician], and that you will cooperate fully with Dr. _____ [name of physician] should
he or she have any questions or need any information regarding the illness or condition of my animal.

_____   _____
Signature of Owner or Authorized Agent   Date

GOVERNANCE AND ORGANIZATION OF SPECIALTY PRACTICE – PART 1

Lloyd S. Meisels, DVM, Hospital Director
Coral Springs Animal Hospital
Coral Springs, FL

In order for a specialty, multi-specialty, or multi-specialty/general practice combination practice to be able to deliver the highest possible levels of both patient care and client (pet owner and rDVM) communications, it must have a defined, written set of guidelines and policies so that the departments within the hospital can work together to consistently and effectively achieve excellent results in both areas.

Economic health of the practice depends upon five major factors:

- Organization
- People
- Technology
- Capitalization and Cost Control
- Marketing

LEADERSHIP

Establish who is in charge. The people in your practice that the leaders are trying to motivate have to believe that this leader has more authority than they have. They can then accept the leader as a figure whose influence can help or hurt them. Ultimately, a leader's results depend on their ability to motivate. Instead of motivating staff by fear of punishment (loss of job), motivate with rewards such as money and benefits (set ranges), bonuses, saying thank you. Create an atmosphere where all staff can show off their talents and skills and get approval, support, loyalty, respect and recognition, continuing education, security, promotions, and public praise. Know what you want each person to accomplish and let them know what you expect.

Punish staff only for breaches of ethics or morality. Errors are not crimes. Rules and regulations that aren't followed lose their meaning. They confuse and demoralize employees. Follow your own rules. Be a role model, "do not do as I say, not as I do.' You need the staff to trust you and believe what you say and do is truthful. Your can earn, not demand, respect for your integrity.

Define goals, long term and short term. Review hospital policies and change them when needed. A good leader listens to what the staff members want for themselves to be sure you both are on the same wavelength.

People

Clients judge our practices subjectively. Their perception of your care of compassion is based on the behavior of the staff they deal with most often. The client's perception is their reality. As practice owners treat the staff, so will the staff treat the clientele.

IBM's company philosophy is *respect for the individual.* Every staff member should be seen as a source of ideas, not just acting as a pair of hands. People are your most important asset. Get incentives right and productivity will follow. Reward top performers, and get rid of dead wood. (Reference: *"Getting the Best Out Of Yourself and Others"* by Buck Rogers, VP of Corporate Marketing at IBM)

People become a Team because of recognition, security, pride, and individuality. Staff members implement and maintain the services a practice provides. They do not implement themselves. The staff must be well trained. Confused staff members confuse clients. Clients do not like that. (Reference: *"Leadership Tools"* by Thomas Cantanzaro, DVM, MHA)

Successful Practices Define their Core Values and their Culture

McDonald's Restaurant's "Q.S.C. & V" (Quality, Service, Cleanliness, and Value) applies to the veterinary practice because we are a service profession whose success relies upon the delivery of unparalleled quality, service, and reliability (in the client's and referring verterinarians' [rDVM's] eyes). From "In Search of Excellence," Tom Peters describes a successful company as loose and tight; that is, they push autonomy down to the staff (loose) while they remain fanatic about their core values (tight).

Management of the Hospital Staff

Teach the staff the practices beliefs, values, and culture (the quality of people you employ, the quality of the work expected). Train the staff and define expectations for the quality of work on patients and the quality of communications with clientele, other staff, and rDVMs. Write detailed job descriptions and set policy to cover every possible contingency (the devil is truly in the details) and specify the organizational structure of your practice, have them understand it.

Control quality (client communications, medical record keeping and staff relationships). Give the staff feedback.

The people and the services and products are the resources to achieve financial results. Of the three it is people that matter most. The best results come from a staff that is properly selected, well trained, and who have overall job satisfaction.

Policies

- Practice solid people management skills. All employees should treat each other with respect, diplomacy, and encouragement. All staff should acknowledge the existence of others (simply by saying hello in the hallway).
- Teach and practice good manners and professional behavior.
- Dress professionally. Define what this means for your hospital. Can Doctors see clients in scrubs or is a lab coat required?
- Insist people come to work on time and work the hours they are paid for (that includes the owners)
- Make sure phones are covered and phone calls are promptly returned.

- Insist that letters and memos are answered promptly. Edit letters of interns and residents.
- Written Sanitation and Safety Procedures must be in place.
- Written Patient Handling Guidelines must be in place
- A policy regarding use of the fee schedule for consistent fee policies must be written.

Examples of Common Sources of Conflict in Specialty and Large Veterinary Hospitals and How to Avoid Them

- In-house case transfers between departments (ie, gastric torsion), when should the case go to the medicine, cardiology, or E/CC service from surgery?
- Which specialist gets the production credit when the case is shared between services?
- Changes that are made in the treatment and diagnostic plan that may undermine the primary doctor's plans, confusing the client and causing the original fee estimate to be inaccurate
- Undefined and unrealistic expectations that each service has of each other
- Personality conflicts between clinicians that catch the client and rDVM in the middle while making the staff uncomfortable
- Inadequate medical records causing communication problems
- Losing medical records
- Doctors leaving early while others stay late and develop resentment
- Work schedule hogs (holidays off, popular CE meetings, etc.)
- Staff hogs (doctors who overuse and hoard "common area" staff)
- Equipment abusers
- Running out of inventory
- Uncooperative, egotistical, condescending behavior by specialists
- Use of ultrasound, endoscope, etc. as diagnostic tools by persons unqualified to do so
- Improper scheduling of the services
- Night staff using surgical packs, and not getting them ready for day service
- Not enough staff, poorly trained staff, etc.

- Nursing not respecting reception and vice versa (ie, not answering the phone or answering it rudely). Phone issues.
- Night staff issues with mislabeled radiographs, inaccurate registration of clients, etc.

Solutions to Common Problems

- Use rounds to eliminate or reduce the miscommunications that are associated with case transfers and to better integrate the practice as a whole
- Case transfer sheets minimize miscommunications
- How to compensate all doctors fairly. Set rules for compensation
- How to change the treatment of a case without looking foolish to the client
- How to use treatment plans (estimates) effectively
- Expectations should be put in writing (see part 2 of this presentation)
- Guidelines for medical records, writing and storing must be in place
- Scheduling of doctors and defining expectations of what gets done and when and by whom
- Show how to efficiently train and utilize staff to minimize wasted time and money
- Guidelines for maintenance and use of expensive equipment
- How to have better communications with rDVMs (see part 2 of this presentation)
- Prohibiting the criticism of other doctors in front of staff (see part 2 of this presentation)
- Getting status reports to reception, calling clients and rDVMs early (see part 2 of this presentation)
- Promoting teamwork and communication among the staff (see part 2 of this presentation)
- Written policies that make the practice work well together (see part 2 of this presentation)
- Phone systems for large hospitals and policies for using them (see part 2 of this presentation)

Meetings

- Have a reason and an agenda
- Prepare for the meeting once the agenda is ready
- Start and end them on time
- Keep minutes
- Have them regularly, not just to put out fires

Problem	Routing	Solution
- Reception has to make 3–4 calls before connecting with a nurse or doctor to get a patient status report - Reception tends to get attitude or sighs and groans, like we are bothering them - Reception should not be afraid to call up regarding a patient - Reports should be readily available	Nurse Manager and Hospital Manager	Eliminate this problem by *"specify date."* Have suggestions ready for meeting regarding this problem on *"specify date."*
- Doctors are not clearly indicating that they have communicated with the rDVM	Hospital Director and Hospital Manager	By *"specify date"* have all doctors filling out communication sheets to indicate their communications with the rDVM

GOVERNANCE AND ORGANIZATION OF SPECIALTY PRACTICE – PART 2

Lloyd S. Meisels, DVM, Hospital Director
Coral Springs Animal Hospital
Coral Springs, FL

Although individual variations in case management and treatments are supported and encouraged, it is important to have certain uniformities among the specialists and services in order to maintain consistent standards for referral veterinarians, clients, and support staff.

SCHEDULING
Maintaining Continuous Coverage
For services with more than one full-time specialist, the Hospital Director will arrange specialist schedules to ensure that (barring an emergency situation), the hospital will be staffed with at least one full-time specialist in each department at all times.

Vacation
Because of continuous coverage requirements, vacation time needs to be coordinated as far in advance as possible. If there are non-resolvable disputes as to time off, preference will be given by seniority. The schedule will be determined by the Hospital Director.

Conferences
Allocation of who gets to go to the national conference in each department will be rotated each year based on seniority. The schedule will be determined by the Hospital Director.

SPECIALTY SERVICE STRUCTURE
A huge amount of responsibility belongs to the specialist for the effective and efficient delivery of patient care and client and referring veterinarian (rDVM) communication related to their service.

Nursing Staff
It is important that nurse roles are standardized within each specialty department. This will minimize variation between services and will prevent conflicts and facilitate cross training.

Each specialty will make a list of expected functions for their nurses and functions that are explicitly not to be given to nurses. For instance, nurses do not need to be nor should they be present with their doctor during exam room consultation after the examination is completed. Nurses should be excused to do other duties as soon as the examination is completed.

Referring veterinarian communication is solely the responsibility of the specialist. Nurses should only be required to take messages from rDVM when the doctor is unavailable.

Nurses and all staff should also be protected from rude or abusive clients by the doctor of their service. Contact the Hospital Manager for assistance.

Examples of coordinating with the nursing staff and using the staff efficiently include:

- In most surgical cases the anesthesia nurse can write up your surgery while you suture the skin
- When your nurse is setting up or cleaning up a procedure is a good time for you to catch up on phone calls or medical record and computer input that doesn't require their help
- Have your first anesthetic patient induced and prepped while you are finishing some other duty
- Working as a team with your staff
- Using nursing staff to take x-rays, as well as lab specimens. A veterinarian's time is best spent educating clients and practicing medicine and surgery. Nurses should place IV catheters, anesthetize and prep patients, prepare prescriptions, do EKGs, and administer medications

Our budget for paraprofessional staff is set at the high end for this profession. We will make every attempt to consistently have enough trained staff to allow you to work efficiently, comfortably, and productively. Learn how to keep everything "moving" so you flow from one procedure to the next.

Expectations of Specialists
The completeness of each case is the sole responsibility of each specialist. The case that you begin is your case from beginning to end, unless direct communication occurs between two specialists to indicate a permanent transfer. If responsibility is to be shared, then the nature of that sharing need is to be made clear to the client, the rDVM, and to both specialists involved.

Each doctor should reevaluate (recheck exam) their own patients. Make sure your clients are instructed to do schedule rechecks with the specialist who is primarily responsible for the case. Similarly, follow-up questions about a case should ALWAYS be referred to the specialist managing that case, not to other specialists. The doctor who submits a laboratory test is responsible for providing results and interpretation to the owner and rDVM in a timely manner. The doctor is also responsible for tracking the laboratory test if the result is delayed.

The specialist should attempt to be the person to talk to clients as much as possible. Avoid giving instructions or interpretations through nurses unless the information is very simple or an echo of previously relayed information discussed by the client and doctor.

All hospitalized patients should be discharged with a typed discharge sheet signed by the specialist. A copy should be signed by the owner and left in the record.

Doctors should determine and calculate all anesthesia protocols (this is not to be done by nursing staff). Before leaving for the day each doctor must:

- Complete the PE/consult forms
- Fill out and submit radiograph reports
- Complete ultrasound reports

- Complete procedure/surgery sheets
- Fill out ICU sheets (current and following day), only DVM may fill these out
- Complete phone logs with owners and rDVM
- Update the invoice and compare invoice with estimate and deposit collected

All phone conversations with owners and rDVM need to be recorded in the record on pink/blue sheets on the left of the chart or on the bottom of the laboratory results sheet.

Desks should be kept organized at the end of each day in case other services need charts of your patients. Charts pending referral letters or lab results should be in one tidy stack. Computers must be locked away when not in use.

Governance of the hospital (ie. setting, overseeing, and enforcement of hospital policy) is the ultimate responsibility of the Hospital Director and his or her staff.

The Hospital Director will have the final authority to determine which animals will be treated by which Specialist and establish policies that determine which veterinarians will be responsible for providing treatments at times when the Employer's practice experiences disparities in case load by specialty, provided that Employee will not be required to provide medical services in situations where the Employee lacks sufficient veterinary expertise to provide competent professional services.

rDVM Communication / Interactions

In all cases the rDVM shall receive the SAME OR HIGHER LEVEL OF COMMUNICATION as the pet owner. Referring veterinarians will always receive immediate attention. Our policy is to have an "open-door" hospital to veterinarians at all times. Phone calls from rDVM are taken immediately whenever possible. If it is not possible to take the call immediately then the call should be returned as soon as possible. Messages should be checked periodically during the day to ensure that rDVM calls are not left waiting.

For each referral case the rDVM should be called the day that the case is received to update them. Even if the client does not allow any further evaluation, the rDVM needs to be updated.

For hospitalized cases, the rDVM needs to updated daily. The rDVM should be contacted prior to contacting the client (often the client will call the rDVM immediately after speaking with the specialist. The rDVM should be kept in the loop by the specialist to ensure accurate communications.

Referral Letters

When significant results become available for a case after its discharge, the rDVM needs to be updated again. All referral cases need to receive a referral letter. The letter may be sent after all significant pending results on the case are available, but it should be sent as soon as possible. The final letter should be sent out but not later than 7 days after discharge.

If a referral cases seen by an emergency/critical care (E/CC) Doctor or general practitioner (GP) has a consultation by a specialist, that specialist must co-sign the letter. All intern letters must be co-signed (by a specialist, E/CC Doctor, or the Hospital Director, whoever is most appropriate to the specific case.)

Patients referred from within our hospital do not require a referral letter but the referring veterinarian within the hospital should receive a voice mail updating them as to the case recommendations and outcome.

Phone Referrals

If an rDVM calls to discuss a case that conversation needs to be documented. We have a system for keeping track of potential future referral cases so that cases that you have consulted with the rDVM with over the phone will end up making their appointment with you rather than someone else. This will ensure continuity. This system will be fine tuned in the future and implemented through the direction of the Referral Coordinator.

If the case needs to be seen by the emergency service the rDVM needs to be made aware that the emergency service is admitting the animal. The specialist is then responsible for updating the emergency service regarding the phone conversations about the case.

For cases that will be seeing the specialist via a regular appointment, we must ensure that the case is scheduled with the specialist who was originally contacted on the phone regarding that case.

Emergency Case and Interactions with E/CC Service

Try to see emergencies that relate to your service primarily if that is possible. Use the E/CC service to admit the patient only if you are unable to see the emergency in a timely fashion. Remember – our policy is to say "yes." The only way to build a strong referral case load is to be convenient and be courteous to rDVM'S (the three A's: available, affable, able). This may require evaluating your time management skills/organization skills. We must avoid the "I'm too busy" excuse.

If the E/CC doctor admits a referral case, try to take over control of the case if it is complicated or if the rDVM is demanding that you be involved. The last option is to oversee the case with the E/CC service being the primary doctor. Even in this situation, try to call the rDVM directly after the consult and notify the rDVM that the case is being managed "together."

Specialists will directly communicate with E/CC doctor(s) involved in a case that they co-manage regarding who will contact rDVM/write the referral letter. As much as possible, the specialist should be the one to call the rDVM and write the letter. At the very least, the specialist will review the referral letter and co-sign.

Most times that rDVMs call, they want to talk to a specialist and send that case ASAP. We have to accept that part of our job means accommodating rDVMs and what they consider to be an emergency referral. Without it, we will not have the strong case load that we currently have. The Hospital Director will set up a schedule as to which specialist within the group will take emergency cases admitted through the emergency service each day. This allocation will be clarified with the emergency service during rounds each day. The Hospital Director will also set up a schedule as to which specialist will primarily take emergency phone calls and referrals each day. Unless the rDVM calls for a specific doctor by name, their call will be directed to the "emergency" specialist of that day. That doctor should make every effort to take that phone call as it comes and to avoid sending it to voice mail. See emergency fit-in appointments as fast as possible. Try not to make these clients wait a long time – try getting them in and hospitalized as fast as possible. Try to avoid long waits because this leads to unhappy clients and ultimately unhappy rDVMs.

The emergency service cannot be expected to provide significant medical advice or changes in therapy for pets being managed by specialists without being able to examine the patient or at least speak directly with the specialist. For instance, if a client calls in wanting additional therapies for their pet they would need to be seen by the emergency service for that service to be able to prescribe new medications or therapies for that pet.

In-House Consults

If there is more than one specialist on duty from the same service, the Hospital Director will make a schedule as to who is doing in-house consults each day.

On Call

The Hospital Director will determine a fair on-call schedule for Specialists, E/CC Doctors, GPs, and interns to call at night or weekends with questions. That clinician must make sure they are available by phone contact within a reasonable time.

Management of Cases When Off Duty (But Not Out of Town)

It is very difficult for another specialist of the same department to step into your case when you are off clinic duty. Therefore, the case will be overseen by an E/CC doctor or intern under your management by phone. The E/CC doctor or intern should communicate with the primary specialist on the case – NOT the on-duty specialist in that department, unless it is a critical emergency.

Management of Cases When Away (Vacation/ Conferences)

Because the complete management of cases started under each doctor is that doctor's responsibility, when you are going to be away, it is important to have taken care of expected follow-up with your cases during that time period. The specialist must make a list of cases that are ongoing and test results that are pending. The specialist needs to identify a person to take care of each case/lab follow-up and directly communicate with that person. The client also needs to be notified as to who they need to call if they need assistance and this information needs to be clear in the record. Contact information needs to be available for the hospital while you are away. Specialists need to update your voice mail as to your absence. Management Staff (Hospital Administrator) needs to be notified of your absence and

your contact information at least several days in advance of your leaving.

Interactions with Other Specialists

Many of our cases require multimodality therapy. Therefore, it is essential that we discuss these cases together as early and as often as possible. WE ARE A TEAM! For cases with multiple specialists involved in their care, those specialists will decide among themselves and directly communicate who will contact rDVM and write thereferral letter for each case.

Referring Cases Outside of Our Hospital

The Hospital Director and specialists as a group will determine specific situations that justify referring a case outside of our hospital. We use our in-house specialists for all specialist consultation, unless that specialist refers the case to another institution. Specialists as a group in rounds will determine when a referral to another hospital is appropriate.

PROFESSIONALISM

We will always treat each other respectfully—no undermining another specialist to a client, rDVM, colleague, or support staff member. This means that there should be no discrediting of other people's opinions, no changing of other doctor's orders in a way that would be embarrassing to the original doctor, and no negative conversation. Complaints and frustrations should not be voiced out loud, creating a negative atmosphere. These issues can be addressed in private and constructively with the Hospital Director. We set an example for the other doctors and staff of the hospital. If we maintain a positive and collegial environment, then the entire hospital will be more productive and peaceful. Do not get caught into the small bickering/complaining that comes from other staff members or doctors.

INTERNS

Interns should NOT be used to communicate with referring veterinarians – this communication must always come from the specialist unless the rDVM is insistent on speaking with a doctor and it is not possible for the specialist to come to the phone. Interns should only perform "routine" conversations with clients on specialist cases.

All specialists are expected to evenly contribute to intern training through lectures/presentations and rounds participation. All specialists are expected to evenly participate in the intern selection process.

An intern coordinator will be selected each internship year. This position will be rotated among all specialists. Tasks include setting up intern lectures/presentations, determining intern mentors, and being the liaison from these mentors to Hospital Director.

ROUNDS

The specialist must try to attend rounds each day that they are scheduled at the hospital. Be punctual. Try to avoid scheduling other appointments or procedures during that hour unless absolutely necessary. Give your complete attention to the doctors presenting. Be respectful of the other doctors if you have a differing opinion. It is fine to share alternative views and to debate alternative opinions as long as this is professional and respectful.

EQUIPMENT AND DRUGS AND SUPPLIES

The need for the hospital to purchase new equipment or drugs and supplies should be discussed at the specialty doctors meeting to determine if there is a need. The request is then submitted to the Hospital Director for budgetary consideration.

REVIEW

The specialists are to be evaluated every 6 to 12 months by the Hospital Director with input from CSR, Nursing, Management, Hospital Director, and appropriate staff DVMs.

FEES

Each specialty will also try to standardize charges for common procedures to minimize as much as possible significant price variation among the group. Estimates for common procedures need to be reasonably consistent even though techniques and medications may vary among the specialists.

MISCELLANEOUS ITEMS
Electronic Medical Records (Paperless)

The practice intends in the very near future (when the software is sophisticated enough) to convert to electronic medical records with medically driven invoicing. Additionally, referral letters will be written through the veterinary communication software to allow convenient access to all needing convenient access to the information.

PHARMACY DISPENSING MACHINES

Lloyd S. Meisels, DVM, Hospital Director
Coral Springs Animal Hospital
Coral Springs, FL

Pharmacy dispensing machines or cabinets are the equivalent of having a "24-hour pharmacist" on the premises. The software associated with these units can be two-way interfaced with veterinary software systems to provide the hospital with a secure cost-effective way of controlling and dispensing inventory and capturing fees for dispensed inventory. Over time these machines, whether leased or purchased, are less expensive than staffing a pharmacy and having to pay staff's salaries, sick time, health insurance, workman's compensation, vacation, etc.

The cabinets (hardware) are custom designed by the company according to the type of inventory stored. There are modules ranging from small compartments for eye ointments up to larger compartments for fluids, catheters, and other bulky items. Most companies have technology that connects to an ordinary refrigerator, and some have remote technology that would help inventory items such as prescription diets that would not fit into the cabinet.

Each person taking an item from the machine must log in using password or thumbprint (preferred) technology. The software allows for certain classes of staff members, ie, doctors to have total access to the unit, whereas an assistant might only be able to open, for example, the shampoo compartment. When the item(s) are removed from the cabinet they are added to the client's invoice immediately and the veterinary software inventory quantity on hand is adjusted at the same time.

MODULARITY FOR VARYING SIZES

The Omnicell Drawer Module (Figure 1) is custom-configurable. The width of each bin can be adjusted to accommodate varying product lengths and the height of bin dividers can be customized for larger and smaller items.

MORE STORAGE IN LESS SPACE

The drawer module increases shelf storage capacity from eight to as many as 24 small items. Multiple drawer modules can be integrated into cabinets for tracking and managing items in space-constrained areas such as the OR, emergency department, and ICU.

We use our system to store important keys that need to be available 24/7 so we know who last used a key to enter an area of the hospital.

Using a system such as this will virtually eliminate the common problem of products that go out without invoicing to a client. It will account from in-hospital inventory transfers from pharmacy to the treatment room, surgery, or intensive care areas. It will eliminate the possibility of drug theft from the machine because every transaction is monitored. If a drawer is left open the user can define "lockdown" time so no one can come behind and extract an item under another user's log-in.

IMPORTANT FEATURES TO CONSIDER

The system needs to provide a field for the patient's name. Many human systems do not have this feature and it is essential for veterinary use. Some may have an alternate ID field that can be utilized for this purpose. The system should provide daily reports including discrepancy reports ideally by blindly (rather than telling the user how many should be there) asking how many items are left in the drawer. There should be at least four levels of security and six is ideal. The company should provide 24/7 support, much of which can be done remotely, but it is important to know how far away a technician is located. This may be problematic away from some urban areas. Consider adequate training of staff by the company and ease of use when buying. Two-way interface is a tremendous advantage over systems that do not interface.

REFERENCES
1. Omnicell, Inc. http://www.omnicell.com/

Figure 1. Examples of commonly used cabinetry.

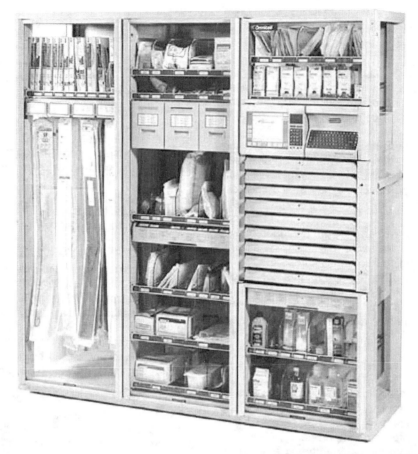

Omnicell ® Three Cell Cabinet

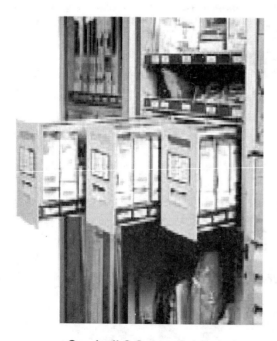

Omnicell ® Suture Cabinet

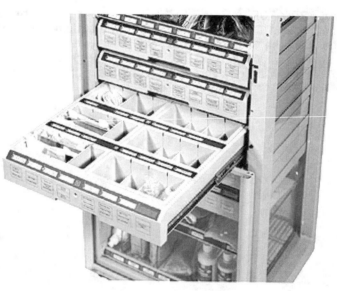

Omnicell ® Drawer Module

USING YOUR COMPUTER TO MAINTAIN MEDICAL RECORDS AND CAPTURE FEES

Lloyd S. Meisels, DVM, Hospital Director
Hospital Director, Coral Springs Animal Hospital
Coral Springs, FL

It is critically important to use the hospital's computer software to its maximum capability in order to conveniently charge fees for all services rendered and products sold. Additionally, the computer can, as described below, save the clinician valuable time in accurate record writing, thereby allowing the doctor to potentially see more patients while creating legible and accurate medical records.

One of the simplest ways to use the computer is to generate estimates, which are better termed treatment and diagnostic plans with a price attached to each line item. For example, if a trauma case comes in to the hospital a user-defined "bundled trauma service group" can be printed in a matter of seconds for the doctor to review with the client. In addition, some veterinary software vendors have "pick lists" which enable the practice to have a subgroup within the estimate from which to pick from. For example, a pick list pop-up group can contain several choices of pain management drugs you might use in a particular trauma case. These treatment/diagnostic plan estimates greatly facilitate remembering everything you normally do in a particular type of medical case. You can easily add and delete items as needed. The estimate should be readily convertible into the final invoice eliminating the need to reenter all the line items a second time.

Medical record writing can be time-consuming, and with many procedures, repetitious. As our society becomes more litigious and veterinarians become more of a target, the medical record as a legal defense can be your best friend or your worst enemy. Veterinarians should write up each record as though a lawyer will be reading them, because one day odds are they will. For outpatient appointments wireless tablets work very well for data entry. They are the approximate size of a clipboard and are much more professional in appearance than having a traditional computer workstation. Some allow you to type, write, or speak into them as a method of data entry.

Templates should be developed for common outpatient and inpatient procedures to minimize the need for writing. Automatically attached to those procedures should be another template of the associated discharge summary and any pertinent client education. Computerized medical records (CMR) have the added advantages of legibility. Accessibility is available from multiple stations on-site and even off-site if desired. This idea has the potential of forever eliminating the frustration and embarrassment connected to the misfiled or lost medical record. Of course, CMRs can be printed out and placed in the medical folder.

A better option is to have electronic medical records (EMRs) to eliminate the medical folder entirely. The EMR is the current and future preferred method of medical record storage. One can access the printed record, all laboratory data, radiographs and ultrasound all at one location. Several national veterinary laboratories already are able to download lab data directly into your patient's records. This procedure minimizes if not eliminates the problem of jammed fax machines, lost printed reports, and errors in written transcription.

Accounting software linked to the veterinary software allows management to "keep score" of what goes on day to day in the practice. One can easily track and assess whether a doctor is seeing more clients then they did in a comparable period previously. The data reveals how much they produce and what their "per client average" is. To further analyze such data, the production report can be user defined by department, ie, surgery, lab, radiology, outpatient, and so on to see what the doctor's strengths and weaknesses are compared with other doctors in the practice.

No piece of equipment in veterinary medicine has more potential to be used in virtually every aspect of practice than the computer. Used properly, a computer can minimize lost income and wasted time by enhancing communications and knowledge between staff members and clientele.

A IS FOR ACUTE, B IS FOR BORDETELLA— RECEPTIONIST MEDICAL TERMINOLOGY TRAINING: PART 1

Christine Merle, DVM, MBA, CVPM
Brakke Veterinary Practice Management Group
Zionsville, IN

WHY LEARN MEDICAL TERMINOLOGY?

Many new employees join a veterinary practice in the position of receptionist/client service. For some, working in a veterinary practice brings many challenges whether it be answering phones, assisting clients, or learning a new software system. On top of all this they must also learn about your practice and the medicine and services that you offer. All of this must occur in a short time period because in many cases they must be an able contributing employee in a very short time. We hope to shorten this time span by hiring "experienced" veterinary employees whether they are pet owners themselves or have experience at another veterinary practice—we assume that their knowledge is exactly what we need. But this is where we make the mistake. CONSISTENCY is one of the most important services that you can offer to your clients—the answer they receive to their pet question should be consistent from one individual to the next whether it is a receptionist, a technician or a doctor. This requires a conscious effort to TRAIN new employees in not only their job duties but more importantly in the terminology of veterinary medicine.

SPELLING

To some spelling comes naturally, to others... well. As part of a pre-interview you may want to have all applicants take a quick spelling test. A sample test is below—be sure that the words you choose to pre-test include common English words, not just veterinary terminology. Word processing programs have become very helpful in regards to spelling and many now recognize common medical terminology as well. Encourage your staff to use the spell check feature when ever possible.

Sample Pre-interview Spelling Test
Circle the correctly spelled word in each group:

1. Veterenarian/ Veterinarian/ Vetarinerian/ Vetarinarian
2. Allargy/ Allergy/ Allergie/ Alergy
3. Suturr/ Sutture/ Suture
4. Diarrea/ Diarrhea/ Diarrhia/ Diarhea
5. Examinasion/ Examenation/ Examination/ Examinnation
6. Vomiting/ Vommitting/ Vomitting/ Vommiting
7. Flem/ Phlegm/ Phlym/ Flim

ACRONYMS

Every profession has their acronyms but I truly believe that veterinary medicine holds the crown for the most. To make it even more confusing, each doctor frequently has their favorites. Acronyms are frequently used in medical records, prescriptions and in patient/client information. Make sure that you have a list of commonly used acronyms and their meanings as part of your training package. Below are just a few to consider for your list.

1. SID – Once daily
2. BID – Twice daily (every 12 hours)
3. TID – Three times daily (every 8 hours)
4. QID – Four times daily (every 6 hours)
5. EOD – Every other day
6. AAHA – American Animal Hospital Association
7. WNL – Within normal limits
8. LGFG – Looks good, feels good
9. BAR – Bright Alert Responsive
10. AVMA – American Veterinary Medical Association
11. PD – Polydipsia (drinking excessively)
12. PU – Polyuria (Urinating excessively)
13. NAVC – North American Veterinary Conference
14. DX – Diagnosis
15. TX –Treatment
16. FX – Fracture
17. RX – Prescription
18. SX – Surgery
19. NPO – Nothing per os, by mouth,
20. HBC – Hit by car
21. V & D – Vomiting & diarrhea
22. E & D – Eating & drinking
23. GI – Gastrointestinal
24. IV – Intravenous
25. IM – Intramuscular
26. SQ – Subcutaneous
27. UA – Urinalysis
28. DOB – Date of birth
29. DVM – Doctor of Veterinary Medicine
30. VMD – Dyslexic DVM (joking ☺) Veterinary Medical Doctor

MEDICAL TERMS TO LAYMEN'S TERMS

Client education is an important part of everyone's role at your practice. Being able to effectively translate medical terms into laymen's terms is essential. For staff, this can sometimes be made easier by teaching them a few commonly used prefixes or suffixes. This encourages them to break down the medical terms. Some commonly used prefixes and suffixes and their meanings are below:

1. Hyper – above
2. Hypo – below
3. Cysto – bladder
4. Hepat – liver
5. Cardio – heart
6. Nephro – kidneys
7. Gastro – stomach
8. Entero – intestinal
9. Hemo – blood
10. Endo – inside
11. Ecto –outside
12. Naso – nose
13. Osteo – bone
14. –itis – inflammation
15. –uria – urine
16. –ectomy – removal
17. –otomy – opening

A IS FOR ACUTE, B IS FOR BORDETELLA—RECEPTIONIST MEDICAL TERMINOLOGY TRAINING: PART 2

Christine Merle, DVM, MBA, CVPM
Brakke Veterinary Practice Management Group
Zionsville, IN

COMMON BREEDS

With many designer dogs becoming the "purebred" breed of the month, it may be difficult for your front staff to identify them. Using the American Kennel Club or the International Kennel Club as your resource, taking the time to teach staff the breed standards of common pets that they see is educational and gives them more confidence in helping determine the designer genes that the new puppy is from. Color patterns are also very helpful for staff to be trained on so that they can tell the difference between a calico and a tabby, too. One more thing about the "designer" dogs—make sure that you are aware of some of these new "breeds"—research some of them online and what ever you do, DON'T call them just a mixed breed or a mutt unless the client calls them that first. Some designer breeds:

1. Labradoodle - Labrador and Poodle
2. Goldendoodle - Golden Retriever and Poodle
3. Puggle - Pug and Beagle
4. Cock-a-poo - Cocker Spaniel and Poodle
5. Schnoodle - Schnauzer and Poodle
6. CoJack - Corgi and Jack Russell Terrier

COMMON PROCEDURES

With the recent changes in vaccination guidelines, it is imperative that time be spent talking to your entire staff regarding the vaccines that you use, the frequency that you recommend and most importantly the "whys" behind that so they can effectively answer clients questions. Regarding vaccinations, recommended vaccine protocols for both puppies and kittens based on age should be discussed. The following is a list of items that should be discussed with any new staff member but especially receptionists/client service specialists.

1. Age when vaccines begin in a puppy and kitten?
2. Frequency of vaccinations in a puppy and kitten?
3. Core vs. non-core vaccines in your practice for both canine and feline:
   a. Distemper
   b. Adenovirus
   c. Parvovirus
   d. Parainfluenza
   e. Leptospirosis
   f. Coronavirus
   g. Lyme
   h. Rabies
   i. Bordetella
   j. Panleukopenia
   k. Viral Rhinotracheitis
   l. Calicivirus
   m. Feline leukemia
   n. FIP
   o. FIV
   p. Other vaccines
4. Brand that you use and why?
5. How it is administered?
6. How often administration is recommended and why?

Surgery is another major area for medical training and discussion. Although spays and neuters are considered routine, it is important for staff be able to communicate the complexity of the procedures that are being performed. Having staff observe a procedure (even through a glass window) will allow them to better understand exactly what is occurring and how the animal is cared for through out the procedure.

Castration: Spay or neuter, recommended age to perform, actual procedure (medical terminology that is translated into laymen's terms), presurgical considerations, postsurgical considerations and why.

Declaw. If performed; recommended age to perform; actual procedure (medical terminology that is translated into laymen's terms), pre- and postsurgical considerations and why.

For practices that may perform other surgeries on a referral basis, receptionists should be educated on those procedures as well.

BASIC ANIMAL FACTS

Despite the internet, not a day probably goes by when a non-client may call with a basic animal question whether it is a pet of theirs or the cute bunny rabbit outside. Being able to answer some common questions regarding animals is helpful to potential clients but also will give your staff some basic husbandry skills that are "assumed" to come with their position.

Here are some basic facts about common animals:

- **Dog**
  - Heart rate: 100–130 beats per minute (110)
  - Temperature: 102°F/38.9°C
  - Gestation Period: 58–70 days (63)
- **Cat**
  - Heart Rate: 110–140 beats per minute (120)
  - Temperature: 101.5°F/38.6°C
  - Gestation Period: 58–65 days (60)
- **Horse**
  - Heart Rate: 23–70 beats per minute (40)
  - Temperature: 100°F/37.8°C
  - Gestation Period: 330–342 (336)
- **Rabbit**
  - Heart Rate: 123–304 beats per minute (205)
  - Temperature: 103.1°F/39.5°C
  - Gestation Period: 30–35 Days

EXTREME CLIENT SERVICE— WAYS THAT YOU CAN MAKE YOUR PRACTICE STAND OUT: PART 1

Christine Merle, DVM, MBA, CVPM
Brakke Veterinary Practice Management Group
Zionsville, IN

Client/Customer Service… you know when it's there and when it's not… well, you just hope that you can go elsewhere next time. Client service is more then just being nice; it requires setting expectations, teaching individuals how to EXCEED those expectations, and holding individuals accountable. Many veterinary practices today do a good job with client service… after all many of us like pets and that is what we see coming through the door everyday. BUT, how do you have your practice take the next step.

To me there are three levels of client service that can be best illustrated through an example: a client picking up a bag of dog food (any size):

- **Level One** – Food is placed next to the client and client is expected to carry it out.
- **Level Two** – Food is placed next to the client and client is asked, "Do you want some help with that?"
- **Level Three** – Food is carried to client's car, no questions asked. You may make a statement such as "Martha will bring that out to your car."

Extreme client service is that Level 3 example—it is just done that way!

SETTING EXPECTATIONS

Think of your reputation. Why do clients choose you? Better yet, find out more about your clients by breaking them down into segments, preferably based on lifestyle demographics. For example, does your practice predominate with "double income–no kids" or suburbanites with young children? What about empty nesters? Are you and your staff of the lifestyle demographic that you serve or is there a big difference between the two? What is your practice's history and culture? What do you want it to be? For example, some practices I walk into give the air of family, others modern, others professional, and still others a bit of country. If I walked into a hospital with marble floors, I wouldn't expect complimentary water to be served from a Dixie Cup. As a staff activity, take the time to discuss what our clients' expectations may be. Review customer surveys from our practice. What are the areas of strengths? What can we do to make them even greater? What are our areas of weakness? What can we do to make them a strength?

TEACHING HOW TO EXCEED

Extreme client service is a direct result of exceeding the expectations that you set. Extreme client service is going beyond what you say you will do OR what you have done in the past. Remember, customers determine satisfaction based on two major factors:

1. Did they find value in the experience based on cost (monetary and non) and
2. Were expectations met?

Consistently exceeding a client's expectations causes you to have to move the bar slightly higher. So teaching your staff to EXCEED is required from the start. Give them concrete examples of how to do this. Some common examples:

- If all pets are scheduled to go home by 5:00 PM, have all of them ready to go by 4:30 PM
- If a test result occasionally is done in 2 days tell the client that they will know in 3 days so that you can exceed their expectation
- Offer to call a client back in 10 minutes rather than putting them on hold— and then call them back in 5 minutes

Key to exceeding especially when time is part of the issue is knowing the average length of time and then adding a buffer to it so that you KNOW that you will always meet the time but hopefully you can exceed it.

HOLDING INDIVIDUALS ACCOUNTABLE

The final step to ensuring extreme client service is holding individuals accountable for their actions. This is tied very strongly to the culture and history of your practice. Accountability includes everyone from the owner veterinarian to the kennel person. Accountability begins first with each other in the practice. You need to have clear understanding of what our jobs/roles are in the practice and how we work together as a team first. One example may be all exam rooms are restocked nightly by the room nurse. First you need to define what a restocked exam room is so that there is no question of what it should look like. All room nurses should then be trained on this. The most important part is that each room nurse now needs to hold the other room nurses accountable. Another example may be with receptionists. The closing receptionist is responsible for making sure all the files for tomorrow's appointments are set aside AND they also release the other receptionists so, if the files aren't done they have two options—have the other receptionist stay and complete it or complete it themselves. Again all receptionists must hold each other responsible for their role's duties.

STAFF ACTIVITY
Documenting your Practice's History

Knowing the history of a practice and its owner will help staff to understand the culture of the practice and the vision for its future. Take the time to answer these questions in a staff meeting. Provide this information to all new employees.

1. Who founded this practice?
2. Why was the practice started?

3. What kind of challenges did the founder face?
4. Was there a time when it looked like the practice was headed for failure?
5. How was the practice able to overcome adversity and survive?
6. How has the practice changed its business over the years?
7. How has the practice responded to new medical technologies and products?
8. How has the practice responded to pet owner demands?

EXTREME CLIENT SERVICE— WAYS THAT YOU CAN MAKE YOUR PRACTICE STAND OUT: PART 2

Christine Merle, DVM, MBA, CVPM
Brakke Veterinary Practice Management Group
Zionsville, IN

MANAGEMENT'S ROLE IN CREATING THE EXTREME CLIENT SERVICE CULTURE

1. **Be an Example.** This is first for a reason— because the first individuals that need to receive extreme client service are the members of your staff! That means that you need to also exceed their expectations of you as an employer... so if you tell them that they will get reviewed annually you should aim to do it biannually. If you expect them to be on time then you should always be 5 minutes early. Management needs to be responsive to staff needs in the same way that you expect them to be responsive to the client needs.
2. **Be Your Own Customer.** When was the last time that you took your pet to a veterinarian? When was the last time you visited your website or walked in your front door? Take the time to be your own customer and truly experience a visit to your practice.
3. **Hire Right.** You've heard it all before, "Hire the 10 and not two 5's." "Don't just hire a warm body." "Hire for attitude." Practices that believe in extreme client service have potential employee's resumes' on hand and are always interviewing and on the look out for good employees. They hire before they are desperate and are willing to grow the practice into another position rather then loose a star.
4. **Develop Your Staff.** Providing a living wage, job security, and advancement is key to allowing individuals to succeed in an extreme client service practice. Develop career paths and incorporate training and development into your practice culture.
5. **Reward the Right Stuff.** Consider offering skill-based pay along with bonuses based on client service. Raises should be based on concrete, achievable, and measurable items. Longevity can be rewarded but only if it is accompanied with strong skills and demonstrable client service examples.

PROVIDING EXTREME CLIENT SERVICE TO CUSTOMERS

1. **Build a Relationship with Owner and Pet.** This is a people business as well as a pet business; being able to relate with owners and their pets is necessary. Spend time working on your interpersonal communication skills especially listening and building rapport. Take time to get to know the clients—don't hesitate in taking notes about the people you see and the pets that they have. Share those notes in the client records so that others can make it a personal touch. Engage and interact with the pet—acknowledge them by name and make sure you use the proper feminine or masculine pronouns. Even in large practices creating a personalized relationship is key to extreme client service. An example for you to consider: If a client mentions that they were taking a vacation to Africa and their pet would be staying with a boarding facility that you recommended, make a note of this in the patient record so that they can be asked about the both the vacation and the pet's boarding experience.
2. **Get Feedback from Customers.** Never hesitate to ask clients for feedback. Even a simple question such as "Did everything go ok with your visit today?" can be asked at the time of checkout or you can let clients know that they will be called within 24 to 48 hours regarding the visit and their feedback would be appreciated. Consider a client comment box or if you have internet savvy clients, consider electronic surveys or feedback forms on your site. Always thank the client for their feedback and if follow up on an issue is required, take personal responsibility and accountability to address the issue.
3. **Be Creative and Share What Works.** An extreme client service culture always is pushing the leading edge and is never content with good enough. Efficiency and creativity should be encouraged. Let's take engaging a client whose pet isn't "happy" to be there. How do you build rapport when the "patient" so obviously doesn't want to be there? What can you do to make both the client and the pet more comfortable? How can you assure the client that the pet will not become any more traumatized?
4. **Be a Positive Team Member.** Being a member of a team requires certain skills. These include 1) taking personal responsibility, 2) encouraging partnerships, 3) establishing a purpose, 4) building trust, and 5) collaborating together. Look for a mentor in your practice and be willing to serve as a mentor to another. When you hear negativity don't participate but focus on positives.
5. **Help Others Succeed.** When a client and their pet receive extreme client service not only do they win but so does the entire practice team. Despite being rewarded individually look at how you can help others. For example, if someone is much better at providing puppy housebreaking tips, ask them to speak to the client in addition to what information you can provide them. If someone is struggling to manage their tasks, step in and help with out being asked.
6. **Be an Advocate for the Pet.** We all have heard about the importance of following up with clients but what about taking the time to follow up with them because of a new product that might interest them or simply to find out if the behavior tips that you provided them helped. Engaging with the client is everyone's responsibility. So if you know that Mrs. Wilson's cat really needs that dental that she didn't schedule before she left, don't just leave the cat in reminder heaven. Actively contact the client and talk to them about dentistry and see if you can find out

what their hesitation may stem from. This should be completely natural and of your own initiative. Of course, know your limitations when it comes to medical options and decisions but contacting a client whose pet you KNOW will benefit from a new service or product you offer is offering EXTREME CLIENT SERVICE.

STAFF ACTIVITY
Getting Client Feedback
1. Make a list of choices that you offer clients
2. Create a list of all the questions that you can ask clients in order to better understand their needs

3. Compare and combine lists. Come up with a master list to promote extreme client service.

Being Creative in our Jobs
Individually, what can we do offer Extreme Client Service? Have each member of your staff do the following:
1. List the duties and requirements of your job
2. List the choices that you have that will help you take care of the client
3. List the options that best fit you, your personality, and how you work
4. List the reasons for your options and how they can work for you and the practice

SMILE — YOU ARE THE RECEPTIONIST STAR!

Christine Merle, DVM, MBA, CVPM
Brakke Veterinary Practice Management Group
Zionsville, IN

It is important to remember that communication is ongoing learning process—learning both about ourselves and then others.

First, communication is a people process not just a language process. Every message contains an interaction of three goals: a task goal, an identity goal and a relational goal. Problems arise because individuals may have different goals.

Second, for every interaction there is both verbal and nonverbal communication. There are several forms of nonverbal interaction: Space, Physical Appearance, Facial Expression, Eye Contact, Vocal Quality, Touch and Body Movement and Gestures. Estimates say that anywhere from 70% to 90% of the meaning in a message is conveyed nonverbally. Miscommunication is the result if verbal and nonverbal actions don't match. REMEMBER the old adage that actions speak louder than words.

Third, there are multiple methods to communicate: written, spoken, visual, gestures, etc. What method works best for you may be different then what works best for another.

Fourth, some communication skills are harder to teach then others. Listening is one of the easier skills to improve.

Finally, values, motivations, priorities and risk level are unique to each individual—as such each individual has a choice. Yes, we can try to influence those choices yet, it is still their CHOICE.

Because many of our interactions are with our "teammates," I would like to review a few individual skills that we must focus on in order to make our participation with teams more successful. Remember we have an individual choice in how successful a team can be. The five skills that individuals should improve are 1) take personal responsibility, 2) encourage partnerships, 3) establish a purpose, 4) build trust and 5) collaborate together.

Difficult clients and noncompliant clients are best confronted by understanding communication styles and learning how to "read people." First it is important to understand that people tend to build rapport with people that are like them. This is especially true in terms of sensory perception. Sensory perception is basically "how we take in the world around us."

There are three main sensory perceptions: **Visual** (the majority of people), **Auditory**, and **Kinesthetic** (the minority). Recognizing an individual's sensory perception will allow you to use words and actions that mimic their preferred sensory which will aid you in building rapport with an individual.

Visual individuals are motivated by what they see. Visuals tend to talk fast and think in pictures. These individuals are concerned with appearances and seem to want control. They will tend to draw a picture for people when they are talking.

In contrast, auditory individuals are motivated by what they hear. These individuals love conversation and use words to express themselves. They will tend to describe what they hear.

Kinesthetic individuals are motivated by what they feel (tactile). They are probably the most likely to be misunderstood as they tend to talk slowly and will think things through before they speak. They are very hands-on individuals.

ADDITIONAL COMMUNICATION TIPS THAT CAN HELP YOU

General Points about People

- We can only remember a few things at a time
- Repetition helps (but... repeat differently)
- We don't want to feel or look stupid
- We sometimes may not know the right questions to ask
- We like to hear positive things, too

Perfecting Communication

- Your attitude sets the tone
- Use positive, open, non-verbal signals
- Ask open questions (when appropriate) and actively listen
- Use visuals and written word to reinforce main points
- Summarize at the end of conversation
- Try to end on a positive note
- Observe the response that you get and make sure it is the one you wanted

Let's practice! Here are some situations:

1. Mrs. B, an existing client, calls in to make an appointment for her new kitten she found at the park in her neighborhood. She wants to know how much it is going to cost. What do you tell her?
2. Mr. R brings his cat Regal in to the practice to be spayed and declawed. You give him the permission form. What do you say next?
3. Mrs. W brings in her dog Doodles to be boarded. She is concerned that Doodles won't be happy there. What do you do next?
4. Mr. M and Patches come in for an annual visit. Patches is now 9 years old. What types of questions might you ask Mr. M?
5. Ms. S wants to bring in her new 8-week-old puppy Toby for its first visit. She wants to know what all Toby needs. What do you say next?
6. Mrs. D calls in the schedule an appointment to get a rabies shot for her dog Butch. What do you do next?
7. Ms. Barker calls to schedule a dental for her senior cat Mystery. What question might you ask her? What information might you want to review in her patient record?
8. Ms. T comes into the practice to pick up some flea medication for her dog Scruffy. What questions do

you ask? What information might you want to review in her patient record?

9. Mrs. R calls regarding a recent article she read regarding the Pet Food Recall; she is concerned that her cat may have eaten one of the recalled foods but she doesn't have a recall list. What do you do next? Where do you look for possible answers to her question?

10. Family F is arriving at the clinic today to euthanize their 23-year-old cat, Sammy. What do you do when you see the family enter the door?

INNOVATIVE HEALTH BENEFIT STRATEGIES FOR VETERINARY PRACTICES

James T. O'Connor, Partner
Egan, Amato & O'Connor
Employee Benefits Consultants
Manasquan, NJ

In this article we will look at innovative ways for small and mid-size employers to control their health benefit costs in both the short and long term. We will look at which approaches are starting to show some promise and which ones still have questions surrounding them. We will also look at what needs to be done over the next one to three years in both the health insurance industry and legislative arena to have a meaningful impact on this dilemma.

Specific areas we will look at will include:

- Latest trends in consumer-driven healthcare plans
- Plan design strategies to reduce costs
- Creating a healthier workforce to reduce costs
- Helping employees become better healthcare consumers
- What should we be asking our legislators to do to help reduce healthcare costs?

As you know by now, President Bush signed the Medicare Prescription and Modernization Act into law on December 8, 2003. With this new law came the introduction of Health Savings Accounts (HSA). The thought behind HSAs is to have employees and their family members become "better healthcare consumers by having them be more involved financially in the purchase of healthcare services." Stated another way, let's move away from the world of copays and modest out of pocket exposure and put in place high deductible plans with a "side account" that employees (and their employer) can put money into. The argument goes that by having to pay now for a substantial portion of the medical bill instead of just a copay the member will be more thoughtful/frugal about what is spent. They will avoid frivolous visits to the doctor, "shop around" for better pricing (Lasix, for example), and over time build up substantial balances in their HSAs such as they do now in their 401(k) plans.

So, is this working? Generally speaking, not yet. Some great strides have been made recently to make these plans more user-friendly, but we have a long way to go. Up until now too much of the discussion has been on the plan design/financial side of the equation – move away from copays and to high deductibles. Simple, right? WRONG. Purchasing healthcare services is a complex equation. Most people do not know what questions to ask or how to assess the answers if the questions are asked.

So is Consumer Driven Healthcare simply a high deductible plan with an HSA? Not exactly!

Let's change the language a bit and call it "Consumer Engagement Healthcare." Philosophically this is a fundamental shift in how health benefits are provided by incorporating:

- Information
- Advocacy
- Ownership

I mentioned earlier that these new plans are not "there yet" in terms of solving the health benefit cost problem but some are making great strides. We, as the buyers of health benefit plans, need to be demanding these types of tools and services from the health insurance carriers who want our business. For those of us who remember the market transition from old-fashioned indemnity plans to managed care 20 years ago we remember how the dialogue changed. We went from talking about claim payment turnaround time and payment accuracy to Physician and Hospital Networks, Gatekeepers, and Preventative Care. While these are not going away, in Consumer Engagement Plans we need to be demanding the following from the health carriers:

- "Gaps in Care" analytical tools to be certain they are identifying members who are not receiving proper care (Information)
- Health Advisors to help those at risk or with chronic conditions use their benefits in the most appropriate manner (Advocacy)
- Plans that provide tools that allow members to become engaged in their own health (Information/Ownership)
- Plans that incorporate Quality and Cost Transparency so members gain access to provider quality information and treatment cost (Information/Ownership)
- Plans that incorporate Disease Management programs for the chronic so the "sick don't get screwed" (Advocacy)
- Plans that when structured properly are not simply "cost shifting" to the members (Information/Ownership)
- Plans that may include a High Deductible Plan with a side fund such as an HSA (Information/Ownership)

So, as you can see, it is much more than simply plan design. It is a strategically thought out program that incorporates many components, plan design being just one, that results in a fundamental behavioral change at the member level.

What about this "Behavior Change" idea? In addition to getting members more involved in the "spend side of the equation" what other behavior are we looking to change? Well, we are looking to influence how members approach their own health:

- Smoking
- Diet
- Exercise
- Alcohol consumption

- Stress
- Health plan compliance
- How care is accessed

It is widely held that modifying employee healthcare behavior is the next significant opportunity to reduce health care costs. The great byproduct of this type of undertaking is that employees and their families' benefit with better health the employer benefits with greater productivity, reduced absenteeism, and ultimately lower health benefit costs. While there is a consensus of opinion that healthy initiatives in the workplace are a "win-win" strategy, the execution of that strategy has long been inconsistent.

As you see in the attached "Healthy Initiatives Spectrum" there are varying degrees of activities that can be performed with the goal of creating a healthier employee population. The spectrum moves from "Minimal" (left) to "Advanced" (right) progressing from the more basic and easier strategies to the more developed. The more fully developed a program becomes the greater the impact it will have on employee behavior resulting in more positive results.

On the left side of the spectrum you will find simple activities such as sending out healthy reminders, newsletters, or articles that focus on the more basic health improvement activities. Employee education campaigns aimed at getting employees to get routine physicals and tests recommended by the medical profession that each person should receive and when they should receive them can help change employee behavior in a more positive way.

As we move to the center of the healthy initiatives spectrum, we encounter more moderate activities that will help to identify specific health issues in a population and/or targeting members for certain diseases. Awareness campaigns, overall improvement goals on a company level, and even going so far as to alerting members seen as "at risk" for certain diseases through a disease management program are used in a program of this kind.

The more advanced stages of a healthy initiatives program will bear greater results as the program matures. An example of an advanced tool in a healthy initiative program would be a Health Risk Assessment (HRA), which is used to identify an individual's risk to certain diseases by looking at family history, lifestyle, etc. The HRA can help map out ways to maximize the individual's health given his/her history and to keep him/her informed of what tests are recommended. Attaching financial incentives such as lower benefit plan contribution amounts for those who comply with the program is a newer strategy being adopted more and more in the marketplace.

For participants who have already been diagnosed with diseases such as diabetes, monitors can be set in place to see compliance rates with certain testing (as recommended by the American Diabetes Association). If the member is not receiving the recommended tests, a reminder system can be put into place to alert them of this and get them back on track.

As you can see, healthy initiative programs take time to develop and should not be implemented without significant forethought. With that having been said, it is clear to most benefit professionals today that putting in the effort to lower the risk of the employee population will create savings in the long-term.

So how do we tie all this together?

First, by understanding that we are at the beginning of this new period in health benefits and the programs and services available today will improve and be more effective in years to come. But we need to make this fundamental shift in how we deliver health benefits and place more emphasis on "Consumer Engagement." _And_, we need the insurance carriers to hear us loud and clear that the actual health-related tools and services they provide must be as good as their marketing materials proclaim. _And_, we want the insurance carriers to give us meaningful pricing discounts for embracing this approach as an employer to lowering healthcare costs. _And_, we want our state and federal elected officials to allow, from a regulatory perspective, for plans to reward employers and employees that proactively work to lower their healthcare costs through lifestyle and health decision-making behavior change.

To be clear, this is not about hurting folks that do not get sick. The dialogue must continue to be about compassionate and comprehensive insurance protection for those in need. However, we also need to add to the equation an increasing focus on disease and injury protection, healthy lifestyle choices, and smarter use of the healthcare system.

If all of the parties in this equation, employers, employees, the healthcare community, insurance companies and government can effectively collaborate on creating a healthier covered population while protecting those in need we will finally reign in our runaway healthcare costs. As a small or mid-sized employer the tools and programs are now available in the marketplace to start. And that is where we are in the journey, at the beginning, but it will accelerate quickly.

EMPLOYEE APPRECIATION

Jerome S. Osteryoung, PhD
College of Business
Florida State University, Tallahassee, FL

"Flatter me, and I may not believe you. Criticize me, and I may not like you. Ignore me, and I may not forgive you. Encourage me, and I will not forget you"
—William Arthur Ward

What is the fundamental need of employees? I am going to suggest that it is to feel appreciated! Employees need to feel appreciated for the work they do, sincere this makes them feel whole and worthwhile. Appreciation is the key to keeping your employees working hard and representing your company in a great manner.

My experience has been that many entrepreneurs feel they appreciate their employees very much and convey that appreciation to them; however, most employees just do not feel the same degree of appreciation. Why does this dichotomy exist? I think the answer is that most entrepreneurs are hearing what they are saying, rather than hearing what their employees need.

Now, obviously, you cannot go around all the time continuously saying great things about all of your employees. Rather, try to observe employees who are doing good things and recognize them on the spot for their effort, perseverance or attitude. The Character Council of Florida (850-482-0001) can help you identify 48 great character traits, which you can praise, ie, creativity, resourcefulness, diligence effort, talent, perseverance, etc.

Two great entrepreneurs whom I have observed doing this on a continual basis are Ron Sachs of Ron Sachs Communications and Matt Brown of Premier Bank. Both of these gentlemen go out of their way to tell each employee how much they appreciate the employee. In fact, you can really sense the great morale of each staff member as you are walking around either business.

I think there are three types of appreciation and you really need to recognize each of these. First, is the recognition when a specific task is done in an incredible manner. The second type of appreciation is of the person himself/herself. Sometimes, it is good to walk up to your staff and say, "You know, I am so happy and thrilled that you are part of my team." The third type of appreciation is an appreciation that each employee has a life outside of work. The more you appreciate each staff member's life outside of the work environment, the more they will appreciate you.

The Jim Moran Institute is lucky to have a great program assistant on our team. I tell her we are fortunate to have her. However, work is not her whole life. She has a family and is also involved in our community. I go out of my way to inquire about her life outside the office and congratulate her on the successes of her family members and on her volunteer work. I just appreciate her as a total worthwhile person and I recognize that she really has so many neat dimensions.

Here are some neat things you can do to show that you really appreciate your staff. First, take a staff member who has really has made a neat contribution to lunch and give that employee a chance to really talk to you. I try to take every staff member who directly reports to me to lunch every month to say, without words, that I really appreciate them. Matt Brown tries to take all of his employees to lunch at least once a year to listen to their concerns.

Another thing to do is the common, "Thank you." I cannot overestimate how important this is. Too, too many times I have heard employees say that there boss never even thanked them for going way beyond the call to duty. A "thank you" is just a neat way to say I appreciate you and is so inexpensive.

At staff meetings, tell the staff of the contributions of various staff members. Everyone likes, but, more importantly, needs, to feel appreciated.

About four years ago, Don Pumphrey, Sr., of Don's Tree Service, took his staff on a Caribbean cruise to say how much he really appreciates them. His employees still talk about this experience because Don put his grateful feelings into action to say to his staff, "I really, really appreciate all that you have done to help my company grow and prosper."

I think that every employee is looking for their boss or supervisor to tell them that they appreciate them working in their business. The more you can make each and every employee feel appreciated, the better the business you will have. Now go out and find ways to make this happen. You can do it!!

HAVE THE COURAGE TO ADDRESS PROBLEM EMPLOYEES DIRECTLY

"To change and to change for the better are two different things."
—German proverb

Changing systems to improve productivity is great. However, it could be a big mistake to change a system to attempt to overcome an employee problem.

Recently an entrepreneur who employed a staff member as a part-time 1099 employee in a key position needed to let her go. She was just was not working out. Ignoring whether this key position should really be a part-time 1099 employee, the entrepreneur decided to change the job to a full-time position, knowing the employee did not want to work full time. It seemed like a simple, non-confrontational way to replace the employee. While there may be many good reasons for switching the job to a full-time position, his primary reason was that the employee was not working out. "So," he thought, "let's just change the system."

Another example of changing systems to overcome an employee problem is the entrepreneur who changed his whole production line just to work around a problem employee. In order to separate quarreling employees, the entrepreneur changed the order of his production line. This change cost the entrepreneur a significant amount simply because he did not have the courage to deal with the employee directly.

While systems or processes need to be modified over time, they should not be changed in order to avoid dealing directly with an employee whose behavior or performance needs to be corrected. Often, an entrepreneur's reaction to a problem employee is to change the system to try to manipulate the employee's behavior instead of going through the discomfort of confronting the employee directly.

Before you consider changing a system or process because of an employee problem, ask yourself these questions:

1. Am I uncomfortable in dealing with this employee directly?
2. Is the system working with for everyone else?
3. Have I sufficiently considered the ramification of the changes I'm considering?

If you have difficulty answering these questions, then spend more time analyzing the situation. However, if the answers to questions 1 and 2 are "Yes," then keep the system and deal with the employee, assuming that the answer to question 3 is also "Yes."

The answer to employee problems is not always a change in systems. It is important to know when you need to deal with a problem employee directly and when you need to make a change in a system or process.

PRESENTEEISM

Employers worry a lot about absenteeism, but new research suggests a bigger threat to productivity is "presenteeism": sick workers who show up at work but are not fully functioning. US companies may lose $150 billion (yes, that's billion) annually because of presenteeism, according to some estimates (Harvard Business Review).

Presenteeism is a newly coined word for the lost of productivity of a worker showing up to work and not fully engaged. This lack of engagement could come from illness or other distractions. Sometimes presenteeism is a function of employees who are burnt out or depressed. I like to say this condition as having a worker physically at work but mentally someplace else.

A study by one firm found that the loss in productivity from workers who come to work ill is significantly higher than a worker who is absent from work. It has been estimated that the cost of a worker showing up for work ill is three times higher than a worker staying home ill.

International Truck tackled this problem head on with a pilot study of employees who had allergy problems. They instituted a study of their employees and found out that 20% to 25% of their staff suffered from allergy and this had a significant impact on each worker's performance. International Truck was able to help these workers get the help they needed and they were grateful for the company's help as they felt so much better and were much more productive.

One common problem that keeps on cropping up in the work place is workers who come in as they do not either want to let their team off or they are worried about losing their PTO (Paid Time Off).

I used to be in favor of PTO, which is a concept that lumps both sick leave and vacation into one pot with a number of days. If an employee does not use any days of sick leave than they can take a very long vacation. With this approach employers never had to make decisions whether an employee had a legitimate illness and PTO seemed a neat concept. However, like many neat concepts the unintended consequences are quite high. That is PTO encourages workers to go to work sick to preserve their PTO time, which just is not good.

Workers who go to work ill tend to affect the entire workforce. I have seen one employee get ill and infect an entire company's work force. If this employee would have stayed home, then almost $100,000 in labor costs would have been saved.

Some of the common ways to address presenteeism are with a corporate wellness program that is designed to help employees stay healthy with both treatment and education. In Leon County, there is a program called, "Working Well Leon County" that is aimed at improving the health of workers in the work force for the entire county.

Some of the other things that you could do to help reduce the amount of presenteeism is to allow a carryover of sick leave from one year to the next. Helping the employee pay for their co-payments to seeing doctors just to encourage them to go when they are not feeling well. Helping them as well with some of their prescription costs including flu shots. Flu shots ought to be one of those things that are provided free as not having this shot can have such a major impact.

Another thing that impacts on presenteeism is just plain boredom on the job. Cross training and periodically changing job assignments really helps here. Keeping the workplace fun and dynamic really do matter in both increasing productivity but avoiding presenteeism.

Now go out and make sure that you have a plan to help presenteeism. Not only is this good for all employees but it just plain good business.

GENERATION Y MANAGING

"Marketers know them and love them as Generation Y or the Echo Boom, a cohort that is more than 50 percent larger than the 45 million strong Generation X."
—Julie Connelly

Eventually, you will have to manage Generation Y staff. These are people who were born after 1978, who will in time become the backbone of our labor force. It will require a real understanding on your part of what causes their behavior and what they want to get out of the work place. Generation Y's behavior and motivation are much different than Generation X and Baby Boomers.

In order to understand Gen Y, you must realize that they are the children of the Baby Boomers, who really value education, so Gen Yers clearly understand the importance of advanced learning. They will want jobs that allow them to grow educationally.

Obviously, this group is way more than tech savvy as they grew up with the continual rapid growth in technology. Just look at how many of these folks get their news off of the web rather than in the print media. In many ways, these employees and future employees consider technology as their birthright: Look at how quickly they jumped on iPods, TiVo, and instant messaging.

They strive for much flexibility, which they just did not have growing up; as their parents (I am so guilty of this) wanted them to be involved in so many different activities. I can remember when our children were going to dance classes, music classes, involved in sports and then having to do homework at night. This type of behavior has made Gen Yers really strive for freedom from fixed constraints. The work environment must change in so many ways to accommodate these types of flexibility demands, by offering things like telecommuting and very flexible working hours.

I think one thing that really does make managing Gen Yers unique is that they want to do work that is meaningful. They do not just want a job so much as they want to work for a company that is going to provide both financial gain and opportunities to ensure that their community is also better off. They are really looking for purpose in their work experience that is significant, but much more than monetarily.

By far, one of the most important things to remember in dealing with Gen Yers is that they are not loyal at all to the company they work for. They are aggressive in their financial and company goals. My son, who has an MBA, moved to Atlanta a year ago with his new bride, and they both worked for same company. Within six months, my son had left this company and moved on to a larger one in a much higher position, and within one year, my daughter-in-law had left the company as well for another improved position. Clearly, many employers are not looking negatively at rapid job movement as they know this is just part of Generation Y.

With the demand for workers increasing over the next 10 years, you really are going to have to understand what motivates Gen Yers and how you are going to take steps necessary to both recruit and retain them. This is a new generation with new goals and aspirations, and we, as much as possible, must change to accommodate them.

EMPLOYEE SUGGESTIONS

"The best way to have a good idea is to have lots of ideas."

—Linus Pauling

It seems like employee suggestion boxes have been around forever. However, there is always a strong need to encourage employees and all related parties to act as consultants and offer improvement ideas. Taking employee improvement ideas seriously is very important. If employees believe there are problems, then there are problems. Perception is reality!

So many neat ideas come from employees. If you stop these employee improvement ideas or problems from flowing up to you, you will stem the tide of some very valuable information.

What seems to turn employees off to submitting ideas is lack of acknowledgment and lack of reward incentives. If an employee submits an improvement idea, they must receive an acknowledgment of their contribution. This is a pretty simple process. An employee who does not get even an acknowledgment is just not going to contribute any more. After all, the role of an employee improvement program is to nurture ideas that will be beneficial to the company. If employees don't receive positive feedback, they will cease their communication of ideas with you.

You probably guessed it. The purpose of this article is to encourage you to establish an employee improvement ideas program. Reward employees for great ideas with a financial reward as well as with a public acknowledgement. The more you reward employees, the more they will contribute. One company gives a cash award to the employee suggestion that is practical, even though bottom of the barrel (just to encourage all improvement ideas).

Employee improvement ideas really do enhance the bottom line. Here are some neat examples.

1. A company received an employee improvement idea involving repairing a leak in a cooling system. The system had leaked for years without anyone thinking much about it. One day an employee submitted a repair proposal that resulted in an annual cost savings of $200,000.
2. Miller Furniture has benefited from employee improvement ideas since the beginning of the early 20th century. It was an employee suggestion that led to the creation of the first cubicle office furniture unit, now one of their best selling products.
3. At Intel, an employee suggestion is responsible for the invention of the first microprocessor, the Intel 4004.
4. A bank in Maryland instituted a program designed to motivate employees to seek out ways to increase revenue or reduce expenses. The program generated $8 million in savings the first year -- an incredible savings for the bank

You can really make a large difference in the morale of your work force and your bottom line by invoking an employee suggestion program.

EMPLOYEE CONFLICT

"No doubt there are other important things in life besides conflict, but there are not many other things so inevitably interesting. The very saints interest us most when we think of them as engaged in a conflict with the Devil."

—Robert Lynd, The Blue Lion

Employee conflict is one of those age-old problems that has always been with us and always will be. If you put enough people together, you will always generate employee conflict as it just part of our human condition.

There are really two things that you must keep in mind when dealing with employees who are not getting along. The first point is to be alert so you very early recognize the symptoms of problems very early . Problems just do not suddenly manifest themselves into all out hostility. Rather, it is usually a slow simmer that gradually builds. The second critical element is how to deal with the problem once it is recognized. You must deal with the problem, because unresolved problems will affect the entire workplace. Employee conflicts never get better unattended, only worse.

Recognizing conflict is key, because it is impossible to take action unless you know there is a problem. One warning sign for potential conflict is when it is well known that two employees just do not like one another. When employees are overheard taking sides with various other employees, the probability for conflict is there. A sure sign is when a staff member comes to the manager and asks him or her to solve the problem.

A sudden change in behavior of an employee in the workplace might signal potential conflict. I once had a staff employee who started coming in late to work and he missed work more and more. I had no idea it was a conflict with another employee till I questioned him as to the cause of the problem.

Once a problem is identified, you must take action. The first step should be to address the employees, first individually, to find out the real issues. If the problem is not solved during individual interviews, meet with the employees jointly. You have to be careful not place any blame or take sides, because this will completely destroy your creditability. Also, you really need to address the specifics about the situation, rather than talking in generalities.

When talking individually, you must acknowledge the conflict exists. Words such as, "Sally, I understand that you and Gayle are not getting along," usually brings everything out in the open. Then you must tell them how this conflict is affecting the entire organization, giving specific examples. And finally, you must mention the consequences of failing to resolve the conflict so your employees clearly understand you intend to follow through. If talking to them individually does not solve the problem, the next step is bringing them together for a meeting.

Bringing both parties in for discussion requires careful monitoring on your part, because it could easily get out of hand. Points to get both parties to agree are that (1) they do actually have a conflict, (2) they will not discuss the conflict with others at work, and (3) what behaviors are acceptable in the workplace and what are not (eg, making faces, asking other staff to take sides, or a disrespectful tone of voice). Create an arbitration process (either formal or informal) to implement when these employees have problems. Also, in this meeting you need to clearly convey how you will monitor their behavior to ensure the conflict is resolved.

Many managers are uncomfortable with employee interventions. Managers can be trained to deal with employee conflicts or you can ask your HR person to help with these sessions.

Employee conflict is just one of those things that will happen in every workplace. Knowing how to remedy the problem is the key to being a great manager and leader.

DEALING WITH DIFFICULT EMPLOYEES

"When I help, I am aware of my strengths and other's weaknesses… Fixing is a form of judgment. It implies something is broken and creates distance. We can only serve which we are profoundly connected to!"
—Sam Dailey-Harris

You can have the greatest workforce in the world, but there will always be some people who are just difficult to get motivated. It is not something that you can raise your magic wand to go fix; rather, you have to work at this problem on a continual basis. If you do not work to remedy this problem, it is only going to remain or get even larger.

Given that a lack of motivated workers is just part of the staffing issues we have to deal with, what can you do? These employees are typically the ones that show up exactly at eight and go home not a second past five. In addition, they are the same staff members who always seem to take the maximum amount of sick leave available. Bottom line is that these staff members are just working for a paycheck and nothing else. They really do not have a strong connection with your business and just put in their time, then go home.

As these types of workers do not have much of a connection with your business, this is what you have to change. One great way to do this is talk to them about what their dreams are. If you can relate to them on a regular basis and show that you care for them not just as workers but also as valuable staff members, then frequently you can turn them around by being connected with them. The more you can show that you see them as a whole person rather than just a worker bee, the higher the probability of success with this strategy.

Another thing that could be happening is that these workers just may not feel comfortable enough, or may even lack the confidence, to take the initiative. One thing you can do here is go to the worker and ask for their advice on pending decisions. The more input you get from them, the more they will be able to reach out further. Additionally, going out of your way to praise these workers will really help them to come out of their protective shells. The whole approach here is to recognize that a nonmotivated employee may just be one that has never been rewarded for this type of motivated behavior.

One additional item you might want to consider, which has worked for me, is to give these unmotivated workers more direction on their work in a positive fashion. Sometimes we just do not expect enough out of these workers, so by giving them very positive instructions, they know exactly what you are expecting, and you can then turn these workers around. Again, it just boils down to ways to improve their confidence in the workplace.

If you have given these things a fair chance and you do not see a real change in behavior, then it is time to evaluate these workers and see if you really want them on your team. Unmotivated workers can destroy the morale in the work place, and this behavior tends to be contagious.

Now go out and make certain that you are doing everything you can to ensure that each of your staff members is a motivated and contributing member of your team.

EXIT INTERVIEWS

"The successful person makes a habit of doing what the failing person doesn't like to do".
—Thomas Edison.

Employee turnover is a business reality and, in many cases, there is very little you can do about it. If an employee finishes college and wants to move on, or has to leave because a spouse takes a job in another part of the country, you're not going change the employee's mind. With an exit interview, however, you can turn the loss into an opportunity.

The exit interview is an information-gathering exercise and should be viewed as a way for the employee to give constructive criticism of your business. You want to find out, first, the real reason the employee is leaving and, second, any ideas he or she might have for improvement of your company.

For example: An employer has a very loyal employee who had been with him for over 20 years. This employee decides to start his own business and go into competition against his old employer. No matter what concessions the employer is willing to make, the employee just wants to go out on his or her own. In this case, a good exit interview would tell the employer what changes might be necessary to improve the business and retain other employees.

Exit interviews are voluntary and you cannot force an employee to participate in one. Nor can you force an exiting employee to fill out a questionnaire about the reasons behind the decision to leave. You should really try to convince each employee to go through these, however, because there is so much information that you will glean.

Ask open-ended questions, such as, "Joe, can you tell me how you reached the decision to leave our company?" Another good question is, "Joe, what have been some of the more frustrating or upsetting events for you during your tenure here?" A great site that has a lot of sample questions for you to ask is at www.businessballs.com/exitinterviews.htm.

After you ask a question, sit back and let the employee talk, and for goodness sake, do not get into an argument, no matter what the employee says. You are after his or her perceptions, not whether those perceptions are wrong or right.

If an employee says that more money is behind the decision to leave, you need to probe this so much deeper. Generally, money is shorthand for something else at a much deeper level that is not right. For most staff, changing jobs is like changing houses, not a pleasant thought (I have lived in the same house for 29 years). Therefore, in the exit interview, you must ask a question such as, "Joe, what are some of the most unpleasant things that you have had to endure around here?" Or, "What changes would we have to make here, to create an environment where you would not even think of leaving?" You can develop a standard set of questions to ask in each exit interview.

Having an exit interview will give you so much more information because your existing staff is just not going to be as frank as departing staff. Now go out and make sure that exit interviews are part of your HR program. You can do this

COMPLACENCY

"To be pleased with one's limits is a wretched state."
—Johann Wolfgang von Goethe

I was talking to an entrepreneur last week and he said that he was so happy as things were going so very well as he wanted all of his employees to continue to work with him. He did not want to do anything that would "rock the boat" for fear that he would not get back to the good feelings he was having now. After I banged on his head for five minutes to wake him up, I started to talk with him how complacency is not a good place to be. Complacency means wanting no change and not willing to risk yourself. Change is the only thing that is constant with business(and life). Not willing to embrace change means you are becoming lethargic and more vulnerable to competition. Additionally, business is risk taking and to become complacent is another way of saying I do not want to risk anything. While this entrepreneur might not of wanted to risk anything, his competitors are lining up ready to take advantage of this complacency.

Sure we like it when our business is running smoothly, but this is not typical and sometimes this is a precursor to not being aware of any underlying problems. Wanting to freeze a business in time is a very dangerous concept. Sure most entrepreneurs want and desire a smooth running business, but this is just not going to happen. You have associates who will be moving on, new products coming on stream and technology changes. All of these changes are normal and part of business. While change is painful, you must embrace change rather than running from it.

I think the real reason for this complacency is fear of change. I know this lady who in my opinion is the bravest lady I know. Why? She faces her fears and then moves through them even though she is scared. I cannot tell you how many times that my fears were so much worse than the actual event (eg, trying to come up with a new idea for this column every week). In the majority of cases that I have seen, most entrepreneurs' fears just do not come about. If they do materialize, however, they are so small compared to what are thoughts were telling us.

Complacency in my opinion is just being not willing to face our fears. However, by facing these fears, we grow, prosper and experience life. President Franklin D. Roosevelt said in his first inaugural address, "We have nothing to fear but fear itself "?

Complacency can be a very harming concept to your business. By facing your internal fears, complacency can never find a home.

COMMUNICATIONS IS EVERYTHING

Communications are what drive every business! Every type of idea, instruction, or interchange is done through communications. By communications, I am talking about either written or oral.

If you think about it, most entrepreneurs and managers spend most of their time communicating to their boss (eg shareholders), customers, and associates. Yet while most of the entrepreneurs time is spent communicating, very little time (if any) is spent on learning how to communicate. For some reason, we all think that we know how to communicate, so that any emphasis on communications is unnecessary. This is just not a valid assumption!

I was invited to attend a staff meeting of a very successful business. Every manager shared honestly how they were doing and everyone was very supportive of everyone else. The owner also shared most of the information from the current financial statement (open book management). The communications were great in this company and you could tell that the associates really liked this process of communications.

Another staff meeting that I attended (folks are just not going to invite me to these meetings anymore) was marked by the entrepreneur talking exclusively about what he wants. There just was no sharing of information. In this meeting, you could tell that the employees just did not feel as involved as the first group I talked about.

So, how do you improve communications in your business? I think there are several things that you need to do. The first is just become aware how you communicate and how you are communicated to. Each person is going to have a unique way of doing this and you need to understand what is going on. I have had one associate who always was incredibly nice and happy when he wanted to request something, but not nearly as nice the other times. For the longest period of time I thought, that when he was happy it was something I did (right!) or something was happening with his home life. Once I was aware of the behavior and what he wanted, it allowed me to use this form of non-verbal communication to understand the behavior.

The Associate Director of JMI (Mrs. Diane Denslow) is very to the point and really does like to waste time with small talk, as she is very busy. I on the other hand, like to have a little bit of an introduction with small talk before we get down to the nitty-gritty. Once we became aware of this (yes, it did take time) we learned to accommodate one another without asking anyone to change. Our communications are much better as we are aware of how to communicate to one another. There is also a series of tests that you and your employees can take to find out the styles of communications that each person prefers.

I once had a secretary that did not like any communication via email. She could never figure out why I would send her an email note, rather than talking

to her as her desk was just outside of my door. It was not till after she had left; that I realized I was just not fully aware of her preferences nor was she willing to accommodate my preferences.

Another thing you need to do is share information. My making yourself vulnerable by this process, it opens the door to great communications. Share the financials; obviously you do not want to show your associates your net profits but show them at least the gross profit. Sometimes associates have the feeling that you are making millions and millions of dollars and this sharing of information really helps in extinguishing all of misinformation which really distorts your associate's perception of you and it, also, builds up trust. Some firms show the limited financials with their managers and then collect this information after the meeting to insure that this information does not get into the wrong hands.

By sharing, this must be two way in that it cannot be just the entrepreneur or manager talking about what they want. Rather this dialog must be two ways. Learning to listen is really a big key in communications. If you are willing to listen (and not just fix the problem) the communications improve so much. Most associates do not want to be judged. If they can come to you or their managers and know they will not be judged, this enables communications to be greatly enhanced.

I frequently have just listened to associates problems and they then comment to me on how great of communicator I am (I just listened).

The final way to increase communications is to clearly share your expectations of where you want to take the company and your expectations about each employee. One entrepreneur we were assisting had a problem employee and was always reprimanding him. However, he never told his employee on how upset he was getting this behavior not was he communicating on how serious of a problem this was. If these expectations were made clear, this little problem would not have become a large problem. By sharing your expectations, you eliminate employees from guessing as to what you want and vastly improve communications.

Communication is the key for a business. By putting emphasis on this process you will improve the bottom line and make your business more fun to work in.

CHECKPOINT CHARLIE

"Nothing in this world can take the place of persistence. Talent will not; nothing is more common than unsuccessful people with talent. Genius will not; unrewarded genius is almost a proverb. Education will not; the world is full of educated derelicts. Persistence and determination alone are omnipotent. The slogan 'press on' has solved and always will solve the problems of the human race."

—Calvin Coolidge

Attention to details is so critical to the success of each and every entrepreneur. Every semester I tell our entrepreneurship students at FSU that the "devil is in the details" and one of the main things an entrepreneur must do is sweat the small stuff. Now, I am not saying that each entrepreneur should be checking on every detail in the business. Rather, an entrepreneur should devise and initiate processes and systems to ensure that responsibility for the details is assigned to a competent and dependable employee(s) and then make sure these systems and processes are monitored.

One neat example of entrepreneurs who really sweat the details is the brotherly team of Grant and Ray Capelouto, owners of Capelouto Termite and Pest Control. They have instituted a Checkpoint Charlie (they actually have a sign at this location) where each of their 38 trucks must stop each day. A supervisor waits at the checkpoint to checkout various details. Some days the inspector might make sure the horns and lights in the trucks work and the next morning make sure the required amount of chemicals is on each truck.

Each truck bay is equipped with a hose and a brush so technicians can wash their trucks each morning. Supervisors check on the appearance of each technician and are vitally concerned with all the details of the business.

Of course, Grant and Ray have managers who oversee the implementation of these policies. What these savvy entrepreneurs have mastered is the execution of systems that make sure each and every detail they consider important is dealt with on a consistent basis.

Systems that guarantee constant attention to details are critical to the success of every entrepreneur. One of the best ways to plan your "micro-awareness system" is to map out the processes that are involved in your business and evaluate what processes are critical to the success of your business and to the betterment of your customers. For example, if restaurant owners want to make sure that the food is delivered in a consistent manner, they first have to figure out each step in the food preparation. They then analyze which steps they should keep, add, or revise to ensure the consistent quality of the food dish. No detail is too small (eg, the amount of seasoning to the size of dish to serve the food on).

Sweating the details is so critical to the success of each and every business. However, even more important is the fact that the Capleloutos understand so well: Attention to detail is not adequate without a monitoring process.

Successful entrepreneurs figure out systems that insure the details of running a business are dealt with and consistently monitored. Now go out and make sure that you are sweating the details!

BE CREATIVE IN MOTIVATING EMPLOYEES
"Our deepest fear is not that we are inadequate- Our deepest fear is that we are powerful beyond measure. It is our light, not our darkness, that most frightens us."
—Nelson Mandela

If there is one common problem all entrepreneurs and managers face, it is motivating employees. Clearly, you want to employee people who are already motivated, but, frequently, that just does not happen.

You must find a way to motivate your employees. This article is about one entrepreneur who faced the challenge of motivating workers in a very creative fashion.

Fred Beshears, owner of Simpson Nurseries in Monticello, along with his management staff have come up with some neat ideas over the years. He invited me to see what he was doing a couple of weeks ago. Simpson Nurseries supplies trees and plants to Home Depot and Lowe's, plus many other retailers throughout the country. Fred has about 150 employees who work outside in the blazing sun in very physical jobs, like loading trucks or repotting plants. The bottom line is that not many of his employees wake up every morning and say, "I really, really want to go work outside today in temperatures of 110 degrees." Therefore, Fred and his two sons, Halsey and Thad, have to really motivate these basic agriculture workers.

Simpson's has come up with the neat concept of "Tree Bucks." Because attendance and punctuality are important to the business, every employee gets $10 worth of Tree Bucks each day they show up for work on time. Additionally, if employees do outstanding work, supervisors can give out additional Tree Bucks as rewards.

Twice a year, the Beshears cook lunch for all their employees. They cook some of the best grilled chicken I have ever tasted (there are perks that come with writing this column). After lunch, employees sit back in their chairs and participate in an auction. Guess what currency they use for the auction! Yep, you guessed it, "Tree Bucks." Fred purchases TV's, barbecue grills, bicycles, goats, Gameboys, and so much more. He even auctions items such as two days off with pay or a three-day vacation trip with pay. Simpson's employees enjoy the bidding and they develop neat strategies to work together to bid higher for the items they really want. Most of the items go for between 300 and 500 Tree Bucks. However, there was a picnic table—complete with tent covering and picnic wear—that sold for $2300 Tree Bucks.

If the employees do not win the bid on items at one auction, they can save their Tree Bucks and bring them back to the next auction in 6 months. As I watched the staff leave the event, I observed that, overall, they seemed to be genuinely pleased.

While Tree Buck auctions may not be for everyone, you can think of some creative way to motivate your staff. You can do this!!

WHAT IS A MANAGER?
"Managing is like holding a dove in your hand. Squeeze too hard and you kill it, not hard enough and it flies away."
—Tommy Lasorda

Every entrepreneur has to manage people. People, as staff, are the lifeblood of every business. The job of every manager must be to look out for each employee. Great managers must understand that they work for their staff and the staff does not work for them. Every employee represents your company to the customer and must be managed so that they present the best image possible.

There are several key elements that characterize great managers. First, managers understand how to communicate effectively. They engage the staff in decisions before they are made so that the staff feels empowered. They listen to the staff because they know the staff has valuable insight into problems. Communication is 70% listening and 30% talking. The more listening you do, the better. It has taken me 35 year of marriage to understand this principle. I really think that you communicate more by being a good listener than by being a good talker.

The second attribute of a great manager is found in how the manager expresses his or her expectations. How can people work for you if you do not lay out your expectations? The more a manger articulates (communication, again) expectations, the better. Spending some time with each employee every month going over expectations is a great process. You must have expectations (goals) and you must communicate these to your staff. However, you must insure that these expectations are met, or "inspect what you expect." Expressing expectations without inspecting is a sure way to lose your credibility.

The last important characteristic of good managers is that they go out of their way to appreciate each and every employee. Thank your employees for the great work they are doing for you. In fact, appreciation is more effective in motivating employees than raises. The after glow of a raise in pay may last a month, but employees carry moments of sincere appreciation with them forever. Fortunately, you can find things employees do well all year long, so your gratitude can be expressed frequently.

The final thing great managers do is that they tell their staff how they are doing. Giving frequent feedback to each member of your staff will insure that they know if they are going on the right path. Too often managers only give feedback when a problem arises rather than recognizing all of the great work each staff member does.

Being a great manager keeps your staff happy, content and stable. Being a great manager by communicating, laying out your expectations, inspecting your expectations, appreciating employees, and giving feedback is a sure way to improve the performance of your business. You can do this!

EMPLOYEE TURNOVER

"The difference between a boss and a leader: a boss says, 'Go!' - a leader says, 'Let's go!'"
—E. M. Kelly, Growing Disciples, 1995

Recently, an entrepreneur whom I am assisting stated that he had 600 W-2's this year and he has a full time staff of less than 50. When I questioned him about this rapid employee turnover, he said it was the nature of the business. At this point I wanted to throttle him by the neck and yell at him, "Employee turnover is bad, bad, bad!" Rather than risk rupturing my vocal cords yelling, I sat down and listened to him talk about this problem. What was most disconcerting about the conversation was that he thought the problem was systemic with today's labor pool and took very little responsibility for this in his own management style.

Most employee turnover is related to poor management practices. Yes, employees are working for wages, but, more importantly, they are working to have their non-financial needs met. It's important to understand that employees are seeking to extract something far more than a paycheck from their work. Most employees need to feel respected, worthwhile and appreciated in their work. Time after time employees leave when they feel underappreciated, sometimes for less money, just to have these more important needs met. The reverse is true as well - when employees are offered a significantly higher salary from another company, they don't leave if they are appreciated at their current workplace.

Most entrepreneurs do not perceive themselves as bad managers. However, a high employee turnover is a telling detail that an entrepreneur may, in fact, be a horrible manager. Asking employees why they are leaving is generally not a good way to tell what the real reason is behind their departure. Instead of evaluating employee satisfaction according to exit interviews, pay attention to the turnover rate. High turnover is the key indicator of employee dissatisfaction. It takes a lot of effort and risk for an employee to change jobs. Resigning is the loudest statement they can make to tell you that your management skills are lacking.

Commit to making every employee feel worthwhile, respected, and revered. You must not be too busy working in your business to recognize the importance of each and every one of your employees. One of the Jim Moran Institute's entrepreneurial clients was also his company's primary salesperson. Because of the huge amount of time he spent selling, he never had enough time to make his fifteen employees really feel needed and, consequently, the company experienced high turnover. Employees can quickly feel less than respected by either abusive bosses or bosses who are just too busy to give the requisite care. One of the things you can do to help is to occasionally, tell employees how much you appreciate them. Even better is to tell your whole company how certain employees have really made a difference. Another thing that really helps is to make sure you go around and ask employees how they are doing. It all just boils down to making each and every employee feel worthwhile.

Employee turnover is a good benchmark to evaluate the effectiveness of your management style. If you are seeing high turnover, your management style may need to be significantly overhauled.

CUSTOMER ABUSE

"Anyone who proposes to do good must not expect people to roll stones out of his way, but must accept his lot calmly if they even roll a few more upon it."
—Albert Schweitzer

Entrepreneurs and their businesses are there to serve clients. Customer service is what allows a business to grow and thrive.

Every business has to survive difficult clients. They are, however, the impossible-to-please or abusive customers who keep entrepreneurs awake at night.

If a customer is using profanity in dealing with any staff member, ask the customer to stop using this language. If it continues, the customer must be asked to leave your premises right then and there. Asking your staff to submit to any abuse for any reason is untenable. No matter how wrongly the customer believes he or she has been mistreated, you just cannot allow any staff member to be abused, period.

If customers yell or using loud voices, they must be told that this behavior is not tolerated for any reason. In this situation, move the customer to a private office if possible. If this does not work, the customer must be asked to leave the premises no matter what his perception of the problem. Customer service is a goal, but protecting your staff from abuse is a higher goal.

Another type of customer abuse comes when the customer is never, ever satisfied. There was an entrepreneur we were dealing with who had a client come in for some very expensive artwork. The client was very demanding when it came to getting the artwork approved, which should have been a warning sign. The work was done exactly to his specifications. The client picked up the artwork and paid the fee. Two weeks later he returned, upset that the work did not meet his specifications.

The staff of the business, who were proud of the work they had done for this customer, were shocked to discover that he was not happy. Efforts to refund a portion of his fee were rejected. The thought of doing the work over was not palatable since this customer could just flat never be satisfied.

In this case the entrepreneur decided that he had taken enough abuse. He had tried to do the right thing with this customer, but nothing would make him happy. The only course of action he had was to keep the funds the customer had paid and cease all communications.

This entrepreneur knows that he might get sued, but he just could not let this customer continue to abuse his staff. The entrepreneur knew that he had given the job 130 percent effort and value but nothing would ever satisfy this customer.

In this case, the entrepreneur did the right thing by trying to appease the customer. When he realized there was nothing he could do, he had to protect his staff and their morale. Sometimes, no matter what you do, you just cannot please a customer.

Make sure you have in place a policy that directs your staff about how to deal with abusive customers. Make sure they know that they should not take any abuse. Additionally, if you have a customer that you know in your gut you cannot please, just take a pass on the work.

EMPATHY

The Encyclopaedia Britannica (1999 edition) defines empathy as: "The ability to imagine oneself in anther's place and understand the other's feelings, desires, ideas, and actions. It is a term coined in the early 20th century, equivalent to the German Einfühlung and modeled on "sympathy." The term is used with special (but not exclusive) reference to aesthetic experience. The most obvious example, perhaps, is that of the actor or singer who genuinely feels the part he is performing. With other works of art, a spectator may, by a kind of introjection, feel himself involved in what he observes or contemplates. The use of empathy is an important part of the counseling technique developed by the American psychologist Carl Rogers."

My wife wanted a new car for her birthday. The car was a 98 Corolla with only 11,000 miles on it. This is true—my wife is a librarian and only drives the car to work and return. Why she wanted really wanted a new car I was unsure, but being a great husband I did get one for her one for her birthday (she forbids me to mention her age, however).

In order to get her a new car and I had to go through the transaction of purchasing a new car. When I walked into the dealership knowing exactly what the new car was going to cost (this was not critical in the discussion), I thought this process was going to be easy and stress free. Boy was I wrong on this one! As we knew what the new car costs (readily available and accurate on the web), the only thing we had to negotiate was the price of the little used car. I checked no less that 5 different sources on the web and they said the value of this "cream-puff" was between 7 to 8 thousand dollars in terms of wholesale value. I went into this process of trying to please my wife and our pocket book by assuming that they would take the new car price and reduce it by 7 to 8 thousand dollars.

When they took my wife's pristine and hardly used automobile out to be evaluated they came back with a price of $3500 claiming that it was damaged (she was sideswiped) and it just was not worth more than that. Now I am finally coming to subject of what I wanted to write about today. The salesman (no used car salesman jokes here) said that I had "wrong" information and only his and the car dealership price was correct. He had no empathy for my situation at all and I wanted to walk out till the dealer's owner came over and smoothed my feathers.

In any sales transaction there can be no win/loose or right/wrong. When I am trying to sell a product to another person, I must have empathy with whatever baggage the customer comes in with. Rather that the salesman saying I was 'wrong" in my valuation of a used car, he should have said something like " I can understand how and why you believe your car is worth between 7 to 8 thousand dollars. With your research, your conclusion is reasonable and I if I was doing the research on the web,

I probably would have reached the same conclusion" This would have made me feel great and not this need to write this article(if you can feel my frustration about this, you are correct). By validating my feelings and having empathy for them, I would have been willing to listen to his compelling points on how misguided I was(which is true). However, the salesman just did not have any empathy for my feelings or my research. He only wanted to be right but in the process of being right he came to a fraction of an inch of losing the sale.

Have empathy with your customers is so critical. Each person has there own set of needs. My expressing empathy for your customers you make them feel as if you are on there side. When we can express or relate to the customers needs in an empathetic way, then we our on our way to having loyal and great customers for our businesses.

DELEGATION

"A manager who avoids delegation cannot possibly hope to complete effectively all of the tasks that find their way onto his or her desk."

—Robert Heller

It is so hard for entrepreneurs to delegate. They have started their businesses and done everything themselves. Micromanaging has been successful for them, so for them to delegate is flat tough.

When they choose not to delegate they get overwhelmed with so many tasks that they no longer have time to spend with their family and to relax and have fun. Delegation is the key that allows any manager freedom to really get things accomplished, things such as developing the vision for their company and planning for its future. When entrepreneurs refuse to delegate, they get bogged down with everyday things that can easily be handled by a staff person. Additionally, delegation promotes employee buy-in, as employees realize they are performing critical work for the success of the business.

Entrepreneurs seem to come from two extremes. There are those entrepreneurs who delegate naturally and feel comfortable assigning work to their staff. Then there are those who don't. They have to hit crises as they try to do it all before they realize that they need to delegate if they are to survive.

Delegation is not only important for the satisfactory operation of a small business, but is absolutely a prerequisite for the firm's growth. Failure to delegate is the reason many small businesses don't grow.

Before you reach a crisis, please consider these reasons to delegate: First, by delegating you are increasing the time you have to do other important things, like spending more time with your family. Second, delegation really reduces the stress of being overwhelmed and simply having too much to do. Finally, delegation empowers employees to take on more of the responsibility of running different aspects of the business. This not only helps owners, but also is advantageous for employees as it expands their job and can prepare them for a higher level position.

Okay, so I need to delegate. How do I do it? The first rule in learning to delegate is to start small. Try delegating some minor tasks (like producing some reports, for example doing a report on sales by type of customer) to employees you think can handle those particular tasks . By starting small you can assess their ability to handle these responsibilities. Also, their small successes will increase your willingness to trust them with even more areas of responsibility in the future.

Because the Jim Moran Institute for Global Entrepreneurship is my baby, I was very reluctant to delegate anything of meaning to my staff. However, I hit the proverbial wall (crisis) and JMI was either going to get stuck or grow. The only way to grow JMI was for me to delegate many of the functions. I wanted JMI to grow and knew that I had to let go and delegate. This process of starting slow and building allowed me to expand JMI while retaining balance in my life.

Another problem with delegation is making sure you control the process. Delegating without control is like trying to steer the car without touching the steering wheel. There are many ways to control delegation, but the one I like the best is to ask the employee to whom you have delegated the work to give you progress reports at certain increments of time. Another way to control is to make sure that you are included in all correspondence about the project (ie, receive copies of all letters and e-mails).

You also need to give the person to whom you have delegated some latitude in carrying out the assignment, otherwise the project has not really been delegated. If you are continuously watching them out of the corner of your eye, you are not really delegating.

One of the complaints frequently I hear from entrepreneurs is that, when they delegate, they never know if the works gets done. To want to know when and how the work gets done is a reasonable. One way to handle this is to make sure you clearly explain your expectations to your employee at the beginning of the assignment. Tell your employee that you want him/her to do the assignment and to keep you posted on his/her progress and to let you know if he/she runs into any stumbling blocks he/she cannot handle. This really does work and is critical in the delegation process.

Robert Heller wrote one great book on the subject called *How to Delegate.* In this very short book, he takes the reader on a very detailed, but very understandable, approach to delegation.

Delegation is one of those concepts that you cannot just talk about, you must do it! I guarantee that increasing the amount of delegation in your business, will make your life much better.

DO NOT BE FRIENDS TO YOUR EMPLOYEES

I am very often so surprised by the many entrepreneurs who want to make their associates or employees their friends. Friends are great and employees are great, but together they are a time bomb.

Sure you want to care about your associates and, sure, you want to help them out. However, this can go too far especially if you have friends working for you. I want my associates to be productive and know that I care about them, but I do not go out of my way to be their friends.

Once you have friends working for you then the line of separation between business and personal becomes so murky. As an entrepreneur and leader you will be called on to make many tough decisions for your business and you must have your mind clear. It is so, so hard to let an associate go and so much harder to let a friend go. You just do need this baggage of friendship when running your business.

Some entrepreneurs that I have seen want to be liked by their associates. However, being liked and being respected are two different things. Being managers, we need to have employees respect us in order to get the work done.

An entrepreneur that we are working with has an employee that was and is her best friend. However, this entrepreneur hired her, as she really needed a job. Being a very good-natured person, she hired her, not because she was qualified, but because of friendship. Now this employee is just not working out and she has to let her go and feeling terribly guilty about this and hoping that she will quit on her own accord. It would have been so much easier for her to have helped this employee find another job, rather than hiring a friend.

Another entrepreneur goes out of her way to make employees her friends. She cultivates this attitude so that she thinks she can manage them better and they will buy into the objectives and goals of the business. This is just not happening as now the employees feel as if they run the company.

While I do not think that friendship fits in a relationship between supervisor and employee, I do think it is perfectly acceptable between fellow employees.

It is very important than you always be kind and concerned with each of your employees but do not stretch this into friendship.

CLIENT APPRECIATION

Jerome S. Osteryoung, PhD
College of Business
Florida State University, Tallahassee, FL

WORDS AND CUSTOMER SERVICE

"Good words are worth much and cost little."
—George Herbert (1593-1633) English
clergyman, writer & metaphysical poet
from *"Jacula Prudentum,"* 1651

Words have meaning, obviously, and their use has to be carefully monitored. How you treat a customer with the words you choose to speak to them has a critical effect on how the customer views your business. If you use the right words, the customer will probably feel wonderful. The wrong words alienate customers and send them to your competitors.

I was going through a bank drive-through and I was in a hurry to take money out of my account to fill my bare wallet. I had filled out the withdrawal slip ahead of time. I sent the slip to the teller in one of those transporters (if someone knows the correct name for those darn things, please let me know). Anyway, the teller gets on the intercom and announces to the whole world, "Sir, I need to see your ID." While I clearly understand the need for photo identification to protect my account, the bank teller's words made me feel as if I had done something terribly wrong. Also, it brought back memories. I hate to admit this, but when I was younger, I had received a few tickets for speeding. Of course, the policemen had always commanded, you guessed it, "Sir, I need to see your ID."

From a teller's perspective, viewing my ID was mandatory. However, her words really alienated me and may potentially offend many other customers in the future. The teller could have softened her request, saying, "Sir, in order protect your accounts, may I please see your ID?" Notice how this request is not only nicer, it also really explains why the teller needs to verify your identification.

One of the things that really drives me crazy is how many times I hear people say, "No problem," after they have provided a service to me. When I thank people for providing services, it invalidates what they did if they say, "no problem." It is so much better to say, "It was my pleasure to be of service to you." Notice how this last statement is warmer and more genuine than, "No problem."

The real point of this article is that you need to pay attention to the words you and your associates speak and how you communicate with your clients and customers. Sometimes sloppiness slips into our vernacular. We must be ever vigilant for requests and responses that need to be modified to make the most of the few precious moments we spend with the people who support our businesses.

Now go out and make sure all your employees are using words that signify warmth and kindness. You can do this!

VARYING CUSTOMER SERVICE

"Advice is like snow — the softer it falls, the longer it dwells upon, and the deeper in sinks into the mind."
—Samuel Taylor Coleridge

Recently I met with an entrepreneur who was getting burned out. He felt that he could no longer meet his customers' expectations. His business had grown; however, he was still treating customers who were placing $200 orders the same as customers who were placing $5,000 orders. Regardless of the size of the order, this entrepreneur (who is also the outside salesman) believed he had to go to the customer's business to go over the order. Even though he had staff members at his retail store who could deal with any and all walk-in traffic, he felt he must visit each customer.

This entrepreneur believed that he had to live up to his own belief that each and every customer should be treated equally. Trying to live up to this belief was completely overwhelming him because he just did not have enough time in the day to service all customers equally.

I saw two important issues regarding this entrepreneur. First, I had to help him find a way to free up more of his time and, second, we had to deal with his belief system towards customer service. Obviously, both of these issues are interconnected.

I asked the entrepreneur if he had ever seen a large company take some of their best customers to sports events or on fishing trips? Of course, he said, "Yes." He then began to see that it is common for entrepreneurs to provide different levels of customer service, depending on the volume of business received from a customer. This is not to say, however, that you should not give excellent customer service to each customer, rather that certain customers should receive higher levels of perks associated with the profits they generate.

This entrepreneur already had the option for customers with small orders to come to his retail location. He could easily change his habit and provide site visits only to customers if he expected their order to be over $200. This idea was difficult to sell to this entrepreneur because I was asking him to change his belief system. Not that his belief system was faulty; rather, it just was no longer serving him and his business!

It is too early to tell how this new customer service policy will work (both in time saved and profitability), but the entrepreneur is heading in the right direction by matching the degree of customer service to the level of financial rewards received from the customer.

Look carefully at your customer service. If you are currently providing the same level of service to all types of customers, you might want to consider adjusting this to fit the profitability provided by each customer. Again, I am not advocating that you *should not* give quality customer service. Rather, I am saying that the level of customer service should correspond to the level of profit provided by the customer.

CUSTOMER GREETINGS

"Words, when well chosen, have so great a force in them, that a description often gives us more lively ideas than the sight of things themselves."

—Joseph Addison

No one can deny the importance of first impressions, and the first words you or your staff members use when greeting customers are instrumental in creating a positive one. Sure, it is important to look professional, but it is even more crucial to ensure that the correct words are used.

One of the most commonly used greetings is, "How may I help you?" Another popular variation is, "May I help you find something?" Many customers, myself included, despise this greeting. Whenever I hear it, I have to suppress the urge to scream, "Get away." Ultimately, I just end up saying, "No thank you. I am just looking."

The problem with this greeting is that it is too broad and it does not address the customer's real need. Customers do not walk into a store just to look around. They are there for one of two reasons: to find information about a product or service or to make a purchase. "May I help you?" is just too general a question to pinpoint the customer's real need. Furthermore, it sends the message that the clerk does not understand why the customer is really there. It also tells the customer that they are not there to buy.

A successful greeting acknowledges why the customer has come to your business. For example, at big box building stores, I often receive the greeting, "What kind of project are you working on today?" Notice how this greeting recognizes why the customer is there and initiates important dialog between the customer and the salesperson. Opening this dialog is essential as it builds trust and elicits the critical information needed for the sale of goods and services.

In addition, whenever possible, customers should be greeted using their name. By remembering their name, you send the message that the customer is important and valued. When I go to my favorite restaurant to eat, the hostess always greets me, "Welcome, Dr. Osteryoung. May I show you to your table?" Along with communicating importance, this greeting also shows an understanding of the customer's real need (in this case, food).

Another example of a great greeting is, "Hello, have you been here before?" If the customer has not, the clerk or server now has an opportunity to quickly share a little about the business. If they have, an appropriate response is, "Welcome back. We appreciate you coming back to visit us." In both of these cases, the customer leaves feeling less like a commodity and more like a valued individual.

Another effective way to greet a customer is to initiate a casual conversation. Choose a topic about which the customer would have similar knowledge – the weather, for instance. A salesperson might ask, "Do you think we are going to get any cool weather soon?" Following the customer's response, the conversation can easily transition to the real reason for the customer's visit. For example, the salesperson might follow with, "What brings you in out of the hot weather today?"

Regardless of what greeting your business uses, customer acknowledgment is of the utmost importance. One research study found that nearly 70% of customers believe that no one cares that they stop in. This is not exactly a great foundation for building loyal customer relationships. Without exception, every customer should be greeted within 30 seconds of their arrival.

Now go out and make sure that your business has an effective plan for greeting customers. Remember, greetings should be delivered within the first few moments of the customer's visit. Pay attention to the words you choose, and make sure that they are sending the right message.

COMMUNICATIONS IS EVERYTHING

Communications are what drive every business! Every type of idea, instruction, or interchange is done through communications. By communications, I am talking about either written or oral.

If you think about it, most entrepreneurs and managers spend most of their time communicating to their boss (eg, shareholders), customers, and associates. Yet while most of the entrepreneurs time is spent communicating, very little time (if any) is spent on learning how to communicate. For some reason, we all think that we know how to communicate, so that any emphasis on communications is unnecessary. This is just not a valid assumption!

I was invited to attend a staff meeting of a very successful business. Every manager shared honestly how they were doing and everyone was very supportive of everyone else. The owner also shared most of the information from the current financial statement (open book management). The communications were great in this company and you could tell that the associates really liked this process of communications.

Another staff meeting that I attended (folks are just not going to invite me to these meetings anymore) was marked by the entrepreneur talking exclusively about what he wants. There just was no sharing of information. In this meeting, you could tell that the employees just did not feel as involved as the first group I talked about.

So, how do you improve communications in your business? I think there are several things that you need to do. The first is just become aware how you communicate and how you are communicated to. Each person is going to have a unique way of doing this and you need to understand what is going on. I have had one associate who always was incredibly nice and happy when he wanted to request something, but not nearly as nice the other times. For the longest period of time I thought, that when he was happy it was something I did (right!) or something was happening with his home life. Once I was aware of the behavior and what he wanted, it allowed me to use this form of nonverbal communication to understand the behavior.

The Associate Director of JMI (Mrs. Diane Denslow) is very to the point and really does like to waste time with small talk, as she is very busy. I, on the other hand, like to have a little bit of an introduction with small talk before we get down to the nitty-gritty. Once we became aware of this (yes, it did take time) we learned to accommodate one another without asking anyone to change. Our communications are much better as we are aware of how to communicate to one another. There is also a series of tests that you and your employees can take to find out the styles of communications that each person prefers.

I once had a secretary that did not like any communication via email. She could never figure out why I would send her an email note, rather than talking to her as her desk was just outside of my door. It was not until after she had left; that I realized I was just not fully aware of her preferences nor was she willing to accommodate my preferences.

Another thing you need to do is share information. My making yourself vulnerable by this process, it opens the door to great communications. Share the financials; obviously you do not want to show your associates your net profits but show them at least the gross profit. Sometimes associates have the feeling that you are making millions and millions of dollars and this sharing of information really helps in extinguishing all of misinformation, which really distorts your associates' perception of you but it also builds up trust. Some firms show the limited financials with their managers and then collect this information after the meeting to ensure that this information does not get into the wrong hands.

By sharing, this must be two way in that it cannot be just the entrepreneur or manager talking about what they want. Rather this dialogue must be two ways. Learning to listen is really a big key in communications. If you are willing to listen (and not just fix the problem) the communications improve so much. Most associates do not want to be judged. If they can come to you or their managers and know they will not be judged, this enables communications to be greatly enhanced.

I frequently have just listened to associates' problems and they then comment to me on how great of communicator I am (I just listened).

The final way to increase communications is to clearly share your expectations of where you want to take the company and your expectations about each employee. One entrepreneur we were assisting had a problem employee and was always reprimanding him. However, he never told his employee on how upset he was getting this behavior not was he communicating on how serious of a problem this was. If these expectations were made clear, this little problem would not have become a large problem. By sharing your expectations, you eliminate employees from guessing as to what you want and vastly improve communications.

Communication is the key for a business. By putting emphasis on this process you will improve the bottom line and make your business more fun to work in.

THE CUSTOMER SERVICE EXPERIENCE: A HOLISTIC APPROACH

Do not be desirous of having things done quickly. Do not look at small advantages. Desire to have things done quickly prevents their being done thoroughly. Looking at small advantages prevents great affairs from being accomplished.

—Confucius

It is great to have a super advertising campaign. Advertising is a very effective way to attract new customers into your business. However, you must make sure that the advertising message you deliver is congruent with the customer service experience you provide alongside your product or service.

I was dealing with a firm that had a very slick and expensive advertising company. This advertising company developed a campaign touting the firm's great customer service with a number of customer testimonials. The ads were super, and since many new customers came in as a result, the campaign was considered a great success.

The rest of the story, however, was not quite as successful. When the customers came in they found that the glowing report given in the ads was anything but accurate. They found sales clerks who thought that servicing the customer was not important, and they had to wait in the checkout line so long that many of them put their products back on the shelves and left the store. Many of the new customers the ads brought in walked out of the stores vowing never to return.

While there are many issues here, the critical one is customer service. It is just not good enough to say that you want all of your staff to smile at customers. Rather, you must clearly define what you want the entire customer service experience to be.

Think of customer service as one overall experience that consists of a series of smaller tasks. Look at your customer service experience in a holistic fashion and then develop a process to create the product you desire. The only way to deliver a great customer service experience is to have a vision of what it should look like in its totality.

For example, say you define the total customer service experience as the great feeling that you want each customer to have when leaving. Having defined the customer service experience in this manner, you know that you must emphasize creating great final impressions for the customer.

However, say you want your customers to feel like royalty from the time they arrive to the time they leave. This customer service experience requires a much more detailed approach. Each customer touch must be outstanding.

What I have found to be useful in getting entrepreneurs through this process is having them close their eyes and just imagine what they would like their customer service experience to be. I then ask them to use feeling words like "wonderful" or "fantastic" to describe what they have imagined.

The point is to develop a description of the type of customer service experience the entrepreneur wants. Once they have this, they can easily ascertain the steps necessary to accomplish this desired experience.

THANK YOU NOTES

I thank you. I am not of many words, but I thank you.
—William Shakespeare from <u>Much Ado About Nothing</u>

I recently purchased a very large item. When I was suffering from buyer's remorse, I received a very kind note from the sales person thanking me for the purchase. My buyer's remorse instantly was transformed into happiness. Simply receiving a thank you note converted me from having doubts about the purchase to a "raving customer."

I think thank you notes are one of the most overlooked items for most entrepreneurs. Too many times, I see customers spend $10,000 to $20,000 without receiving a thank you note. Sure, it takes a few minutes to write these notes, but they are worth it! Each of these notes needs to be personal with the common theme of thanking customers for their purchases and of letting the customer know how much they mean to you.

Sometimes, it's just a good idea to send a thank you note to customers once a year expressing what they mean to you and your business. Thank you notes do not have to be reserved for only customers. Employees, business associates, and special people in your life (including your significant other) really appreciate receiving these notes.

I don't have customers per se, but I try to send notes when someone that I have observed has done a wonderful thing, when someone wins a very special award, when someone is promoted, when someone does something very special, and when someone goes way beyond what is expected. I just try to send these out to thank the people for going the "extra mile" to make our world a better place.

There are three some important points to remember about thank you notes. First, they should be very personal with specifics mentioned. Second, they should be brief. Third, they must be very sincere. Finally, and I can't emphasize this enough, they must be handwritten — e-mail thank you notes just won't cut it!

My champion thank you note writer is Glen Davidson, who is Chairman of the Board of PATLive. He sends wonderful notes and also includes a relaxing CD. Another extreme example is Nic's Toggery—they send out thank you notes to customers who have bought nothing, but just walked in one of their shops to look around.

Examples of some great thank you notes can be found in *The Thank You Book: Hundreds of Clever, Meaningful, and Purposeful Ways to Say Thank You* by <u>Robyn Freedman Spizman</u>.

Thank you notes will improve your customer service, your employee morale, and might also improve your family relationships. Everyone wants to be thanked and appreciated.

CLIENT SATISFACTION

Jerome S. Osteryoung, PhD
College of Business
Florida State University, Tallahassee, FL

NEVER BLINDSIDE A CUSTOMER

"What you do speaks so loudly that I cannot hear what you say."

—Ralph Waldo Emerson

Blindsiding a customer is one of the best ways to run them off. Customers have certain expectations. Meeting those expectations, whether the expectations are reasonable or not, is absolutely critical to the success of any business.

I think the people who are most guilty of blindsiding customers are in the medical profession. One time I was placed in an examining room, not in the waiting lounge, while I waited to see a doctor for 3 hours. Obviously, I was simmering mad, especially when the physician did not apologize or even recognize the scope of the problem.

I think most customers understand problems when they come up, but they need to be notified and told about the delay. If a nurse or other staff member had come in and said, "An emergency has come up and the doctor has gone to the hospital to deal with it, but he will be back in an hour and a half," I could have dealt with it. What happens in this case is that the patient, me, just assumed, "I am not important to them. If I were important, they would not keep me waiting for 3 hours."

If this was just an isolated case, I could understand, but everyone I talk to about this subject has his or her own horror story about dealing with a physician. In my case, I refused to go back to see this specialist, but went, instead, to Mayo Clinic in Jacksonville. I now travel all the way to Jacksonville to see a physician, just to get away from this awful customer service.

Another industry that seems to relish in blindsiding is the construction industry. I cannot tell you how many times I have called for a plumber or carpenter and had them show up days after their appointment with me. Again, what is communicated to customers is that they are not important.

Well, the point of this article is not to throw harpoons at various professions, but to make the point that it is a realistic expectation to assume people will show up at the time they said they would. If things come up, and they will, then a telephone call telling the customer what is going on is paramount. I like the 10-minute rule: If you cannot meet with a customer within 10 minutes of the appointment time, then you must, really must, call the customer to tell what is going on and when you will be there.

What drives me crazy is to sit in the waiting room, waiting for a doctor (with a preset appointment) and not be told when I will be able to see the physician. All the staff has to do is to say that the physician is running late and he should be able to see you in a certain amount of time. It is so much better to communicate what is happening rather than having customers think that you really do not care about them. Yes, patients are customers, too.

All your customers have the basic assumption that they are worthwhile and they need to feel respected. By blindsiding customers, you are affecting them in a deep psychological way. A customer should never, ever be blindsided and you avoid this by communicating any problems you may encounter while meeting in their expectations of your services.

Now go figure out a mechanism to ensure that you never blindside any of your customers!

CHECKPOINT CHARLIE

"Nothing in this world can take the place of persistence. Talent will not; nothing is more common than unsuccessful people with talent are. Genius will not; unrewarded genius is almost a proverb. Education will not; the world is full of educated derelicts. Persistence and determination alone are omnipotent. The slogan 'press on' has solved and always will solve the problems of the human race."

—Calvin Coolidge

Attention to details is so critical to the success of each and every entrepreneur. Every semester I tell our entrepreneurship students at FSU that the "devil is in the details" and one of the main things an entrepreneur must do is sweat the small stuff. Now, I am not saying that each entrepreneur should be checking on every detail in the business. Rather, an entrepreneur should devise and initiate processes and systems to ensure that responsibility for the details is assigned to a competent and dependable employee(s) and then make sure these systems and processes are monitored.

One neat example of entrepreneurs who really sweat the details is the brotherly team of Grant and Ray Capelouto, owners of Capelouto Termite and Pest Control. They have instituted a Checkpoint Charlie (they actually have a sign at this location) where each of their 38 trucks must stop each day. A supervisor waits at the checkpoint to checkout various details. Some days the inspector might make sure the horns and lights in the trucks work and the next morning make sure the required amount of chemicals is on each truck.

Each truck bay is equipped with a hose and a brush so technicians can wash their trucks each morning. Supervisors check on the appearance of each technician and are vitally concerned with all the details of the business.

Of course, Grant and Ray have managers who oversee the implementation of these policies. What these savvy entrepreneurs have mastered is the execution of systems that make sure each and every detail they consider important is dealt with on a consistent basis.

Systems that guarantee constant attention to details are critical to the success of every entrepreneur. One of the best ways to plan your "micro-awareness system" is to map out the processes that are involved in your business and evaluate what processes are critical to the success of your business and to the betterment of your customers. For example, if restaurant owners want to make sure that the food is delivered in a consistent manner, they first have to figure out each step in the food preparation. They then analyze which steps they should keep, add, or revise to insure the consistent quality of the food dish. No detail is too small (eg, the amount of seasoning to the size of dish to serve the food on).

Sweating the details is so critical to the success of each and every business. However, even more important is the fact that the Capleloutos understand so well: Attention to detail is not adequate without a monitoring process.

Successful entrepreneurs figure out systems that insure the details of running a business are dealt with and consistently monitored. Now go out and make sure that you are sweating the details!

CLEAN DESKS

"Regardless of past efforts and intentions, today's consumers recognize only what they feel, and if your good intentions and accompanying actions don't give them the feeling that you care and are providing excellent service, they won't be happy."

—Lee Pemberton

Let me start out this article to say by saying that I am not a neat freak or anything like that, but I have my limits. Occasionally, my desk does get messy, but I just cannot tolerate this for long as it does drive me crazy. This is just me!

My wife wanted (really, insisted) on a new front door as it had large gaps around the base. Being the dutiful husband (she would question this) that I am, I went to purchase this door from a store that specializes in these types of products. When I arrived and was looking around the floor room, I could see that all of the desks of the sales staff were in plain view. Several of the desks looked like Hurricane Katrina had hit them this morning, and I felt very uncomfortable in ordering from this store. Here's why. I thought that if the desks were that messy, then the entire business must not be organized. Not the best of logic, but for so many people share this belief. Many, many customers assume that a messy desk or office means that the entire organization is haphazard, if not completely dysfunctional.

Sure, staff needs some flexibility as to how they keep their personal space; however, if this affects customer service or the customer's perception, than it just shouldn't be tolerated. Perception is reality, and customers just perceive that a messy desk signifies a poor business; as a manager or business owner, you'll want to nip this problem in the bud immediately.

I just know that I am going to get a ton of e-mail saying that each employee has had a right to keep their desks anyway, they want. Also, folks are going to argue that messy people are more creative, which may or may not be true. However, when a messy desk influences customer perception, that this is just not acceptable as it is not good business practice.

I used to work with a fellow professor who kept not his desk, but his whole entire office, not just his desk, was so messy that the janitorial staff refused to clean it. When you went to visit him in his office, you had to stand up to converse as because he had 3 three feet (this is not an exaggeration) of files, old exams, and notes on his desk. There was no room to sit in his office as all the chairs had mountains of journals stacked on them. Students knew when they took him for a course one of his courses there was a good chance that he was going to lose their papers. Obviously, as the word got out, they avoided his classes like the plaque plague, even though he was a very good educator.

Even if staff do not have contact with the public, I think it is still so very important to that they keep their offices clean. Managers frequently perceive assume that a messy desk is not an efficient one and tend to evaluate these folks workers lower because of this habit.

Now go out and encourage your staff to have clean and orderly look work areas. You may encounter resistance at first, but they will thank you in the end. You can do this!

COMMUNICATIONS IS EVERYTHING

Communications are what drive every business! Every type of idea, instruction, or interchange is done through communications. By communications, I am talking about either written or oral.

If you think about it, most entrepreneurs and managers spend most of their time communicating to their boss (eg, shareholders), customers, and associates. Yet while most of the entrepreneurs time is spent communicating, very little time (if any) is spent on learning how to communicate. For some reason, we all think that we know how to communicate, so that any emphasis on communications is unnecessary. This is just not a valid assumption!

I was invited to attend a staff meeting of a very successful business. Every manager shared honestly how they were doing and everyone was very supportive of everyone else. The owner also shared most of the information from the current financial statement (open book management). The communications were great in this company and you could tell that the associates really liked this process of communications.

Another staff meeting that I attended (folks are just not going to invite me to these meetings anymore) was marked by the entrepreneur talking exclusively about what he wants. There just was no sharing of information. In this meeting, you could tell that the employees just did not feel as involved as the first group I talked about.

So, how do you improve communications in your business? I think there are several things that you need to do. The first is just become aware how you communicate and how you are communicated to. Each person is going to have a unique way of doing this and you need to understand what is going on. I have had one associate who always was incredibly nice and happy when he wanted to request something, but not nearly as nice the other times. For the longest period of time I thought, that when he was happy it was something I did (right!) or something was happening with his home life. Once I was aware of the behavior and what he wanted, it allowed me to use this form of non-verbal communication to understand the behavior.

The Associate Director of JMI (Mrs. Diane Denslow) is very to the point and really does like to waste time with small talk, as she is very busy. I on the other hand, like to have a little bit of an introduction with small talk before we get down to the nitty-gritty. Once we became aware of this (yes, it did take time) we learned to accommodate one another without asking anyone to change. Our communications are much better as we are aware of how to communicate to one another. There is also a series of tests that you and your employees can take to find out the styles of communications that each person prefers.

I once had a secretary that did not like any communication via email. She could never figure out why I would send her an email note, rather than talking to her as her desk was just outside of my door. It was not till after she had left; that I realized I was just not fully aware of her preferences nor was she willing to accommodate my preferences.

Another thing you need to do is share information. My making yourself vulnerable by this process, it opens the door to great communications. Share the financials; obviously you do not want to show your associates your net profits but show them at least the gross profit. Sometimes associates have the feeling that you are making millions and millions of dollars and this sharing of information really helps in extinguishing all of misinformation which really distorts your associate's perception of you, but it also, builds up trust. Some firms show the limited financials with their managers and then collect this information after the meeting to insure that this information does not get into the wrong hands.

By sharing, this must be two way in that it cannot be just the entrepreneur or manager talking about what they want. Rather this dialog must be two ways. Learning to listen is really a big key in communications. If you are willing to listen (and not just fix the problem) the communications improve so much. Most associates do not want to be judged. If they can come to you or their managers and know they will not be judged, this enables communications to be greatly enhanced.

I frequently have just listened to associates' problems and they then comment to me on how great of communicator I am (I just listened).

The final way to increase communications is to clearly share your expectations of where you want to take the company and your expectations about each employee. One entrepreneur we were assisting had a problem employee and was always reprimanding him. However, he never told his employee on how upset he was getting this behavior not was he communicating on how serious of a problem this was. If these expectations were made clear, this little problem would not have become a large problem. By sharing your expectations, you eliminate employees from guessing as to what you want and vastly improve communications.

Communication is the key for a business. By putting emphasis on this process you will improve the bottom line and make your business more fun to work in.

CUSTOMER GREETINGS

"Words, when well chosen, have so great a force in them, that a description often gives us more lively ideas than the sight of things themselves."

—Joseph Addison

No one can deny the importance of first impressions, and the first words you or your staff members use when greeting customers are instrumental in creating a positive one. Sure, it is important to look professional, but it is even more crucial to ensure that the correct words are used.

One of the most commonly used greetings is, "How may I help you?" Another popular variation is, "May I help you find something?" Many customers, myself included, despise this greeting. Whenever I hear it, I have to suppress the urge to scream, "Get away." Ultimately, I just end up saying, "No thank you. I am just looking."

The problem with this greeting is that it is too broad and it does not address the customer's real need. Customers do not walk into a store just to look around. They are there for one of two reasons: to find information about a product or service or to make a purchase. "May I help you?" is just too general a question to pinpoint the customer's real need. Furthermore, it sends the message that the clerk does not understand why the customer is really there. It also tells the customer that they are not there to buy.

A successful greeting acknowledges why the customer has come to your business. For example, at big box building stores, I often receive the greeting, "What kind of project are you working on today?" Notice how this greeting recognizes why the customer is there and initiates important dialog between the customer and the salesperson. Opening this dialog is essential as it builds trust and elicits the critical information needed for the sale of goods and services.

In addition, whenever possible, customers should be greeted using their name. By remembering their name, you send the message that the customer is important and valued. When I go to my favorite restaurant to eat, the hostess always greets me, "Welcome, Dr. Osteryoung. May I show you to your table?" Along with communicating importance, this greeting also shows an understanding of the customer's real need (in this case, food).

Another example of a great greeting is, "Hello, have you been here before?" If the customer has not, the clerk or server now has an opportunity to quickly share a little about the business. If they have, an appropriate response is, "Welcome back. We appreciate you coming back to visit us." In both of these cases, the customer leaves feeling less like a commodity and more like a valued individual.

Another effective way to greet a customer is to initiate a casual conversation. Choose a topic about which the customer would have similar knowledge – the weather, for instance. A salesperson might ask, "Do you think we are going to get any cool weather soon?" Following the customer's response, the conversation can easily transition to the real reason for the customer's visit. For example, the salesperson might follow with, "What brings you in out of the hot weather today?"

Regardless of what greeting your business uses, customer acknowledgment is of the utmost importance. One research study found that nearly 70% of customers believe that no one cares that they stop in. This is not exactly a great foundation for building loyal customer relationships. Without exception, every customer should be greeted within 30 seconds of their arrival.

Now go out and make sure that your business has an effective plan for greeting customers. Remember, greetings should be delivered within the first few moments of the customer's visit. Pay attention to the words you choose, and make sure that they are sending the right message.

CUSTOMER ABUSE

"Anyone who proposes to do good must not expect people to roll stones out of his way, but must accept his lot calmly if they even roll a few more upon it."
—Albert Schweitzer

Entrepreneurs and their businesses are there to serve clients. Customer service is what allows a business to grow and thrive.

Every business has to survive difficult clients. They are, however, the impossible-to-please or abusive customers who keep entrepreneurs awake at night.

If a customer is using profanity in dealing with any staff member, ask the customer to stop using this language. If it continues, the customer must be asked to leave your premises right then and there. Asking your staff to submit to any abuse for any reason is untenable. No matter how wrongly the customer believes he or she has been mistreated, you just cannot allow any staff member to be abused, period.

If customers yell or using loud voices, they must be told that this behavior is not tolerated for any reason. In this situation, move the customer to a private office if possible. If this does not work, the customer must be asked to leave the premises no matter what his perception of the problem. Customer service is a goal, but protecting your staff from abuse is a higher goal.

Another type of customer abuse comes when the customer is never, ever satisfied. There was an entrepreneur we were dealing with who had a client come in for some very expensive artwork. The client was very demanding when it came to getting the artwork approved, which should have been a warning sign. The work was done exactly to his specifications. The client picked up the artwork and paid the fee. Two weeks later he returned, upset that the work did not meet his specifications.

The staff of the business, who were proud of the work they had done for this customer, were shocked to discover that he was not happy. Efforts to refund a portion of his fee were rejected. The thought of doing the work over was not palatable since this customer could just flat never be satisfied.

In this case the entrepreneur decided that he had taken enough abuse. He had tried to do the right thing with this customer, but nothing would make him happy. The only course of action he had was to keep the funds the customer had paid and cease all communications.

This entrepreneur knows that he might get sued, but he just could not let this customer continue to abuse his staff. The entrepreneur knew that he had given the job 130 percent effort and value but nothing would ever satisfy this customer.

In this case, the entrepreneur did the right thing by trying to appease the customer. When he realized there was nothing he could do, he had to protect his staff and their morale. Sometimes, no matter what you do, you just cannot please a customer.

Make sure you have in place a policy that directs your staff about how to deal with abusive customers. Make sure they know that they should not take any abuse. Additionally, if you have a customer that you know in your gut you cannot please, just take a pass on the work.

THE CUSTOMER SERVICE EXPERIENCE: A HOLISTIC APPROACH

"Do not be desirous of having things done quickly. Do not look at small advantages. Desire to have things done quickly prevents their being done thoroughly. Looking at small advantages prevents great affairs from being accomplished."

—Confucius

It is great to have a super advertising campaign. Advertising is a very effective way to attract new customers into your business. However, you must make sure that the advertising message you deliver is congruent with the customer service experience you provide alongside your product or service.

I was dealing with a firm that had a very slick and expensive advertising company. This advertising company developed a campaign touting the firm's great customer service with a number of customer testimonials. The ads were super, and since many new customers came in as a result, the campaign was considered a great success.

The rest of the story, however, was not quite as successful. When the customers came in they found that the glowing report given in the ads was anything but accurate. They found sales clerks who thought that servicing the customer was not important, and they had to wait in the checkout line so long that many of them put their products back on the shelves and left the store. Many of the new customers the ads brought in walked out of the stores vowing never to return.

While there are many issues here, the critical one is customer service. It is just not good enough to say that you want all of your staff to smile at customers. Rather, you must clearly define what you want the entire customer service experience to be.

Think of customer service as one overall experience that consists of a series of smaller tasks. Look at your customer service experience in a holistic fashion and then develop a process to create the product you desire. The only way to deliver a great customer service experience is to have a vision of what it should look like in its totality.

For example, say you define the total customer service experience as the great feeling that you want each customer to have when leaving. Having defined the customer service experience in this manner, you know that you must emphasize creating great final impressions for the customer.

However, say you want your customers to feel like royalty from the time they arrive to the time they leave. This customer service experience requires a much more detailed approach. Each customer touch must be outstanding.

What I have found to be useful in getting entrepreneurs through this process is having them close their eyes and just imagine what they would like their customer service experience to be. I then ask them to use feeling words like "wonderful" or "fantastic" to describe what they have imagined.

The point is to develop a description of the type of customer service experience the entrepreneur wants. Once they have this, they can easily ascertain the steps necessary to accomplish this desired experience.

CUSTOMER SERVICE

"In the United States, you say the customer is always right. In Japan, we say the customer is God. There is a big difference."

—Japanese Businessman

I was going on a business trip to London and then take some time to relax and enjoy this wonderful city and country. I was so excited about the trip and could not wait to get to the airport. When I got to the Tallahassee airport I found out that my travel agent had my first name recorded on the ticket as "Jerry," but my passport said "Jerome." Now I have traveled with this name difference before all over the world, to Sweden, Jamaica, Australia and many more places, and there has never been a problem. In fact, I never even noticed the name difference. However, this time when I arrived at the airport 2 hours early, the ticket agent would not let me get on the plane. She said that since the names did not match (Jerry and Jerome); I might have stolen the ticket. Of course, I was upset as I really wanted and needed to go to London..

Clearly, the ticket agent did not handle this well as she only viewed her position that I might have stolen the ticket and that I was not Jerry in that all of my ID said Jerome (I should have shown her my picture in this column). Her position was that I was the enemy and I that was very wrong plus there was nothing that she was going to do to help as it was all my fault! In fact, when I thought I was not going to make it on the plane with my wife, I offered to buy a ticket under the Jerome name

and she said that the cost would be $3,000 (the original ticket only cost $1000).

While we were going through this lengthy discussion, we tied up the ticket line for over 30 minutes. Clearly, the problem was not the employee but rather the lack of customer service training in this airline. While the ticket agents have to put up with terrible abuse, they cannot and should not assume the customer is the enemy. In fact in any business, when the customer becomes the enemy, it is time to find a new line of work.

With the 9/11 scare the airlines and security need to make sure that everything is done to protect our country. Clearly, the name difference problem was a significant problem and I had to deal with it, but it was the way the ticket agent treated me as not a wonderful customer, or a customer, but the enemy that so infuriated me. I know that to be successful you must deliver bad news in a kind a genuine way and not assume the customer is the enemy. All, she had to say in a kind way is that "We are not allowed to let anyone travel unless their ID and ticket match for their protection and ours. I am sorry about this problem but here are some things that might help."

With customer service it is the attitude of the employee that determines the effectiveness of customer service. You need to make sure that all of your employees that have interaction with the public have the attitude of wanting to serve and be helpful to any all customers.

CUSTOMER SERVICE THROUGHOUT THE ORGANIZATION

"Knowing is not enough; we must apply. Willing is not enough; we must do."

—Johann von Goethe

I went to see a banker friend (of course he may not be a friend after he reads this article) about a committee we serve on together. As I walked into the bank, there was not a greeter and the two customer service representatives were servicing other customers. They did not even acknowledge my presence. As I had never been to his office before, I was not even sure if I was in the right location. Of course, I should have asked him where his office was.

I wandered around the central area of the bank over and over again. wearing a path in the carpet. It seemed like an eternity before someone noticed that I had a very lost look on my face. This lady came out of her office and pointed me in the right direction. She, also, promised not to charge me for the carpet damage.

When I reached my friend's office, his assistant was on a personal phone call to a friend. I heard her say, "Let me put you on hold, while I deal with this person." This was not a warm and friendly greeting at all. She took the information that I wanted to see the banker and she said he would be with me shortly. Immediately afterwards, she resumed her phone conversation with her friend. Never did she offer me a drink or a cup of coffee or anything to demonstrate a warm welcome. She was only concerned with her personal issues.

When the banker was free he came out and got me, which I appreciated. When I left the bank, he walked me to the front doors, a very personable and welcome gesture.

Now in all fairness, I just might have hit an unusual time in this bank, but, from that one encounter, I felt that the bank does not enforce customer service as a high priority to low-level employees.

Customer service simply cannot be rendered at a high level but must be pervasive throughout the entire organization. Who do most customers interact with on a daily basis? It is the employees— eg, tellers and waiters—who sit on the lower rungs of the corporate ladder.

If an organization really wants to have great customer service, they must make sure that each and every employee is trained in great customer service and then management must make sure this training is continuously reinforced and rewarded. Just a slip here or a slip there in customer service can really make a difference.

Now go out and make sure that you have a program in place to train and continuously monitor all employees for customer service.

DEALING WITH DIFFICULT EMPLOYEES

"When I help, I am aware of my strengths and other's weaknesses… Fixing is a form of judgment. It implies something is broken and creates distance. We can only serve which we are profoundly connected to!"
—Sam Dailey-Harris

You can have the greatest workforce in the world, but there will always be some people who are just difficult to get motivated. It is not something that you can raise your magic wand to go fix; rather, you have to work at this problem on a continual basis. If you do not work to remedy this problem, it is only going to remain or get even larger.

Given that a lack of motivated workers is just part of the staffing issues we have to deal with, what can you do? These employees are typically the ones that show up exactly at eight and go home not a second past five. In addition, they are the same staff members who always seem to take the maximum amount of sick leave available. Bottom line is that these staff members are just working for a paycheck and nothing else. They really do not have a strong connection with your business and just put in their time, then go home.

As these types of workers do not have much of a connection with your business, this is what you have to change. One great way to do this is talk to them about what their dreams are. If you can relate to them on a regular basis and show that you care for them not just as workers but also as valuable staff members, then frequently you can turn them around by being connected with them. The more you can show that you see them as a whole person rather than just a worker bee, the higher the probability of success with this strategy.

Another thing that could be happening is that these workers just may not feel comfortable enough, or may even lack the confidence, to take the initiative. One thing you can do here is go to the worker and ask for their advice on pending decisions. The more input you get from them, the more they will be able to reach out further. Additionally, going out of your way to praise these workers will really help them to come out of their protective shells. The whole approach here is to recognize that a nonmotivated employee may just be one that has never been rewarded for this type of motivated behavior.

One additional item you might want to consider, which has worked for me, is to give these unmotivated workers more direction on their work in a positive fashion. Sometimes we just do not expect enough out of these workers, so by giving them very positive instructions, they know exactly what you are expecting, and you can then turn these workers around. Again, it just boils down to ways to improve their confidence in the workplace.

If you have given these things a fair chance and you do not see a real change in behavior, then it is time to evaluate these workers and see if you really want them on your team. Unmotivated workers can destroy the morale in the work place, and this behavior tends to be contagious.

Now go out and make certain that you are doing everything you can to ensure that each of your staff members is a motivated and contributing member of your team.

WORDS AND CUSTOMER SERVICE

"Good words are worth much and cost little."
—George Herbert (1593-1633) English clergyman, writer & metaphysical poet from *"Jacula Prudentum,"* 1651

Words have meaning, obviously, and their use has to be carefully monitored. How you treat a customer with the words you choose to speak to them has a critical effect on how the customer views your business. If you use the right words, the customer will probably feel wonderful. The wrong words alienate customers and send them to your competitors.

I was going through a bank drive-through and I was in a hurry to take money out of my account to fill my bare wallet. I had filled out the withdrawal slip ahead of time. I sent the slip to the teller in one of those transporters (if someone knows the correct name for those darn things, please let me know). Anyway, the teller gets on the intercom and announces to the whole world, "Sir, I need to see your ID." While I clearly understand the need for photo identification to protect my account, the bank teller's words made me feel as if I had done something terribly wrong. Also, it brought back memories. I hate to admit this, but when I was younger, I had received a few tickets for speeding. Of course, the policemen had always commanded, you guessed it, "Sir, I need to see your ID."

From a teller's perspective, viewing my ID was mandatory. However, her words really alienated me and may potentially offend many other customers in the future. The teller could have softened her request, saying, "Sir, in order protect your accounts, may I please see your ID." Notice how this request is not only nicer, it also really explains why the teller needs to verify your identification.

One of the things that really drives me crazy is how many times I hear people say, "No problem," after they have provided a service to me. When I thank people for providing services, it invalidates what they did if they say, "no problem." It is so much better to say, "It was my pleasure to be of service to you." Notice how this last statement is warmer and more genuine than, "No problem."

The real point of this article is that you need to pay attention to the words you and your associates speak and how you communicate with your clients and customers. Sometimes sloppiness slips into our vernacular. We must be ever vigilant for requests and responses that need to be modified to make the most of the few precious moments we spend with the people who support our businesses.

Now go out and make sure all your employees are using words that signify warmth and kindness. You can do this!

THANK YOU NOTES

"I thank you. I am not of many words, but I thank you."
—William Shakespeare from <u>Much Ado About Nothing</u>

I recently purchased a very large item. When I was suffering from buyer's remorse, I received a very kind note from the sales person thanking me for the purchase. My buyer's remorse instantly was transformed into happiness. Simply receiving a thank you note converted me from having doubts about the purchase to a "raving customer."

I think thank you notes are one of the most overlooked items for most entrepreneurs. Too many times, I see customers spend $10,000 to $20,000 without receiving a thank you note. Sure, it takes a few minutes to write these notes, but they are worth it! Each of these notes needs to be personal with the common theme of thanking customers for their purchases and of letting the customer know how much they mean to you.

Sometimes, it's just a good idea to send a thank you note to customers once a year expressing what they mean to you and your business. Thank you notes do not have to be reserved for only customers. Employees, business associates, and special people in your life (including your significant other) really appreciate receiving these notes.

I don't have customers per se, but I try to send notes when someone that I have observed has done a wonderful thing, when someone wins a very special award, when someone is promoted, when someone does something very special, and when someone goes way beyond what is expected. I just try to send these out to thank the people for going the "extra mile" to make our world a better place.

There are three some important points to remember about thank you notes. First, they should be very personal with specifics mentioned. Second, they should be brief. Third, they must be very sincere. Finally, and I can't emphasize this enough, they must be handwritten – e-mail thank you notes just won't cut it!

My champion thank you note writer is Glen Davidson who is Chairman of the Board of PATLive. He sends wonderful notes and includes a relaxing CD. Another extreme example is Nic's Toggery—they send out thank you notes to customers who have bought nothing, but just walked in one of their shops to look around.

Examples of some great thank you notes can be found in *The Thank-You Book: Hundreds of Clever, Meaningful, and Purposeful Ways to Say Thank You* by <u>Robyn Freedman Spizman</u>.

Thank you notes will improve your customer service, your employee morale, and might also improve your family relationships. Everyone wants to be thanked and appreciated.

HOW TO MAKE A WIN–WIN PRACTICE SALE

Karl Salzsieder, DVM, JD
Salzsieder Consulting and Legal Services
Kelso, WA

A win–win practice sale means the buyer and seller both win and the practice sells. It may be obvious that win–win is best, but sales are made that are not win–win if there has been an unfair price or unfair sale terms in a practice sale closing. The practice sale may be to an independent third party or to an inside person, usually an associate doctor. The practice sale can be 100% cash out from the buyer's cash savings or cash from financing. Even with cash from financing, it could be 100% cash out with no down from the buyer. This is because today's specialty lenders are willing to make those 100% loans even when veterinary practices generally have a sale price including 60% to 80% goodwill. The reason lenders make these high leverage loans is because veterinarians are a good credit risk. Losses nationally are only in the 1% to 4% range.

A practice sale can be a partial sale to an associate or a 100% sale to the associate or a third party. If the sale is a partial sale, unless the buyer has cash, the seller will have to finance the sale. Only if the seller will subordinate 100% of the practice as security to the bank, will the bank lend on a partial sale. Most banks will not lend for a partial sale.

Other than financing issues, the main win–win issues have to do with the sale price and (if it is a partial sale) with the timing of when the partial buyer may be able to purchase more shares or even to purchase controlling interest.

The next main area of issue for a buy out win–win is: was the price fair? To have a fair price the price should be the fair market value (FMV) based on a practice valuation by a practice valuator or appraiser. This person should have experience with the valuation methods used in the current market place to arrive at a practice value based on earnings. A practice valuation is to be based on the excess earnings of the practice after the seller's (and any other veterinarian's) compensation has been adjusted to a production basis with earnings set at about 22% of their production.

Another important adjustment that is commonly needed in the practice profit and loss statement, before the valuation is complete, is that the rent for the physical facility must be imputed, if needed, so that it is at fair market rent. This rent is based on any other commercial building in the same geographical area, as determined by a third party person in the real estate field.

The rest of the valuation will require the valuator to look at nonrecurring costs and other expenses sometimes listed as private expenses for automobile or excess continuing education travel or personal items taken from the practice and paid for by the practice.

The records are reviewed on a cash basis and non-cash expenses like depreciation and equipment amortization are removed. Leases for equipment are removed because it is presumed the buyer would be a cash buyer unless it is an associate buying only a minority portion. After all the adjustments are made, an excess cash earnings calculation is made. There is a deduction for return on the investment in capital that is to be invested for the tangible assets. The final excess earning is usually calculated in a growing practice by giving more credit to the more current years, by using a weighted average method for calculating the excess cash earnings that predict future earnings.

After these future cash earnings are calculated, there is an analysis of subjective risk factors made by the valuator to determine what a potential buyer's return on investment should be as compared with the risk factors. This return on investment rate, after also considering the growth rate of the practice, will allow the valuator to arrive at a capitalization rate usually in the 33.3% to 20% range resulting in a multiplier of the excess earnings being 3 to 5 for the calculation of the good will.

If the non-win–win practice sale occurs, because the practice value was not properly determined, there is a much higher likelihood that the buyer may fail or not be able to pay for the practice from proceeds of the practice earnings after paying himself an adequate compensation for being the onsite veterinarian or one of many.

In practices with a low excess cash earnings the practice value may be only computed based on a post sale cash flow basis which is heavily calculated from the loan payments that exist on closing. This method of calculating value may work in the short run for a practice purchase that is in a growing area but has much higher risk to the buyer. The above issues and terms are the important items in helping a buyer and seller arrive at a win–win practice sale and understanding how to raise the practice value.

The buyer should take the first step to begin a discussion on purchasing a practice. The buyer should with the help of an attorney draft a letter of intent. This is a multi page document that is non-binding on either party, but sets out the terms of the potential purchase, from the buyer's perspective including any pre-agreed terms from the seller.

The terms of the letter of intent include most of the terms of the subsequent binding purchase and sale agreement with the exception of some of the representations and warranties of both parties.

The letter of intent will include the time of the purchase, the price and percentage of the practice that is to be purchased and how the purchase price is to be paid. It will include the details about whether the purchase is to be a stock purchase or an asset purchase. Most buyers prefer to buy only assets so they have a tax depreciation future write off. If the practice is a corporation or LLC and the buyer is a partial buyer, they will not have a choice, but will have to purchase a specific amount of shares of the corporation or a specific number of membership units of the LLC. Depending on the price negotiations and the tax consequences to a seller, occasionally a seller may demand the sale is a stock sale even with a 100%.

Once the letter of intent is delivered to the seller, the negotiation can begin. This will result in changes to the letter of intent, hopefully resulting in agreed upon terms. These final agreed terms are then transferred to a more formal and binding purchase and sale agreement. It will almost always include a purchase subject to financing contingency. Once the purchase and sale agreement or stock sale agreement (for a corporation) or membership unit sale agreement for a LLC is finalized by signatures, it can be presented to lending institutions for soliciting financing offers from lenders.

When the offers to the buyer are received from lenders, the buyer can select one and make plans for the sale closing. Most lenders will require adequate disability insurance and life insurance on the buyer. This requirement may hold up the closing if there are any health issues with the buyer. The buyer needs to plan ahead and apply for these insurance coverages early. It may take 6 to 12 weeks to get the insurance necessary before the sale can close.

Whenever there is a sale for less than 100% of the shares, there must be an agreement that includes the following contingencies, to allow one of the owners to get out (sellout) upon one of the following trigger events. Otherwise all owners would have to sell the whole practice, while attempting to work together if possible while waiting for the sale. These major buy-sell agreement areas have to do with the following:

- When a buyer or seller just wants to get out
- When there is a disability
- When there is a marriage
- When there is a divorce
- When there is a death
- When there is a bankruptcy
- Upon retirement

It is obvious that any time there is more than one shareholder, there is always the risk that the relationship will not work out and one or the other shareholder just wants to get out because it is not working out. This should be reason enough, that there is an agreement to provide how one or the other of the shareholders shall remain and what they will pay and what terms they will use in closing that final sale to the departing shareholder. This means there must be a provision describing how the future value will be determined.

If there is a disability of one of the parties, then that party may have to get out if they are unable to continue working as a practicing veterinarian. They will need to be bought out.

If there is a marriage of an owner there needs to be an agreement spelling out whether or not there are any rights of ownership going to go to the new spouse, and if yes or no, what would be done in that situation.

If there is a divorce by an owner, there obviously are issues of whether the practicing spouse or the non-practicing spouse shall be able to remain an owner. The remaining owner (if any) needs to know how if they want would they be paid off to have their shares purchased by the remaining owners.

If there is death, it is obvious there should be a pay off to the estate. Sometimes the terms of a buy out of a veterinarian's estate, might be different than the terms for another type of buy out.

If there is a bankruptcy, by one of the shareholders, obviously there are issues of how to pay out the bankruptcy shareholder, because their money will be needed to settle the bankruptcy rather than own part of a business.

Upon retirement, a seller may want a long-term buy out to assist with retirement income.

In retirement, there are many issues about whether or not the retired person can work part-time. If they work what would the compensation be? Can they own and most importantly, can they have management or voting rights in the business if they are only working part-time or not working at all?

If all the above issues are considered there is no reason a practice sale can't be a win–win transaction and experience for all parties.

HOW TO INCREASE PRACTICE VALUE $100,000 IN 1 YEAR

Karl Salzsieder, DVM, JD
Salzsieder Consulting and Legal Services
Kelso, WA

Increasing practice value is very easy in most practices, once the practitioner understands how a practice value is determined and what changes in management will affect the bottom line. When the bottom line (also known as the earnings or practice profit on a cash basis) is increased the practice value rises markedly.

Generally today in most practices for every additional dollar added to the cash basis bottom line the practice value increases from $3 to $5. Therefore, if we set our goal to increase the practice value $100,000 in one year, all we have to do is to manage the practice so in a year's time there will be an additional $20,000 to $33,000 additional cash available at the end of the year. This is only about $2,000 to $2,750 per month.

A practice valuation is to be based on the excess earnings of the practice after the seller's (and any other veterinarian's) compensation has been adjusted to a production basis with earnings set at about 22% of their production.

Another important adjustment that is commonly needed in the practice profit and loss statement, before the valuation is complete, is that the rent for the physical facility must be imputed, if needed, so that it is at fair market rent. This rent is based on any other commercial building in the same geographical area, as determined by a third party person in the real estate field.

The rest of the valuation will require the valuator to look at nonrecurring costs and other expenses sometimes listed as private expenses for automobile or excess continuing education travel, or personal items taken from the practice and paid for by the practice.

The records are reviewed on a cash basis and non-cash expenses like depreciation and equipment amortization are removed. Leases for equipment are removed because it is presumed the buyer would be a cash buyer unless it is an associate buying only a minority portion. After all the adjustments are made, an excess cash earnings calculation is made. There is a deduction for return on the investment in capital that is to be invested for the tangible assets. The final excess earning is usually calculated in a growing practice by giving more credit to the more current years, by using a weighted average method for calculating the excess cash earnings that predict future earnings.

After these future cash earnings are calculated, there is an analysis of subjective risk factors made by the valuator to determine what a potential buyer's return on investment should be as compared to the risk factors. This return on investment rate, after also considering the growth rate of the practice, will allow the valuator to arrive at a capitalization rate usually in the 33.3% to 20% range resulting in a multiplier of the excess earnings being 3 to 5 for the calculation of the good will.

If the non-win-win practice sale occurs, because the practice value was not properly determined, there is a much higher likelihood that the buyer may fail or not be able to pay for the practice from proceeds of the practice earnings after paying himself an adequate compensation for being the onsite veterinarian or one of many.

In practices with a low excess cash earnings, the practice value may be only computed based on a post sale cash flow basis, which is heavily calculated from the loan payments that exist on closing. This method of calculating value may work in the short run for a practice purchase that is in a growing area but has much higher risk to the buyer. The above issues and terms are the important items in helping a buyer and seller arrive at a win-win practice sale and understanding how to raise the practice value.

There are many ways to manage a practice or make changes in management that will result in $2,000 to $2,750 per month additional cash to the bottom line at the end of the month. Obviously, one of those main issues is to look at pricing of individual items on the fee schedule. There is the question of whether to raise the fee or to just charge for the services that are being delivered. Every practice is unique in its pricing needs, dependent on the style of medicine that is practiced, the volume of practice, and the overhead costs and the current fee schedule. The reason that the pricing or the fee schedule is unique to a practice is because the cost for the facility, equipment and overhead costs, and the cost of outside services and staff have a unique charge for the geography where the practice is located. There are also important issues besides the price of each service. That is to deal with the medical issues of the practice. The following is a list of issues that can be managed in addition to price changes. These non-cash change items include but are not limited to the following present and historical data items of the practice:

- The quality of medicine practiced
- The acceptance or compliance of clients with doctor's recommendations
- The percentage of pets current or not, on all medical recommendations
- The number of clients using the practice including return visits
- The number of new clients coming in each week or month
- The number of pets and/or clients exiting the practice each week or month
- The hours the practice is open and available to provide the client service
- The training levels of staff presently and ongoing
- The current style of practice versus the future style to be implemented. Here we can show medical metrics (the number of injections, prescriptions, x-rays and lab tests) vary from one doctor to another and from one practice to another. This variation can be as much as three times, thus a drastic income difference.
- The cash flow of the practice versus expenses and accounts receivable, Including:

o The current team staffing levels and costs versus plan
o The current doctor quality of medicine versus plan (see metrics)
o The current doctor client contacts versus plan
o The current staff client contacts versus plan
o The current rent versus plan
o The current management costs versus plan
o The prices of services rendered, compared with costs
o The estimated costs of renovation and equipment
o The costs of the practice versus the needed net return

To further explain the effect of the above items, we will explain the minimum benchmarks to be met to maximize the bottom line.

The quality of medicine practiced determines the ultimate success of the practice relative to client satisfaction, doctor satisfaction and facility and staff utilization. The practice must offer what's best for the pet's health for each and every patient. This is the first practice protocol.

The knowledge of the clients compliance with medical recommendations, determines the potential to practice quality medicine for all pets. Our goal is for over 80% to 90% of the pets to be current to recommendations, if there is an adequate system for scheduling care and if some time payments are available to meet clients' needs.

The percentage of pets current on preventive medical care (vaccinations, stool and blood tests, etc.) recommendations, may explain client compliance or doctor and/or staff quality relative to client education or the clients' ability to pay. The existence or lack of a reminder system will also have a big effect on compliance. This compliance like above, predicts deliverable care and should be at a minimum of 80% to 90% current for our regular loyal full service clients.

The number of clients using the practice must be in line with the capacity of the facility, the number of doctors available and the staffing levels. The client count should be increasing each year. Clients should be returning to our hospital one point five to three times per year on average.

The number of new clients must at a minimum be greater than the number of exiting clients and/or patient deaths. We prefer to have a net gain of at least 10% per year in client numbers. The number of new clients will also be determined by staff, doctors and facility availability and what the practice does for get acquainted visits. New clients should be 25 to 30 or more per doctor per month.

The hours the practice is open and available to provide client service should now, depending on the location, be approaching 7 days per week at least for part of each day.

The training levels of staff must be high and always continuing with staff meetings at least every 2 weeks. In larger practices this may have to be handled by departments.

The cash flow of the practice must have a net positive value after the appropriate compensation, rent expense, staffing and purchase payments for practice or equipment replacement are made or the practice demise is near.

The team staffing levels and costs also affect the cash flow to the bottom line. Generally, the doctors should produce over $400,000 of revenue per doctor each year. This requires an average patient charge over $100.

The non-veterinary staff costs must be below 20% of practice gross revenue before taxes and benefits.

In order to improve the doctor's ability to produce more, there should be some leverage of the doctors by increasing staff utilization. The staff can take histories and do basic treatments upon the direction of the doctor. Staff should spend more time with the client and the patient than the doctors do. Generally this will average two times the doctor exposure to clients. Staff should spend 20 to 40 minutes with clients when counting check in, history taking and patient release instructions. The doctor should only spend 7 to 12 or 15 minutes with the clients on average. Some may spend 20 minutes if they do much surgery or do many discharge appointments.

The facility rent should be at the market rate. The rent rate is a factor in managing a practice and having adequate fees to cover the same. Rent should be at least one percent or less per month of the value of the facility plus triple net costs.

There should be some management expenses of 2% to 4% or gross whether they are paid to lay staff or the owners.

If the above benchmarks are followed and fees are appropriate, it should be easy to raise monthly excess cash earnings by $2,000 to $2,750 and raise practice value by $100,000.

VETERINARY TECHNICAL STAFF NEED PAY BONUSES BASED ON MEDICAL CARE AND/OR BENCHMARKS

Karl Salzsieder, DVM, JD
Salzsieder Consulting and Legal Services
Kelso, WA

Veterinary technical staff members deserve more than a fixed compensation plan. To be fair, technical staff should also include reception staff. If the veterinary profession is to adequately recruit and retain technical staff there must be some incentive compensation to keep them enthusiastic and supportive of practice growth, whether growth comes in those chaotic spurts or by gradual year-to-year growth. The veterinary technical staff must be able to be appreciated when they work harder or stay later due to the diversity of our caseload and the variability of our work schedules. The author would expect most readers would agree that the technical staff members are not over paid in any demographic or geographic setting in our profession.

Therefore, any measurement of change in a practice would certainly be a wonderful excuse to add compensation to our staff members for being part of the solutions for the occasional stressful situations. The author, over 30 years time, has lost several great veterinary technical staff persons to the nursing profession, usually for lack of compensation, prior to having more incentive compensation possibilities for staff, even though we may never be able to equal the nursing profession's compensation.

Therefore, staff members should be given incentive compensation based on the practice reaching or maintaining benchmarks preset by owners. One incentive compensation would be to pay some share of the increase in gross revenue as compared with the same period the year before. Some staff may also be able to earn incentives based on their production data.

Some choices of the incentive compensation areas the author would include are discussed below.

PRODUCTION INCENTIVES FOR INCREASED MEDICAL CARE GIVEN AND INCREASED PATIENTS SCHEDULED

- **A set amount for each blood draw by the technical staff.** Usually this should be $1 per draw given to the blood drawing staff member or it could be divided between the patient-restraining person and the blood-drawing person. The records of these blood draws can be either computerized or kept on a tabulation sheet in the treatment area.
- **A set incentive amount for a preset percentage of fully booked days by the reception staff.** Here there should be a set dollar amount or a percentage of the gross (0.5–1%) divided as follows. If the front office books all appointments 90% full or more, they get three-quarters of this amount. If they book only 80% or more they get a half of this amount, or if they book less than 70% they only get a fourth of this amount. Of course these incentives would be divided between the whole reception staff. And this would assume that the reception staff supervisor would make sure all members assisted in filling the appointment book, and possibly find some work in other departments for those who are not.
- **A set amount for meeting or exceeding a specified number of dentals per day for the dental technician staff.** In this case, depending on the hospital, one can set a minimum of 3 or 4 dentals per day and if that minimum is exceeded, then 10% of the additional dentistry revenue could go into an incentive package.

MANAGEMENT BENCHMARKS WHICH MUST BE MAINTAINED BY THE STAFF TO ASSIST IN CONTROLLING COSTS

- 5% (or some other preset amount) of the savings on labor cost, when the labor cost (before taxes and benefits) is maintained below a preset benchmark (eg, 20% of gross revenue). This incentive would be shared with all leaders working on staff schedules.
- 5% or 10% of the savings of cost of goods sold (COGS) to assist in controlling purchases and to maintain them below a preset amount (eg, 20% of gross revenue). This incentive pool of funds is shared by the inventory ordering staff. It could also be shared with those who receive or take inventory before the inventory order is made, so that the orders prevent out-of-stock inventory items.
- 10% of the increase in the hospital gross revenue over the same period one year ago. Obviously this amount is affected by not only the work and the production that is done by the doctors and staff, but also by the changes in pricing. If a hospital feels a large percentage of any increase in hospital revenue is due to price changes, rather than real growth, this percentage could be decreased or limited. Of course, it can be monitored, if there are management statistics showing client and patient counts to confirm the growth is real and not just from price increases.

A limitation should be set on all incentive compensation so that in any month when there is not an excess cash flow or profit to the practice on a cash basis (before depreciation and before payments to purchase the business or equipment), there will be no cash payment of incentives. This teaches staff that the practice must be in the black before money can be shared.

Staff are very appreciative of any incentives when paid monthly. In the author's experience, it is common for the staff to request that these extra checks (even though given at pay time) be written separately. It is assumed they spend them differently from the paycheck, possibly as fun money. It is recommended that all staff should share in the success of a practice, whether by individual efforts or by the general success of the practice's gross increasing. Your staff will appreciate your offering these above incentives as part of their compensation.

VETERINARY PRACTICE LIABILITY AUDIT

Karl Salzsieder, DVM, JD
Salzsieder Consulting and Legal Services
Kelso, WA

A practice liability audit is very important management practice that should be done at least once a year in every practice. The practice liability audit a very broad topic intended to cover the liability risks of most all practices, including issues about business entity, landlord liability risks, and many of the business and practice operation liability exposures that go on every day when a practice is open for business. Ownership risks can be decreased by the proper business entity being formed. The business entity can be a proprietorship, partnership, corporation, or limited liability company.

The proprietorship is a matter of an individual opening the doors and getting a business license. No official business entity is formed other than getting a business license. The proprietorship then has all liability passed to the owner if a risk is not covered by insurance. A partnership is the same in that all risks are passed the owners. However, a partnership is made up of two or more individuals in ownership.

The corporation is a separate business entity that when properly formed and maintained, protects the shareholders from liability of the business other than their own negligence. This is a common business entity for veterinary practices. The main issue other than the normal maintenance of corporate minutes and annual meetings and so forth is that the shareholders have to decide whether they wish the entity to be taxed as a corporation thereby having the owners get paychecks from the corporation and get dividends, or whether they desire the corporation to elect to be taxed as a partnership hence being called an S-corporation. If the shareholders decide to have an S-corporation, they do not take paychecks from the corporation but rather take distributions like owners do in the proprietorship and the partnership. The decision to elect to have a paycheck with payroll taxes and dividends for the remaining money or to be taxed as an S-corporation is a question to be deliberated between the shareholders and the CPA depending a lot on the amount of profit that is generated by the business.

A limited liability company (LLC), or (in some states) a professional limited liability company (PLLC), is equally protective of the liability exposure of a business to the shareholders or in this instance the membership unit holders. This entity protects the owners from liability except for their own negligence. The membership unit holders have the choice of whether to be taxed as a partnership or a corporation. The same rules would apply that apply if they elected to be taxed as a corporation where they could get a paycheck with payroll deductions and they could get proceeds at the end of the year as profit. If they do not elect to be taxed as a corporation, they would be taxed like a partnership and the money would flow through to the owners to be taken as distributions. At this time in our history, most new business formations for veterinary hospitals are being opened as limited liability companies.

Another ownership issue has to do with the real estate. The real estate also should be owned as a separate entity and preferably as a limited liability company to protect the owners from liabilities of the public. Certainly, the minimum recommendation is that the real estate would be separate from the veterinary business ownership even if it is the same owners. This allows for the business to pay the proper rent and set their fees accordingly to be able to afford the rent. Not only does this give a fair return on investment to the real estate owners, but it reinforces the practice management techniques to require the business to have fees high enough to pay market rate rent. When market rent is paid there will be increased practice value because that's what is imputed in a proper practice valuation. There will be increased real estate value because the return on investment value will the there and if there is a separate entity for the ownership, like an LLC, there will be less liability passing to the owners.

Other business risks should be reduced by insurance coverage and proper internal management. For insurance coverage, the main areas are in the malpractice arena and in the business, operations, liability, and fire and casualty type insurance.

In the malpractice arena, the owner should be sure to have large enough limits relative to their patients' value. They should be sure to have license board defense insurance. It should include special coverage for associates, so that each associate will be provided their separate defense attorney in addition to the hospital having their own defense attorney.

The other insurance for business and operations should include building and contents and make sure that the values are high enough on the insurance policy. Some insurance companies require 80% coverage or you will be deemed a co-insurer in a loss. If you only cover for 60% of the value you may be liable for 40% in the loss. If your insurance coverage is for 80% or more, the company will pay all the loss subject to a deductible.

There are other insurance coverages available including equipment breakdown, business income and property loss, overhead expenses, earthquake coverage, flood insurance, outdoor sign coverage, and animal loss coverage.

The animal loss coverage should include when one animal injures another, when there are stolen pets, and product liability if pet toys, leashes, etc. are sold.

There is also personal liability insurance for the client slip and fall coverage that should be maintained in every hospital. There is employer business liability to cover things that are not covered by Worker's Compensation. In the Worker's Compensation area, an issue that is not covered would be sexual harassment, which is now a high-risk exposure for employers.

Be sure there is also insurance coverage for tenants if there are any in the building and for non-owned automobiles to cover any staff members taking a business automobile usage.

In the insurance area of animal loss, be sure that you realize there is a bailment legal issue to be covered. Some jurisdictions allow mechanic or agister liens for clients not paying bills. The author recommends you never keep a pet for a bill not paid. Beyond the business and liability insurance area, one must understand there are practice protocol ways to reduce the liability exposure.

In a court of law, under malpractice, there are four elements that must be met by the plaintiff's attorney. They include duty of care, breach of that duty (where the veterinary medical standards are not met), proximate cause of the injury by the breach of the veterinarian, and lastly there has to be some damages to the plaintiff to get a settlement.

Under the duty of care, the DVM defendant must have imputed knowledge of a reasonable prudent DVM having and exercising the knowledge and skill of another member of the veterinary profession in good standing in the same or similar locality. They must have met with this knowledge the medical standard of care. The duty of care also involves getting informed consent from the owner before procedure is completed.

This informed consent means informing the client of reasonable risk associated with the recommended procedure. If the client is not adequately informed of these risks, they can be deemed to have not given proper authorization to do the work.

Another major risk area for exposure to liability, brought about by a client's complaint to the license board, would be in the area of record keeping. In keeping medical records one must realize that included in the records are all of the documentation from the appointment book through the treatment records, surgery records, DEA records, and x-rays.

When there is a complaint to the state licensing board, the records will be requested. Even if the complaint is dismissed, there commonly is found a record violation. Therefore, complete and timely records must be kept. Documentation of client communication should be included.

If there are any unorthodox or nonstandard methods of diagnosis or treatment to be provided, the medical record must include the client's written consent. If the client declines an examination and you choose to continue to treat it, note that also in the medical record that an exam was offered.

To limit the risk relative to a patient's treatment and medical records there must be a balancing of the vendor invoices regarding DEA shipments and all the usage charts for DEA and legend drugs in the hospital at least on a monthly basis.

This requires that there is a separate file for copies of invoices for the legend drugs and that these invoices can be matched to the DEA records. The DEA records should include a separate unopened inventory and a separate open inventory that then would show the surgery use or the dispensing of the legend drugs.

In following the client processing, patient examination, diagnosis and treatment, there are many risks to be concerned with. The first of course would be checking in the client and getting the accurate ownership or agency relationship. One must find out that the owner is at least 18 years of age or older and hopefully there is some confirmation of ownership; 18 years of age is required to make a binding contract.

When the pet record is created, there should be some adequate pet identification. There may be an issue of whether every pet should be scanned or not for the microchip. At least scanning may be required for stray or lost pets or emergency treatment cases.

The client needs to sign the authorization granting the veterinary hospital the right to do an examination. The examination should include all systems of the body based on a checklist and maybe even including a temperature on every pet, even if a well pet, depending on the Practice Act's specificity. In the state of Oregon a temperature being taken is required even if the condition of the pet is normal.

After the examination is complete, the doctor and/or technician must provide the recommended diagnostic steps needed. These diagnostic recommendations for testing or radiology, etc. must be explained in detail to the clients' level of understanding. If there is not adequate explanation and delivering of information then a legal authorization is not obtained. There needs to be the potential tests explained. Differential tentative diagnosis needs to be explained. There needs to be proposed or recommended treatments, either based on the current information or deferred until the laboratory results are done. The client must be given some idea of reasonable alternative treatments. Then the client can grant informed consent to proceed to the next diagnostics and possible treatments. It is always best to have the client sign especially the estimate and/or pet care health plan to confirm they have the proper information and understanding. It is also good to make a confirmed contract by having them make a deposit before the work is done.

Many of these alternative choices of diagnostics and/or treatments may be waived by the client but again should require signing of a form confirming the authorization waiver or denial. There should be forms signed and handouts given and explanations made regarding any zoonotic disease that may exist from the condition of the patient or of parasite possibilities. If all informed consent is given, all authorization is granted and the possible outcomes have been explained, your practice liabilities will be much decreased.

MOST COMMON PRACTICE ACT VIOLATIONS FROM MEDICAL RECORDS

Karl Salzsieder, DVM, JD
Salzsieder Consulting and Legal Services
Kelso, WA

The major areas associated with medical record liability for license board violations can be costly. The overall picture of what legally is part of a patient's record goes from the appointment schedule to the examination, the laboratory, the x-ray room, and all that has been performed in the treatment and surgery areas, plus information about all the time the patient was in the hospital. This should cover food offered and consumed, lodging behavior and any other body intakes or body discharges, actions and reactions.

Medical malpractice lawsuits against veterinarians are few in number currently due to the damages not being sufficient to warrant most attorneys taking the case. As most readers know this is due to the fact that the courts award damages for the loss of a pet only up to the economic value of the pet. At this time there are only a few states that have legislated some non-economic damages and those are larger when a case includes a defendant's "intentional" harm to the patient.

A malpractice case against a veterinarian is a case in negligence not requiring any intent on the part of the defendant. A case in medical malpractice requires the following four elements.

First the veterinarian has a duty of care, which is a given in doctor–patient relationships. Next the doctor must have breached that duty, and third the breach of duty must have "proximately" caused the harm. Last, as referred to above, there must be damages.

When a client calls or writes a complaint to the license board the elements of negligence in malpractice are not needed. Also no attorney is needed, so there is no cost to the client. Therefore, as consumer awareness increases (and it is with the world wide internet web) more complaints are filed with the state veterinary license boards as violations of the State's practice act. With the practice acts having broad definitions of "unprofessional conduct" and specific requirements for medical records there are numerous license board violations against veterinarians.

When a veterinary licensing board sees a complaint, they must investigate that complaint, which will include requesting copies of all records pertinent to the case. If the board sees no written documentation, incomplete or illegible records, it will be difficult for them to discern the veterinarian's intent or treatment. Most all practice acts include proper record keeping as part of the required administrative rules. So when the records are deficient and/or illegible, there will be a practice act violation, even if the complaint was without merit. Some states have over 90% of complaints that end with a records violation.

Practitioners must have a copy of the practice act from their state to confirm the required detail of records required. It may seem surprising that some states require a specific list of body systems and detail checks that every pet must incur to be deemed to have had a complete examination. In Oregon, this includes that every pet must have a temperature taken, unless of course a patient owner would waive that requirement. Good records will also require documentation of client consent for service.

Part of the owner's consent for treatment or hospital admittance or surgery for other procedures requires that the owner be informed of many different aspects of the case. This is the part of the consent that is deemed "informed" consent. To have "informed" consent, there must be information given that must be followed by getting the consent.

The information should include any information a reasonable and prudent client would consider material in making a medical care decision. This must include necessary and potential tests, diagnosis, whether differential or tentative, with the knowledge available at the time to make the proposed and recommended treatments and any reasonable alternatives that might benefit the patient.

Finally, there should be some probability of success or failure explained with each treatment that is given. When the client needs this information, they need to be informed of the purposes of the procedure, the risks of the procedure and the expected outcome. It should be noted that this information given to clients should be noted in the medical record. It must be delivered to the client at the level of the clients' ability to understand. This information made available to the client cannot just be handouts. There must be a discussion between staff persons or the doctor and the client to allow for clients' questions and to allow for some collaboration with the client that would allow them to reach a decision.

Part of this information would include the cost of the proposed treatments, the possible consequences of refusing some of the recommended treatments and the consequences of not utilizing any medical therapy. After this information is given, the client should be ready to give consent which is the actual permission for the veterinary staff to proceed. It is best to have to clients sign giving this authorization. If they refuse, then a note should still be made in the record that the information was delivered and the client accepted or declined, but refused to sign.

There should also be a plan for payment that is discussed with the client followed by the clients' agreement. This can include a minimum percentage of the plan or estimate being required for deposit and the agreement of when the final amount will be paid or the use of the available credit plan at the hospital. Further, depending on the case, clients need to be informed if there needs to be any referral to a specialist or emergency clinics for continued or follow-up care.

In addition to the information being required to inform the client, there also is a very important public health requirement issue about informing the clients of any zoonotic diseases. The most common zoonotic diseases that must be part of a veterinary practice's every day information available to clients that should be documented in the record would be about the parasite issues that are currently being disseminated by the Companion Animal Parasite Council (CAPC), an independent council that has a liaison with the US government.

In this basic parasite information, there should be information about *Toxocara* and other parasites. The CAPC is informing the public that millions of human infections of *Toxicara* larva migrans are suspected in the United States annually. CAPC wants the public to be informed on animal and human health through recommendations on diagnosis, treatment, prevention, and control of parasitic infections. The goal is to preserve and strengthen the human-animal bond while minimizing the risk of zoonotic infection.

The veterinary practice should be recommending the CAPC guidelines that "all family pets should be treated year round with broad spectrum heartworm and/or other anthelmintic that will also protect against intestinal nematodes." Further, CAPC recommends that patients get preventive flea and/or tick products the year round. CAPC further recommends that fecal examinations be conducted 2 to 4 times during the first year of life and then 1 to 2 times per year for adults depending on the patient health and lifestyle factors. CAPC recommends administering anthelmintic treatment for puppies 2, 4, 6 and 8 weeks of age plus followed by monthly preventative. They also recommend administration biweekly of anthelmintic treatment for kittens between 3 and 9 weeks of age followed by monthly preventative care. These guidelines could be deemed standards of care due to their publicity and availability. The veterinary license board defense is commonly determined, in addition to record keeping, on the basis of whether or not the practitioner met the standard of care. Standards of care are formed from references like CAPC and from what other veterinarians do in similar situations.

Any information, about zoonosis, that is delivered to the client in word and handout should be documented in the medical record. The record should also include copies of what has been given as follow-up care instructions. The record should note any attempts to contact the client for further needed consent for condition and treatment changes.

If unorthodox or nonstandard methods of diagnosis and treatment are provided the medical record, they must include the client's written consent. If the client declines an examination and you choose to continue to treat, it must be noted in the medical record that an exam was offered.

Even in urgent care situations, where maybe only emergency care is rendered, the medical record must include at a minimum:

- Name, address and phone number of the owner and/or client
- Name, number of identification and/or the number of other identification of the animal and/or group of animals
- Species, breed, age, sex and color or distinctive markings of the animal
- Beginning and ending dates of the custody of the animal.

The medical records must be contemporaneous and never have erasers. If an error is made it is okay to write an addendum. If the records are electronic they must have a lock-up (security) and lock-out at a non-alterable time. The original records should stay at the clinic of origination except when there is an emergency transfer for health of the pet, then the original records should be required to be returned. Records do not belong to clients even though most Practice Acts require that owners may get copies, even if there is a fee.

Another major area that can be a serious license threat, whether before the license board or directly before the DEA are the controlled substances records. First of all, every veterinarian working in a practice should have their own DEA license. This should include owners, associates and relief veterinarians. The DEA records should be kept specifically to show all shipments received and all dispensing of the controlled substances. This means vendors, shipping slips and invoices should be kept separate from the billing department so that an inventory can be balanced based on invoices and receipts versus the legend drug inventory in stock at any given time. These would have to include an "unopened record" of controlled drugs received and the controlled drugs dispensed to a patient or to other departments of the hospital when they are "opened". This would be the opened DEA drug inventory record that can show the controlled substances that were used in surgery or dispensed through the pharmacy. These records that are kept of opened drugs must include the client's name, the pet's name, the quantity used, the date used, the user and the wasted amount. All of these inventories should be balanced weekly or no later than monthly to show the remaining inventory that should balance with the received inventory minus the used inventory. There should be no greater than 10% loss on injectables without some special explanation.

A small list of items should be excluded from medical records. Do not include in the patient's record any derogatory statements about any clients, patients, and/or other doctors—no negative notes about the owner,s personality, credit rating, chemical addictions, or other personal data. There should be no records about any equipment malfunctions or deficiencies in the hospital related to a particular case. Most of these issues may be suspected but not completely confirmed without a service technician making the finding.

Medical records are a major component in practice act violations that come before the veterinary license boards in all states. When a client complains to the license board, the medical record is always part of the investigation to confirm the doctor's intent or actions taken and to see whether they match the complaint from the client. A good medical record is not only a prevention of liability before the practice act, but also a good defense to offset some of the false claims made by clients against veterinarians to the veterinary license board.

LEGAL CODE OR EMPLOYEE CODE OF HONOR

Karl Salzsieder, DVM, JD
Salzsieder Consulting and Legal Services
Kelso, WA

Staff management can be a fun cooperative project or it can be a daily drudgery depending on the cooperation and staff participation in discussions and agreements on the staff attitude and behavior or some would say "corporate culture." Staff culture can be affected by staff participation in drafting a hospital code of honor for acceptable behavior. Without a staff developed code of honor, the negative interactions will continue to deteriorate the morale or staff culture over time as the staff grows and is required to live and work through stressful times in the work place.

If there is not a code of honor, all any practice has for behavior guidelines or minimum standards is the inherent abilities and backgrounds of the team members and the other minimum standards as spelled out in the law. This is not to say there are not some super staff teams that may do well without the time and effort spent to develop the code of honor. But usually those consistently positive teams would be small staff teams, where there may be some natural leaders that uphold a given standard and set the example, while others follow without a plan.

This article includes employee law review and methods and contents of ideas to help the hospital develop an employee code of honor that establishes minimum standards of behavior for team members and doctors to use daily in respecting and interacting with each other. The team members should strive to include at least 10 minimum behavior traits they can agree on that they would like to maintain as characteristics of their team.

Usually the traits should center around respect, honesty, timeliness, accountability, and the golden rule of treating others as they would want to be treated. The code of honor should be printed and posted in staff areas, so all can see and review daily as they pass by the posting. With this standard and posting, staff members can hold each other accountable for those characteristics in each other.

If a staff is left to only live by the law, there certainly are minimum standards of not having theft, assault, or sexual harassment, but these are not self-drafted, or necessarily bought into by team members, hence there is likely to be much less holding each other accountable for them, or more importantly for the higher standards of character desired.

Without the code of honor, the standards of behavior may be set to the minimum standards of the law. The minimum laws to be upheld in the office would be including at least the following:

- Theft must be prohibited. The code of honor would include honesty as a minimum standard. Veterinary hospitals have the right to screen and check references for honesty in staff members. If they do not check for this trait, they are not upholding the requirements of the doctors as DEA license holders, which are required for the clients and the hospital operations.
- Assault must be prohibited. That's the law. But even though assault can be an attack under the law, it can also be a threat of "substantial harm." That means threats alone are not an assault, but a threat combined with the suggestion an attack is likely to occur is an assault.
- If there is an honor code standard for treating staff members with respect in words and staff members agree to avoid all gossiping, then threats would not be acceptable behavior between staff members.
- Staff members should not be defamed under the law. That means someone cannot slander a person by speaking words that lower one's reputation. Also, someone cannot libel another person by writing something that would lower one's reputation. A code of honor could again cover this by agreeing everyone should respect others in conversation and writing. It seems simpler in the code format. Alternatively, the code could say staff members will treat each other under the golden rule of treating others like they would like to be treated.
- Laws may protect the privacy of employees, depending on the state the business is in. But most privacy laws are to protect government employees. However, if there are provisions in the code of honor that require the respect and privacy of the records and property of others, then staff members may hold others accountable for this behavior.
- There are laws that prevent discrimination in the work place. The two main laws are the Title VII of the Civil Rights Act of 1964, and the Age Discrimination restrictions in the Employment Act (ADEA). Together they ban discrimination because of race, sex, color, national origin, religion, or age (if over 40). However, a code of honor can cover this in the having respect for team members section.
- Sexual harassment is against the law. It may be under Title VII or some specific state law as a form of illegal sex discrimination. Some states treat sexual harassment as a separate offense. The big issue in most cases the violation is in the perception of the victim, which means it's a high-risk behavior. If the code of honor provides for respectful behavior to the other staff persons, this behavior problem may also be curbed.

To keep your team happy, productive, and employed long term, the author recommends you develop and use the code of honor method to develop your "corporate culture" and raise the morale in your hospital. Developing a code of honor may take months or even years in some cases, but keep this topic as an important item on the staff meeting agenda. Even once it is completed, there will need to be updates or changes as staff members change. Best of all, staff behavior will change when a code of honor is built by the team.

STAFF EMPOWERMENT (DOCTOR LEVERAGE) INCREASES VETERINARY PRACTICE SUCCESS

Karl Salzsieder, DVM, JD
Salzsieder Consulting and Legal Services
Kelso, WA

Veterinary practice success today is about relationships between the client and the veterinary practice team. The client wants a caring team of staff and doctors to take the time to do a detailed examination, diagnosis, and treatment combined with getting an adequate history. The clients want the close relationship, with the veterinary practice to build confidence that someone at the practice is caring for their pet. Yet the doctor must see 15 to 24 or more patients per day to generate the revenue to support the hospital overhead, including the high cost of the high tech equipment needed to maintain the high quality of medicine to meet the standard of care.

The benchmarks today for veterinarians show production needed at $400,000 to $500,000 per year per doctor. At 22% of production, this will generate $88,000 to $111,000 for doctor compensation. If the average patient charge is $150 per patient, the doctor will have to average 15 patients or more per day per year, including doing surgery, diagnosis, and treatment. In most practices that means some days the doctors will see 30 patients and some days the doctor will see 10 patients. On the busy days, the doctor will have to limit the contact time with the client and patients to 15 to 20 minutes maximum. In order to also complete the needed surgery, staff will have to assist seeing patients and answering clients' questions.

For the practice to be "high tech" and "high touch" or "high in caring" the increased contact time must come from our team support along with empathetic doctors. In order to continue to raise the standards of the hospital with "high tech" and its equipment requirements, the costs go up. The support staff must be able to comfort and build the client relationship while at the same time delivering high quality care and the perception of the same by the client. In the author's experience when the staff members can take a complete history before the doctor enters the examination room, the doctor can do the examination in 7 to 12 minutes and order the diagnostic tests and/or treatments and move to the next room.

To build the relationship and get client compliance, the staff person can explain the needed tests and/or treatment and answer most client questions.

To accomplish this, we must have more doctor leverage and more staff contact time with the client. This will require training of staff members and providing staff members with the tools (whether on paper or on the computer) so they can be consistent and thorough in communication with the client to get adequate history by body system and explain the needed care plan. The staff member taking the history will have a body system, history-taking sheet to discuss each system with the owner to confirm and question any abnormalities known by the owner. This history taking by the staff person will take up to 10 to 15 minutes.

After client compliance with recommended diagnostic tests and treatment is attained by the team member, there comes a time for the patient to be discharged. Here again the team members must be able and trained to deliver the discharge instructions and medications to a level of client understanding and cooperation so the patient gets the proper care. The team member going over the treatment and go home instructions usually will spend 10 to 15 minutes with the client.

Now the client has spent 20 to 30 minutes with the staff person and only 7 to 12 minutes with the doctor. Yet upon client surveys, the client perceives they have spent 30 minutes plus with the doctor.

Of course, even though the client has no perception of the time needed for the staff members to draw body samples and run the tests, these procedures are also performed by the staff members completing the patient's cycle to total another 10 to 15 minutes at the least, of contact with the patient by the staff person..

Therefore, the staff members have spent 30 to 45 minutes on each patient, while the doctor only spent the examination time of 7 to 12 minutes plus the review of tests time and client results presenting time of 10 to 12 minutes to add to a total doctor's time of 17 to 24 minutes. The staff has spent 30 to 45 minutes with the patient, which is twice or more the amount of time the doctor has spent with the client and patient. All parties win, with leveraged doctors and properly trained and empowered team members. Clients will also perceive more relationship building and a higher quality of medicine.

IS YOUR PROFIT TRICKLING AWAY?

Denise L. Tumblin, CPA
Wutchiett Tumblin and Associates
Columbus, OH

Owners of Well-Managed Practices[SM] (WellMP) realize that keeping expenses in line is an integral part of practice management. If you don't pay attention, it's easy for costs to spiral out of control and harm profitability. Careful expense management keeps your checkbook balanced and your stress lower, helps you offer high-quality care, and ensures that you receive a fair return on your investment when you sell your practice.

Most people think careful expense management means cutting expenses. Overspending certainly occurs in certain areas of practice and cutting costs is warranted. However, careful expense management also means planning the amount of spending you need to promote continued practice growth.

1. **Develop a budget.** Defining your goals for spending is the foundation for effective expense management. Use the WellMP targets and your prior year expenses as a starting point to set your expectations for the coming year (Table 1).
2. **Communicate your plan.** Once you've set expense targets, share them with the team members who'll help you achieve them. Typically this would include a hospital administrator, practice manager, bookkeeper, and the team leaders in the client and patient care departments.
3. **Measure and analyze your performance.** Create an organized, systematic approach for your monthly review of practice results. Understand which items are important for short-term cash flow and long-term sustenance and growth. Create action plans to respond to problems or opportunities that you identify during this review.
4. **Invest your time and energy managing the highest cost areas.** Good management and control of expenses in the major expense categories will have a higher bottom-line impact than great management of smaller expense categories. While all costs should be managed well, your available time is the limiting factor.

DRUGS AND SUPPLIES

It's common that this expense runs $15,000 to $30,000 high. Use these strategies to ensure a well-managed inventory. Think lean—but not too lean; you don't want the frustration of running short on commonly used items.

- Identify three to four suppliers who consistently provide the most favorable pricing.
- Don't let vendor price increases slip by—make note of current costs and adjust fees accordingly.
- Monitor your markups closely—target an average markup of 140% to 175%.
- Include a $9 to $12 dispensing fee when pricing dispensed medications that are handled.
- Carry a reasonable inventory level—target 8 to 12 inventory turns per year and take a complete physical inventory count at least annually.
- Periodically check to make sure you're billing clients for all drugs and supplies you provide during a pet's treatment.
- Implement controls to discourage inventory theft.

STAFF COSTS

Managing this expense is simple—staff members must be efficient, effective, and productive. What's not so simple is making it happen. Here are five investments that are critical to well-managed staff costs:

- **Hire right.** Find people who exemplify your practice standards. Outline the steps to fill any open position and follow them every time you hire. List the qualifications that team members must demonstrate to succeed. Offer competitive compensation packages to draw stellar candidates.
- **Invest in training.** Write a balanced training program for each position. Designate a trainer who is patient, responsible, organized and a good communicator. Set a reasonable pace so new employees don't become overwhelmed.
- **Continue staff education.** Design an annual, written continuing education schedule for all positions. Hold regular in-house CE meetings and provide opportunities for external CE to recharge your staff's enthusiasm.
- **Provide regular feedback.** Define the responsibilities of each position so team members know what you expect. Offer sincere positive reinforcement every day. Conduct timely evaluations that focus on positive, future-oriented thinking.
- **Conduct staff meetings.** Often, practice owners rely on word of mouth to spread information to staff members, creating confusion and ultimately affecting client service and patient care. Meetings create time to think together. They keep everyone on the same page, enhance consistency throughout the practice, create a more cohesive team, and reduce turnover.

Table 1. Operating Expenses as a Percentage of Total Revenue*

Variable expenses

Drugs and medical supplies	9.0%
Heartworm/flea and tick products	5.0%
Laboratory	3.2%
Diets (therapeutic and retail)	3.1%
Over the counter retail products	0.3%
Credit card fees	1.2%
Total	21.8%

Fixed expenses

Health insurance	2.2%
Workers compensation insurance	0.6%
Liability insurance	0.2%
Advertising	1.0%
Office supplies/postage	1.1%
Computer supplies/support	0.3%
Equipment repairs/maintenance	0.5%
Continuing education/travel	0.7%
Legal, accounting, & business consulting	0.8%
Payroll service	0.1%
Telephone	0.6%
Miscellaneous	0.5%
Licenses, dues and subscriptions	0.3%
Business meetings/entertainment	0.2%
Uniforms	0.1%
Total	9.0%

Staff compensation

Wages	23.2%
Payroll taxes	2.0%
Total	25.2%

Facility expense

Rent	5.5%
Utilities	0.8%
Repairs/maintenance/lawn care	0.6%
Real estate taxes	0.4%
Property insurance	0.2%
Janitorial	0.4%
Total	8.0%

*Source: Benchmarks 2007 – A Study of Well-Managed Practices^{SM} by Wutchiett Tumblin and Associates and Veterinary Economics.

VALUING YOUR PRACTICE IN TODAY'S MARKET

Denise L. Tumblin, CPA
Wutchiett Tumblin and Associates
Columbus, OH

The value of a veterinary practice is management's report card and a forewarning of most owners' future financial security.

Dr. Steve Bailey owns a two-doctor companion animal practice in Maryland. Working with his financial advisor, he recently learned that he would need to sell his practice for $1,100,000 if he is going to be financially secure when he retires in five to six years. He knows he needs to get his 'ducks in a row' to be ready for the sale. So, he's decided to have his practice valued and at the same time learn what he can do to be sure that he reaches his financial goal.

Dr. Bailey isn't alone. Even with so much riding on the outcome, many practice owners have never had their practice valued. If you had a similar amount invested in your retirement plan, wouldn't you be checking the value every day? It's time to face the facts—a practice's value is not equal to one year's gross; a practice's mere existence is no assurance of value; and the owners' management decisions control the practice's value.

So, let's look at the value of Dr. Bailey's practice and see how his everyday decisions will control the final outcome.

The excess earnings method is the standard method used to value veterinary practices. The principal components are the practice's net assets and goodwill. Net assets include working capital such as cash, accounts receivable, and drugs, hospital, and retail supplies. Values are obtained from the practice's Balance Sheet and then adjusted, as necessary, to reflect fair market value. For example, the valuator adjusts accounts receivable to reflect only collectible accounts.

Net assets also include tangible assets such as office supplies, furniture, medical and office equipment, and vehicles. They are also valued at fair market value—the price a buyer would pay for each item in its current condition. Then the balance of all outstanding debts (accounts and taxes payable, notes, leases, etc.) is subtracted to arrive at net asset value.

In companion animal Well-Managed Practices[SM], the net asset value usually represents 15% to 20% of the total value. The percent is higher in equine and food animal practices and lower in referral practices.

Goodwill makes up the balance. Its fair market value is tied directly to the practice's excess expected earnings. These are the earnings after all normal operating expenses and a fair return on the practice's net working capital and tangible assets have been paid.

The calculation of excess expected earnings begins with taxable income for the prior three years. Then, adjustments are made for:

1. Income and expenses that are on the tax return which are not included in the calculation of earnings such as interest expense and the gain on the sale of equipment.
2. Expenses that are not on the tax return which are included in the calculation of earnings such as non-deductible entertainment expense and owners' health insurance premiums.
3. Non-recurring expenses such as architectural fees, litigation costs, and repairs due to flood damage.
4. Rent expense if the rent paid is not the fair market rent.
5. Under-spending on items such as repairs and maintenance to the facilities, continuing education for doctors and staff, and services provided by the owner or the owners' family at no cost to the practice.
6. Veterinary pay to reflect fair market compensation of the services provided by all doctors—owners, associates, contractors, etc.
7. Management compensation to reflect the fair market value of the owners' management services.

The adjustments for the fair market value of veterinary and management services are two of the most critical. The adjustments do not count bodies; they consider medical services and management provided to the practice and apply a fair compensation rate to determine the practice's true cost for these services.

In companion animal practices, veterinary compensation of 18% to 24% of medical services and 2% to 12% of medical products will be applied to medical revenue to determine the fair market value for veterinary compensation. In an equine practice, compensation rates depend on how services are provided. Compensation rates for fieldwork commonly range from 25% to 28%. For outpatient services provided at the practice, the range is 22% to 24% and for surgical services, it's 18% to 22%. Fair market compensation will be higher than the actual paid if doctors have been underpaid in the short term because of cash flow concerns. It will be lower if owners have been including their owner earnings as part of their veterinary salary or when associates have been sharing in owners' profits.

The fair market value of management compensation is based on a percent of revenue, typically 2% to 3%. The total cost, plus payroll taxes, replaces amounts actually paid.

Adding and/or subtracting adjustments to income results in the valuator's estimate of the practice's expected earnings for each year. Then, the earnings are averaged using a weighted average. For example, if three years of practice operations are included, the weighting will be 3, 2, and 1. This has the effect of basing 3/6 or 50% of the goodwill value on the most recent year's earnings.

Next, the weighted average expected earnings are reduced by an investment return on net working capital and tangible assets. This is the final adjustment in the excess expected earnings calculation; these are the earnings that are capitalized to arrive at goodwill value.

The multiple used to capitalize earnings is the inverse of the return on investment in the practice's goodwill. It is based on several factors including general market risk, veterinary industry risk, and the specific risk of owning the practice being valued. In recent years, required returns on goodwill have generally ranged from 20% to 25% in companion animal and equine practices resulting in multiples ranging from 5 to 4.

Why does one practice carry more risk than another? The valuator considers several factors including the practice's expected revenue and profit growth, competitive position, demographics, management systems, fee structure, staffing, revenue from dispensing, revenue from ancillary services and products, transferability of goodwill, ability to cover expenses and debt payments, and compliance with federal and state laws.

In summary, here are the key components of the excess earnings formula:

- Revenue
  - o Normal, ongoing operating expenses
  - o Fair market value of veterinary compensation
  - o Fair market value of owners' management compensation
     = Expected earnings; calculated as a weighted average
  - o Investment return on working capital and tangible assets
     = Excess expected earnings
     x Capitalization multiple
     = Goodwill value
     + Net asset value
     = Total practice value

Now, for Dr. Bailey's practice. The value is currently $600,000:

Net Asset Value	
Accounts Receivable	$ 10,000
Inventory	20,000
Equipment	80,000
Total	$110,000
Goodwill Value	$490,000
Total Practice Value	$600,000

Dr. Bailey is $500,000 below his target of $1,100,000 and wants to learn what he can do to build value and, at the same time, continue to raise his standards of patient care. We'll need to take a close look at how his management decisions are affecting his practice's value. Since goodwill is the predominant component of value, we began with an analysis of the practice's excess earnings and capitalization multiple.

The analysis revealed that earnings are being negatively affected primarily by the practice's fee structure and low client visitation.

FEE STRUCTURE

Dr. Bailey's exam fee is $35, a reasonable level given the economics of his community. His average charge per doctor transaction (ADT) is $90. Study results show that in Well-Managed Practices[SM] the ADT averages 3.2 to 3.4 times the exam fee. This means that the doctors' ADT should be at least $112.

Dr. Bailey and I took a close look at the practice's fee schedule. The medical progress exam fee is low; we raised it to 80% of his exam fee. He isn't charging for electronic monitoring or hospitalized patient exams. Several of his fees for internal laboratory services and nonelective surgeries are low. Making these few adjustments increased the doctors' ADT to $100. This increase will provide more cash flow for doctor salaries, staff salaries, and reinvestment in new technology. Here's the impact on practice value:

ADT	Practice Value
$90	$600,000
$100	$900,000

Action Step: Is your ADT 3.2 to 3.4 times your exam fee (4.0 to 4.4 for general equine practices)? If not, look closely at your fee schedule. Are your value-based services consistent with other Well-Managed Practices[SM] in similar communities? (Refer to 2007 Benchmarks - A Study of Well-Managed Practices[SM] and the AAHA Hospital Fee Reference Guide.) Are you billing for all services provided including IV catheters, fluid pumps (daily), and medical progress exams? Low fees and unbilled services will eventually hinder your ability to provide the best medical care for your patients. As cash flow dwindles, your ability to hire the best and the brightest and keep up to date with medical technology declines.

CLIENT VISITATION

Clients visit Dr. Bailey's practice for veterinary services an average of 2.0 times per year. Study results show that in companion animal Well-Managed Practices[SM], client visitation ranges from 2.6 to 3.4 times per year.

To get a closer look at the scheduling process, I talked with Dr. Bailey's receptionists. I learned that scheduling medical progress exams is usually left to the client's discretion and there is no effort to contact clients that do not respond to written reminders. In talking with Dr. Bailey's associate, I learned that a practice philosophy for ongoing, lifelong client education has not been established; clients are not being prepared for the changes in medical care that can be expected as their pet ages. Proactive scheduling will increase client visits to 3 times a year. Here is the impact on practice value:

Visitation	Practice Value
2.0 Per year	$600,000
3.0 Per year	$800,000

Action Step: When client visitation is low, the source is frequently the client communication (or lack of) during outpatient and/or discharge appointments. Are you proactively scheduling medical progress exams or do you rely on your clients to call if they perceive that all is not well? Do you spend a few minutes of every outpatient appointment educating your client on the next steps in their pet's lifelong care? Or, are you just too busy thinking about waiting clients crowding your reception area? As a pet owner, the last thing I want is for my veterinarian to rely on my observations to diagnose my pet's recovery—what if I guess wrong?

OPERATING EXPENSES

I reviewed the practice's operating expenses and found them generally in good order. However, when reviewing the inventory purchases for the prior year, I found that the time spent each week seeking the lowest prices on each item, was eliminating the savings of lower prices.

Dr. Bailey reduced his purchase cost by working closely with fewer suppliers and negotiating lower prices on the higher volume. His annual expense dropped from 19% of medical revenue to 18% for an annual savings of $6,000.

Here's the impact on practice value:

Drug and Medical Supplies	Practice Value
22%	$600,000
21%	$628,000

Action Step: If you spend hours each week seeking the lowest prices from 8, 10 even 12 suppliers, you have tipped the cost/benefit scale. Select three or four suppliers and work with them to get the best in price and service.

STAFFING

Reviewing the capitalization multiple, Dr. Bailey's practice shows higher risk in two areas, the primary being staff turnover. The practice has significant turnover. More than half of the staff has been with the practice for less than two years.

Dr. Bailey and I looked closely at the reasons for staff turnover. Here's what we learned. The hiring process is not well defined; the interview questions change from applicant to applicant, and there is no rating system to qualify and differentiate applicants. Second, there is no written training program to help get new employees quickly up to speed. As a result, his core staff is spending hours every day training new hires, some that don't stay more than a few weeks! This is frustrating his core employees and also bright, energetic, willing-to-learn new hires who get discouraged at their inability to do things right.

I gave Dr. Bailey a training program outline for each position in his practice. It lists the training steps by day, week, and month for the first three months of employment. It also requires a check off of completion by the trainer and the trainee—both are equally responsible for the new hire's learning. It will take 12 to 18 months to see the effect of these changes. A better-trained staff will not only increase earnings, the reduction in ownership risk alone will increase the practice's capitalization multiple. Dr. Bailey and I also discussed the 'hidden expense' of staff turnover. The time spent training new employees and the duplication in staffing to cover inexperienced new people easily cost the practice $20,000 in profit and $92,000 in value.

Here's how changing the capitalization affects value:

Capitalization	Practice Value
4.0	$538,000
4.6	$600,000
5.0	$645,000

Action Step: Often practice owners expect their staff to be at their level of commitment and interest; sometimes even expecting them to know everything the first day. It just doesn't work that way. Start with a clear idea of your ideal team and then put the hiring, training, evaluating, promoting, and compensating process in writing. Knowing what you want is the first step. The second is learning how to focus on doing what only you as a veterinarian and owner can do, and training others to do the rest. The final step is getting excited about your staff's learning and growing and making it happen for their sake.

Completing all of these changes will increase the one-year value of Dr. Bailey's practice to over $1,100,000 within 18 to 24 months. Now Dr. Bailey's goal is to maintain his focus to keep his management and medical standards high and his practice operating efficiently.

You, too, have considerable control over your practice's value. If your goals include receiving fair value for your practice and providing the highest standard of medical care, focusing your attention on management as well as medicine must be part of your plan.

This information is intended to provide the reader with general guidance in practice succession matters. The materials do not constitute, and should not be treated as, appraisal, tax, or legal guidance or technique for use in any particular succession situation. Although every effort has been made to assure the accuracy of these materials, Wutchiett Tumblin and Associates does not assume any responsibility for any individual's reliance on the information presented. Each reader should independently verify all statements made in the material before applying them to a particular fact situation and should independently determine whether the succession technique is appropriate before recommending that technique to a client or implementing such a technique on behalf of a client or for the reader's own behalf.

COMMON QUESTIONS REGARDING THE VALUATION OF A VETERINARY PRACTICE

I am Hiring a Valuator to Value my Practice. What Should I Expect in Terms of the Process?

When potential clients call our office, we have a 30-minute conversation to better gauge where they are in their planning process. Questions we may discuss include: What is the purpose for the valuation? When do you want to retire? Who's buying your practice? These answers give us a better idea of how we can help accomplish their goals.

To begin, we send out an engagement letter and document request. The engagement letter states the purpose of the valuation, valuation date, and the cost to complete the work. The client is required to sign the engagement letter so the intent of our work is clear to both parties. The document request lists financial information such as tax returns, financial statements, a depreciation schedule, an equipment list, and an employee census form.

Typically, we estimate 8 to 12 weeks to complete the report. The client controls the time and cost by the accuracy and timeliness of the information we receive.

When we've received all the documents and information, we start the valuation analysis. Two to three phone calls are scheduled with the client to ask questions and discuss the current operations of the practice. These conversations are critical to the valuator's professional opinion of the practice.

Once we've finalized our analysis and conclusion, we send the client a draft report and schedule a conference to discuss in detail how we arrived at the value. This conference provides an opportunity for the owner to ask questions about the valuation and the next steps involved in the selling process. After the conference, we make any necessary changes and send out a final Valuation Report.

What Does a Valuation Report Include?
The Statement of Value
The statement of value identifies the property to be valued (assets and liabilities or stock), the name and tax structure of the practice entity, the date of the valuation, the valuation method, the purpose and intended use of the report, the primary sources of information used by the valuator in arriving at value, items that should be brought to the attention of the reader that impact the opinion of value, a statement attesting to the independence of the appraiser, and the valuator's opinion of net asset value, goodwill value, and total value.

The Net Asset Value
This section details the values of all assets and liabilities included in the opinion of value. Each asset and liability is footnoted, explaining the source of the information (for example, financial statement, computer report, representation of management) and an explanation of any adjustments made to arrive at fair market value.

The Goodwill Value
The calculation of goodwill begins with practice income and shows every adjustment the valuator makes in arriving at the earnings stream to be capitalized. Each adjustment is footnoted with an explanation of why and how it was determined. This section also includes the calculation of the fair market cost of veterinary and management services, the return on asset deduction, and application of the capitalization multiple.

Assumptions and Limiting Conditions
This section details the limiting conditions on the use of the report and on the scope of the valuator's responsibility.

Qualifications of the Appraiser
This is a summary of the appraiser's qualifications and experience relevant to valuing veterinary practices.

Certification
The appraiser certifies the opinion of value, his or her independence, the limited conditions and uses of the report, and names those involved in the preparation of the Valuation Report.

Supporting Schedules
Here we include schedules and illustrations that provide further explanation of the methods, assumptions, calculations, and values used in arriving at the opinion of value.

Does the Valuation Report Need to be Updated as of the Sale Date?
Yes. The fair market value of assets and liabilities should be updated as of the sale date. Goodwill value is constant for one year because it is based on a tax year (12 full months of operation).

For example, a practice valuation is completed as of December 31, 2006. The seller and buyer establish a sale date of June 30, 2007. At that time, the assets and liabilities are updated to reflect fair market value as of June 30, 2007. This means completing an actual count of inventory, updating collectible accounts receivable, adding 2007 equipment purchases, and subtracting practice debt.

Should I Have my Practice Valued if I'm Not Selling Right Away?
Yes. A valuation should be viewed as a planning tool. While the motive is to ensure that when it comes time to sell you will be fairly paid for the practice you have built, there is a significant fringe benefit. When you go through the valuation process, your attention is focused to the operations of your practice. Because the value of your practice is directly tied to operating efficiency, your attention will result in growing a successful Well-Managed Practice[SM].

When are Practice Valuations Mandatory?
- Buying or selling a practice
- Buying or selling a partial interest in a practice
- Writing or updating a buy/sell agreement
- Planning for financial security
- Retirement planning
- Estate planning
- Third party financing
- Mergers
- Property settlements

Why do I Need to Hire a Professional Appraiser to Value my Practice?

It is important that you hire a professional who specializes in the valuation of veterinary practices. These professionals have extensive experience in the profession and perform their work with objective, unbiased, professional judgment. Valuation is scientific, but it also includes an element of art. It is quite like a surgery. A veterinarian may follow certain procedures as he or she begins a surgery, but the art of surgical skill and experience plays an important role in the outcome. No two surgeries are the same, and the same is true for valuations.

The valuator is faced with many decisions throughout the valuation process. This is not a task for the inexperienced. An inflated value is of no use when it is rejected by all potential buyers. It can easily result in a seller receiving less than the practice is worth, as overvalued practices that remain unsold for an extended period of time grow stale like overpriced real estate. An under-valuation jeopardizes you and your family's financial security.

If no valuation is completed and the buyer relies on your representation of value, the liability for misrepresentation falls solely on your shoulders. This can lead to the potential for future litigation.

Is Taxable Income the Same Thing as Excess Earnings?

NO. Taxable income is determined for tax purposes as reported on the practice's tax return. Owners of C Corporations often express concern about their tax strategy of withdrawing all profits at year-end to avoid taxes. Because of the adjustment process, they needn't be concerned. Adjustments are made to taxable income to arrive at excess earnings including fair market rent, fair market veterinary compensation for owners and associates, and economic depreciation. Even so, it is best to keep your financial records clean. Pay personal expenses from your personal checking account and business expenses from your business checking account.

What Makes one Practice Riskier Than Another?

Let's consider staffing, the product/service mix, the facilities and equipment, and transferability as examples. When it comes to staffing, there's higher risk of ownership when staff turnover is high, wages are low, or there are inadequate or nonexistent training protocols. When you consider the service/product mix, there's higher risk associated with a higher percent of revenue coming from dispensing and retail sales and non-medical services such as boarding and grooming. Why? Because many of these products and services can be obtained from sources other than a veterinary practice. With facilities and equipment, owners face higher risk if the building is outdated or is at 100% capacity without the ability to expand because of property constraints. Transferability of goodwill becomes a higher risk in one-doctor, niche practices that are being sold to an outside buyer.

Are Practice Values Declining?

The answer is YES if you compare practice value to gross revenue. An historical review of value versus revenue shows startling changes in the age-old relationship:

	WellMP	National Average
1970s	100%	80%
1980s	110%	70%
1990s	80%	60%
2000+	85%	50%

Caution: the application of a gross revenue multiplier is not a reliable method for determining a practice's value.

The reason for the decline is that owner profit, as a percent of revenue, is declining. In 1992, the amount available to owners after all operating expense have been paid and before reinvestment was averaging 18% to 21% of revenue in general equine and companion animal Well-Managed Practices[SM]. By 2006, this percent had declined to 13% to 16%. As goodwill value is tied to profitability, the decline in profit, as a percent of revenue, has resulted in a decline in value, as a percent of revenue.

The answer is NO if you look at values in dollars. Dollar values are on the rise in Well-Managed Practices[SM]. Owners are paying closer attention to profit variables such as fees, staff retention, client retention, and advances in patient care. They are also gaining a better understanding of the concept of ownership risk and are putting management systems in place to reduce owner risk for themselves and for future buyers.

BUYING A PRACTICE: THE ISSUE IS AFFORDABILITY

Denise L. Tumblin, CPA
Wutchiett Tumblin and Associates
Columbus, OH

Dr. Laura Lars, a 1998 graduate, has been practicing in a three-doctor practice for the past 6 years and has decided it's time to strike out on her own. Earlier this year, she prepared a list of requirements to help her narrow down the type and locations of practices she would consider for purchase. She's finally found a practice that fits her needs with one exception: the purchase price is $600,000, excluding the cost of the real estate, which is $200,000 higher than she originally intended to invest. "Can I afford to buy this practice?" asks Laura. She contacted her financial advisor for assistance and here are the steps they took to answer Laura's question.

STEP 1: DEFINE AFFORDABILITY. WHAT CAN I AFFORD?

The affordability of a practice depends on three things: 1) the practice's excess earnings, the earnings available to the owner after all practices expenses have been paid, 2) the after tax cost of the annual loan payments, and 3) the personal financial resources of the buyer.

If the excess earnings are greater than the buyer's loan payments, then cash flow from sources outside of the practice will not be needed to cover the buyer's payments; the investment will pay for itself. As Dr. Lars has limited personal financial resources, this measure of affordability is the one that is most important to her.

STEP 2: SCRUTINIZE THE VALUATION REPORT

A Valuation Report prepared by an experienced, professional valuator will contain most of the financial information that Laura and her advisor will need to assess affordability. From reading the Report, Laura learns that the appraised value of $600,000 represents $100,000 of working capital and tangible assets and $500,000 of goodwill value. The excess earnings available to her after all operating expenses have been paid will be $112,000 assuming that the practice continues to produce the annual earnings that it has averaged over the past 3 years.

Laura's advisor explains that excess earnings are a crucial number in the determination of affordability. Excess earnings is the amount remaining after all practice expenses have been paid; it is the amount that she will have available to make loan payments and invest in new equipment. Practice expenses include all variable, fixed, staff compensation, associate compensation, and rent expenses and fair compensation for Laura's veterinary services and her management responsibilities. Laura looks closely at the amount specified as fair veterinary compensation. The valuator used a split-rate formula based on medical revenue produced by doctors of 24% of medical services and 8% of medicine dispensed. This is the amount that will be available to Laura and her associate as compensation for their veterinary services. Laura knows that in the last two or three years, Split-Rate Compensation™ has become a common method of compensating doctors for their veterinary services and she believes that a 24/8 split is reasonable. Management services were valued at 3% of total revenue. This will be Laura's compensation for her management responsibilities once she assumes her role as owner. After studying the practice's revenue, operation expenses, and fair compensation for veterinary services and management, she believes that the earnings remaining for her as the practice owner (her return on investment) will also be fair.

The Report also documents the valuator's opinion of the risk and the investment return to be expected by the owner of the practice. Together, these factors significantly impact the valuator's opinion of value. In fact, all other variables being equal, the higher the risk, the lower the practice's value. Laura will rely on this information in deciding if the risk in owning this practice is within her comfort zone.

STEP 3: EVALUATE PAYMENT OPTIONS

The down payment, interest rate, and repayment period determine the buyer's annual payments. Laura has several payment options. The following illustration is a sample of the options available to her for a $600,000 purchase and shows annual payments ranging from $68,000 to $144,000 (Table 1).

While option D would give Laura the lowest annual cost, it would also mean that over the life of the loan, her payments would total $1,020,000 versus $707,000 under Option A. Her advisor has cautioned her to measure affordability based on payment terms that are most realistic for the type of investment she is buying. For a veterinary practice, that means a repayment period of no more than 10 years. Then, if she selects a longer payment term (and can do so without a prepayment penalty), she'll give herself a little breathing room but still have the option of repaying the loan faster. Laura decides to base her measure of affordability using the payment terms in options A and C.

Table 1. Example of Payment Options

Payment Options	A	B	C	D
Down payment	10%	5%	10%	10%
Term	7 yrs.	5 yrs.	10 yrs.	15 yrs.
Interest rate	8%	9.5%	8.5%	9.5%
Annual payment	$101,000	$144,000	$80,000	$68,000

STEP 4: INCLUDE THE COST OF TAXES

How will income tax affect Laura's excess earnings and debt payments? Laura's advisor explains that tax liability can add significantly to her cost and must be considered in her calculation of affordability. The tax cost will depend on whether Laura buys assets or stock and, if stock, whether the stock represents a C Corporation or an S Corporation.

The interest she pays on the loan will be tax deductible if she buys assets or S Corporation stock. If she buys C Corporation stock, the amount of her interest expense deduction will be limited to the amount of her investment income. Laura, like many young veterinarians, has limited investments and buying C Corporation stock will result in little if any tax deduction for interest paid.

The second tax issue is the availability of a deduction for depreciation. When buying assets, all depreciable (or amortizable) assets such as medical equipment, office equipment, vehicles, and goodwill can be depreciated/ amortized over the life of the asset and the annual depreciation expense is generally tax deductible. When buying stock, no depreciation deduction is available.

The following illustration shows the total cash required to cover the first year's payments plus tax associated with the payments when: 1) both interest and depreciation are tax deductible, and 2) when neither deduction is available to the taxpayer. Calculations assume an effective income tax rate of 35%. Employment taxes have not been considered (Table 2).

Now Laura can compare each payment option, including taxes, with the practice's excess earnings of $112,000. She sees that her original selection of Options A and C are still the most attractive provided she buys assets and not stock. And, where else could she make an investment that will pay for itself in seven years?

Dr. Lars has learned that there is much to consider in evaluating the affordability of a practice. However, with careful planning and assistance from her financial advisor, realizing her dream of owning her own practice won't keep her awake at night! As she re-evaluates her prospects as future owner, she is confident she is making the right decision.

THE VALUATION REPORT

A Valuation Report typically includes the following:

- **The Statement of Value**
  The statement of value identifies the property to be valued (assets and liabilities or stock), the name and tax structure of the practice entity, the date of the valuation, the valuation method, the purpose and intended use of the report, the primary sources of information used by the valuator in arriving at value, items that should be brought to the attention of the reader that impact the opinion of value, a statement attesting to the independence of the appraiser, and the valuator's opinion of net asset value, goodwill value, and total value.

- **The Net Asset Value**
  This section details the values of all assets and liabilities included in the opinion of value. Each asset and liability is footnoted explaining the source of the information (for example, financial statement, computer report, representation of management, etc.) and an explanation of any adjustments made to arrive at fair market value.

- **The Goodwill Value**
- The calculation of goodwill begins with practice income and shows every adjustment made by the valuator in arriving at the earnings stream to be capitalized. Each adjustment is footnoted with an explanation of why and how it was determined. This section also includes the calculation of the fair market cost of veterinary and management services, the return on asset deduction, and application of the capitalization multiple.

- **Assumptions and Limiting Conditions**
  This sections details the limiting conditions on the use of the report and on the scope of the valuator's responsibility.

- **Qualifications of the Appraiser**
  This is a summary of the appraiser's qualifications and experience relevant to valuing veterinary practices.

Table 2. Total Cash Required to Cover the First Year's Payments Plus Tax Associated with the Payments When 1) Both Interest and Depreciation are Tax Deductible, and 2) When Neither Deduction is Available to the Taxpayer

Payment Options	A	B	C	D
Down payment	10%	5%	10%	10%
Term	7 yrs.	5 yrs.	10 yrs.	15 yrs.
Interest rate	8%	9.5%	8.5%	9.5%
Annual payment	$101,000	$144,000	$ 80,000	$ 68,000
Total Cash Required:				
Interest and depreciation Deductible	$107,000	$162,000	$ 77,000	$ 59,000
Interest and depreciation Non-deductible	$155,000	$222,000	$123,000	$105,000

- **Certification**
  The appraiser certifies the opinion of value, his or her independence, the limited conditions and uses of the report, and names those involved in the preparation of the valuation report.

- **Supporting Schedules**
  Here, schedules and illustrations that provide further explanation of the methods, assumptions, calculations, and values used in arriving at the opinion of value are included.

SELLING TO AN ASSOCIATE IS NOT AN EVENT: PREPARING FOR OWNERSHIP TRANSITION

Denise L. Tumblin, CPA
Wutchiett Tumblin and Associates
Columbus, OH

Do you have your exit strategy mapped out? Do you plan to sell a part interest to an associate, continue to practice for a few years, and then sell your remaining share of the practice? Do you have your practice valued every 2 to 3 years as part of your planning process until you're ready to sell, and then plan to present the most recent valuation report to your associate and ask for an answer in 2 to 3 weeks?

Unfortunately, the above strategy doesn't do much to prepare your associate for a buy-in. You haven't considered where the associate is in his or her thinking. And sometimes because of a lack of knowledge, training, and preparation for ownership, the associate is overwhelmed and backs off. If this sounds familiar, read on.

The sale of an interest in a veterinary practice is not an event; it is a process that starts 4, 5, even 10 years before the sale. The time frame depends on the readiness of the practice and the people involved. For example:

- Moving into a tax structure that minimizes your tax on the sale proceeds may require 10-year advance planning. The benefits of planning can mean hundreds of thousands of dollars of tax savings.
- Timing the sale to catch the peaks in value as the practice goes through its growth phases. Even 12 months can make a sizeable difference in the selling price.
- Preparing an associate for the financial responsibilities of ownership takes 5 or 6 years and is a critical part of the process, particularly if you are financing the purchase.

How do you prepare an associate for ownership? Let's look at the steps Dr. Steve Bailey and Dr. Meg Jones took to assure Meg would be ready for ownership.

Meg joined Steve's companion animal practice in Maryland two years ago. She brought 5 years of medical experience, a special interest in feline and senior wellness, and a desire to become a practice owner. Meg and the practice proved to be an excellent match. Now, she and Steve are ready to begin her transition into a management role with the intention of a 30% buy-in in the year 2008.

Steve knew developing a plan for the buy-in would give Meg time to get used to the idea of ownership, provide an opportunity for her to learn about management, and assure the buy-in would be a positive, successful experience for both. With Meg's input, Steve created the following four-year action plan.

2007
Transition Meg into Management

Steve divides his ownership responsibilities in management into five areas – Employee Development, Financial Management, Client Development, Medical Development, and Facilities, Equipment and Technology Management—and receives management compensation of 3% of total practice revenue.

Steve and the practice's management consultant identified the specific responsibilities and related implementation for each management area, and then allocated the management compensation among the five areas based on time and effort required for each:

• Employee Development	30%
• Financial Management	15%
• Client Development	30%
• Medical Development	10%
• Facilities, Equipment, & Technology Management	15%

Meg reviewed the management responsibilities for each area and agreed to assume responsibility for Medical Development. Meg's schedule will be modified to reflect 4 hours of management time: 2 hours for management planning on Tuesdays, and 2 hours for management meetings on Wednesdays.

Involve Meg in Weekly Management Meetings

Steve and Meg will conduct management meetings on Wednesdays. From 12:30 to 1:30, they will discuss short- and long-term medical and management planning for the practice, with each leading the discussion for their own management area.

Then, from 1:30 to 2:30, they will meet with the Client and Patient Care Coordinators to discuss items for consideration from the 12:30 meeting, and challenges (and recommended resolutions) the directors identify from their respective departments. Together they will make final decisions, determine how the decisions will be implemented, who will implement the decisions, and a target date for completion.

Increase Meg's Management Knowledge and Awareness

Steve and Meg mapped out the medical and management continuing education programs each would attend during 2007. Their plan included 8 to 10 hours of management programs for Meg, and she will begin reading management journals.

Compensate Meg for Management

Steve and Meg agreed the current compensation allocation for each management area was reasonable. Once Meg satisfactorily completes a 6-month management orientation period, she will begin receiving 10% of the management compensation for her management role in Medical Development.

They also plan to adopt Split-Rate Compensation[SM] for veterinary pay in 2007 and will seek guidance from their practice management consultant to create the appropriate formula for their practice.

2008

Expand Meg's Management Involvement

Steve will begin involving Meg in financial decisions such as setting fees, establishing the annual spending budget, setting salaries for staff members, etc. She will also assume responsibility for an additional area of management, Client Development. After satisfactorily completing a 6-month orientation period, Meg will receive 40% of the management compensation (10% for Medical Development and 30% for Client Development).

Enhance Meg's Involvement in Developing Current and Long-Range Practice Goals

Steve recognizes Meg has goals and visions for the practice, too, and wants to involve her in shaping the future. Developing practice goals will be part of their weekly management meetings.

First, they plan to address the potential growth areas identified by the practice's valuator during the valuation process—restructure fees, increase client visitation, reduce their annual drug expense, and improve staff retention—to accomplish their mutual goals of enhanced patient care and improved profitability.

Begin Educating Meg About Financial Statements and Production Reports

The practice's management consultant will facilitate a discussion about the purpose of and use of financial statements and production reports. Steve's goal is to guide Meg's understanding about the financial reports, the key revenue and expense components they track, and explain where to find and how to interpret the information they need to manage the practice. Then, once a month, they will discuss selected revenue and expense components during their management meeting.

Steve is aware the buy-in will be Meg's largest monetary transaction to date. He wants their advisor's help in guiding Meg to an understanding of how her cash flow will change once she becomes an owner, so she sees the benefit of ownership.

Continue Conducting Weekly Management Meetings

When conflicts come up down the road, Steve and Meg know they will be in a much better position to reconcile them favorably if they've established a pattern of meeting regularly and have learned how to communicate and co-work with each other through some of the easier challenges.

Continue to Expand Meg's Management Knowledge and Awareness

Steve and Meg's continuing education plan for 2008 plan includes 12 to 16 hours of management programs. Meg will continue to read management journals, and she and Steve will update their list of management books outside of veterinary medicine they each plan to read.

Begin Meg's Education About the Valuation Process

The practice valuator will facilitate a discussion with Steve and Meg about the valuation method that will be used to value the practice and explain the buy-in process in detail. The valuator will discuss the compensation formula for practice owners (Figure 1) and how it will affect Meg as a future owner, as well as the affordability of the buy-in.

Veterinary Compensation – Based on individual production:
- 24% of medical services
- 6% of medical products

Management Compensation – Based on total practice revenue:
- 3% of revenue
- Divided among five management areas

Owner Return – Based on ownership share:
- Amount available to owners after all operating expenses have been paid (including veterinary and management compensation)

Figure 1. Sample owner compensation formula.

2009

Share All Practice Financial and Production Reports with Meg

Steve and Meg will discuss the results of the monthly financial statements and production reports during their management meetings. Their goals—continue their progress with enhancing patient care, improving profitability, and enhancing Meg's knowledge about the business side of practice.

Discuss Financing Arrangements for Meg's Buy-in and the Portion of the Practice that will be Available for Purchase

Currently, Meg is planning to purchase 30% of the practice, and Steve will finance the deal. Meg plans to pay 10% down, with the balance financed over 7 years at prime plus 2 ½% to 3% interest, and loan payments will be paid quarterly. Meg will also explore outside financing options.

Meg and Steve will re-evaluate the portion of the practice she will purchase and the financing terms and make a final decision during this stage in the process.

Ask the Practice's Valuator to Value the Practice

Steve's valuator will value the practice at the tax year-end of December 31, 2008, which will take approximately 8 to 10 weeks. Once the valuation is complete, Meg will sign a Confidentiality Agreement, drafted by Steve's attorney, and receive a copy of the Valuation Report. She will have 4 to 6 weeks from the date of receipt to respond with her intent to proceed (or not proceed) with the purchase. Meg will ask her own advisor to review the Valuation Report on her behalf.

Determine the Owner's Compensation Formula

Currently, Steve and Meg plan to utilize Split-Rate Compensation for veterinary pay, divide the 3% management fee 60% Steve and 40% Meg, and divide owner return based on share of ownership. They will re-evaluate this and make a final decision during this stage in the process. Their valuator will prepare a written summary of Meg's after-tax/after-loan payment income.

Ask the Practice's Attorney to Draft the Buy/Sell Agreement

The attorney will guide Steve and Meg through the legal steps and documents that are necessary to complete the transaction.

Steve and Meg will also inform their tax accountants of the pending buy-in for advice about tax issues that should be addressed before the sale is completed.

Ask the Valuator to Update the Valuation Report as of the Closing Date

Steve and Meg know it will take some time for the attorney to finalize all of the necessary legal documents. They will ask their valuator to update the Valuation Report as of the closing date, which will primarily consist of an update to the Net Asset Value.

Steve and Meg are confident their four-year plan will smooth Meg's transition into ownership. They may make some revisions to the plan along the way, but the co-working relationship they develop will assure a positive, successful experience for both.

But what happens if midway through the process Steve or Meg decides the future partnership isn't a good fit? They've agreed to discuss it and determine the necessary adjustments to keep the buy-in moving forward if possible. If the differences are too great to overcome, Meg will likely leave the practice and Steve will begin the search for a new associate who has the potential for becoming an owner.

Use the above guidelines as a starting point for developing your own transition plan. Seek counsel from your advisors (practice management consultant, practice valuator, tax accountant, tax attorney, etc.) to create the best exit strategy for you and your practice.

This information is intended to provide the reader with general guidance in practice succession matters. The materials do not constitute, and should not be treated as, appraisal, tax, or legal guidance or technique for use in any particular succession situation. Although every effort has been made to assure the accuracy of these materials, Wutchiett Tumblin and Associates does not assume any responsibility for any individual's reliance on the information presented. Each reader should independently verify all statements made in the material before applying them to a particular fact situation and should independently determine whether the succession technique is appropriate before recommending that technique to a client or implementing such a technique on behalf of a client or for the reader's own behalf.

CAN YOU AFFORD NOT TO SELL TO AN ASSOCIATE?

Denise L. Tumblin, CPA
Wutchiett Tumblin and Associates
Columbus, OH

Dr. Bob Beckett is the sole owner of Heritage Veterinary Hospital, an equine and companion animal practice in the Northeast. He started the practice 15 years ago and recently expanded his facility to include a treatment and haul-in area for his equine practice. He came to the area shortly after graduation and has never regretted his decision. "I love this part of the country and feel blessed every day for making the decision to relocate here."

Dr. Beckett has three associates. Dr. Amy Rice joined the practice in 2001 and Dr. David Thompson was hired in 2005. Both are full-time associates. A third associate works only during the breeding season.

For two years, Dr. Beckett had been thinking about the advantages of sharing some of the risks and responsibilities of ownership with Dr. Rice, a hard-working, smart associate who's well-liked by clients and staff. "While I don't plan on abdicating all of my owner responsibilities, it would sure be nice to spend a little more time fly fishing in Montana knowing that someone was back at the practice maintaining momentum," says Dr. Beckett.

In September 2005, Dr. Beckett decided to offer Dr. Rice a 20% interest in the practice. When I talked with him in October, I recommended that we start the process with a valuation. I wanted to be sure that the value was where it needed to be for him to be comfortable going forward with the buy-in. He was hoping for a value of at least $1,000,000. If it came in above $1,000,000, he would take the next steps in the sale process. If it came in lower than a $1,000,000, I'd determine what areas of the practice were holding down the value and he would spend 2006 making the necessary management changes to get his value back on track. Then, with a revaluation at the end of 2006, the sale would take place in early 2007.

The practice valuation came in at $1,100,000, $100,000 higher than Dr. Beckett's minimum. So he began the next steps in the sale process.

Two weeks before the agreements were to be signed, Dr. Beckett got 'cold feet.' He'd been thinking about how his share of the owner profits will decrease once Dr. Rice becomes a partner. When Dr. Rice buys 20%, she'll start receiving 20% of the profits and she'll use these profits to make payments to Dr. Beckett. He called in a panic: "Cynthia, it looks like I'm giving Dr. Rice the money to buy my practice. Why should I sell? Wouldn't I be better off keeping the practice and all of the profits until I'm ready to leave the practice for good?"

A few days later Dr. Rice called in a panic: "Cynthia, it looks like I'm paying a lot of money to buy a 20% interest in this practice. Wouldn't I be better off leaving and starting my own practice for a lot less money?"

WHY SELL TO AN ASSOCIATE?

Why did Dr. Beckett initially decided to sell a part interest to Dr. Rice? Do his goals support his decision?

Goal #1 – The Continuation of the Practice

After starting it from scratch and seeing it grow in size and reputation year after year, Dr. Beckett wants his practice to continue to prosper. And, while there are certainly no guarantees, he'd like to think that the practice will exist 25 or even 50 years from now. He knows that no one else will run it exactly the way he does but he also knows that under Dr. Rice's direction, the practice philosophy will remain focused on what's best for the patient. He realizes that growing owners from within is the best way to accomplish this—it allows for a smooth transition over time.

Goal #2 – Financial Protection for Himself and His Family

As part of Dr. Rice's buy-in, she'll sign a Shareholder's Agreement that requires her to buy the rest of Dr. Beckett's ownership interest in the event of his death or disability. And, she'll commit to paying the fair market value. No fire sales for his practice! While he may be able to protect himself and his family in the event of his death with life insurance, the cost of disability, buy-out insurance is prohibitive.

Goal #3 – A Planned Exit Strategy

While Dr. Beckett has no plans to retire anytime soon, the Shareholder's Agreement also requires Dr. Rice to buy Dr. Beckett's remaining interest at the appraised value when he retires. He knows of colleagues who waited until retirement to sell. Some found it took years to find a buyer. Others witnessed buyers using the leverage of the seller's retirement to negotiate a deeply discounted price. He's also witnessed the winding down of a nearby practice as the seller approached retirement age, which sharply cut the value by the time the owner actually retired and sold.

"Yes, my goals do support my decision to sell a part interest to Dr. Rice," says Dr. Beckett, "But what about the immediate and long term financial impact? What is the immediate change in my income? Will I make less than I am making now?"

To start, Dr. Beckett will finance Dr. Rice's buy-in. If she has a 20% down payment, Dr. Beckett will set the interest rate at 1.5% over prime. In today's market, that's an attractive return that will increase as the prime rate increases.

The gain on the sale of Dr. Beckett's stock will be taxed at the federal, capital gains rate of 15% versus his ordinary income rate, which is 33%. His after tax income on the sale proceeds would be greater than his after tax income on owner profits of the same dollar amount.

A seller's affordability analysis shows Dr. Beckett how much better or worse off he'll be over the next seven and ten years if he sells versus keeps the 20% interest for himself.

"This was by far, the biggest eye opener for me," noted Dr. Beckett. "If owner profits grow by only 3%

more with Dr. Rice as a co-owner, in ten years, my added value from selling is $198,000 and I've accomplished my original goals." In fifteen years, his added value will grow to $792,000!

While Dr. Beckett is confident that Dr. Rice's increased involvement, commitment, and efforts as an owner will mean greater owner profits, it's wise to look at what needs to change, financially, to achieve these results. Dr. Rice's average charge per doctor transaction is currently about $12 lower than Dr. Beckett's. Reviewing their appointment schedule shows that their outpatient, inpatient, and surgery caseloads are fairly balanced. If the difference in Dr. Rice's ADT is due to missed charges, her ADT will need to increase by $2 to achieve the 9% (vs. 6%) increase in owner profits. If the difference is due to the level of care, her ADT will need to increase by $3 to $6. Is this doable?

SHOULD I BUY A PART INTEREST?

Why did Dr. Rice initially decide to buy a 20% interest in Heritage? Do her goals support her decision?

Goal #1 – A Practice Philosophy that Revolves Around What's Best for the Patient

Dr. Rice supports and values Dr. Beckett's philosophies regarding patient care, client care, and staff development. "While there are a few things I'd change if I owned the practice, maybe I should share some of my management ideas with Dr. Beckett," says Dr. Rice. "He's always been receptive to my ideas regarding patient care."

Goal #2 – A Reasonable Balance in her Personal and Practice Life

She knows that practice ownership requires a greater personal investment and that the time involved in starting her own practice would be extensive. At Heritage, the infrastructure is in place—a steady stream of patients, experienced staff, and fully equipped exam rooms, treatment areas, and surgical suites.

Also, sharing ownership allows time away from the practice and shared on-call time. This would be more challenging as a sole owner. If she starts her own practice, she'll work solo for several years until the practice grows large enough to support an associate. She knows a colleague who started his own mixed animal practice last year and his workweeks easily exceed 60 hours. She could limit her new practice to either equine or companion animal, but she really enjoys doing both.

Goal #3 – Share in the Value Created by her Efforts

She doesn't want to remain an employee forever. If Dr. Beckett doesn't want a partner, she'll begin to look elsewhere. She sees the investment value of a practice as being necessary for her future financial security and she likes the idea that the value of her interest will grow with her efforts.

"Yes, my goals support my decision to buy a part interest." says Dr. Rice, "But what about the immediate and long term financial impact? What is the immediate change in my income? Will I make less than I am making now?"

A buyer's affordability analysis helps answers Dr. Rice's questions. It can show her how her income will increase as a result of receiving her 20% share of owners' profits and her one-third share of the owners' practice management fee; how her income will decrease by the cost of her quarterly principal and interest payments; and how income taxes will affect the bottom line.

If she finances her buy-in with a 20% down payment, over seven years at prime plus 1.5%, her after tax cash flow will increase by $19,500 in seven years and more as time goes by.

Like Dr. Beckett, Dr. Rice has a vested interest in growing owner profits and practice value. Her added value as an owner of Heritage helps make her decision. In seven years, after her payments are finished, her added value grows to approximately $398,000. If she remains a 20% owner for another three years, her added value grows to $575,000. Says, Dr. Rice, "That's how associates who become new owners build value!"

As a seller, your added value over time changes based on the percent that you sell and your practice's ability to grow profits at a faster rate with co-owners than with one owner. What about your practice? Can you afford *not* to sell?

This information is intended to provide the reader with general guidance in practice succession matters. The materials do not constitute, and should not be treated as, appraisal, tax, or legal guidance or technique for use in any particular succession situation. Each reader should independently determine whether the succession technique is appropriate before recommending that technique to a client or implementing such a technique on behalf of a client or for the reader's own behalf.

HOW DO YOU KNOW WHEN YOU HAVE THE RIGHT PERSON?

Ranked in order of importance, here are the factors to weigh most heavily when considering an associate's ownership potential:

1. Personality traits
2. Interest in ownership
3. Communications skills
4. Medical skills
5. Career goals
6. Business skills

Study participants also identified the skills and attributes that are most important in screening associates for ownership:

- Philosophy compatible with owners
- Respect for co-workers, pets, and clients
- Positive interaction with staff members
- Ability and interest in educating others

- Progressive attitude: Good long-range vision with courage to stay the course; continuing efforts to advance the practice
- Integrity and high ethical standards
- Excellent practitioner
- Leadership qualities
- Financial responsibility and economic knowledge

Source: The 2004 Well Managed Practice[SM] Study: An Associate Guide by Veterinary Economics and Wutchiett Tumblin and Associates.

WHAT ARE THE TOP THREE BENEFITS OF OWNERSHIP, IN ORDER OF PRIORITY?

Owners Say

1. Voice in the direction and growth of the practice; the ability to set the standard of care and model the practice culture.
2. Greater earning power and financial return.
3. Long-term financial security; an investment that pays dividends now and provides value when you're ready to sell.

Associates Say

1. Increased income; financial gain.
2. Authority to make decisions regarding the practice's future including ethical standards, standards of care, and employees. The ability to make changes, try new things.
3. Ability to set own schedule and address quality of life issues.

Source: The 2004 Well Managed Practice[SM] Study: An Associate Guide by *Veterinary Economics* and Wutchiett Tumblin and Associates.

APPRECIATING A LONG-TERM ASSOCIATE

Denise L. Tumblin, CPA
Wutchiett Tumblin and Associates
Columbus, OH

What would you do if you won the lottery? It would be fun to *spend* some money—buy a stylish sports car or the latest plasma big screen TV for your family room. It would also be great to *invest* some of that money. What's the difference between spending and investing?

When you spend money, it's gone. While you may enjoy what you buy, whether it is food, a nice vacation, or even that fancy sports car, your purchase will be gone sooner or later, consumed or depreciated. When you invest, you're anticipating that your purchase will increase in value, or appreciate.

When you hire an associate, you're making an investment in your practice, with the expectation that the associate's value will increase. Which investment should you make? Do you need to hire a potential new owner, or does your practice need an associate who will stay with the practice long term, but not buy in?

The truth is, you may not be completely sure when you hire which you're really getting. After all, the potential associates you interview don't have a crystal ball either. But hiring a long-term associate may offer more benefits than you realize.

WEIGHING THE VALUE

Each year, the consultants with Wutchiett Tumblin and Associates and *Veterinary Economics* team up to develop a study and benchmark results to help practitioners take their businesses to the next level. In *The 2004 Well-Managed Practice Associate Management Guide*, we asked owners, "What are the most valuable benefits of having a long-term associate, and why?"

Respondents most frequently cited continuity of care, which builds and maintains strong relationships among the doctor, patient, and client. Clients feel better when the doctor caring for their beloved pets knows them and their pets, and a long-term associate brings this stability to the practice.

Owners also said they develop confidence in the associate's medical ability and people skills. Over time, with good training and mentoring, the long-term associate will hone his or her skills and provide consistent care that reflects the practice's medical philosophy. The benefit is less management, which leaves you more time for other responsibilities.

Staff members also benefit, because they know what to expect from the doctor. Like any good team, the more you practice together, the better you become at working together.

A less obvious benefit is that a long-term associate provides balance. With a dependable associate, you can afford to exercise your entrepreneurial spirit—which is likely part of the reason you became a practice owner. Rather than focusing exclusively on the day-to-day effort of providing services, you can step back and look at the practice's direction. With this big-picture view, you may find more creative solutions to persistent challenges.

Of course, long-term associates also bring unique management issues. For example, approximately 45% of owners surveyed said long-term associates do hit a salary ceiling. Their compensation peaks at around $80,000 (estimated at $90,000 to $95,000 in 2007 dollars). Owners said the primary limitation on compensation is the associate's behavior—the depth of case workup, average transaction charge and production, staff utilization, hours worked, and participation in activities that increase his or her skills and knowledge.

One way to help raise an associate's salary is to compensate the associate based on production so that his or her salary keeps pace with fee increases. You could also create opportunities to increase production by adding new services or technology to the practice.

Then consider such nonfinancial rewards as continuing education benefits, more days off, and flexible scheduling, which the associate may enjoy as much or even more than a salary increase. Quality of life improvements and consideration for the associate's priorities can buy more loyalty than any financial consideration.

SHOW YOUR APPRECIATION

Appreciation means both a rise in value or price, especially over time, and also recognition of the quality, value, significance, or magnitude of people and things according to *The American Heritage Dictionary of the English Language*, Fourth Edition. Recognizing the value of your long-term associate helps you more genuinely show your appreciation for all that he or she brings to the practice.

Responses from owners and associates alike show that to build a successful long-term relationship with an associate, owners need to nurture the relationship and communicate openly; value and respect the associate's opinions, commitment, and other contributions; and be fair, honest, and consistent.

If you're fortunate enough to have a long-term associate adding value to your practice every day, be thankful. And be sure to tell your associate how much you respect him or her and appreciate his or her contributions.

LOW OR NO? DEALING WITH LOW-COST COMPETITORS

Ernest E. Ward, Jr., DVM
Seaside Animal Care, PA and E[3] Management, Inc.
Calabash, NC

It's every practice owner's nightmare: a new clinic opens less than a mile away offering much the same services at a fraction of what you've been charging for years. You need a strategy to beat these low-ballers. The question is: what's the best way to proceed? All you need to do is drop your prices and clients will continue to flock to your doors. Even better, you reason, you'll probably gain more clients in the process. Unfortunately, this approach will deposit you in a price war. There are NO winners in a price war—only survivors. Even if you do beat your competitor and run them out of business, you may not have much of a business left when the fight is over. That doesn't sound like much of a victory.

A different approach is to simply ignore the new competitor. Keep delivering your services in the same manner at the same price and quality. Economic research clearly demonstrates that this is usually a fatal mistake. Eventually most businesses must abandon entire market segments as customers seek out the lower priced products or services offered by a rival. Does this sound remarkably similar to what has happened to the average product sales of a practice after online stores started appearing ten years ago?

Another option is to differentiate your clinic from the low-cost provider. While this approach seems simple and direct, it is surprisingly challenging for the average business or veterinary clinic. This strategy holds some promise as long as you meet several conditions discussed later.

Finally, some businesses choose to set up a low-cost business of their own to compete head-on with the new clinic. An example of this is providing a "vaccine clinic" or "low-cost spay and neuter services" on certain days to directly compete with the new clinic. This strategy, known as a "dual strategy," is also unlikely to succeed long-term unless synergy can be created between the existing business model and the new low-cost offering. In other words, it confuses the consumer or client and they tend to de-value higher-priced offerings ("If they can provide vaccines and spays cheaper, why aren't they lowering their prices on x-rays and ear cleanings?").

DO LOW-COST BUSINESSES SUCCEED?

The most important question you must ask yourself when confronting a low-cost competitor is: Are low-cost businesses a lasting, long-term threat? Can that new clinic's low-cost strategy succeed for years or more? The prevailing wisdom for several decades has been that low-cost business can't sustain itself long-term, that a business that charges significantly less than existing businesses will go bankrupt. Business experts cite the destruction of low-cost airlines after the deregulation if the industry in the 1980s. People Express, anyone? What they don't talk about is the re-emergence and success of low-cost airlines in the 1990s. Jet Blue and Southwest Airlines have become serious market share holders and, incidentally, are making lots of money.

Successful low-cost businesses employ several tactics to stay ahead of their bigger rivals: 1) they focus on a small line of goods or services; 2) they deliver that small number of services or goods or provide one benefit better than their rivals; 3) they develop super-efficient systems to keep costs low and profits high.

Trader Joe's is owned by the German retailer Aldi. They operate 4100 stores in Germany and 7500 worldwide and have hit the radar of every student of success in the past ten years. Trader Joe's advantages are straightforward and brimming with logic: 1) they stay small—Trader Joe's and Aldi's stores are generally 15,000 square feet and carry 700 products – 95% of which are store brands – compared with the 25,000-plus products that traditional supermarkets carry; 2) the chains carry none of the products that their rivals do, giving them competitive advantage and a strong negotiation platform; 3) the small number of products simplifies the supply-chain thereby decreasing shipping and inventory management costs; 4) Aldi and Trader Joe's seek outside streets and lower cost retail spaces to further decrease operating and start-up costs.

Aldi doesn't go out of its way to provide their customers with great service. In fact, Aldi was one of the first retailers to require its customers to pay a refundable deposit to use its shopping carts (you read that correctly). Shoppers must return the carts to the cart storage areas, saving employee time and energy to round them up. While they shave every corner, they get the basics of business right. They have numerous check-out lanes to minimize wait times even during the busiest times. They have the fastest scanning machines to process customers quickly.

Most retailers follow local pricing. Prices for certain items may be more at a Wal-Mart in San Francisco than in Charlotte, North Carolina. Aldi sets the same prices for all of its stores, regardless of location. This reinforces the company's image as the customer's ally in the war on outrageous prices. In fact, a 2006 poll found Aldi to be Germany's third most trusted brand, behind Siemens and BMW. Not bad for a small, cheap retailer. And they are cheap. The company adds about 8% to the supplier's cost to cover transportation, rent, marketing and other overhead costs and another 5% for employee costs. That's a 13% average mark-up compared with 28% to 30% of most European retailers. Accordingly, 89% of Germans made a trip to an Aldi at least once in 2005 and Aldi owned 20% of the German supermarket business.

So the new answer is that yes, low-cost businesses can succeed long-term, if they carefully structure their business to capture a specific consumer segment. By adhering to a strictly disciplined diet of small consumption of resources and high asset turnover rates, these businesses can create high operating margins and thus high market capitalizations. (If that bored you or sounded alien, don't fret. You're in the veterinary profession, not a trained business analyst.) On *Forbe's* richest people of 2006 list, 12 of the top 25 richest people in the world had made their fortune in the low-cost world. The list included the five heirs of Sam Walton (Wal-Mart), Aldi's two founders, IKEA's Ingvar Kamprad, Mittal Steel's owner, Michael Dell, and the founder's of Zara and Wipro (if some of those names are unfamiliar to you, remember there's a big world out there with lots of people looking for low prices) .

IS LOW-COST A STRATEGY?

Aldi, JetBlue, market capitalizations—what does that have to do with my veterinary practice in Alabama? More than you might think. For starters, this issue concerns people's behaviors and buying trends. Consumers are becoming used to paying relatively less and less for many goods and services. Sure, inflation is real but the average American (and this is occurring globally) has more buying power than ever before. The profit margins of most veterinary businesses are very low. We must become better business owners and managers if we want to do better.

In 1980, the great business expert Michael Porter wrote a seminal work on generic business-level strategies. He described "overall cost leadership, differentiation, and focus." Each of these represents, Porter argues, "a fundamentally different approach to creating and sustaining a competitive advantage." "Usually a firm must make a choice between them or it will become stuck in the middle." Ah, the dreaded "middle" management experts persistently warn us about. And rightly so. The middle is the least profitable and most vulnerable to failure. That doesn't mean that your practice will go bankrupt or you won't make any money if you're in the middle (well, you may not make very much). It just means it's not a very good business and will have little resale value if and when you decide to sell.

Porter's musings led to these often-quoted business maxims:

- "If you want to be a bad product manager, have a low-cost strategy."
  - o Customers are price sensitive and if you can deliver a product for less than your competition, you'll generate more sales. Even if you have an inferior product or service, if it's cheaper, people will buy it.
- "If you want to be a good product manager, do not pursue a low-cost strategy unless you truly are offering a commodity product that cannot be differentiated at all from the competition."
  - o Instead, you should create a strategy to differentiate your product or service from the competition and consider low price to the consumer as part of that strategy.

Unfortunately, Porter's work has been misunderstood and misinterpreted. Many people take these maxims to believe that low-cost is a strategy unto itself when, in most cases, it is not. Low-cost, in Porter's dictum, refers to the cost from the company's perspective to produce the good or service. Experts may mistakenly interpret Porter and advocate developing a strategy around providing the lowest cost to the consumer. If this occurs without regard to operating costs and profitability, the business will fail. Many have and will continue to do so. Low-cost to the consumer is not the strategy of Aldi or JetBlue, despite what they may want consumers to believe. Their objective is to provide a limited good or service as cost effectively as possible: 13% average markup for Aldi's goods and JetBlue's 4.7 cents per available seat-mile compared with 8 cents for Delta, Northwest, and United. These low-cost companies make more money and are more valuable because they are more efficient and therefore more profitable. This is what Porter meant in his generic business strategies treatise of 1980.

STEPS TO RESPONDING TO A NEW LOW-COST PROVIDER

The minute a low-cost (low price) clinic opens in your area, ask yourself: "Is the new clinic targeting a segment we don't serve or will it take away sales?" If the new clinic hopes to serve clients that no one else is currently serving or providing services or selling products you don't want to compete with, you shouldn't worry – for now. A wait-and-see approach may work, especially if you're already positioned as a premiere medical practice providing unequaled service.

If you are unsure or feel threatened by your new rival, don't launch into a price war. Don't match or try to beat the competitor's prices. The odds are against the existing company prevailing in a price war. Keep in mind that low-cost business models are designed to make money—a fact that many business owners forget when a client confronts them about matching a competitors price. In a race to the bottom, challengers always come out ahead of the existing businesses. In the late 1980s, Aldi, Dell, E*Trade and Southwest Airlines won their respective wars when Carrefour, Compaq, Fidelity, and United entered price wars that were supposed to drive their opponents out of business.

Even if you copy the critical elements of a low-cost clinic's business model, you're unable to effectively match their prices. That's because the individual elements don't matter as much as how they interact in the business. Take the example of low-cost airlines and internet-based ticketing. The low-cost players generate up to 98% of their bookings online while traditional airlines book about 20% of their trips over the internet. Internet bookings are more attractive to leisure travelers with flexible schedules and one destination than business travelers with tight schedules and multiple destinations. When traditional airlines set up internet booking systems, they experience limited uptake of the service since they don't lower their operating costs significantly. Further, online bookings work best when the airline has one type of aircraft and one class of service. It is extremely challenging for a large traditional airline to create an online experience due to the multitude of aircrafts and different levels of service. This complexity drives many customers to resort to their normal method of booking air travel through a travel agent or by calling the airline directly. Even more complicating is the fact that many of the established airlines participate in industry-wide reservation systems such as Sabre, which control how they can perform booking and which the newer companies have opted not to join. Finally, there is a large network of travel agents who have worked with specific airlines for many years who would revolt if the airline took away their ability to book trips directly. The net result is that while all of the major airlines have duplicated Southwest's and JetBlue's online booking service, they have yet to see reduced operating costs resulting in improved profits.

But you're a small veterinary clinic in Alabama, not a huge airline like Delta. What has this got to do with my business when Mrs. Jones comes in screaming that she can get her dog's pills for half of what I charge down the road? Everything, if you want to remain a financially sound business enterprise. If you think that the new clinic will take away clients and you've taken the advice of not entering a price war, what do you do? You try to differentiate your clinic to co-exist with the low-cost player. This is a consultant's favorite strategy and works, in certain situation and under certain conditions.

- Design cool products such as Apple and Bang & Olufsen
- Continually innovate in the way that Gillette and 3M do
- Offer a unique product mix like that of Whole Foods and Sharper Image
- Brand a community like Harley-Davidson and Red Bull
- Sell experiences like Four Seasons, Nordstrom and Starbucks

These tactics succeed when three additional conditions apply. First, smart companies don't solely rely on these tactics. Bang & Olufsen is able to compete with low-cost electronics manufacturers because it designs cool new products, creates an upscale brand, and invests time and money to create hip, contemporary retail outlets. As veterinarians, we should make sure our clinics reflect what today's pet owners desire: a modern, high-tech and caring staff and facility.

Second, the business must be able to persuade consumers that they need additional features or benefits and pay a premium for them. For 20 years Gillett has succeeded in selling men a "closer shave" at ever higher prices. We must market the justification for better equipment such as lasers, laparoscopic tools, and digital x-rays and commensurate higher prices to our clients. Clients who want the "closest shave" have no qualms about forking over $8 for the latest shaver—if they

believe it's worth it and their face feels smoother. You have to deliver or you fail.

Finally, you must bring costs and benefits in line before implementing it. You can't charge a lower price of your costs are too high nor can you charge a premium if the quality isn't there. This is about good business stewardship and forces you to become a better manager—or else.

If you can't differentiate yourself, you really have two options: become a low-cost business (a profitable one—albeit at a lower profitability than before the competition began) or become a smaller business. Both require radical restructuring of your business model and may take considerable time. If you become smaller, you may be able to merge with other smaller clinics. These aren't attractive options for many practice owners, but they are viable options if we are truly interested in the long-term success of our practice. The really horrible news is that we largely create these competitive pressures ourselves.

In the final analysis, there are mainly two profitable models of veterinary clinics. The first is a low volume, high quality, high cost, and high priced practice. High tech diagnostic and medical equipment is provided in an atmosphere of warmth and compassion. An emphasis on education and the total client and patient "experience" is the driving principle behind every action. Staff members often are paid a high salary with exceptional benefits and have high demands placed on their abilities. These practices serve a niche market made up of clients who value highly their pets and are willing to pay for premium service. They may or may not be financially successful; they simply value their dogs and cats and set no foreseeable limit on what they are willing to spend—as long as they get what they desire.

The second successful model is the high volume, low cost, and low price clinic. These profitable businesses focus on a limited number of services: vaccinations, preventives and products, basic surgery and medical care, traditional diagnostics and modalities. They are less concerned with the "experience" and more concerned with getting clients and patients in and out in a timely manner. Their clients also span the economic strata with the difference being these clients view veterinary services as ubiquitous and undifferentiated and aren't willing to pay any more than the lowest price in a community, even if they have to travel some distance to find it. Individual staff members and their abilities become less important in this model as opposed to having adequate numbers.

Be cautious about entering into a price-matching or price-slashing war. Ultimately, the entire profession suffers. While there are no easy solutions, by adopting a strategy, not a reaction, you have a better chance of long-term success.

WHERE DID MY STAFF GO? GETTING THE MOST OUT OF THE MINIMUM

Ernest E. Ward, Jr., DVM
Seaside Animal Care, PA and E[3] Management, Inc.
Calabash, NC

According to a 2006 University of Wisconsin study, the number one concern of all business owners was simply "finding and retaining good employees." Forget "doing a good job" or "providing the best service", it's much more basic than that. It's "I need help!" While this isn't news to anyone who has been involved with hiring employees or managing a business in the past, say, thousand years or so, it doesn't mean that we're making any progress. My goal as a business owner is to hire individuals with the best potential, exhaustively train and test them and then reward them generously for a job well done. Further, my goal is to study my business and develop systems that allow me to deliver veterinary medical services as efficiently and effectively as possible.

WHERE ARE ALL THE WORKERS?

The number one question I get as a management consultant and business owner is "where do you get such great staff?" My standard answer goes something like this: you don't "get" great staff, you develop them. Sure, we discover individuals who are phenomenal, but we don't stop there. We aim to make everyone better. Most staff members share one quality: they love dogs and cats. From that starting point we submerse them in a positive and challenging learning environment with the sole purpose of producing team members who 1) know the information we want them to know; 2) know how to effectively communicate with each other and clients; 3) fully understand what is expected of them with regards to their behavior, responsibilities and work duties. This requires significant effort on our administrative team as well as our senior staff members, but in order for us to deliver the quality of veterinary medical services we desire, we must possess a capable and caring team.

The reality is that the US job market is tightening. The number of available workers diminishes each year as baby boomers age out of the work force. Examine the latest data from 2005 presented in the table below from the US Bureau of Labor Statistics:

The labor force is declining at an alarming rate. This means our profession will be competing for fewer available employees in upcoming years.

Moreover, the face of the workforce is changing. These charts are from the 2006 Secretary of Education's Commission on the Future of Higher Education Issue

Table 2. Civilian labor force by sex, age, race, and Hispanic origin, 1984, 1994, 2004, and projected 2014

[Numbers in thousands]

Group	Level				Percent distribution				Annual growth rate (percent)		
	1984	1994	2004	2014	1984	1994	2004	2014	1984–94	1994–2004	2004–14
Total, 16 years and older	113,544	131,056	147,401	162,100	100.0	100.0	100.0	100.0	1.4	1.2	1.0
16–24	23,989	21,612	22,268	22,158	21.1	16.5	15.1	13.7	–1.0	.3	.0
25–54	74,661	93,898	102,122	105,627	65.8	71.6	69.3	65.2	2.3	.8	.3
55 and older	14,894	15,547	23,011	34,316	13.1	11.9	15.6	21.2	.4	4.0	4.1

NOTE   Age of baby boomers is 20–38 in 1984, 30–48 in 1994, 40–58 in 2004, and 50–68 in 2014.

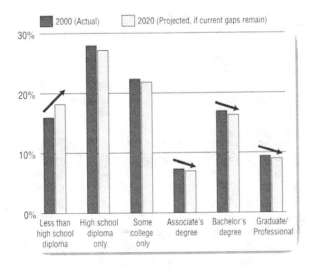

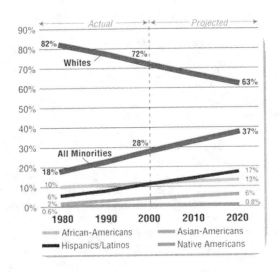

Paper. The study clearly demonstrates that minorities, especially Hispanics /Latinos, are the fastest growing segment of the US workforce. This will be a consideration in our future employment strategy and will potentially change the ways we train our staff. More interestingly, if our profession is successful in capturing increased numbers of minorities in our profession, something that we have had little success with historically, we may find that we attract increasing numbers of minority pet owners into our businesses.

The unfortunate news from the Secretary of Education's report is that fewer US citizens are acquiring advanced education. This will result in lower personal income for many Americans. At first, you may rejoice, "If there are fewer people seeking college and professional degrees, I'll have a larger applicant pool and all of this 'job shortage' stuff won't affect me." And you're right –

but in the worst possible way. What this really means is that fewer people may have enough money to pay for high quality veterinary medical care. This is definitely a frightening trend and must be closely watched. Of course, if the US economy grows at exaggerated rates, this problem won't manifest because the average income of all workers, regardless of education, will increase. Think in terms of "a rising tide floats all ships" theory. My concern, and that of many business owners, is what happens if that tide isn't as high as we wish?

Another fact to consider is how long the average employee stays at a given job. This 2006 data from the Bureau of Labor Statistics reveals that most employees stay at a job for a little less than five years. Unfortunately, this is not the case for the average veterinary practice staff member.

Median years of tenure with current employer for employed wage and salary workers by age and sex, selected years, 1996-2006

TOTAL						
20 to 24 years	1.2	1.1	1.1	1.2	1.3	1.3
25 years and over	5.0	4.7	4.7	4.7	4.9	4.9
25 to 34 years	2.8	2.7	2.6	2.7	2.9	2.9
35 to 44 years	5.3	5.0	4.8	4.6	4.9	4.9
45 to 54 years	8.3	8.1	8.2	7.6	7.7	7.3
55 to 64 years	10.2	10.1	10.0	9.9	9.6	9.3
65 years and over	8.4	7.8	9.4	8.6	9.0	8.8
Men						
20 to 24 years	1.2	1.2	1.2	1.4	1.3	1.4
25 years and over	5.3	4.9	4.9	4.9	5.1	5.0
25 to 34 years	3.0	2.8	2.7	2.8	3.0	2.9
35 to 44 years	6.1	5.5	5.3	5.0	5.2	5.1
45 to 54 years	10.1	9.4	9.5	9.1	9.6	8.1
55 to 64 years	10.5	11.2	10.2	10.2	9.8	9.5
65 years and over	8.3	7.1	9.0	8.1	8.2	8.3
Women						
20 to 24 years	1.2	1.1	1.0	1.1	1.3	1.2
25 years and over	4.7	4.4	4.4	4.4	4.7	4.8
25 to 34 years	2.7	2.5	2.5	2.5	2.8	2.8
35 to 44 years	4.8	4.5	4.3	4.2	4.5	4.6
45 to 54 years	7.0	7.2	7.3	6.5	6.4	6.7
55 to 64 years	10.0	9.6	9.9	9.6	9.2	9.2
65 years and over	8.4	8.7	9.7	9.4	9.6	9.5

US Bureau Labor Statistics September 08, 2006

EXAMINING THE STAFF REQUIREMENTS OF THE VETERINARY WORKPLACE

Regardless of your position on these issues, a simple fact remains: it's challenging to staff a veterinary hospital. The first step to improving your workplace starts with you, the owner. You must determine what the objective of your business is. "To be a veterinarian and practice high quality medicine" you instantly respond. Correct – except for that whole "business" thing. The objective of any business is to make profit. Now how that business creates profit is determined by the type of business it is: a paint store sells paint and associated accessories, a dentist cares for your teeth and so forth. In order for the enterprise to survive it must be profitable. Blah, blah, blah you think to yourself. As long as I'm paying the rent and the staff and making a comfortable living, I'm doing just fine, thank you very much. You are, but you're not a successful business owner – you're a successful job owner. The first step is that you must re-

frame and re-define what it means to own and run a successful business. It goes beyond merely having a place to call your own and being able to practice medicine. It transcends the day-to-day and has a long-term success strategy with goals and direction and a clear sense of purpose. Sit down with a pen and paper (or computer and keyboard) and write down what your top priorities in your practice are. Define what you and your practice stand for. This isn't some existential or new-age exercise, this is about discovering who you are what it is that you want to contribute to this world. No worry about grammar or spelling or if it's profound – just put it down. Then reflect on it. Some of it will be silly or even absurd but you need to focus of what makes you *you* and what makes your practice *your practice*. This exercise is beneficial to all stages of veterinary practices

The point of defining the purpose of your practice is the foundation for how you build, staff and deliver it. Too many practices from a lack of identity and the consumer isn't able to differentiate it from other available offerings. A vet is a vet is a vet.

Once you define the purpose of your practice, you can begin creating roles for your staff. In a high quality setting with a low-volume caseload and a high-touch factor, you'll need to strategically position positive, energetic staff to interface with your clients. In a high-volume, lower-touch setting, the emphasis still should be on courtesy but you'll require systems that allow for faster processing for getting clients in and out quickly. An example would be one front-desk receptionist or greeter in a low-volume clinic whose primary responsibility is to greet everyone by name and assist with billing and telephones when necessary and two to four receptionists/billing assistants in a high volume clinic whose sole job is to bill and get people in and out in a timely fashion.

The role of veterinary technicians and assistants will vary with your objective. In low-volume clinics the emphasis is on staff-to-client interaction so you'll need to have adequate well-trained team members (in the manner that you want your services delivered, not just in their ability to obtain laboratory samples or perform diagnostic tests). These staff will generally cost you more and therefore require a higher fee schedule to maintain profitability. In a high-volume clinic where low operating cost and consumer price is the objective, there is less time for detailed one-on-one interactions and an associated decrease in the need for well-trained or highly skilled employees.

The role of the veterinarian is also different based on the practice niche. In the low-volume model, the veterinarian may have ten to fifteen minutes to perform a physical examination and discuss the pet's needs in addition to another fifteen to twenty minutes of staff-to-client time. This requires a veterinarian who understands how to optimize that opportunity, doesn't needlessly pratter on about the weather or current events but really listens to a client and provides valuable tactics for preserving health. There is little time to do anything but perform physical examinations and surgery. The highly skilled staff is able to complete all but the most challenging technical tasks leaving the doctor free to spend the majority of her time with clients or in surgery. In a high-caseload practice, the veterinarian will have limited time to interact with the client; she performs her duties as efficiently and politely as possible and moves on to the next case. Since the staff may be less trained (and less costly), she may have to assist with technical procedures when the need arises.

The problems begin when veterinarians and their practices become trapped in the "middle." They share attributes with both models yet never commit exclusively to either. These practices are the least profitable and often experience the highest employee turnover because this "inbetween-ness" is terribly frustrating. Some clients demand a lot of attention and others want it for less money. Additionally, the veterinarians often work the longest hours and struggle with true contentment because they're never quite practicing in their best style. They try to serve too many masters and fail to fully please anyone, least of all themselves.

While this brief article can never provide you with specific details on how to better run your practice, you can create a process to improve your workflow. Define your practice, create processes and develop systems that allow you to consistently create your dream and build a successful business.

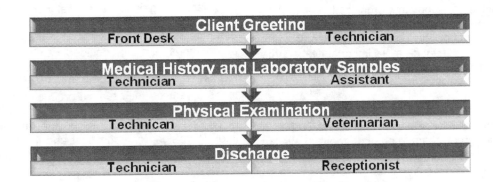

WHY WOULD ANYONE WANT TO WORK HERE?

Ernest E. Ward, Jr., DVM
Seaside Animal Care, PA and E[3] Management, Inc.
Calabash, NC

The number one question I am asked as a business owner and management consultant is "How do you get such great employees?" While there is no simple answer, the key message I try to convey is that you don't just *find* great team members, *you make great teams.* That's a critical distinction that practice owners and managers must make if they are to seize control of their businesses and develop systems to not only constantly improve their business and profitability but also retain "A" employees. As the job market tightens, we will have to make our workplaces more inviting and rewarding and increase the pain of leaving.

THE TRADITIONAL EMPLOYEE ACQUISITION AND RETENTION STRATEGIES

In the manner of "keeping up with the Joneses," the traditional technique for businesses to attract and retain top employees has been to match competitors' offers, ensuring that their wages, health care benefits, continuing education allowances are in-line with the rest of the industry. While this strategy may be effective at getting candidates in the door, it may not effectively elevate the right people into the next level—great team members who will be passionate about their work and intensely loyal to the organization and its mission.

Further, simply matching industry benchmarks and standards fails to force practices to consider what is unique about their business and values or their employees' attitudes about the organization and their work. Of course reasonable pay and benefits matter to prospective hires, as do the jobs they'll have to perform. But people also choose jobs—more importantly, become engaged with their work—on the basis of how well their personal preferences and aspirations connect with the business.

The need for a unique employee experience becomes apparent when a business recognizes that in order to retain great team members they'll have to provide more than just a paycheck. This isn't just business jargon and noise; this is a fundamental element of the most successful companies. The organization stands for something and the employees are aligned in supporting that mission. Businesses that do not have a clearly defined mission and active leadership tend to falter and experience swings in productivity, employee turnover, and profitability. When your business stands for something, you attract like-minded individuals who share your passion and these individuals are often loyal and produce exceptionally well as long as they are positively led and feel connected to the organization.

THE FIRST 90 DAYS

After the practice has clearly defined itself and the owners and managers have created a vision and roadmap for the future of the company, it's time to develop a hiring strategy. While there is no "perfect" or "right" method of hiring, there is universal agreement that the most successful businesses have a strategy. Here are three hiring and first 90 days strategies to consider (your future employees are):

As a new hire, the employee works closely with the team and when 90 days are up, the team members, not management, decide who stays or goes.

A new hire works on several new tasks or develops new skills under the close scrutiny of a manager. At the end of 90 days, the new hire must demonstrate an area that she has become qualified and exceptional in and desires to pursue that area within the company. The decision to hire or not is made by management.

The new hire undergoes extensive training during the first 90 days, learning how the practice operates. After 90 days, if the candidate is selected by management, she would further train as an apprentice under a senior staff mentor.

Each system appeals to different organizations and prospective hires. For example, people who enjoy collaborative work seek out and thrive in the first example, whereas an individual who like fast-paced and a bit of ambiguity and risk would prefer option two and perhaps feel stifled by the third option. You should develop a system that most closely reflects your philosophies and you will attract more like-minded employees. My own practice involves using a hybrid of all three that exemplifies what we stand for and how we conduct business and behave as an organization.

Let's examine some interesting real-world examples of the above new hire strategies:

Whole Foods Market

Team hiring is an essential part of the culture of Austin-based Whole Foods Market. It is explained to potential hires that each department is a small autonomous team that decides who stays or goes. After 4 weeks, the team must vote two-thirds in favor of a new hire to remain employed. Each team is evaluated 13 times a year on their team's productivity, so each team selects its members carefully. Raises and bonuses are given based on productivity so the team has a vested interest in hiring only the best and the ones with whom they believe they can work most effectively (and profitably) with.

Trilogy Software

Another Austin-based company on the rise is Trilogy software. The company was founded in 1989 and is valued at over one billion dollars today. Founder Joe Liemandt bases his hiring philosophy on allowing the new hire to experience lots of areas of the company and then decide where they feel most valuable. Additionally, during the third month of employment, the new hire must embark on a new project for the company and demonstrate that they can bring value to the company. Based on that new project and their experience with management, they are hired or let go. And its profitable: recruits' projects have produced more than $25 million in direct revenues and led to over $100 million in new business. While it's easy to initially dismiss this strategy for the veterinary industry, are we asking our new hires to innovate and create before we've "trained" or frightened the creative urge through our micromanagement?

The Container Store

The Container Store sells everything from five dollar Tupperware tubs to home storage solutions for thousands-of-dollars. Because the storage systems can be expensive and complex, the company understands that they must train their staff to give the best advice—or the customer may waste thousands of dollars and numerous hours in returns and clarifications and headaches. Their first 90 days consists of immediate and intense training. In fact, their first week includes Foundation Week—5 days dedicated to information training about their products, processes and company values. Even more impressive is the 235 hours of formal training each employee receives during their first year. This compares to the retail industry average of 7 hours. More than 40% of new employees are recommended by friends who work for the company and 97% of employees agree with the statement: "People care about each other here."

THE CHANGING ROLE OF JOBS

As our society becomes more affluent, more and more people have the luxury of allowing work to fill a variety of roles in their lives. Research published in the March 2007 Harvard Business Review identifies six types of employees based on psychodemographic characteristics (Table 1)

The benefit of these characterizations is to allow an employer to recognize that their workforce will made up of individuals who are attracted to these criteria. Therefore, if an employer is unhappy with the "type" of employee they attract, they should restructure their hiring and training and retention strategies to better entice their preferred employee type. In this manner the employee can create better alignment with her employees by designing a program for the best team member.

Southwest Airlines has consistently attracted outgoing, friendly, customer-oriented employees since its inception in 1967 (it changed its name from Air Southwest to Southwest Airlines in 1971). They understand their target market and seek out only individuals who agree with their philosophy. Even in a competitive marketplace such as the airline industry, Southwest has always put potential and attitude above

Table 1. Six Types of Employees Based on Psychodemographic Characteristics

Employee Type	Expressive Legacy	Secure Progress	Individual Expertise and Team Success
The Role of Work	*Work is about creating something with lasting value.*	*Work is about improving one's lot in life and finding a predictable path.*	*Work is about being a valuable part of a winning team.*
What Appeals and Engages	- Autonomy - Entrepreneurial opportunities - Creative opportunities - Stimulating tasks that enable continual learning and growth	- Fair, predictable rewards - Concrete compensation, solid benefits and retirement package - Stability - Structure and routine - Career training	- Collaboration - Fun - Stability and structure - Opportunity to gain competence - Opportunity to leverage personal strengths

Employee Type	Risk and Reward	Flexible Support	Low Obligation and Easy Income
The Role of Work	*Work is one of multiple opportunities to live a life filled with change and excitement.*	*Work is a source of livelihood but not yet (or not currently) a priority.*	*Work is a source of immediate economic gain.*
What Appeals and Engages	- Opportunity to improve personal finances - Flexibility - Opportunity to choose tasks and positions from a long menu of options - Open-ended tasks and approaches to getting work done	- Flexibility - Well-defined vacation and family benefits - Well-defined work routines – the ability to plug in and out of tasks and assignments with ease - Virtual, asynchronous tasks and assignments - Fun	-- Jobs that are relatively easy to come by - Well-defined work routines - Lucrative compensation and benefits packages - Stability and security - Recognition

experience and credentials. From the minute a prospective employee submits their application, every Southwest employee is eyeing them closely. Are they friendly to receptionists and support staff? Are they outgoing and quick with a smile. Each applicant must give a 3-minute speech about themselves in front of as many as 50 other applicants. But it's not just about the presenter. Southwest managers are trained to watch the applicants in the *audience* as well. Are they bored or disinterested? "We want to see how they interact with people when they think they're not being evaluated," Southwest recruiter Michael Burkhardt told Business 2.0 in April 2006. Their screening methods keep turnover low (5.5% annually) but, more importantly, helps select employees who keep customers happy, resulting in the fewest number of passenger complaints of any airline every year since 1987.

Here are some final tips for creating a great workplace:

- **Define your business** – Take the time to thoroughly determine what you and your business *really* stand for and communicate that clearly to your current and prospective employees as well as your clients

- **Understand the type of employee you desire** – By knowing what type of employee fits with your practice philosophy, you can set out to create an workplace that meets everyone's needs and attracts those who agree with your beliefs

- **Create systems for employee development** – Based on your type of business, ensure that you have in place well-understood and communicated steps to develop like-minded employees into your dream employee. This is time-intensive but allows you to produce the type of employees that will benefit your business the most.

- **Share your story** – What is your history? Why did you become a veterinarian and why do you own a practice? Sharing your story with new and prospective hires can transform the traditional employer-employee hierarchy into a team-oriented experience. People want to understand the motivation behind their leaders. If left unspoken, most employees assume that the "boss is in it for the money."

- **Praise in public, reprimand in private** – While this seems logical, all too often employers take an immediate approach to reprimand, regardless of who's around.

- **Don't be afraid to demand an employee's best** – "A" employees want, and need, to be pushed. When you observe an employee failing to perform at their potential, take them aside and simply (and non-threateningly) tell them you've noticed. Generally that's all the pushing you'll ever have to do.

- **Exemplify** – The best leaders know that they're constantly being watched by their employees. How they behave is often directly reflected in the behavior of their organization. Align what you want from your employees with how you conduct your life and you'll be surprised at how closely they mimic each other. Your practice is a direct reflection of your beliefs, behavior, and attitude. The owner has no one to blame other than themselves if they don't like the way their practice is performing, how their staff is behaving, or how their clients are treated. The buck stops somewhere—and it is always with the person or persons on top. The team is never any better than its leadership. 54% of NFL Championship WINNING teams have been coached by coaches with at least two wins (9 coaches, 22 wins, 41 Super Bowls). That means that most of the time, the best professional football team is being coached by an individual who has won their before. Who says leaders aren't important?

HEALTHY MIND, HEALTHY BODY, HEALTHY BOTTOM LINE:
IS YOUR HEALTH AFFECTING YOUR PERFORMANCE?

Ernest E. Ward, Jr., DVM
Seaside Animal Care, PA and E[3] Management, Inc.
Calabash, NC

"Good medicine equals good business." Check, heard that one a million times. "If you take care of the customer the business will take care of itself." True, true, also familiar with that one. "The key to a productive and profitable business is a healthy workforce." What's that? Run that by me again. I'm afraid I don't understand…

The business literature is littered with platitudes and clichés that fail to address the core of any activity – your ability to perform at a peak level. In fact, everything assumes you *are* performing optimally. Sorry to burst your bubble, but nothing could be further from the truth. The reality is that very few people, in any profession or lien of work, are performing at their best. Why do I say this? Part based on observation and anecdote and part based on scientific studies. The purpose of this discussion is to inspire you to carefully evaluate your personal well-being and that of those surrounding you. As employers and leaders, I believe it is our duty to maintain fitness and health and help those that we work with do the same so that we can live longer, more fulfilling and more productive lives. If you're not operating at 100%, it may be costing you more than you realize.

THE NUMBER ONE HEALTH THREAT TO OUR ECONOMY

Let's start by examining some of the facts concerning health and productivity. Since overweight/obesity is the number one health threat in this country, most of the research over the past decade has dealt with this issue.

- An estimated 65% of US adults over the age of 20 are obese or overweight and obesity now affects 29% of US workers. The cost to US employers is staggering – approximately 9% of all US healthcare costs or about $123 billion – are attributed to obesity and excess weight, and the productivity loss associated with obesity is even higher than what has been reported for tobacco use.[1] Obesity is strongly associated with chronic medical conditions such as hypertension and type 2 diabetes and ranks second, only to tobacco use, as a cause of preventable morbidity and mortality in the United States.

- Obesity is estimated to account for 43% of all healthcare spending by US businesses on coronary heart disease, hypertension, type 2 diabetes, hypercholesterolemia, stroke, gallbladder disease, osteoarthritis of the knee and endometrial cancer combined.

- Medical costs for obese employees are 77% higher than for healthy weight employees. Obesity-related disabilities cost employees $8,720 per claimant per year.

- Compared with their healthy-weight counterparts, medical costs and absenteeism costs increased on average by $917 among men and women 30 to 60 pounds overweight and by $2, 256 among men and women 60 to 100 pounds overweight.

- A BMI at risk (≥27) yields an average productivity loss of 5.79 hours per week in absenteeism, disability costs and worker productivity, which is even higher than productivity loss related to smoking. The total productivity loss per employee with an "at risk" BMI, factoring in an average salary of $17.25 per hour over 48 weeks equates to approximately $4,794 per year.

- Obese employees are more than twice as likely to experience high-level absenteeism (seven or more absences due to illness over six months) compared to low risk, healthy-weight employees.

- Labor time lost due to health reasons represents lost economic output totaling $260 billion per year.

- Employees earning $10 to $15 per hour were more likely to miss work due to illness or report that they were unable to concentrate at work because they were not feeling well or worried about a sick family member.

There are two ways to look at this data: 1) overweight/obesity issues impact our clients' productivity and earnings which potentially negatively impacts our practice revenue; 2) our employees' health status determines how productive and consistent our service delivery is. An overweight/obese workforce will likely result in reduced productivity and inefficiency leading to decreased profitability. Either analysis is generally undesirable.

TIPS AND FACTS FOR IMPROVING YOUR HEALTH

- **Ratio of Waist to Hip Size**
  - Fat that pushes your waist out in front is the most dangerous kind of fat you can have in your body.
  - Exercise reduces abdominal fat, so the more you have, the less likely it is that you get a healthy amount of exercise.
  - Measure your waist at the narrowest point and your hips at the widest (around your buttocks).
  - Divide waist by hips
  - Goal is less than 0.92
- **Know your numbers**
  - Height, weight and Body Mass Index (BMI)
  - Total cholesterol (fractionated is best)
    - (Keep total below 240; less than 200 ideal; HDL above 40 and LDL below 130)
- **Blood Pressure**
  - 120/80 or Below
  - 140/90 or Higher – Increased Risk for Heart Attack, Stroke, Kidney Failure, Organ Damage
- **Resting Heart Rate**
  - Average is 72 bpm (40–60 ideal)

Classification of Overweight and Obesity by BMI, Waist Circumference, and Associated Disease Risks

	BMI (kg/m²)	Obesity Class	Disease Risk* Relative to Normal Weight and Waist Circumference	
			Men 102 cm (40 in) or less Women 88 cm (35 in) or less	Men > 102 cm (40 in) Women > 88 cm (35 in)
Underweight	< 18.5		-	-
Normal	18.5 – 24.9		-	-
Overweight	25.0 – 29.9		Increased	High
Obesity	30.0 – 34.9	I	High	Very High
	35.0 – 39.9	II	Very High	Very High
Extreme Obesity	40.0 +	III	Extremely High	Extremely High

* Disease risk for **type 2 diabetes**, **hypertension**, and **CVD**.
\+ Increased waist circumference can also be a marker for increased risk even in persons of normal weight.
SOURCE: National Heart, Lung and Blood Institute

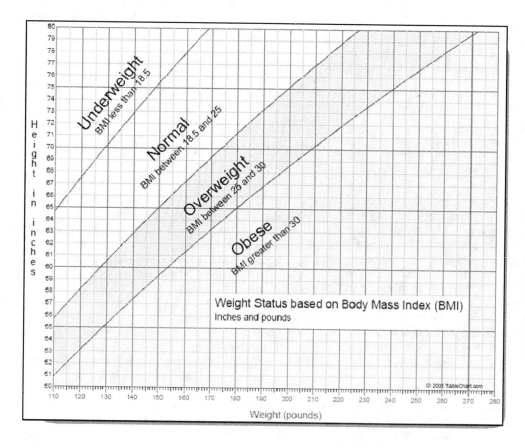

Healthy Weight Ranges According to CDC, NIH and BMI Index	
Height	Weight (lbs.)
5'0"	97-123
5'2"	104-131
5'4"	110-140
5'6"	118-148
5'8"	125-158
5'10"	132-167
6'0"	140-177

- **Mammogram, Prostate Specific Antigen (PSA), rectal exam, colonoscopy**
- **Improve Cardiovascular Health**
  - Treadmill Stress Test
  - Walk/Run 2 miles under 25 minutes
  - 40% of Obese People Report They Do "Vigorous" Exercise at least 3 times a week
  - Exercise for 30 minutes at least 5 times a week
    - Brisk walk
    - Cycling or Swimming
    - Sustained aerobic activity is the goal
    - Wear a pedometer (buy one for each employee)
- **Improve Your Flexibility**
  - Yoga, Pilates, stretching
  - More flexible individuals report decreased severity of injuries post-trauma and falls
- **Get Adequate Sleep**
  - 7–9 hours for most people
  - Do you need an alarm clock to wake up?
  - Do you require coffee to get going?

GETTING YOUR TEAM ON BOARD

Once you've decided to embark on improving your health, it's certainly acceptable to enlist your team in the effort. Good leaders understand that the team must observe the leaders undertaking change if they are going to do it themselves. Let's be honest, this type of change is both challenging and frightening for most of us. Before asking someone else to do it, first ask them to help you do it. Set a goal but avoid setting a weight objective. If you are "chasing a number" you are only dieting as opposed to changing your lifestyle and improving your health and well-being. The purpose of losing weight is to enable you to do the things you once did: run and play with your kids or grandkids, possess energy and vitality and enthusiasm, be a more productive worker and more attentive loved one. In fact, you'll probably first notice that you've forgotten just how much fun physical activity and breaking a sweat is. Many people have "normalized" their current couch-potato status and think that "this is how everyone feels." You shouldn't be feeling run-down, tired all the time, stressed out and a persistent I'm-at-my-wits-end. 25, 35, 45, 75 – they're just numbers or calendar dates. In this modern time, we are re-defining what it means to age – and yet record numbers of Americans report that they don't feel as physically able as their parents.[9] It's never too late to

seize control of your life and re-claim health and vitality. It requires dedication, hard work and honesty.

After you achieve your first fitness goal (ie, completing a 5K race), approach your team members individually and ask them to join you on your next endeavor. Offer to pay for the registration fee, buy them new running shoes, or pay for gym membership. I have utilized (and continue to do so) all three of these tactics and have found my staff to be extremely appreciative. My goal as a practice owner is to help improve my staff member's lives through training, income, motivation, and exemplifying a healthy lifestyle.

Whatever the reason you choose – economic, social, or philosophical – it pays to get healthy. I want to stay fit for my loved ones. I want to be as active and productive for as long as possible. Healthier people are fun to be around. Remember, you're only as good as you feel and how you feel is largely dictated by how fit and healthy you are.

REFERENCES

1. RAND Corporation study, March 2004.
2. The National, Heart, Lung, and blood Institute Expert Panel on the Identification, Evaluation and Treatment of Overweight and Obesity in Adults. Executive summary of the clinical guidelines on the identification, evaluation, and treatment of overweight and obesity in adults. J Am Diet Assoc. 1998; 98(10): 1178-1190.
3. Thompson D, Edelsberg J, Kinsey KL, Oster G. Estimated economic costs of obesity to US business. Am J Health Promot. 1998;12(2):120-127.
4. Finkelstein E, Fiebelkorn C, Wang G. The costs of obesity among full-time employees. Am J Health Promot. 2005;20(1):45-51.
5. Burton WN, Conti DJ, Chen CY, Schultz AB, Edington DW. The role of health risk factors and disease on worker productivity. J Occup Environ Med. 1999;41(10): 863-77.
6. $17.25 = Average hourly earnings from U.S. Bureau of Labor and Statistics Hourly wage was augmented by 25% for benefits and tax burden.
7. Tucker LA, Friedman GM. Obesity and absenteeism: an epidemiologic study of 10,825 employed adults. Am J Health Promot. 1998;12(3): 202-207.
8. Davis K, Collins S, Doty M, Ho A, Holmgren A. Health and Productivity Among US Workers. Commonwealth Fund. August 2005.
9. Gallup Poll study, 2006.

EXCELLENT CUSTOMER SERVICE—THE TEAM APPROACH

Jeffrey Werber, DVM
Century Veterinary Group
Los Angeles, CA

Did you ever stop to think why clients come to your hospital? Although we would all love to think that they come to us, sometimes passing a number of other hospitals along the way, because we are such great care providers, the truth is they are traveling to us because of the overall SERVICE and QUALITY MEDICAL CARE we provide. There are many great veterinarians around, but just being a competent clinician does not guarantee success in today's very competitive marketplace. Success will come when, in addition to excellent patient care, we start treating our clients as gold by providing excellent service!

Treating your clients (and, of course, your patients) well should be the mission of the entire "practice team." This means that it is equally as important for your receptionists, technicians, and kennel help as it is for the veterinarians on your staff. It is imperative that common practice goals are established and shared among the entire staff and that everyone is aware of his or her responsibilities. It helps to have a clear mission statement, which the staff knows, understands, and agrees with. If your hospital does not currently have a mission statement, I encourage you to sit down with your staff veterinarians and write one, then share it with the entire staff and with your clients. The truly successful team is properly trained, educated, communicates well with each other as well as the clients, and shows respect for clients and the entire staff.

Proper training is so important to the success of any hospital team. Although in most hospitals everyone has fairly clear job descriptions, I always recommend that employees become cross-trained and spend time in other areas of the hospital. Technicians should go up front on a busy morning and see what the receptionists have to work through to check patients and clients in, answer the phones, and check clients out. Likewise, receptionists should spend time in the treatment or surgery areas during the hours when most of the surgeries and procedures are being done. By doing this, everyone develops a better understanding of what their co-workers go through in a day, which will hopefully increase everyone's level of patience when things start to get a little hectic. To further promote good training and cross training, continuing education is a must—and needs to be on going. It is critical that continuing education programs be as specific as possible for any given position. A final ingredient to develop and promote mutual respect and admiration among staff members, and to resolve any potential negative issues, is regular **mandatory** staff meetings.

One of the most important aspects to a successful team and to treating clients as special as they really are, is communication. This involves communication via both character or personality traits, as well as physical traits.

Essential personality traits for successful communication are displaying compassion and care, patience, humility, having good listening skills, flexibility, and tolerance and respect for others. I can't stress enough the positive feedback I get from clients when my staff members comfort a client whose pet is very ill or has just been euthanatized. You or a team member spending a little extra time with a client in an examination room to explain all the medication they will be using on their pet, or to show them the tricks about giving pills or brushing a pet's teeth, is an invaluable service tool. When clients become a little upset about something and sometimes need to "vent," there is nothing more effective than to listen to them, humble yourself, be flexible, and try to resolve the issue at hand calmly. I have found that most clients are pretty reasonable, so when they do get upset about something, they are usually right. Arguing with a client is so counterproductive because even if you "win" (the argument), you still "lose" (the client). Do not forget one of the more basic rules of a service business—the client is (almost) always right! After listening to a client's complaint, I use some basic "active listening" techniques to acknowledge their disappointment or dissatisfaction, and, if appropriate, I will try to at least explain why or how the error occurred. Then, whether or not I agree with the client, I will apologize (either for the incident or for the way they feel about it) and ask the client what we can do to make them happy. You would be surprised that most clients actually want less to satisfy them than what you were willing to give!

When trying to resolve a conflict or help a client through a difficult time or when you simply want to impress a new client, communication's physical traits are of utmost importance. Make sure to maintain eye contact, stay relaxed, and speak slowly and clearly. It is wise to express interest and concern and make sure that any facial expressions or gestures are appropriate for the situation. Verbally, always be polite and address people by their appropriate name or title.

Although technicians and doctors should always practice these communication skills and try to keep clients' needs, feelings, and expectations in mind, the hospital team members who are under the most pressure to "perform" are your personnel working the reception area. Whereas a patient's needs are best met by veterinarians and the technical staff, the client's needs are usually in the hands of the receptionists. There is nothing more frustrating than doing a great job on a case, feeling great about it and impressing the client, only to have the client move on to "elsewhere animal hospital" because of a problem with your front staff. Of course, having a fantastic front staff with substandard medical/surgical patient care is not any better! Once your team truly realizes and believes that your clients, and not you, are the ones who actually sign your paycheck (because in essence, they do!), then you will begin to put as much emphasis on client care as you do patient care. I always tell my staff to try to treat our clients as if they are doing us a major favor by coming to us—because they are! And we can return the favor by servicing them well and taking great care of their precious pets.

Have you ever wondered why you have the clients that you do? Do your clients choose your hospital, or does your hospital choose your clients? My theory is that the clients we have are not there by accident, but rather come to us, or stay, because of the hospital and team that we've established. Think about where your clients come from and what it is about your facility, which keeps them coming back. This especially holds true once your hospital has a solid mature client base, where many of your new clients are being referred by your more established ones. Most people tend to socialize and "hang" with others who are in the same social class and circles. So, once you establish a style in how the hospital is run, how your fellow employees function together as a team, and how you treat your clients, the clients who you appeal to will most likely refer more clients just like them. Understand that once this pattern or "style" is established it can be changed, but it may not be easy. Early on, when a practice is young, new clients come to your hospital because of location, marketing tools you have chosen to implement (yellow pages, direct mailers, print advertising, ancillary pet business associations, etc.), and some word of mouth. This immature, growing client base will most likely be extremely eclectic and very "moldable." I recommend you work closely with your hospital's team and office or practice manager to carefully evaluate and determine which of the many different types of client personalities you want to see more of in the practice, and start pouring on the charm to these clients. Find out exactly what they want—and give it to them! Now, I'm not implying that you should offer inferior service to anyone, but do try to concentrate your efforts and "go the extra mile" on the clients and relationships you choose to cultivate.

Veterinary clients, like anyone else, want to be treated well. They want to know that their pets, their four-legged or winged "children," are as important to you as they are to them. They want you to care for them and their pets, to respect them, and to cater to them. If you do this well, willingly, and truly enjoy it, your clients, for the most part (there are always fickle ones everywhere), will remain very loyal and will be a great source of new referrals. Let's face it, if your clients are miserable then they will make you miserable and you'll be destined for an early burn-out. But, if you work hard as a team to attract the clients you want, practice will continue to be fun and productive!

AUTOMATION IN PRACTICE—BALANCING HI-TECH WITH WARMTH AND COMPASSION

Jeffrey Werber, DVM
Century Veterinary Group
Los Angeles, CA

The James Herriot books have done a lot to promote the beauty of our profession, although some may argue that they, in a way, hurt us a little. There's no doubt that he often oversimplified our medicine and surgery and led many to believe that we should be able to diagnose a problem just by looking at the patient, and that our recommended treatments should be just as uncomplicated. I am afraid, however, that many of our colleagues have moved to the opposite extreme, becoming almost too technical, too advanced, have too many toys, and have lost sight of why we entered this great profession in the first place. Think about it for a second. What made you choose to become a veterinarian? The money? Hardly! The great hours? Not! I hope most of us would agree that a love for our animal friends was a prime motivating factor. Do you truly love animals? I would hope so, but I know from years of experience and talking with pet companions and parents (owners), that many of us forget to show how much we love our four-legged, scaly and winged creatures. We are actually pretty lucky, because if pediatricians were caught doing to their patients what we are allowed and should be doing to ours, they would be arrested! Why is it that when I walk into an exam room with a new client and patient, and get down on the floor to smooch with and play with my new friend, the client inevitably says that she's never seen a veterinarian do that? They usually go on to say that, they would expect to see it—they just haven't. What happened to all the "animal loving" veterinarians of the world? This is the part of James Herriot that we shouldn't forget. We shouldn't forget the compassion, the warmth, and the true appreciation that we should have and display towards our animal friends.

Here's one: "I became a veterinarian because I enjoy working with animals but dislike dealing with people." Oh, that will get you far in this business! (I actually had an associate who came to me with that revelation just 6 months out of an internship, and is now doing emergency work exclusively.) When our patients become talented enough to bring themselves in to our offices and write their own checks or sign their own credit card slips, then you might do okay with this attitude. Don't hold your breath! We need to spend more time bonding to our clients as well as to our patients. We are in a terrific position in that when we do our jobs well (and there is no reason why we shouldn't) we actually receive double the appreciation. Our patients love us (at least most of them) and can't wait to come and see us again, and our clients adore us for helping their pet companions feel better and stay healthy. It is such a high to get the strokes that we get all day long—something that most people rarely get from their jobs on a day-to-day basis.

These relationships are not easy to develop. It can take years of work to achieve that level of trust and respect from a client, but once you have, it takes a lot to destroy it. I find that too many veterinarians today spend way too much time on some of the less important issues and not enough trying to develop these lasting bonds. I've recognized the importance of cultivating these bonds years ago, and in my practice, I've become the most popular veterinarian. Why? Am I the least expensive? Not even close—I have the highest per patient average and I generate the highest revenues. Do I spend more time with my clients than my associates? Not necessarily—although I try! My schedule is the most solidly booked so this is often difficult. I wish I could spend more time with them. Am I the best, most talented, or most accomplished veterinarian in my practice? No way! I have a boarded surgeon in the practice and two other associates who are much sharper than I am. So what is it? It's simple. I truly love what I do, I adore my patients and my clients (at least most of them) and work hard to develop those lasting bonds, and I remain very committed to all of them. My clients know that I am always there for them and can be reached 24 hours a day. I try to never allow a client to leave my office dissatisfied. Have I made mistakes? Of course I have, but when clients know how sincere you are and how much you really care, they tend to be much more forgiving.

The true elements that lead to success in practice have considerably less to do with medical, surgical, and technical skills than they do with "people" skills! Ouch! Just how good are we? How good do our clients think we are? The reality is, our clients don't really know, but their perception is more important than the true reality! As long as you don't really mess up (consistently), you deliver results, and your clients and patients adore you, you are going to do very well as a practitioner. As long as you continually show them that you truly care and that you love their precious pet companions, you will be a winner.

One problem I continually see in practice is that many new graduates and interns really lack confidence! Its one thing to be new and a little green, but displaying any sense of indecision or a lack of confidence can mean the "kiss of death" for that developing client–doctor relationship. The new graduate or the DVM who has completed an internship program is definitely ready to start meeting the challenges of practice; he or she simply needs to know what they don't yet know. When you exude confidence, there is no detriment in telling a client that you are not sure about something, as long as you get the correct information to them in a very timely fashion. You definitely need a game plan though, so when you walk into that exam room, you can present your plan to the pet guardian. Depending on the case, it may be totally appropriate to offer more than one plan (especially if finances are an issue), but even the alternative treatment or diagnostic options should be offered with confidence. The problem I often notice is the veterinarian having very little clue about something, so they basically ask the pet's parent(s) what they would like to do. "Well, gee," the client would say, "I thought YOU were the doc!"

Communication is key! I'm sure this is no surprise! As with any successful relationship, trust and open communication are paramount. Without a doubt, 95% of problems in a hospital setting, be they staff issues, patient care issues, or client issues, result from breakdowns in communication. To prevent these problems, make sure your clients truly understand your game plan, your post-visit instructions, estimated fees, and so on. Make sure all your support staff is also very aware and familiar with your hospital cases and that they understand all of the doctor's orders. And, almost more important than trying to avoid these problems and communication breakdowns, is how you deal with them when they arise. How good of a listener are you? How HUMBLE are you? How badly do you want to keep the client/patient? Putting these client "fires" out is a true art—one that is certainly worth developing. Mistakes will happen, so the better you are at this skill, the less permanent client relationship damage you will experience. Never challenge a client, especially in the reception area. The last place you want an angry or upset client to be is in the reception area. Once alone with the client, find out from him/her what the problem is, and what, if anything, has been done to rectify it. One valuable (and financially sound) lesson I've learned over the years is to let the client do the talking first, and you simply do the listening. Try to practice **active listening** where you repeat what you've just heard, or at least what you think you've just heard: "Let me make sure I understand, you're upset because..." This allows the client to actually hear what they've just said. After listening, sympathize/empathize with your client, let them now how you understand why they are so upset or disappointed (this does not admit guilt or necessary wrongdoing on you or your staff's part), then let them know how much you value their relationship and how important it is to you that they leave happy or satisfied, and ask what you can do for them to ensure that happens. Let them tell you what will make them happy; don't start offering them the world. I've found that most people are fairly reasonable and will ask for less than you would have been willing to give. Try to resolve all issues! Evaluate the trade-off and determine both the financial and goodwill "worth" to each client's relationship to your practice. Remember, a dissatisfied client will tell at least seven people of their negative experience!

Unless this particular client has a history of being difficult or rude to your staff, it is generally not worth allowing them to leave with unresolved issues. Conversely, when a client sees how much you've gone out of your way to make sure they leave happy, the bond they have with your practice actually strengthens.

It's been a while since I've been in school, but seeing many new graduates over the years, I'm a bit concerned over what is been stressed as "important" to our new colleagues. It seems that many graduates are led to believe that unless they join multi-doctor "specialty" group hospitals, their practical skills will suffer. They need this type of practice environment or they won't become good doctors! Where did this nonsense come from? I guess that means that most of us here today must not be very good doctors! I think the opposite is more true—that you become a better general practitioner when you work in an environment where you don't have access to all the high tech "toys," an environment which forces you to think, reason, get a thorough history, and, using your hands, ears, and head, perform a better physical exam. This approach also keeps things more personal with your client and patient, which, once again, enhances the bond! I'm not saying that having the great ultrasound machines, lasers, endoscopes, video otoscopes, and tonometers is bad, I just don't think we should rely so heavily on them. After all, not all of our clients can afford to allow us to use them. Besides, I'm not so sure that all of us can afford to buy them in the first place.

Lately, I've begun to wonder whether our schools in their admission processes, or we for that matter in our interview and hiring practices, are actually using the wrong criteria to select the best candidates to enter our wonderful profession. Does a stellar academic record ensure success as a practitioner? Do outstanding clinical skills also guarantee the same? In my opinion, they don't. Furthermore, how important are these for a new graduate? How much should we expect our new grads to know just entering practice for the first time? Even if they had great clinical and academic records, are you going to let them loose with your patients and clients unsupervised? Well, I sure wouldn't! And I'm sure most of you wouldn't either. Do I really care about these qualities? Not really. Why? Because these skills can be taught! Some catch on more quickly than others, but basically, anyone able to get through the very challenging academic and clinical programs which our US schools offer can learn and develop the skills required to become a competent veterinarian. Competent? Most definitely. Successful? Not necessarily! As I'm sure most of you have learned over the years, success in practice is much more strongly dependent on communication skills, compassion, empathy, confidence, organizational and management skills, and in developing strong relationships with your clients and patients—and, unfortunately, these qualities cannot always be taught!! If someone has the basic personality, these qualities can be perfected and fine-tuned, but personality cannot be taught. It's time our veterinary colleges and universities take a closer look at who they want representing them in the future!

In conclusion, I encourage all of you to take a good look at yourselves in the mirror and try to become a bit more introspective about why you chose to become veterinarians, then get out some of those old James Herriot books to help you realize what's really important for us as healers and as protectors of that wonderful bond which exists between us and our animal companions. Who knows, you might become even more successful!

INTERNAL MARKETING: THE KEY TO KEEPING CLIENTS WHERE THEY BELONG—IN *YOUR* PRACTICE!

Jeffrey Werber, DVM
Century Veterinary Group
Los Angeles, CA

We're sure by now many of you have mastered certain techniques aimed at attracting new clients into your offices. However, due to our current economic trends and an extremely competitive marketplace, these new clients are unfortunately not tearing our doors down. Furthermore, during lean times clients seem to be even more demanding, possibly because they know they may have the upper hand. Because of this, it has become painfully evident to us that we must develop strategies geared at nurturing all of our new and existing client base. After all, what is the point of spending time, effort, and energy trying to attract new clients to your practice if you haven't developed methods to keep them there? We feel that this "Internal Marketing" is the key to staying afloat in the future!

When looking to start a business, realtors and consultants will tell you that the three most important considerations are "location, location, and location!" We feel that the three most important components to attracting and maintaining a client base is "service, service, and service." Killing 'em with **kindness** is certainly okay but killing 'em with **service** is even better. Certainly we don't mean to underplay the import of quality medical care, but we hope it is a given that this is something all of you are already providing. The truth is that most clients don't really know how to measure or recognize quality care as long as they see results, but service is something they can definitely measure and seem to respond to.

Here are some of the sure-fired methods, which have proven so successful for us in keeping our clients loyal and happy.

1) Ask your clients what they want! It's often difficult to provide clients with a service if you're not sure exactly what service they'd like to be offered. There may be certain services you are currently not providing to your clients that they may want, such as early drop-offs, late pick-ups, a system for hassle-free prescription refills, a particular product, etc. You may never find this out if you don't ask. Provide questionnaires to your clients for comments, suggestions, criticisms and recommendations. Also, have meetings with your staff and make sure they understand that you need their help in gathering client feedback. Often a client will make a passing comment to one of your staff members, so make sure your staff members report back to you!

Oh yes, one more thing—it doesn't help to collect these comments if you don't act upon them. Clients want to know that their voices are being heard.

2) Show your clients that you care. Don't be afraid to display affection to your patients. This seems to be very difficult for many veterinarians and quite frankly, we don't understand why. It really shouldn't be that difficult for an animal lover to pick up a small dog or cat and hold it or give it a hug, or to kneel down and play or roughhouse with a large dog. One thing for sure is that clients love to see their veterinarian hug, kiss, or play with their pets. News of this type of behavior definitely travels quickly through your client's circle of friends.

3) Call backs! If you, your associates, or your staff members are currently not making these, you are missing the boat. There is little more appreciated by a client to show that you truly care than a phone call from you or a staff member checking up on their pet. We try to call back every surgical, major medical, and dermatological case, and all new clients within 1 week after being seen or released. If your client is not home, leave a message for them, or better yet, leave it for their pet. Our clients really appreciate these phone calls. Try it—you'll be amazed at the feedback you get.

4) Correspondence. Internal marketing is everything! Communicating with your clients means educating your clients. You want them to become information dependent! Once educated, your clients will be more apt to respond to the special programs you may design in the future. Correspondence may be in the form of a personal letter, monthly newsletters, postcard mailers, over the counter fliers, or give-aways. Whichever marketing plan you choose, the goal is to keep your clients informed about up-to-date trends in veterinary medicine, and changes or additions to your practice and staff, such as any new diagnostic equipment you may have purchased or new personnel you may have hired. Did you know that most clients have no idea that veterinarians use the same dental equipment as their own dentists? When communicating with your clients, always try to maintain a "one big happy family" atmosphere. You'd like to be treated like a member of their extended family. Remember, clients look to their veterinarian just like parents look to their pediatrician!

5) We can't all have a house-call practice, so it's therefore very important to always "be available." If you offer emergency service, great, but if you don't, at least be available to your clients in their time of need. Make arrangements with a local emergency facility that will work with you and will make sure you get your case back in the morning. Have the emergency report immediately faxed to your office so that you can promptly attend to your client's pet upon its arrival. Even if the pet doesn't need any further medical attention, still have the emergency report faxed to your office so that you can call your client ASAP to discuss the condition of their pet. Remember, clients appreciate the attention you give to their "children." Availability also means **promptly** returning your clients' phone calls. Any delays may send the wrong signal that you are either too busy for them or that their pet is not a high priority. Create a daily phone log so that if your day is hectic you can have your receptionist or technician call your clients to inform them that you will personally call them later in the day. This will send your clients the message that you are on the ball and that you truly are concerned about them and their pets.

6) Custom-tailored target marketing. As we mentioned earlier, try to stay aware of your clients' demands for various services. This information will prove invaluable when creating a strong detailed internal marketing plan. Based on your clients' feedback, programs such as dental, grooming and bathing, or deworming specials can be implemented. For example, in September we created the *B, B, & B*, or *Bath, Brush and Back to School* special. In September, as most schools are getting back in session, and the weather is cooling down, we seem to experience a quiet time, so we created our *B, B, & B* special to combat this quiet period. With a creative postcard mailing which we began about a month earlier, we targeted patients ranging from 5 to 10 years of age. We offered a free bath with every dental prophy and polish. The response to our special was overwhelming, as we averaged 7 prophy and polish procedures per day during the month of September. Actually, we were forced to extend the special into the second week of October. The results of our special left us with a remarkable revenue increase through pre-anesthetic lab tests, dental prophies, extractions, and other ancillary procedures such as ear cleanings, growth removals, and vaccinations. Everybody "won" with this promotion—our patients, our clients, and our hospital. Also, keep an eye out for what might be happening in your town as far as holidays and monthly events. Try to tie in some sort of special or promotion to these celebrated events. Some examples might be a grooming special on Valentine's Day to keep your patients "Lovingly Cute" or a boarding special over the Christmas holiday.

Lastly, everyone loves receiving birthday cards! Not only should you be sending your patients a birthday card and sometimes even a gift, but you can impress the heck out of your clients by sending them a card on their birthday—from their pet(s)!

We are sure that for some of you just getting started in this area, all of this may sound great, but is rather overwhelming. This type of intensive marketing doesn't come easy, or cheap. It is, however, very efficient and effective. If you are the creative type, you need to sit down and devote some time to gather some client feedback, come up with some ideas, and then plan your marketing strategy. Although your first project need not be very elaborate, expensive, or time consuming, it should always remain focused and look professional. A simple postcard mailer offering some special or educational message, possibly tied in to a calendar event or something going on in your community, might be the ticket. Other than the computer time, postage, and some staff time bundling and mailing the postcards, this effort shouldn't set you back very much either. If you are like me and only partially creative, or like many others who don't have a creative bone in their bodies, then you may need to enlist the help of a marketing specialist to help you develop and implement you marketing plan. These professionals are usually available to consult on a per project basis, and need not be hired full-time. Fortunately, one of my colleagues has such a background and actually consults with other veterinarians on this subject, which has made it relatively easy for us. Don't sell your staff short though! You might have some extremely talented and creative people under your employ who can write well, draw well, develop catchy slogans, and come up with phenomenal marketing and promotional ideas, while others who might be able to stuff a mean envelope or be very quick at sealing and stamping 4,000 mailers (especially for a nice incentive!) Except for some large-scale printing, rarely have we had to look beyond our office for help to get the job done.

Hopefully, you now understand a little bit more about this fascinating form of marketing. Next time you sit down to plan your budgets, ease up a little bit on your Yellow Page ads, your print ads, or your direct mail campaigns, and plan to spend a little more on the marketing, which will bring you an even greater return on your dollar—***Internal Marketing!***

I'M A GREAT VETERINARIAN—WHY AREN'T I MAKING ANY MONEY?

Jeffrey Werber, DVM
Century Veterinary Group
Los Angeles, CA

When it comes to achieving financial success as practicing veterinarians, we are definitely our own worst enemies. I can't believe that according to national averages, a pharmacist and an optometrist earn more than a veterinarian! That is really sad! Why? Because most of us are afraid to charge what we are truly worth. Afraid that a client will balk or reject our recommendation and treatment plan if we charge what we feel we deserve. We seem to lack the confidence to look clients in the eye and comfortably let them know what our diagnostics and treatment plan will cost. We need to feel proud about what we do, what we know, how hard we work, how nice our facilities are, and we need to start charging accordingly for our time and services.

I've always been a strong proponent of the notion that financial success often follows personal success. You've got to believe in yourself. When you are really happy at what you do, you begin to exude a certain air of confidence that is contagious to all around you. You become a more competent salesperson, selling yourself, your hospital, and your diagnostic and treatment plans. Don't kid yourselves into thinking that we don't have to sell ourselves all day long! I know I'm a good salesman, but the truth is, by being good at selling what I do, I'm given the opportunity to do what I love to do. One of my younger associates complained that I always got the good cases. He would go into a room and never be able to convince the client to allow him to run the appropriate diagnostics. I remember one day that I was about to go into an exam room to see a patient and he said to me "good luck—they're not going to spend anything on that dog." I proceeded into the room and, I guess, performed my magic. Ten minutes later the dog and I came out of the exam room, marched into the main treatment room, and I proceeded to do a complete physical exam, including blood and urine analyses, radiographs, ECG, tonometry—the works. Am I a better doctor than my associate? No, but I'm obviously a better salesperson, or I exude more confidence, or the clients simply believed that my motivation was strictly to provide better health care for their four-legged child. No wonder why I have so much fun practicing—I get to practice good medicine, I have great clients and patients, I am continuously faced with new case challenges, and because of all this, I make a very nice living. Most importantly, I delegate all the parts of practice that I don't like.

I know that many practice managers hate this—but it works for me. I LOVE going out into the reception area, the more crowded the better! The "expert's" objections have a lot to do with the potential disruption up in front, adding to delays as clients see you and want to grab your attention. This often leads to conflicts and the doctor inadvertently giving information contrary to what the receptionist may have just given. I do appreciate all these objections, but I still love to do it. Since, for me, the client and patient bond is what I find to be the most enjoyable part of practice, it's an amazing feeling to walk out there and be bombarded by wagging tails, active canine tongues licking passionately, purring cats, and smiling clients often displaying their adoration for you and/or the hospital. I often say that when new clients witness this first hand, they seem to become bonded to the practice almost immediately. You couldn't pay for better PR! I can almost guarantee that they are missing this at their current, or prior, veterinary offices. For me, it adds to the practice "high" I continually try to achieve, which, of course, adds to the "fun!"

More of us have to learn that a higher salary is not necessarily the answer to improving job satisfaction. We are very fortunate in that we can enjoy our true passion on a daily basis. I know many people who may make a lot of money at their jobs or careers, but are miserable. I'd rather earn less, but love my work! Or better yet, I'd like to do what I love to do—practice veterinary medicine—and earn even more! Is it possible? Absolutely! I know many veterinarians earning very healthy incomes. How? Some own multiple practices. Others have used their strong business acumen to build huge, high-grossing operations. Still others have found different ways to make money while continuing to work with pets, through pet spas, ancillary services, or pet supplies. Your only limiting factor is your own creativity. Before you embark on such a pursuit, make sure that the price you pay through time, effort, money, and energy spent will truly be worth it. Another option would be to hire more staff, delegate well, and have them help you take your hospital to the next level saving you from having to do much more work. Your staff can take a lot of pressure off of you and with training can usually take over the tasks that you hate to do. I have found that many practitioners who seem to be losing their love and enthusiasm for practice become disenchanted with specific things—not practice in general. The key to maintaining job satisfaction is to identify what it is that you dislike and delegate it to other team members. The reason that I still love practice so much after 20 years is that I make sure to spend a lot of time doing the things I love, and very little to no time on the things I don't. I am forever thankful that I have such a terrific, talented staff!

Now, the challenge is to keep your staff as passionate about your practice and their roles within it, as we discussed earlier. Accomplish this and you'll either need to start turning business away, extend your hours, or hire another veterinarian (or, if you're great at delegating, hire even more technicians).

In conclusion, I hope you realize and agree that we are members of the greatest profession known to man. It offers us so much versatility and variety, and empowers us to enjoy as many facets as we desire. In my mind, there's no excuse for not being able to discover many of the joys which veterinary medicine can bring to your professional lives. I urge you to go out and find, or simply rediscover these passions, and continue to nurture and promote that wonderful bond which exists between us and our four-legged friends.

CAN I RETIRE? HOW MUCH DOES IT TAKE?

Fritz Wood, CPA, CFP®
Lake Quivira, KS

When money is tight, it's easy to understand why retirement doesn't loom large on your horizon. Focusing on making ends meet this month takes priority over the long-distant future. Many people wage a constant battle between saving, investing and paying off debts. Others are focused on near-term goals like a car or home purchase, saving for college, or putting money aside for that long-awaited and much-deserved vacation.

ORDERING YOUR PERSONAL FINANCIAL PRIORITIES

Just as veterinarians examine before diagnosing, and diagnose before prescribing, your financial life must also follow a logic path. Before investing for retirement, it's smart to make sure you have other priorities covered first:

- **Adequate insurance coverage** – Certain catastrophic risks must be transferred to insurance companies. If you lack health insurance and become seriously ill or involved in an accident, your financial future may be ruined. If you become disabled and lack disability insurance, your financial future may be ruined. If you lack adequate insurance and your car is totaled or stolen, your home is badly damaged, or you harm another (eg, a car accident, someone slips and falls at your home), your financial future may be ruined. If others—your parents or your kids—depend on you or your spouse financially, and you lack adequate life insurance and one of you dies, it may ruin your financial future. The financial downside of these risks is so great that you cannot bear them alone—you must transfer the risk to an insurance company. Before investing, make sure these risks are covered via adequate insurance.
- **Extinguish credit card and other bad debt** – It's almost always a good idea to get rid of credit card and other high-interest rate loans before you invest for retirement. When you retire debt, you effectively earn the rate you'd otherwise have paid. For example, by paying off that 20% credit card, you're making a guaranteed, risk-free 20%. That makes it a no-brainer priority over investing for retirement. There is one exception to that rule: if your employer offers a retirement plan that will match your contributions up to a certain level, fund it up to that level—even if you have credit card debt—because you're getting a 100% guaranteed, risk-free return on your investment. It very rarely makes financial sense to accelerate mortgage and student loans at the expense of investing for retirement. These debts typically carry a reasonably low interest rate and have income tax advantages.
- **Accumulate a modest cash cushion** – Financial emergencies happen. Your car will break down, the tires and brakes will need replaced, your heater or air conditioner or plumbing will one day need repair. If you have a modest cash cushion to fall back on, you won't need to put these inevitable but unexpected expenses on a credit card. To establish this emergency fund, have money transferred from your checking account to a savings account, putting it a bit further out of reach of everyday expenses.

SAVING AND INVESTING FOR RETIREMENT

When you first think about investing, one of the biggest obstacles is figuring out where you'll find the money to start. Perhaps coming up with a couple hundred bucks will require a lot of diligence and cost-cutting. You might feel as though you'll never be able to accumulate enough to begin. But rest assured, you don't need a big bankroll to start investing. A wide range of options are available for those of modest means. There are ways for beginners to invest with the amount of money most people spend on soda or coffee every month.

Start Small

This is a wealth-creating habit. Just as a huge oak tree springs forth from a miniscule acorn, a money tree can grow from a tiny bit of seed capital. Starting small works for both saving and investing.

Let's start with saving. If you spend as much as your earn—and most people do—you need to slowly decrease your spending. Each month, choose one way to decrease spending. For example, if you spend $5 a day on lunch, brownbag it a couple days a week. Instead of hitting the local coffee shop, bring your java from home. Drop cable and magazine subscriptions. Instead of going to the movie theater, check out movies from your local public library. Are you saving a ton? No, but you ARE saving, and that's what's important. If you consistently spend less each month, you will make cumulative progress and begin to feel in control over your finances. This habit is guaranteed to help you get out of debt faster and you'll develop wealth slowly but constantly. Starting small and being patiently methodical is far better than not starting at all.

Now, let's examine starting small with investing. This is where your Maltese can grow in to a Mastiff over time.

Your first investing priority is at work. If your employer provides a retirement plan, start there. Many employers match some portion of your contribution to encourage participation. That's free money. And since your contribution is automatically subtracted from your paycheck, it's out of reach and out of mind. Another bonus—this money goes in to the retirement plan before it's taxed, so less of your income will be taxed now. Finally, the money grows over the years without being taxed, allowing it to grow faster. It will be taxed upon withdrawal, but that may be decades away.

If your employer doesn't have a retirement plan—and unfortunately most private practices don't—it's up to you. But you can still save in a tax-smart way by investing in a Roth Individual Retirement Account (IRA). You'll fund this with money that's already been taxed, but money withdrawn later is tax free. Many mutual fund companies (eg, Schwab, T. Rowe Price, Vanguard, American Century) offer you the option of having a pre-set sum—usually $50 or more—automatically deposited from your checking account each month. This autopilot approach eliminates the chance that you'll "forget" to save or spend the money on less worthy items.

Compounding – Time is on Your Side

The most important thing is to start early. Albert Einstein was famously quoted as saying "Nothing is more powerful than the power of compound interest. It is the eighth wonder of the world."

The U.S. Securities and Exchange Commission has published a helpful consumer resource titled "*Get the Facts on Saving and Investing – A Roadmap to Start You on a Journey to Financial Security Through Saving and Investing*" which you can access for free at www.sec.gov/pdf/facts.pdf.

You're never too young or too old to worry about your financial future. Even a little money can go a long way toward building a secure retirement. Simply put, you want to invest in order to create wealth and make work optional at some point in your life. It's relatively painless, and the rewards are plentiful. How can you become a successful investor? By making investing a habit—by making it a part of your everyday life. You can seize control of your financial future. Start small, start now.

Consider this scenario: An investor who starts saving at age 32 and contributes $100 a month to a Roth IRA will have about $340,000 at age 65, assuming a 10.4 percent annual return (the long-term average of large company stocks in the US). But an investor who starts saving at 22 and contributes $100 a month will have about $980,000—a quantum difference. Since compounding helps your money grow over time, even small contributions can have a big impact when you're ready to retire. And by opening an account early in your career, and making periodic, if small deposits, you're developing good investing habits that will last a lifetime. Einstein was right—start now!

Tenets of Investing Success

1. Start small—you don't need a ton of cash to begin. Often you can get started for less than the cost of an iPod.
2. Start now—let compounding work to your great advantage
3. Pay yourself first, not last—don't try to save what's left at the end of the month after all the bills have been paid—that's futile regardless your income level. Instead, have money deducted from your paycheck or your bank account before you have a chance to spend it frivolously. Experts recommend you invest 10% of your gross (before tax) pay, but it's okay to start with a lower amount and work your way up over time.
4. Invest regularly—like every time you get paid
5. Let Uncle Sam help—take full-advantage of your employer's retirement plan or a Roth IRA.
6. Broadly diversify—a mutual fund allows you to own a small piece of hundreds or thousands of different companies. You don't want all your eggs in one basket.
7. Adopt a long-term perspective—don't obsess or worry about day-to-day, week-to-week, month-to-month, or even year-to-year volatility—you're in it for the long-haul.
8. Invest frugally—choose low-cost investments over high-cost investments. Before investing in a fund, read about it at www.morningstar.com. Know what you're buying—make sure you understand the fund's objectives and that it's right for you. Specifically, I recommend you consider broad-based index funds, or funds targeted to your retirement date.

INFLUENCE — GETTING YOUR CLIENT TO SAY "YES"

Fritz Wood, CPA, CFP
Lake Quivira, KS

KEY POINTS

- Practitioners can—and should—employ tactics and strategies to augment compliance.
- Your communication skills—ie, getting your clients to "Yes"—is equally important to your clinical, diagnostic, and surgical skills
- Compliance rates today are inferior. A minority of your clients receive the care you know to be in their best interest.

OVERVIEW

Compliance is a most-serious quality of care issue. Today, millions of cats and dogs do not receive the level of care you believe is best for them. The opportunity to provide more and better care to your patients is omnipresent. The business opportunity inherent in improved compliance is staggering. The untapped potential in your patient base may be double your current production

Most practice teams judge their level of compliance by "gut feel" rather than measuring actual compliance rates, and they think their compliance rates are quite high. But a comprehensive, in-depth study by AAHA showed that in almost every single case, the level of compliance is significantly lower than what practice teams believe (AAHA's "The Path to High-Quality Care – Practical Tips for Improving Compliance," copyright 2003, back cover)."

The profession's failure to consistently and confidently make recommendations—with conviction—for what is truly in the pet's best interest has resulted in low compliance. The quality of care delivered today is significantly less than what is possible. My personal challenge is that within 48 hours of reading this, you would take at least one action step to begin improving compliance in your practice. Pets benefit, clients benefit, and the entire veterinary health care team benefit!

THE BOTTOM LINE

- Your existing clients represent a huge, untapped resource.
- The greatest opportunity in your practice is with existing clients.

- Extraordinary revenue potential walks through your front door each day—and those clients already know your name, address, phone number, and have even given you money before.

THE OPPORTUNITY

Even in high-performing veterinary practices, hundreds of thousands of dollars "walk out the door" each year in terms of services and products that never got recommended or delivered, or if they where provided, were never charged for. These are existing clients, with existing pets. Doing more with existing clients is easier—and more productive and cost-effective than attracting new clients. Consider the following untapped profit centers:

- Laboratory (including pre-anesthetic testing, offering screens as part of the annual wellness examination, and following-up with chronically dispensed, long-term medications)
- Dentistry
- Senior care
- Behavioral care
- Strategic deworming
- Nutrition
- Flea/tick control
- Heartworm preventive

SUMMARY

- Sharpening your communication skills will jumpstart your practice.
- If you communicate better, more pets (and pet owners) will benefit from your clinical, diagnostic, and surgical skills.
- There exists a body of knowledge which—if studied and practiced—can and will save pets lives and contribute to their health and longevity.
- Today, practitioners capture only a minor fraction of the opportunities that present each day.
- The opportunity to double your gross income resides within your existing client base—if you capture the everyday opportunities that present each day.

REFERENCES/SUGGESTED READING

1. *Influence,* Robert Cialdini, PhD.
2. *The Path to High-Quality Care,* AAHA Press.
3. Wayner CJ, Heinke ML. Complicance: Crafting quality care. Vet Clin North Am. 2006;36(2):419-436.
4. www.ncvei.org

TENETS OF PERSONAL FINANCIAL SUCCESS

Fritz Wood, CPA, CFP
Lake Quivira, KS

Personal financial planning is the process of organizing your financial goals into a workable plan so that you can live with financial security in the style you desire. It involves proper handling of cash flow, assets, and liabilities. Financial planning is the way to get from where you are now to where you want to be. It brings the future into the present, while there's still time to do something about it. To quote Peter Drucker, "the best way to predict the future is to create it."

The planning process is straightforward:

- Determine what you *have.*
- Determine what you *want.*
- Determine how to get what you want, *using* what you have.

Determining what you have involves preparing a Personal Financial Statement. This document lists your assets, liabilities, and net worth. Also, a Cash Flow Statement may be prepared. This document tracks your personal cash receipts and disbursements over a period of time.

What do you want to achieve? Do you have short-term financial goals (eg, eliminating credit card or other high-cost consumer debt, building an emergency fund, buying a car or home, starting a regular investment plan)? What about your long-term objectives? What are your lifetime goals? What must you accomplish in life? How do you enjoy spending free time? What are your hobbies? Are there hobbies you've not pursued, or that have gotten rusty from inactivity over the years? Visualize how you would spend time if money were of no concern. Where are you? What are you doing? Although each of us conjures up a unique picture, we often have many of the same thoughts:

- Financial independence (you are not dependent on the state or federal government, your children, your parents, or your paycheck)
- No financial worries
- Own a nice home
- Help children get a college education
- Own a nice vacation property
- Travel

Many people find their vision of the future is unrealistic, given their modest level of saving and investing. Many find they need to modify their expectation of the future. Although this process may be a bit humbling, it should not discourage you. It's far better to modify you expectations, and have an accurate picture of the future, than to have no idea whether or not your picture is feasible. If you remember nothing else, remember that it is never too late to begin. Start today.

What are the biggest threats to your future financial security?

- Doing nothing
- Waiting
- Inflation
- Failing to diversify
- Investing too little
- Investing too conservatively
- Failing to insure against catastrophic risks

Why doesn't everyone plan for their financial future? Common reasons given include:

- "I don't make enough money. My income level doesn't warrant planning."
- "The future will sort itself out."
- "I've already waited too long. It's too late to start now."
- "I'm afraid of what I might find. The truth might be painful."
- "When I win the lottery, it won't matter anyway."

In fact, retirement planning is probably more critical for people with modest income than for the very wealthy. I'm sure we can all think of people in their 'golden years' who are not enjoying an idyllic existence. What's the good news? Each of us has the power and ability to profoundly influence our personal financial future. We can do something about it.

The first, and most important rule of retirement planning is to pay yourself first. If you're under age 40, set aside at least 10% of your income each year. If you're older and haven't started investing, you may need to set aside a higher percentage. The easiest way to do this is to set up an automatic withdrawal or transfer from your bank or checking account. On a certain day each month, have 10% (or more) of your monthly income subtracted from your account and transferred to a high quality, no-load, low-cost mutual fund. The idea is simple—you can't spend what you don't have. After all, it's human nature to spend all our disposable income. For proof, recall how quickly your expenses increased the last time you got a pay raise! All of the sudden, it was time to buy that new car or bigger house.

According to an American Animal Hospital Association (AAHA) Veterinary Career Survey, retirement potential ranked above average in terms of importance, and below average in terms of satisfaction. Increasingly, people are focused not just on how to meet this month's payments, but also on their longer-term financial goals and objectives. Common examples include funding a child's college education, and achieving financial independence. Financial independence is that point in time when you have acquired sufficient assets to spend time however you choose. It doesn't matter whether you choose to continue working, or hang it up and travel the world.

Having sufficient resources allows you the *freedom* to do whatever you want. With the aging baby boom generation, unprecedented numbers of people are closely considering their financial future.

BEFORE YOU INVEST

Don't even consider investing until your financial house is in order. For example:

- Are potential catastrophic risks covered by insurance? Do you maintain adequate health, life, disability, long-term care, property and casualty, and professional liability insurance?
- Do you have an ample emergency fund? Have you arranged access to cash totaling 3 to 6 months of living expenses? Have you considered any large expenses you might incur in the next year or two? Do you have any tax payments due soon? Will you have to replace that old car in a year or two? When is the next tuition payment? You don't want to be caught short of cash and be forced to liquidate a long-term investment to pay for a short-term need.
- Do you carry a zero balance on all your credit cards?

If you thoughtfully and honestly answered 'yes' to these questions, investing may be suitable for you at this time.

BASIC PRINCIPLES FOR SUCCESSFUL INVESTING

1. What do you want to achieve with this money?

Are you setting this money aside for a child's college education? Is it for your retirement? Are you saving for a new car? A new home? Will it be used to buy into a partnership, or to start your own practice? You shouldn't invest until you know what you plan to buy with this money—albeit that may change as time passes. Ultimately, your objectives for this investment will boil down to safety, current income, long-term growth, or some combination thereof. Once you know your purpose in making the investment, you'll quickly eliminate many inappropriate alternatives.

2. Diversify Your Assets

Have you prepared a personal financial statement recently? If you're a practice owner, when was your practice last valued? What percentage of your total assets are tied to the practice, including the land, building, equipment, leasehold improvements, furniture and fixtures, and goodwill? If you're like most veterinarians, the vast majority of your eggs are in one basket. This exposes you to inordinate and unnecessary risk. Also, recognize that your practice is an illiquid asset, it is not easily or quickly converted to cash. By diversifying into more liquid assets such as stocks, bonds, and cash reserves, you can mitigate this risk. I don't infer that you should hesitate to invest in your practice, I believe you must do so continuously to be successful. However, it's critically important that you spread your assets among more than one basket.

Next, determine an initial investment allocation among stocks, bonds, and cash reserves. The proportions that you choose (your "asset mix") should depend on your objectives, time horizon, and risk tolerance. Time is particularly critical since the longer you have to invest, the more risk you can accept. Keep in mind that your asset mix, not your individual investment choices, tends to have far greater long-term impact on your investing success. Unbelievably, one renowned study showed that 94% of investment performance depended upon the asset mix. Only 6% of investment performance depended upon which specific investment was selected or when the investment was made. Why is asset mix so important? Consider the following historical performance:

Compound Annual Returns (1926-2006):

Small Company Stocks	12.7%
Large Company Stocks	10.4%
Long-Term Government Bonds	5.4%
Treasury Bills	5.3%
Inflation	3.7%

Source: Ibbotson Associates, 2007
Past performance is no guarantee of future results.

Over the past 80 years, commons stocks have clearly outperformed the other asset classes.

How much of your liquid assets should be devoted to equities (stocks or stock mutual funds)? A rule-of-thumb is to subtract your age from 120, and place that percentage in stocks, or stock mutual funds. For example, a 40-year-old might place 80% of his or her liquid assets in equities. But, depending on your investing temperament, you may be comfortable with more or less risk. In addition, your particular financial situation may dictate a higher- or lower-risk approach. This rule-of-thumb also assumes that you are willing to tolerate short-term ups and downs in the stock market in pursuit of higher returns over time. Note that as you move closer to actually spending your money, your emphasis should gradually shift from growth-oriented investments (stocks) to income-oriented investments (bonds and cash reserves).

How much risk can you accept? This is one of the toughest questions for investors to answer. Risk doesn't bother any of us until we begin to lose some money. As you study an investment, find out the worst it has ever performed. A stock or mutual fund with one great year can look good even if performance before and after that were miserable. That impressive 3, 5, or 10-year performance record may be masking some real ugly years. Does the investment you're considering give a smooth ride or fluctuate wildly from year to year? Picture yourself in this investment after it has lost some of your hard-earned money. How do you feel? If this thought makes you uneasy, nauseous, or unable to sleep at night, it's time to find another candidate. If you invest outside of your risk tolerance or comfort zone, you'll probably be tempted to dump the fund at the worst possible time—after a big fall. On the other hand, many people invest too conservatively and will find it difficult or impossible to meet their long-term goals and objectives. This is especially true in Individual Retirement Accounts and employer sponsored retirement savings plans, where the money is typically out of grasp until you reach age 59 $^{1/2}$.

3. Distinguish Between Saving and Investing

Saving is short-term, investing is long-term. Saving may guarantee you a specific dollar amount by a certain date, investing most surely will not. Saving will usually result in a loss of purchasing power over time, investing should result in increased purchasing power over the long haul.

Very often, having money in a 'safe' refuge has actually resulted in no real gain in purchasing power. Not that you shouldn't have money in the bank, just don't expect that it will outpace inflation on an after-tax basis. However, money that you anticipate needing in the short-term (less than 5 years) should definitely be stored in a safe haven.

I am often asked whether it makes more sense to buy individual stocks or rather, to buy stock mutual funds. In almost all cases, I have a strong preference for stock mutual funds. The reasons are many, not the least of which is that credible research indicates that one would need between $2 and $3 million dollars in liquid assets in order to adequately diversify by purchasing individual stocks. Needless to say, few enjoy this enviable position.

4. Start Investing as Soon as Possible

Time in the market matters—timing the market does not. Timing the market is an unqualified myth, yet reasonable people will survey overall market conditions before investing (as in, "the market is awfully high right now, I think I'll wait until it comes down a bit before I invest my hard-earned money"). This research, even if nothing more than a gut-feel, is a colossal waste of time. Think of the millions of frustrated investors who maintained that mindset and sat on the sidelines from 1995 through 1999—arguably the best 5-year period in the history of the US stock market. The truth is very simple—no one, repeat no one, knows the near-term future of the stock market. To guess is futile and humbling. So we consistently believe that "now" is always a good time to invest.

Of course, there are many hundreds of investment newsletters and market-timing services which purport to know the unknowable. Before heeding the advice of these heresy publications (we call them financial pornographers), ask yourself a few questions: Why do they need to sell subscriptions to their timing service if they have it all figured out? Is 100% of their personal money invested as they advise? Was the company yacht and airplane purchased on astute market timing, or subscription revenue from the newsletter's trusting followers? Suffice it to say that there is no credible research indicating that market timing is possible or profitable. Market timing is a fool's errand. No one now

living or dead has ever consistently guessed the market's next move.

Time in the market is THE SINGLE most important factor in terms of investment success. Time can be your greatest ally, or your worst enemy. No matter the existing market conditions, today is a good day to invest—not as good as yesterday, but much better than tomorrow. Lost time is never found.

5. Invest Regularly

Sure and steady wins the race. It matters less where you start. It matters more that you start. Starting is what counts. As you choose your investments, consider a dollar-cost averaging strategy of investing a set dollar amount on a fixed schedule, regardless of market conditions. This strategy will allow you to acquire more shares at lower prices than at higher prices. Of course, the practice of dollar-cost averaging does not ensure a profit or protect against a loss in declining markets. You must also consider your ability to continuously invest through periods of low price levels.

An easy way to invest regularly is to establish an automatic investment plan with a mutual fund company whereby a certain dollar amount is transferred from your checking account, your savings account, or your paycheck to a mutual fund account on a fixed schedule (eg, weekly, bimonthly, monthly, or quarterly). The beauty of this approach, in addition to all the benefits of dollar cost averaging, is that it makes budgeting unnecessary. This investment is on remote-control; it is regular, constant, automatic, disciplined, and unconscious. In short, it works!

This strategy is sometimes known as "paying yourself first." You effectively treat yourself like any other creditor. It's human nature to spend at least 100% of our income. Most of us have too much month at the end of our money. However, you can't spend what you don't have. If you consistently set aside 10% of your paycheck (more if you're older and haven't started investing yet) for long-term growth (invest in vehicles that will outpace inflation on an after-tax basis), you will have applied the Golden Rule of investing—your personal financial future should be bright and your worries few. If you think living on 90% of what you make would cramp your lifestyle, just think back to how quickly you adjusted to your last 10% pay raise!

6. Have Realistic Expectations and a Long-Term Perspective

According to the great American philosopher Dolly Parton, "If you want the rainbow, you have to put up with the rain." Unfortunately, conventional wisdom tells us that stocks are risky investments. No doubt, this is due to their day-to-day volatility and the fact that they are not FDIC insured. However, for the long-term investor, stocks are the only option you have to increase purchasing power. For the long-term investor, what could possibly be riskier than bonds and cash reserves where you are virtually guaranteed to lose purchasing power after taxes and inflation? Of course, if you need the money soon (in 5 years or less), or if you think you might bail out in a storm, you are not a good candidate for the stock market.

7. Invest Frugally

Like all companies, mutual funds incur operating expenses. With mutual funds, however, those expenses are passed on directly to you—in effect, lowering your rate of return by the amount of the expense. Therefore, it is important to use efficient funds, those with lower than average expense ratios. This information is easily found in the prospectus. The average expense ratio for a diversified stock fund is around 1.5%. Does the fund you are considering operate more or less efficiently? When the stock market is up 20% or 30% per year or more (as it was in the late 1990s), a 2.5% expense ratio doesn't bother you much. However, in a year when the market returns only 5%, fully half your profits disappear. Which is the least costly mutual fund family? Without a doubt, that honor belongs to Vanguard, the second largest fund family. Their no-load mutual funds are notoriously cost efficient. In fact, in his book *Mutual Fund$ For Dummie$*," author Eric Tyson argues that if you've found a mutual fund you like, compare it to a similar fund offered at Vanguard. You're decreasing your chances of success if you choose similar performing, but higher cost funds elsewhere.

There are more immutable laws of investing success:

- Avoid load funds
- Buy and hold—don't actively trade
- Take advantage of tax-deferred investing when possible
- Know what you're buying
- If it sounds too good to be true...it is
- Don't let the "tax" tail wag the "investment" dog
- Insurance is not an investment...refuse to invest in insurance products

MANAGING DEBT

A new car comes with an operator's manual. Even a simple wristwatch has a detailed "how-to" booklet. However, no one is handed instructions with a paycheck. Managing money is not a skill commonly taught in even the best business schools. You probably will have to learn for yourself, often making the same mistakes as those before you. Just as there are absolute principles about anatomy, physiology, and our physical world, there are a few personal financial "truths" which you would be unwise to violate. Unfortunately, most people ignore the immutable laws of personal financial success. Instead, they search in vain for the elusive - and mythical - holy grail of wealth building. Here are a few time-tested rules that you can learn and apply, no matter your age, fiscal situation, or financial literacy.

- Maintain an ample emergency fund to avoid credit card debt
- Prioritze/pay off debts in order (either smallest debt to highest, or highest interest rate to lowest)
- Leverage can work to your great benefit—or your great detriment
- Don't borrow money to buy depreciable assets (eg, cars)
- It may make sense to borrow money for things that:
  o Increase your income
  o Increase in value
- Good debt
  o Low interest rate
  o Tax deductible
- Bad debt
  o High interest rate
  o Not tax deductible
- Student loans
- Home mortgage
- Other consumer debt

Are you in over your head?
- www.nfcc.org
- Consumer Credit Counseling Service
- http://www.usdoj.gov/ust/eo/bapcpa/ccde/index.htm

To learn more, visit:
- www.fritzwood.com
- www.vanguard.com
- www.aicpa.org/financialliteracy
- www.annualcreditreport.com
- www.garrettplanningnetwork.com

ACUTE UPPER AIRWAY PRESENTATION IN CATS: NOTHING TO SNEEZE AT

Leah A. Cohn, DVM, PhD, Diplomate ACVIM (SAIM)
College of Veterinary Medicine
University of Missouri, Columbia, MO

Eleanor C. Hawkins, DVM, Diplomate ACVIM (SAIM)
College of Veterinary Medicine
North Carolina State University, Raleigh, NC

Upper respiratory infections (URI) are quite common in cats. Mortality due to common URI is very rare. However, these infections are not trivial. In group settings, and especially when young or unvaccinated cats congregate, URI can spread easily and affect large proportions of the population. In animal shelters especially, these infections can result in tremendously increased costs and decreased ability to place animals in homes. Although a causal link remains unproven, it is entirely possible that acute URI can predispose to later development of chronic rhinosinusitis, a problem in cats which is difficult to manage and usually impossible to cure. Additionally, more virulent strains of the common calicivirus infection can and does result in significant mortality as well as morbidity.

CAUSATION

Feline URI is multifactorial. Multiple risk factors are involved, as are multiple pathogens. Pathogens may cause infection in isolation, or in combination. Particularly, secondary bacterial infection may follow primary viral URI. Evidently, viral pathogens are the most common cause of URI in cats. Feline calicivirus (FCV) is perhaps more prevalent, but feline herpesvirus-1 (FHV-1; aka feline rhinotracheitis) often causes a more severe clinical disease (with virulent calicivirus infection proving the exception to the rule). Primary bacterial pathogens involved in feline URI include *Bordetella bronchiseptica* and *Chlamydophila felis*. Secondary bacterial infection with a variety of pathogens can complicate either viral or primary bacterial URI. Each of the primary causes of feline URI will be addressed briefly.

FCV: Typical (FCV) and Virulent Systemic Strains (VS-FCV)

Typical FCV infection is a very common cause of URI in cats throughout the world. There are numerous strains of FCV resulting in variable disease manifestations and varied antigenicity. Depending on strain and host factors, infected cats may remain healthy or may develop fever, oral ulcerations, nasal discharge and sneezing, and sometimes lameness. The typical oral/respiratory disease is most severe in unvaccinated kittens after maternal antibody has waned (~10 to 14 weeks). The virus is shed via oral, nasal, and ocular secretions, and although more stable in the environment than other causes of feline URI, probably remains infectious for only a week. The greatest viral shedding occurs in the weeks during and after clinical infection, but apparently recovered cats may shed virus persistently for months to years. These recovered carriers may be widespread in localized populations of cats making it nearly impossible to eliminate exposure altogether in large group settings.

VS-FCV results from hypervirulent viral mutants. Unlike typical FCV, these virulent strains seem to cause more severe disease in adult (and often in FCV vaccinated) cats than kittens. VS-FCV results in a disease presentation quite distinct from that of typical FCV infection. Infected cats develop high fevers; swelling (edema) of the face and limbs; alopecia, crusting, and ulceration of the skin (especially the face, ears, and feet); and death. Mortality rates approach 50% even with supportive care. The virus is shed through feces and sloughed skin/hair as well as nasal, oral, and ocular secretions. Mildly affected cats (often kittens) can pass a virulent and potentially fatal form of VS-FCV, so all exposed cats must be considered potentially contagious. The virus itself is readily spread by fomites, and may be carried by veterinary personnel to other cats in the facility or even to their own pets at home. Facilities with documented cases of VS-FCV may need to temporarily shut down feline admissions to stop the spread of infection. Fortunately, this disease is rare.

FHV-1

Most cats are likely exposed to the single serotype of FHV-1 at some point in their lives. Exposure in susceptible cats can result in moderate to severe respiratory and ocular infection, although vaccinated or older cats may be infected but display minimal clinical signs. The most severe infections typically occur in kittens shortly after maternal antibody wanes (~9 weeks) and young, unvaccinated cats. Viral shedding in nasal, oropharyngeal, and ocular discharges is responsible for cat-to-cat and fomite-transmission; aerosol transmission is uncommon and the virus itself does not persist long in the environment. Two to six days after initial exposure, fever, anorexia, nasal discharge and sneezing, and ocular discharge develop. Many cats hypersalivate. Ulcerative and interstitial keratitis, corneal sequestrum formation, and anterior uveitis may be seen. Rarely, viral pneumonia and dermatologic symptoms are seen. Mortality rates are low, with most affected cats improving spontaneously in 10 to 20 days. As with all herpesviral infections, although clinical signs may resolve on their own, the immune system does not eliminate the infection. Instead, viral latency develops. Reactivation of virus can occur at any point later in life, generally in association with stress or immune suppression.

Bordetella bronchiseptica

This gram-negative coccobacillus is an important cause of respiratory infection in dogs, but only recently it has been given attention as a primary respiratory pathogen of cats. Kittens are no more likely to be infected than adult cats, but may show more severe clinical signs. Clinical signs following experimental infection of cats included sneezing, oculonasal discharges, submandibular lymphadenopathy, and cough. The organism has also been isolated from naturally infected cats with a range of respiratory signs, including pneumonia. Spread of infection may be through cat-to-cat contact or via infectious discharges, and shedding can occur for weeks after infection from recovered cats. The organism is also found in healthy cats; it is more likely to cause disease in conditions of stress or overcrowding. The same bacterium can be transmitted between dogs and cats, and can also infect immunocompromised humans.

Chlamydophila felis

This bacterial species is predominantly an ocular pathogen. The organism is labile in the environment and is spread primarily through cat-to-cat contact. From 5 to 10 days after exposure, serous ocular discharge may be seen from one or both eyes. This progresses to bilateral mucopurulent discharge and chemosis, sometimes with sneezing and nasal discharge. Although not a commonly recognized problem, there is evidence that the infection may be transmitted from cats to people resulting in human conjunctivitis. Infected cats may continue to shed organisms for months after recovery.

Mycoplasma

The true role of these fastidious organisms in URI of cats is unknown. Mycoplasma species may be found in the upper airways and oropharynx of both healthy dogs and cats, and can be detected during lower and upper respiratory infections. They may be simply secondary pathogens, or may have a more important but yet undefined primary role in disease. Because they lack a cell wall, they are not cultured with routine methods nor are they killed with beta lactam type antibiotics.

DIAGNOSIS

Clinical findings associated with URI due to any pathogen are similar (sneezing, nasal/ocular discharge, hyporexia), but particular manifestations are more likely with one type of infection than another. For example, Chlamydophila is more likely to cause severe conjunctivitis with milder nasal signs, B. bronchiseptica is more likely to cause cough, FCV is likely to result in oral ulcerations, and cats with FHV-1 infection are often more severely lethargic and demonstrate marked nasal signs and possible keratitis. In many situations (especially kittens or cats recently adopted into single cat households), specific etiologic diagnosis is unnecessary. However, confirmation of a specific diagnosis can sometimes be helpful in settings such as catteries or animal shelters. Sometimes, a simple test such as microscopic evaluation of a conjunctival scraping may identify inclusions suggestive of Chlamydophila, or characteristic ocular lesion such has dendritic ulcers may strongly suggest FHV-1 infection.

Often, confirmation of disease diagnosis is complicated. For example, although the best way to confirm infection with B. bronchiseptica via positive culture, it can be isolated from the upper airways of healthy cats. Serologic evidence of exposure to the pathogens associated with URI may be associated with infection, simple past exposure, or even vaccination. For organism with latency or carrier states, detection of nucleic acids via PCR methods may not imply active infection. Confirmation of VS-FCV depends on isolation of identical viral strains (usually from oropharyngeal swabs or necropsy specimens) from more than one affected cat. No test can differentiate VS-FCV from typical FCV in a single cat.

When bacterial infections are suspected culture can be used to identify pathogens. For any of the primary pathogens (Bordetella, Chlamydophila, or Mycoplasma) the laboratory should be notified of the clinical suspicion so that appropriate culture media and procedures can be used. Oropharyngeal, tracheal or deep nasal culture swab samples should be collected into charcoal Amies transport medium when B. bronchiseptica is suspected. Chlamydophila can be cultured after vigorous conjunctival sampling; swabs should be placed in special media and kept refrigerated prior to timely laboratory submission.

Recently, panels of real-time PCR assays have been offered to detect common causes of URI. Feline URD panels offered by at least one commercial and another university laboratory include assays for feline herpesvirus-1 (FHV-1), feline calicivirus (FCV), Chlamydophila felis, Mycoplasma felis, and Bordetella bronchiseptica. Such panels offer advantages in real-life situations such as animal shelters where multiple different pathogens may be present. However, as mentioned previously, detection of nucleic acid sequences from a given pathogen cannot be assumed to prove disease causation.

THERAPY

In most cases, cats with URI will recover without specific treatment. Basic nursing care is usually best provided in a home situation, rather than in hospital, both to minimize exposure of other cats to a contagious infection and to minimize stress and likelihood of secondary infection in the affected cat. Hyporexia/anorexia is common, but can sometimes be overcome with simple measures such as feeding foods with strong odors such as fish-based cat food or by warming the food. Rarely, forced feeding is required (eg, via nasoesophageal tube). Adequate systemic hydration should be maintained (subcutaneous or intravenous fluids are seldom required), and humidification of the environment can help keep respiratory secretions moist.

Although ineffective against the most common causes of URI (viral infection), antibiotics are often employed empirically. Amoxicillian-clavulanic acid is a good broad spectrum empiric choice for control or prophylaxis of secondary infection. For treatment of specific bacterial infections, other antibiotics may be indicated. Doxycycline has good efficacy against Bordetella, Chlamydophila, and Mycoplasma but may be associated with discoloration of teeth in kittens (including developing feti) and with esophagitis. Other reasonable choices include trimethoprim-sufamethoxazole, fluoroquinolones, and erythromycin-type compounds such as azithromycin and clarithromycin. In cats with C. felis conjunctivitis, ophthalmic chloramphenicol or tetracycline ointments should also be applied. These same ophthalmic ointments may be useful in cats with corneal ulcers due to FHV.

Antiviral drugs are not generally used to treat URI. Acyclovir, used to treat herpes infections in humans, does not seem to have good efficacy against FHV-1. Other antiviral drugs are potentially toxic in cats. The one antiviral medication in common usage is L-lysine. Available as a nutricutical, L-lysine (500 mg/PO BID) is believed to interfere with herpes viral replication. In cats with corneal ulcers resulting form FHV, topical antiviral drugs such as trifluridine, idoxuridine, or adenine arabinoside are also used.

PREVENTION

Prevention of feline URI is dependant on both management practices to minimize exposure and vaccination. Minimization of crowding and stress, cleanliness, and routine disinfection are all crucial when cats are housed in groups, such as in catteries or shelters. A thorough discussion of shelter design and management is beyond the scope of this talk. A valuable resource with more detail on this topic can be found at the University of California, Davis Koret Shelter Medicine Program Web site (http://www.sheltermedicine.com/ portal/is_cleaning.shtml#top3). As an undeveloped virus, FCV is resistant to many routine disinfectants but is susceptible to a 5% bleach solution diluted 1:32 (1/2 cup per gallon) or potassium peroxymonosulfate. It should be noted that there are no disinfectants that work in the presence of organic debris, so basic cleaning must precede disinfection.

Vaccinations are available for FCV, virulent FCV, FHV-1, Chlamydophila, and B. bronchiseptica in cats. For individual pet cats, recommendations from the 2006 American Association of Feline Practitioners Feline Vaccine Advisory Panel suggest that vaccination against both FCV and FHV-1 should be considered core vaccines. However, it is important to understand that vaccination does not prevent infection or development of a carrier state, but rather minimizes disease severity. In addition, there may well be resistant strains of typical (and of course, virulent) FCV. Both FCV and FHV-1 vaccines can be found as modified live (MLV) and killed vaccine for parenteral injection, or as a MLV for intranasal (IN) administration. Occasionally, respiratory signs follow IN vaccination. Killed vaccines may be preferred for pregnant queens and cats with concurrent retroviral infection, but otherwise use of MLV is standard. After initial vaccination and booster vaccination at one year, duration of immunity is likely at least 3 years so revaccination need not be carried out more frequently. Both Chlamydophila and Bordetella vaccines are considered "non-core" and are generally not suggested for use in pet cats.

Vaccination in shelters has a different set of consideration than individual pet vaccination. Unless records are available to prove otherwise, cats are assumed to be unvaccinated and vaccinated immediately upon shelter entry. Because intranasal (IN) vaccination can induce mild clinical signs, this can serve as a source of confusion in shelters deciding which cats should be isolated, or even culled. However, even injectable MLV vaccine occasionally induce clinical signs, IN vaccines may offer more rapid protection than injectable vaccines, and at least one paper suggests that IN vaccination in addition to injectable vaccination for FCV/FHV-1 offers increased protection (Edinboro, 1999). Vaccination against Chlamydophila is reserved for shelters with a demonstrated problem with the infection. Even then, vaccination does not prevent infection or shedding. Because there is some risk of zoonotic transmission, some shelters prefer to cull infected cats. The importance of Bordetella in causing URI in sheltered cats is unclear, but the infection can be transmitted between species (dogs and cats). In shelters with a demonstrable problem with Bordetella infection, IN vaccination of cats may be warranted.

Recently, a vaccination for virulent systemic FCV has become available (CaliciVax®, Fort Dodge Animal Health). This killed virus vaccine incorporates one of several strains of FCV known to cause severe systemic disease. Generally, hypervirulent strains of FCV have arisen from new genetic mutations in each group of cats infected. Although the new vaccine demonstrated protection from challenge with the same virulent strain used in its development, to our knowledge challenge has not be attempted (and therefore protection has not been demonstrated) with any other virulent strain.

SELECTED REFERENCES

1. Bannasch MJ, Foley JE. Epidemiologic evaluation of multiple respiratory pathogens in cats in animal shelters. J Feline Med Surg. 2005; 7:109-19.
2. Helps CR, Lait P, Damhuis A, et al. Factors associated with upper respiratory tract disease caused by feline herpesvirus, feline calicivirus, Chlamydophila felis and Bordetella bronchiseptica in cats: experience from 218 European catteries. Vet Rec. 2005;156:669-73.
3. Hurley KE, Pesavento PA, Pedersen NC, et al. An outbreak of virulent systemic feline calicivirus disease J Am Vet Med Assoc. 2004;224:241-9.
4. Pedersen NC, Sato R, Foley JE, et al. Common virus infections in cats, before and after being placed in shelters, with emphasis on feline enteric coronavirus. J Feline Med Surg. 2004;6:83-88.
5. Stiles J, Townsend WM, Rogers QR, et al. Effect of oral administration of L-lysine on conjunctivitis caused by feline herpesvirus in cats. Am J Vet Res. 2002; 63:99-103.
6. The 2006 American Association of Feline Practitioners Feline Vaccine Advisory Panel Report. http://www.aafponline.org/resources/guidelines/2006 Vaccination_Guidelines_JAVMA.pdf.

WHAT TESTS SHOULD I PERFORM IN THIS RESPIRATORY PATIENT?

Janice A. Dye, DVM, MS, PhD, Diplomate ACVIM
National Health & Environmental Effects Research
Laboratory
Research Triangle Park, NC

Diagnostic efforts are directed towards identifying a specific, hopefully treatable, underlying cause of the respiratory disease. However, many common respiratory diseases in companion animals are idiopathic conditions, and are therefore primarily diagnoses of exclusion. Recognizing that there are many causes of respiratory disease in dogs and cats, and that within the syndrome of upper vs. lower airway disease, parenchymal diseases, pleural space diseases, and cardiovascular disorders, the spectrum of disease is great; each patient should be treated as a new and unique case. A complete evaluation should be performed not only to rule out potential underlying disease(s), but also to establish a data base which can be used to monitor the effectiveness of subsequent treatments as well as to assess disease progression.

HISTORY

Acquisition of an accurate patient history is an important first step. It is used initially to localize disease and to characterize the type, frequency, and severity of clinical signs. For example, coughing is the most common presenting complaint for cats with bronchopulmonary disease and dogs with chronic bronchitis. However, coughing is not pathognomonic for a particular diagnosis as it may result from tracheobronchial inflammation, excessive airway secretions, or bronchoconstriction. Other common presenting complaints include dyspnea, sneezing, wheezing, noisy or abnormal breathing, retching or vomiting. Although one clinical sign may predominate, several signs are often present.

Historical assessment is limited by the accuracy of the owners' observations and the amount of time they are able to observe the patient. Intermittent signs or subtle changes in respiratory pattern or effort are often difficult for the owner to appreciate; and may in fact go unrecognized for long periods. Respiratory signs with illness (ie, fever, dyspnea, or weight loss) should be approached with urgency; while the occasional cough, sneeze, or "weird sound from the throat" may relate to more insidious and ill-defined condition(s).

Further questioning may reveal that some signs appear to be exacerbated by certain seasons (suggestive of allergies), or certain activities (eg, exercise, exposure to cold air) or changes in the animal's living conditions (eg, home construction, exposure to irritants such as cigarette smoke). Careful attention should be given to documenting previous or concurrent illnesses, especially upper respiratory tract infections, and/or rhinitis and sinusitis conditions.

In addition, questions pertaining to recent changes in the bark or meow are suggestive of laryngeal paralysis. Similarly, worsening of cough with drinking or eating is suggestive of a swallowing disorder or again, laryngeal paralysis. Routine questioning should also confirm whether the pet's vaccination status is current, whether parasite and heartworm preventatives are used, and whether there has been any recent exposure to potentially ill animals (eg, boarding, dog parks, new puppies or kittens) which may increase the likelihood that one is dealing with a respiratory infection. Certainly, unexplained or progressive cough in the geriatric pet should alert to the possibly of underlying lung or thoracic neoplasia.

PHYSICAL EXAMINATION

The examination should begin from a distance. Prior to handling the pet, try to assess its stance, respiratory pattern, rate and effort. Also try to assess its level of anxiety because fear can readily influence the normal breathing pattern. By combining this information with the signalment and history, a priority scale of probable rule outs can be developed. For example, cats or dogs with bronchial disease frequently cough, while cats with hypertrophic cardiomyopathy seldom do; cough is a variable finding in parenchymal disorders (eg, pulmonary fibrosis) and in pleural space disease. Moreover, cardiac disease should always be considered in animals presenting with lethargy and respiratory problems, but no history of coughing. Careful auscultation of the heart may detect murmurs or arrhythmias which would further support cardiac disease and guide the diagnostic work up accordingly (ie, thoracic radiographs, EKG, and echocardiography). Tachypnea in conjunction with respiratory distress and right-sided heart changes may indicate pulmonary hypertension. Estimates of pulmonary arterial pressure are used to obtain this diagnosis.

Concurrent respiratory and gastrointestinal signs may be indicative of underlying parasitic disease (eg, ascarids or heartworms). Persistent tachypnea may be indicative of restrictive lung disease where parenchymal infiltration, pleural, or mediastinal disease are limiting the ability of the animal to adequately expand the lungs. The presence of pleural effusions (eg, chylothorax, FIP), thymic lymphosarcoma, and other possibilities can also result in a patient exhibiting tachypnea.

Open-mouthed breathing is an ominous sign and should always warn of the possibility of severe respiratory distress; including that associated with marked bronchoconstriction. Because distal airways normally narrow during expiration, signs of small airway obstruction may be most evident on expiration. Some cats with presumed bronchoconstriction appear tachypneic and exhibit subtle expiratory pushes at the end of each breath. Alternatively, other cats, especially those with long-standing airway inflammation and remodeling, tend to breathe slowly and deeply, with marked abdominal efforts. Open-mouthed breathing may also be observed in very "nervous" animals or may be related to upper airway obstruction associated with brachycephalic airway syndrome, nasopharyngeal polyps, or occluded nasal passageways (eg, severe rhinitis, fungal balls, nasal adenocarcinoma).

The ability to adequately assess lung sounds depends on the cooperation of the patient and the persistence of the veterinarian. A quality stethoscope and a quiet examining room are essential. Regardless of where you start, one should be thorough. One should always compare both sides and determine whether sounds are diminished on one side relative to the other. Absence of breath sounds in a distressed pet may indicate bilateral pleural space involvement, or in a cat, the presence of severe bronchoconstriction. In the latter situation, the cat is often cyanotic and may have a sinus bradycardia.

Even in cats and dogs with significant pulmonary disease, it is not uncommon for normal breath sounds to be present, especially if the animal is breathing quietly. In this situation, a deeper breath can often be induced by temporarily occluding the external nares. Repeat until all lung fields are assessed. Tracheal sensitivity should be assessed by application of firm, not crushing, pressure over the trachea until the animal begins to cough. In cats or dogs with bronchial disease, a deeper, moist cough is often elicited; after which loud adventitial sounds (crackles and wheezes) may be appreciated. Occasionally, in cases with excessive mucous secretion or severe tracheal collapse, tracheal palpation may elicit paroxysmal coughing and result in obvious dyspnea. Be prepared to initiate emergency steps if dyspnea persists.

MINIMUM DATA BASE

If a thorough history and physical examination were able to be obtained, one should be able to formulate a list of likely differential diagnoses that "fit" or are consistent with the animal's signalment and primary presenting problem(s) and other findings. This list will guide you in selecting additional diagnostic tests to better understand what your patient has. Because many of the common diseases in dogs and cats are idiopathic syndromes, what you do NOT find can be as important as what you do find.

Specific causes of respiratory disease can only be diagnosed if one looks for specific causes. To this end, fecal analyses (Baerman preparations, flotation and/or sedimentation), and select serologies are useful to diagnose pulmonary parasitic disease. Detection of pulmonary parasites often requires several fecal analyses to be performed. Parasites such as lung worms (*Aelurostrongylus abstrusus*, *Capillaria aerophilia*), lung flukes (*Paragonimus kellicotti*) and ascarids can cause lung disease. In epizootic areas, an occult heartworm test for *Dirofilariasis immitis* should be performed in dogs and in cats. In cats, heartworm disease is associated with signs ranging from coughing and difficulty breathing, to vomiting, weight less and fainting (eg, feline heartworm). Seemingly, larvae forms are the main cause of the problem, resulting in significant pathology in the pulmonary arteries and arterioles.[1]

Quality thoracic radiography is essential in evaluating the dogs and cat with respiratory disease. For maximal radiographic interpretation, short exposure times and high detail film/digital image acquisition are required. Both lateral views and a ventrodorsal (or dorsal ventral) view should be obtained. Specific findings will be discussed in case examples reviewed. Fluoroscopy is useful to assess functional or dynamic changes such as tracheal or main stem bronchial collapse.[2]

Airway cytology can help to identify the presence of inflammation and to characterize the types of inflammatory cells present.[3] On occasion, neoplastic cells or organisms (eg, Blastomyces) can be observed. Of note, results obtained from cytology can vary tremendously depending on the depth of the airways sampled (trachea vs. alveoli), the method used to obtain the sample (washings, brushings, or lavage techniques), the method used to process the sample, not to mention the patient's airway pathology itself.

Positive bacterial cultures occur in approximately one third of the cats and dogs with bronchial disease. It can be difficult, however, to determine whether growth of small numbers of bacteria reflects innocuous colonization or true infection. A variety of organisms may isolated in low numbers from the airways of clinically healthy pets. With chronic lung disease, mucociliary clearance mechanisms may be impaired due to ineffective cough reflexes and changes in the viscoelastic properties of the airway secretions. Hence, in animals with chronic bronchial disease, bacteria could set up more permanent residence in the diseased airways. Although antibiotic treatment is indicated if positive bacterial cultures are obtained from animals with bronchial disease, clinical signs may not necessarily resolve completely even though follow up cultures prove negative. This is due to the presence of ongoing airway pathologic changes such as mucus hypersecretion and remodeling. Increasingly, molecular testing (PCR, multiplex PCR strategies) is being used, often in conjunctional with routine microbiological examinations, to assess emerging or more complex infectious disease situations (eg, methicillin-resistant *Staphylococcus aureus* (MRSA), Bartonella species, pathogenic feline herpesvirus or calicivirus isolates, canine influenza). Only reputable laboratories using validated protocols and other controls should be used.

An arterial blood gas analyses analysis evaluates how effectively the lungs are delivering oxygen to the blood and how efficiently they are eliminating carbon dioxide from it. The test also indicates how well the lungs and kidneys are interacting to maintain normal blood pH (acid-base balance).

Although not specific for respiratory disease, a CBC, biochemical profile, and urinalysis are important to evaluate concurrent systemic abnormalities (eg, hyperadrenocorticism with pulmonary interstitial changes or mineralization).

ADDITIONAL OR ADVANCED DIAGNOSTICS

If the clinical signs are less clearly localizable or the signs worsen despite appropriate treatment, additional diagnostic steps may be indicated. Since these steps entail more risk to the patient and/or call for specialized equipment, referral may be warranted and should be discussed as an option.

Cranial CT scans with rhinoscopic exam, and mucosal biopsies are needed to diagnose nasopharyngeal disease (polyps, neoplasia, webbing) or occluded nasal passageways (eg, severe rhinitis, fungal balls, nasal adenocarcinoma).

For conditions such as suspect laryngeal paralysis, a direct visual examination under anesthesia is required. Combined use of laryngoscopy and bronchoscopy may allow detection laryngeal paralysis and other specific airway changes (eg, tracheal collapse, mucosal reddening, intraluminal masses). The increased availability of fiberoptic technology and video-endoscopy has enhanced recognition of the benefits gained from visualization of the lower airways, in part because sampling of a grossly abnormal area may increase the likelihood of obtaining a diagnostic sample.[4] Alternatively, if interstitial disease is prominent, fine-needle aspirates may yield more information (eg, fungal organisms, neoplastic cells) than intraluminal sampling alone.

In select veterinary institutions or referral centers, advanced pulmonary function testing and specialized imaging (ie, fluoroscopy, CT scans, high-resolution CT scans) are available to more thoroughly assess upper airway abnormalities as well as pulmonary disease, especially reactive airway diseases or interstitial lung diseases.[5] Computed tomography can also be used to guide fine-needle lung aspirates or to obtain tissue-core biopsies of intrathoracic lesions.[6]

Although not related to the lung per se, endoscopic ultrasonography can be used in a variety of thoracic applications including examination of the mediastinum, bronchial lymph nodes, and esophagus. Depending on the size and location of pulmonary lesions, ultrasonography can also be useful in performing fine needle aspiration of pulmonary masses.[7] When less invasive measures fail to adequately explain the signs of animals with atypical disease progression, an open lung biopsy may provide a definitive diagnosis. This is particularly useful in animals with interstitial lung disorders.[8]

REFERENCES

1. Browne LE, Carter TD. Levy JK, Snyder PS, Johnson CM. Pulmonary arterial disease in cats seropositive for *Dirofilaria immitis* but lacking adult heartworms in the heart and lungs. Am J Vet Res 2005; 66:1544-9.
2. Macready DM, Johnson LR, Pollard RE. Fluoroscopic and radiographic evaluation of tracheal collapse in dogs: 62 cases (2001-2006). J Am Vet Med Assoc.. 2007; 230:1870-76.
3. McCullough S, Brinson J. Collection and interpretation of respiratory cytology. Clin Tech Small Anim Pract. 1999; 14:220-6.
4. Johnson L. Small animal bronchoscopy. Vet Clin North Am Small Anim Pract. 2001; 31:691-705.
5. Johnson VS, Corcoran BM, Wotton PR, Schwarz T, Sullivan M. Thoracic high-resolution computed tomographic findings in dogs with canine idiopathic pulmonary fibrosis. J Small Anim Pract. 2005; 46:381-88.
6. Zekas LJ, Crawford JT, O'Brien RT. Computed tomography-guided fine-needle aspirate and tissue-core biopsy of intrathoracic lesions in thirty dogs and cats. Vet Radiol Ultrasound. 2005; 46:200-4.
7. Gaschen L, Kircher P, Lang J. Endoscopic ultrasound instrumentation, applications in humans, and potential veterinary applications. Vet Radiol Ultrasound. 2003; 44:665-80.
8. Reinero CR, Cohn LA. Interstitial lung diseases. Vet Clin North Am Small Anim Pract. 2007; 3:937-47.

INTERSTITIAL LUNG DISEASE: WHAT DOES IT MEAN?

Janice A. Dye, DVM, MS, PhD, Diplomate ACVIM
National Health & Environmental Effects Research
Laboratory
Research Triangle Park, NC

Interstitial lung disease (ILD) represents a heterogeneous collection of diffuse pulmonary parenchymal disorders. The pathology of ILD centers on the pulmonary interstitium, in particular, that of the alveolar region. Anatomically this refers to the space between the alveolar epithelial cells, the adjacent capillary endothelial cells, and their shared basement membrane. In health, the thinly walled, flexible alveolar units allow for (a) ease of lung distention during inspiration, and (b) extensive surface area for efficient gas exchange. In ILD, it appears that Type II pneumocytes, lung fibroblasts, and certain other cell types engage in an anomalous healing response that ultimately leads to loss of significant functional alveolar space. In so doing, the normally compliant lung becomes progressively stiff and inelastic. Physiologically, diffuse parenchymal thickening (ie, fibrosis) results in a restrictive breathing pattern.

In animals and humans, a variety of conditions have been associated with development of interstitial lung disease. Conditions range from metabolic disorders (eg, hyperadrenocorticism) and infectious diseases (eg, herpesvirus, calicivirus, feline immunodeficiency virus [FIV], toxoplasmosis); to toxicant (eg, paraquat), drug (eg, bleomycin), and occupational exposures (eg, silica, talc, asbestos). In most instances, however, the cause remains unknown. Collectively, parenchymal lung disorders have an insidious onset and are often quite resistant to treatment.

The goal of this article is to increase awareness of ILD in small animals and to assist veterinarians in its recognition. We will review what is currently known about ILD in dogs and cats, focusing on common clinical and pathophysiologic changes, but emphasizing their unique underlying pathologic features. Diagnostic options and therapeutic limitations are discussed. Because many of diagnostic algorithms used in dogs and cats are based on analogous conditions in humans, recent advances in ILD in people are also discussed.

ILD IN HUMANS

A number of related, somewhat confusing terms have been used to describe ILD in people. Certain terms reflect clinical designations for lung disease involving the interstitium, while other terms are more specific pathologic subclassifications. Until recently, if an underlying cause was not apparent, the term *idiopathic pulmonary fibrosis* or IPF was used clinically to describe any and all "fibrotic lung disease of unknown origin." In 2000, however, a consensus statement was published by the ATS/ERS in which IPF in humans was classified as a distinct diagnosis separate from other types of ILD. Use of the term IPF is currently restricted to individuals exhibiting rather specific histologic changes on lung biopsy. Key features include interstitial fibrosis with fibroblast/myofibroblast foci, metaplasia of the alveolar epithelium (honeycomb lung), and interstitial smooth muscle metaplasia/hyperplasia. The term *usual interstitial pneumonia* or UIP is the pathologic subclassification given to this collection of changes. Rarely, however, UIP-like changes can occur as a result of collagen vascular disorders or as end-stage changes associated with environmental or toxicant exposure.

Despite attempts to better define IPF, in humans IPF remains a poorly understood yet prevalent type of ILD. Presenting complaints of individuals with IPF include progressive exercise intolerance, shortness of breath, and cough, although the latter is not always present. IPF can be found concurrently with pulmonary neoplasia. Of all interstitial lung disorders, IPF is notable for its progressive nature and resistance to therapeutic intervention. The prognosis for IPF is on par with that of aggressive pulmonary malignancies, with a median survival after diagnosis of less than three years. Thus, in human medicine, early and accurate diagnosis of IPF is vital to allow early referral for lung transplantation, the only effective treatment available to date.

ILD IN ANIMALS

Do dogs or cats develop IPF as it is currently defined in people? If not, what types of interstitial diseases have been recognized in companion animals? How should one attempt to diagnose ILD in animals? What prognosis does ILD in animals carry? Besides lung transplantation, are there any recommended treatments for ILD in animals? In the remainder of this article, we will attempt to address these questions. Be forewarned, however, that in veterinary medicine, inconsistencies in the diagnosis of ILD have contributed to a rather poor understanding and characterization of ILD in animals. Much remains to be determined regarding the incidence/prevalence of ILD in animals, basic knowledge of underlying disease mechanisms, and efficacy (if any) of specific therapeutic approaches with regard to fibrotic disease progression.

First, as mentioned above, although uncommon, fibrotic ILD has long been recognized in companion animals. ILD has been sporadically reported in both dogs and cats in association with infectious agents, toxicant exposure (eg, paraquat), drug or vaccine reactions, inhaled particles, and as a component of immune-mediated (polyarthritis) or neoplastic disorders.

Interestingly, over the last decade, several independent case and case series reports have also described an idiopathic fibrotic lung condition in **dogs**, most notably in terrier breeds (eg, West Highland White Terriers). As discussed above, although the term *idiopathic pulmonary fibrosis* has long been used in veterinary literature—and was used to describe these dogs—classic histologic features of UIP were not identified. Rather, based on distinct alveolar ultrastructural changes, Norris and colleagues hypothesize that terrier dogs may have a genetic predisposition to aberrant collagen regulation.

Clinically, these dogs present for chronic coughing, dyspnea, and tachypnea. On auscultation, inspiratory crackles and wheezing are commonly noted. Radiographic changes often include mild to severely increased interstitial markings, with and without additional bronchial markings. Right-sided cardiomegaly (cor pulmonale) is also present in many dogs. Bronchoscopic findings may reveal normal airways or mild airway mucoid reactions. The mean survival time after diagnosis is approximately 1.5 to 2 years. The predominant histopathologic abnormality is alveolar septal fibrosis. Treatment with prednisolone, with or without bronchodilators, is most commonly used, but with variable response. In summary, dogs can develop significant pulmonary interstitial fibrosis of unknown etiology, which clinically resembles IPF in humans.

In **cats**, until recently, only sporadic reports of spontaneous ILD existed. In these instances, histologic findings were likely more compatible with distinct forms of ILD (eg, cryptogenic fibrosing alveolitis) rather than UIP, hence IPF. In 2004, Williams and colleagues published a case series report in cats demonstrating pathologic lung changes that closely mimicked UIP in humans. In a related clinical report, Cohn and colleagues summarized the clinical features of these cats. Unfortunately, similar to people, the majority of cats with IPF-like disease had generally poor response to therapy and thus poor outcome.

Specifically, the cats with histologic criteria of UIP tended to be middle aged to older, with no apparent sex or breed predisposition. Presenting complaints included respiratory distress and less commonly, cough. Physical exam abnormalities included notable tachypnea, with inspiratory or combined inspiratory/expiratory effort, and generalized adventitial lung sounds. Radiographic abnormalities included diffuse or patchy interstitial changes, bronchial patterns, and alveolar infiltrates, often in combination. Occasionally, based on bronchial lavage fluid findings, mild neutrophilic inflammation was present. Of note, several cats did poorly after what seemed to be an uneventful lavage procedure or after undergoing other minimally invasive diagnostic procedures. These cats seem to have very limited respiratory reserve and should be considered extremely labile. Coincident pulmonary neoplasia was identified in several cats. Response to therapy (which included corticosteroids, antibiotics, bronchodilators, and even diuretics) was generally poor, and most cats died within days to months of their initial diagnosis. In all, cats with histologic changes compatible with UIP had signs that closely mimicked that of IPF in humans. Likewise, current treatment attempts were similarly unrewarding.

FUTURE DIRECTIONS

The concept that ILD stems from an exaggerated inflammatory and subsequent reparative response related to prior (or possibly ongoing) alveolar insult have led to routine use of immunosuppressive agents (eg, glucocorticoids) in ILD, with relatively inconsistent results. IPF, however, may actually represent more of an alveolar fibroproliferative disorder wherein select alveolar epithelial cells become "activated," again possibly due to previous or ongoing injury. Hence, more recent therapy approaches have attempted to alter interactions between alveolar epithelial cells and fibroblasts (eg, use of interferon gamma or antagonists of growth factors such as TGF). These approaches have been hindered by the magnitude of and chronicity of fibrotic changes already in place by the time a definitive diagnosis of IPF is obtained. However, improvements in thoracic imaging, especially high-resolution CT imaging, have provided a means diagnosing cases much earlier in the course of disease, and have obviated the need for surgical biopsy in many patients. In so doing, non-invasive imaging has allowed for easier assessment of therapeutic outcomes in clinical trials, and more clinical trials have been initiated. High-resolution imaging has also shown that pulmonary hypertension is an underappreciated co-morbid condition that should be specifically addressed. A preliminary study in dogs suggests that high-resolution CT may also be useful in diagnosing, staging and even therapeutically monitoring fibrosis in dogs.

REFERENCES

1. Dungworth DL. Interstitial pulmonary disease. Adv Vet Sci Comp Med. 1982; 26:173-200.
2. Gross TJ, Hunninghake GW. Idiopathic pulmonary fibrosis. N Engl J Med.. 2001; 345:517-525.
3. Mason RJ, Schwarz MI, Hunninghake GW, et al. NHLBI workshop summary. Pharmacological therapy for idiopathic pulmonary fibrosis. Past, present, and future. Am J Resp Crit Care Med. 1999;160:1771-1777.
4. Noth I, Martinez FL. Recent advances in idiopathic pulmonary fibrosis. Chest. 2007; 132:367-650.
5. King TE, Costabel U, Cordier JF, et al. Idiopathic pulmonary fibrosis: diagnosis and treatment. International consensus statement. American Thoracic Society (ATS), and the European Respiratory Society (ERS). Am J Resp Crit Care Med. 2000; 161:646-664.
6. American Thoracic Society/European Respiratory Society International multidisciplinary consensus classification of the idiopathic interstitial pneumonias. Am J Resp Crit Care Med. 2002; 165:277-304.
7. Longstaffe J, Humphreys D, Hayward A, et al. Paraquat poisoning in dogs and cats-differences between accidental and malicious poisoning. J Small Anim Pract. 1981; 22:153-156.
8. Corcoran BM, Cobb M, Martin MWS, et al. Chronic pulmonary disease in West Highland white terriers. Vet Rec. 1999; 144:611-616.
9. Lobetti RG, Milner R, Lane E. Chronic idiopathic pulmonary fibrosis in five dogs. J Am Anim Hosp Assoc. 2001; 37:119-127.
10. Norris AJ, Naydan DK, Wilson DW. Interstitial lung disease in West Highland White Terriers. Vet Pathol. 2005; 42:35-41.

11. Rhind SM, Gunn-Moore DA. Desquamative form of cryptogenic fibrosing alveolitis in a cat. J Comp Pathol. 2000; 123:226-229.

12. Williams K, Malarkey D, Cohn L, Patrick D, Dye J, Toews G. Identification of spontaneous feline idiopathic pulmonary fibrosis. Morphology and ultrastructural evidence for a type II pneumoncyte defect. Chest. 2004; 125: 125: 2278-2288.

13. Cohn LA, Norris CR, Hawkins EC, Dye JA, Johnson CA, Williams KJ. Identification and characterization of an idiopathic pulmonary fibrosis-like condition in cats. J Vet Intern Med. 2004; 18: 632-641.

14. Johnson VS, Corcoran BM, Wotton PR, Schwarz T, Sullivan M. Thoracic high-resolution computed tomographic findings in dogs with canine idiopathic pulmonary fibrosis. J Small Anim Pract. 2005; 46:381-88.

THE COUGH THAT WON'T QUIT

Janice A. Dye, DVM, MS, PhD, Diplomate ACVIM
National Health & Environmental Effects Research
Laboratory
Research Triangle Park, NC

Chronic cough, a common condition in companion animals, is often a diagnostic challenge. Although common, it does not represent a specific diagnosis or disease. Coughing is simply a clinical sign related to one of more of the following underlying conditions:

1. Development of airway injury, inflammation, or excess mucous secretions
2. Excessive bronchoconstriction or airflow limitation
3. Stimulation of irritant (rapidly adapting stretch receptors, RARs) or chemo- (C-fibers) receptors within the airways and airspaces.

In and of itself, the cough reflex can be beneficial. A cough is generated by a sudden expiratory effort, initially against a closed glottis. This effort produces a noisy expulsion of air, thus clearing mucus or trapped foreign material from the lungs. Coughing becomes problematic, however, if it is too severe or persists for too long. Chronic cough typically starts out as an acute condition that fails to resolve completely. Put another way, most owners will relate that they noticed their pet "started coughing one day" and although the cough may have since waxed and waned, the main reason for seeking veterinary attention is that the cough itself "just won't quit." The inciting condition (eg, a transient viral infection, a dead or dying heartworm, a prior dental cleaning with bacterial embolism) may no longer be present, much less be definable. What should a veterinarian do?

A systematic approach to diagnosis and treatment can be effective for many cases of chronic cough. As one seeks to identify specific underlying factors (eg, pulmonary parasites, bacterial pneumonia, congestive heart failure [CHF]) one can best "treat any treatable" underlying condition. However, ancillary supportive care to suppress ongoing airway inflammation, relieve airway constriction and collapse, and directly suppress the cough reflex may be necessary. The initial examination and diagnostic approach should seek to rule out more ominous causes of chronic cough. Cough with illness (ie, fever, dyspnea, or weight loss) should be approached with urgency; while cough as the "only" sign may relate to more insidious and ill-defined condition(s). The same basic principles of *airway supportive care* become the mainstay for managing chronic cough when a specific cause cannot be identified.

It should be noted that chronic cough can be a frustrating problem for the owner/patient and veterinarian. However, a *shotgun* or polypharmaceutical drug trial is NOT a substitute for a systematic approach to its diagnosis and treatment. Herein, we will review: (1) the pathophysiology of cough in relationship to lung and extrapulmonary inflammation and mechanical stimulation; (2) conditions commonly associated with cough in dogs, cats, and humans, and (3) rational approaches to treatment.

COUGH REFLEXES

In human pulmonary medicine, coughing is considered chronic if it occurs on most days for at least 3 months of the year for a 2 or more year period. Because dogs and cats have shorter life spans, in veterinary medicine, coughing is generally considered chronic if it occurs for 2 or more consecutive months.

Despite being one of the most frequent complaints for which people seek medical attention, relatively little is known about the pathogenesis of chronic cough. As a primary defensive reflex, in health, cough protects the airways from inhaled, potentially harmful stimuli. In disease, the cough reflex threshold is seemingly lowered and coughing may become excessive. Largely transmitted via vagal afferent pathways, select airway receptors mediate and influence activation of the cough reflex. Stimuli converge on the brain stem respiratory network and supramedullary brain centers. Central or conscious control of cough is also involved. In long-standing disease, plastic changes in the intrinsic and synaptic excitability of cough increase at the brain stem, spinal, and even ganglionic level, such that cough can be more easily induced. Chronic exposure to irritants or to certain inflammatory mediators (eg, tachykinins) also contribute to the neurogenic plasticity of this reflex network.

In the airways, RARs are the primary afferent nerve fibers evoking the defensive cough. Experimental findings suggest that, via RAR activation, a variety of conditions elicit cough. Conditions include smooth muscle constriction, mucous accumulation, mechanical irritation, and mucosal application of tussive agonists (eg, capsaicin, bradykinin, citric acid). However, other mediators (eg, leukotrienes, histamine, methacholine) are capable of stimulating RARs, but they are *ineffective* at inducing cough. Additionally, there exist chemically responsive afferent fibers throughout the airways and lungs. Typically quiescent in health, these pathways may be recruited during conditions of inflammation. Extrapulmonary (laryngeal, tracheal, and main stem bronchial) low threshold mechanosensors have also been described and are exquisitely sensitive to touch.

Airway pathologic changes occurring in association with chronic cough commonly include mucosal changes (epithelial denudation and increased inflammatory cells of various types) as well as increased airway vascularity, increased goblet cells, and sub-basement membrane thickening. These remodeling changes reflect repair attempts in response to chronic inflammatory insult, or deranged airway epithelial-mesenchymal units. Alternatively, generic epithelial damage elicited by severe cough itself (ie, repetitive mechanical and physical trauma) may stimulate epithelial cells to increase production of growth factors (eg, nerve growth factor) and expression of surface receptors (eg, TRPV-1, the capsaicin receptor).

It is difficult to prove whether chronic cough promotes airway wall remodeling or airway wall remodeling leads to chronic cough. Regardless, once airway remodeling becomes established, both mechanisms likely contribute to a positive feedback loop that culminates in *"a cough that just won't quit."* Used alone, current antitussive agents are largely ineffective at suppressing cough. Cough challenge testing may help define cough hypersensitivity states and allow for more effective antitussive agents to be developed in the future.

CAUSES OF COUGH

Causes of cough in **animals** can be subdivided into the following categories:

- **Inflammatory** – Feline bronchopulmonary disease or asthma, eosinophilic pulmonary disease syndromes, chronic bronchitis and/or chronic obstructive pulmonary disease, and interstitial lung diseases
- **Infectious** – Tracheobronchitis or pneumonia related to a host of viral, bacterial, fungal, or protozoal organisms
- **Parasitic** – Related to direct effects or secondary to immune responses to migrating or dying parasites including Dirofilaria, Aelurostrongylus, Paragonimus, Capillaria, Filaroides, Ascarids, and miscellaneous organisms
- **Injury-related** – Airway or parenchymal damage due to inhalation of irritants (smoke inhalation, environmental tobacco smoke) or aspiration of foreign material (plant material, food, gastric acid; often comorbidity with laryngeal paralysis or megaesophagus)
- **Neoplastic** – Primary lung, tracheal, laryngeal, or metastatic disease, or compression by enlarged lymph nodes, thymus, or heart-base tumors
- **Cardiovascular** – Left atrial enlargement, pulmonary edema, and pulmonary embolism
- **Congenital or acquired conditions/ malformations** - Brachycephalic airway syndrome, chondromalacia of tracheal or bronchial cartilage, tracheal stenosis, ciliary dysfunction, and mucosal (IgA reductions) or systemic (feline immunodeficiency virus [FIV]) immunodeficiencies. Although the actual defect may be congenital, cough may not develop until later in life as secondary changes such as airway remodeling or bronchiectasis develop.

Chronic cough occurs commonly in **humans** with asthma and eosinophilic bronchitis, chronic bronchitis/COPD, gastroesophageal reflux disease (GERD), rhinosinusitis or postnasal drip syndrome (recently renamed upper airway cough disorder), and less commonly due to bronchiolitis and bronchiectasis, lung neoplasia, medication (ACE inhibitor), interstitial lung disease, exposure (often occupational) to nonallergic irritants (dusts, cold air, endotoxin, molds), and idiopathic or psychogenic cough disorders.

The remaining discussion focuses on **chronic bronchitis (CB)**, a condition common to dogs, cats, and people, which clearly exemplifies the complex interplay between airway pathologic changes and persistence of cough. In people, CB is diagnosed clinically by a chronic (mostly productive) cough. It is thought to develop owing to bacterial colonization and resultant airway inflammatory responses (ie, generation of cytokines and chemotactic stimuli) by the airway epithelium, which propagates airway injury and inflammation. The diseased airway is less capable of clearing bacteria, so colonization persists. Over time, bronchial gland hyperplasia, goblet cell metaplasia, and peribronchiolar fibrosis develop. These changes further impair host clearance of pathogenic or even opportunistic bacteria. As mononuclear cells infiltrate the airway walls, and neutrophils (with their collagenase, elastase, and protease byproducts) increase within the airway lumen, the airways are further compromised.

Although not as well characterized in animals, similar changes appear to occur in dogs and cats. Moreover, in dogs, tracheal or bronchial collapse often coexists with these changes, possibly due to breed-related chondromalacia or simply to long-standing airway remodeling. In advanced cases, cor pulmonale (right heart failure) may develop as sequelae to chronically increased pulmonary vascular resistance.

Initial diagnosis of CB in animals is a largely *rule out* process. It involves a thorough "bug and cancer" hunt. It requires a complete physical exam including careful auscultation of all lung fields and assessment of airflow decrements in conducting air passageways. Radiographic/fluoroscopic assessment of the airways, lung parenchyma, and cardiovascular system is essential. Airway cytological and microbial evaluation via bronchoscopy or other techniques to obtain airway wash/brushing/biopsy samples, fecal parasite testing, serology, and so forth are necessary to *rule in* specific causes of cough as listed above. During such a workup, what you do *not* find can be as important as what you *do* find. Hence in the absence of more specific disease findings, middle-aged dogs or cats presenting for cough in conjunction with neutrophilic/monocytic lung inflammation, are typically diagnosed as having CB.

CASE MANAGEMENT

The next step is to *"treat the treatable."* In people with chronic bronchitis/COPD, several controlled studies have shown that combination therapy with long-acting beta$_2$-adrenergics and inhaled corticosteroids can significantly improve symptoms and reduce clinical exacerbations. Limited studies in dogs and cats suggest that a similar combination approach (ie, suppress ongoing airway inflammation and relieve airway constriction) is likely to be of benefit. More limited data suggests that certain antibiotics (macrolides) or other bronchodilators (methylxanthines) may be beneficial owing to immunomodulatory effects and reduction of mucous production. In dogs with overt tracheal collapse, placement of intraluminal self-expanding wall stents can dramatically reduce cough. Depending on airway culture results, antimicrobial therapy may be beneficial. It is, however, difficult to determine whether growth of small numbers of bacteria reflects innocuous colonization or true infection. Generic recommendations also include maintaining current vaccination status, limiting exposure to infectious agents (dog parks, boarding), and minimizing irritant exposure (eg, cigarette smoke). Lastly, in dogs with chronic cough due to significant airway collapse or for patients who simply cannot sleep due to cough, direct cough suppression, especially at night, is warranted. In dogs, narcotic antitussives such as hydrocodone bitartrate appear most effective.

Ultimately, successful management of chronic cough requires a team effort by the owner and veterinarian. It is beneficial at the onset of the case to discuss in depth the most likely cause(s) of the cough, how diagnostic testing will help to rule in or out such causes, and risks/benefits of certain lesser versus more invasive diagnostic procedures to obtain this information. Good client rapport is important because many of the conditions associated with chronic cough are incurable, ultimately progressing to cardiac or pulmonary insufficiency. Treatment trials with follow-up examination and diagnostic testing are often necessary to refine drug dosages and to effectively manage (although rarely cure) conditions related to chronic cough.

REFERENCES

1. Mazzone SB. Cough. An overview of the sensory receptors regulating cough. Cough. 2005;1:2
2. Nimi A, Torrego RS, Nicholson AG, et al. Nature of airway inflammation and remodeling in chronic cough. J Allergy Clin Immunol. 2005; 116:565-70.
3. Boulet L-P. Future directions in the clinical management of cough. ACCP Evidence-based clinical practice guidelines. Chest. 2006; 129:287S-292S.
4. Nelson S, Mason CM. The inflammatory response in chronic bronchitis. Semin Respir Crit Care Med. 2000; 21:79-86.
5. Padrid PA, Hornof W, Kurpershoek C, et al. Canine chronic bronchitis: A pathophysiologic evaluation of 18 cases. J Vet Intern Med. 1990; 4:172-180.
6. Hawkins EC, Rogala AR, Large EE, et al. Cellular composition of bronchial brushings obtained from healthy dogs and dogs with chronic cough and cytologic composition of bronchoalveolar lavage fluid obtained from dogs with chronic cough. Am J Vet Res. 2006; 67:160-7.
7. Corcoran BM, Foster DJ, Fuentes VL. Feline asthma syndrome: a retrospective study of the clinical presentation in 29 cats. J Small Anim Pract. 1995; 36:481-8.
8. Dye JA, McKiernan BC, Rozanski EA, et al. Bronchopulmonary disease in the cat: Historical, clinical, radiographic, clinicopathologic, and pulmonary functional evaluation of 24 affects and 15 health cats. J Vet Intern Med. 1996; 10:385-400.
9. Sin DD, Johnson M, Gan WQ, et al. Combination therapy of inhaled corticosteroids and long-acting beta$_2$-adrenergics in management of patients with chronic obstructive pulmonary disease. Curr Pharm Res. 2004; 10:3547-60.
10. Kuehn NF. Chronic bronchitis in dogs. In King LG, editor: Textbook of Respiratory Disease in Dogs and Cats. 1st ed., St. Louis: Saunders, 2004.
11. Kirschvink N, Leemans J, Delvaux F, et al. Inhaled fluticasone reduces bronchial responsiveness and airway inflammation in cats with mild chronic bronchitis. J Feline Med Surg. 2006; 8:45-54.
12. King P. Is there are role for inhaled corticosteroids and macrolide therapy in bronchiectasis? Drugs. 2007; 67:965-74.

AIR QUALITY FOR RESPIRATORY PATIENTS

Janice A. Dye, DVM, MS, PhD, Diplomate ACVIM
National Health & Environmental Effects Research
Laboratory
Research Triangle Park, NC

Concern over the quality of indoor residential as well as outdoor environmental air has been growing. Accordingly, concerned pet owners may approach their veterinarians to inquire about the possibility of air pollutants causing disease or cancer in their pets. They may also inquire as to methods to improve the purity of the air in the home if they have a pet with chronic respiratory disease.

This article is intended to provide a brief overview of the potential adverse health effects associated with commonly encountered air pollutants, irritants, and allergens (eg, cigarette smoke, endotoxin, excessive dampness, nitrogen dioxide). Since many dogs and cats spend virtually all of their lives within the family domicile, the focus of the review will be on indoor air pollutants and select environmental (ie, outdoor) air pollutants. Owners should be cautioned about use of certain ionizing air purifiers which have been shown to increase indoor ozone concentrations well in excess of levels considered safe.

REFERENCES

1. Dye JA, Costa DL. A brief guide to indoor air pollutants and relevance to small animals. In: Kirk, RW, Bonagura JD (eds.): Current Veterinary Therapy XII. Philadelphia: WB Saunders, 1995; pp 252-257.
2. Costa DL, Gavett SH, Kodavanti UP, et al. Ambient particulate matter and health: what are the animals telling us? In: Mohr U (ed.): Relationships between Respiratory Disease and Exposure to Air Pollution. Washington, DC: ILSI Press, 1999; pp 185-194.
3. Osman LM, Douglas JG, Garden C, et al. Indoor air quality in homes of patients with chronic obstructive pulmonary disease. Am J Respir Crit Care Med. 2007; 176:465-72.
4. Britigan N, Alshawa A, Nizkorodov SA. Quantification of ozone levels in indoor environments generated by ionization and ozonolysis air purifiers. J Air Waste Manag Assoc 2006; 59:601-10.
5. Hope AP, Simon RA. Excess dampness and mold growth in homes: an evidence-based review of the aeroirritant effect and its potential causes. Allergy Asthma Proc 2007; 28:262-70.

COUGHING DOGS: DETERMINING WHY

Eleanor C. Hawkins, DVM, Diplomate ACVIM (SAIM)
College of Veterinary Medicine
North Carolina State University, Raleigh, NC

Some clients with coughing dogs would like to simply receive medication to stop the cough. However, treatment is most likely to provide long-term relief if an accurate diagnosis of the underlying cause is made. A cough is an explosive release of air from the lungs through the mouth. It is generally a protective reflex to expel material from the airways, but inflammation or compression of the airways can also stimulate cough. Thus, cough is associated with many lower respiratory tract and cardiac diseases. A complete discussion of the evaluation of the coughing dog would necessitate detailing all aspects of the diagnosis of cardiopulmonary disease. In this article, selected components that have been particularly useful in my own clinical experience are highlighted.

Disease outside of the lower respiratory tract and cardiovascular systems may also cause cough. Although not well documented in dogs, gastroesophageal reflux and post-nasal drip are common causes of cough in people.

HISTORIC CHARACTERIZATION

Because the list of differential diagnoses for cough is long, prioritization through a careful history is quite useful and a thorough systemic review is always indicated. Questions to explore in depth with the client include:

- How would you describe the cough (including quality and loudness)?
- How long has the cough been present?
- How frequent does the cough occur, when does it occur, and what is its pattern?
- Who smokes in the house or around the dog?
- Has there been any change in bark quality or intensity?
- Has there been any vomiting or regurgitation?
- Has there been a change in attitude or appetite?

Productive Versus Nonproductive Cough

Classically, differential diagnoses for cough are divided into those that cause productive cough and those that cause nonproductive cough. A productive cough results in the delivery of mucus, exudate, edema fluid, or blood from the airways into the oral cavity. A moist sound can often be heard during the cough. Animals rarely expectorate the fluid, but swallowing can be seen after a coughing episode. If expectoration occurs, clients may confuse the cough with vomiting. In human medicine, categorizing cough as productive or nonproductive is rarely difficult because the patient can report the coughing up of secretions. In veterinary medicine, recognition of a productive cough is more difficult. If the owner or veterinarian has heard or seen evidence that the cough is productive, it usually is. *However, not hearing or seeing evidence of productivity does not rule out the possibility of its presence.* Productive coughs are most commonly caused by inflammatory or infectious diseases of the airways or alveoli or by heart failure. Differential diagnoses include pulmonary edema (cardiogenic or noncardiogenic), canine infectious tracheobronchitis, canine chronic bronchitis, allergic bronchitis, bacterial bronchitis or pneumonia, aspiration pneumonia, parasitic disease, and severe fungal pneumonia.

Hemoptysis is the coughing up of blood. Blood-tinged saliva may be observed within the oral cavity or dripping from the commissures of the mouth after a cough. Hemoptysis is an unusual clinical sign that most commonly occurs in animals with heartworm disease or pulmonary neoplasia. Less common causes of hemoptysis are mycotic infections, foreign bodies, severe congestive heart failure, thromboembolic disease, lung lobe torsion, and some systemic bleeding disorders, such as disseminated intravascular coagulation.

Intensity of Cough

Cough associated with airway inflammation (tracheitis and/or bronchitis) or large airway collapse is often loud, harsh, and paroxysmal. The cough associated with tracheal collapse is often described as a "goose-honk." Cough associated with pneumonias and pulmonary edema is usually soft.

Acute Contagious Cough

Dogs presented with acute cough, particularly with a history of exposure to group housing or to other dogs with cough, should be considered to have a potentially infectious cause until proven otherwise. Canine contagious cough is discussed in detail in a separate article.

Timing of Cough

Cough resulting from tracheal disease is exacerbated by pressure on the neck, such as pulling on the animal's collar. Cough caused by airway inflammation (bronchitis) tends to occur more frequently upon rising from sleep or during and after exercise or exposure to cold air. Cough caused by heart failure tends to occur more frequently at night. The client's perception of frequency may be biased by the times of day during which they have the most contact with their pets, often in the evenings and during exercise.

Other Frequently Useful Historic Information

Exposure to smoke or other irritants can exacerbate any inflammatory airway disease and while obtaining such a history does not lead to a specific diagnosis, significant relief of clinical signs can often be achieved by eliminating the irritant from the dog's environment. A history of voice change is suggestive of laryngeal disease, usually laryngeal paralysis. A history of vomiting or regurgitation increases suspicion for aspiration pneumonia. Diseases such as infectious tracheobronchitis and canine chronic bronchitis are not associated with a decrease in attitude or appetite.

CHARACTERIZATION BY PHYSICAL EXAMINATION

As with history, a complete physical examination is always indicated and can provide helpful information in prioritizing differential diagnoses. Some particularly useful components of the physical examination for dogs with cough include heart rate and heart sounds, lung sounds, induction of cough, and fundic examination. Body temperature is also valuable and the presence of fever suggests inflammatory or infectious disease. However, a normal body temperature cannot be used to rule out infection.

Heart Rate and Heart Sounds

A critical component of the evaluation of dog with cough is determining whether the patient is in heart failure. Heart rate is extremely useful for assisting in making this determination because dogs in heart failure are nearly always tachycardic. Patients that are bradycardic are unlikely to be in failure. The presence of a new or recently intensified heart murmur can be supportive of advancing heart disease and possibly failure. Cough due to left atrial enlargement is unlikely in a dog without a murmur of mitral insufficiency.

Lung Sounds

Auscultation is a fairly insensitive means of detecting lung disease; however the detection of crackles, wheezes, or decreased lung sounds provides very valuable information. Crackles are usually associated with diseases that result in edema or an exudate within the airways such as pulmonary edema, pneumonias and bronchitis, as well as some interstitial pneumonias, particularly pulmonary fibrosis. Wheezes are less commonly heard in dogs, compared with cats, but can be associated with bronchoconstriction, bronchial wall thickening, exudate or fluid within the bronchial lumen, intraluminal masses, or external airway compression. Wheezes caused by an intrathoracic airway obstruction are loudest during early expiration. Sudden snapping at the end of expiration can be heard in some dogs with intrathoracic tracheal collapse.

Decreased lung sounds over one or both sides of the thorax can occur with pleural effusion, pneumothorax, diaphragmatic hernia, or mass lesions. Consolidated lung lobes and mass lesions can result in enhanced lung sounds because of the improved transmission of airway sounds from adjacent lobes. Therefore, the most important finding is asymmetry to the intensity of lung sounds between right and left sides.

Induction of Cough

It is very useful to attempt to induce a cough in the examination room by applying pressure to the trachea. If a cough can be induced, first ask the client if "that" cough is the cough they are concerned about. Some dogs may have long standing chronic cough due to tracheal collapse or chronic bronchitis that is distinct

from the current presenting complaint. Assuming the induced cough is the presenting problem, a more accurate characterization can be obtained. Watch the patient carefully following cough to observe swallowing efforts suggesting productivity. A cough that is easily induced by tracheal palpation is suggestive of tracheobronchitis, though secondary tracheitis can occur as a result of coughing.

Fundic Examination

Fundic examination is frequently overlooked in veterinary practice despite its lack of invasiveness and low cost. Although usually unremarkable, the presence of lesions such as chorioretinitis can immediately change the prioritization of differentials. For instance a puppy with cough and chorioretinitis is much more likely to have distemper than infectious tracheobronchitis.

SYSTEMIC SCREENING

A complete blood count, serum biochemical panel, and urinalysis are often part of the initial evaluation of a sick patient. Useful information about the systemic health of the dog can often be obtained. It should be remembered, however, that the complete blood count is insensitive with respect to inflammatory lung disease. For instance, half of dogs with bronchopneumonia have no leukocytosis or neutrophilia. Similarly, an absence of eosinophilia cannot be used to eliminate parasitic or allergic disease from the differential diagnoses. Polycythemia is suggestive of chronic hypoxemia and suggests long standing, severe disease.

THORACIC RADIOGRAPHY

Findings on thoracic radiographs, in close conjunction with information obtained through the history and physical examination, are often used to determine the subsequent steps in evaluating dogs with cough.

Radiographs Consistent with Heart Failure or Heart Disease

Heart failure is often documented radiographically. Typical abnormalities such as increased size of pulmonary veins and perihilar infiltrates in dogs with a supportive presentation are highly suggestive of a diagnosis of heart failure and appropriate treatment is initiated. An electrocardiogram (ECG) and echocardiogram may provide additional useful information about the etiology of the failure.

For dogs whose presentation or radiographs are suggestive of a possible diagnosis of failure, further testing can include trial treatment with furosemide or measurement of plasma B-type natriuretic peptide (BNP), N-terminal pro-B-type natriuretic peptide (NT-proBNP), or N-terminal pro-atrial natriuretic peptide (NT-proANP). Increased levels of these peptides have been associated with congestive heart failure, and the extent of elevation may correlate with severity of disease.[1] An NT-proBNP assay is available commercially.

Left atrial enlargement can also be identified radiographically. Left atrial enlargement due to mitral insufficiency with impingement on the mainstem bronchus appears to be associated with cough in some dogs. Treatment with a salt-restricted diet and an afterload reducer, such as enalopril, can be administered in an attempt to decrease pressure left atrial pressure.

Pulmonary Parenchymal Abnormalities

In some cases the history and physical examination of a patient along with classic radiographic abnormalities will be highly supportive of a particularly diagnosis. Some examples are typical cases of heartworm disease or blastomycosis. More often, differential diagnoses can only be prioritized based on radiographic changes and further evaluation is needed. For patients that are sufficiently stable and whose differential diagnoses include diseases for which there are specific noninvasive tests, such tests are performed next. Examples include fecal examinations for pulmonary parasites, heartworm tests, and tests for mycotic disease. For patients in respiratory distress, it may be useful to determine if other organs are involved. It may be possible to collect specimens for cytologic or histologic examination from other organs more safely than from the lung in such unstable dogs. Examples include concurrent lymphadenopathy or hepatopathy in diseases such as lymphoma or mycotic disease. Computed tomography of the lungs has been shown to be superior to thoracic radiographs for the characterization of parenchymal disease.

For most dogs presenting for cough with radiographic abnormalities of the pulmonary parenchyma, collection of pulmonary specimens for cytologic, microbiologic, and, in some cases, histologic evaluation is indicated. Specimen collection techniques include tracheal wash, non-bronchoscopic bronchoalveolar lavage, transthoracic lung aspiration, bronchoscopy and bronchoalveolar lavage (or other specimen collection methods as indicated), and lung biopsy by thoracotomy or thoracoscopy.

Selection of the most appropriate specimen collection technique depends upon the stability of the patient, the financial abilities of the client, the primary differential diagnoses, and the location of radiographic lesions. While it is impossible to detail the approach to all combinations of the above, the following are some common situations. Tracheal wash often provides a representative sample in patients with signs of airway inflammation, aspiration pneumonia, or broncho-pneumonia. Additional information concerning airway collapse or other concurrent or complicating conditions may be obtained by bronchoscopy with bronchoalveolar lavage. Masses or with reticulonodular interstitial infiltrates that are adjacent to the body wall and can be identified ultrasonographically can often be evaluated by ultrasound guided transthoracic lung aspiration. Lung aspiration is relatively contraindicated in dogs with cavitary lung lesions or pulmonary hypertension because the risk of pneumothorax or hemothorax is higher than usual. Dogs with diffuse, reticular interstitial lung disease can be evaluated by bronchoalveolar lavage or lung aspiration. Some of the diffuse interstitial diseases (eg, pulmonary fibrosis, some neoplasias, and some infectious diseases) can be diagnosed only through lung biopsy.

Pleural or Mediastinal Abnormalities

Chylothorax is associated with cough. Pleural disease may also cause cough if there is primary lung disease with secondary pleural involvement, as may be seen with spontaneous pneumothorax or pyothorax. Pleural effusions are evaluated initially by the cytologic analysis of pleural fluid. Bacterial culture, measurement of fluid triglycerides, or thoracic ultrasound may also be indicated. Mediastinal disease can be difficult to characterize radiographically. Lesions in the region of the heart are often evaluated by echocardiography. Computed tomography may be necessary for further characterization.

Normal Thoracic Radiographs

It is not uncommon for dogs with chronic cough to have normal thoracic radiographs. The most common differential diagnoses are tracheal collapse and chronic bronchitis, with or without tracheobronchomalacia. A bronchial pattern with increased interstitial markings is typically seen on thoracic radiographs of dogs with chronic bronchitis, but changes are often mild and difficult to distinguish from clinically insignificant changes associated with aging. In one study, thoracic radiographs had a sensitivity of 50% to 65% for the diagnosis of chronic bronchitis. Detection of airway collapse requires obtaining radiographs of the thorax during expiration and of the neck during inspiration, fluoroscopy, and/or bronchoscopy. Because collapse is dynamic, it is difficult to ever rule out the diagnosis. Rather, detection of collapse can be used to rule in its presence.

Considerations for dogs with acute cough but normal thoracic radiographs include canine infectious tracheobronchitis, influenza, acute aspiration, and acute foreign body inhalation. Careful investigation of the recent history often allows prioritization of these differential diagnoses.

Gastroesophageal reflux is one of the most common causes of cough in people. The two problems often exacerbate each other, with the efforts of cough causing reflux and the presence of reflux leading to cough. The relationship between reflux and cough in dogs is not well established. Recent studies of brachycephalic dogs showed a strong association with concurrent gastrointestinal signs such as ptyalism, regurgitation, and vomiting. If thorough evaluation has failed to identify respiratory or cardiac disease, treatment with omeprazole and metaclopromide may be tried. In people, a beneficial effect may not be seen for many weeks, making it difficult to attribute improvement in signs directly to therapy.

REFERENCES

1. DeFrancesco TC, et al. Prospective clinical evaluation of an ELISA B-type natriuretic peptide assay in the diagnosis of congestive heart failure in

dogs presenting with cough or dyspnea. J Vet Intern Med. 2007;21:243-250.

2. Prosek R, et al. Distinguishing cardiac and noncardiac dyspnea in 48 dogs using plasma atrial natriuretic factor, B-type natriuretic factor, endothelin, and cardiac troponin-I. J Vet Intern Med. 2007;21:238-242.

3. Mantis P, et al. Assessment of the accuracy of thoracic radiography in the diagnosis of canine chronic bronchitis. J Small Anim Pract. 1998;39:518-520.

4. Poncet CM, et al. Prevalence of gastrointestinal tract lesions in 73 brachycephalic dogs with upper respiratory syndrome. J Small Anim Pract. 2005;46:273-279.

MANAGING BACTERIAL BRONCHOPNEUMONIA: IMPROVING OUTCOME

Eleanor C. Hawkins, DVM, DACVIM (SAIM)
College of Veterinary Medicine
North Carolina State University, Raleigh, NC

Bacterial bronchopneumonia occurs much more frequently in dogs, compared with cats, and this discussion focuses on this disease in dogs. Successful management of dogs with bacterial pneumonia includes three key components: appropriate antimicrobial therapy; adequate supportive care; and identification (and management, where possible) of the underlying cause.

IDENTIFICATION OF THE UNDERLYING CAUSE

This key component is being considered first because information can be obtained during the presentation of the patient that can lead to the identification of an underlying cause. Dogs may develop bacterial bronchopneumonia following exposure to primary pulmonary bacterial pathogens, particularly *Bordetella bronchiseptica*. Most other cases of bacterial bronchopneumonia are secondary. General categories of underlying disease for consideration include: primary respiratory viral infection, aspiration, impaired airway clearance, immune compromise, and, less frequently, neoplasia and fungal or parasitic infection. The role of *Mycoplasma* sp. as a primary or secondary pathogen is poorly understood.

Primary Bacterial Pathogens

Bordetella can result in pneumonia, particularly in puppies. A recent study found that of 65 puppies with community acquired infectious pneumonia, 49% had infection with *Bordetella*. There is often a history of exposure within the previous 2 weeks to another dog with cough or a group housing situation (eg, boarding, pet store, or shelter). A practical method for obtaining a definitive diagnosis of *Bordetella* infection is by tracheal wash cytology and culture. Cytology is expected to show septic, neutrophilic inflammation, with small gram-negative rods. Organism identification is confirmed through routine bacterial culture, and important antibiotic sensitivity information is obtained. Polymerase chain reaction (PCR) testing is also available but does not provide antibiotic sensitivity information. The specificity and sensitivity of PCR testing in a clinical population has not been reported.

Primary Respiratory Viral Infection

Bacterial bronchopneumonia can be a complication of dogs with distemper or the severe form of canine influenza. Most dogs with the severe form of canine influenza are from concentrated housing (eg, greyhound tracks and shelters) and likely have a second underlying factor: immune compromise due to stress. Dogs with a history that is consistent with influenza should be immediately isolated until a diagnosis can be confirmed.

Rising serum antibody titers provide the most sensitive and specific results, but involve a prolonged time delay awaiting the 2- to 3-week period to obtain the second specimen. Nasal or pharyngeal swabs can be collected for PCR, but are consistently positive only early in the course of disease. Therefore, specimens should be collected as soon as the differential diagnosis is considered. A bedside antigen test for people has been used for testing in dogs, again using nasal or pharyngeal swabs for collection of specimens (Directigen Flu A, Becton, Dickinson). In this preliminary study, the sensitivity is less than that of PCR. The specificity is not known for dogs. Distemper occurs most often in unvaccinated puppies. Evidence for disease in other organs (ophthalmologic, gastrointestinal, or neurologic disease) along with an appropriate history are highly suggestive of the diagnosis. Confirmation can be attempted through various means (eg, immunofluorescence assay [IFA], PCR, virus isolation), all requiring that virus be present in the specimen at the time of collection.

Aspiration

Aspiration of a foreign body is an uncommon cause of pneumonia. More often the culprit is overt aspiration of esophageal or stomach contents due to: esophageal disease, such as megaesophagus, reflux esophagitis, or esophageal obstruction; localized or systemic neuromuscular disease affecting normal swallowing reflexes; depression of swallowing reflexes due to anesthesia or other cause for decreased consciousness; and abnormal pharyngeal anatomy, such as occurs with laryngoplasty, brachycephalic airway syndrome, mass lesions, or cleft palate; and iatrogenic causes, such as overly aggressive force feeding, mineral oil administration, and malposition of feeding tubes. Bronchoesophageal fistula is quite rare. Identification of these causes requires a careful history and physical examination. Thoracic radiographs are scrutinized for evidence of esophageal disease. Additional tests may be indicated including: oral and pharyngeal examination, contrast-enhanced radiographic studies to evaluate the esophagus, or specific neuromuscular tests

Impaired Airway Clearance

The most dramatic instance of impaired airway clearance occurs in dogs with ciliary dyskinesia. Initial infections are most often diagnosed at a young age. Nasal discharge, bronchiectasis, otitis externa, situs inversus, or abnormal sperm motility may be present. Support for the diagnosis is possible by measuring the clearance of a drop of radionucleotide from the distal trachea, presuming infection with an organism known to cause ciliary dysfunction (such as *Bordetella*) has been ruled out. More specific confirmation requires electronmicroscopy or ciliogenesis. Impaired airway clearance also plays a role in patients with bronchiectasis due to other causes. Airways that fail to taper are generally identified by careful examination of radiographs. Abnormalities in airway clearance, such as mucosal damage and alterations in the amount and quality of mucus present, may contribute to the development of bacterial infection in dogs with chronic bronchitis.

Immune Compromise and Other Causes

Some causes of immune compromise are readily apparent through history and physical examination, such as chronic glucocorticoid excess, ongoing chemotherapy, or suboptimal housing conditions. Other pulmonary pathology can potentially create a situation that impairs airway clearance, normal blood flow, or other protective mechanisms of the lung, allowing for the development of overt infection.

ANTIBIOTIC THERAPY

A wide variety of bacteria can infect the lungs. Common bacterial isolates from dogs with pulmonary infections include *Bordetella bronchiseptica, Streptococcus* spp., *Staphylococcus* spp., *Escherichia coli, Klebsiella* spp., *Proteus* spp., *Pasteurella* spp., and *Pseudomonas* spp. Anaerobic organisms can be part of mixed infections, particularly in dogs with aspiration pneumonia or with lung lobe consolidation. *Mycoplasma* organisms have been isolated from dogs with pneumonia, but their exact role is not known.

The antibiotic sensitivity of the involved organisms is difficult to predict, particularly because gram-negative infections and infections with multiple organisms are common. Tracheal wash is indicated for all animals that can tolerate the procedure to obtain antibiotic sensitivity data. Antibiotics are initially selected based on severity of clinical signs and, when available, the morphology and gram-staining properties of organisms found in tracheal wash fluid. Antibiotic selection is subsequently modified, as needed, based on the sensitivity data from bacterial cultures and clinical response.

The extent to which an antibiotic can penetrate into the airway secretions does not need to be a major consideration in patients with bacterial pneumonia. Antibiotics generally achieve concentrations within the pulmonary parenchyma equal to those in plasma. Nebulization of antibiotics is rarely indicated and should not be performed without concurrent administration of systemic antibiotics.

For dogs with mild or moderate clinical signs, antibiotics to consider for initial administration include amoxicillin-clavulanate (20 to 25 mg/kg q8h), cephalexin (20 to 40 mg/kg q8h), or chloramphenicol (50 mg/kg q8h). Fluoroquinolones are reserved for patients with resistant gram-negative infections.

Dogs with severe clinical signs or possible sepsis should be treated initially with intravenous antibiotics. Broad-spectrum coverage in dogs with life-threatening infections can be achieved with meropenem (8 mg/kg q8h) or the combination of either ampicillin with sulbactam (22 mg/kg of ampicillin intravenously q8h) and a fluoroquinolone or ampicillin with sulbactam and an aminoglycoside (eg, amikacin, 5 to 10 mg/kg q8h). Sulbactam is a beta-lactamase inhibitor, as is clavulanate, and the combination of ampicillin with sulbactam provides a drug with similar activity as amoxicillin-clavulanate in an intravenous formulation.

Antibiotic treatment should be continued for at least 1 week beyond the time when the clinical signs resolve. Recommendations for patient monitoring are discussed below.

SUPPORTIVE CARE
Critical Care

Dogs in severe respiratory distress should be treated with fluid therapy and oxygen supplementation. Fluids are administered intravenously at high rates to treat shock and should be continued after initial stabilization of the animal's condition to maintain systemic hydration, which is necessary to maximize the effectiveness of airway clearance mechanisms. However, overhydration must be avoided because of a tendency for pulmonary edema.

Oxygen supplementation is initiated immediately in compromised animals. Positive-pressure ventilation is required for animals in severe respiratory distress that is unresponsive to oxygen therapy.

Trial treatment with bronchodilators can be attempted to potentially decrease bronchospasms (more common in cats than dogs), improve mucociliary clearance, and decrease ventilatory muscle fatigue in patients that are failing to respond to oxygen supplementation alone. Bronchodilators can potentially exacerbate ventilation: perfusion (V/Q) mismatching, worsening hypoxemia. They are discontinued if no improvement is seen or clinical signs appear to worsen following their administration.

Rapid-acting glucocorticoids are administered for the treatment of shock. Some clinicians advocate their use in patients with aspiration pneumonia, though this application is controversial. The antiinflammatory effects of glucocorticoids can be beneficial, but they can interfere with normal defense mechanisms in tissues that have been severely compromised. Low doses of short-acting formulations can be given during the first 24 hours to control severe clinical signs but should then be discontinued.

Airway Hydration

The drying of secretions results in increased viscosity and decreased ciliary function, which interfere with the normal clearance mechanisms of the lung. Thus, the water content of airway secretions must be maintained and airways must be hydrated in animals with pneumonia. Animals with any evidence of dehydration should receive fluid therapy. Diuretics can cause dehydration, and their use is contraindicated in such animals.

Additional moisture for the airways can be provided through humidification or nebulization. Such therapy is particularly recommended for animals with areas of consolidation or with suspected decreased airway clearance, such as those with bronchiectasis. *Humidification* refers to the saturation of air with water vapor. Depending on the temperature, the volume of water that remains as vapor is limited. The moisture reaches only the nasal cavity and the proximal trachea. Vaporization is not effective in hydrating deeper regions of the lungs. However, the more proximal effect can still provide some relief, particularly in animals with nasal discharge. Humidification is convenient and can be achieved simply by placing the animal in a steamy bathroom or in a small room with an inexpensive vaporizer, readily available at pharmacies.

Nebulization is necessary to provide moisture deeper into the airways. Nebulizers generate small, variably sized droplets, with a diameter ranging from 0.5 to 5 μm being required to reach the deeper airways. Several types of nebulizers are available. Disposable jet nebulizers are inexpensive, and they can be attached to bottled oxygen or an air compressor. Effective, inexpensive portable compressors are commercially available if needed for home use. The nebulized oxygen is delivered to the animal through a face mask. The particles can be seen as a mist.

Sterile saline solution is used as a nebulizing solution because it has mucolytic properties and is relatively nonirritating. Premedication with bronchodilators has been suggested as a way to reduce the bronchospasms, although I have not encountered problems using saline alone in dogs. It is recommended that nebulization be performed two to six times daily for 10 to 30 minutes each time. Nebulization should be followed immediately by physiotherapy to promote the expectoration of exudate that may have increased in volume with rehydration. Nebulizers and tubing should be replaced after no more than 24 hours of use in actively infected patients, and face masks cleaned and disinfected.

Physiotherapy

Animals that are recumbent must be turned at least every 2 hours. Lying in one position impairs airway clearance, and lung consolidation can occur if one side remains dependent for prolonged periods. Animals that are in a sufficiently stable condition and can tolerate the oxygen demands should be mildly exercised. Activity causes animals to take deeper breaths and to cough, which promotes airway clearance,

Physiotherapy is indicated after nebulization to promote coughing and to facilitate the clearance of exudate from the lungs. Mild exercise is used when possible. Otherwise, coupage is performed. To perform coupage, the person strikes the animal's chest over the lung fields with cupped hands. The action should be forceful but not painful and should be continued for 5 to 10 minutes if tolerated by the patient. Coupage may also be beneficial for animals with lung consolidation that are not receiving nebulization.

Other Treatment

Expectorants are of questionable value and are not recommended. Some clinicians have noted improvement in patients with increased respiratory efforts and tenacious secretions with oral or intravenous

N-acetylcysteine. This drug is most often recognized as a mucolytic administered by nebulization. Nebulization of the drug is NOT recommended because it is an irritant. If efficacious by systemic administration, the mechanism of action is likely through its antioxidant and anti-inflammatory effects. This use of the drug has not been studied in dogs, so a specific dosage cannot be recommended. The dosage of 70 mg/kg q4–6h has been suggested for treatment of acetaminophen toxicity, and has been used by some clinicians in the setting of bacterial pneumonia. Dosages used in clinical trials in people with chronic obstructive pulmonary disease include 600–1200 mg/person/d, a much lower dosage per kilogram.

Patient Monitoring

Patients with bacterial pneumonia should be closely monitored for signs of deteriorating pulmonary function. Respiratory rate and effort and mucous membrane color are monitored at least twice daily. Thoracic radiographs and CBC are evaluated every 24 to 72 hours. If the dog's condition does not improve within 72 hours, it may be necessary to alter treatment or perform additional tests. Patients showing improvement are sent home and re-evaluated every 10 to 14 days. Once clinical and radiographic signs have resolved, antibiotic treatment is continued for an additional week. Many dogs with bacterial pneumonia require treatment for 4 to 6 weeks or longer.

The evidence of infection on initial radiographs can obscure that of focal disease processes such as neoplasia or foreign bodies, and focal opacities may not be apparent while a dog is receiving antibiotics. Therefore, radiographs should be re-valuated approximately 1 week after antibiotic therapy has been discontinued in dogs with recurrent infection or suspected localized disease. Persistence of localized disease after long-term antibiotic therapy is an indication for bronchoscopy, thoracoscopy, or thoracotomy.

Prognosis

Bacterial pneumonia responds readily to appropriate therapy. The prognosis is more guarded in animals with underlying problems that predispose them to infection, and the likelihood of eliminating these problems must be taken into consideration.

REFERENCES

1. Radhakrishnan A, et al. Community-acquired infectious pneumonia in puppies: 65 cases (1993-2002). J Am Vet Med Assoc. 2007; 230:1493-1497.
2. Spindel ME, et al. Detection and quantification of canine influenza virus by one-step real-time reverse transcription PCR (Abstract), J Vet Intern Med. 2007;21:576.
3. Clercx C, et al. Use of ciliogenesis in the diagnosis of primary ciliary dyskinesia in a dog. J Am Vet Med. Assoc 2000; 11:1681-1685.

MANAGING CANINE CHRONIC BRONCHITIS: SUCCESS WITH THE BASICS

Eleanor C. Hawkins, DVM, Diplomate ACVIM (SAIM)
College of Veterinary Medicine
North Carolina State University, Raleigh, NC

Canine chronic bronchitis is defined as cough occurring on most days of two or more consecutive months in the past year *in the absence of other active disease*. Changes associated with long-standing inflammation are present histologically and include fibrosis, epithelial hyperplasia, glandular hypertrophy, and inflammatory infiltrates. Some of these changes are irreversible. Excessive mucus is present within the airways, and small airway obstruction occurs. Chronic bronchitis is strongly associated with smoking in people. It is presumed that canine chronic bronchitis is a consequence of a long-standing inflammatory process initiated by infection, allergy, or inhaled irritants or toxins. A continuing cycle of inflammation likely occurs as mucosal damage, mucus hypersecretion, and airway obstruction impairs normal mucociliary clearance, and inflammatory mediators amplify the response to irritants and organisms.

PRESENTING SIGNS

Chronic bronchitis occurs most often in middle-aged or older, smaller breed dogs. Terriers, poodles, and Cocker spaniels are over-represented among dogs with chronic bronchitis. Smaller breed dogs are also predisposed to collapsing trachea and mitral insufficiency with left atrial enlargement causing compression of the mainstem bronchi. These causes for cough must be differentiated, and their contribution to the development of the current clinical features determined, for appropriate management to be implemented.

Dogs with chronic bronchitis are typically presented for loud, harsh cough. The cough is expected to be productive because mucus hypersecretion is a component of the disease. However, dogs cannot report the productive nature of their cough and hearing "wetness" in a cough is a very insensitive measure. The cough has usually progressed slowly over months to years, although clients will usual report the initial onset as acute. There should be no systemic signs of illness. As the disease progresses, exercise intolerance becomes evident; then incessant coughing, with or without overt respiratory distress, is seen.

Dogs with chronic bronchitis are often presented because of a sudden exacerbation of signs. The change in signs may result from transient worsening of the chronic bronchitis, perhaps after a period of unusual excitement, stress, or exposure to irritants or allergens; from a secondary complication, such as bacterial infection; or from the development of a concurrent disease, such as left atrial enlargement and bronchial compression or heart failure. In addition to obtaining a routine complete history, the client should be carefully questioned about the character of the cough and the progression of signs. Detailed information should be obtained regarding environmental conditions, particularly exposure to smoke, other potential irritants and toxins, or allergens; exposure to infectious agents, such as boarding or exposure to puppies; and all previous and current medications and the response to treatment.

On auscultation, increased breath sounds, crackles, or occasionally wheezes are heard. End-expiratory clicks caused by mainstem bronchial or intrathoracic tracheal collapse may be heard in animals with advanced disease. A prominent or split second heart sound occurs in animals with secondary pulmonary hypertension. Dogs with respiratory distress (end-stage disease) characteristically show marked expiratory efforts because of the narrowing and collapse of the intrathoracic large airways. The presence of a fever or other systemic signs is suggestive of other disease, such as bacterial pneumonia.

MAKING THE DIAGNOSIS

The diagnosis of chronic bronchitis requires not only the presence of chronic cough, but also the absence of other active disease. Therefore, it is necessary to eliminate other diseases from the list of differential diagnoses before the diagnosis can be made. Disease considerations include bacterial infection, mycoplasmal infection, bronchial compression (particularly due to left atrial enlargement), pulmonary parasites or heartworm disease, allergic bronchitis, neoplasia, foreign body, and chronic aspiration. The possibility of secondary disease complicates this simple definition. Potential secondary diseases include bacterial or mycoplasmal infection, airway collapse, bronchiectasis, and pulmonary hypertension.

Thoracic radiographs are most useful for ruling out other active disease and identifying concurrent or secondary disease. A bronchial pattern with increased interstitial markings is typically seen on thoracic radiographs, but changes are often mild and difficult to distinguish from clinically insignificant changes associated with aging. In one study, thoracic radiographs had a sensitivity of 50% to 65% for the diagnosis of chronic bronchitis. Neck films obtained during inspiration and thoracic films obtained during expiration, or fluoroscopy, are useful for identifying airway collapse.

Tracheal wash or BAL fluid should be collected at the time of the initial presentation and after a persistent exacerbation of signs. Neutrophilic or mixed inflammation and increased amounts of mucus are usually present. The finding of degenerative neutrophils indicates the possibility of a bacterial infection. Although not a specific finding, the finding of eosinophils is suggestive of a hypersensitivity reaction, as can occur with allergy, parasitism, or heartworm disease. Slides should be carefully examined for organisms. Bacterial cultures are performed. Although the role of *Mycoplasma* infections in these cases is not well understood, *Mycoplasma* cultures are also considered. Bronchoscopy, with specimen collection, is performed in selected cases, primarily to help rule out other diseases. The maximum benefit of bronchoscopy is obtained early in the course of disease, before severe permanent damage has occurred and while the risk of the procedure is minimal.

Further diagnostic procedures are indicated to rule out other potential causes of chronic cough, and the selection of these depends on the presenting signs and the results of the previously discussed diagnostic tests. Diagnostic tests to be considered include systemic evaluation (ie, CBC, serum biochemical panel, urinalysis), tests for heartworm tests and for pulmonary parasites, and echocardiography. Echocardiography may reveal evidence of pulmonary hypertension secondary to chronic hypoxemia, including right heart enlargement.

TREATMENT

Each dog with chronic bronchitis is presented at a different stage of the disease, with or without concurrent or secondary cardiopulmonary disease. Therefore, each dog must be managed as an individual. If the dog is clinically stable and the cough not too severe, medications can initiated one at a time to better assess the most effective combination. Once the cough has been controlled for several weeks, it may be possible to decrease the amount of medication needed. However, with progression of disease the medications may need to be added or the dosages of ongoing medications increased.

Minimizing Exposure to Potential Irritants or Allergens

Exacerbating factors, either possible or proven, are avoided. It is difficult to make a definitive diagnosis of allergic disease, so potential allergens are considered in all dogs with chronic bronchitis and particularly in dogs with eosinophilic inflammation in airway specimens. Where possible, trial elimination is pursued. Irritants such as smoke (from tobacco or fireplace) and perfumed products should be avoided in all dogs. Motivated clients can take steps to improve the air quality in their home, such as cleaning or eliminating carpet, furniture, and window treatments; cleaning the furnace and regularly replacing air filters; and using an air cleaner. The American Lung Association has a useful website with nonproprietary recommendations for improving indoor air quality (www.lungusa.org).

Maintaining Airway Hydration

Maintaining airway hydration will facilitate mucociliary clearance. Adequate airway hydration is best achieved by maintaining systemic hydration. Therefore, diuretic therapy is avoided in these patients. In severely affected dogs, placing the animal in a steamy bathroom or in a room with a vaporizer daily may provide symptomatic relief, although the moisture does not reach far into the airways. Nebulization of saline will allow moisture to reach deeper in the lungs.

Nebulizers generate small, variably sized droplets, with a diameter ranging from 0.5 to 5 µm being required to reach the deeper airways. Several types of nebulizers are available. Disposable jet nebulizers are readily available and inexpensive, and they can be attached to bottled oxygen or an air compressor. Effective, inexpensive portable compressors are commercially available if needed for home use. The nebulized oxygen is delivered to the animal through a face mask. The particles can be seen as a mist.

Sterile saline solution is used as a nebulizing solution because it has mucolytic properties and is relatively nonirritating. Premedication with bronchodilators has been suggested as a way to reduce the bronchospasms, although I have not encountered problems using saline alone in dogs. Once or twice daily nebulization for 10 to 15 minutes may be helpful, particularly in dogs with reduced clearance due to bronchiectasis. Nebulizers and tubing should be replaced after no more than 24 hours of use in actively infected patients, and face masks cleaned and disinfected.

Other General Management Strategies

Excitement or stress can cause an acute worsening of signs in some animals, and *short-term tranquilization* with acepromazine or sedation with phenobarbital can be helpful in relieving the signs. Routine *dental prophylaxis* and *teeth brushing* will help maintain a healthy oral flora and may decrease any contributions of the normal aspiration of oropharyngeal bacteria to ongoing airway inflammation.

Patients that are overweight and/or unfit can benefit from *weight loss and exercise*. Exercise should be tailored to the dog's current fitness level and degree of pulmonary dysfunction to avoid causing excessive respiratory efforts or even death. Observing the dog during specific exercise, such as a short walk, while in the client's presence may be necessary to make initial recommendations. Instructing the client in the measurement of respiratory rate, observation of mucus membrane color, and signs of increased respiratory effort will improve their ability to assess their dog's status during exercise.

Theophylline

Theophylline is a methylxanthine bronchodilator that has been used for years for the treatment of chronic bronchitis in people and dogs. This drug became unpopular with physicians as newer bronchodilators with fewer side effects became available. However, recent research in people suggests that theophylline is effective in treating the underlying inflammation of chronic bronchitis even at concentrations below those resulting in bronchodilation (thus, reducing side effects), and that the anti-inflammatory effects may be synergistic with those of glucocorticoids. Theophylline may also improve mucociliary clearance, decrease fatigue of respiratory muscles and inhibit the release of mast cell mediators of inflammation. The potential beneficial effects of theophylline beyond bronchodilation may be of particular importance in dogs because their airways are not as reactive as those of cats and people. However, theophylline alone is rarely sufficient to control the clinical signs of chronic bronchitis.

Other advantages of theophylline are the availability of long-acting preparations that can be administered twice daily to dogs and that plasma concentrations of drug can be easily measured by commercial diagnostic laboratories. A disadvantage of theophylline is that other drugs, such as fluoroquinolones and chloramphenicol, can delay its clearance and cause signs of theophylline toxicity if the dosage is not reduced by one third to one half. Potential adverse effects include gastrointestinal signs, cardiac arrhythmias, nervousness, and seizures. Serious adverse effects are extremely rare at therapeutic concentrations.

Variability in sustained plasma concentrations has been found for different long-acting theophylline products. Dosage recommendations are currently available for a generic product from a specific manufacturer (Theochron or TheoCap, Inwood Laboratories 10 mg/kg q12h). If beneficial effects are not seen, the patient is predisposed to adverse effects, or adverse effects occur, plasma theophylline concentrations should be measured. Therapeutic peak concentrations for bronchodilation, based on data from people, are 5 to 20 µg/mL. Plasma is collected during peak concentrations, generally 4 to 5 hours after administration of a long-acting product or 1.5 to 2 hours after administration of immediate-release products. Measurement of concentrations immediately before the next scheduled dose might provide useful information concerning duration of therapeutic concentrations.

Theophylline and related drugs that are not long-acting are useful in specific circumstances but must be administered three times daily. (eg, theophylline base, 9 mg/kg q8h; aminophylline, 11 mg/kg q8h). Palatable elixirs of theophylline derivatives (eg, oxtriphylline, 14 mg/kg q8h) are convenient for administration to toy breeds. Therapeutic blood concentrations are reached more quickly following the administration of tablets or capsules that are not long-acting.

Sympathomimetic Bronchodilators

Sympathomimetic drugs are preferred by some clinicians as bronchodilators. Terbutaline and albuterol are selective for β2 adrenergic receptors, lessening their cardiac effects. Potential adverse effects include nervousness, tremors, hypotension, and tachycardia. The clinical use of bronchodilators delivered by metered dose inhaler, such as albuterol and ipatropium (a parasympatholytic), has not been reported in dogs with chronic bronchitis.

Glucocorticoids

Glucocorticoids are often effective in controlling the signs of chronic bronchitis in dogs and theoretically may slow the development of permanent airway damage by decreasing inflammation. Potential negative effects include an increased susceptibility to infection in dogs already impaired by decreased airway clearance; a tendency toward obesity, hepatomegaly, and muscle weakness that may adversely affect ventilation; and pulmonary thromboembolism. Therefore short-acting products are used, the dose is tapered to the lowest effective one (when possible, 0.5 mg/kg q48h or less), and the drug is discontinued if no beneficial effect is seen. Prednisone is initially given at a dose of 0.5 to 1.0 mg/kg every 12 hours, with a positive response expected within 1 week.

Dogs that require relatively high dosages of prednisone, have unacceptable adverse effects, or have conditions for which glucocorticoids are relatively contraindicated (such as diabetes mellitus) may benefit from local treatment with fluticasone propionate (Flovent, GlaxoSmithKline) administered by metered-dose inhaler (MDI). Advantages are minimizing systemic side effects and relative ease of administration in some dogs compared with pilling. To date, however, it is still not known how much drug is deposited in the lower airways, how much remains in the oral and nasal cavities, and how much is absorbed systemically in dogs. Theoretical concerns about the oronasal deposition of the potent glucocorticoid in dogs, compared with people, include the high incidence of periodontal disease and the inability to effectively rinse the mouth with water after use. However, some veterinarians have been using glucocorticoid MDIs to treat idiopathic *feline* bronchitis for many years without frequent, obvious adverse effects. A recent clinical report of treatment of chronic bronchitis (10 dogs) and eosinophilic broncho-pneumopathy (3 dogs) with glucocorticoids administered by MDI cited no side effects in dogs treated with MDI glucocorticoids alone, and reduced side effects in dogs treated also with a decreased dosage of previously prescribed systemic glucocorticoids.

I prefer to obtain a clinical remission of signs using orally administered drug first, except in dogs with relative contraindications for systemic glucocorticoid therapy, such as having diabetes mellitus. Dogs that require a relatively low dose of oral glucocorticoids to control clinical signs, have no noticeable adverse effects, and that can be pilled without difficulty are often well maintained with oral therapy. Otherwise, once signs are in remission, treatment by MDI is initiated and the dosage of oral prednisone gradually reduced.

A spacer must be used for effectively administering drugs by MDI to dogs, and the airflow generated by the patient must be sufficient to activate the spacer valve. Padrid[4] has found the Optichamber (Respironics, Inc) to be effective for cats, and we have used this spacer for dogs. A small anesthetic mask, with rubber diaphragm, is attached to the spacer. Widening of the adapter of the anesthetic mask that is inserted into the spacer is necessary to create a snug fit. This is achieved by wrapping adhesive tape around the adapter. Home made spacers, such as toilet paper tubes, are not recommended because of potential interference with drug delivery due to drug adherence.

The dog is allowed to sit or lie down on the floor or in the client's lap. The client steadies the head. The MDI, attached to the spacer, is actuated (pressed) twice. The mask is placed immediately on the dog's face, covering the mouth and nose completely, and it is held in place while the dog takes 7 to 10 breaths.

No dosing studies have been performed in dogs. The following treatment schedule has been recommended for cats, and could theoretically be applied to dogs. For cats with mild daily symptoms: 220 µg of fluticasone propionate by MDI twice daily and albuterol by MDI as needed. The maximum effect of fluticasone is not expected until 7 to 10 days of treatment. For cats with moderate daily symptoms: treatments with MDI as described for mild symptoms; in addition, prednisone is administered orally for 10 days (1 mg/kg every 12 hours for 5 days, then every 24 hours for 5 days). For cats with severe symptoms: dexamethasone is administered once (2 mg/kg IV), albuterol is administered by MDI every 30 minutes for up to 4 hours, and the cat is administered oxygen. Once stabilized, these cats are prescribed 220 µg of fluticasone propionate by MDI every 12 hours, and albuterol by MDI every 6 hours as needed. Oral prednisone is administered as needed.

Cough Suppressants

Cough suppressants are often quite effective in the management of chronic bronchitis, but are used cautiously because cough is an important mechanism to clear airway secretions. In some dogs, however, the cough is incessant and exhausting, or ineffective because of marked tracheobronchomalacia and airway collapse. Cough suppressants can provide significant relief in such patients and may even facilitate ventilation and decrease anxiety. A narcotic cough suppressant, such as butorphanol (0.5 mg/kg q6–12h, orally) or hydrocodone (0.25 mg/kg q6–12h, orally) is generally required. Limiting administration to times of the day when coughing is most severe may preserve some beneficial effect of cough. For dogs with severe cough, hydrocodone may provide the greatest relief and the dosage can be increased to effect while monitoring for side effects.

Management of Complications

Management of secondary infections, airway collapse, and pulmonary hypertension are discussed in a separate presentation.

REFERENCES

1. Mantis P, et al. Assessment of the accuracy of thoracic radiography in the diagnosis of canine chronic bronchitis. J Small Anim Pract. 1998;39:518-520.
2. Bach JF, et al. Evaluation of the bioavailability and pharmacokinetics of two extended-release theophylline formulations in dogs. J Am Vet Med Assoc. 2004;224:1113-1119.
3. Bexfield NH, et al. Management of 13 cases of canine respiratory disease using inhaled corticosteroids. J Small Anim Pract. 2006;47:377-382.
4. Padrid P: Feline Asthma: diagnosis and treatment. Vet Clin North Am Small Anim Pract. 2000;30:1279-1293

CHRONIC BRONCHITIS: CONFOUNDING ISSUES

Eleanor C. Hawkins, DVM, Diplomate ACVIM (SAIM)
College of Veterinary Medicine
North Carolina State University, Raleigh, NC

Treatment recommendations for canine chronic bronchitis are generally based on a combination of environmental control, weight loss, and glucocorticoid and bronchodilator administration. This overall approach is successful in the control of cough and improvement of breathing for many dogs with chronic bronchitis. However, some dogs fail to respond well to "routine" management. There are numerous challenging issues that may arise in these patients and preclude a successful outcome.

DIFFICULTY IN MAKING AN ACCURATE DIAGNOSIS

Chronic bronchitis in dogs was defined by Wheeldon as chronic or recurring cough occurring on most days of two consecutive months in the preceding year in the absence of other specific bronchopulmonary disease. The cough history is readily obtained from the owners. Notice that while mucus hypersecretion is a component of chronic bronchitis, a productive cough was not considered in the original definition because it is not possible to correctly identify a cough as productive in many dogs. An accurate diagnosis is largely dependent on ruling out other disease, yet it is difficult to prove a "negative." How extensive of a work-up is required to comfortably reach the diagnosis? *The initial evaluation of dogs with chronic cough should be very thorough.*

A thorough evaluation will strengthen the diagnosis and increase the likelihood of identifying concurrent or complicating conditions that can confound therapy. Thorough diagnostic testing may again be necessary as persistent exacerbations occur. Although each case must be considered as an individual, general recommendations include: a history, including interrogation for exposure to cigarette smoke or other potential environmental irritants; physical examination, including observation for signs of concurrent or complicating conditions; complete blood count; thoracic radiographs, which include the usual two views of the thorax during full inspiration, a lateral view during expiration, and a lateral cervical film during inspiration (or fluoroscopy where available); and collection of an airway specimen for cytology and culture. Ideally, bronchoscopy is performed. There is much more to be gained by performing bronchoscopy early in the course of disease when the procedure is quite safe and the identification of any active process may spare the lung further permanent damage, than as a "last resort" when the patient is a high anesthetic risk and the likelihood of significant improvement of lung structure and function is quite poor. However, if not feasible, a good tracheal wash is sufficient for most cases. Arterial blood gas analysis is valuable for objective monitoring of disease progression. Echocardiography may provide useful information regarding concurrent or complicating conditions. A controlled study has demonstrated that thoracic radiography has only 50% to 65% sensitivity in the diagnosis of chronic bronchitis. Therefore, radiographs are useful to support a diagnosis of bronchial disease and to rule out other causes of cough, but cannot be used to eliminate chronic bronchitis from consideration.

CONCURRENT CONDITIONS

Left Atrial Enlargement

Left atrial enlargement secondary to mitral insufficiency can cause a bronchial cough in some dogs through pressure on the bronchi. Many small breed dogs appear to be predisposed to both chronic bronchitis and valvular endocardiosis. Assessment of bronchial impingement can be made with radiographs or bronchoscopy, though the degree of impingement does not appear to correlate with degree of signs. Airway compression in many dogs with left atrial enlargement does not seem to contribute to cough. Treatment to reduce atrial size should be attempted in affected dogs that fail to respond to appropriate management of their chronic bronchitis. For most dogs, a low salt diet is instituted and enalapril is begun (0.5 mg/kg/d, then increased to twice daily if response is not adequate). It is often necessary to add amlodipine in these patients (0.1 mg/kg/d, then increased if necessary, with monitoring). Potential adverse affects due to systemic hypotension are monitored by measuring systemic blood pressure and a renal panel a few days after any treatment change; response to therapy is monitored by change in cough frequency and radiographic assessment of atrial size.

Concurrent Respiratory Tract Disease

Other concurrent conditions that can exacerbate clinical signs include disorders affecting any other component of the respiratory tract that increase the work of breathing or result in exaggerated airway pressures. Brachycephalic airway syndrome and soft palate elongation are examples of confounding conditions whose potential role should not be overlooked.

COMPLICATING CONDITIONS

Major complicating conditions include intrathoracic large airway collapse, pulmonary hypertension, and infection.

Intrathoracic Large Airway Collapse

Intrathoracic large airway collapse is likely a consequence of chondromalacia and small airway obstruction. It is possible that underlying genetic factors are involved. Direct trauma to the mucosa because of collapse during cough or shear forces from air movement can perpetuate a cough–cough cycle. Collapse can occur in advanced cases during expiration, impairing ventilation. Collapse may be suspected on the basis of an end expiratory push during observation of breathing or an end expiratory snap on auscultation. Severe cases have a loud, audible expiratory cough/wheeze.

There is no known means of reversing chondromalacia. Treatment is aimed at decreasing cough and small airway obstruction. Ideally, these goals are achieved through the routine management recommendations for chronic bronchitis. Practically, cough suppression is often necessary. Although one is classically taught to avoid cough suppression when a cough is productive, it is not clear that cough is an effective clearance mechanism in dogs where cough results in complete airway collapse. Progress is being made in the use of intraluminal airway stents. In selected cases, dramatic improvement of clinical signs may be seen. However, in many cases of advanced chronic bronchitis, airway collapse continues out into the main stem bronchi, beyond the reach of currently available stents. The response in such cases may not be great or long lasting. Only increased experience will allow accurate prognostication for specific cases.

Pulmonary Hypertension

Pulmonary hypertension is another potential complication of chronic bronchitis. As primary and secondary pulmonary hypertension has been studied in greater depth in people in recent years, it is apparent that neither the pathophysiology nor the treatment of pulmonary hypertension is straightforward. Although commonly considered to be a result of vasoconstriction secondary to hypoxemia, endothelial dysfunction and vascular remodeling appear to play major roles. Species differences in pathophysiology are likely, and studies in people are complicated by the potential direct affect of cigarette-associated toxins because the majority of people with chronic bronchitis are smokers. In people, pulmonary hypertension secondary to chronic obstructive pulmonary disease (COPD) is rarely severe.

Clinical signs of pulmonary hypertension include exercise intolerance, weakness, syncope, and respiratory distress. Unfortunately, these signs can be difficult to distinguish from signs due to underlying cardiac or pulmonary disease. Physical examination may reveal a loud split S2 heart sound. Radiographic evidence of pulmonary hypertension may be present in severely affected patients and includes pulmonary artery enlargement and right-sided cardiomegaly. The diagnosis of pulmonary hypertension is most often made through Doppler echocardiography. Use of this modality to estimate pulmonary artery pressure requires the presence of pulmonary or tricuspid regurgitation and a highly skilled echocardiographer.

Treatment to improve oxygenation by managing chronic bronchitis through traditional means is clearly indicated. Long-term oxygen therapy is a major component of treatment in people, rarely practical for pets. It is not entirely clear whether dogs with secondary pulmonary hypertension should have direct treatment for pulmonary hypertension. There is obvious theoretical benefit, but there are potential disadvantages as well. Unfortunately, little is known about the treatment of pulmonary hypertension of any cause in dogs and adverse consequences can occur through worsening of ventilation: perfusion (V/Q) matching or other drug-related side effects. Therefore, careful monitoring of clinical signs and pulmonary artery pressures is indicated. The drug most commonly used to treat pulmonary hypertension in dogs is sildenafil citrate (Viagra, Pfizer), a phosphodiesterase V inhibitor that causes vasodilation through a nitric oxide pathway. Dosage and toxicity studies have not been published, but a dosage range from 0.5 to 2.7 mg/kg (median 1.9 mg/kg) orally every 8 to 24 hours has been reported. A dosage of 0.5 mg/kg orally every 12 hours can be used initially and increased to effect.

Infection

The role of infection with bacteria or *Mycoplasma* in chronic bronchitis is another issue that needs further study. Many dogs with chronic bronchitis or an exacerbation of signs do not have infection. Yet some dogs have active infection either as a presumed underlying cause (eg, chronic *Bordetella* infection) or as a consequence of diseased mucosa. Although the incidence may not be high, it is one of the few factors that can be directly treated. Therefore, I recommend cytology and culture of airway specimens at the time of original diagnosis and during persistent exacerbations of signs *prior to the arbitrary initiation of antibiotics*.

It is important to document that infection does exist. Results of trial treatment with antibiotics are extremely difficult to interpret. An apparent positive response could occur as a result of the normal waxing and waning of signs or a coincidental decrease in inhaled irritants. An apparent negative response could occur as a result of the unpredictable resistance patterns of the commonly involved gram-negative organisms or a failure to achieve therapeutic mucosal concentrations of drug. Unfortunately, it is not obvious in every case what constitutes a true infection even with specimen collection and culture. The trachea is not normally sterile, and people with chronic bronchitis have increased bacterial numbers in the large airways presumably as a result of decreased clearance and not necessarily infection. However, there is some evidence in people that the chronic low levels of organisms may contribute to ongoing inflammation, although whether antibiotic treatment in such cases is beneficial is debatable. Quantitative cultures from guarded bronchial brushings or bronchoalveolar lavage fluid are used in making the diagnosis of true infection in people. One study in dogs suggests that bronchoalveolar lavage fluid resulting in growth of greater than 1.7×10^3 CFU/mL by culture or more than two intracellular bacteria in any of 50 oil immersion fields on gram stain of a concentrated slide preparation (cytospin) is consistent with true infection. The role of *Mycoplasma* in respiratory infections remains uncertain. Accurate *Mycoplasma* cultures can be difficult to obtain and require weeks before results are known. Testing by PCR may allow a more rapid diagnosis, but reports of its use in clinical situations are lacking. Trial treatment is considered for dogs that are responding poorly to appropriate management for chronic bronchitis.

The penetration of antibiotics into the airways is probably of little consequence for dogs with pneumonia.

The ability to reach the mucosa may be of greater significance in dogs with infection of the airways. Fluoroquinolones and azithromycin reach good concentrations in the airways. However, azithromycin is generally not a good choice for chronic bronchitis because of its poor activity against gram-negative organisms and fluoroquinolones are generally better reserved for resistant infections. Further, if theophylline is being used the addition of a fluoroquinolone can lead to decreased theophylline clearance and signs of toxicity. If the combination is necessary, reduce the theophylline dose by 30% to 50% and monitor plasma concentrations. Although doxycycline has been recommended in the past because of its airway concentrations in people and in vitro effectiveness against *Bordetella* and *Mycoplasma*, recent work suggests that the drug is highly protein bound in dogs and may not reach the airway lumen as well as previously thought. Amoxicillin-clavulanate does not reach high airway concentrations in people, but the drug has a high therapeutic index and given at the high end of the dose range three times daily may be sufficient for susceptible organisms, particularly while active inflammation disrupts the normal blood–bronchus barrier. The spectrum of amoxicillin-clavulanate is reasonably broad and it is often effective against *Bordetella*.

REFERENCES

1. Wheeldon EB, et al. Chronic bronchitis in the dog. Vet Rec. 1974;94:466-471.
2. Mantis P, et al. Assessment of the accuracy of thoracic radiography in the diagnosis of canine chronic bronchitis. J Small Anim Pract. 1998;39:518-520.
3. Barbera JA, et al. Pulmonary hypertension in chronic obstructive pulmonary disease. Eur Respir J. 2003;21:892-905.
4. Hida W, et al. Pulmonary hypertension in patients with chronic obstructive pulmonary disease: recent advances in pathophysiology and management. Respirology. 2002; 7:3-13.
5. Bach JF, et al. Retrospective evaluation of sildenafil citrate as a therapy for pulmonary hypertension in dogs. J Vet Intern Med. 2006; 20:1132-1135.
6. Peeters DE, et al. Quantitative bacterial cultures and cytological examination of bronchoalveolar lavage specimens from dogs. J Vet Intern Med. 2000; 14:534-541.
7. Bidgood T, et al. Comparison of plasma and interstitial fluid concentrations of doxycycline and meropenem following constant rate infusion in dogs. Am J Vet Res. 2003; 64:1040-1046.

HOW I TREAT FELINE BRONCHITIS

Eleanor C. Hawkins, DVM, Diplomate ACVIM (SAIM)
College of Veterinary Medicine
North Carolina State University, Raleigh, NC

STRENGTHEN THE DIAGNOSIS OF IDIOPATHIC DISEASE

Although most cats with bronchitis have idiopathic diseases, a search for specific causes of bronchitis is highly recommended. Identifying a specific etiology for clinical signs may allow for specific treatment and even cure of an individual cat. Differential diagnoses for cats presenting with signs of bronchitis include allergic bronchitis, pulmonary parasites (*Aelurostrongylus abstrusus*, *Capillaria aerophila*, and *Paragonimus kellicotti*), heartworm disease, bacterial bronchitis, and mycoplasmal bronchitis. Occasionally cats with typically interstitial lung diseases can present with signs suggestive of bronchitis. Additional differential diagnoses to consider include carcinoma, toxoplasmosis, and idiopathic pulmonary fibrosis.

EMERGENCY STABILIZATION

Emergency stabilization includes administration of a bronchodilator and rapid-acting glucocorticoids, and providing supplemental oxygen. For cats in severe distress, terbutaline (0.01 mg/kg SC, repeated in 10–15 min if necessary) is administered subcutaneously. Onset is rapid and stress is minimized. If distress is less severe, aminophylline (5 mg/kg PO q12h) or theophylline base (immediate release; 4 mg/kg PO q12h) can be administered orally. Do not administer long-acting theophyllines for emergency stabilization because they require a longer period to reach therapeutic concentrations.

Albuterol can be given by metered-dose inhaler (MDI) or by nebulization in cats that fail to respond to systemic bronchodilators. This route of administration can be stressful for cats that are not used to a face mask. It is possible to nebulize a chamber (oxygen hood or oxygen cage), but large volumes of drug will be needed for a therapeutic effect in a large space and the mist created in the process can result in a wet patient. During episodes of distress, constriction and obstruction of airways may preclude the travel of drug deep into the lungs. Multiple, repeated treatments may be needed for effect. Unfortunately, a maximum tolerable dose has not been established. Careful attention is paid to heart rate and attitude for any sign of toxicity.

Prednisolone sodium succinate is the recommended glucocorticoid for a life-threatening crisis (up to 10 mg/kg IV). If intravenous administration is too stressful, the drug can be given intramuscularly. Alternatively, dexamethasone sodium phosphate (up to 2 mg/kg IV) can be given.

As soon as appropriate drugs are administered, the cat is placed in a cool, stress-free, oxygen-enriched environment. Respiratory rate should be recorded and monitored for objective evidence of progress.

MANAGEMENT OF STABLE PATIENTS
Environment

Any patient with inflammatory airway disease can benefit from improvement of air quality. Some cats with a diagnosis of idiopathic bronchitis may have allergic airway disease, as the latter diagnosis is difficult to confirm. More importantly, irritants in the environment will exacerbate any ongoing inflammation. Potential sources of allergens or irritants are determined through careful owner questioning. Smoke can be particularly irritating and should be eliminated from the cat's environment. The effect of litter perfumes can be evaluated by replacing the litter with sandbox sand or plain clay litter. Indoor cats may show improvement in response to measures taken to decrease the level of dusts, molds, and mildew in the home. Such measures include carpet, furniture, and drapery cleaning; cleaning of the furnace and the frequent replacement of air filters; and the use of an air cleaner. The American Lung Association has a useful website with non-proprietary recommendations for improving indoor air quality (www.lungusa.org). Any beneficial response to an environmental change is usually seen within 1 to 2 weeks.

Glucocorticoids

Most cats with idiopathic bronchitis require glucocorticoid treatment for control of signs. Results can be dramatic. However, drug therapy can interfere with environmental testing; therefore the ability of the animal to tolerate a delay in the start of drug therapy must be assessed on an animal-by-animal basis. Glucocorticoids will relieve the clinical signs in most cats and may protect the airways from the detrimental effects of chronic inflammation. Short-acting products such as prednisolone are recommended because the dose of drug can be tapered to the lowest effective amount.

Prednisolone is recommended, rather than prednisone, based on anecdotal experience and a preliminary study suggest that prednisolone may be more effective in cats than prednisone. An initial dosage of 0.5 to 1 mg/kg every 12 hours is prescribed initially. If signs are not controlled within 1 week, the dosage is doubled. Once the signs are controlled, the prednisolone is tapered to the least effective amount. A reasonable goal is to administer 0.5 mg/kg or less every other day. Depot steroid products, such as methylprednisolone acetate (10 mg/cat intramuscularly is effective for up to 4 weeks), are not ideal for long term management but can be an effective alternative for cats that spend prolonged periods out of door or are difficult to handle due to temperament.

Alternatively, glucocorticoids, such as fluticasone propionate (Flovent®, GlaxoSmithKline), can be administered locally to the airways by MDI. This means of drug delivery is routine for treating airway disease in people. Advantages of administration by MDI are a decrease in systemic side effects and relative ease of administration in some cats, compared with oral administration. To date, however, it is still not known how much drug is deposited in the lower airways, how much remains in the oral and nasal cavities, and how much is absorbed systemically in cats. Theoretical concerns about the oronasal deposition of the potent glucocorticoid in cats, compared with people, include the high incidence of periodontal disease and latent herpesvirus infections and the inability to effectively rinse the mouth with water after use. However, some veterinarians have been using glucocorticoid MDIs to treat idiopathic feline bronchitis for many years without frequent, obvious adverse effects.

I prefer to obtain a clinical remission of signs using orally administered drug first, except in cats with relative contraindications for systemic glucocorticoid therapy such as having diabetes mellitus. By beginning with oral therapy I can determine the steroid responsiveness without adding the variable of unknown drug delivery. Cats that require a relatively low dose of oral glucocorticoids to control clinical signs, have no noticeable adverse effects, and that can be pilled without difficulty are often well maintained with oral therapy. Otherwise, once signs are in remission, treatment by MDI is initiated and the dosage of oral prednisolone gradually reduced.

A spacer must be used for effectively administering drugs by MDI to cats, and the airflow generated by the cat must be sufficient to activate the spacer valve. Padrid[2] has found the Optichamber (Respironics) to be effective. A small anesthetic mask, with rubber diaphragm, is attached to the spacer. Widening of the adapter of the anesthetic mask that is inserted into the spacer is necessary to create a snug fit. This is achieved by wrapping adhesive tape around the adapter. Alternatively, a mask and spacer specifically designed for use in cats is available (Aerokat, Trudell Medical International). The use of homemade spacers should be discouraged because they introduce another variable into the amount of drug delivered to the patient. Commercial spacers are designed specifically to minimize retention of drug on the spacer walls.

In my experience, cats are more tolerant of receiving drugs by MDI if they are acclimated to the device in advance. I recommend having the owner start by simply placing the face mask over the cat's nose for a brief period, associating the experience with a period of low stress followed by a favorite treat or game. Gradually, the additional steps required to actually administer drug are added. The cat is allowed to rest comfortably on a table or in the client's lap. The client places their arms on either side of the cat or gently steadies the cat's neck and head to provide restraint. The MDI, attached to the spacer, is actuated (pressed) twice. The mask is placed immediately on the cat's face, covering the mouth and nose completely, and it is held in place while the cat takes 7 to 10 breaths, inhaling the drug into its airways.

The following treatment schedule has been recommended. For cats with mild daily symptoms: 220 µg of fluticasone propionate by MDI twice daily and albuterol by MDI as needed. The maximum effect of fluticasone is not expected until 7 to 10 days of treatment. For cats with moderate daily symptoms: treatments with MDI as described for mild symptoms; in addition, prednisone is administered orally for 10 days (1 mg/kg every 12 hours for 5 days, then every 24 hours for 5 days). For cats with severe symptoms: dexamethasone is administered once (2 mg/kg IV), albuterol is administered by MDI every 30 minutes for up to 4 hours, and the cat is administered oxygen. Once stabilized, these cats are prescribed 220 µg of fluticasone propionate by MDI every 12 hours, and albuterol by MDI every 6 hours as needed. Oral prednisone is administered as needed.

Bronchodilators

Cats that require relatively large amounts of glucocorticoids to control clinical signs, that react unfavorably to glucocorticoid therapy, or that suffer from periodic exacerbations of signs can benefit from bronchodilator therapy. Albuterol administered by MDI is a convenient for the immediate, at-home, treatment of acute respiratory distress (asthma attack). Cats with idiopathic bronchitis are routinely prescribed an albuterol MDI, spacer, and mask to be kept at home for emergencies. As described for MDI glucocorticoids, it is helpful to acclimate the cat to the procedure *before* it is needed in an emergency situation.

For cats that require constant treatment with a bronchodilator, theophylline can be prescribed. Theophylline is effective and inexpensive, can be given to cats once daily and plasma concentrations can be easily measured for the monitoring of difficult cases. Theophylline has been used for years for the treatment of chronic bronchitis in people. This drug became unpopular with physicians as newer bronchodilators with fewer side effects became available. However, recent research in people suggests that theophylline is effective in treating the underlying inflammation of chronic bronchitis even at concentrations below those resulting in bronchodilation (thus, reducing side effects), and that the anti-inflammatory effects may be synergistic with those of glucocorticoids. Theophylline may also improve mucociliary clearance, decrease fatigue of respiratory muscles and inhibit the release of mast cell mediators of inflammation. The possibility of these additional benefits beyond bronchodilation have not been explored in cats.

A disadvantage of theophylline is that other drugs, such as fluoroquinolones and chloramphenicol, can delay its clearance and cause signs of theophylline toxicity if the dosage is not reduced by one third to one half. Potential adverse effects include gastrointestinal signs, cardiac arrhythmias, nervousness, and seizures. Serious adverse effects are extremely rare at therapeutic concentrations.

The pharmacokinetics of theophylline products are different in cats compared with dogs, resulting in different dosages. Variability in sustained plasma concentrations in both species has been found for different long-acting theophylline products. Further, the individual metabolism of all of the methylxanthines is variable. No studies have been performed in cats using currently available products, but based on extrapolations from a study in dogs we currently use a dosage of 10 mg/kg q24h of a specific generic drug (Theochron,

Inwood Laboratories). Plasma theophylline concentrations are monitored in cats that respond poorly, are predisposed to adverse effects or show signs of adverse effects. Therapeutic peak concentrations, based on data from people, are 5 to 20 µg/mL. Plasma for the determination of these concentrations should be collected 12 hours after the evening dosing of the long-acting products and 2 hours after short-acting products. Measurement of concentrations immediately before the next scheduled dose might provide useful information concerning duration of therapeutic concentrations.

Sympathomimetic drugs can also be effective bronchodilators. Terbutaline is selective for beta-2 adrenergic receptors, lessening its cardiac effects. Potential adverse effects include nervousness, tremors, hypotension, and tachycardia. Note that the recommended oral dose for cats (one eighth to one fourth of a 2.5-mg tablet) is lower than the commonly cited dose of 1.25 mg/cat.

Other Potential Treatments

A therapeutic trial with an antibiotic effective against *Mycoplasma* is considered because of the difficulty in documenting infection with this organism. Either doxycycline (5 to 10 mg/kg every 12 hours) or chloramphenicol (10 to 15 mg/kg q12h) is administered for 14 days. For cats that are difficult to medicate, azithromycin (5 to 10 mg/kg q24h for 3 days, then every 72 hours) can be tried. Remember that administration of doxycycline should always be followed with a bolus of water to minimize the incidence of esophageal stricture.

Antihistamines are not recommended for treating feline bronchitis because histamine in some cats produces bronchodilation. However, an in vitro study has shown that the serotonin antagonist, cyproheptadine, has a bronchodilatory effect. A dose of 2 mg/cat orally every 12 hours can be tried in cats with signs that cannot be controlled with routine bronchodilator and glucocorticoid therapy. This treatment is not consistently effective.

Much interest has been shown among clients and veterinarians for the use of oral leukotriene inhibitors in cats (eg, Accolate®, Singulair®, and Zyflo®). However, the clinician should be aware that in people, leukotriene inhibitors are *less* effective in the management of asthma than glucocorticoids, and they are not used in the emergency management of the disease or for refractory cases. Their advantage for people lies in decreased side effects, compared with glucocorticoids, and ease of administration. To date, toxicity studies have not been performed on these drugs in cats. Further, several preliminary studies suggest that leukotriene inhibition in the cat would not be expected to have efficacy comparable to that in people. Therefore, their routine use in cats is not currently advocated. Further investigation into their potential role in treating feline bronchitis is certainly indicated.

REFERENCES
1. Graham-Mize CA, et al. Bioavailability and activity of prednisone and prednisolone in the feline patient (abstract). Vet Dermatol. 2004; 15(Suppl 1): 9.
2. Padrid P. Feline asthma: Diagnosis and treatment, Vet Clin North Am Small Anim Pract. 2000;30:1279-1293.
3. Bach JF, et al. Evaluation of the bioavailability and pharmacokinetics of two extended-release theophylline formulations in dogs. J Am Vet Med Assoc. 2004; 224:1113-1119.
4. Padrid PA, et al. Cyproheptadine-induced attenuation of type-I immediate hypersensitivity reactions of airway smooth muscle from immune-sensitized cats. Am J Vet Res.1995; 56:109-115.

HOW I TREAT IDIOPATHIC CHRONIC RHINITIS

Eleanor C. Hawkins, DVM, Diplomate ACVIM (SAIM)
College of Veterinary Medicine
North Carolina State University, Raleigh, NC

FELINE IDIOPATHIC CHRONIC RHINOSINUSITIS

Feline chronic rhinosinusitis has long been presumed to be a result of viral infection with herpes or calicivirus. However, studies have failed to show an association with persistent viral infections and chronic rhinitis based on measurements of serum antibodies (indicating exposure) or tests for the viruses. It is possible that infection with these viruses results in damaged mucosa that is more susceptible to bacterial infection or that mounts an excessive inflammatory response to irritants or normal nasal flora. Preliminary studies have also failed to find an association with chronic rhinitis and infection with *Bartonella*.

No one treatment is effective for all cats. Options include facilitating drainage of discharge, decreasing irritants in the environment, controlling secondary bacterial infections, treating possible *Mycoplasmal* or feline herpesvirus (FHV) infection, reducing inflammation and, as a last resort, turbinectomy and frontal sinus ablation.

In my experience, cats can often be managed very well with long-term chronic antibiotic therapy with a single agent. Antibiotic strategies that seem likely to ultimately fail are those based on short-courses (eg, 2 weeks), with a different drug instituted every time that signs return. If a deep-seated bacterial infection is contributing to signs, such as with infection of obstructed sinuses, osteomyelitis, or infection of damaged or even necrotic turbinates, treatment for 4 to 6 weeks or longer would be expected to be necessary to have prolonged benefit. Changing antibiotics every time clinical signs recur may increase the likelihood of the development of an organism with marked antibiotic resistance.

First line, broad-spectrum antibiotics such as amoxicillin (22 mg/kg q12h) or trimethoprim-sulfadiazine (15 mg/kg q12h) are often successful. I reserve fluoroquinolones for cats with documented resistant gram-negative infections. If a beneficial response to antibiotic therapy is seen within 1 week of its initiation, the antibiotic should be continued for at least 4 to 6 weeks. If a beneficial response is not seen, the antibiotic is discontinued. Cats that respond well during the prolonged course of antibiotics but that relapse shortly after discontinuation of the drug despite 4 to 6 weeks of relief are candidates for continuous long-term antibiotic therapy. Often treatment with the previously used antibiotic can be successfully re-instituted. Amoxicillin administered twice daily is often sufficient.

If no improvement is seen with the above protocol, chloramphenicol (10 to 15 mg/kg q12h) or doxycycline (5 to 10 mg/kg q12h, followed by a bolus of water) can be prescribed. These drugs have activity against many bacteria and *Chlamydophila* and *Mycoplasma* organisms and can be effective in some cats when other antibiotics have failed.

Some clinicians prefer to prescribe azithromycin for cats with chronic rhinitis. This drug also has activity against *Mycoplasma* organisms and requires infrequent dosing. A study comparing the clinical response to amoxicillin or azithromycin in shelter cats with signs of rhinitis (typically acute rather than chronic disease) found no significant differences between these treatments. Certain antibiotics, such as azithromycin, may be beneficial in chronic inflammatory disease because of antioxidant or anti-inflammatory properties rather than through the treatment of pathogens.

Drainage is facilitated by keeping secretions moist, performing intermittent nasal flushes, and judicious use of topical decongestants. Keeping the cat in a room with a vaporizer for part of the day or during the night can provide symptomatic relief by keeping secretions moist. Alternatively, drops of sterile saline can be placed into nares. Some cats have marked improvement in clinical signs for weeks after flushing of the nasal cavity with copious amounts of saline or dilute betadine solution. General anesthesia is required, and the lower airways must be protected with an endotracheal tube, gauze sponges, and positioning of the head to facilitate drainage from the external nares. Topical pediatric decongestants, such as 0.25% phenylephrine or 0.025% oxymetazoline, may provide symptomatic relief during episodes of severe congestion. A drop is gently placed in each nostril daily for a maximum of 3 days. If longer therapy is necessary, the decongestant is withheld for 3 days before beginning another 3-day course to prevent possible rebound congestion after withdrawal of the drug (based on problems with rebound congestion that occur in people).

Irritants in the environment such as smoke (from tobacco or fireplace) and perfumed products should be avoided. Any inhaled irritant will exacerbate mucosal inflammation. Motivated clients can take steps to improve the air quality in their home, such as carpet, furniture, and drapery cleaning; cleaning of the furnace and the frequent replacement of air filters; and the use of an air cleaner. The American Lung Association has a useful website with non-proprietary recommendations for improving indoor air quality (www.lungusa.org).

Treatment with lysine may be effective in those cats with active herpesvirus infections. It has been postulated that excessive concentrations of lysine may antagonize arginine, a promoter of herpesvirus replication. Because the specific organism(s) involved is rarely known, trial therapy is initiated. Lysine (500 mg/cat q12h), obtained from health food stores, is added to food. A minimum of 4 weeks is necessary to assess success of treatment.

Anecdotal success in occasional cats has been reported with treatment with the second-generation antihistamine cetirizine (Zyrtec, Pfizer). A pharmacokinetic study of this drug in healthy cats found a dosage of 1 mg/kg orally every 24 hours to maintain plasma concentrations similar to those reported in people.[4] No efficacy studies are available.

Another unproven option to decrease the severity of clinical signs is the supplementation of the diet with omega 3 fatty acids. The effectiveness of this approach may, in part, be dependent on the amount of omega 3 fatty acids already present in the patient's diet.

Cats with severe, persistent signs despite the previously described methods of supportive care may benefit from glucocorticoids to reduce inflammation. Risks are involved. Glucocorticoids may further predispose the cat to secondary infections, increase viral shedding, and mask signs of a more serious disease. Glucocorticoids should be prescribed only after a complete diagnostic evaluation has been performed to rule out other diseases. Prednisolone is administered at a dose of 0.5 mg/kg every 12 hours. If a beneficial response is seen within 1 week, the dose is gradually decreased to the lowest dose that is still effective. A dose as low as 0.25 mg/kg every 2 to 3 days may be sufficient to control clinical signs. If a clinical response is not seen within 1 week, the drug should be discontinued. Anecdotal reports have been made of success in some cats using inhaled glucocorticoids, such as fluticasone propionate (Flovent®, GlaxoSmithKline) administered by metered-dose inhaler (MDI).

Cats with severe or deteriorating signs despite conscientious care are candidates for turbinectomy and frontal sinus ablation, assuming a complete diagnostic evaluation to eliminate other causes of chronic nasal discharge has been performed. Turbinectomy and frontal sinus ablation are difficult surgical procedures. Major blood vessels and the cranial vault must be avoided, and tissue remnants must not be left behind. Anorexia can be a postoperative problem; placement of an esophagostomy or gastrostomy tube provides an excellent means for meeting nutritional requirements if necessary after surgery. Complete elimination of respiratory signs is unlikely, but signs may be more easily managed. For cats with persistant mild to moderate signs, surgical intervention is not recommended, and a number of these cats will have spontaneous clinical improvement after many months.

CANINE IDIOPATHIC CHRONIC RHINITIS

Idiopathic chronic rhinitis in dogs is often characterized by the inflammatory infiltrates found in nasal biopsies. Thus, the disease lymphoplasmacytic rhinitis has been described. It was originally reported to be a steroid responsive disorder, but a subsequent report and clinical experience suggest that corticosteroids are not always effective. Neutrophilic inflammation is also commonly found, predominantly or along with lymphoplasmacytic infiltrates.

The most important step in the management of these patients is to be as confident as possible in the diagnosis of "idiopathic." Many specific lung diseases, such as foreign bodies, neoplasia, and fungal infections, result in a concurrent inflammatory process.

Several investigations have been carried out to find an underlying cause for dogs with chronic rhinitis without a specific diagnosis following routine diagnostic evaluation including nasal imaging, rhinoscopy and biopsy. Windsor et al performed multiple polymerase chain reaction (PCR) assays on paraffin-embedded nasal tissue from dogs with idiopathic chronic rhinitis and failed to find evidence for a role of bacteria (based on DNA load), canine adenovirus-2, parainfluenza virus, Chlamydophila spp. or Bartonella spp. in affected dogs. High amounts of fungal DNA were found in affected dogs, suggesting a possible contribution to clinical signs. Alternatively, the result may simply reflect decreased clearance of fungal organisms from the diseased nasal cavity. Although not supported in the previously quoted study, a potential role for Bartonella infection has been suggested based on a study that found an association between seropositivity for Bartonella spp. and nasal discharge or epistaxis and a report of three dogs with epistaxis and evidence of infection with Bartonella spp. Preliminary results of an ongoing study in our laboratory have failed to find an obvious association between bartonellosis and idiopathic rhinitis.

Treatment of idiopathic canine chronic rhinitis is similar to that described for feline idiopathic chronic rhinosinusitis. Dogs are treated for secondary bacterial rhinitis using long-term therapy with a single antibiotic as described above for cats. Improvement in indoor air quality can decrease the severity of clinical signs. Like cats, some dogs will benefit from efforts to facilitate the draining of nasal discharge by humidification of air or instillation of sterile saline into the nasal cavity. And supplementation with omega 3 fatty acids may be beneficial in some cases.

Burgener et al reported successful treatment of dogs with lymphoplasmacytic rhinitis using immuno-suppressive doses of prednisone (1 mg/kg q12h). A positive response is expected within 2 weeks, at which time the dose of prednisone is decreased gradually to the lowest effective amount. If no response to initial therapy occurs, other immunosuppressive drugs such as azathioprine can be added to the treatment regimen. Unfortunately, immunosuppressive treatment is not always effective. In the event that clinical signs actually worsen during treatment, corticosteroids should be immediately discontinued and the dog carefully reevaluated for underlying disease.

Other treatments that may be effective in some dogs include antihistamines or itraconazole. According to a preliminary study by Kuehn, administration of itraconazole (5 mg/kg q12h) resulted in dramatic improvement in clinical signs in some dogs with idiopathic chronic rhinitis. Treatment was required for a minimum of 3 to 6 months. The rationale for this treatment may be supported by the previously mentioned findings of increased fungal load in affected dogs. Dogs with severe or nonresponsive signs are candidates for rhinotomy and turbinectomy for both diagnostic and therapeutic purposes.

REFERENCES

5. Berryessa NA, et al. The role of Bartonella spp. in feline chronic rhinosinusitis (abstract). J Vet Intern Med. 2007;21:608.

6. Ruch-Gallie R, et al. Efficacy of amoxicillin and azithromycin for the empirical treatment of cats with upper respiratory infections (abstract). J Vet Intern Med. 2004;18:385.

7. Maggs DJ, et al. Effects of L-lysine and L-arginine on in vitro replication of feline herpesvirus type-1, Am J Vet Res. 2000;61:1474-1478.

8. Papich MG, et al. Cetirizine (Zyrtec) pharmacokinetics in healthy cats (abstract). J Vet Intern Med. 2006;20:754.

9. Burgener DC, et al. Lymphoplasmacytic rhinitis in five dogs. J Am Anim Hosp Assoc. 1987;23:565-568.

10. Windsor RC, et al. Idiopathic lymphoplasmacytic rhinitis in dogs: 37 cases (1997-2002). J Am Vet Med Assoc. 2004;224:1952-1957.

11. Windsor RC, et al. Molecular detection of microbes in nasal tissue of dogs with idiopathic lymphoplasmacytic rhinitis. J Vet Intern Med. 2006;20:250-256.

12. Henn JB, et al. Seroprevalence of antibodies against Bartonella species and evaluation of risk factors and clinical signs associated with seropositivity in dogs. Am J Vet Res. 2005;66:688-694.

13. Breitschwerdt, et al. *Bartonella* species as a potential cause of epistaxis in dogs. J Clin Microbiol. 2005;43:2529-2533.

14. Kuehn NF. Prospective long term pilot study using oral itraconazole therapy for the treatment of chronic idiopathic (lymphoplasmacytic) rhinitis in dogs (Abstract). British Small Animal Veterinary Association Annual Congress, Prague, Czech Republic, 2006.

THE CONUNDRUM OF THE CONTAGIOUS CANINE COUGH

Eleanor C. Hawkins, DVM, Diplomate ACVIM (SAIM)
College of Veterinary Medicine
North Carolina State University, Raleigh, NC

Leah A. Cohn, DVM, PhD, Diplomate ACVIM (SAIM)
College of Veterinary Medicine
University of Missouri, Columbia, MO

The list of differential diagnoses for acute cough in dogs includes numerous cardiac and respiratory diseases. Infectious causes are also many, and include viruses (eg, canine influenza virus, distemper virus, parainfluenza virus, adenovirus 2), bacteria (eg, *Bordetella bronchiseptica*, *Mycoplasma* spp, *Streptococcus equi* subsp *zooepidemicus*), protozoa, mycoses, and parasites.

Bordetella bronchiseptica and the respiratory viruses are particularly contagious organisms and infection in a dog presented to your hospital has important implications not only for that patient and client, but also for other patients in your hospital and other dogs who have contacted the coughing dog. Infections with respiratory viruses, other than distemper and influenza, are generally mild and short-lived if uncomplicated by co-infections. Vaccination against infection with distemper is widespread and generally effective. Therefore, this discussion will focus on infections with *Bordetella* and influenza virus.

PRESENTATION

A history of recent exposure to other dogs with cough or to group housing situations is supportive of a diagnosis of infection with either *Bordetella* or influenza because they are both highly contagious. Influenza has a shorter incubation period (usually less than 1 week, compared with up to 2 weeks for *Bordetella*) and because most dogs are naïve to influenza antigens, evidence for spread of disease may be more rapid in cases of influenza. Most dogs diagnosed with influenza infections are from dense, group housing situations.

Cough is often the presenting sign of dogs with either *Bordetella* or influenza infections. Either infection can result in a loud, harsh cough that is readily induced by tracheal palpation (more typical of tracheobronchitis), or a soft, moist cough (more typical of pneumonia). *Bordetella* most often causes a loud, harsh cough, while influenza most often results in a soft, moist cough. Nasal discharge is more commonly noted in dogs with influenza, compared with dogs with *Bordetella*.

Either infection can result in signs of overt pneumonia, such as soft cough, tachypnea, increased respiratory efforts, auscultable crackles, or fever. This more severe form of influenza has been identified most often in stressed patients, such as dogs from race tracks or animal shelters. A peracute, hemorrhagic pneumonia due to influenza has been reported in race track greyhounds. *Bordetella* can result in pneumonia, particularly in puppies. A recent study found that of 65 puppies with community acquired infectious pneumonia, 49% had infection with Bordetella.

DIAGNOSTIC EVALUATION

Systemic screening tests (complete blood count [CBC], serum biochemical panel, urinalysis) and thoracic radiographs are indicated in all patients with signs suggestive of pneumonia. Even in patients without overt signs of pneumonia on physical examination, a CBC and thoracic radiographs will increase the sensitivity of identifying the presence of pneumonia. It should be noted that neither a normal CBC nor body temperature can be used to rule out a diagnosis of pneumonia because only half of patients with pneumonia have a fever or leukocytosis on presentation.

If thoracic radiographs confirm the presence of bronchopneumonia and the patient is sufficiently stable, then a tracheal wash is performed prior to initiating antibiotic therapy. Bacterial culture can confirm a diagnosis of bordetellosis. Most importantly, antibiotic sensitivity information for *Bordetella* organisms or for secondary bacteria in cases with influenza can be invaluable in guiding the treatment of these potentially fatal infections.

Patients with mild clinical signs due to either *Bordetella* or influenza will not likely benefit directly from a definitive diagnosis because these infections are usually self-limiting. However, a definitive diagnosis may be useful for the treatment of patients with more severe clinical signs, and for developing recommendations for the monitoring and management of previously exposed dogs in a shelter or kennel setting.

Bordetella bronchiseptica

A practical method for obtaining a definitive diagnosis of *Bordetella* infection is by tracheal wash cytology and culture. Cytology is expected to show septic, neutrophilic inflammation with small gram negative rods. Organism identification is confirmed through routine bacterial culture. Polymerase chain reaction (PCR) testing for multiple respiratory pathogens, including *Bordetella bronchiseptica*, is available commercially and through certain university-based laboratories. Deep pharyngeal swabs are suggested for testing, although *Bordetella* can be found in the pharynx of some healthy dogs by culture of pharyngeal swabs, so tracheal wash specimens may be more specific. The sensitivity and specificity of PCR testing for a clinical population has not been established, nor has the effect of prior treatment with antibiotics. Tracheal wash culture for the diagnosis of bordetellosis is preferred over testing by PCR because important antibiotic sensitivity data is obtained concurrently. In outbreaks, it may be prudent to obtain both bacterial cultures and a PCR panel because the panel has the potential to also identify nonbacterial pathogens. Examples of other pathogens for which PCR testing is available include canine influenza virus, canine distemper virus, canine adenovirus type 2, canine parainfluenza virus type 3, canine herpesvirus and canine respiratory coronavirus.

Canine Influenza

Serology, ELISA for antigen detection, virus isolation, and PCR can be used to confirm a diagnosis of influenza, but each has its strengths and weaknesses. Advantages of serology are that blood is a simple specimen to collect and infection can be detected even after viral shedding has ceased. The main weakness of serology is that confirmation must be delayed pending collection of convalescent serum to confirm rising antibody titers. More timely results are possible with antigen detection and PCR. Preliminary data using nasal swabs for specimens indicates that PCR is much more sensitive in detecting virus than antigen detection by ELISA or virus isolation. Other specimens that can be submitted for virus isolation or PCR are pharyngeal swabs, tracheal or nasal wash fluid, or lung tissue. Results from any test for viral detection can be falsely negative because of the relatively short period of shedding after the development of signs in most patients. For best results, samples are collected from febrile dogs very early in the course of disease. When shelters are affected, multiple dogs should be sampled (at least 3 to 5 dogs, or 10% of affected dogs).

TREATMENT
Mild Disease

Dogs with mild disease due to either *Bordetella* or influenza infection generally have self-limiting disease. No specific treatment is clearly beneficial. As a bacteria, *Bordetella* should theoretically be responsive to antibiotic therapy. While antibiotics may shorten the duration of clinical signs, no antibiotic protocol is known to eliminate the organism. Further, some antibiotics may not reach the site of infection in therapeutic concentrations. *Bordetella* organisms can be found on the surface of the epithelial cells and to reach these organisms antibiotics would need to reach adequate concentrations in epithelial lining fluid. However, other factors may influence the ability of antibiotics to reach the airway lumen, including the presence of airway inflammation and the potential for some drugs to be delivered to the site of infection within inflammatory cells.

Sensitivity of *Bordetella bronchiseptica* to antibiotics is not predictable and published reports have shown an evolution in sensitivity over time. In reports within the past 10 years, most isolates were sensitive to doxycycline, chloramphenicol, enrofloxacin, and amoxicillin/clavulanate. Fewer isolates were sensitive to trimethoprim-sulfa, and much resistance was found to first generation cephalosporins and ampicillin. Although amoxicillin/clavulanate is not thought to reach high concentrations in the epithelial lining fluid of healthy dogs, it has a high margin of safety and is a reasonable consideration for dogs with non-life-threatening infection. However, in order to increase its concentrations in the airways it should be administered three times daily at the high end of the dosage range, making it inconvenient for many owners. Fluoroquinolones reach high concentrations in the epithelial lining fluid but should generally be reserved for more significant infections. Chloramphenicol reaches reasonable airway concentrations and is a rational choice for puppies where fluoroquinolones and tetracyclines may be relatively contraindicated. Doxycycline reaches reasonable airway concentrations in people, but is more highly protein bound in dogs and may not penetrate into the epithelial lining fluid as readily. It also has the disadvantage of potential dental staining in puppies, although this occurs less commonly with doxycycline than tetracycline. Azithromycin can achieve high airway concentrations, is convenient for owners, and is used to treat *Bordetella pertussis* in people, but sensitivity to *B. bronchiseptica* has not been reported. Also be aware that the spectrum of azithromycin is quite narrow. Another strategy to reach high airway concentrations is by nebulization of antibiotics. Some veterinarians report success in controlling signs and kennel outbreaks with nebulized gentamicin, but no controlled studies have been published. As with oral antibiotic therapy, it has been shown that nebulized antibiotic therapy does not eliminate *Bordetella* from the airways of infected dogs. Unless stringent disinfection is applied, nebulization has the potential to spread infection from dog to dog.

Specific treatment for influenza in people is with oseltamivir phosphate. To be effective, the drug must be given within 12 to 48 hours of the onset of signs, and the major benefit is a decrease in the median duration until improvement of signs by just over 1 day. No controlled efficacy trials are available for dogs. To our knowledge dose and toxicity studies have not been done in dogs, although the drug has been used by individuals to treat dogs with upper respiratory tract signs and parvo virus infection. It is unlikely that a sufficiently early diagnosis will be possible in most cases. Appropriateness of use of a sometimes scarce human resource must also be considered, particularly in the absence of more supportive data and in the situation of mild clinical signs.

Effectiveness of nonspecific treatments for mild, infectious cough has not been extensively explored. One limited field study of dogs with infectious tracheobronchitis found no benefit to the administration of steroids. Cough suppressants are often prescribed. Potential benefits are reducing secondary inflammation caused by persistent coughing and allowing rest for the patient and owners. A potential disadvantage is decreasing an important clearance mechanism in a patient who likely has disruption of normal ciliary function. In the authors' experience cough is best controlled by minimizing stimuli that induce cough, such as excitement or pressure from a collar, combined with the judicious use of narcotic cough suppressants on an as needed basis.

Severe Disease: Pneumonia

Dogs with pneumonia due to influenza are typically infected with secondary bacteria. As discussed with mild disease, virus specific drugs are not known to be effective. Therefore, dogs with severe pneumonia due to either bordetellosis or influenza are treated according to general recommendations for treating bacterial bronchopneumonia. Initially, antibiotics should be broad-spectrum. Modification to treatment is then based on results of cultures of airway specimens and response to treatment. Reported sensitivity results for *Bordetella* isolates were discussed above, but occasionally dogs with severe pneumonia due to *Bordetella* may have infection complicated by other bacteria. A variety of bacteria have been isolated from dogs with influenza, including *Streptococcus equi* subsp *zooepidemicus* and gram-negative organisms that are resistant to commonly prescribed antibiotics. Antibiotics to consider for initial treatment of severe pneumonia include the combination of ampicillin with sulbactam and either a fluoroquinolone or an aminoglycoside, or meropenem.

PROTECTING OTHER DOGS

Bordetella may persist in the airways of dogs for up to 3 months, although dogs do not appear to be particularly infective for this prolonged period. This early study, based on experimentally induced infection, found that bacterial counts were related to clinical signs, decreasing with the resolution of signs. Resolution of coughing may also decrease the physical spread organisms. Vaccination against bordetellosis likely decreases the duration of shedding of organisms if administered *prior to* exposure, based on more rapid clearance of the organism as detected by culture. Influenza may be shed for as long as 10 days in infected dogs, and can be shed by dogs prior to development of clinical signs. However, by the time of presentation it is often difficult to isolate virus from pharyngeal swabs.

In a hospital, shelter, or other group housing environment, it is critical to immediately isolate any acutely coughing dog and to clean and disinfect all areas of contact. Both *Bordetella* and influenza are killed by routine disinfectants. Because disinfectants do no work in the presence of organic debris, thorough cleaning is essential.

Dogs with either disease potentially can be shedding organisms prior to the onset of classic clinical signs. Therefore, it is essential that routine infection control procedures be consistently followed for every animal. Examples of common failures in hospital infection control include: not washing hands between every patient, not removing all debris before disinfecting, not allowing sufficient contact time for disinfectants, not disinfecting muzzles between use, having insufficient air exchange and humidity control, allowing coughing dogs to wait in the waiting room, allowing patients to sniff each other as walking past each other or past cages, neglecting to consider people and clothing as potential fomites, and housing patients with insufficient distance between cage fronts (allowing spread by aerosol). The AVMA has a useful website entitled: Recommendations for managers and workers of kennel facilities that can be found at www.avma.org/public_health/influenza/canine_guideline s.asp.

PREVENTION

There is no vaccine available for canine influenza. Early studies of the equine product have not been promising. Vaccines are available for *Bordetella*, but are effective only in decreasing clinical signs and duration of shedding. Therefore, the most important means of

prevention of infection with either of these agents is to avoid exposure. Measures to maintain systemic health and prevent concurrent infection (eg, adenovirus 2, CDV) may not prevent infection with bordetellosis or influenza but may minimize disease severity.

Vaccines that are currently available for *Bordetella* in dogs include modified live intranasal products and a subcutaneously administered antigen extract product. Comparison of vaccine efficacy is difficult for several reasons. Protection with respect to *Bordetella* vaccines means a decrease in severity and duration of clinical signs. These important endpoints for the client introduce subjectivity into scientific studies. In addition, because host, environmental, and organism (strain) factors play large roles in severity of clinical signs and efficacy of vaccines, vaccination efficacy will likely be different under different experimental situations. Manufacturers continually aim to improve their product, and the products reported in refereed journals are not always the currently available products. Lastly, vaccine efficacy studies are extremely difficult and expensive to perform.

The different routes of administration of vaccine stimulate the immune system in different ways. Local immunity (eg, secretory IgA) would be expected to have more robust stimulation with intranasal administration; systemic immunity (eg, IgG) would be expected to have more robust stimulation with subcutaneous administration. Limitations of the studies conducted thus far are such that is too early to conclude that sequential administration of both types of vaccine is necessary in a clinical setting.

Onset of duration of protection may be an important consideration in shelters or for controlling outbreaks. One study showed that protection was provided by intranasal vaccination at 72 hours (3 days) post vaccination, but not at 24 or 48 hours. *Seropositive* dogs (dogs previously vaccinated or exposed to natural infection) which were vaccinated with a subcutaneous product developed rising specific serum IgG concentrations between 4 and 5 days of vaccination.

Based on the 2006 AAHA canine vaccine guidelines, the recommendation continues to be for either type of vaccine to be administered to dogs with expected exposure, given at least 1 week in advance. Yearly boosters are given. The exception to yearly boosters is the situation where boarding or other likely high level exposure may occur after 6 months from the previous vaccine, in which case a booster is suggested. This is outside of the manufacturers' recommendations. Puppies at risk for exposure are vaccinated according to manufacturers' recommendations (generally two subcutaneous vaccines or one intranasal vaccine is administered, depending on the age at first vaccination).

REFERENCES

1. Crawford PC, et al, Transmission of equine influenza virus to dogs. Science. 2005; 310:482-485.
2. Crawford C, Canine influenza virus (canine flu), University of Florida College of Veterinary Medicine

Veterinary Advisory, www.vetmed.ufl.edu/pr/nw_story/CANINEFLUFACTSHEET.htm, 2005.

3. Yoon K-J, et al. Influenza virus in racing greyhounds. Emerg Infect Dis. 2005;11:1974-1976.

4. Thrusfield MV, et al. A field investigation of kennel cough: incubation period and clinical signs. J Small Anim Pract. 1991; 32:215-220.

5. Radhakrishnan A, et al. Community-acquired infectious pneumonia in puppies: 65 cases (1993-2002). J Am Vet Med Assoc. 2007;230:1493-1497.

6. Spindel ME, et al, Detection and quantification of canine influenza virus by one-step real-time reverse transcription PCR (Abstract). J Vet Intern Med. 2007;21:576.

7. Speakman AJ, et al. Antibiotic susceptibility of canine *Bordetella bronchiseptica* isolates. Vet Microbiol. 2000; 71:193-200.

8. Foley JE, et al. Molecular epidemiology of feline bordetellosis in two animal shelters in California, USA. Prev Vet Med. 2002;54:141-156.

9. Bidgood T, et al. Comparison of plasma and interstitial fluid concentrations of doxycycline and meropenem following constant rate intravenous infusion in dogs. Am J Vet Res. 2003;64:1040-1046.

10. Miller CJM, et al, Gentamicin aerosolization for the treatment of infectious tracheobronchitis (abstract). Proceed Am Coll Vet Intern Med, 2003.

11. Bemis DA, et al, Aerosol, parenteral, and oral antibiotic treatment of Bordetella bronchiseptica infections in dogs. J Am Vet Med Assoc. 1977;170:1082.

12. Thrusfield MV, et al. A field investigation of kennel cough: efficacy of different treatments. J Small Anim Pract. 1991;32:455-459.

13. Bemis DA, et al, Pathogenesis of canine bordetellosis. J Infect Dis. 1977;135:753-761.

14. Jacobs AAC, et al. Protection of dogs for 13 months against *Bordetella bronchiseptica* and canine parainfluenza virus with a modified live vaccine. Vet Rec. 2005;157:19-23.

15. Davis R, et al, Comparison of the mucosal immune response in dogs vaccinated with either an intranasal avirulent culture or a subcutaneous antigen extract vaccine of *Bordetella bronchiseptica*. Vet Therap. 2007; 8:32-40.

16. Ellis JA, et al. Effect of vaccination on experimental infection with *Bordetella bronchiseptica* in dogs. J Am Vet Med Assoc. 2001;218:367-375.

17. Crawford PC, et al. Cross-reactivity of canine and equine influenza antibodies (Abstract). Proc Am Coll Vet Intern Med, 2006.

18. Gore T, et al. Intranasal kennel cough vaccine protecting dogs from experimental *Bordetella bronchiseptica* challenge within 72 hours. Vet Rec. 2005;156:482-483.

19. Ellis JA. Comparative efficacy of an injectable vaccine and an intranasal vaccine in stimulating *Bordetella bronchiseptica*-reactive antibody responses in seropositive dogs. J Am Vet Med Assoc. 2002; 220:43-48.

20. Gore T, et al. Intranasal kennel cough vaccine protecting dogs from experimental *Bordetella bronchiseptica* challenge within 72 hours. Vet Rec. 2005;56:482-483.

BRACHYCEPHALIC AIRWAY SYNDROME, PART 1: A NEW UNDERSTANDING – IT IS AN INTRANASAL PROBLEM!

Gerhard U. Oechtering, Prof.Dr.med.vet., Dipl. ECVAA
Ingmar Kiefer, Dr.med.vet.
Claudia Noeller, Dr.med.vet.
Department of Small Animal Medicine
University of Leipzig, Germany

In brachycephalic dogs, wrong breed selection has led to overemphasis of brachycephalia and almost complete loss of the nose. This structural deformity causes severe malfunction of the airway, often resulting in brachycephalic airway syndrome (BAS).

ANATOMY

BAS is a well-described combination of upper airway disorders in these breeds. Symptoms can vary broadly as well in intensity as in frequency of dyspneic episodes. We examined the anatomic specifics of the brachycephalic nose by computed tomography (CT) and compared them with those of the normocephalic nose (Figures 1, 2, and 3). The phenotypic appearance of the brachycephalic head depends on the shape of the skull and is strongly related to breed specific skeletal features. Such short-headed or round-shaped breeds are characterized by a short face, open orbitae, and display childlike traits.

The main problems in brachycephaly arise from the highly shortened facial bones and the resulting dislocation of nasal structures caused by the dorso-rotation of the teeth. Concomitant with increased stages of brachycephaly, the nares and the nasal entry get narrower; the

rostral ending of the respiratory duct (meatus nasi ventralis), the nasal conchae and the whole ethmoidal bone are pushed into an increased upright position; and the nasolacrimal drainage system is characterized by an increased angle and a steeper course. Nasal conchal material is pushed into the respiratory duct in some animals with higher degrees of brachycephaly and hinders respiratory air flow.

MORPHOMETRIC MEASUREMENTS

Morphometric measurements of the skull revealed characteristic differences among the brachycephalic dog breeds (Figure 2). The pug had an even shorter craniofacial skull than the French and English Bulldogs.

ABERRANT CONCHAE

Extreme shortening of the craniofacial skull, and thus of the nasal cavity, leads to abnormal configuration of the conchae. Two main types of aberrant conchal growth can be described:

1. Rostral, aberrant conchae obstructing the nasal passage (RAC) and
2. Caudal aberrant conchae obstructing the choanae (CAC, Figure 3, B-4a).

Furthermore, these conchae are characterized by a low degree of branching and crude lamellae. The severe intranasal deformities in brachycephalic dogs described here are the basis for a new pathophysiologic understanding of BAS. Detailed structural analysis of aberrant, stenosing conchae (RAC, CAC) is an indispensable prerequisite for the development of an intranasal surgical therapy of BAS in the form of partial laser-assisted turbinectomy (LATE therapy).

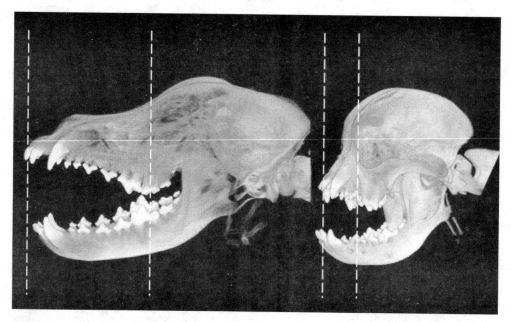

Figure 1. Three-dimensional CT-reconstruction of a normocephalic (*left*) and brachycephalic (*right*) skull.

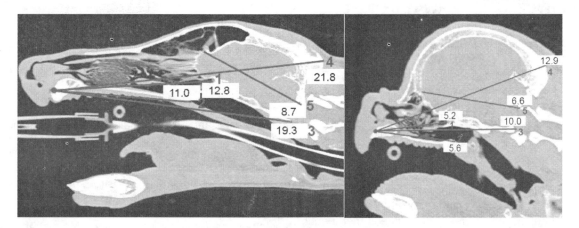

Figure 2. Examples for morphometric measurements of a normo- and brachycephalic skull. From Oechtering TH, Oechtering GU, Nöller C. Structural characteristics of the nose in brachycephalic dog breeds analysed by computed tomography, Tieraerztl Prax. 2007;35(K):177-187; with permission.

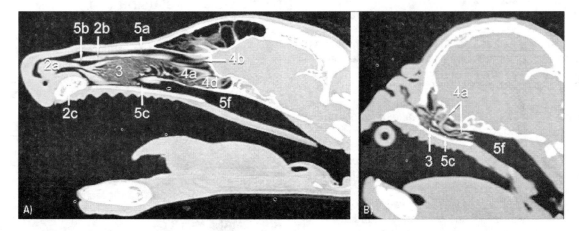

Figure 3. Sagittal CT scans of a normocephalic and a brachycephalic head. 2a = Plica alaris, 2b = Plica recta, 2c = Plica basalis; 3 = Concha nasalis ventralis; 4a = Concha nasalis media (Endoturbinate II), 4b = Concha nasalis dorsalis (Endoturbinate I), 4d = Endoturbinate IV; 5a = Meatus nasi dorsalis, 5b = Meatus nasi medius, 5c = Meatus nasi ventralis, 5f = Meatus nasopharyngeus. From Oechtering TH, Oechtering GU, Nöller C. Structural characteristics of the nose in brachycephalic dog breeds analysed by computed tomography. Tieraerztl Prax. 2007;35(K):177-187; with permission.

THERMOREGULATION

It is a very well known fact that brachycephalic dogs also suffer from severe heat susceptibility. If it is hot outside, humans begins to sweat and the evaporating water will cool the large surface of our skin and with that our blood. Dogs cannot sweat. Nevertheless, they also use the mechanism of evaporation cooling – they have their large surface inside the nose: an anatomic marvel of nasal turbinates. Panting is the most important element of thermoregulation in dogs. Both a patent intranasal airway for inspiration and an undisturbed oral expiration are essential for effective cooling.

Brachycephalic dogs lost their nose, not by chance but due to intentional breeding. With our recent research, we concentrated on the nasal influx and demonstrated severe obstruction of the intranasal as well as the rostral nasopharyngeal airways (choanae) in brachycephalic breeds. In the course of our recent investigations, we had strong indications that there is a substantial impairment of the oral (expiratory) airflow as well. These findings support the assumption that heat and stress susceptibility in brachycephalic dogs is a primary failure of peripheral thermoregulation and not of central mechanisms. More basic research on brachycephalia is needed to investigate the relation between anatomic malformation and functional impairment.

BRACHYCEPHALIC AIRWAY SYNDROME, PART 2: LASER-ASSISTED TURBINECTOMY (LATE) – A NOVEL THERAPEUTIC APPROACH

Gerhard U. Oechtering, Prof. Dr.med.vet., Dipl. ECVAA
Johanna P. Hueber, DVM
Claudia Noeller, Dr.med.vet.
Department of Small Animal Medicine
University of Leipzig, Germany

The brachycephalic airway syndrome (BAS) is a well-described combination of upper airway disorders in predisposed breeds. Reports on the difficulty in breathing of short-nosed breeds of dogs and therapeutic suggestions date back to the 1930s. Symptoms can vary widely as well in intensity as in frequency of dyspneic episodes. Snoring is the most common manifestation. In the worst cases, severe dyspnea with life-threatening asphyxia and syncope can be seen.

Most authors focus on the same specific anatomic features if they want to characterize BAS and if they want to explain reasons for the respiratory problems: narrow nostrils, elongated soft palate, and everted lateral ventricles. It is remarkable that all these anatomical structures are located either rostrally or caudally to the nasal cavity itself. But the fundamental eye-catching difference between brachycephalic and normocephalic dogs is the "missing" or extremely short nose.

Despite of the fact that today's treatment has remained generally unchanged over the past few decades, the results are not very satisfactory. Stimulated by clinical experience along with endoscopic and computer-tomographic examinations, we hypothesized that internal structures of the extremely reduced nasal cavity obstruct the main intranasal airways.

Our objectives were to evaluate intranasal airway stenosis in brachycephalic dogs and to introduce a surgical procedure, laser-assisted turbinectomy (LATE), with the purpose of creating patent nasal airways in form of a re-established meatus nasi ventralis (MNV).

MATERIAL AND METHODS

In a prospective study we examined and treated 80 brachycephalic dogs with severe respiratory insufficiency. Exclusion criteria were severe laryngeal or tracheal collapse. Three different breeds were represented: Pug, French Bulldog, and English Bulldog. Endoscopic examination, CT scans, and measurement of intranasal airflow resistance (impulse oscillometry, excluding influence of nares and palatum molle) were performed preoperatively to evaluate endonasal obstruction and as a basis for planning the surgical pathway. Endoscopically, a Diode-Laser fiber was used to remove obstructive parts of the conchae thus creating a new MNV. Postoperative controls followed with endoscopy, CT scans including virtual CT-endoscopy, and measurement of intranasal airflow resistance.

RESULTS

Abnormal conchal growth obstructing the nasal meatus was obvious in all dogs. In 49 dogs, the choanae and the meatus nasopharyngeus were also obstructed by parts of the concha nasalis ventralis (CNV) or the concha nasalis media (CNM). With LATE, we could resect the blocking structures and succeeded in creating a patent MNV. This was verified with conventional endoscopy and with virtual CT-endoscopy. Intranasal airflow resistance was reduced by approximately 50%.

The beginning and end of the surgical pathway was strongly influenced by the expression of aberrant conchae. The presence of rostral aberrant branches of the middle conchae made it necessary to resect them together with the ventral parts of the concha nasalis ventralis. Intense mineralization of rostral aberrant conchae aggravated laser vaporization. Caudal aberrant conchae had to be removed regardless whether they were branches of the concha nasalis media or ventralis.

DISCUSSION/CONCLUSION

The severe intranasal obstruction we were able to demonstrate in all dogs in our study allows us to reason that brachycephalic dogs suffer—in addition to the "classic" problems of BAS like stenotic nares and elongated soft palate—from a severe intranasal obstruction with consecutive impaired nasal airstreams and abnormal high airflow resistance.

With CT, endoscopic investigations, and measurement of intranasal airflow resistance we could clearly show that conchal tissue obstructs the nasal airway in varying manner and intensity. LATE is an appropriate technique to create a new patent and functional endonasal airway in brachycephalic breeds.

RHINOMANOMETRY

In order to evaluate surgical success objectively, intranasal airway resistance excluding influence of nostrils and soft palate was measured before and after LATE surgery. In addition, the long-term effect on airway resistance was investigated.

Nasal airway resistance of each nasal cavity was measured in anesthetized and spontaneously breathing patients both pre-operatively, one week post-LATE surgery, and 6 months after surgery. By inserting plastic tubes into the nostrils, influence of these structures on airway resistance could be eliminated. The influence of the soft palate on airway resistance was eliminated by retraction of this structure using a hook-shaped instrument or measuring after staphylectomy. The upper airways of all patients were subsequently investigated by endoscopy and CT.

A mean decrease of 69% in resistance could be shown. Pre- and postoperative intranasal airway resistance in pugs was significantly higher than in French bulldogs.

CONCLUSION

Partial turbinectomy (LATE) results in a significant decrease of intranasal airway resistance in dogs with BAS. Differences between breeds are probably due to differences in body size or/and length of nose. LATE surgery reducing intranasal airway resistance shows an immediate short-term effect and stable long-term effects.

The results of this study indicate that LATE is an effective and reliable therapy for intranasal airway obstruction.

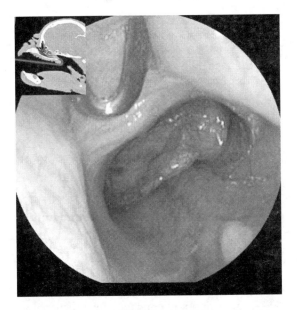

Figure 1. Post-rhinoscopic view of aberrant endochoanal conchae in a Pug obstructing the meatus nasopharyngeus

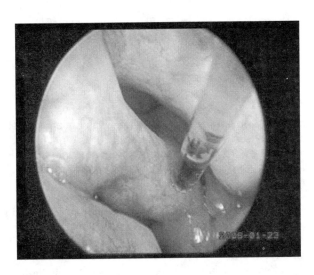

Figure 2. Beginning of LATE surgery: Endoscopic view of the diode laser fiber.

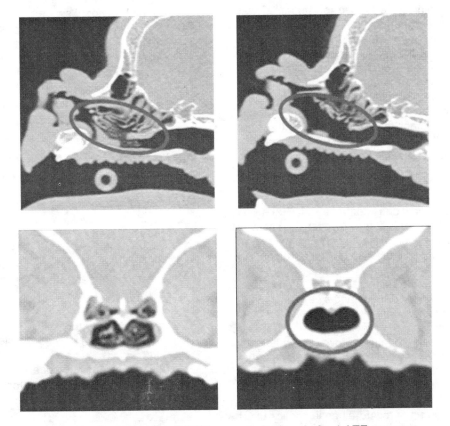

Figure 3. Sagittal and axial CT scans before and after LATE-surgery.

BRACHYCEPHALIC AIRWAY SYNDROME, PART 3: SUCCESSFUL ANESTHESIA AND RECOVERY

Gerhard U. Oechtering, Prof.Dr.med.vet., Dipl. ECVAA
Michaele Alef, Dr.med.vet., Dipl. ECVAA
Claudia Noeller, Dr.med.vet.
Department of Small Animal Medicine
University of Leipzig, Germany

In human anesthesia, "difficult airways" are a common problem for anesthetists and intubation is often challenging. In small animal medicine, problematic upper airways are a rare condition and in general, intubation is easy to perform – with one major exception: brachycephalic breeds.

Partial to subtotal obstruction of the upper airways is common in all these animals, although in varying intensity. The majority of these obstructions are clearly visible and easy to detect (Table 1), while others remain hidden and are unlikely detected during examination with the naked eye (Table 2). To aggravate the situation, a number of animals are very susceptible to any form of stress. Even minor necessary manipulations during preanesthetic evaluation, induction, or recovery can lead to critical situations.

PREANESTHETIC EVALUATION

To judge the clinical relevance of upper airway obstruction, even a thorough clinical evaluation might not provide a true picture of the situation. Specific questions aiming at symptoms in the context of the brachycephalic airway syndrome may be of additional value (Table 3).

Auscultation of heart and lungs may be difficult due to stridulous breathing. Some animals react even on the stress of the examination with respiratory signs. In these cases, we should restrict the examination to the bare essentials. If there is a known history of syncope, a thorough cardiologic examination is advisable to distinguish respiratory from cardiovascular causes.

PREMEDICATION

A sedative premedication is controversial. Too much sedation can lead to a reduction of respiratory reactivity towards hypoxia and hypercapnia and also can cause an increased collapsibility of the nasopharyngeal region. An intravenous catheter is mandatory but can also present a challenge of its own with an increasingly excited animal with worsening respiratory distress and a very tough skin covering small peripheral veins.

While restraining these animals, it is an absolute must to avoid all pressure or tension towards the neck or throat as well as any flexion of the neck that could compromise oral, nasopharyngeal, or laryngeal airways.

INDUCTION

Generally speaking, we regard all anaesthetics used in modern small animal medicine as suitable. Safety in brachycephalic anaesthesia in our opinion is not primarily a question of selecting the "right" drug but depends on experience of the anesthetist with the particular drug and above all on the appropriate and correct handling of the brachycephalic animal in every stage of the procedure.

Table 1. Upper Airway Obstructions in Brachycephalic Breeds that are Easy to Detect

- Stenotic nares (cranial stenosis)
- Macroglossia
- Overlong soft palate
- Enlarged tonsils
- Everted lateral laryngeal ventricles (Laryngocele)
- Collapsed or dysplastic larynx

Table 2. Hidden Upper Airway Obstructions in Brachycephalic Breeds

- Stenotic nares (caudal part, at the transition from vestibulum to the cavum nasi)
- Hyperthrophic and dysplastic turbinates obstructing the main intranasal airways
- Caudal aberrant conchae – obstructing the choanae and the postnasal space
- Hypertrophy of the middle and rostral parts of the palatum – obstructing the nasopharyngeal space
- Hyperplastic and oedematous mucous membranes of the nasopharynx – resulting in marked collapsibility of the nasopharynx
- Tracheal obstructions: Hypotrachea or collapsed trachea
- Bronchial obstructions – Bronchial collapse

Table 3. Anamnesis in Brachycephalic Animals

- At what age did you observe the first respiratory symptoms?
- Describe the amount of exercise that is needed to provoke respiratory signs or signs of exhaustion.
- Describe the amount of excitement or stress that is needed to provoke respiratory signs.
- At which temperature range do symptoms begin to aggravate?
- Is there evidence of syncope - during exercise or even at rest?
- Is there snoring only during sleep or all day long?
- Is there evidence of sleep apnea?
- Describe the worst respiratory situation so far.

Improper positioning during induction or recovery can easily cause dramatic airway occlusion. For example, a "normal" sternal position in the unconscious unintubated animal with its head and chin on the table can kill the patient. In these dogs, even slightest external pressure against the base of the tongue or throat can occlude oral and nasopharyngeal airways completely.

INTUBATION

Intubation in brachycephalic animals is not without its problems. A procedure that is comparatively easy in normocephalic dogs can be challenging even for the experienced. The relatively large outer diameter of the head-neck transition stands in sharp contrast to the inner diameters of pharynx, larynx, and trachea. To make the situation worse, these narrow regions seem to be filled with redundant soft tissue originating from palatinal, pharyngeal, and laryngeal mucosa. In addition to that, the huge root of the tongue occupies vital space of the airways, predominantly in bulldogs. Table 4 lists some helpful points for intubation of brachycephalic dogs.

Table 4. Points for Successful Intubation in Brachycephalic Dogs
• Plane of anesthesia deep enough
• Fully straightened neck (trained assistant)
• Laryngoscope with long and curved blade (large base of tongue)
• Bright light source
• Suction device for saliva and mucus (gentle negative pressure to avoid damage to vocal folds)
• Tubes of different sizes, also those supposed to be too small – better a small one in place than failed with the proper one

VENTILATION

Especially in critical patients, it is advisable to ventilate the animal. This can be performed manually or with ventilators via the conventional endotracheal tube; the use of masks is not recommended. A very interesting alternative to conventional ventilatory techniques is the use of jet ventilation, either with automatic ventilators or a manual device (http://www.vbm-medical.de/cms/108-1-jet-ventilation.html). This enables the use of very small endotracheal catheters (10 F) both during intralaryngeal surgery and also during recovery. One has to keep in mind, that this technique provides no protection against aspiration and if laser surgery is used, particular attention has to be paid that oxygen concentration does nor exceed 40 Vol%.

MONITORING

Continuous monitoring of expired carbon dioxide (capnography) and oxygen saturation (pulse oximetry) are very useful tools for respiratory monitoring. In brachycephalic breeds, sudden episodes of bradycardia are not uncommon; therefore, continuous ECG monitoring is also advisable.

MAINTENANCE

Maintenance of anaesthesia does not differ appreciably from anesthetic techniques in normocephalic dogs.

RECOVERY (Table 5, Figure 1)

Table 5. Recovery from Anesthesia in Brachycephalic Dogs
• Extubate as late as possible.
• Use a maxillary sling (Figure 1) or spread jaws with simple bite block.
• Avoid any external pressure against the base of the tongue or throat.
• Be prepared for emergency re-intubation.

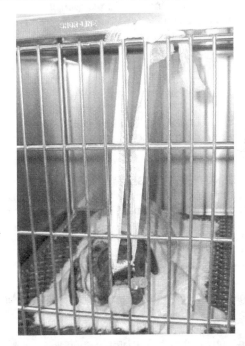

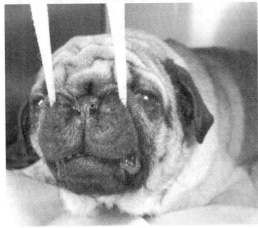

Figure 1. Maxillary sling during recovery.

RESPIRATORY DISEASE: WHAT IS THE SOURCE?

Elizabeth Rozanski, DVM
Diplomate ACVIM (SA) and ACVECC
Cummings School of Veterinary Medicine
Tufts University, North Grafton, MA

OVERVIEW

Evaluation of the pet with respiratory disease may be challenging. The best approach to problem solving usually reflects first an assessment for immediate intervention, and then careful evaluation to localize the problem, and then finally determination of the specific problem and the available options for controlling or curing it. Immediate intervention is warranted in any pet that is having difficulty breathing. Respiratory distress may be appreciated by observing loud or noisy breathing, labored breathing, discolored (pale pink, gray or bluish) mucous membranes or by difficulty laying down or on one's side (orthopnea). Respiratory distress may be a life-threatening emergency and should be treated promptly. The appropriate immediate therapy will reflect the underlying cause, and may include supplemental oxygen, thoracocentesis, or sedation and intubation.

LOCALIZING THE PROBLEM

All causes of true pulmonary problems may be traced to abnormalities in the upper airway, the lower airway, the pulmonary parenchyma or the pleural space. Occasionally, pets with either marked metabolic acidosis or pain may have tachypnea which may be misinterpreted as respiratory distress.

Most effective localization relies on pattern recognition, which is an appreciation of a conglomerate of historical and physical findings that are linked with a specific condition. Most successful clinicians incorporate pattern recognition as a method of problem solving in most day to day clinical challenges.

UPPER AIRWAY OBSTRUCTION

Causes of upper airway obstructions include brachycephalic airway syndrome (specifically elongated soft palate, laryngeal collapse and everted laryngeal saccules), laryngeal paralysis, pharyngeal foreign bodies, and neoplasia. Recently nasopharyngeal turbinate have also been described as a component of upper airway obstruction in brachycephalic airway syndrome. All upper airway obstructions are magnified in heat, humidity and with exertion. Clinically, upper airway obstruction may be suspected with loud or noisy breathing and longer inspiratory times.

Clinicians should be familiar with normal upper airway anatomy and function and be prepared to deal with any number of crises, including the ability to deal with challenging intubations and the potential for urgent tracheostomies.

Management of upper airway obstruction may include surgical or medical therapy. Surgical therapy includes soft palate resection, stenotic nares resection, arytenoids lateralization and in rare cases permanent tracheostomies. Medical therapy includes sedation, anti-inflammatory agents (steroids), harnesses and weight loss. Dogs that have laryngeal paralysis may have concurrent neuromuscular disease or esophageal motility disorders, including megaesophagus

Table 1. Common Characteristics of Upper Airway Disease

Condition	Signalment	Age	Co-Morbidity	Treatment
Brachycephalic airway syndrome	Brachycephalic breeds of dog and less often, cat	Middle age and older	Obesity, cardiac disease	Surgical Sedation Weight loss
Laryngeal paralysis (bilateral)	Retrievers Setters Large breed dogs	Older	Neuromuscular disease Arthritis	Palliative surgery (lateralization) Sedation Harness
Laryngeal collapse	End-stage tracheal collapse, brachycephalic breeds, some lar par dogs	Older dogs	End-stage tracheal collapse, brachycephalic	Permanent trach Lateralization? Sedation
Pharyngeal foreign bodies	Any	Young,	None; acute onset	Remove; tracheostomy?
Laryngeal neoplasia	Older cats > dogs	Older	Varies, slowly progressive	Biopsy, resect, chemotherapy, radiation, palliative

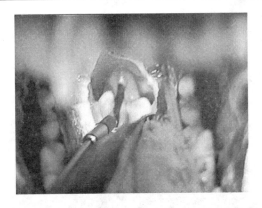

Figure 1. Laryngoscopic view of the larynx in dog with laryngeal paralysis.

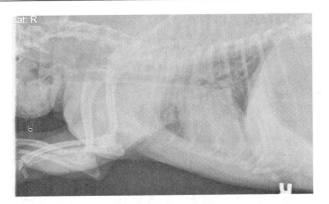

Figure 2. An intraluminal tracheal stent, which was placed to provide support for collapsing trachea. This bichon also has chronic bronchitis and obesity.

LOWER AIRWAY DISEASE

Lower airway disease is common in cats and smaller breed dogs (particularly Cocker spaniels). Intra-thoracic tracheal collapse can be a specific form of lower airway disease, while cervical collapse will result in signs of upper airway collapse. Signs of lower airway disease include cough, wheeze and occasionally shortness of breath. Some affected dog have a marked expiratory push, similar to heavey horses. Lower airway disease may be either acute, such as infectious tracheobronchitis or chronic. Chronic bronchitis is defined as cough most days of the previous 2 months without other underlying cause. Thoracic radiographs from dogs with chronic bronchitis may be relatively normal or may reveal a heavy broncho-interstitial pattern and/or evidence of bronchiectasis. Bronchoscopy is considered the gold standard to evaluate airways. Appropriate therapy involves addressing inflammation, attempting to limit airway remodeling and controlling cough. This might include glucocorticoids, antibiotics (for secondary infections), bronchodilators, and cough suppressants.

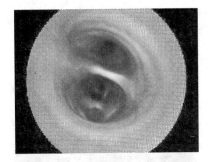

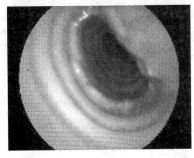

Figure 3. Bronchoscopic image from a Chih X with severe cough. The lower airways were normal, but a stricture was identified in the cervical trachea (shown in the lower image)

Table 2. Common Characteristics of Lower Airway Diseases

. Condition	Breed	Age	Co-Morbidity	Treatment
Chronic bronchitis	Any, cockers	Older	Obesity Mitral regurgitation	Weight loss, cough suppression, glucocorticoids, bronchodilators
Feline lower airway disease	Any, Siamese?	Young to middle aged	Exclude Heartworm	Glucocorticoids, Bronchodilators Aerosol therapy?
Eosinophilic bronchitis	Any	Younger	Heartworm infection, may have parenchymal infiltrate as well	Glucocortucoids, de-worm
Intra-thoracic tracheal collapse	Yorkie, Poms, Poodles	Middle age to older	Obesity, chronic bronchitis	Weight loss, anti-inflammatories, cough suppressants, stent (palliative)

PULMONARY PARENCHYMAL DISEASE

Parenchymal pulmonary disease will cause respiratory distress on both inspiration and expiration. Patients will commonly seem very distressed. Thoracic radiographs will document interstitial to alveolar infiltrates. Common sources of parenchymal disease include pulmonary edema (cardiogenic and non-cargiogenic), pneumonia, pulmonary contusion, pulmonary fibrosis and neoplasia. Treatment is directed at the underlying cause. In some cases, multiple sources may co-exist.

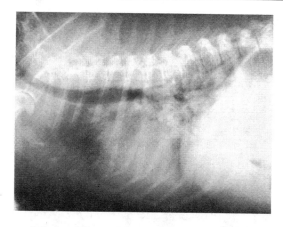

Figure 4. Lateral thoracic radiograph from a Westie with pulmonary fibrosis.

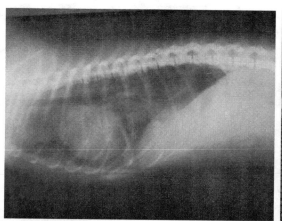 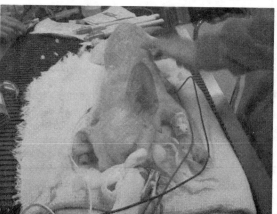

Figure 5. Lateral thoracic radiograph and the actual Chihuahua, after severe thoracic trauma.

Table 3. Common Characteristics of Parenchymal Lung Disease

. Condition	Breed	Age	Co-Morbidity	Treatment
Cardiogenic pulmonary edema	Small Doberman, Boxer Male cats	Middle aged to older	Urinary disease in cats?	Diuretics ACE-inhibitors Beta-blockers
Non-cardiogenic pulmonary edema	Any	Young > Older	Seizures, airway obstruction	Rest
Pneumonia	Any Cats RARE	Older	ALWAYS	Antibiotics (community versus hospital-acquired)
Neoplasia	Any	Older	Primary tumor	Palliative, chemotherapy, surgery
Fibrosis	Westies, terriers	Older	None	Unknown
Trauma	Any	Young >older	Possible	Supportive

PLEURAL SPACE DISEASE

Pleural space disease is characterized by a short and shallow ventilatory pattern, often with increase abdomen effort. Auscultation may document a quiet thoracic cavity with louder sounds dorsally. Small volume pleural effusions may be helpful as diagnostic aids, but less so therapeutically. Treatment of pleural effusion is directed at removal of the effusion and specific therapy directed at the underlying cause.

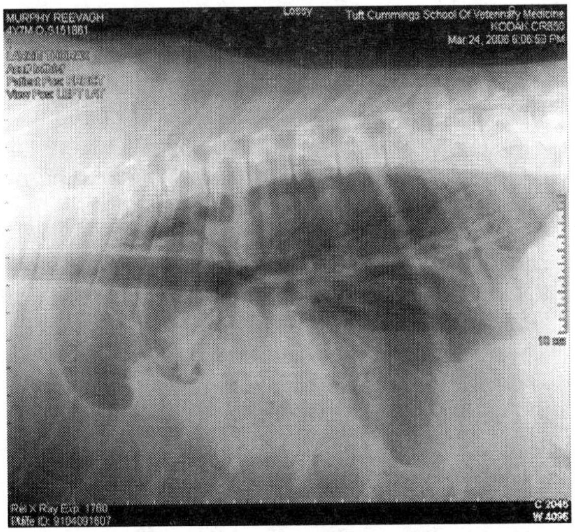

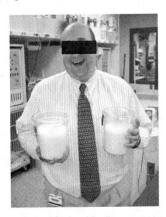

Figure 7. This clinician has just removed almost 3 liters of a chylous effusion from a Labrador

Figure 6. This Irish wolfhound had pleural effusion due to a lung lobe torsion.

Table 4. Common Characteristics of Pleural Effusion

Condition	Breed	Age	Co-Morbidity	Treatment
Heart failure	Small breed, chronic valvular disease, cats	Older	Left heart failure	Thoracocentesis, increased diuretics
Pericardial effusion	Retrievers/shep	Older	Splenic disease	Pericardiocentesis
Neoplasia	Any	Older	Primary tumor	Intra-cavitary chemotherapy, other palliative
Pyothorax	Any, hunting breeds, cats	Young	Sepsis	Surgery Chest tubes Antibiotics
Pneumothorax	Trauma-Any Spontaneous-Northern breeds	Trauma-young Spontaneous-any	Trauma- any Spontaneous-uncommon	Trauma- medical Spontaneous-Surgical
Chylothorax	Afghan Hounds, cats	Middle to older	Lung lobe torsion in some	Resection of affected lobe, thoracic duct ligation, pericardiectomy

References are available from the author upon request.

ACUTE AND CHRONIC DISEASE OF THE PLEURAL SPACE

Elizabeth Rozanski, DVM
Diplomate ACVIM (SA) and AVECC
Cummings School of Veterinary Medicine
Tufts University, North Grafton, MA

Identification of pleural space disease in a patient represents a major diagnostic and therapeutic target for the clinician. Pleural space disease may consist of an effusion, pneumothorax, or a space-occupying mass (eg, contents of a diaphragmatic hernia). Pleural effusion develops when there is an altered balance between the normal production and drainage of pleural effusion. In the normal individual, a few milliliters of pleural effusion coat the visceral and parietal pleura, and serve to lubricate the serosal surface and permit normal respiration. Pneumothorax describes the presence of air within the pleural cavity, and may be traumatic, spontaneous or iatrogenic in origin.

Pleural effusion may be suspected based upon physical examination, and confirmed via thoracic radiographs or ultrasonography. Computed tomography is also a useful method of identifying pleural effusion, but rarely the first diagnostic step. Thoracocentesis is useful for both as a diagnostic and therapeutic procedure. In some cases, thoracocentesis may be performed prior to documentation of pleural effusion by diagnostic imaging, particularly in cases of severe distress. In many cases, if ultrasonography is not readily available, a single dorsoventral (DV) radiograph, even improperly positioned, can highlight the presence or absence of effusion. Properly positioned thoracic radiographs may be performed following removal of effusion.

TIPS FOR SUCCESSFUL THORACOCENTESIS

- Determine if you anticipate a diagnostic or therapeutic centesis. In almost all cases, as much effusion as possible should be removed, which is often in contrast to abdominocentesis.
- In a young dog with pleural effusion, evaluate the clotting time PRIOR to tapping the chest. Anticoagulant rodenticide toxicity is a common cause of pleural effusion (usually with a widen mediastinum as well) and thoracocentesis should be either entirely avoided in this situation or postponed until after correction of the coagulopathy.
- Anticipate, based upon imaging results, the volume of effusion that is present. An average sized cat may have 200 to 300 mL of effusion (30–50 mL/kg) while a retriever-sized dog may easily have 2 to 3 liters of effusion. This step is important, as removing 50 mL from a Labrador may help your diagnostic efforts, it would not be expected to therapeutic. In addition, if you remove a greater volume that anticipated, that may suggest either ongoing leak (in cases of pneumothorax) or inadvertent drainage of the abdomen (in cases of bi- or tri-cavitary effusion).
- Prepare supplies and determine need for sedation, For dogs with large volume effusions, sedation with either butorphanol and diazepam or propofol [recall this a **potent** cardiovascular depressant] is often beneficial for patient comfort and for decreasing the time required. For example, removing 3 liters of effusion is about 5 to 10 times faster with a 16-gauge catheter than with a 22-gauge needle. For most cats, a butterfly catheter is adequate, but in very large cats a longer needle may required.
- Recall that for animals with chronic effusions, there is an increased risk of iatrogenic pneumothorax so taps with a catheter fed into the chest may be less traumatic than needles.
- Dogs and cats have fenestrated mediastinums, so the specific side that the effusion is removed from is less important than often given credit for.
- Save adequate volumes of the effusion for analysis and record the total volume removed.
- If desired, perform post-tap radiographs or other imaging.
- Monitor patient's recovery, in most cases marked improvement in respiratory rate and effort is evidence immediately. Thus if respiratory distress persists or worsens, it is concerning that either iatrogenic pneumothorax has developed, or that there is underlying parenchymal or airway disease. Following removal of a large volume of effusion, a dog may cough for the next 12 to 24 hours as previously atelectatic lung re-inflates.
- Don't delay performed centesis for pets that are short of breath; this is an urgent/emergent procedure.

DISEASE PROCESSES ASSOCIATED WITH PLEURAL EFFUSION; GUIDELINES FOR RECOGNITION AND MANAGEMENT

Pleural effusions typically develop because of increased hydrostatic pressure, decreased oncotic pressure, lymphatic leakage or increased vascular permeability. In some cases, a combination of two or more causes may co-exist. Often, evaluation of the patient's signalment, history and physical examination can directed the diagnostic efforts. Additionally, evaluation of the effusion itself, both grossly and microscopically may provide important clues as to the source of the effusion. The most common effusions are discussed below.

MODIFIED TRANSUDATES
Cardiac Disease

Right-sided cardiac disease and pericardial effusion are two common causes of pleural effusion in small animals.

Cardiac disease, specifically cardiomyopathy is a particularly common cause of effusion in cats. Other physical examination findings that are supportive of cardiomyopathy include a murmur and/or gallop and a low rectal temperature. Cats with pleural effusion associated with cardiomyopathy tend to be older, and the clinician should recall that a cat that has previously had effusion, a recurrence of shortness of breath is often (always?) associated with recurrent effusion. In dogs, pleural effusion is seen in end-stage valvular disease and cardiomyopathy. Occasionally, isolated right-sided defects may also result in effusion. Echocardiography is the diagnostic test of choice to evaluate cardiac structure and function. Analysis of brain natriuretic peptide (BNP) is emerging as a patient-side test for evaluation of atrial stretch. Fluid analysis is a modified transudate and/or occasionally chylous. Treatment of cardiac disease induced pleural effusion involves treatment for the underlying disease, draining as much effusion as possible, and increasing the furosemide dose and/or adding another diuretic such as spironolactone or spironolactone-hydrochlorothiazide.

Pericardial effusion is another common cause of pleural effusion. Physical examination findings consistent with pericardial effusion include muffled heart sounds, jugular venous distention, and pulsus paradoxus. Echocardiography is diagnostic. The pleural effusion is a modified transudate. Pericardiocentesis will result in rapid re-absorption of the pleural effusion (by removing the right-sided heart failure component). Treatment of pericardial effusion reflects the underlying cause of the pericardial disease and may include pericardiectomy.

Malignant Pleural Effusion

Malignant pleural effusion (MPE) is a another cause of a modified transudate. Neoplasia may be divided into lymphoma and non-lymphoma in regards to treatment options.

Lymphoma commonly results in MPE and an associated anterior (cranial) mediastinal mass. In cats, the cranial aspect of the chest is usually uncompressible and in dogs, hypercalcemia is common (most are T-cell lymphoma). Treatment of MPE associated with lymphoma involves standard chemotherapeutic protocols, and is usually associated with a good short-term outcome.

Non-lymphoma neoplasia may also result in pleural effusion. Thymoma is common in older dogs and cats. Metastatic neoplasia (carcinoma) is also possible, such as with primary lung tumors, mammary tumor or other carcinomas. Treatment of a suspected metastatic effusion usually shifts to palliative care, and may include periodic centesis, and/or infusion of local chemotherapy, such as carboplatin. In moderately effusive states, a reasonable quality of life main be maintained for many months. Recently, the concept of a pleural-port has been introduced and to date met with fair to good reviews.

EXUDATES
Chylothorax

Chylous effusion may also have properties of a modified transudate. Chylous effusion is rich in triglycerides and tends to look milky or pinkish ("strawberry milkshake'). Chylous effusion may be either primary [idiopathic] or secondary to a variety of conditions such as congestive heart failure, heartworm infestation, or an anterior mediastinal mass. Appropriate work-up involves evaluation for an underlying cause, and specific therapy if possible. If not possible, then therapy may be surgical (thoracic duct ligation, ± pericardiectomy and omentalization). Surgical therapy has a success rate of 50% to 70%, so it is essential that a "cure" is not promised. Long-standing effusion may result in restrictive pleuritis, with on-going respiratory difficulties.

Pyothorax

Pyothorax represents a collection of infected material within the thorax. Most cases are thought to be due to penetrating wounds (including bite wounds) or foreign bodies. In dogs, pyothorax is considered a surgical disease, while in cats, medical management is often adequate. Infection is common anaerobic, and broad-spectrum antibiotics are warranted. For animals treated medically, pleural lavage is occasionally employed, using 10 to 30 mL/kg of warm heparinized (10 IU/mL) saline infused and withdrawn every 4 to 8 hours.

Hemothorax

Hemothorax is most commonly associated with trauma or anticoagulant rodenticide intoxication; however in these cases thoracocentesis may not be performed. In cases where hemothorax is detected, the most common cause by far is neoplasia (eg, rib tumor), although other causes such as lung lobe torsion or pancreatitis may also be responsible.

PNEUMOTHORAX

Pneumothorax may be classified as traumatic, spontaneous, or iatrogenic. **Traumatic** pneumothorax is the most common and usually easily recognized due to other signs of trauma. Some animals have concurrent pulmonary contusions, or other thoracic trauma. Animals presenting emergently with respiratory distress following trauma should under urgent thoracocentesis. Auscultation may document decreased lung sounds, but this may be masked by correspondingly louder sounds from pulmonary contusion. For animals with a known history of injury, needle thoracocentesis may be performed as guided clinically. Due to the high density of tissue thromboplastin, the previously healthy injured lung will heal rapidly, thus chest tubes are not commonly required in the trauma patient. A good guideline is that three or more thoracocenteses ("three strike rule") within 24 hours is sufficient justification for placement of the chest tube in the traumatic pneumothorax. It is exceedingly rare to have a patient with trauma require a thoracotomy for resection of the traumatized lung.

Spontaneous pneumothorax is defined as pneumothorax that develops without evidence of trauma. Historically, dogs will present with signs of either shortness of breath or difficulty "settling down." Northern breeds are predisposed. Causes include bulla and blebs, as well as neoplasia or foreign bodies (quills). Cats with lower airway disease may also develop spontaneous pneumothorax, as may patients with heartworm disease. Primary spontaneous pneurnothorax associated with bulla or bleb is considered a surgical disease, even if the air leak spontaneously stops, it is still likely to recur without surgical resection.

Iatrogenic pneumothorax is a pneumothorax created by the veterinary professional. These are most commonly associated with thoracocentesis in a patient with abnormal pleura. The normal pleura will heal rapidly if inadvertently punctured; however, if the diseased pleura is punctured, the normal rapid sealing will not occur. This is a big risk in particular with chylous effusions, or any exuduative process.

OTHER PLEURAL SPACE CONDITIONS

Other conditions may affect the pleural space, these include most commonly diaphragmatic hernia, thoracic bite wounds and a variety of neoplasia. **Diaphragmatic hernias** (DH) are usually traumatic in origin, although congenital disease has been described. DH should be surgically repaired as soon as the patient is stable. Older literature initially suggested that a delay of 24 hours was associated with a better outcome, but later studies have suggested that early repair is preferable. Chronic DH is associated with a high peri and post-operative complication rate, including the development of re-expansion pulmonary edema (Non-cardiogenic/high protein) and/or pneumothorax.

Thoracic bite wounds commonly penetrate the chest, even if the puncture site seems small. Thus, all thoracic wounds should be cleaned and completely explored, and the surgeon prepared to enter the chest as needed for further repair. Broad-spectrum antibiotics are warranted. **Chest wall and rib neoplasia** may also present with signs of pleural effusion. Advanced imaging is often required to highlight the lesion and to determine if a surgical option exists. CT scanning is evolving as an invaluable tool in surgical and oncological planning.

References are available from the author upon request.

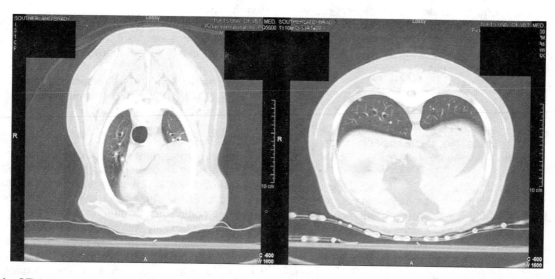

Figure 1. CT images of an 18-month-old Labrador, who presented for evaluation of shortness of breath and a palpable mass. The biopsy of the mass confirmed osteosarcoma, and the CT highlighted not only the mass, but also evidence of metastasis (seen at the periphery of the lung in the right hand image at the top left lung), which altered the treatment plan.

RESPIRATORY INFECTION IN PEDIATRICS PATIENTS

Elizabeth Rozanski, DVM
Diplomate ACVIM (SA) and ACVECC
Cummings School of Veterinary Medicine
Tufts University, North Grafton, MA

Infectious diseases of the respiratory system are common in small animals, particularly the pediatric patient. The most commonly observed infectious diseases include feline upper respiratory tract infections, tracheobronchitis, and pneumonia. It is important to be vigilant, as occasional other conditions may mimic pulmonary infection, including diaphragmatic hernia, congestive heart failure and pyothorax. Most treatment is supportive.

CANINE INFECTIOUS TRACHEOBRONCHITIS/ PNEUMONIA

Infectious tracheobronchitis ("kennel cough," ITB) is a term that may be applied to the clinical syndrome caused by a variety of bacteria and viruses. Commonly implicated organisms include Bordetella bronchiseptica, parainfluenza, and Mycoplasma. Recently, canine influenza has emerged as a new infection and been implicated in some canine respiratory disease. Other bacteria such as E. coli, Klebsiella, and Pseudomonas may also colonize airways after an initial insult with a viral disease. Occasionally, it may be difficult to distinguish kennel cough complex from canine distemper virus. Pet store puppies are at increased risk, and in fact in our hospital, due to the lack of available puppies at shelters, the increase in pet store purchases has made ITB far more common than parvovirus. In Massachusetts, many puppies are sold with a "little cough" which may progress in to severe pneumonia. ITB in adult dogs, with the exception of the emerging canine influenza, tends to be mild and more commonly an irritating cough rather than critical illness.

Specific breeds of puppies, including bulldogs and toy breeds (eg, Yorkies) appear to be at an increased risk of infection and even death.

Clinical signs include a cough, lethargy, and difficulty breathing. Physical examination is occasionally unremarkable, although many puppies have mild fevers (103°F range) and seem depressed. Some puppies will have other congenital defects such as hernias, undescended testicles or congenital heart disease. Usually, tracheal palpation will trigger a paroxysm of coughing. Routine laboratory testing is usually normal for a pediatric patient although an inflammatory leukogram may be present and characteristic serum chemistry profile results of puppies are observed. Puppies, particularly toy breeds, may be hypoglycemic if they have been anorexic and often appear to be outwardly ill.

Initial Therapy

Initial therapy should be focused on determining in the puppy should be discharged home or hospitalized. These decisions will reflect the degree of illness of the puppy, as well as practical constraints, such as a hospital staffing, isolation facilities, and owner finances. Owner should be advised as to the unpredictable nature of pet stores in helping either finance hospitalization or return the puppy's purchase price. Most clients grow very fond of individual puppies very rapidly, and are often reluctant to return them to suboptimal environments. However, the hospitalization costs for such puppies can be significant, particularly if oxygen or intensive nursing care is required. The primary therapy focuses on supportive care, including fluids (subcutaneously or intravenously), antibiotics, and monitoring appetite and blood glucose levels. Nebulization and gentle coupage may be very helpful in clearing infection. Antibiotic choices are usually empiric, even if a tracheal wash is performed, it is several days until bacterial culture and sensitivity data are available. Antimicrobials with good activity against Bordetella include aminoglycosides, fluoroquinolones, chloramphenicol, trimethoprim-sulfa and tetracyclines. Systemically ill puppies should receive parenteral antibiotics. Puppies with cough alone may be treated effectively with aerosolized gentamicin.

Diagnostic Imaging

Thoracic radiographs are a good practice in clinically puppies. While the extent of the infiltrates may lag behind clinical signs (as well as the later resolution), radiographs are helpful to assess the extent and distribution of the pneumonia, and to exclude other more rare causes of distress.

Laboratory Investigation

Monitoring and supplementing glucose is advisable. A complete blood count and chemistry profile, as mentioned above, are useful but not necessarily diagnostic. A tracheal wash should be performed at the discretion of the attending clinician. The advantages of knowing the sensitivity pattern of the infection are obvious; however, the risk to a small or compromised patient is real. In recent years, polymerase chain reaction (PCR) testing for a variety of disease have become available; these may be warranted in larger outbreaks in specific kennels or in particularly valuable puppies. In addition, if infection with distemper virus is considered a possibility, PCR may be used to support or refute that diagnosis. Serology for canine influenza is also available; this appears to be a regionally important disease.

Future Directions

As the pet store industry continues to flourish, it is likely very important to continue to develop and support guidelines for safe and healthy puppies and to help limit the shipping and distribution of unwell puppies. Prevention should include quarantine of puppies at risk, and careful tracking of shipping of unwell puppies. Within a hospital, coughing young dogs should be consider contagious and isolated as much as possible from other dogs. However, critically ill puppies should not be discharged home, nor should they be treated completely out of sight of clinic personnel. Vaccination against *Bordetella* should be performed in dogs at risk of exposure.

MISCELLANEOUS CONDITIONS IN PUPPIES

As pediatric pulmonary infections are common, it is crucial to avoid tunnel vision when treating patients with respiratory complaints. Perhaps up to 5% of puppies and kittens suspected of having isolated respiratory infection may have other disease. Other conditions may co-exist with infection or may masquerade as pulmonary infection. Specific areas to completely evaluate include cardiac structure and function, evidence of pleural space disease (pyothorax, diaphragmatic hernia) or esophageal dysfunction. If a patient is not recovering quickly or if the scenario seems odd, it is worth future investigation.

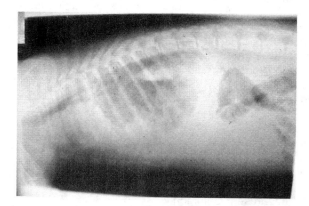

Figure 1. Lateral thoracic radiograph from a Golden retriever puppy that had apparent failure to respond to antibiotics for presumptive pneumonia. Repair of the diaphragmatic hernia was uneventful.

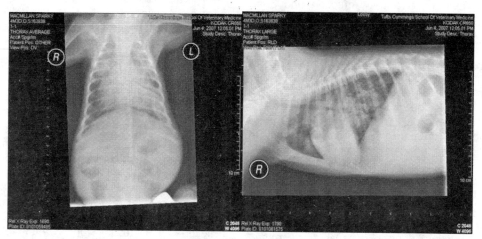

Figure 2. Lateral and dorsoventral (DV) thoracic radiographs from a 4-month-old Springer puppy. *Bordetella bronchiseptica* was cultured from a tracheal wash, and the puppy hospitalized for 4 days.

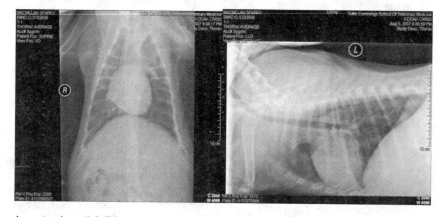

Figure 3. Lateral and ventrodorsal (VD) radiograph from the same puppy as shown in Figure 2. The puppy's coughing had relapsed, and *B. bronchiseptica* was again cultured from a tracheal wash sample.

KITTENS

Respiratory infections are very common as well in kittens. In contrast to the puppy situation, there are plenty of kittens born every where in the US. Thus, most kittens are obtained from shelters, neighbors, or found as strays.

Most respiratory infections in kittens are initially viral in origin. Herpes (rhinotracheitis) and calicivirus are the most common. Kittens with herpes usually have ocular lesions as well. A particularly virulent calici virus strain was described several years ago, but thankfully appears to be rare. Treatment of viral disease is primarily supportive. Lysine is popular for chronic ocular changes but not helpful acutely. Some clinicians have used acyclovir or interferon, but reports of success are limited. Kittens with viral respiratory infections may have marked fevers (104–106°F; 40–41.1°C) and may be dehydrated and potentially hypoglycemic. Secondary bacterial infection is common and may be associated with a variety in infecting organisms. Kittens will develop a mucopurulent nasal discharge, and progressive lethargy and anorexia. Anorexia is often worsened by oral ulcers and lack of the sense of smell. Kittens with signs of systemic illness should be hospitalized in isolation or treated aggressively as outpatients. Fluids and parenteral antibiotics are very useful, and should be used until the kitten is eating and drinking adequately. In cases of severe ocular damage, enucleation may be warranted if the eyes have ruptured. This may be postponed until the kitten is an adequate anesthetic risk, although the clinician is reminded that eye injuries may be very painful. Enucleations should be performed rapidly to prevent hypothermia, and atropine should be available or given due to vagal nerve stimulation and resultant bradycardia.

Kittens that were found as strays with cough should be considered at risk of lung worm in part of the world where it is endemic. The snails that serve as the intermediate host at easily caught and consumed by feral kittens. Larvae may be seen in a Baermann fecal sedimentation or in a tracheal wash specimen.

Table 1. Antibiotics and Dewormers Commonly Used in Pediatric Pulmonary Infections

Drug name	Route	Dose	Indications	Comments
Fenbendazole	Orally	50 mg/kg daily	Lung worms	Cats > dogs
Amakacin	IV	15 mg/kg q 24 hours	Severe bacterial infection	Potentially nephrotoxic
Clavamox®	Orally	12.5–25 mg/kg q 12 hours	Bacterial infection	
Chloramphenicol	Orally	10–15 mg/kg q 12 hours	Bacterial infections	Human- aplastic anemia
Doxycycline	Orally IV	5–10 mg/kg q 12–24 hr	Mycoplasma Bacterial infections	Gi upset possible
Enrofloxacin	Orally Slow IV (off-label) IM	10–20 mg/kg q 24 hr (Dog) 2.5–5 mg/kg q 24 (Cat)	Bacterial infection	Not for anaerobes or Strep Blindness in cats
Trimethoprim-sulfa	Orally	15 mg/kg q 12 hours	Bacterial infection	Rare immune effects
Zitromax (Azithromycin)	Orally	5–10 mg/kg q 24 hours	Bacterial infection Atypical organisms	Pricey

REFERENCES

1. Crawford PC, et al. Transmission of equine influenza virus to dogs. Science. 2005; 21;310(5747):482-5.
2. Radhakrishnan A, et al. Community-acquired infectious pneumonia in puppies: 65 cases (1993-2002). J Am Vet Med Assoc. 2007; 230(10):1493-7.
3. Ellis J, et al. Comparative efficacy of an injectable vaccine and an intranasal vaccine in stimulating Bordetella bronchiseptica-reactive antibody responses in seropositive dogs. J Am Vet Med Assoc. 2002;220(1):43-8.
4. Gaskell R, et al. Feline herpesvirus. Vet Res. 2007;38(2):337-54.
5. Helps CR, et al. Factors associated with upper respiratory tract disease caused by feline herpesvirus, feline calicivirus, Chlamydophila felis and Bordetella bronchiseptica in cats: experience from 218 European catteries. Vet Rec. 2005 May 21;156(21):669-73.
6. Hurley KE et al. An outbreak of virulent systemic feline calicivirus disease. J Am Vet Med Assoc. 2004;224(2):241-9.

EMERGENCY MANAGEMENT OF AIRWAY OBSTRUCTION

Elizabeth Rozanski, DVM
Diplomate ACVIM (SA) and ACVECC
Cummings School of Veterinary Medicine
Tufts University, North Grafton, MA

Airway obstruction is a true emergency. Successful resolution requires a rapid combination of pattern recognition, excellent judgment and technical acuity. Airway obstruction may be divided into several categories, including laryngeal paralysis, brachycephalic airway syndrome (BCAS), allergic reactions, neoplasia, and foreign objects both in and around the airway (eg, sticks/abscesses). In the first three categories in particular, the obstruction will be magnified by tissue edema created by high flow rates as the patient tries to breath around the obstruction. In addition, hyperthermia is common as effects to cool by panting are thwarted, and increased muscle activity is associated with aggressive respiratory efforts.

PATTERN RECOGNITION

Airway obstruction caused by anatomic abnormalities is most common on hot and humid days, or following some sort of exertion. Most anatomic airway obstruction dogs have historical or physical examination evidence of pre-existing disease. Dogs with laryngeal paralysis are usually older large breed dogs, with a preponderance of Labrador retrievers. Most dogs have been "noisy" breathers for awhile (months to years), with a relatively sudden onset of severe distress. In contrast, brachycephalics are immediately recognizable by their physical appearance. Overweight Bulldogs and Pugs seem over-represented in specific crisis, although any brachycephalic breed may be affected. Brachycephalics are also seemingly commonly affected when hospitalized for other conditions, such as corneal ulcers or knee disease. Knowledge of this is vital to the practitioner, because while some dogs (eg, Beagles) may bark and whine for hours seemingly without consequence, the anxious whiny Bulldog is a potential disaster waiting to happen. Dogs with allergic reactions typically are apparent on physical examination, and intra-airway foreign bodies typically are rapidly appreciated. Upper airway obstruction can either be life-threatening or rapidly progress to such.

EXCELLENT JUDGMENT

As clinicians, we all strive for excellence in judgment. The decision making in upper airway obstruction involves answering the following questions:

- Should I give sedation? Should I give steroids?
- Do I need to intubate?
- What is likely to happen if I do that?
- Do I need to do a tracheostomy?
- Where are "we" going long term?

Mild sedation is warranted for many dogs with upper airway obstruction, particularly those with chronic and dynamic conditions. As the respiratory inspiratory flow rates increase, mobile soft tissues are "sucked" into the lumen of the airway, resulting in increased obstruction to flow as well as edema of the tissues themselves. Laryngeal saccules will evert, and as well decrease the laryngeal diameter, which will increase the airway resistance. Acepromazine in low doses ± butorphanol is often very helpful to limit the dynamic component. Dogs that are hyperthermic should also be actively cooled with room temperature intravenous (IV) fluids and wet down with tepid water. A single dose of rapidly acting glucocorticoids is often warranted due to extreme tissue edema. Hyperthermia in dogs serves as a strong incentive to pant, and this will further increase airway edema. For dogs that have severe obstruction (evidenced by cyanosis, or extreme distress), sedation alone is not enough and the pet should be anesthetized and rapidly intubated. DO NOT WATCH A DOG WITH MARKED DISTRESS WAITING FOR IT TO GET BETTER.

Intubation is often life-saving. Most clinicians and technician are proficient at intubating dogs and cats with normal anatomy. The challenges that accompany airway obstruction reflect the underlying disease. Pets with laryngeal collapse or paralysis are easy to intubate, as their obstruction is far more dynamic. If the pet is only moderately distressed, it is reasonable to take a few seconds to evaluate function (abduction/collapse) but if there is severe distress this may be postponed until a future date. Brachycephalics are often challenging to intubate under the best of circumstances. Useful aids include a long laryngoscope blade, and multiple tube sizes. Clinicians should consider learning to intubate blindly using digital palpation only, to use a bronchoscope which is primarily advanced into the trachea and then the tube is advanced past that, or intubating first with a long polypropylene catheter and then advancing the tube over that. If you are unable to intubate within ~ 20 to 30 seconds, an urgent tracheostomy should be performed, although if you are prepared this is relatively unlikely. As a side note, you should not plan to do an oral examination on a pet with a potential upper airway obstruction without having all the supplies needed handy. This is because sedation for examination may result in the collapse of the residual airway lumen.

Following intubation, the next step is to support the pet and to decide what to do next. The next step with reflect the disease process. It is important to decide between leaving the pet sedated and intubated versus performing a tracheostomy. The step chosen typically reflects the underlying disease. The following are my biases from the Northeast part of the US, clinicians in other parts of the world may have other choices.

LARYNGEAL PARALYSIS

Most laryngeal paralysis dogs are older retrievers. In most, sedation and cooling are adequate. The owners should be advised regarding palliative surgical options, with the understanding of the risk to benefit ratio, and particularly of the real potential for aspiration pneumonia. If the dog is intubated, following sedation and cooling, extubation should be attempted. If not possible, and surgical palliation is not immediately available, a tracheostomy should be performed. My rationale for this is that these dogs are at an already increased risk of aspiration and leaving them intubated will greatly increase the risk of this. Additionally, these tend to be older and occasionally decrepit dogs, and arthritis and other consequences of prolonged immobility are rapidly apparent. Consideration should be given to performing a tracheal wash for evaluation of airway cytology and bacterial culture.

BRACHYCEPHALIC AIRWAY SYNDROME

While BAS is multi-factorial, most often elongated soft palate and subsequent eversion of the laryngeal saccules are responsible for the crisis situation. Intubation even for a day or longer until either the swelling can be reduced or palliative surgery may be performed is a reasonable option. Bulldog tracheostomies are not to be taken lightly. They have small trachea overall and thick necks, these features combined with a tracheostomy may prove fatal. Ultimately, it important to evaluate the larynx for concurrent laryngeal collapse. As a preemptive strike, it is wise to evaluate and surgical palliate the upper airway of brachycephalics prior to a crisis developing.

ALLERGIC REACTIONS

Most allergic reactions cause hives (uticaria) and little more. True anaphylactic reactions appear to be exceeding rare in dogs and cats. A number of dogs develop facial swelling and edema, with occasionally airway obstruction following the chewing on sticks or other objects. Treatment should involve glucocorticoids, antihistamines, and rest. If airway occlusion is present, a tracheostomy is advised.

FOREIGN OBJECT

Most foreign object airway obstructions are only partial, as complete obstructions would also certainly result in the patient's death prior to arrival. Methods of removing obstruction include a modified Heimlich maneuver, hemostats or long towel clamps, or bronchoscopy. A temporary tracheostomy may be advised if the object is not rapidly removed. Dogs with severe qullings (porcupine) may be very challenging to treat, as, when the porcupine is attacked, quills often fill the larynx making intubation contra-indicated.

NEOPLASIA

Suspected neoplasia airway obstruction is less common, but may develop over weeks to months. Thyroid and laryngeal neoplasia are particularly common. The clinician should recall that the thyroid is a very vascular structure, and hemorrhage may occur after aspiration of a neck mass, potentially resulting in airway obstruction. If a laryngeal mass is identified and biopsied, it is uncommon to not require a temp tracheostomy as post-procedural swelling often reduces the lumen of the airway even further.

CATS

Upper airway obstruction is less common in cats than in dogs. In young cats (particularly purebred cats), nasopharyngeal polyps may develop and result in airway obstruction. In older cats, neoplasia is relatively common. In cats in particular have a predisposition to laryngospasm, and placement of a tracheosomy tube should be considered prior to the recovery from anesthesia. It is not a good plan to "see how they do," as asphyxiation is likely.

TECHNICAL ACUITY

As with all procedures, experience breeds comfort. Clinicians and technicians should evaluate multiple airways and prepare for emergencies. Digital and sylet guided intubation should be attempted in "non-crisis" settings, so that they are not impossible in the crisis setting. Tracheostomies should be practiced on cadavers if possible. Equipment for the difficulty airway should be carefully maintained, and kept in a convenient location.

References are available from the author upon request.

EFFECTIVE OXYGEN SUPPORT

Elizabeth Rozanski, DVM,
Diplomate ACVIM (SA) and ACVECC
Cummings School of Veterinary Medicine
Tufts University, North Grafton, MA

OVERVIEW

Supplemental oxygen is beneficial in a variety of situations, including hypoxemia, head trauma, and critical illness. There are multiple methods of providing supplemental oxygen, with various advantages and disadvantages. It is prudent for the clinician to be prepared to provide supplemental oxygen via several routes and to be able to recognize the pros and cons of the different methods. Options for providing supplemental oxygen include facemask or flow by, oxygen hood, nasal oxygen, transtracheal or nasolaryngeal oxygen, oxygen cage and mechanical ventilation. Patient factors to consider include: species, nasofacial confirmation (eg, brachycephalic), degree of compromise, breathing pattern, complexity of patient care treatment, and other possible causes of respiratory distress. Oxygen is most often available in tanks, although in larger facilities there may be a central source of oxygen. Oxygen tanks come in a number of sizes, but most commonly the smaller E tank, which contains about 660 liters of oxygen and the larger tanks (H), which contain 6900 liters. Busy practices should ensure that they have enough oxygen in stock to get through a busy weekend. Practices with a central supply should be sure to have in-house several back-up canisters in case of oxygen system malfunction. An oxygen tank, which requires a large amount of oxygen to fill and maintain a cage, may go through an H tank every 24 hours. For oxygen administered by other routes, most often, oxygen flow rates are set at about 50 to 100 mL/min, thus for a 30 kg (66 pound) Labrador, this translates to 3000 to 4000 Liters/day. When oxygen is going to be administered for more than a few minutes, humidification is warranted to prevent the drying effects of forced air.

The percentage inspired oxygen contact obtained is dependant upon both flow rate and the respiratory rate and strategy of the patient. For example, oxygen sources typically are set at 50 to 100 mL/min, while inspiratory flow rate are often in the order several hundred mL/SECOND. Thus, if you provide the above 30-kg dog with 2.5 liters/minute of supplemental oxygen, you are providing him with ~40 mL/minute of 100% oxygen. If his inspiratory flow rate is an average of 300 mL/second, you are providing 40 mL (100% oxygen) and 260 mL (21% oxygen) for a sum total of any FiO_2 of 32%. [40 mL of 100% oxygen, plus 55 mL (0.21 x 260 mL) = 95 mL of 100% oxygen within 300 mL/sec = 32% oxygen]

Conversely, if the patient is panting, with a flow rate of 800 mL/sec, you will have 40 mL 100% oxygen plus 760 mL of 0.21% oxygen (160 mL), so 200 mL of oxygen in 800 mL of air flow/sec for a FiO_2 of 25%. Panting dogs in particular may have a very hard time benefiting from nasal oxygen, as it very hard to get supplemental oxygen flow rates high enough to be beneficial.

Face Mask

In very compromised pets or those recovering from anesthesia, it is simple and effective to provide oxygen by a facemask. Dogs and cats will typically not tolerate a face mask if they are not very sedate or ill. It is important to counsel support staff and new clinicians not to fight with the patient to hold the facemask, as this dramatically increases energy expenditure on the part of the patient.

Supplies: Face mask, tubing, oxygen $

Flow by Oxygen

Occasionally, in order to avoid the struggles associated with facemask placement, individuals will hold oxygen tubing near a patient's face with the hopes of increasing the FiO_2. The likelihood of significant improvement is slight, and if oxygen is truly needed, a different route is preferred.

Supplies: Tubing, oxygen $

Nasal Oxygen

A red rubber or other soft plastic tubing may be placed with the nasal passages to permit the delivery of supplemental humidified oxygen. Animals in extreme distress will often not tolerate the restraint required to suture (staple) in nasal lines. Nasal oxygen is relatively contraindicated in brachycephalic pets, pets with excessive panting, and may be more challenging in cats or very small dogs. The oxygen flow rate will reflect the diameter ("French") of the tubing, thus with very small pets, with only a 3.5 or 5 Fr catheter being tolerated, the relative flow rate may be quite low.

Procedure: Select nasal catheter: choose the largest size that will be tolerated by the patient — cats 3.5–5 Fr, small dogs 5–8 Fr, medium dog 10–12 Fr, large dogs 10–14 Fr. Instill local anesthesia into nostril, use either lidocaine or proparacaine. Pre-measure the catheter to the medial canthus of the eye. Put a piece of white tape at the desired location. Pre-load the needle driver with suture (or use a stapler). Insert the tube, and promptly secure in place. Consider placement of an e-collar to prevent dislodgement of the tube. Place bilaterally if desired. Connect to humidified oxygen source.

Supplies: Nasal catheter, tubing, suture, scissors, oxygen, local anesthetic $

Oxygen Hood

An oxygen hood may be either commercially purchased (eg, Jorgenson Laboratories, others) or made with cellophane wrap and an e-collar. The collar is secured around the patient's neck and oxygen is introduced into the hood. The hood is vented to prevent carbon dioxide retention.

Supplies: Hood, oxygen and tubing $-$$

Transtracheal Oxygen

Oxygen may be delivered transtracheally via a tracheostomy tube or with a catheter placed directly into the trachea. This technique does not work well in very small pets, as it is very challenging to safely pass a catheter into the lumen of the trachea without damaging the tissues.

Procedure: The neck is sterilely prepped. If the patient is not obtunded, a local block may be performed. A through the needle catheter (eg, Intracath®) is passed into the trachea to the thoracic inlet and supplemental oxygen is provided at a lower flow rate (10–50 mL/kg). The catheter should be bandaged in place. Successful placement in the trachea should be confirmed (free aspiration of air, similar to a transtracheal wash).

Supplies: Through the needle catheter, oxygen, tubing, bandage materials, prep supplies $-$$.

Nasotracheal Oxygen

Oxygen may also be delivered directly in to the trachea by placement of a nasotracheal oxygen catheter. This technique is particularly helpful to by-pass the pharynx and/or larynx.

Procedure: This technique may be performed two ways. The first way is to simply pass nasal oxygen tubing farther in through the pharynx and attempt to advance further during inspiration. This may take a few attempts, as the tendency of the tube is to go down the esophagus. The second, which is my preference, is to place under sedation to evaluate the upper airway obstruction. In this scenario, the obstruction is first classified (eg, dynamic, fixed) and then if not immediately treatable, the nasal catheter is fed into the back of the nasopharynx and then grabbed with hemostats and directed into the trachea. A bit of dexterity may be required.

Supplies: Red rubber catheter, suture, tubing, oxygen, ± laryngoscope and sedation. $-$$

Oxygen Cage

Supplemental oxygen may also be delivered by placing the pet within an oxygen-enriched chamber or cage. This technique is particularly helpful for animals that are too stressed to undergo any other form of supplemental oxygen (eg, cats, small dogs) as it is very well tolerated. The disadvantages of an oxygen cage include that it is a relatively inefficient use of oxygen and, when the cage is opened, the oxygen concentration will re-equilibrate quickly with the room air.

Supplies: Oxygen cage, source of oxygen $$$-$$$$

Mechanical Ventilator

Positive pressure ventilation (PPV) with a mechanical ventilator provides the most control over the percentage oxygen, and the breathing pattern of the patient. In animals that are expected to be hypoventilating for more than a few minutes (eg, some intoxications, neurologic disease) or those with respiratory failure (PaO_2 < 50 mmHg on supplemental oxygen), PPV may be life-saving. The decision to provide PPV is beyond the scope of this brief discussion, but should be considered warranted in some cases. Practitioners associated with busy ER or critical care services typically find PPV invaluable in caring for critically ill or injured pets.

Supplies: Mechanical ventilator, adequate technical and professional staff to monitor pet.

Recommendations for further reading are available from the author upon request.

UPDATE ON FELINE ASTHMA

Rhonda L. Schulman, DVM, Diplomate ACVIM
Southern Arizona Veterinary Specialty
and Emergency Center
Tucson, AZ

Feline bronchopulmonary disease (FBPD), often referred to as "feline asthma," actually encompasses a group of common, but poorly understood, airway diseases. It is estimated that bronchopulmonary disease affects 1% of the general cat population and > 5% of the Siamese breed. Cats of any age can be affected and there is no clear gender predisposition.

PATHOPHYSIOLOGY

Airways have a limited number of ways of responding to inhaled irritants or immunologic stimuli. The airway walls can become thickened and edematous. These thickened airways then experience a greater degree of narrowing in response to a given amount of smooth muscle contraction. Submucosal glands may become hyperplastic and secrete excessive amounts of thick mucus. In humans, hyperreactivity of the airways is a hallmark of clinical asthma; this has been documented in some cats. These physiologic changes result in narrowed airways and increased airway resistance. Initially, reversible airflow obstruction may be seen (which can respond to medications); however, with time, airway remodeling may occur, resulting in a "fixed" airway obstruction.

True asthma results from an IgE mediated hypersensitivity to airborne allergens. Helper T cells produce a variety of interleukins and direct the release of inflammatory mediators. In humans, asthma often has a genetic component.

Infection with Mycoplasma may also have a role in the generation of feline bronchopulmonary disease. Mycoplasma is an extracellular pathogen which attaches to and destroys ciliated epithelial cells. Mycoplasma infection has been shown to produce airway inflammation and hyperreactivity in mice. In humans, infection with M. pneumoniae has been found to be significantly associated with asthma. Studies have shown that 50% of children experiencing their first asthmatic attack were also infected with M. pneumoniae. Furthermore, those children suffering from mycoplasmal infections were far more likely to suffer from recurrences of asthma. In cats, approximately 25% of feline patients evaluated for bronchopulomonary disease culture positive for Mycoplasma.

Another potential cause of feline bronchopulmonary disease is the use of bromide to treat seizures. Two separate studies found that approximately one third of feline patients treated with bromide began coughing and showing evidence of lower airway disease. In some of these cats, the bronchopulmonary changes were so severe as to result in euthanasia. In cats receiving bromide, eosinophilia was found in the bronchoalveolar fluid.

CLINICAL SIGNS

Affected cats typically have intermittent respiratory distress and may be without clinical signs between episodes. In some cats, FBPD can result in severe, potentially fatal respiratory distress. With time, progressive airway changes can develop that result in more severe clinical disease and diminished quality of life. Cats typically display coughing and wheezing. Owners may mistake coughing for gagging or vomiting. An increase in respiratory rate and/or effort is usually present during episodes. Signs may progress to more overt dyspnea wherein the cat may become cyanotic and display open-mouth breathing.

During the physical examination, harsh lung sounds, crackles or wheezes may be auscultated. The clinician may note a prolonged expiratory phase to respiration. An abdominal effort may be noted during respiration. During more severe episodes, the cat may be cyanotic and open-mouth breathing.

Differential Diagnoses

There are many differential diagnoses to consider for a cat presenting for coughing, wheezing or respiratory difficulty. In addition to feline asthma and other inflammatory, noninfectious bronchopulmonary disease, infectious causes including viral, fungal, protozoal, bacterial or parasitic agents; cardiac disease, pleural space disease (chylothorax, pyothorax, pneumothorax, hemothorax), neoplasia, upper airway disease, respiratory tract foreign bodies and pulmonary thromboembolism should be considered. Clinicians should also keep in mind that the cat may actually be vomiting or gagging and the client is mistaken in presenting the cat for coughing.

DIAGNOSIS

A minimum database (CBC, chemistry profile, urinalysis) may be more beneficial for ruling out causes other than asthma for coughing and respiratory distress. In feline bronchopulmonary disease, the CBC may reveal eosinophilia in approximately 20% of the cases. Neutrophilia and/or a stress leukogram may also be present. Hyperproteinemia or hemoconcentration may also be noted. Fecal analysis is recommended to rule out parasites.

Thoracic radiographs usually display many abnormalities in cats suffering from bronchopulmonary disease. A bronchial pattern, described as "doughnuts" and "tramlines," is frequently present. Peribronchial cuffing is also present. Other radiographic findings may include flattening of the diaphragm, atelectasis of the right middle lung lobe and air trapping. Rarely, radiographs may be normal.

Airway cytology, obtained through either tracheal wash or bronchoscopy, reveals inflammation. In healthy cats, the predominant cell type (80% to 90%) is the alveolar macrophage. In cats suffering from bronchopulmonary disease, increased numbers of eosinophils and/or neutrophils are found. Airway eosinophilia is considered to be more consistent with true asthma whereas airway neutrophilia may be seen more with chronic bronchitis. It is important that samples are handled appropriately and in a timely manner. A recent study by DeClue and Reinero found that storage of samples for greater than 48 hours affected the cellular composition.

Either bronchoalveolar lavage fluid or tracheal wash fluid can be submitted for bacterial and *Mycoplasma* culture. It can be difficult to distinguish between true bacterial infections versus colonization of the airways. Growth of a single organism without the use of enrichment broth is consistent with a true infection. Isolation of *Mycoplasma* is always of clinical significance because *Mycoplasma* is not recovered from the airways of healthy cats. Additionally, the destructive effects of *Mycoplasma* upon the respiratory epithelium make isolation of it of note.

Bronchoscopy allows visualization of the airways. Increased secretions as well as edema may be seen. Complication rates for bronchoscopy in cats range from 25% to 40%; however, most complications are considered minor.

In humans, pulmonary function testing is usually done as part of the work-up for a suspected asthmatic or bronchitic patient as well as in monitoring the response to treatment. In veterinary medicine, pulmonary function testing is usually limited to teaching hospitals and large referral centers. Noninvasive tests such as tidal breathing flow volume loops and barometric whole body plethysmography have been used in cats. Tidal breathing flow volume loops (TBFVL) measure air flow and volume during both inspiration and expiration. In healthy cats, peak flow occurs during late inspiration and early expiration. Decreased expiratory flow rates are seen in feline bronchopulmonary disease, resulting in a flattening of the curve. Barometric whole body plethysmography (BWBP) is another noninvasive measurement of pulmonary function that can be done on nontrained cats. The patient is placed into an airtight, ventilated chamber. Pressure changes are measured as the cat inspires and expires. During bronchoconstriction, the major alteration is seen in early expiration.

TREATMENT
The Acute Crisis

Asthmatic cats may present in true respiratory distress (open-mouth breathing, cyanotic) which may prove to be fatal. It is crucial to stabilize these cats without causing them undue stress. Oxygen needs to be supplemented in a fashion that does not make the cat anxious or induce panic. If it is available, the cat should be placed into an oxygen cage. Both bronchoconstriction and inflammation need to be addressed. Bronchodilators include both beta-2 agonists such as terbutaline and methylxanthines such as aminophylline and theophylline. If available, inhalational bronchodilators such as the beta-2 agonist albuterol may provide more immediate relief than if given by injection. If an inhalational bronchodilator is not available, injectable bronchodilators should be used. Epinephrine should be considered as a last resort. A systemically acting corticosteroid such as dexamethasone should be administered during the acute

attack as inhalational corticosteroids do not reach full efficacy for a period of time.

CHRONIC THERAPY
Glucocorticoids

Glucocorticoids (GC) are an *essential* tool in the management of feline bronchopulmonary disease. GC are necessary for treating the inflammatory component, thus preventing progression of the disease. Oral GC should be used in the initial management of cats with bronchopulmonary disease. GC should be tapered to the lowest effective dose to minimize side effects if possible. In minimally affected cats, i.e. very intermittent clinical signs, GC therapy may be halted when clinical signs are not present (after an appropriate period of tapering off of medication).

An alternate delivery method of GC is via inhalation. This allows for more immediate delivery to the target organ with fewer systemic side effects. It has been proven that untrained cats will have deposition of inhaled materials in their lower airways. Inhaled GC have been shown to reduce bronchial reactivity and eosinophilia. Minimal impact on the immune system is seen with inhaled GC. They do produce some changes in the hypothalamic-pituitary-adrenal axis, but the clinical significance of these alterations is not known. Inhalational GC therapy should initially be administered concurrently with oral GC because it can take up to 10 days for the inhaled medication to reach full effect. Fluticasone (Flovent) 110 µg/actuation is a commonly used inhaled GC in veterinary patients.

Bronchodilators

Bronchodilators are also available in both oral and inhaled formulations. Bronchodilators such as albuterol are crucial during the acute asthmatic crisis. Inhaled albuterol can be administered every ½ hour for up to 4 hours during a crisis. Bronchodilators are also useful in the management of chronic disease but should not be used as the sole therapy. Bronchodilators are not anti-inflammatory and do nothing to prevent airway remodeling. There is some concern that chronic albuterol administration can actually result in airway inflammation. Bronchodilators should be administered during times of increased symptoms or to decrease the amount of GC administered, not as a monotherapy.

Antibiotics

Antibiotics are rarely indicated in the treatment of feline asthma, with the exception of treating *Mycoplasma* infections. If *Mycoplasma* is isolated, an appropriate antibiotic such as doxycycline should be administered at the usual dose. Other bacterial infections only warrant treatment if culture suggests a true infection (growth of a single agent) rather than colonization of the airways.

Serotonin Inhibitors

Cyproheptadine, a serotonin inhibitor, has been advocated as an additional therapeutic for asthma. Serotonin mediates smooth muscle contractility in feline airways. Studies have not shown consistent benefit. It may be that higher doses are necessary.

Cyclosporine

Asthma is mediated by T-helper 2 cells so suppressing T cells may be of benefit. Cyclosporine decreases interleukin 2 (IL-2) production resulting in inhibition of T-cell proliferation. Experimentally, cyclosporine reduces airway reactivity and remodeling. However, cyclosporine is very expensive and can cause gastrointestinal upset. Further investigation into the use of cyclosporine for treating feline asthma is necessary.

Immunotherapy

"Allergy shots," such as are used to treat atopic skin disease, are another consideration in the treatment of feline asthma. The mechanism by which immunotherapy works is still poorly understood. There is little correlation between allergens determined by skin tests and allergens seen on blood panels. There is also no correlation between the number of reacting allergens (a high number suggesting a very allergic patient) and the amount of airway eosinophilia. When compared with normal cats, cats with airway disease do have a greater number of positive allergen reactions, regardless of the test methodology. Immunotherapy involves exposing the patient to a known allergen and thus carries the risk of inducing an anaphylactic reaction. Studies on cats with naturally occurring disease are needed before this therapy can be safely recommended.

Omega 3 Fatty Acids

Omega 3 fatty acids as found in fish oil have received a lot of attention due to their potent antioxidant and anti-inflammatory effects. One study did not find any decrease in bronchial reactivity or change in airway cytology. A decrease in pulmonary oxidative stress was noted however.

Environmental Modification

One of the simplest yet most often overlooked as aspects of managing feline asthma is modifying the environment. Inhaled particles can act as irritants as well as potentially inducing allergic reactions. If an offending allergen can be identified and removed from the cat's environment, then the asthma could be potentially be completely resolved. Unfortunately, it is usually impossible to remove all allergens from the environment even if the allergen(s) can be identified. It is still important to reduce the amount of airborne allergens and irritants. HEPA filters and air cleaners should be used. Common household airway irritants include dusty cat litter, tobacco smoke, and aerosols.

HOW TO USE INHALANT MEDICATIONS IN CATS

Rhonda L. Schulman, DVM, Diplomate ACVIM
Southern Arizona Veterinary Specialty
and Emergency Center
Tucson, AZ

Inhalant medications are being used more frequently in the treatment of feline asthma and other bronchopulmonary disease. Inhalants are chosen for a variety of reasons including local application to the organ of interest, fewer systemic side effects, and potentially more rapid onset of action. Additionally, it is often difficult for owners to administer medications orally to cats, resulting in poor compliance. It has been shown that nontrained cats will inhale material presented to them via a facemask and that these particles will reach the lower airways. As with any method of drug delivery, the medication will only work if administered appropriately. It is recommended that veterinarians give owners detailed instructions on the appropriate method and necessary equipment for use of inhalant medications.

EQUIPMENT

The two major classes of medications used in the treatment of feline asthma, corticosteroids and bronchodilators, are available as metered-dose inhalers (MDI). MDI deliver a specific amount of medication per actuation (puff). The actuation of the MDI is supposed to be coordinated with a slow, deep inhalation. The timing of this breath has proven difficult in humans and impossible in veterinary patients. For this reason, the use of a *spacer* is strongly recommended. In humans, spacers have been shown to potentially double the amount of medication reaching the lower airways. Additionally, in humans with asthma, the use of spacers appears to reduce the systemic effects of inhaled glucocorticoids. The spacer serves as a storage area for the medication until the patient breathes it in. A veterinary specific spacer, Aerokat®, is available (www.aerokat.com). The Aerokat has a built-in facemask that will fit most cats and small dogs on one end and an opening on the other end that fits the MDI device. Spacers meant for human use can also be used. They will need to be used with an appropriate facemask.

TECHNIQUE

1. Shake the MDI 3 to 4 times, then remove the cap and insert the MDI into the appropriate end of the spacer.
2. Place the facemask gently over the cat's face, making sure the nose is covered.
3. Actuate the MDI.
4. Hold the mask in place for 7 to 10 seconds.
5. If two actuations of the same medication are prescribed, wait 30 to 60 seconds in-between repeating administration. Start again at step 1, shaking the MDI.
6. If using both a bronchodilator and a corticosteroid, use the bronchodilator first, wait for 5 minutes, then administer the corticosteroid. The bronchodilation achieved will allow for deeper deposition of the corticosteroid into the lungs.
7. Follow manufacturers' recommendations for cleaning.
8. The owner needs to monitor the number of actuations administered to know when the MDI needs to be replaced. The number of actuations contained within the MDI is listed on the canister. The owner can divide the total number of actuations by the number to be administered daily to know how many days the MDI will last for. Fluticasone at 1 actuation twice daily will last for 2 months. It is inaccurate to see if the MDI floats in water as a judge of whether or not the canister is empty.

MEDICATIONS

Formulations of both glucocorticoids (GC) and bronchodilators are available in MDI. Inhaled GC have been shown to reduce bronchial reactivity and eosinophilia. Minimal impact on the immune system is seen with inhaled GC. They do produce some changes in the hypothalamic-pituitary-adrenal axis, but the clinical significance of these alterations is not known. Inhalational GC therapy should initially be administered concurrently with oral GC because it can take up to 10 days for the inhaled medication to reach full effect. A frequently used glucocorticoid (GC) in veterinary patients is fluticasone 110 µg/actuation (Flovent®).

Bronchodilators

Albuterol, a beta-2 agonist is widely available as a MDI (Ventolin®, Proventil®). Albuterol is best used during the acute crisis and during times of increased symptoms. Within 5 minutes of administration, albuterol relaxes bronchial smooth muscle, decreasing bronchoconstriction and improving airflow; its effects last 3 to 6 hours. There is some concern that chronic albuterol administration can actually result in airway inflammation. Bronchodilators should be administered during times of increased symptoms or to decrease the amount of GC administered, not as a monotherapy.

References are available from the author upon request.

WHOOPS! SPAY / NEUTER COMPLICATIONS AND HOW TO AVOID THEM

Mark Bohling, DVM
College of Veterinary Medicine
University of Tennessee
Knoxville, TN

Complications can be part of any surgical procedure, and spay and neuter are no different. The beginning of complication management is to know all of the potential complications and their causes. Only then can one make plans to avoid and/or treat the complications. With few exceptions, complications begin or are caused during surgery, but may not become apparent until the postoperative period, sometimes even weeks or months after surgery. This fact makes careful surgical technique all the more important, and the primary avoidance strategy.

OPERATIVE COMPLICATIONS
Hemorrhage

Hemorrhage can be divided into two categories; serious hemorrhage and continuous oozing. The former is usually caused by a failure of ligation, most commonly due to technical errors. The ligature must be 100% reliable in all situations. Measures that will help with this include:

1. Obtain adequate pedicle length
2. Place ligature far enough proximal to be able to cut off the pedicle at least 6 mm distal to the ligature
3. Proper suture size (too small may cut through the pedicle, too large may not enclose tightly enough)
4. Ensure that the second knot throw doesn't loosen the first throw
5. Don't rely on inspection/manipulation after ligation (tends to loosen the ligature, creates false sense of security)

The problem of oozing can be technical error in ligation but is more commonly patient related. Bitches in heat or recently in heat may ooze; estrogens may be at least partly responsible. Ingestion of anticoagulant rodenticides, aspirin, and several other drugs may result in bleeding; treatment is based on etiology. Certain breeds (especially Dobermans) are more likely to present with inherited disorders of coagulation (eg, von Willebrand's disease). History will not always reveal these patients and screening (buccal mucosal bleeding time) should be employed when the index of suspicion for a possible bleeding disorder is high. Blood products should always be available in spay/neuter as in any other primary surgical practice (this can be achieved with blood on hand, or ready access to a donor)

Iatrogenic Ureteral Trauma

Iatrogenic ureteral trauma usually occurs during efforts to deal with a dropped ovarian pedicle, when the ureter is traumatized during attempts to grasp the ovarian artery. Although caused in surgery, this complication may not be apparent until later, when the patient re-presents with uroabdomen if the ureter has a leak, or lumbar pain in the event of ureteral stricture leading to hydroureter and hydronephrosis. In most cases, nephroureterectomy must be performed because the location of ureteral trauma is too proximal for neoureterocystostomy. In the event of a dropped ovarian pedicle, increasing the exposure, and availability of self-retaining retractors, can greatly improve visualization and help reduce the risk of this complication.

POSTOPERATIVE COMPLICATIONS
Dehiscence

Dehiscence most often seen secondary to self-trauma; dehiscence can have catastrophic consequences, although thankfully it usually does not. This complication is frequently (though not always) due to technical error, as a patient will usually leave a comfortable closure alone. Too-tight skin sutures are commonly to blame here; intradermal closure or very loose skin sutures should be used, and any suspect patient sent home in an e-collar, rather than wait for a problem. Sometimes, an otherwise adequate closure is stressed beyond the limits of tissue and/or sutures by an extremely active patient, and minor herniation or even more serious dehiscence can result. While the surgeon cannot control the patient's behavior at home, good discharge instructions should specify limited activity for 2 weeks or until suture removal. More rarely, incisional dehiscence may result from severe surgical infection or impaired wound healing such as may be seen with Cushing's disease or diabetes.

Incisional Infections

Of course surgical infections occur for a variety of reasons, some of which are not under the control of the surgeon (the patient that goes home to a filthy, wet environment, for example). Adherence to Halstead's surgical principles is the best plan for avoidance of incisional infections. This does not necessarily mean gowning and full surgical regalia, however. Attention to the creation of a healthy surgical wound (gentle tissue handling, hemostasis, minimization of dead space, reduction of anesthetic and operative time, and use of only the minimum number of sutures of the smallest possible gauge) should be the focus. Even the areas not under the surgeon's direct control should still be addressed in the discharge instructions (importance of clean, dry housing).

Reactions to Buried Sutures and/or Surgical Adhesives

These problems are best avoided by minimizing the amount of implanted foreign material. Intradermal sutures should be fine gauge and knots compact (avoid unnecessary use of extra throws) and deeply buried. PDS suture, while not particularly inflammatory, is very long lasting, and poorly buried knots often crop up later as suture granulomas. If a surgical tissue adhesive is used, it should be restricted to skin only and a minimum amount used.

Scrotal Swelling and Discoloration

This is usually caused by oozing from small cutaneous or subcutaneous vessels rather than leakage from the testicular pedicle. Attention to hemostasis and subcutaneous closure, and postoperative exercise restriction (particularly for very active dogs) can help reduce the incidence of this problem. If the scrotum should begin to swell, cold compresses may help reduce the severity of the problem if applied within the first 48 to 72 hours; after that time, warm compresses should be used.

Postoperative Vaginal Bleeding

This is a fairly uncommon but potentially quite serious complication. Vaginal bleeding has been noted to begin anywhere from 4 days to 3 weeks after spay. Usually it is mild and self-limiting, but on rare occasion, it will become life threatening. What appears to happen in these cases is that the uterine body ligature erodes through the uterine vessel(s), leading to vaginal bleeding. Any serious vaginal bleed post-spay is an indication for abdominal exploration. The uterine stump is re-excised and double ligated with Miller's knots. A two-pass uterine ligature (such as one of the modifications of the Miller's knot) may reduce the risk of this complication when compared with a single-pass ligature.

Sinus Tracts and Stump Granulomas

These complications are created during surgery, due to poor aseptic technique, excess remaining stump tissue, or use of nonabsorbable ligature material. Occasionally a uterine stump granuloma can become so large that it causes fecal or urinary obstruction. Sinus tracts can develop with the use of nonabsorbable ligatures or the use of non-surgical ligating materials such as nylon cable ties. Treatment consists of exploration and correction of the cause.

Ovarian Remnant Syndrome

Except in the very rare case of accessory ovarian tissue (reported in cats), or exogenous sources of progestins, this condition is an iatrogenic issue. Failure to remove the entire ovary is a technical error and is avoided by obtaining adequate exposure of the ovarian pedicle and checking the removed reproductive tract for two entire ovaries. In the rare developmental anomaly of uterus unicornis, there may still be an ovary on the side lacking the uterine horn. This ovary may be located as far cranially as the diaphragm and is easy to miss if a complete abdominal exploration is not performed. Ovarian remnant(s) may cause signs of estrus beginning as early as 2 weeks to as late as years after ovariohysterectomy.

Urinary Incontinence

Urinary sphincter incontinence is a potential physiologic consequence of the loss of estrogens following ovariohysterectomy and may affect as many as 10% to 20% of spayed bitches. This condition, while not a true "complication" of surgery, is still an undesirable outcome and should be discussed with the clients before surgery. More rarely, adhesions may form between the uterine stump and urinary bladder and cause incontinence. The accidental placement of the uterine body ligature around the vagina and a ureter has also been reported to cause ureterovaginal fistula with ensuing incontinence.

SPAY / NEUTER SURGICAL & TIME-SAVING TECHNIQUES

Karla Brestle, DVM
Medical Director, National Spay/Neuter Response Team
Humane Alliance, Asheville, NC
www.humanealliance.org

Although cost is consistently a factor in high-volume high-quality spay/neuter, the "quality" portion of our procedures must always come first. Quality is routinely defined as "a degree of excellence." This definition is consistent with the evaluation that we as spay/neuter surgeons should afford our patients the finest care possible. Specifically, we should address each aspect of patient care with this concept in mind.

The quality of our procedures should encompass not the surgery alone, but all portions of presurgical and postsurgical care. This begins with use of suitable monitoring equipment (such as pulse oximeters) and proper cleaning, sanitizing, and sterilization of surgical instruments and drapes. For example, it would be standard operating procedure to disallow cold sterile be used in the clinic. In addition, the surgeon must be willing to cap, glove, and mask, as well as gown if deemed necessary for more intensive procedures.

These standards provide for much more than ensuring the well being of our patients. They enhance both the client and veterinary community perception, which is an extremely important tool in promoting the reputation and acceptance of high-volume, high-quality spay/neuter clinics. In addition, we consistently recognize an augmentation of efficiency and reduction of complications with this approach.

High-volume, high-quality spay/neuter (HVHQSN) programs are efficient surgical initiatives that meet or exceed veterinary medical standards of care in providing accessible, targeted sterilization of large numbers of dogs and cats in order to reduce their overpopulation and subsequent euthanasia. In pursuit of this effort, surgeons become extremely proficient at performing sterilization procedures and develop techniques unique to the field or utilize existing less well-known techniques that lead to increased efficiency.

Several of the existing techniques are performed in private practice across the country, but depending on where you attended veterinary school, you may or may not be aware of their use. The modified Miller's knot, for example, is an extremely efficient and secure knot that is used by many veterinarians, while just as many have never even heard of it. Similarly, the figure 8 knot has an analogous story. A distinctive knot that has a small but dedicated following is the feline ovarian pedicle tie. This knot is accomplished as an instrument self tie and is not only extremely secure, but leaves no potentially reactive suture behind.

HIGH-VOLUME SPAY / NEUTER CLINICS: WHAT DO THEY MEAN TO A COMMUNITY?

Karla Brestle, DVM
Medical Director, National Spay/Neuter Response Team
Humane Alliance, Asheville, NC
www.humanealliance.org

The Humane Alliance Spay/Neuter Clinic in Asheville, North Carolina, has been making a tremendous impact on the animal overpopulation problem in the western North Carolina (WNC) region since the spring of 1994. William H. McKelvy founded the organization with the mission to provide low-cost spay/neuter services, the non-lethal, responsible solution to pet overpopulation. We recognized that the best defense against the stray, unwanted, and abandoned pet population is sterilization. What began as a local effort escalated into a regional endeavor.

More than 200,000 companion animals have been spayed and neutered at the Humane Alliance Spay/Neuter Clinic since the program started in May 1994. We sterilized over 25,000 companion animals in 2006. These regional programs do not create themselves. They require the planning and coordination of many talented people. We, as a community of citizens concerned about animal welfare, are faced with the challenge of finding a home for every pet. It takes a cooperative partnership of the entire community to solve pet overpopulation. Competent prevention and intervention programs are the key to driving down euthanasia rates in our shelters. Humane Alliance of WNC has addressed this community effort to create a region where no pet would be without a home by working hand-in-hand with all of the animal welfare organizations throughout the region.

We provide a free transport service in addition to our local public services. It is an effective and innovative service that has been implemented through the coordinated efforts of many dedicated individuals. The transport system accommodates delivery of homeless pets for rescue organizations, pets belonging to low income residents of WNC, and county shelter pets to our facility for sterilization. This service is provided for 34 non-profit animal welfare organizations in 23 counties, and five county shelter facilities. These groups have a demonstrated history of cooperative participation with the clinic. The clinic belongs to the region.

The animal welfare organizations provide comprehensive programs that support adoption, guarantee comprehensive medical treatment through local practitioners, transfer animals from animal control agencies, create foster home networks, and promote an aggressive spay/neuter component. By 1996 mandatory pre-adoption sterilization was one common goal of animal welfare organizations within WNC. The participating organizations have raised hundreds of thousands of dollars to assist in the cost of spay/neuter since 1995. The partnership of these organizations in WNC has been integral to the success of this program. All of the partners agree that spay/neuter is the responsible solution to pet overpopulation and the choice that saves lives. Their purposes are proactive and have served to change the public's perception of their rights and responsibilities regarding their pets. The public has to know that sterilization of companion animals is a responsible solution to pet overpopulation. It is imperative that we educate and motivate individuals to choose to be a part of the solution to the homeless pet population.

The Humane Alliance is privileged to work with supportive local veterinarians who recognize the value of the clinic's services. These veterinarians and their participation in a free postoperative exam program are invaluable to the clinic and the cause of animal welfare. Cooperation between the private veterinarians and animal welfare organizations is absolutely pivotal to the well being of companion animals.

Fundamental to all preventive work is sterilization. Neutering is recognized as our best defense against all the sources of shelter overpopulation. This regional spay/neuter facility is an efficient, effective means of accomplishing an aggressive, targeted sterilization campaign. It is a catalyst in uniting organizations with separate missions to a common purpose. Community coalitions are critical to the success of proactive programs.

The success of this model has been demonstrated in the reduction of intake and euthanasia rates in Buncombe County (where the clinic is located). In fact, the intake has decreased by 70% since the Humane Alliance opened. To address this epidemic nationally, the Humane Alliance has created the National Spay/Neuter Response Team (NSNRT).

The NSNRT is a strategic training program designed by Humane Alliance Spay/Neuter Clinic to address a national epidemic; "There is no disease or condition of companion animals that takes as many of their lives as euthanasia," according to Janet M. Scarlett, DVM, MPH, PhD, who is Associate Professor of Epidemiology at Cornell University. Clearly, our nation's best defense against all of the sources of shelter intake is targeted, aggressive, high-volume, high-quality, low-cost sterilization. This is an urgent need that will require a skilled, dedicated and well-organized team to train organizations to open and operate strategically placed high-volume, high-quality, low-cost spay/neuter clinics in areas of need across the nation.

STANDARDS OF CARE FOR HIGH-QUALITY, HIGH-VOLUME SPAY/NEUTER

Brenda Griffin, DVM, MS
Diplomate ACVIM (Small Animal Internal Medicine)
College of Veterinary Medicine
Cornell University, Ithaca, NY

Historically, negative perceptions of "high volume" or "low cost" spay/neuter surgery have been many and common. I have heard and read comments such as: "There is no such thing as 50% off safe or 50% off sterile" and "If you are making a small incision, you can not possibly be removing the entire reproductive tract." Many have expressed concerns and sentiments that those doing high volume surgery cannot possibly be doing a good job—that the standards of care must be below those that are acceptable. Despite the success and outstanding track records of numerous programs (Table 1), these perceptions continue to exist today. Consequently, many veterinarians who work in spay/neuter clinics and shelters worry about their professional reputations: for instance, they may worry about how they are viewed by other veterinarians or how their employment or association with the humane field will affect their professional resumes or future employment opportunities. For me personally over the course of my own career, I have encountered countless comments about my chosen field of interest: "Why are you interviewing at a shelter...that's not the only job you can get, is it?" "That crazy Dr. Griffin, who knows what she is doing..." "Shelter medicine is a no-brainer: no special knowledge or experience is needed." "What are you doing with your (ACVIM) credentials?" "For you to work at the shelter would be a waste."

Personal annotations aside, a national effort to address these negative perceptions was recently undertaken by the American Society for the Prevention of Cruelty to Animals (ASPCA) and PETsMART Charities. In order to address such concerns surrounding high volume spay/neuter and to advance this extremely important and valuable practice area, they convened a panel of 19 veterinarians for a Summit to Advance Spay/Neuter in December 2006. Participants included experienced veterinary practitioners from spay/neuter programs (including stationary clinics, mobile clinics, feral cat programs and MASH-style programs), academic veterinarians board-certified in surgery, anesthesiology, and small animal internal medicine, and a veterinary epidemiologist.

The first goal and accomplishment of the participants of the Spay/Neuter Summit was to establish a formal definition of large-scale spay/neuter programs: High-volume, High-quality Spay/Neuter (HVHQSN) programs are efficient surgical initiatives that meet or exceed veterinary medical standards of care in providing accessible, targeted sterilization of large numbers of dogs and cats in order to reduce their overpopulation and subsequent euthanasia. Participants also set specific objectives and formed a national task force to accomplish the following: development of professional guidelines for performing high volume/high quality spay/neuter, epidemiologic studies to demonstrate the impact of such programs on pet overpopulation, and development of recruitment strategies and training opportunities for veterinarians and veterinary students in HVHQSN.

Higher volume (or lower cost) is NOT obtained by lowering quality. Support teams, equipment, and protocols are geared towards safety, efficiency and humane quality care of large numbers of companion and feral cats and dogs. In pursuit of this effort, surgeons become extremely proficient at performing sterilization procedures and develop techniques unique to the field or utilize existing less well-known techniques that lead to increased efficiency.

The task force has developed standards of care for High Volume/High Quality Spay/Neuter Programs including recommended surgical, anesthetic and peri-operative practices. These standards are based upon accepted principles of research in surgical asepsis, surgical technique, and microbiology, as well as review of the scientific literature and expert opinions. These surgical practices are intended as achievable,

Table 1. Mortality Rates at HVHQSN Clinics

Program Name	Number of Surgeries Performed	Number of Deaths (for any reason)	Mortality Rate
Angels of Assisi Dr. Kelly Farrell, Roanoke, VA	6,885 in 2006	3	0.044
Spay-Neuter Assistance Program, Inc. (SNAP Texas) Dr. Jim Weedon, Houston and San Antonio, Texas	21,478 in 2006	8	0.037
Feral Cat Spay/Neuter Project Dr. Christine Wilford Seatlle, WA	8,592 in 2006	15	0.175
Shelter Outreach Services (SOS) Dr. Leslie Appel Finger Lakes Region, NY	21,000 since clinic opened	19	0.09
EmanciPET Dr. Ellen Jefferson, Spay/Neuter Clinic Austin, TX	69,000 total since clinic opened	19	0.028

and represent what is believed to be an acceptable standard that is obtainable in programs that practice high volume/high quality spay/neuter. The task force plans to publish their recommendations later this year.

Note: Little comparative information exists in the literature regarding mortality rates associated with spay/neuter surgery of dogs and cats. A retrospective study from a teaching hospital examining the mortality rates of cats and dogs undergoing elective S/N and declaw surgeries found them to be 0.10% (1/1,016) and 0.14% (2/1,459), respectively.[1] Another retrospective study of cats (n=935) and dogs (n=646) undergoing the same procedures in private practice revealed a 0% mortality rate.[2]

REFERENCES

1. Pollari, et al. Postoperative complications of elective surgeries in dogs and cats determined by examining electronic and paper medical records. J Am Vet Med Assoc. 1996;208:1882-1886.
2. Pollari, et al. Evaluation of postoperative complications following elective surgeries of dogs and cats in private practice using computerized records. Can Vet J. 1996;37:672-678.

THE FUTURE IS NOT FAR AWAY: NONSURGICAL STERILIZATION

Brenda Griffin, DVM, MS
Diplomate ACVIM (Small Animal Internal Medicine)
College of Veterinary Medicine
Cornell University, Ithaca, NY

Julie Levy, DVM, PhD
Diplomate ACVIM (Small Animal Internal Medicine)
College of Veterinary Medicine
University of Florida, Gainesville, FL

OVERVIEW

For over 30 years, researchers have been studying methods to control reproduction. Tremendous advances have been made in recent years with many successes in the human and wildlife fields. During this time, a few scientists have been working to apply these technologies to cats and dogs. In 2000, the Alliance for Contraception in Cats and Dogs (ACCD) was established in order to focus and direct these efforts in order to expedite the development of contraceptive drugs and vaccines specifically for cats and dogs.

Since then, ACCD has held three international symposia to facilitate interaction of interested individuals and to encourage exchange of ideas and research results. The Third International Symposium on Non-Surgical Contraceptive Methods of Pet Population Control was held in November 2006 with 120 individuals in attendance along with 38 speakers from nine countries. Speakers presented the latest data and information on contraceptive drugs and vaccines under development, discussed the market for contraceptive products, and explored the role of veterinarians in acceptance and effective introduction of contraceptives and non-surgical sterilants. Participants developed action plans and formed collaborative teams to respond to challenges and opportunities in the field. Symposium proceedings are available at www.acc-d.org.

With over 4 million companion animal deaths each year, shelter euthanasia remains the leading cause of death of healthy cats and dogs in the US. Controlling their reproduction represents a critically important strategy for decreasing shelter euthanasia. Indeed, addressing the welfare of surplus pets begins by not allowing the surplus to develop in the first place. Low-income communities and feral/free-roaming cats represent leading sources of animals that are euthanized in shelters: the provision of accessible and affordable sterilization for these animals is critical to success. The development of nonsurgical methods of sterilization would provide a practical alternative to surgical sterilization; these products have the potential to greatly increase the numbers of dogs and cats that are sterilized since they will not require the technical expertise, equipment and time that surgical sterilization requires. In its position statement on Dog and Cat Population Control, the AVMA encourages research into the development and use of nonsurgical methods of sterilization.

Contraceptive drugs and vaccines work by exerting a targeted pharmacological effect or prompting an immune response that inhibits or blocks some component of the animal's reproductive system, resulting in infertility. The ideal contraceptive product would rapidly induce permanent sterilization, eliminate breeding behavior as well as fertility, and provide at least as many health benefits as surgical sterilization, while requiring only a single dose. Furthermore, the ideal product would be effective in dogs and cats of both sexes and all ages, and be safe and easy to administer. At this time, no single product is able to fulfill all of these criteria; however, several promising products are under development. Even if the ideal formulation cannot be produced, safe products that induce sterility in dogs or cats, male or female, will be valuable tools in the fight against pet overpopulation.

For veterinary practitioners, the availability of safe and effective contraceptive products will create opportunities to meet the needs and interests of pet owners who decline anesthesia, are averse to surgical castration, or that seek temporary contraception. As consumers increasingly expect veterinary products and practices that mirror human options, the ability to provide the most technologically advanced and least invasive interventions is an advantage to any practice. Because nonsurgical contraceptives can be administered more quickly and easily, and perhaps less expensively than surgery, these alternatives may have a higher profit margin and free up time and space for other clients and procedures.

Thorough investigation of products is time-consuming and expensive and requires substantial investment not only from the scientists, but also from pharmaceutical companies and investors. The fact that little is available after all this time points to the need for those who feel this is an important opportunity to get involved. Veterinarians can play key roles in advancing development of nonsurgical tools. The exciting news is that one nonsurgical sterilant (Neutersol®) is expected to be re-released in the US in 2009 and long-acting contraceptive products are already available in Australia, and New Zealand, and will soon be available in Europe. Information on contraceptive products currently available or under development is summarized here. Additional information may be found at the ACCD Web site (www.acc-d.org).

Nonsurgical methods of sterilization will be safe, effective alternatives to surgical sterilization that can be used to increase the number of dogs and cats sterilized. It is of paramount importance that these products be accepted by veterinarians and by the public in order for them to have a reaching impact. The scientists, pharmaceutical companies and funding agencies behind these products are to be applauded.

NEW PRODUCTS: CONTRACEPTIVE DRUGS AND VACCINES

New pharmaceutical agents that have received regulatory approval in one or more countries include Neutersol® (Abbott Animal Health, USA), Suprelorin®

(Peptech Limited, Australia), Gonazon® (Intervet, France), and Canine Gonadotropin Reducing Factor Immunotherapeutic (conditional approval, Pfizer Animal Health, USA).

Neutersol is the first permanent, nonsurgical method of sterilization for companion animals. It is currently licensed for use in the US for chemical castration of puppies 3 to 10 months of age, although it has been shown to be effective in adult dogs and cats as well. It is an intratesticular injection of a zinc compound (zinc gluconate neutralized by arginine), which results in sclerosis of the testes and permanent sterility. It is 99% effective and very safe. The precise mechanism of action is unknown; the testicles atrophy over weeks to months following injection, resulting in a 70% to 90% reduction in testicular size in very young puppies and 50% in older dogs (atrophy may not be symmetrical). Sterility may take up to 60 days in postpubescent males. In most cases, Neutersol can be administered without sedation. An insulin syringe or a TB syringe with a long, fine needle is used to administer a single injection into each testicle and patient discomfort is minimal. FDA studies showed that Neutersol reduces but does not abolish testosterone production, and its effects on hormone-dependent diseases and behaviors have not been established. However, studies have revealed a significant decrease in prostate size in Neutersol-injected dogs versus controls. The only significant safety concern which was reported in field use is the development of scrotal ulcers at the injection site in a very small percentage of dogs. This appears to be most commonly observed in large adult dogs (an off-label use) and may be related to poor injection technique allowing some of the chemical to contact the scrotal skin and connective tissues. Injection site reaction rates are similar to rates of wound complications in surgically castrated dogs, but use of Neutersol avoids adverse events or deaths associated with the use of anesthesia.

This product is a useful option in veterinary practice as well as animal shelters. The obvious advantage is that it eliminates the need for anesthesia and surgery and saves substantial time. While available previously for a short time from Addison Laboratories, Neutersol was used successfully by programs in the US (including one event in which 200 dogs were sterilized in one day) and abroad (including a 10,000 dog study conducted by the head of the Mexican VMA which demonstrated safety and efficacy of Neutersol use in dogs over 10 months of age). Originally introduced by Addison Laboratories, Abbott Animal Health is currently contracted to manufacture and distribute the product, anticipated to be available in early 2009.

Suprelorin is a deslorelin implant that is approved and available for use in male dogs in Australia and New Zealand. Suprelorin is expected to be launched in Europe in 2008. Deslorelin is a GnRH agonist. When GnRH agonists are given continually at low doses, they suppress pituitary function. This action results in safe, reversible contraception. Regulation of GnRH receptors at the gonadotropin-producing cells of the anterior pituitary reversibly blocks the production and release of the gonadotropins LH and FSH. Without their stimulating effects, gonads cease to produce gametes (egg cells and sperm) and female and male sex hormones. Therefore, all related body functions and behavior cease until the block is removed. This method was discovered over 30 years ago, and has since been used to treat human prostate cancer patients. An implant containing 5 mg deslorelin provides contraception for 12 months. As in human subjects, adverse effects have not been observed in dogs and cats. However, one complication of GnRH agonists that is not observed with GnRH antagonists is that they may trigger a single estrus cycle when first implanted due to an initial stimulatory effect on GnRH receptors. The duration of contraception may vary beyond one year among individuals. Treatment can be safely repeated.

Intervet's Dr. Marc-Antoine Driancourt presented data on a new canine contraceptive, Gonazon®, which received approval in the European Union in November 2006. This product is a one-year, reversible contraceptive implant for female dogs. While this does not fit the profile of a permanent or long-term tool for dog population management programs, Dr. Driancourt announced some limited data in cats showing that queens had suppression of estrus over an extended period of time (nearly three years at the date of his presentation). This raises the possibility that the product might be useful in the control of feral cat populations, although the expense involved in manufacturing GnRH agonist implants may be a limiting factor.

Canine Gonadotropin Releasing Factor Immunotherapeutic is a new anti-GnRH vaccine from Pfizer that has conditional FDA approval. Created and licensed for treatment of benign prostatic hyperplasia (BPH), the product results in suppression of testosterone release in of male dogs for at least six months and can be repeated.

OTHER APPROACHES UNDER DEVELOPMENT

Contraceptive and sterilant technologies currently under exploration but that have not yet completed the regulatory process include GonaCon™ (NWRC-USDA, Colorado, USA) and ChemSpay™ (Senestech, Flagstaff, Arizona, USA).

Dr. Kathleen Fagerstone from the National Wildlife Research Center of the USDA presented data on the GnRH vaccine GonaCon, developed and tested for use in several wildlife species. Data are being submitted to the EPA initially for approval for use in deer and other cervids. Pilot studies in dogs by Drs. Brenda Griffin and Henry Baker at Auburn University revealed severe injection site reactions and inconsistent suppression of fertility in male beagles. Evaluation in cats by Dr. Julie Levy at University of Florida has yielded more promising results and a majority of female cats responded to a single injection with more than three years of infertility Injection site reactions consisting of a small subcutaneous lump occurred after two years in a few cats, several of these resolved spontaneously.

Dr. Loretta Mayer of Senestech/Northern Arizona University presented early stage technology for permanent sterilization of female dogs with ChemSpay. The drug is an industrial chemical that has been shown to deplete the ovarian follicles and cause sterility in rodents, and there are some preliminary data showing this effect may also occur in dogs. This is a totally new approach and is exciting for its potential for permanent sterility. Dr. Mayer is currently working on dose levels and formulation for single-treatment application. Dr. Levy is currently investigating the use of this compound in female cats.

ACKNOWLEDGMENT

The authors would like to thank Ms. Karen Green, Project Manager of the Alliance for Contraception in Cats and Dogs, for her assistance in the preparation of this manuscript.

IS SHE SPAYED? IS THERE ANOTHER TESTICLE?

Brenda Griffin, DVM, MS
Diplomate ACVIM (Small Animal Internal Medicine)
College of Veterinary Medicine
Cornell University, Ithaca, NY

DISTINGUISHING BETWEEN SEXUALLY INTACT AND SPAYED QUEENS AND BITCHES

Accurate identification of queens and bitches that have been spayed represents a longstanding and sometimes frustrating clinical dilemma. Pets with unknown histories are commonly presented to veterinarians and animal shelters for determination of reproductive status. Various methods of identification have been utilized to identify surgically sterilized cats and dogs, including application of special tattoos, application of tattoo paste in the surgical incision to "mark" the surgical scar, feline ear cropping (removal of an ear tip in free-roaming cats), and implantation of microchips. Unfortunately, none of these methods are uniformly widespread in their use. Furthermore, evidence of an abdominal incision from previous ovariohysterectomy may be lacking, particularly if the animal was spayed at a very young age or if a flank approach was used (a common practice in cats in European countries). In many instances, cats and dogs undergo unnecessary anesthesia and surgery, only to reveal that previous ovariohysterectomy has been performed. This translates into unnecessary trauma for pets, expense for owners, and frustration for practitioners.

Clinical Evaluation

A complete physical examination should be performed. The overall body condition should be noted. Metabolic rate has been shown to significantly decrease and a tendency towards obesity has been well documented in spayed cats compared to reproductively intact queens. If the cat is overweight, a clinical suspicion that she has been previously spayed is warranted. Changes in metabolic rate following ovariohysterectomy have not been well defined in bitches.

If the patient will allow it, the ventral abdomen should be shaved from the umbilicus to the pubis, and the skin of the midline should be carefully inspected for the presence of a scar. In the author's experience, palpation is not a reliable indicator of the presence of a spay scar. Some intact females have a prominent linea alba that may be mistaken for a scar, and spayed cats and dogs frequently have scars that are not readily palpable, yet may be visualized once the overlying hair is removed.

Careful inspection of the mammary glands should also be performed. Spayed cats and dogs typically have atrophied mammary glands and very small teats subjectively, compared to the well-developed glands and prominent teats of intact females. The inguinal area is also a common location for tattoos, which are more readily visualized once the hair is removed. The pinnae should also be examined for the presence of tattoos or cropping (in the case of cats), and the patient should be scanned for the presence of a microchip.

The owner should be questioned carefully regarding behavioral signs of estrus. Most cats experience winter anestrus; therefore time of year should be considered when assessing the presence of estrus signs. Cat owners may confuse normal affiliative or greeting behaviors such as head rubbing or tail waving with signs of estrus. Lordosis and treading can usually be induced in estrual queens by stroking the back or dorsal rump. This can be done during the course of an exam to help verify the presence of behavioral signs of estrus. In cases where the presence of behavioral estrus is present, vaginal cytology can be performed for confirmation. In dogs, signs of estrus are accompanied by more dramatic physical changes including enlargement of the vulva and bloody discharge, facilitating recognition.

If reproductive status can not be determined based on physical examination, hormonal evaluation is recommended prior to consideration of exploratory surgery. Alternatively, owners may elect to wait and see if signs of behavioral estrus appear. Whenever possible, definitive determination of reproductive status should be made.

Hormonal Evaluation

Tests for measuring serum concentrations of luteinizing hormone (LH) may be used to distinguish spayed and sexually intact animals since serum concentrations of LH increase after ovarian removal as a result of the lack of negative feedback from the gonads. In the reproductively intact cat or dog, the normal sequence of endocrinological events is such that LH concentrations remain at low basal concentrations, except for very brief periods when ovulation occurs and gonadotropin-releasing hormone stimulates LH release. After this sudden spike, LH returns to basal concentrations in less than 24 hours in most cases. Negative feedback control of LH results from ovarian estradiol secretion and maintains LH at basal concentrations. Following ovariohysterectomy, this negative feedback control is removed, and LH concentrations remain increased indefinitely. Commercially available LH test kits will be "positive" in spayed animals, while negative results are consistent with the need for surgery.

TOMCATS: CRYPTORCHID OR NEUTERED?

Bilateral cryptorchid cats and unilateral cryptorchid cats in which surgical removal of the scrotal testicle has been performed may be mistaken as neutered cats due to the absence of scrotal testes. Such cats may present for sexual behaviors including spraying, fighting and mounting or for urine odor. Demonstration of penile spines is consistent with a diagnosis of the presence of a testicle. An increase in serum testosterone concentration following administration of hCG or GnRH may be used for diagnosis of retained testicle(s) in the cat, but is not necessary. Penile spines are reliable external indicators of the presence of testosterone in male cats, and are present in unilateral and bilateral cryptorchid cats. Penile spines (Figure 1A) begin to appear in kittens as early as 12 weeks of age and are obvious by 6 months of age. They regress within 6 weeks following castration, and the mucosal surface of the penis becomes flat and smooth (Figure 1B). The presence of penile spines may be considered diagnostic for the presence of a testicle.

When compared to scrotal testicles, retained testicles are generally grossly smaller. Testicles located in the inguinal region are frequently very difficult to palpate and may not be readily palpable due to the large inguinal fat pad in many cats. Furthermore, irregular deposits of fat may be mistaken for retained testicles.

In addition to development of penile spines, there are other androgen-dependent physical changes that occur as cats mature to puberty. These include secondary sex characteristics such as the formation of jowls, widening of the neck and thickening of the skin. Although most tomcats do not develop distinct jowls before 2 years of age, their skin may subjectively appear "tougher" or more difficult to puncture with a hypodermic needle.

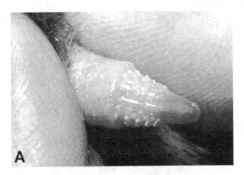

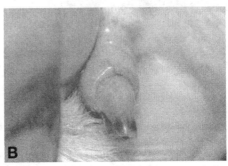

Figure 1. Penile spines (A) begin to appear in kittens as early as 12 weeks of age and are obvious by 6 months of age. They regress within 6 weeks following castration, and the mucosal surface of the penis becomes flat and smooth (B). The presence of penile spines may be considered diagnostic for the presence of a testicle.

YIKES! HOW TO HANDLE FERAL CATS SAFELY

Julie Levy, DVM, PhD, Diplomate ACVIM
College of Veterinary Medicine
University of Florida, Gainesville, FL

OVERVIEW

Nonlethal control of feral cats via trap-neuter-return (TNR) programs is an increasingly popular approach taken by humane groups and municipal animal control agencies. As these programs grow in popularity, veterinarians are likely to be asked to participate by sterilizing feral cats in their practices. While this can be a rewarding activity, it can also be extremely dangerous for both cats and personnel if special precautions are not adhered to.

SAFETY FIRST

One of the dominant concerns about working with feral cats is safety. Feral cats have an uncanny ability to escape during handling, and can inflict serious injury during recapture attempts. A loose cat can thoroughly damage a clinic in its frantic efforts to escape. It is recommended that anyone who works with stray animals, including feral cats, receive prophylactic rabies immunizations. Gloves should be worn at all times to reduce exposure to body secretions from cats. The most common health risks for individuals working with feral cats are bites and scratches.

Even semi-tame cats may bite defensively if they are startled, as in the attempt to place a cat in a carrier for transportation. For these reasons, it is imperative that safe cat handling techniques be developed and enforced. Not only does this guarantee the safety of personnel, but it also prevents the unfortunate situation in which public health officials require the euthanasia of biting cats for rabies examination.

The safest method for handling feral cats is to admit them in wire humane traps or other escape-proof containers which permit anesthetic to be injected through the wire mesh (Figure 1). The trap should not be opened until the cat is recumbent. At the completion of surgery, the cats are returned to their traps before awakening. With this system, cats are never handled awake. Handling systems that involve transferring cats from one container to another or opening a container to restrain a cat only invite escapes and injuries.

If cats must be housed for several days, they may be released into a secure cage. Cats should always be transferred in a secure room with solid ceilings, secure doors and windows, and without hiding places. Special feral cat boxes can be purchased which have "portholes" that may be latched closed after the cat has hidden in the box (Figure 2). These boxes allow safe and minimally stressful movement of the cat to other areas and the front sliding door permits relatively safe transfer to other carriers. If a feral cat escapes from its cage, the safest method of capture is with a net on a pole (Figure 3). Attempts to catch a feral cat by hand, or with a blanket are extremely dangerous for personnel. Catch poles are very dangerous for cats and only serve to cause more panic. If a cat has entered an inaccessible site, it may be necessary to retrap it.

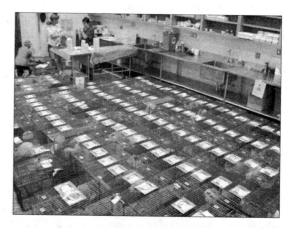

Figure 1. Using techniques which eliminate handling of conscious cats, such as requiring that cats arrive in wire traps, allows the safe handling of 200 or more feral cats in a few hours.

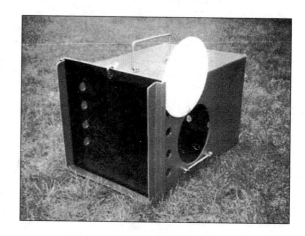

Figure 2. Feral cats will naturally seek to hide in a "feral cat handler box." The porthole door can be closed to confine the cat for cage cleaning or for transport.

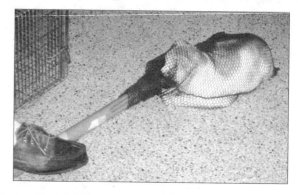

Figure 3. Catching an escaped feral cat with a net allows a "hands-off" capture. The netted cat can be moved back to its enclosure or can be injected with anesthetic through the net.

ANESTHESIA

Injectable anesthetics are preferred for feral cats because they can be administered to cats still in their traps and there are no waste gases. A cocktail of Telazol (1 vial, 500 mg) reconstituted with ketamine (100 mg/mL, 5 mL) and large animal xylazine (100 mg/mL, 1.25 mL) instead of water is just one of many that have been used in feral cats. "TKX" has several advantages for large-scale cat anesthesia. A small injection volume (0.2–0.25 ml for average adult cats, 0.1–0.15 mL for kittens) can be administered "intracat" through the wire of the trap, eliminating the need to handle conscious cats (Figure 4). Time to recumbency is generally 3 to5 minutes, and vomiting is uncommon. General anesthesia is usually adequate for abdominal surgery. The xylazine component of the cocktail is reversed with yohimbine administered intravenously at the same volume as the TKX. The major disadvantages of TKX include hypothermia, prolonged recovery time, and poor postoperative analgesia. Buprenorphine (0.03 mg per

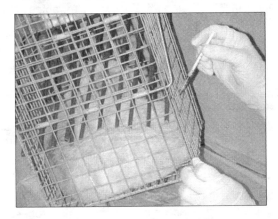

Figure 4. The safest method for managing feral cats in the clinic is to inject anesthetic through the sides of the trap and to remove the cat only after it is immobilized.

average adult cat SC) can be added to improve analgesia. Cats should be returned to their traps prior to recovering from anesthesia and should be closely monitored until fully awake. Cats generally return to sternal position within 2 hours, but frequently are not fully recovered from anesthesia until the following morning. Faster recovery times may be achieved by using a lower dose of TKX for immobilization and then using gas anesthesia by mask or endotracheal tube to obtain a surgical plane.

TKX has been used on more than 20,000 feral cats in a Gainesville trap-neuter-return program with a remarkable safety record. Considering that these are often unthrifty, parasitized animals of unknown background, highly stressed, and unsuited for preanesthetic examination, the observed rate of 3 deaths per 1,000 cats compares favorably with reports of anesthetic death rates of pet animals in private practices.

RESOURCES

1. Tomahawk Trap Company, www.livetrap.com: Feral Cat Handler ($56.93), Cat Single Door Trap ($50.08), TD10 Trap Divider for confining trapped cats for injection ($16.45), volume discounts available.
2. Levy JK. Feral cat management. In: Miller L, Zawistowshi S (eds.): Shelter Medicine for Veterinarians and Staff. Blackwell Publishing, 2004, pp 377-388.
3. Williams LS, Levy JK, Robertson SA, Cistola AM, Centonze LA. Use of the anesthetic combination of tiletamine, zolazepam, ketamine, and xylazine for neutering feral cats. J Am Vet Med Assoc. 2002;220:1491-1495.

HOW MANY DOGS OR CATS DO WE NEED TO STERILIZE TO GET ZERO POPULATION GROWTH? IT DEPENDS....

Margaret R. Slater, DVM, PhD
College of Veterinary Medicine and Biomedical Sciences
Texas A&M University, College Station, TX

This article will discuss the 70% figure for sterilization that is commonly cited as the threshold to successfully decrease pet populations, describe the commonly used population dynamics models for dogs and cats, and present examples from the literature in dog and cat populations. These examples will illustrate the usefulness of models as well as why we don't always need to aim for 70% sterilization.

WHERE DID 70% COME FROM?

The 70% figure for sterilization to successfully control dog or cat populations has been discussed in the last 10 or 15 years. Originally, it seems to have come from 13th century agriculture. It was discussed by a gentleman named Fibonacci who used it in the context of animal population growth or reduction. This work was cited by Lewis Plumb and popularized extensively by Merritt Clifton and, later, by Marvin Mackie.

It seems that 70% has also been cited as the percentage of animals needing to be vaccinated against rabies to prevent an outbreak. Coleman and Dye reported that the figure appeared in New York State among veterinarians in the 1940s. However, recent advances in modeling have demonstrated that 70% isn't always appropriate and the percentage depends on animal density, social structures, disease spread, and other factors.

WHY POPULATION DYNAMICS MODELS?

Do we always need to get 70% of all free-roaming cats spayed or castrated to control their population? Do we need to get 70% of all owned dogs sterilized in countries with dog problems? It depends....and population dynamics models can help us decide.

These percentages depend on models: simplified representations of a complex ecological system. The population of animals is dynamic: animals find and defend territories, they select mates, reproduce and rear young, find food and shelter and avoid predators during some period of time. For dogs and cats, "ecology" may involve local ordinances and policies, cultural beliefs, and human interventions. Our conceptual model of dog and cat populations becomes a mathematical model when we represent it with mathematical equations.

Biologically, a population of animals is a group of the same species, who live together and reproduce. However, a population from a modeling or epidemiologic (or veterinary) perspective is much more narrowly defined. We might talk about only owned dogs or unowned, free-roaming cats or abandoned animals, dogs in shelters or a single colony of feral cats. Each population will grow or decrease in different ways for different reasons. Each may or may not interact with one of the other populations, which is especially important for community level population models. Studies in the early 1980s illustrated the complex interrelationship of the populations. More recent work has also used these diagrams to help visualize a set of subpopulation and demonstrate where additional data are needed. In general, in population dynamics modeling, males are ignored. This is fine as long as there are enough males in the population of interest to inseminate all the females and the vital rates for males are the same as females.

A population dynamics model has to have a clear objective before it is built. There are many purposes models can serve: 1) simple descriptions of a biological process or situation; 2) synthesis of current knowledge and understanding to see where the gaps are; 3) guidance for future experimental work; 4) evaluation of different interventions and their effects; 5) risk analysis or decision support; and 6) predictions of future changes in the population. In the animal protection field, we are most often interested in #4, but there are published examples of #1, #2, and #6. For example, rabies control in dogs was accomplished by vaccination and sterilization of neighborhood dogs. In eight years, 65% of females were sterilized and vaccinated and the total population of dogs decreased 28%. And human cases of rabies dropped to zero.

There are many types of models. Demographic models (aka structured population models) take into account the affects that demographic variables like age or life stage might have on population growth and are a little more commonly used for dogs and cats. They make fewer assumptions about the population and allow more flexibility in modeling. If age is important, it can be accounted for, most commonly by dividing the ages of the population into classes or groups. Sometimes, stage of life is more important than actual age: kitten, reproductive adult or non-reproductive adult, for example. These models use matrices to summarize the calculations. Fertility or fecundity tables (which indicate average reproduction for females in each age class or stage) and survivorship tables (life tables) which provide data on mortality for each class or stage are crucial information for these models. One study found that euthanasia of 50% was equivalent in control to sterilization of 75% of the fertile cats. However, survival data were sparse, survival was the most influential variable in the model and the model assumed a closed population.

WHAT DATA ARE NEEDED?

Changes in populations are based on four "vital statistics." Birth (aka fertility, fecundity) and death (mortality, survival) depend on the size and success of the current population. Immigration and emigration depend on the movement of animals in or out of the population (due to the animals' own movements or the intervention of humans). Births and immigration increase the population and deaths and emigration decrease it. If there are more births and/or immigration than deaths and emigration, then the population will increase, and vice versa. In a closed population, immigration and emigration are zero and only birth and death rates influence population size.

To use the demographic matrix model approach, more detailed data are needed. For fecundity, we need the average number of female young born to a female of a particular age class or stage in a particular time period (often a year). We also need the age or stage specific mortality. There are three common ways to calculate this: 1) follow a group (cohort) of individuals across time and see what their life span is; 2) collect data across a shorter time span on all animals that died during that period and their age at death (also requires growth rate of the population; 3) use cross-sectional data (often from a questionnaire) to estimate survival for each age class or stage. These methods are listed from best to least reliable.

Getting good data for the model is the most difficult part for dog and cat populations. First, the populations of interest can vary substantially from place to place. Second, we don't often have funding or ability to collect detailed data in the populations of interest. And third, sometimes it is just very difficult to actually obtain the data. For example, how do we estimate the number of dogs abandoned? Do all the animal shelters in the city of interest keep records on the numbers of kittens who enter the shelter? It is crucial that the investigators making the model clearly document where they obtained their data and exactly what data they used so that it is easy to decide if the data seem realistic and similar to a population to which we might want to apply the model.

So far, all the models discussed are deterministic: we use our one best estimate for fecundity or mortality and the model gives us one single answer in terms of population change. Stochastic models allow us to incorporate variability into our vital statistics. For example, we can include data in the model that incorporates the range of litter size in bitches. Stochastic models also allow us to include the role of chance in influencing populations.

So a model is created that seems to be appropriate for the population and incorporates natural variability and chance. What if our estimates aren't very accurate? What if we are just giving our best education guess? Actually, even if we are sure of our estimates, it is important to do a sensitivity or elasticity analysis. This means that we change the value of our vital statistics and see how this influences the model and the overall conclusions from the model. It also allows you to see which of the vital statistics has the greatest effect on the model. This might be useful to know if fecundity is the most important and we are talking about a sterilization plan. Sensitivity analysis changes the vital statistics by a fixed amount that makes sense for the population. Elasticity analysis changes the vital statistics by the same proportion. The choice depends on the population and what seems logical, but one of these analyses should be done for any model.

How do we tell if our model is valid? The simplest way is to compare the model to the existing data or a subset of existing data. The harder way is to compare the model results and projections to a new independent data set. The latter is generally considered to be more rigorous, but new data sets may be hard to find. And depending on the objective of the model, we may not need to be able to generalize the model's results to other data sets. Even if the models don't match, the comparisons may provide valuable insight into the knowledge gaps or to times or locations where unusual events occurred and generate hypotheses to be tested.

SOME RECENT EXAMPLES

A Ricker model was used to study free-roaming cats in counties in Florida and California with high volume spay/neuter programs. This type of model focuses on the growth rate of the populations, the effect of population density on growth and the idea that carrying capacity limits growth rate. The model used birth and death rates and assumed a closed population. This type of model can show changes in population size either by slowing growth or by modifying the environment to decrease the carrying capacity. The authors' primary interest was the impact of sterilization on population growth. There were limitation in the data used (from programs in the counties and from published data) and in the assumptions. However, several of their conclusions are worth further consideration. First, they calculated that 94% and 71% of cats in the FL and CA counties, respectively, would need to be sterilized to decrease growth. At the county level thousands or tens of thousands of cats would need to be sterilized. Second, targeting smaller populations should make it possible to reach high levels of sterilization. And third, data on cats trapped again as part of the sterilization efforts could help with population size and sterilization percentage estimates to evaluate success.

A demographic model for owned dogs in the Teramo region of Italy was used to estimate population growth based on current dog data from a telephone questionnaire. Fertility and immigration were estimated from the questionnaire data. Survival was estimated based on life tables of purebred dogs in the US. Emigration was based on dogs abandoned and taken to shelters in the area. Using the current 30% spay frequency, the population of dogs was estimated to grow by about 3% per year in the next 20 years if the average age of sterilization was three years. However, if bitches under one year of age were targeted, the population growth could be stabilized or decreased with only 26% of bitches needing to be spayed. Sensitivity analysis indicated that age-specific death rates of the dogs were the most important vital statistic in the model.

A stage-structured model was used to evaluate several methods of controlling free-roaming cat populations. The data came from a radio-collar study of 54 cats in a small Texas town. Based on that cat population, sterilizing 75% of the females and returning them was the most effective method to decrease the population over a 10-year period (by 82%) and required handling the fewest cats. Euthanizing 75% of female cats resulted in a 69% decrease in population over the same time period.

CONCLUSIONS

- Population dynamics models can be very useful in studying pet populations. Contact a nearby college or university to see if an ecologist or wildlife biologist can help build the models with you.
- The data for the models can be difficult to find. Search the scientific literature but also seek organizations or individuals who keep detailed records on the population of interest.
- Understand that some of the assumptions of models and the data used cause serious limitations. Still, learn what you can from what has been done.
- Target a manageable population of interest. Often we have based this on human locations (eg, zip codes with the largest number of kittens brought to the shelter) or socioeconomic status (such as low-income families for subsidized sterilization). However, we should also consider dog or cat based targets such as a colony of cats, dogs living around a dump, etc. This may dramatically change the percentage of animals that need to be sterilized.
- Population dynamics modeling is a tool that can help us plan or evaluate a potential intervention and help us decide if 70% (and of what population!) really is our goal…or not.

REFERENCES

1. Colman PG, Dye C. Immunization coverage required to prevent outbreaks of dog rabies. Vaccine. 1996; 14:185-186.
2. Gotelli NJ, A Primer of Ecology. Sinauer Associates, Inc. Sunderland MA, 3rd ed., 2001.
3. Anderson MC, Martin BJ, Roemer GW. Use of matrix population models to estimate the efficacy of euthanasia versus trap-neuter-return for management of free-roaming cats. J Am Vet Med Assoc. 2004; 225:1871-1876.
4. Owen-Smith N. Introduction to Modeling in Wildlife and Resource Management. Blackwell Publishing, Malden MA, 2007.
5. Nassar R, Fluke J, Pet population dynamics and community planning for animal welfare and animal control. J Am Ved Med Assoc. 1991;198:1160-4.
6. Patroneck G, Glickman L. Development of a model for estimating the size and dynamics of the pet dog population. Anthrozoos. 1994;7: 25-42.
7. Frank J. An interactive model of human and companion animal dynamics; the ecology and economics of dog overpopulation and the human costs of addressing the problem. Human Ecol. 2004; 32: 107-130.
8. Foley P, Foley JE, Levy JK, Paik T. Analysis of the impact of trap-neuter-return programs on populations of feral cats. J Am Vet Med Assoc. 2005; 227: 1775-81.
9. Di Nardo A, Candeloro L, Budke CM, Slater MR. Modeling the effect of sterilization rate on owned dog population size in central Italy. Prev Vet Med, in press.
10. Hill PM, Population dynamics and management of free-roaming cats. Masters Thesis, May 2006, Texas A&M University.

FERAL CATS 101: LET'S GET WILD

Christine L. Wilford, DVM
Feral Cat Spay/Neuter Project
Seattle, WA

This article will enable you to positively impact the lives of individual free-roaming cats while working to humanely reduce the free-roaming cat populations to extinction. Discussion of the ethics surrounding free-roaming cats and trap-neuter-return (TNR) are beyond the scope of this lecture.

FERAL VERSUS FREE-ROAMING

For my purposes, the term *free-roaming* describes cats that are not living as pet cats with a traditional home, and the term *feral-behaving* describes cats that appear unsocial with people. In private practice, we see feral-behaving cats in the clinic that act fully socialized at home. Being unable to distinguish a cat's social standing under duress is the reason to avoid labeling an unknown cat as feral. In most shelters, "feral" = death, even for frightened, tame cats.

WHY DEAL WITH FERAL CATS ANYWAY?

People are compassionate. Millions of people are compassionate and do not ignore animals in need. Some people spend hundreds of dollars feeding wild birds, squirrels, and raccoons. Others people feed free-roaming cats.

We gain pleasure interacting with non-human species. People enjoy contact with species other than humans. Ask a fancier to remove their bird feeders, because the droppings attract rats. Tell your neighbor that his raccoons may carry rabies and should be removed. It won't happen, nor will people stop feeding homeless cats.

Veterinarians are essential to ending overpopulation. Vets improve the lives of free-roaming cats through spay/neuter while preventing more homeless kittens and growth of cat colonies. People desperately seek spay/neuter services for these cats. Because veterinarians are the only source, we are essential to reducing free-roaming cat populations.

Free-roaming cats are the largest source of kittens entering shelters. Millions more cats die in shelters than die from any single infectious disease. An estimated six million cats are killed in shelters *each year* awaiting homes that never come. From where do they come? According to a study by Julie Levy, DVM,[1] the sterilization rate of owned cats is 85% compared with free-roaming cats at 2%. When applied to the estimated total cat population, Levy projects that owned cats create 33 million kittens annually while free-roaming cats create 147 million, a convincing argument that free-roaming cats are the most significant source of homeless kittens. *To reduce shelter kill rates requires preventing overpopulation at its source by altering free-roaming cats.*

VETERINARY SERVICES

Minimum services to provide. Minimum services are scanning for microchip, spay/neuter, ear tip, and rabies vaccination. Most trappers/caretakers deal with dozens, if not hundreds, of cats, because they trap colonies for other people. Veteran trappers often request minimal services while individuals feeding a single cat or colony may request more, eg, flea control, ear mite treatment, ear cleaning, FeLV test, FIV test, FVRCP vaccine, FeLV vaccine, and so forth.

Keep to the mission. Many individuals struggle between doing what is best for each cat versus focusing on the big picture: overpopulation and spay/neuter. If you aim to reduce overpopulation through spay/neuter, then offer minimal services. If you believe that all cats should receive comprehensive care, then realize that translates into less money for spay/neuter.

SAFE HANDLING: EQUIPMENT

Video demonstrations are available at www.feralcatproject.org in the Our Clinic Model section.

Do no harm: to you or the cat. Do not treat feral-behaving cats without preparation. Do not pose risks to yourself, your staff, or the cats. A calm, organized atmosphere with fast, efficient handling is a symphony.

Traps or plastic carriers only. Do not allow feral-behaving cats to arrive in cardboard carriers or top-opening carriers: you will have escapes. Require plastic carriers or traps and require that they remain covered to reduce stress. Some clinics prohibit carriers altogether and only accept traps. However, many caretakers cannot afford many traps and can only bring a few cats at a time.

Trap divider. Buying your own trap divider allows easy restraint for IM sedation before examination.

Squeeze cage. For cats in plastic carriers, use a squeeze cage to inject sedation. (You'll use it on pet cats, too!) With the right steps, cats transfer easily to the squeeze cage. We prefer the OMNI Cage.

Capture net. You need this, if a cat escapes. (Pet cats may require a capture net from time to time, as well.) We prefer the Freeman Cage Net.

The right atmosphere. When a cat escapes, it typically tries to escape vertically, climbing anything in its path. Before transferring any cat from carrier to squeeze cage, prepare for escape. Block the door, so that no one can unexpectedly open it. Clear items from counters, shelves, etc. Be sure there are no holes in the walls or cabinets and that the ceiling tiles are secure. Have the capture net in the room. Always use the quietest voices and slowest movements to reduce stress and fear.

ANESTHETIC SELECTION

Many anesthetic regimens are available. The ideal anesthetic is one with the fewest risks, intramuscular administration, rapid onset of action, and appropriate duration.

The most common anesthetic used on free-roaming cats is "TKX," a cocktail of tiletamine HCl and zolazepam HCl (Telzaol®) reconstituted with large animal xylazine and ketamine. Peer-reviewed journal articles describe the safety and use of TKX on tens of thousands of free-roaming cats.[2]

Variations of TKX include using atropine to prevent second-degree heart block and using the lower concentration of xylazine for clinics needing a shorter duration. Large-scale, MASH-type clinics require a longer duration of anesthesia. In more efficient clinics, using small animal xylazine reduces the incidence of vomiting and bradycardia while still providing sufficient duration.

We typically use a low induction dose to achieve restraint and augment with isoflurane by mask, if needed. In circumstances of poor health or prolonged recovery, we reverse xylazine with yohimbine.

We approach each cat as a high anesthetic risk, so that we provide the safest anesthetic experience for each.

MINIMAL SERVICES TO PERFORM

Physical exams. Our veterinary technicians triage cats after sedation. Veterinarians follow up. The goal of our physical exam is to determine whether the cat can humanely return to a feral lifestyle. We ask, "Can this cat find shelter, food, water and escape predators?" although many are being fed and have shelter. The vast majority appear healthier than my private practice patients.

Spay and neuter. Besides the obvious reproductive benefits, studies show weight gain and increased health of free-roaming cats after spay/neuter.

Pregnant cats. We spay any pregnant cat unless it is in labor. We do not euthanize live birth kittens. One can argue incongruity, but our policy satisfies our clinic. When shelters have more homes than cats, we will stop spaying pregnant cats.

We handle these spays quietly and discreetly to avoid distress to people who are not like-minded. We are accustomed to our own angst. Perhaps misconstrued as callousness, we've agonized over many difficult decisions and have become efficient at the decision-making process.

Surgical technique for pregnant cats. Most vets are inexperienced at late-term spays. Proper technique is vital or cats will hemorrhage. We suggest ligating the uterine arteries individually as well as using two transfixing ligatures around the uterine body. The clamp should be removed when tightening the ligature on the uterine stump. I have posted several cats that hemorrhaged after inexperienced volunteer veterinarians did not sufficiently tighten the ligatures around the uterine body.

Rabies vaccination. All free-roaming cats over 4 pounds receive a three-year rabies vaccine. We use 4 pounds as an age estimate knowing that most kittens below 4 months will be socialized and adopted into pet homes. For public health considerations, all free-roaming cats must be vaccinated for rabies.

Ear tipping. The ear tip, removing the top 1 cm of ear, *protects the cat!* An ear tip only means the cat is altered, not that the cat is feral or homeless. If an ear tip cat is trapped, it should be released on the spot to avoid transport, sedation, and stress. If an ear tip cat is presented for spay/neuter, it can be sent home without sedation and surgery. Performing the ear tip is simple and cheap.

Euthanasia. Obvious cases require euthanasia, such as emaciation, tiny kidneys, and fresh fractures, but some cases are less clear. Making a decision with very little information is a challenge. Many vets toil over wanting lab work or radiographs, but a decision must be made without those aids. Season and weather are considerations because they affect food supply and the ability to stay warm and dry.

In some cases, we allow select caretakers to take cats home for veterinary care. Sickly, adult cats that receive antibiotics (doxycycline), shelter, and food for a week often become robust, free-roaming cats again. Some caretakers administer injectable medications and subcutaneous (SQ) fluids through a capture net.

OPTIONAL SERVICES

FVRCP vaccination. In field studies, an estimated 50% to 60% of free-roaming adult cats had no detectable antibodies to feline panleukopenia. Previous assumptions were that adult, unvaccinated cats must have had exposure, survived and thus, have immunity. Now we know that assumption was incorrect, and vaccines could be beneficial.

FeLV-FIV testing. Overpopulation kills more cats than any single infectious disease. People working with populations, eg, public health, recognize that needs of individuals are often not the same as needs of populations. Viral testing is expensive, of variable accuracy, and does not prevent overpopulation. To save the most lives, money should be directed toward spay/neuter and not toward viral testing. In 1997 we FeLV tested our first 500 cats and found a 1% incidence of positives costing approximately $350 to find each positive. We stopped FeLV testing in 1998.

Ear mites/ear cleaning. We no longer clean ears or treat ear mites. We found that offering more procedures led to more confusion, stress and mistakes in the clinic. We KISS—Keep It Simple Stupid—so that we provide high quality spay/neuter and remain focused on our goal. Also keep in mind that an ear cleaning-induced vestibular problem is a death sentence for a free-roaming cat.

Flea treatment. We do not routinely treat for fleas; however, we apply flea treatment to small or thin cats with heavy flea loads. We also offer flea treatment to caretakers as an option and request a donation.

Additional surgical procedures. *Tails.* If we find an otherwise healthy cat with a severely traumatized tail, we amputate. The procedure is quick, simple and means the difference between euthanasia and life.

Polydactyle nails. Extra nails of polydactyle cats can grow become ingrown into the foot. We examine polydactyle cats for ingrown or potential problem nails. We declaw *only* the problem nail.

Enucleation. We see several ruptured eyes each year. If we have time, we enucleate the cat. If we are too busy, we release the cat only with assurance that the caretaker will pursue treatment and recovery before release. These cats have been living with one visual eye, and they do well when released.

Abscesses. We truly don't see very many abscesses. Big tomcats often have scars and healing abscesses. For an active abscess, we lance, flush and leave an opening to provide drainage. We request caretakers provide antibiotics for 5 to 7 days until they are certain healing is progressing.

Extractions. We occasionally extract loose teeth, if time allows. Free-roaming cats seem to present with less dental disease than pet cats.

Oddballs. Other things we see quite regularly include congenital angular limb deformities, blind eyes, pododermatitis, embedded collars, stomatitis unrelated to dental disease, fleas, lice, and healed and unhealed fractures.

KITTENS

Pediatric spay/neuter is Heaven. Easy, fast, inexpensive and the ultimate prevention of overpopulation! Kittens recover very quickly from anesthesia and surgery. We ear tip feral-behaving kittens, if there are no resources for socialization. We tattoo the tame kittens and those entering socialization.

RESOURCES

www.feralcatproject.org (videos and product information)
www.sheltervet.org

REFERENCES

1. Levy JK, Crawford PC. Humane strategies for controlling feral cat populations. J Am Vet Med Assoc. 2004;225(9):1354-1360.
2. Williams LS, Levy JK, Robertson SA, et al. Use of the anesthetic combination of tiletamine, zolazepam, ketamine and xylazine for neutering feral cats J Am Vet Med Assoc. 2002;220(10):1491-1495.

INTESTINAL SURGERY: NEW APPROACHES TO OLD PROBLEMS

Ronald M. Bright, DVM, MS, Diplomate ACVS
VCA-Veterinary Specialists of Northern Colorado
Loveland, CO

HEALING CHARACTERISTICS OF THE BOWEL

For the first 4 to 5 days following surgery on the bowel (enterotomy, end-to-end anastomosis), there is no intrinsic strength and the bowel is supported primarily by suture. The small intestine regains 75% of its strength within 14 days of injury. Large bowel heals more slowly, taking 21 days to regain 75% of its original strength.

THE ROLE OF THE SURGEON

The surgeon is largely responsible for ensuring a successful outcome in intestinal surgery. Hypoproteinemia, suture selection, and needle choices are important considerations but appear to be less important than gentle tissue handling, preservation of the blood supply, strict asepsis, a tensionless suture line, and meticulous placement of sutures. Increased risks of leakage following intestinal surgery include surgical removal of foreign bodies, presence of infection at the time of surgery (peritonitis), and enterotomies versus anastomoses. Interestingly, enterotomies are associated with a higher rate of dehiscence and leakage peritonitis.

Suture selection today is made easier by the availability of first-rate suture material. Monofilament absorbable sutures are very close to being the "ideal" suture material. Polypropylene is also acceptable but be careful when using this for continuous suture patterns as some recent case reports describe problems with intestinal obstruction With the advances that have been made in needles and suture materials, I don't believe there is ever any indication for using anything but a swaged-on needle. Silk and chromic gut should be considered obsolete.

The size of the suture material for intestinal surgery in dogs and cats, regardless of size, should be limited to 3/0 or 4/0. Acceptable needles include taper-cut, reverse-cutting, or taper point. The author prefers the RB-1 needle, which is available on most sutures.

Sutures should always incorporate the submucosa layer and to ensure this always happens, contact with the lumen is necessary. Any attempt to prevent going into the lumen may compromise the procedure because the submucosa may not be engaged. This is a serious technical error, which will likely lead to dehiscence of the bowel repair.

Packing off segments of bowel with a saline-soaked towel or laparotomy pads will act as a barrier to contamination of the entire peritoneal cavity. Intestinal contents should be "milked" away from the site of incisions where appropriate. This will decrease the amount of spillage of intestinal contents.

Following surgery, the surgical site should be gently irrigated with warm saline and suctioned dry. Routine irrigation of the entire abdomen is discouraged unless there is gross contamination outside of the isolated area of packed off bowel or if there is peritonitis present upon entering the abdomen. I like to thoroughly irrigate the subcutaneous layer after linea Alba closure as well.

There are a number of factors that assist in minimizing failure of the intestinal repair:

- Careful manipulation of the bowel aimed at preserving its blood supply
- Tension-free closures of enterotomy incisions or anastomoses
- Selection of proper sutures which excludes chromic gut or silk suture
- Use of suture that is not too large for delicate intestinal surgery
- Precise and discriminating use of electrocautery
- Sharp dissection whenever possible
- Careful suture placement that approximates tissue gently
- Correct use of perioperative antimicrobial prophylaxis
- Begin feeding the animal within 18 to 24 hours of the surgery if possible

PERIOPERATIVE ANTIMICROBIAL PROPHYLAXIS

I prefer a simple approach to the use of antibiotics during the perioperative period. Ideally, the antibiotic chosen should always be given intravenously to achieve maximum plasma/tissue levels at the time of incising into the bowel. It has been shown that the optimum time to give the drug is approximately 20 to 30 minutes prior to surgery. Giving the drug more than 2 hours after the initiation of surgery will diminish the benefit of giving perioperative antibiotics.

A first-generation cephalosporin, such as cefazolin, would be an acceptable choice, except for its poor coverage against important anaerobes such as *Bacteroides fragilis*. Anaerobes greatly outnumber aerobes in the distal small bowel, colon, and rectum.

My preference is cefoxitin, a second-generation cephalosporin, because it provides excellent coverage against all of the pathogens we are likely to encounter with bowel surgery in small animals.

HOW MUCH BOWEL CAN BE RESECTED?

For decades, we have been taught that removing more than 50% to 60% of the small intestine results in short bowel syndrome (SBS). Animals with SBS typically have a number of nutritional and metabolic derangements that often lead to death. Malabsorbtion, weight loss, intractable diarrhea, and fluid and electrolyte abnormalities are the most important concerns related to SBS. SBS, although talked about a lot in veterinary medicine, has only been reported in 7 dogs No cases involving cats have been described. A recent study[1] provides us with information on 13 dogs and 7 cats that had an average of 68% of the small intestine removed most often related to foreign bodies. The range was 50% to 90%. Seventeen of the animals were discharged from the hospital. Median survival time was 828 days. In 12/15 animals where long-term follow-up was available, the outcome was considered good. In this report, the percentage of bowel resected did not have a significant impact on survival time and outcome.

ANASTOMOSIS TECHNIQUES

The anastomosis of two segments of bowel should be kept simple. Everting and inverting patterns are generally unacceptable in companion animals. Disruption of the blood supply especially during the critical postoperative days 1 to 5 influences my decision to avoid these suture patterns. The simple interrupted or continuous appositional patterns are excellent in preserving the blood supply. Most surgeons today prefer a simple-interrupted or continuous appositional suture patterns. Appositional suture patterns when used in intestinal anastomoses should be limited to the adult dog and cat.

LUMEN DISPARITY

Lumen disparity associated with an intestinal resection usually requires some form of correction. Various methods are available including spatulation of the smaller bowel segment, cutting the small diameter segment of bowel at a sharp angle, or suturing the lumen of the larger bowel until its diameter matches that of the other segment. Optimal control of correcting lumen disparity in my hands is best achieved using the lumen-decreasing technique.

OMENTAL OR SEROSAL PATCHING TECHNIQUES[2]

Omental or jejunal serosal patching (using a segment of jejunum) should be used to augment primary suture lines or, in some instances, as a full-thickness "patch." I recommend a "wraparound" omental patch on all of my anastomoses or enterotomies. I now employ a skin stapler for quick and safe placement of the wraparound patch, being careful to avoid major mesenteric vessels. The jejunal serosal patch is used when a more substantial augmentation of an enterotomy or anastomosis is required, ie, when infection is present at the time of surgery or if there are some minor concerns about viability of the bowel following an enterotomy or end-to-end anastomosis.

The segment of bowel that is most difficult to resect and reestablish bowel continuity with an end-to-end anastomosis is the proximal duodenum. This is an ideal site where partial resection of a lesion can be accomplished and the bowel integrity restored using a segment of jejunum as a *full thickness* "patch." This is also an area where a "patch" using a peritoneal-musculature flap can be utilized.

FOREIGN BODIES

Linear foreign bodies (LFBs) are most often seen in cats but in my more recent experiences, I have seen a comparable incidence in dogs. The average age of cats seen with thread +/- needle was 2.7 years in one study. The needle is involved in less than 10% of the cases.

The effect of a linear foreign body initially results in partial obstruction. The pathogenesis of the obstruction results from the object becoming "fixed" somewhere cranially in the GI tract, most notably under the tongue or

within the pylorus. Normal smooth muscle contraction of the small intestine continues to propel the object aborally but due to its fixation, it will begin to do serious damage to the mesenteric border of the bowel. Continuing peristalsis against the pressure of the fixed linear object will eventually result in a perforation of the gut with leakage and peritonitis quickly following. This provides us with a huge incentive to diagnose and treat this problem as soon as possible.

Historically, the owner will recall (but not always) seeing the cat or dog playing with thread or string and may even notice it being missing shortly after the cat becomes ill. Dogs are less helpful in this regard since the source of their linear foreign body is so varied. Vomiting with regularity combined with anorexia and depression are the most common signs seen with LFBs. Weakness and dehydration may eventually result from vomiting. Some melena or blood-tinged stool may be seen.

On physical examination, some degree of dehydration is usually detected. The base of the tongue may reveal a loop of string/thread. In cats, approximately 50% of the time the LFB is found tethered under the tongue. The anus should also be examined for the presence of string. Abdominal palpation will often reveal tenderness and a "bunching up" effect of the small bowel in the cranial abdomen.

The diagnosis relies on the history and physical examination findings combined with diagnostic imaging. Abdominal radiography will usually reveal a pleated pattern sign and multiple gas bubbles appearing eccentrically throughout the affected loops. Barium contrast studies will reveal shortening of the bowel and eccentric pleating throughout the bowel. Sometimes the linear object can be seen after the barium clears portions of the bowel because it retains some of the barium contrast material. A close look at serial films will reveal that the position of the bowel remains fixed on successive films. Early peritonitis may also be verified by the loss of serosal detail. In 14% of cases radiography may be of no help in the diagnosis of LFB. Ultrasound would then be indicated to help confirm the diagnosis.

Surgery is the recommended treatment. If the string is under the tongue, it can be cut (same with string protruding from the anus) and occasionally this will alleviate the signs. Conservative management in one study (cutting the sublingually positioned string) was successful in 9 of 24 cats.

A gastrotomy combined with multiple enterotomies is the traditional method of removing LFBs. However, I prefer a technique described by Anderson, who described the possible removal of a linear object with a gastrotomy alone or combined with limited enterotomies (usually only one). The LFB is sewn to a red rubber tube cut to a length of approximately 12 to 13 cm starting at the closed tip end of the tube. The catheter is passed through the pylorus with the foreign body attached to it and is gently massaged throughout the bowel until the placations are relieved. It can either be passed completely through the bowel and be retrieved by an assistant from the anus, or it is removed through a single enterotomy incision. Although it may be tempting to primarily close a rent or tear in the mesenteric side of the bowel that may be present, I prefer to resect that segment.

If perforation and peritonitis are present at the time of surgery, then the prognosis is considerably worse for the patient. This again stresses the need for prompt and accurate diagnosis and subsequent surgery.

BIOPSIES

Intestinal biopsies may be necessary to assist in the diagnosis of bowel disease. A longitudinal incision with a side-to-side closure or a longitudinal incision followed by a transverse closure is an acceptable biopsy technique. I believe in keeping it simple: longitudinally oriented biopsies with side-to-side closure. We now routinely close these enterotomy incisions with a continuous suture pattern starting and ending just beyond the margins of the incision.

REFERENCES

1. Gorman SC, Freeman, LM, Mitchell, SL, Chan DL. Extensive small bowel resection in dogs and cats. J Amer Vet Med Assoc 2006;228:403-407.
2. Crowe DT The serosal patch: Clinical use in 12 animals, Vet Surg. 1984:13: 29-34.

GASTRIC DILATATION-VOLVULUS (GDV) – AN UPDATE

Ronald M Bright, DVM, MS, Diplomate ACVS
VCA–Veterinary Specialists of Northern Colorado
Loveland, CO

SIGNALMENT, PATHOPHYSIOLOGY, AND RISK FACTORS

Gastric dilatation-volvulus (GDV) is most commonly seen in large and giant breed dogs and occasionally in cats. Acute GDV results in an overdistention of the stomach with fluid, gas, and ingesta and is accompanied by a clockwise (rarely counterclockwise) rotation of the stomach. The distention of the stomach results from the animal's impaired ability to empty gas from the stomach.

RISK FACTORS

Recent articles published by Glickman and associates have uncovered some important information related to risk factors These risk factors can have both a positive and negative impact on a dog's chances of having a GDV episode.

Personality Traits

There appears to be a direct relationship between temperament and the tendency to develop GDV. Animals with a fearful or "unhappy" personality are more likely to develop GDV and stress plays a role in precipitating GDV as well. Hyperactive animals have a predisposition for GDV. Some families of large and giant breed dogs are at greater risk for developing GDV especially when it can be documented that a first-degree relative (parent, offspring, sibling) has had at least one confirmed incident of GDV.

Body Condition and Anatomical Factors

A thin or lean body condition (moreso in giant breeds), high abdominal depth (large and giant breeds), high thoracic depth-to-abdominal depth ratio (large breeds) and Irish Setters with an exaggerated depth-to-width ratio are factors increasing the risk for GDV.

Dietary Factors

Intake of a large amount of dry food per meal, especially when fed only once daily, is a significant risk factor for developing GDV. A rapid rate of eating and eating out of a raised feed bowl also increase the risk. Additional risks are feeding a dry food diet with fat being one of the first four ingredients. Likewise, citric acid contained in dry foods that are moistened prior to consumption increase the risk. Decreasing the risk can be accomplished feeding a dog food that has rendered meat meal with bone as one of its first four ingredients.

Other Risk Factors

Risks of dying with GDV increase fourfold when the dog is presented recumbent, threefold if depressed, 11 times if gastric perforation has occurred, and 30-fold if presented in a comatose state. Other risks factors include a lean body condition and a first-degree relative (parent, offspring, sibling) that has had a GDV event.

PATHOPHYSIOLOGY

The etiology of GDV appears to be multifactorial. Gastric distention probably results in some degree of functional or mechanical obstruction. Aerophagia is responsible for most of the gas accumulation. Fluid sources include ingesta, gastric secretions, and eventually transudate from venous obstruction due to the volvulus. The ability to relieve distention through eructation or passage of gastric contents aborally through the pylorus is impaired. The stomach usually rotates in a clockwise direction when viewing the animal from behind. The short gastric vessels may become twisted with resultant thrombosis or avulsion. The latter may contribute to the hemoabdomen within hours of GDV occurring. Over time, increased intragastric pressure eventually results in decreased blood flow to the stomach wall, which can lead to necrosis. Gastric distention eventually becomes so great that occlusion of the caudal vena cava and portal vein occurs resulting in decreased venous return from the abdomen to the heart leading to decreased cardiac output, myocardial hypoxia, hypovolemic shock, and hypotension. The cardiac-related problems may lead to arrhythmias and hypotension and decreased portal blood flow can lead to an increased rate of endotoxin release by gram-negative bacteria. These bacteria and their associated enteric toxins move across the mucosal barrier and enter the circulation via the intestinal or diaphragmatic lymphatics or peritoneal surfaces. Concurrent portal vein occlusion decreases the ability of the reticuloendothelial system to handle toxins and absorbed (translocated) bacteria.

Hypoventilation can result from decreased movement of the diaphragm. The spleen can become congested and thrombosed, and necroses and splenic torsion can occur. One report describes GDV occurring **after** splenic torsion in two dogs. It appears that reperfusion injury may be associated with GDV secondary to significant tissue damage.

CLINICAL SIGNS

The signs of GDV include recent episodes of self-limited mild to moderate gastric distention, anorexia, or occasional vomiting. Restlessness, retching, and excessive eructation or flatulence may be reported. Dogs with GDV for a lengthy period may present with depression, shock-like state, and some degree of abdominal pain.

Signs observed on physical examination include a grossly distended (tympanic) abdomen, abdominal pain, splenomegaly, and evidence of circulatory shock. Hyperpnea and dyspnea may also be observed.

Most laboratory findings are nonspecific for GDV. Hemoconcentration is commonly seen. Hypokalemia usually occurs but is often seen after the initial fluid resuscitation efforts. Plasma lactate concentration has been reported as a predictor of gastric necrosis and survival among dogs with GDV.

Various degrees of weakness may be associated with hypotension and/or cardiac arrhythmias.

TREATMENT CONSIDERATIONS (INITIAL)

Treatment traditionally consisted of rapid decompression of the stomach with an orogastric tube. If this was unsuccessful, then trocarization of the stomach was necessary. Trocarization is usually done on the left side with a 14- to 18-gauge hypodermic needle because of the movement of the spleen to the right side in most cases. However, the left side should not be used if a "ping" is not heard at the site of penetration. This may indicate the presence of the spleen or transverse colon. Following trocarization and some degree of decompression, another attempt at orogastric decompression is usually successful.

Recently, I have begun to perform the trocarization technique **first** as it is more efficient, is not as cumbersome in an awake dog, and decreases any chance of injury to the distal esophagus or stomach from the orogastric tube. It may diminish the possibility of reperfusion injury which is thought to negatively influence mortality rates. I prefer to use a 14- or 16-gauge over-the-catheter needle to accomplish this. If gastric lavage is going to be done with an orogastric tube, it can be done safely now because the stomach has been decompressed and usually derotates simultaneously. Two large-bore intravenous catheters are placed in the front legs concurrent with gastric decompression. Rapid administration of a balanced electrolyte solution (100 mL/kg the first hour) or hypertonic saline alone (4–5 mL/kg over 15 minutes) is done. If hemodynamic restoration is done with hypertonic saline or crystalloids, I routinely give 10–20 mL/kg of Hetastarch (spread out over 24 hours and usually started during surgery).

Managing these patients for pain is of paramount importance. I prefer a strong analgesic such as fentanyl (given initially after IV catheter placement at a dose of 0.005 mg/kg). A constant-rate infusion (CRI) of fentanyl is continued at a rate of 0.02–0.05 µg/kg/minute. A loading dose of ketamine (0.5 mg/kg IV) can also be given followed by the addition of 60 mg of ketamine/liter of crystalloids. If surgery is elected, the addition of lidocaine can be added to the CRI protocol. This helps manage pain while decreasing the amount of injectable or inhalant anesthesia needed during surgery. The infusion dose (CRI) is 10–50 µg/kg/min (using 2% lidocaine). When giving multiple drugs as a CRI for pain management, I prefer to have one of the drugs (fentany) administered using a syringe pump.

A broad-spectrum antibiotic (cefoxitin 20 mg/kg q8h) is given for a 48-72 hour period. Oxygen is given as needed throughout the perioperative period via a nasal cannula (when not under anesthesia). Continuous ECG monitoring is routinely done while the animal is in the hospital since cardiac dysrhythmias occur at a high rate (42%) in GDV patients. Blood pressure measurements should be taken during the perioperative period. Catheterization of the urinary bladder is done when indicated to closely monitor urine output. I routinely add 40–60 mEq/L of KCl to fluids after surgery to attempt to maintain normokalemia. Serial potassium and magnesium levels are repeated multiple times during the hospitalization period; Mg or K deficits are corrected to help prevent cardiac rhythm disturbances

With a recurrence rate of 75% to 80% following medical management, definitive treatment with a gastropexy is highly recommended. Because of the risk for aspiration pneumonia, administration of injectable metoclopramide (0.3 mg/kg SC) is given preoperatively as famotidine (0.5–1.0 mg/kg IV). Both drugs are continued for one week to protect against aspiration pneumonia and gastric ulcer/perforation.

TREATMENT (DEFINITIVE)

Some type of right-sided gastropexy is recommended after repositioning of the stomach. I prefer an incisional gastropexy due to its simplicity, speed, and predictable results. If the stomach is filled with ingesta, performing a gastrotomy and emptying the stomach is an option, I rarely do this even when the stomach contains a significant amount of ingesta. I do not believe the time and additional morbidity (contamination, failure of suture line) is justified in these patients. A splenectomy and/or partial gastrectomy may be indicated depending on the degree of pathology to these structures. An alternative to partial gastrectomy, especially if the damage to the stomach is limited to a relatively small area, is invagination of normal stomach tissue over the devitalized area. However, this **must** be followed by a period of systemic antacid therapy to prevent ulcer formation and severe hemorrhage.

PROPHYLACTIC GASTROPEXIES

Recently, the risk factors identified for GDV have stimulated a number of veterinarians to begin to offer a "prophylactic" gastropexy in those animals considered to be at a significant risk for GDV. The signalment (eg, Great Dane), temperament, and in particular, the identification of a first-degree relative with at least one episode of GDV all contribute to the decision to perform a prophylactic gastropexy. Although this can be done by standard "open" laparotomy techniques, laparoscopic or laparoscopic-assisted techniques are now being used successfully. These minimally invasive techniques allow a gastropexy to be an "in-patient" type procedure. We also recommend a prophylactic gastropexy in dogs that have been diagnosed with a chronic or partial torsion form of GDV or following surgery for a splenic torsion.

REFERENCES

1. Glickman LT, Glickman NW, Schellenberg DB, et al. Incidence of and breed-related risk factors for gastric dilatation-volvulus in dogs. J Am Vet Med Assoc. 2000;216:40-45.
2. Glickman LT; Glickman NW, Schellenberg DB, et al. Multiple risk factors for the gastric dilatation-volvulus syndrome in dogs: A practitioner/owner case-control study. J Am Anim Hosp Assoc. 1997; 33:197-202.

3. Glickman LT, Glickman NW, Schellenberg DB. Non-dietary risk factors for gastric dilatation-volvulu in large and giant breed dogs. J Am Vet Med Assoc. 2000;217:1492-1499.

4. Raghaven RM, Glickman LT, Schellenberg DB, et al. Predisposition to gastric dilatation-volvulus in relation to genetics of thoracic conformation in Irish Setters. J Am Anim Hosp. 1997;33:379-383.

5. Glickman LT, Emerick T, Glickman NW, et al. Radiological assessment of the relationship between thoracic conformation and the risk of gastric-dilatation-volvulus in dogs. Vet Rad Ultrasound. 1996:37:174-180.

6. Millis, DL, Nemzek, J, Riggs C et al. Gastric dilatation-volvulus after splenic torsion in two dogs. J Am Vet Med Assoc. 1995; 207: 314-318.

7. Badylak SF, Lantz GC, Jeffries M. Prevention of reperfusion injury in surgically-induced gastric dilatation-volvulus in dogs. Am J Vet Res. 1990:51:294-299.

8. de Papp E, Drobatz KJ, Hughes D. Plasma lactate concentration as a predictor of gastric necrosis and survival among dogs with gastric dilatation-volvulus: 102 cases (1995-1998). J Am Vet Med Assoc. 1999; 215:49-52.

9. Wagner AE, Dunlop CI, Chapman, PL. Cardiopulmonary measurements in dogs undergoing gastropexy without gastrectomy for correction of gastric dilatation-volvulus. J Am Vet Assoc. 1999;215: 49-52.

10. Parton AT, Volk SW, Weisse C. Gastric ulceration subsequent to partial invagination of the stomach in the dog with gastric dilatation-volvulus. J Am Vet Med Assoc. 2006;228:1895-1900.

11. Hardie RJ, Flanders JA, et al. Biomechanical and histological evaluation of a laparoscopic stapled gastropexy technique in dogs. Vet Surg. 1996;25: 127-132.

12. Wilson ER, Henderson RA, et al. A comparison of laparoscopic and belt-loop gastropexy in dogs. Vet Surg. 1996;25:221-224.

13. Rawlings, CR; Foutz,TL et al. A rapid and strong laparoscopic-assisted gastropexy in dogs. Am J Vet Res. 2000; 62: 871-875.

PRACTICAL RECONSTRUCTIVE SURGICAL TECHNIQUES

Ronald M Bright, DVM, MS, Diplomate ACVS
VCA-Veterinary Specialists of Northern Colorado
Loveland, CO

INITIAL MANAGEMENT OF WOUNDS

Regardless of the cause of a skin wound (iatrogenic, traumatic), reconstructive techniques can be considered after the recipient site is properly prepared. For excisional biopsies, in the case of neoplasia, reconstruction can usually be done during the same surgery. However, when tissue damage results from accidental trauma, proper preparation of the wound is mandatory to facilitate repair by a reconstructive technique.

Regardless of the circumstances surrounding the wound, the first step is to attempt to decontaminate the wound by extensive debridement and lavage. Sometimes this can be done and the wound prepared for reconstruction immediately. However, when there is extensive tissue trauma, contamination, or infection, a delayed repair is in order.

Suturing a wound within a few hours of injury is called **primary closure**. Waiting a few days before closing a wound (before the presence of granulation tissue) is termed **delayed primary closure** (usually within 4 to 5 days of injury). Closing a wound after granulation tissue has appeared is **delayed secondary closure**. Wounds left to heal by contraction and epithelialization is termed **second intention** healing and often require long periods of bandaging. Second intention healing is a less desirable way to manage larger wounds

The ideal situation for wound management is to close the wound immediately after preparation of the tissue. This is acceptable when there is little chance of a wound infection and dehiscence after closure. The decision to close a wound should be based on the integrity of the local tissue defense mechanisms and the estimation of the number and virulence of bacteria present. Wounds with excessive tissue destruction, heavy bacteria, and the presence of foreign bodies, are unsuitable for primary closure even if done within a short time after injury. Conversely, it is possible to have primary closure of wounds regardless of the time between injury and repair when there is minimal bacterial contamination and tissue destruction is not severe. If there is any doubt about the decision to primarily close a wound, it should be managed as an open wound until a more accurate assessment can be made.

Protection of the wound should be done while preparing the surrounding skin for surgery. Packing the wound with sterile saline-soaked sponges or filling the wound with sterile water-soluble jelly are acceptable methods of protecting the wound. Following a surgical scrub of the surrounding skin, the jelly or sponges can be removed by mechanical removal of the sponges or vigorous irrigation of the water-soluble jelly within the wound.

Once the wound and surrounding skin have been prepared, the entire wound must be inspected to accurately assess the extent of damage. The extent of trauma is not always obvious and requires close observation of deeper tissues, especially when encountering bite wounds.

DEBRIDEMENT

This is defined as the removal of devitalized tissue and foreign material from the wound. The goal is to convert a contaminated or infected into a surgically "clean" wound. It is difficult to standardize the methods of debridement, since the technique will vary depending on the type, location, and duration of the wound and the manner of injury. There are two basic types of debridement, *layered* and *en bloc*. **Layered** is most commonly used and involves removing devitalized tissue and foreign material beginning at the level of the skin and proceeding to the wound depths.

Badly damaged skin lacking any bleeding should be removed initially. Although skin is important for eventual wound closure, it is preferable to remove devitalized skin and graft the wound later. After removal of damaged skin, all of the deeper tissue that is devitalized, has a poor blood supply, or is heavily contaminated should be removed. This is particularly true for subcutaneous fat and muscle. Muscle that is friable or soft, has dirt ground into it, does not bleed when cut or contract when stimulated is removed. It is better to remove muscle of questionable viability than to experience the consequences of liquefaction necrosis and possible clostridial infection.

En bloc debridement is the most certain method of removing devitalized and contaminated tissue in areas where there is excess tissue. This type of debridement has limited application to extremities or in wounds with exposed nerves, blood vessels or tendons. En bloc excision is done by packing the wound with sterile gauze and suturing the overlying skin to hold it in place. The wound is then excised like a tumor including a margin of surrounding skin so the gauze in the wound is never exposed.

LAVAGE

Lavaging wounds remove foreign material and separated particles of tissue while diluting or decreasing the number of bacteria. Sterile isotonic saline is routinely used. A very large volume of lavage solution decreased the incidence of infection. Continuous and pulsatile high-pressure lavage is more effective then conventional bulb-syringe lavage although the latter is okay in most wounds.

PRIMARY VERSUS DELAYED OR SECONDARY CLOSURE

Following debridement and lavage, the surgeon must then decide if the wound can be closed. The decision to close the wound is based on the amount of devitalized tissue and contamination that remains, time interval between injury and repair, and the assurance that careful observation of the wound will be possible.

Primary closure is performed under ideal conditions and the surgeon should be convinced that healing would progress uninterrupted. If delayed closure is elected, the wound is not closed until infection has been controlled (usually 3 to 5 days after debridement and lavage). Delayed closure allows daily observation of the wound to assess the progression of healing. It also will help the surgeon decide if more debridement is necessary. Delayed closure reduces the chance of infection because it allows new blood vessels to grow into the wound bed. For the first 3 to 4 days, wet-to-dry dressings are preferred by the author using 0.5% chlorhexidine solution or saline alone. When the gauze is removed during daily (in some cases twice daily) bandage changes, nonviable tissue adheres to the gauze. After the fourth day, I prefer to change to a non-adherent pad placed on the wound that has topical application of a triple antibiotic ointment. Closure of the wound ultimately is done when the tissue appears healthy, the wound is bright red (indicating blood vessel ingrowth), and any exudate present is minimal, nonodorous, and serous in nature.

Delayed secondary closure is done <u>after</u> the formation of granulation tissue (after the fifth or sixth day). Delaying closure for an extended period of time is indicated when the wound is infected or dirty and there is a large amount of damaged tissue deep within the wound. A rim of tissue around the skin margin should always be removed just prior to closing the wound. When doing a secondary closure, the skin edges can be closed over granulation tissue. Some surgeons prefer to excise exuberant granulation tissue before closing the skin.

Wounds must be closed after minimum tension. If not, dehiscence may result due to tissue strangulation or sutures tearing through the tissue. If the wound cannot be closed without excessive tension, then a reconstructive surgical procedure should be considered. Only when all signs of infection are gone, can a skin flap or graft be performed.

PRIMARY CLOSURE USING A "WALKING" SUTURE PATTERN

This is classified as a tension-relieving suture pattern. It always surprises me how large a defect can be closed using the "walking" suture pattern. This can be used on "fresh wounds" but I primarily use it on delayed primary closure or delayed secondary closure wounds that are well vascularized. It is imperative that a cutting needle be used as the needle must engage the dermis (on the skin side) because of the tension placed on each suture. I prefer to use a monofilament suture 000 size (Biosyn, Monocryl) that has a shorter time of absorption but good initial tensile strength.

Several "rows" of sutures can be placed depending on how big the defect is and how viscoelastic the skin is surrounding the defect. The needle should first engage the dermis deep into the "cul-de-sac" and then into the tissue within the wound (Figures 1 and 2).

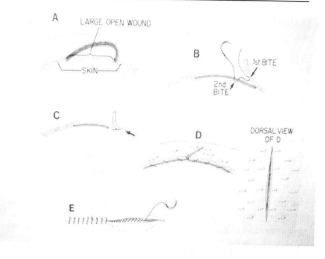

Figure 1.

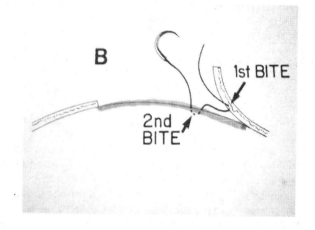

Figure 2.

SEED GRAFTS (PINCH, PUNCH, ISLAND GRAFTS)

Seed grafts are small pieces of full-thickness skin placed in a granulation tissue bed with regular spacing between the grafts. These grafts arfe harvested by elevating a piece of skin and cutting it free (pinch) or cutting is as a plug (punch). The indications for this type of graft include small wounds on limbs, contaminated wounds or low-grade infected ones, or wounds in an area where surrounding tissues may rub on the graft (axillary space) or where there is some movement.

These grafts are placed in a bed of healthy granulation tissue after removing any debris, necrotic tissue, and chronic or exuberant granulation tissue. They are usually harvested from the mid-thoracic area where the skin is thin and hairy. The top portion of the tented piece of skin is cut off at a right angle to the direction of traction with a scalpel blade. The piece of skin is approximately 2 to 4 mm in diameter. A 4-mm skin punch instrument can be used as well. On subcutaneous tissue is transferred with the piece of skin (Figure 3).

Small slit-like pockets are made with a scapel blade in the granulation tissue (see Figure 3). The pockets are 2 to 4 mm deep and 5 to 7 mm apart. A graft is placed in

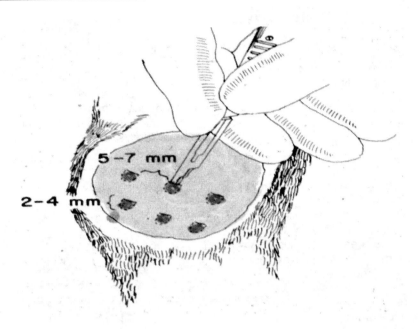

Figure 3.

each pocket. If bleeding is brisk and the graft floats out of the pocket, it can be held in place by forceps for 2 to 3 minutes or by direct digital pressure. It is best to work from dorsal to ventral when placing the grafts into the pockets. The donor site is left to heal as an open wound and covered with a bandage.

The recipient site is covered with a nonadherent bandage impregnated with an antibiotic ointment. The area is wrapped with padded cotton and gauze followed by some type of bandaging tape. The bandage is not changed the first time until the third or fourth postoperative day. These wounds will need to remain bandaged for 14 to 21 days.

The seed grafts serve as a source of epithelium that grows from each graft edge and will eventually cover all of the surfaces of the granulation tissue. Some epithelium will also migrate inwardly from the edges of the wound.

PRACTICAL RECONSTRUCTIVE SURGERY— HOW WOULD YOU CLOSE IT?

Ronald M Bright, DVM, MS, Diplomate ACVS
VCA–Veterinary Specialists of Northern Colorado
Loveland, CO

AXIAL PATTERN SKIN FLAP

An axial pattern flap has a single neurovascular trunk that allows a segment of skin to be moved to an adjacent site while remaining viable. A number of these have been used and identified in the dog for reconstruction purposes with excellent results.

A 6-year-old Schnauzer is presented with a "dirty" margin related to incomplete excision of a soft tissue sarcoma. It involves the stifle area located just slightly medial to the patella. A wide (3-cm margin) excision is required. What are some viable options?

    a. Full-thickness free mesh graft
    b. Sliding graft (pedicle graft)
    c. Island ("seed") graft
    d. Other?

This location is ideal for an axial pattern graft and in this case, a caudal superficial epigastric graft was used. This graft has a major vessel (caudal superficial epigastric artery) that supplies a segment of skin and subcutaneous tissue. Depending on the conformation of the dog (long-legged retriever vs. dachshund or corgi), this graft can be used to reconstruct defects in the flank, inner thigh, and inguinal areas. In the short-legged/long body breeds, it may reach distally as far as the knee or hock.

Technique

1. The surgeon doing mastectomies in either the dog or cat should be comfortable with this technique since there are many similarities. The second through fifth mammae is the maximum amount of skin that can be moved to repair a defect. The flap can be placed on a fresh or granulating bed. A measurement should be made from just behind the last mammary gland to the most cranial mammary gland needed to form a flap that is of the desired length to fill the defect (Figure 1).
2. A superficial epigastric axial pattern flap is started making two parallel incisions starting 2 to 3 cm caudal to the last mammary gland. The incisions are carried cranially to the desired length and joined. The end of this axial flap will only remain viable if the cranial limit stops at the 2nd mammary gland. Subcutaneous tissue is bluntly excised and the flap is raised from the muscle fascia underneath.
3. The flap is now rotated to cover the wound defect (Figure 1).
4. The flap is sutured in place.
5. The donor site is closed by undermining the skin and advancing the edges together with a "walking" suture pattern. To get a longer and somewhat more mobile flap, the flap can be made into a four-sided "island" flap by connecting the medial and lateral flap incisions behind the last mammary gland. When this is done, the incision should be limited to the SKIN only to avoid cutting the epigastric vessels (Figure 2).
6. Sterile sponges are placed over the wounds and bandaged with multiple layers of soft bandaging material. The bandage should be changed at least daily the first 3 days.

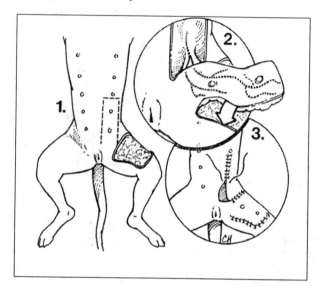

Figure 1.

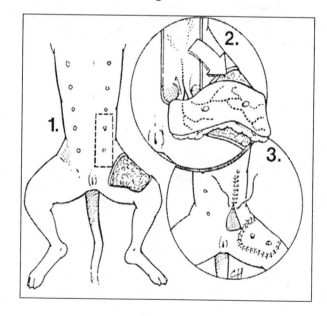

Figure 2.

DIRECT FLAPS

We have very few options when dealing with distal limb injuries. Most of the time direct flaps are applicable to injuries involving the carpus/tarsus area and areas distal to this. Alternative reconstructive techniques are iimited but could include island ("seed") grafts, full-thickness mesh grafts, and partial thickness grafts.

These flaps are distant flap development and transfer type grafts. This is a two-stage technique. The limb with the defect is moved to the flap and secured to it for 12 to 14 days before the pedicle(s) can be divided and the transfer complete.

The donor site is located over the lateral or ventrolateral surface of the thorax or abdomen. The width of the flap is made to match the width of the defect. The length of the flap is determined by the length of the defect and the additional length needed to position the flap over the recipient site. The flap base is positioned dorsally or ventrally depending on where the defect is located on the limb. Once the skin flap is sutured in place, two sutures, one above and below the graft site, are placed between the leg and body wall skin to assist in keeping the leg immobile under the bandage.

Lateral defects on the limb are easiest to repair whereas medial or circumferential defects are more challenging. The medial and circumferential defects are closed by wrapping the transected pedicle(s) of the flap around the medial aspect of the wound during the second stage procedure (Figure 3).

Warning! This technique is generally NOT suitable for large, old, or arthritic animals. When the leg is bandaged to the body wall for the 12 to 14 days between surgeries, the animal must be able to walk on three legs. Obviously, it is most suitable for use in small dogs or cats.

These distant flaps, as depicted above, can be either single or bipedicle grafts. The single ("hinge") flap is adequate for 90- to 180-degree lesions and the flap is sutured along three sides. During the second-stage surgery 12 to 14 days later, the fourth side is sutured.

The bipedicle flap requires making a "belt-loop" on the body wall as seen in Figure 3. This can cover a wound involving the entire circumference of the leg. Initially, it is sutured on two sides to the body wall (cranial/caudal).

When the pedicle is divided and the remainder of the wound covered, revascularization between the recipient bed and the donor piece of skin has occurred. Sometimes if the length of donor skin is great, it may be necessary to transect the pedicles in stages, ie, half of the width of the pedicle every 2 to 3 days starting on the 10th day. After the transection is complete and the recipient defect covered, the donor defect is closed.

Bandages are necessary to secure the leg to the trunk (along with the two sutures between the body wall and leg. The bandage over the leg and flap is usually changed every **3 days** until th e second stage transfer is complete.

MOVING LOCAL TISSUES TO CLOSE SURFACE DEFECTS

Random-based flaps are flaps based on numerous small blood vessels and take advantage of recruiting adjacent skin into wound defects. These flaps take advantage of the viscoelasticity characteristics of skin. Depending on the location of the defect, a random-based flap (also referred to as a subdermal plexus flap)

can be either single or double pedicle. (Figures 4, 5, 6) These flaps require redundant tissue adjacent to the wound. The flap maintains a point of attachment at the donor site and is nourished by a random blood supply via the subdermal plexus. These flaps are also classified according to the shape and movement of the flap.

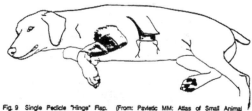

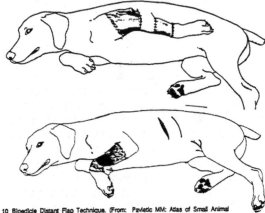

Fig. 9 Single Pedicle "Hinge" Flap. (From: Pavletic MM: Atlas of Small Animal Reconstructive Surgery. Philadelphia, J.B. Lippincott, Co., 1993)

Fig. 10 Bipedicle Distant Flap Technique. (From: Pavletic MM: Atlas of Small Animal Reconstructive Surgery. Philadelphia, J.B. Lippincott, Co., 1993)

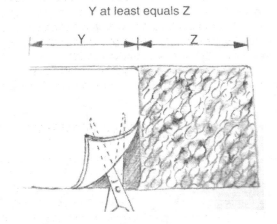

Figure 3.

Y at least equals Z

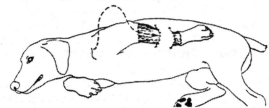

Figure 4.

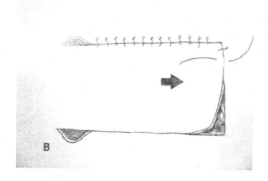

Figure 5.

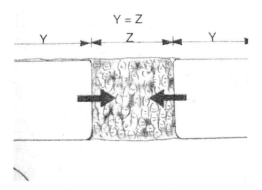

Figure 6.

I prefer to have the suture emerging at both ends so traction can be applied daily from either end. Intravenous fentanyl is given prior to pulling the skin together as this manipulation appears to be painful. Once the edges meet, I place a continuous suture to keep the edges apposed. These skin sutures and the intradermal suture are removed in 10 to 12 days.

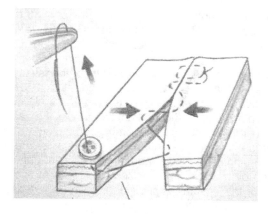

Figure 7.

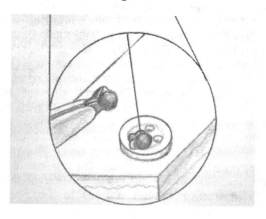

Figure 8.

The closure is accomplished with walking type sutures. The triangles in Figure 5 are used when there is a "dog ear" formation.

ADJUSTABLE HORIZONTAL MATTRESS SUTURE

This is an intradermal suture that is tightened periodically to gradually pull together the edges of a wound. I use these mostly in fresh wounds but can be used or wounds that already have begun to contract. An intradermal mattress suture starts at one end and continues to the end of the wound in a continuous placement fashion (Figure 7). The final bite allows the needle to emerge through the full thickness of the skin and pass through a button. A split shot is then placed on the suture while placing a small amount of tension on the suture (Figure 8).

ACKNOWLEDGMENTS
1. Figures 1, 2, 4, 5, 6, 7, and 8 reprinted with permission from Swaim SF, Henderson RA. Small Animal Wound Management, 2nd ed. Baltimore: Williams & Wilkins, 2007.

HOW I USE OMENTUM

Ronald M Bright, DVM, MS, Diplomate ACVS
VCA-Veterinary Specialists of Northern Colorado
Loveland, CO

BACKGROUND

The omentum has proven to be an organ of exceptional versatility. Until the 1800s, its role and function remained a mystery. Its ability to seal perforations, hernias, and fight infections has been demonstrated. It has been used to help achieve hemostasis, neovascularize devitalized structures, and provide lymphatic drainage. It has earned the nickname, deservedly, of the "abdominal policeman." Since the early 1900s, omentum has been used in a variety of surgical situations most notably in gastrointestinal and urogenital operations in people.

Extra abdominal uses of the omentum were first reported in the 1930s in humans and for chest reconstruction in animals in the 1980s. The omental lengthening procedures described by Ross and Pardo in the dog gave new impetus for further exploration into the extraabdominal uses of omentum.

ANATOMY AND PHYSIOLOGY

The greater omentum varies in size and texture between animals. It originates from the greater curvature of the stomach and extends caudally to the pelvic inlet. It serves a number of important functions but animals can survive without it. It increases serosal surface area for fluid production and absorption. It protects the abdominal viscera and aids in the localization and resolution of peritonitis.

CLINICAL USES OF OMENTUM

The omentum is rich with vascular and lymphatic plexuses and has great mobility. It can adhere to a site of contamination or injury with the peritoneal cavity and help contain infection. It also contributes neovascularization and increases oxygen tension to tissue that may be partially devascularized. The omentum participates directly in bacterial and foreign material absorption and in the transport of phagocytes into the peritoneal cavity.

Over the last 100 years, human surgeons have used omentum in reconstructive surgery in virtually all areas of the body. In the late 19th century, it was used to close perforated gastroduodenal ulcers

Reported Uses in People
Intra-abdominal:
- Repair of vesicovaginal and vesicocolic fistulas
- Augmentation of bowel anastamoses
- Augmentation of wound closures involving the urinary bladder
- Repair of defects of the abdominal wall

Extra-abdominal:
- Support of primary suture lines of the esophagus
- Closure of full-thickness defects of the esophagus
- Repair of thoracic wall defects
- Palliation of lymphedema of an extremity
- Revasularization of tissue that is ischemic
  - Brain of stroke victims
  - Myocardial ischemia
  - Non-healing wounds of the skin
- Resurface scalp defects
- Reconstruct facial deformities
- Repair of bronchopleural fistulas

Uses Reported in Literature (Veterinary)
Intra-abdominal
- Augment intestinal surgery wounds (enterotomy, end-to-end anastomosis)
- Prostatic abscesses and cysts
- Augment urinary bladder incision lines
- Pancreatic abscesses
- Liver biopsy sites

Extra-abdominal
- Thoracic wall defects created by "en-bloc" excision of rib tumors/abscesses
- Non-healing wounds (mostly in cats)
- Diaphragmatic repair
- Primary lymphedema
- Drainage of chylothorax

CHARACTERISTICS OF OMENTUM AND ITS USE IN RECONSTRUCTIVE SURGERY

The unique characteristics of omentum make it useful for reconstructive surgery. Its pliability can allow it to fill deep, irregular, and rigid spaces and be spread and distributed over wide flat defects. It may be lengthened to cover defects. When it is detached from the stomach and based on the right or left gastroepiploic pedicle, it reaches the axillary and inguinal regions in most instances. More specialized lengthening procedures in the dog will allow it to extend to the hock or elbow and possibly further (see below).

On occasion, an animal will present with a wound that will not heal in spite of excellent wound management, primary wound closure, and an attempt at treating an underlying cause. If all causes of impaired wound healing are eliminated but the wound continues to not heal, omentum can be mobilized and moved to the site of the wound in an attempt to provide new arterial, venous, and lymphatic communications. This will hopefully alter the mileau of the wound so it can eventually undergo primary healing. In particular, this has been a method used successfully in cats with chronic non-healing wounds.

The omentum can be lengthened by various methods and mobilized to the desired intraabdominal or extra-abdominal locations. When used extra-abdominally, it is tunneled subcutaneously to reach the desired location.

LENGTHENING PROCEDURES

A cranial ventral abdominal midline incision can be used to gain access to the omentum and its attachments. Other lengthening procedures may or may not be necessary for some intraabominal techniques (pancreatic abscesses, liver biopsies, prostatic abscesses/cysts and urinary bladder). Depending on the use of the omentum, it may be advisable to use a paracostal approach to free up the omentum while forming a pedicle. This approach is usually reserved for extra-abdominal uses of omentum.

When a length of an omentum is too short to reach the desired location, a left or right gastroepiploic pedicle can be developed (Figure 1).

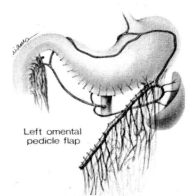

Figure 1.

Alternatively, freeing up the dorsal leaf of the omentum can develop increased length of the omental pedicle. This is done by separating and dividing the omentum from its short epiploic vessels and from a few vascular attachments to the spleen and pancreas. This immediately doubles the length of the omentum that is available (Figures 2 and 3). An inverted "L" shaped incision will allow further lengthening of the omentum (Figures 4 and 5).

The omentum is then moved to the desired location within the abdomen (pancreas, bladder, prostate). If the omentum is moved extraabdominally, it is tunneled subcutaneously to the site of the wound. The omentum exits a defect created ventrally or paracostally in the abdominal wall. In the case of chest wall reconstruction a paracostal incision is ideal. (Figure 6)

After the tunneling is complete, the omentum is placed within the wound and gently tacked to the underlying subcutaneous tissue or fascia. The skin adjacent to the wound is now apposed over the omentum. Drains may or may not be used, depending on the discretion of the surgeon. In most cases, a drain is not necessary.

The full-thickness wound created to allow the omentum to exit the abdomen is closed sufficiently to prevent any evisceration while preserving the blood supply of the pedicle. Is it necessary to go back and completely close the wound at a later date? For paracostal wounds, this is not necessary. If the exit wound is ventral in location, however, I recommend that the amputation of the omental pedicle at the level of the body wall be done followed by complete closure of the wound. This should not be done until 4 to 6 weeks after the initial surgery.

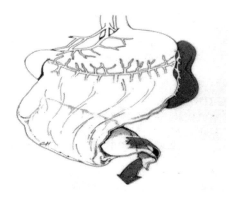

Figure 2.

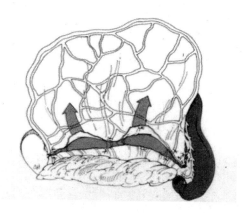

Figure 3.

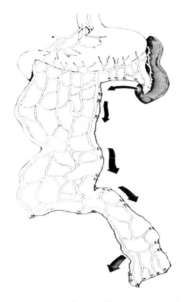

Figure 4.

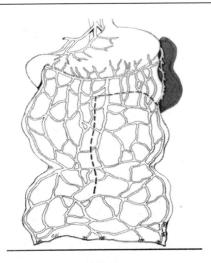

Figure 5.

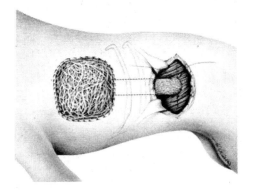

Figure 6.

References

1. Brockman DJ, Pardo, AD et al. Omentum-enhanced reconstruction of chronic nonhealing wounds in cats: techniques and clinical use. Vet Surg. 1996;25:99-104.

2. Roa DM, Bright RM, et al. Microvascular transplantation of a free omental graft to the distal extremity in dogs. Vet Surg. 1999;28:456-465.

3. Lascelles BDX, Davison L. Use of omental pedicle grafts in the management of non-healing axillary wounds in 10 cats. J Small Anim Pract. 1998;39:475-480.

4. Ross WE, Pardo AD. Evaluation of an omental pedicle extension technique in the dog. Vet Surg. 1993;22:37-43.

5. Johnson MD, Mann FA. Treatment of pancreatic abscesses via omentalization with abdominal closure versus open peritoneal drainage in dogs: 15 cases (1994-2004).

BRACHYCEPHALIC AIRWAY DISEASE

Daniel J. Brockman, BVSc, CVR, CSAO,
Diplomate ACVS and ECVS, FHEA, MRCVS
Royal Veterinary College, University of London
Hatfield, Hertfordshire, United Kingdom

Brachycepahlic airway disease is a group of conditions commonly found among brachycephalic breeds. Skull foreshortening has not been accompanied by changes in the soft tissues of the head, in these breeds. Although invariably present to a greater or lesser extent the upper airway abnormalities do not always warrant attention. Owners become used to the noise their dogs make when breathing. In addition, despite the fact that the abnormalities are present at birth, clinical disease may not be a problem until middle age; do not rule this out just because the animal has not had a problem for the first 4 years of its life.

The primary pathology includes:

- Stenotic nares
- Long soft palate

Secondary pathology includes:

- Secondary pathology includes:
- Eversion of the lateral ventricles
- Laryngeal collapse

In addition, many brachycephalic dogs have some degree of tracheal hypoplasia, redundant pharyngeal mucosa, and scrolling of the epiglottis, compounding their poor conducting airway function.

CLINICAL FEATURES

With mild disease these dogs may only show exercise intolerance or dyspnea following periods of stress or excitement. The condition may be exacerbated by extreme heat and other forms of stress so as to precipitate an acute obstructive crisis resulting in cyanosis and collapse. Acute exacerbations of this condition require emergency measures such as sedation, oxygen supplementation, intravenous fluid administration, and emergency intubation or tracheostomy. Affected animals usually make a loud noise during both inspiration and expiration (louder than normal!) and have visibly small external nares. When these animals become distressed, laryngeal and pharyngeal edema develops, worsening the obstruction. Impaired heat dissipation, along with increase muscular effort, results in pyrexia and a vicious cycle develops.

INVESTIGATION/DIAGNOSIS

These are aimed at ruling out other causes of inadequate ventilation/tissue perfusion. A full physical examination should help rule out cardiovascular disease and pulmonary disease, although auscultation is notoriously difficult in these animals because of referred upper airway noise.

- Hematology and serum biochemistry
- Thoracic radiography – Often normal, but occasionally demonstrates alveolar disease (presumptive post-obstruction pulmonary edema and/or aspiration pneumonia) and will give information regarding tracheal diameter
- Lateral radiograph of the larynx – See large, full soft palate, extending caudally and occupying almost all the common pharynx. There may also be air shadows present in the area of the lateral ventricles.

Definitive diagnosis of the soft palate and laryngeal deformity is made under general anesthesia. It is easier to examine the larynx without an endotracheal tube in place but be prepared to place one at any time; also be ready to place a temporary tracheostomy to allow recovery from anesthesia whether surgery has been performed or not. A large edematous soft palate along with edematous folds of pharyngeal mucosa will obstruct the view of the larynx. The soft palate should normally end just caudal to the tonsillar crypts. As a rule, if the soft palate is not edematous, it is probably not causing an immediate problem. The larynx will appear closed dorsally (collapse of the arytenoids) and may be full ventrally (everted ventricles) and generally edematous.

TREATMENT

This must be planned carefully. Whenever possible, airway surgery should be performed at the beginning of the day so that the patient can have constant supervision for the first few hours following surgery (the most critical time). A single large dose of short-acting corticosteroids should be administered prior to surgical manipulation of the airways (dexamethasone 0.5–1 mg/kg IV). It is best to follow examination of the upper airways with surgical treatment if necessary rather than have to give a second anesthetic.

Once the decision to perform surgery has been made, some surgeons like to place a tracheostomy tube to allow manipulation of instruments inside the oral cavity (see later). The dog is placed in ventral recumbency and the nares, if stenotic, are treated by removing a small wedge of the parietal cartilage as shown in Figure 1. The mouth is then held open using tape suspended between two drip stands. The caudal edge of the soft palate is grasped with Allis tissue forceps and drawn forward. Two mosquito forceps are placed across the palate at the level of the caudal tonsillar crypt. The redundant soft palate is excised and with the forceps still in place a continuous suture is loosely placed to oversew the ends of the cut palate. The forceps are then removed and the suture pulled tight, minimal bleeding should occur. The laryngeal ventricles are removed quite simply by grasping them with Allis tissue forceps and carefully cutting them out using Metzenbaum scissors; be careful not to damage the vocal folds caudal to these as excessive scar tissue production (webbing) may result.

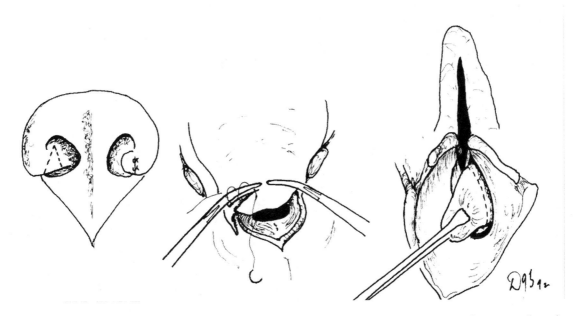

Figure 1. With the dog in ventral recumbency, the nares, if stenotic, are treated by removing a small wedge of the parietal cartilage.

Postoperative Care

Postoperative care consists of routine tracheostomy management. This can generally be removed 12 to 24 hours after surgery. Antibiotics are not necessary. The animal should be kept as quiet as possible for the following 7 to 10 days.

TRACHEAL HYPOPLASIA

A condition common in bulldogs, tracheal hypoplasia is characterized by a narrowed trachea. There is no surgical treatment for this condition. Generally, affected animals can live a normal life, providing their upper airway is in good condition.

TRACHEOTOMY
Temporary Tracheostomy

A temporary tracheostomy is performed as a routine precaution prior to some upper airway surgery or in the emergency situation to bypass life-threatening upper airway obstruction. Any animal that has a tracheostomy tube in place needs constant supervision! A selection of tracheostomy tubes is available; if they are to be used to maintain anesthesia, cuffed ones are best. If they are to be used to maintain an airway for longer periods of time, the type that has removable central cannulas that facilitate cleaning is probably better. Have a selection of tube sizes available and select a tube for the patient that will allow good flow of air both through and around it.

Placement

If at all possible, this procedure should be performed under aseptic conditions; however, some emergency situations will prevent all but cursory cleanliness. A ventral midline skin incision is made in the neck 2 to 4 cm caudal to the larynx. The sternohyoid/sternothyroid muscles are separated in the midline to reveal the ventral trachea. Long stay sutures of 2-0 monofilament nylon are placed around tracheal rings with two tracheal rings separating them (Figure 2). An incision is made between the fourth and fifth tracheal rings between the stay sutures and the tube placed into the tracheal lumen. The skin is closed around the tracheostomy tube and the tube is secured by passing umbilical tape or similar around the dog's neck. The pre-placed stay sutures are tied in a loose bow.

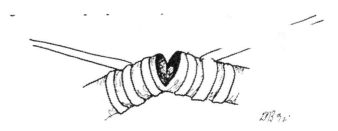

Figure 2. Placement of a temporary tracheoastomy tube.

CARE OF A TRACHEOSTOMY TUBE

As previously stated, animals with tracheostomy tubes in place require constant monitoring. The lumen of the tube will become occluded by tracheobronchial secretions and blood if it is not cleaned regularly. Thus tubes with insert sleeves are recommended for all but very short periods of time. If the tube is the correct size the animal will breathe around it when the proximal airway is patent. This will be a good indicator as to when a tube can be removed. In the event that the tube becomes removed prematurely, the stay sutures will allow the trachea to be gently pulled up to the skin incision, permitting easy replacement of the tube. Once the tube can be safely removed it is simply pulled out leaving the hole to heal by secondary intention. Keep animal quiet for several days following tube removal. If the skin heals prior to the tracheal defect sealing, subcutaneous emphysema can develop, which in the extreme situation could lead to pneumomediastinum, pneumothorax, and death.

Permanent tracheostomy is a satisfactory salvage procedure.

OUTCOME

The prognosis for these dogs is good in general. Dogs presented while young typically do better following surgical therapy than dogs that do not present until later in life. Theories that might explain this revolve around fatigue and atrophy of the pharyngeal musculature, producing untreatable pharyngeal obstruction in older dogs.

BASIC CARDIAC SURGERY

Daniel J. Brockman, BVSc, CVR, CSAO,
Diplomate ACVS and ECVS, FHEA, MRCVS
Royal Veterinary College, University of London
Hatfield, Hertfordshire, United Kingdom

VASCUAR RING ANOMOLIES

Vascular ring anomalies are congenital (developmental) abnormalities of the great vessels. These conditions are rare. Different forms exist, including persistent right aortic arch, double aorta, aberrant left subclavian, aberrant right subclavian, and persistent right ductus with a left aortic arch.

PERSISTENT RIGHT AORTIC ARCH

This anomaly accounts for approximately 95% of all "vascular ring" anatomic variants. It commonly occurs along with an aberrant left subclavian. Breeds commonly affected include German Shepherd dogs and Irish setters but many other breeds have been reported.

Pathogenesis and Pathophysiology

Development of the aorta from the right fourth rather than the left fourth aortic arch results in confinement of the esophagus between the right-side aorta and the ligamentum arteriosum (which develops from the left sixth aortic arch). The left subclavian artery can also constrict the esophagus as it crosses from right to left. The esophagus cranial to the confinement becomes dilated and dysfunctional. The degree of compromise to swallowing is probably inversely proportional to the size of the residual esophageal lumen through the area of narrowing in addition to esophageal function oral to this site. Regurgitation of especially solid food meals may result in aspiration pneumonia. The inability to pass sufficient nourishment beyond the heart base results in malnourishment despite a ravenous appetite.

Diagnosis
History and Physical Examination

Affected animals typically demonstrate intolerance of solid food around the time of weaning. The severity of regurgitation varies, however, according to the diameter of the esophageal lumen. Physical examination can reflect changes that range from extreme ill thrift and aspiration pneumonia, to a normal animal. Occasionally, air-filled cervical megaesophagus can be appreciated during physical examination.

Radiographic Evaluation

Plain film radiographs may reveal cranial thoracic megaesophagus, and a right-sided aorta causing the trachea to deviate abruptly in the mid-thorax and evidence of pulmonary alveolar disease (pneumonia). Barium swallow usually confirms megaesophagus cranial to an esophageal constriction at the heart base along with a normal esophaus aboral to this location.

Treatment

Stabilize medically prior to surgery (antibiotics for pneumonia, nutritional support: feeding tube). For a left fourth or fifth intercostal thoracotomy, isolate and divide the ligamentum between ligatures, and divide any other constricting fibrous tissue. Check for retroesophageal left subclavian artery and divide between ligatures if present. Check esophageal patency by passing a large bore stomach tube, and follow with routine closure.

Postoperative treatment includes continued therapy for pneumonia (if present), and feeding gruel from an elevated platform.

Outcome

Prognosis is fair to good. Clients should be aware that it may be necessary to continue to feed the pet from an elevated platform indefinitely. Occasionally megaesophagus never resolves

PATENT DUCTUS ARTERIOSUS (PDA)
Pathogenesis

Eccentric distribution of smooth muscle and elastic tissue in the intima of the ductus prevents postnatal closure of this structure. If the rest of heart and lung development is normal, left to right shunting of blood occurs. If fetal pulmonary circulation persists, right to left shunting is more likely.

Treatment

Left to right shunting PDAs should be occluded. A right to left shunting PDA is not amenable to surgical treatment.

PDA Occlusion

Although many centers are now occluding PDAs with transarterial vascular coils and embolization devices, traditional surgical occlusion still predominates. The ductus is approached through a left fourth intercostal thoracotomy (left fifth is occasionally better in dogs and commonly better for cats). The ductus is identified and carefully dissected free from its mediastinal attachments so as to allow passage of a ligature around the vessel. Extreme care and considerable skill is required for this dissection since the craniomedial aspect of the ductus shares a common adventitia with the aorta and is very delicate at this site. In addition, inadvertent puncture of the pulmonary artery can occur during dissection of the medial ductus. The surgeon must have the expertise or backup to attempt salvage of a ruptured ductus before embarking on this surgical procedure. Once encircled, the ductus is ligated with one ligature on either side of a transfixed ligature (ie, three ligatures). Chest closure is routine.

Outcome

Successful ligation gives excellent results in young dogs with return of cardiac changes to normal. Dogs presented as adults may not have complete resolution of atrial enlargement or mitral regurgitation (if present) but will still enjoy improved quality of life. Five to 10% of dogs undergoing this procedure will have rupture of the ductus during surgery. In inexperienced hands, these patients frequently exsanguinate and die. For experienced surgeons, the fatality rate is less than 1%.

PERICARDIAL EFFUSION
Pathogenesis

Pericardial effusion can develop secondary to trauma, neoplasia, viral or bacterial infection, right heart failure, and rupture of the left atrium. Primary idiopathic pericardial effusion also occurs

Surgical Management (Subtotal Pericardectomy)

This procedure can be curative in some cases of recurrent (presumed) idiopathic pericardial effusion (recurred three or more times) and infective pericarditis. It may be palliative in the treatment of slow-growing intrapericardial neoplasia (chemodectoma). Finally, it may be used as a diagnostic procedure.

Technique

Subtotal pericardectomy may be performed through a right lateral (fifth intercostal), a left lateral (fifth intercostal) or mid-line sternal approach depending on the pathology suspected and surgeon preference. In addition, thoracoscopic pericardial windows may provide good palliation for animals known to have neoplastic pericardial effusions.

The pericardium is emptied of fluid, the phrenic nerves are identified and gently elevated from the pericardium (this may be difficult from a lateral approach and is, therefore, not done on the side opposite the thoracotomy). The pericardium is removed as close to the heart base as is safe. Some animals with idiopathic and infective effusion will have markedly thickened pericardium with neovascularisation. Electrocautery is often needed to limit the haemorrhage from the incised pericardial surface.

Closure is routine but thoracostomy tubes frequently need to be maintained for extended periods of time to manage excessive effusion.

HOW I TREAT URETHRAL SPHINCTER MECHANISM INCOMPETENCE

Daniel J. Brockman, BVSc, CVR, CSAO,
Diplomate ACVS and ECVS, FHEA, MRCVS
Royal Veterinary College, University of London
Hatfield, Hertfordshire, United Kingdom

URETHRAL SPHINCTER MECHANISM INCOMPETENCE

Urethral sphincter mechanism incompetence (USMI) has also been called: estrogen-responsive/dependent incontinence, pelvic bladder incontinence, and short urethra incontinence. It may be analogous to urge or stress incontinence in women. This type of incontinence arises when the sphincter mechanism of the urinary bladder becomes overwhelmed and permits "overflow" of urine. The sphincter mechanism of the bladder is found at the trigone and the proximal urethra. It has active smooth muscle and skeletal muscle components and passive elastic components within the wall of the distal bladder and proximal urethra. The sphincter mechanism is under autonomic and somatic neural control and is, therefore, under conscious and unconscious control. In addition, the sphincter mechanism is influenced by changes in intrabdominal pressure as well as intravesicular pressure. Sphincter mechanism incompetence may be congenital but most commonly it is an acquired form of incontinence that becomes evident in older female dogs and occasionally in male dogs. Risk factors for the development of this form of incontinence appear to be breed, age when ovariohysterectomy was performed, and overall age.

HISTORY AND CLINICAL FEATURES

Historically, affected patients have a "postural" incontinence and/or leak urine at times of rest or, occasionally, excitement. Classically, dogs with this condition will leave puddles of urine after sleeping or when lying down. The incontinence may be intermittent and inconsistent. Physical examination of the animal is nonremarkable.

DIAGNOSIS

Diagnostic investigations are aimed at ruling out other causes of incontinence. Serum chemistry, complete blood count, urinalysis, and radiographic imaging (excretory urography, retrograde vaginourethrography), and cystoscopy will help rule out other pathology that could explain incontinence. Attempts to make urethral pressure profilometry a "test" for USMI have not been successful but a urethral pressure profile is considered useful information by many investigators. Sphincter mechanism incompetence is, therefore, a diagnosis by exclusion.

THERAPY
Medical

The mainstay for therapy is medical. Alpha adrenergic agents such as phenylpropanolamine can be cuarative for many patients. Judicious use of estrogens alone or in combination can help control animals who fail alpha-adrenergic therapy. Caution must be used in prescribing prolonged estrogen therapy because of the potential side effect of bone marrow suppression.

Surgical/Invasive Treatments

If medical therapy fails, surgical therapy may be indicated. Some of the treatments that have been advocated for management of USMI are summarized in Table 1.

Of the procedures that have been reported, colposuspension has undergone the most rigorous scientific investigation. Research on this procedure has shown it to be helpful in 90% of affected dogs and unhelpful in the remaining 10%. The procedure has only been used in the female dog and involves sutures passed through the vaginal stump and around the prepubic tendon on either side of the bladder neck. This procedure has the effect of pulling the bladder into a more intra-abdominal position, thereby allowing an increase in the influence of intra-abdominal pressure over the urethral sphincter mechanism. In addition, it will gently entrap the proximal urethra. It has been shown that this technique increases the overall length of the effective urethra and the maximal urethral closure pressure. A variation on this operation has been used in male dogs with USMI with some good effect. Fixation of the deferent ducts to the lateral body wall can also draw the male urinary bladder into a more intra-abdominal position. This procedure has not been evaluated in as many animals as colposuspension.

Table 1. Surgical Procedures Advocated for the Management of USMI

Procedure	No. Treated	Cured	Improved	Failed
Colposuspension	183	53%	37%	10%
Polytef/collagen injections	22	77%	----	23%
Cystourethropexy	10	60%	30%	10%
Urethropexy	100	62%	30%	8%

Retropubic Vaginopexy (Colposuspension)
Technique

The patient is clipped and prepared for surgery in a routine manner. A Foley urethral catheter is placed. The perivulval skin should be included in the prepared surgical field and the vagina should be lavaged with dilute chlorhexidine solution. The dog should be positioned in dorsal recumbency in a "frog-leg" position. The sterile drapes must be positioned to allow access to the vulva but the vulva should be covered during the parts of the procedure that don't require its access.

Caudal mid-line abdominal skin incision from just cranial to the umbilicus to just beyond the cranial pubis is made. The prepubic tendons are exposed by dissection. The abdominal cavity is entered, abdominal retractors positioned, and a "traction" suture is placed in the cranial pole of the urinary bladder. Gentle traction on the bladder will maintain an intra-abdominal bladder position and minimize the risk of iatrogenic urethral injury. The surgeon must then place a lubricated finger through the vulva into the vaginal body. With this finger in position the vaginal wall should be exposed, on either side of the urethra, in the caudal abdomen by blunt dissection. Once exposed, the vaginal wall is grasped by Allis tissue forceps on either side of the urethra. The surgeon should then remove the finger from the vagina and change surgical gloves. The vulva should be draped out of the field of surgery again. Two sutures of 2-0 or 0 polypropylene are preplaced around the prepubic tendon and through the vaginal body on each side. The suture needle should pass through the ventrolateral vaginal wall in either a craniocaudal or caudocranial direction rather than a lateromedial direction. Once all the sutures are placed, they are securely tied. The surgeon should ensure that it is possible to pass a "little finger" through the space between the sutures and the pubic bone, to ensure that the urethra is not obstructed. Abdominal wall closure is routine. The urethral catheter should be maintained for 12 hours.

Dogs undergoing this procedure must be kept quiet for several weeks after surgery. Strenuous physical activity must be avoided for 4 to 6 weeks, so as to avoid avulsion of the sutures.

HOW I TREAT ECTOPIC URETERS

Daniel J Brockman, BVSc, CVR, CSAO,
Diplomate ACVS/ECVS, FHEA, MRCVS
Royal Veterinary College, University of London
Hatfield, Hertfordshire, United Kingdom

URETERIC ECTOPIA AND URETEROCELE

Ectopic ureters are ann anomaly resulting from abnormal development of the metanephric ducts from the mesonephric buds that arise from the mesonephric ducts resulting in caudal displacement of the ureteric openings. One or both ureters enter the urethra or vagina of female dogs and the prostatic urethra or seminal vesicles of the male dog. Breed and familial predisposition for Siberian huskies and Golden retrievers have been suggested.It is commonly associated with other congenital abnormalities such as hydronephrosis, short urethra, disorders of the bladder sphincter mechanism, renal hypoplasia, and hydroureter. Most ectopic ureters follow an intramural (within the wall of the bladder and proximal urethra) course but occasionally will be entirely separate (extramural). Ureterocele is a dilation of an intracystic portion of the (usually ectopic) ureter. This may be associated with a duplex urine collection system (ie, two renal pelves and two ureters from the same kidney) The condition is usually treated in a similar manner to other cases of ectopia but may require excision of the redundant collection system.

HISTORY AND CLINICAL FEATURES

This is most commonly diagnosed in female dogs that have had a dribbling incontinence since birth. Affected animals commonly can void small amounts of urine normally but often dribble constantly and have staining of the perivulval skin and hair and occasionally dermatitis on the ventrum. It has also been seen in aged female dogs with late onset incontinence, and in the cat. It is relatively infrequently diagnosed in males but may be just as common. Ectopia causes incontinence less frequently in males probably because of the length of the urethra and urethralis muscle (and therefore the sphincter mechanism). If incontinence does not occur, hydronehrosis and or pyelonephritis may be the presenting disease.

DIAGNOSIS

A cystocentesis or catheter urine sample should be obtained for urinalysis, culture and sensitivity. Routine CBC and serum chemistry should be performed. The diagnosis of ureteric ectopia is confirmed radiographically, under general anesthesia, by excretory urography (fluoroscopy is helpful) and/or retrograde vaginourethrography. Remember to prepare the patient adequately for this study (ie, several enemas). Urethrocystography may also aid diagnosis of ureteric ectopia in female dogs.

SURGICAL OPTIONS

- Ureteronephrectomy is advised when severe hydronephrosis and hydroureter exist or if the associated kidney is aplastic.
- Neoureterocystostomy is recommended for animals with intramural ureteric ectopia
- Ureteral transection and neoureterocystostomy is recommended for animals with extramural ureteric ectopia.

Prior to surgery any infection in the bladder should be appropriately treated. A caudal ventral midline coeliotomy incision is performed and the urogenital tract examined. Stay sutures in the cranial pole of the bladder will help with subsequent exposure and manipulations. A ventral cystotomy incision is made and extended across the trigone into the proximal urethra. Again, stay sutures are placed along the edges of this incision to facilitate exposure and limit the amount of instrument manipulation of the bladder wall. Intramural ectopic ureters usually join the bladder wall in a normal position and tunnel caudally in the submucosa to open in the distal urogenital tract. The trigone and proximal urethra are carefully examined for ureteral orifices. If found the ureter(s) should be catheterized using a soft rubber catheter. Occasionally two ureteric openings will be present, one in the bladder and one more distal; the ureteric orifice should therefore be probed in both directions. Any ectopic ureteral opening discovered in the proximal urethra shoud be opened with scissors, cutting through the urothelium and submucosa, such that the new ureteric opening is positioned in the bladder trigone. The distas (ectopic) ureter segment should be excised leaving approximately 1cm of ureter attached at the trigone. The new orifice is created using simple interrupted sutures of 5-0 polydioxanone in a simple interrupted pattern so as to appose the ureteric urothelium to the vesicular urothelium. The resulting distal urethral mucosal defect is closed with a simple interrupted appositional pattern using the same suture material. If a distal ureteric opening cannot be found, the neoureteral stoma is created in the trigone by direct incision into the submucosal tunneling ureter in this location. It is opened distally with scissors and the neostoma created as above. The author prefers to remove a segment of the intramural ureter and ablate the mucosal defect with sutures as above, with particular attention to closing the distal end of the ureter.

Technique for Ureteronephrectomy

Generous ventral midline incision from just caudal to the xiphoid to beyond the umbilicus. The left kidney is found by elevating the colon thereby reflecting the remaining small intestine to the right which is held in place by the mesocolon. The right kidney is found by locating the descending duodenum and using the mesoduodenum to reflect the other abdominal structures in a similar way. The kidney is packed off with moist laparotomy towels and the perirenal fascia stripped from the capsule by blunt dissection. The renal vessels and ureter are identified and the renal artery is dissected free and ligated close to the aorta (prevents blind sac for thrombus to form) the renal vein is treated similarly. Both should be double ligated with silk or PDS. The ureter is then dissected free as close to it's attachment to the bladder as possible and divided between ligatures (prevent blind sac as focus for infection) Gentle traction on the kidney should then pull the ureter out to complete the removal. Abdominal closure is routine.

Postoperative Complications

1. **Persistent urinary tract infection (UTI):** Requires careful monitoring and therapy; if it persists, it could be hydroureter and hydronephrotic kidney acting as a reservoir for infection; therefore, ureteronephrectomy will be needed.
2. **Persistent incontinence:** Could be due to re-canalization of a submucosal tunnel or a poor sphincter mechanism, occasionally poor vaginal conformation causes pooling of urine at urination which then slowly leaks out. A repeat radiographic study may help determine the problem also a voiding cystogram will show any functional abnormality of the vagina.

DOES MY GDV PATIENT NEED ALL THOSE FLUIDS? MAYBE NOT!

Daniel J. Brockman, BVSc, CVR, CSAO,
Diplomate ACVS and ECVS, FHEA, MRCVS
Royal Veterinary College, University of London
Hatfield, Hertfordshire, United Kingdom

Gastric dilatation–volvulus syndrome (GDVs) patients are commonly presented as emergencies. Treatment protocols based on best current evidence regarding the pathophysiology resulting from GD and GDV have resulted in good survival rates. It is likely that any future improvements in the treatment of this condition will be as a direct result of a better understanding of the disease mechanisms involved. The most profound functional changes that occur are associated with GD and GDV and vary according to the extent of gastric dilation, the degree of gastric rotation, and the duration of each. Although it is often helpful to consider the pathophysiology on an organ or body system basis, the changes that occur are complex and interdependent. For the body as a whole, the consequences of GDVs are reduced oxygen delivery to tissues. These changes can be so mild that they are barely evident or they can be so severe that they result in irreversible "sepsis syndrome," either through uncontrolled infection (sepsis) or non-infectious systemic inflammatory response syndrome (SIRS).

PATHOANATOMY

Dilation of a normally positioned stomach results in a 90 degree counter-clockwise gastric rotation around the gastroesophageal junction. The majority of dogs affected with GDVs undergo simultaneous dilation and clockwise rotation (between 180 and 360 degrees) of the stomach about the gastroesophageal junction. From a pathophysiologic perspective, GD and GDV can create similar systemic effects, but there is evidence that the deleterious effects to the blood supply of local organs (stomach and spleen) are greater when volvulus has occurred. Splenic displacement has been documented in many patients with GDVs and is considered inevitable because of its close anatomic association with the greater curvature of the stomach. The magnitude of displacement should, in theory, have a direct relationship with the degree of splenic vascular compromise.

EXPERIMENTAL MODELS OF GDV

Attempts to precisely recreate the pathoanatomy of dogs with naturally occurring GDV have failed. In addition, all of the experimental models of this disease require general anesthesia, abolishing any conscious influence (such as release of endogenous catecholamines and cortisol) over events in these dogs. It seems that it is impossible to rotate the stomach of an otherwise normal dog and dilate it with air and have it remain in that state without additional "devices." Passi et al[3] ligated the thoracic esophagus around an orogastric tube, via thoracotomy, and ligated the pylorus through a right subcostal laparotomy; they inflated the stomach to a mean pressure of 25 +/- 11 mmHg to create a model of GD. Merkley et al[4] used the experimental model of GD that was predominant at that time, using an intragastric balloon inflated to 80mm Hg. Orton and Muir[5] argued that such high intragastric pressures (80 mmHg) should not be used since the intragastric pressure in dogs with naturally occurring disease varied from 9 to 62 mmHg. They favored, therefore, using an intragastric balloon inflated to a pressure of 30 mmHg. In addition, these workers created a small celiotomy to allow concurrent rotation of the dilated stomach to create GDV. Subsequently, models of GDV have involved umbilical tape ligatures placed at the gastroesophageal junction and at the pylorus, in such a way that branches of the vagus nerve and the gastric vasculature are not compromised, to create an air-tight seal. The stomach is then inflated via a Foley catheter in the pyloric antrum to a pressure of 30 mmHg and the stomach is sutured in a rotated position to create GDV. The length of time that these models of GD or GDV were maintained varied between 90 and 180 minutes. In addition to these models of GD and GDV, Lantz et al[13] studied the effect of gastric volvulus alone by suturing the nondistended stomach in position after rotating it 360 degrees. All models of GD or GDV that required celiotomy for their creation had the celiotomy closed before any measurements were made.

In summary, none of these models perfectly recreate the natural disease. In addition, anesthetic drug protocols have varied from model to model and this could have a significant effect on results. Because of the careful use of control animals, however, experiments using these models have provided a valuable insight into the events that follow GD and GDV.

CIRCULATORY PATHOPHYSIOLOGY

The results of experiments using the models mentioned above together demonstrated that acute gastric dilation, using intragastric pressures equivalent to those seen in dogs with natural disease, cause mechanical obstruction to the caudal vena cava with predictable consequences with respect to cardiac output. Typically, systemic arterial pressure fell and heart rate increased in all these models. Finally, since simply decompressing the stomach was not always enough to return hemodynamics to control levels, data from these experiments contains the clue that additional factors were mediating prolonged systemic hypotension in animals recovering from GD and GDV and endorsed the need for additional intravascular fluid therapy.

Clinical Evidence

Good objective clinical data regarding the pre-fluid resuscitation circulatory status of dogs with GDVs is not contained in any of the large reports of this condition. One small prospective study by Wagner et al (1999) evaluated cardiopulmonary variables in six dogs that underwent gastropexy without partial gastrectomy, for GDV. Unfortunately, four of these six dogs had intravenous fluid therapy before any measurements were made and all had intraoperative fluid therapy "according to the perceived needs of the patient, made by the attending clinician and anaesthetist." These workers concluded that not all dogs with naturally occurring GDVs have severe circulatory derangements. The study population did not include any dogs that required partial gastric resection, creating study population bias, and with so many uncontrolled variables such as degree of gastric distention and fluid administration, and the small sample size, it is difficult, therefore, to interpret these data as being sound scientific evidence. Other evidence of the degree of systemic hypoperfusion was provided indirectly by De Papp et al[1] who retrospectively evaluated venous plasma lactate concentration as a predictor of gastric necrosis and survival in 102 dogs. In this study, the dogs with gastric necrosis were compared with dogs that did not have gastric necrosis; mean venous plasma lactate were 6.6 mmol/L and 3.3 mmol/L, respectively. Originally, these workers hypothesized that the gastrointestinal tract was the source of the lactate; but ultimately they concluded that any ischemic tissue in the body could contribute to the venous plasma lactate concentration, especially if the sample was retrieved prior to gastric decompression and release of the splanchnic (portal venous) reservoir of gut-derived lactate. In their discussion these authors suggested that high lactate was more likely to reflect systemic hypoperfusion rather than gut production alone and as such should be considered a marker of disease severity rather than a direct indicator of gastric wall ischemia. In addition, dogs with naturally occurring GDVs frequently have rupture of the short gastric vessels and hemoperitoneum, both of which can affect regional organ blood flow (see later) and systemic hemodynamic parameters.

The prevalence of cardiac arrhythmias in dogs recovering from GDVs has been well documented). Evidence of myocyte injury in the form of serum cardiac troponin I (cTI) and cardiac troponin T (cTT) has been demonstrated in dogs clinically affected with GDVs. In the absence of the identification of a direct myocardial depressant factor, other cardiotoxic element, or electrolyte derangements in the plasma of dogs affected with GDVs, reduced coronary blood flow and increased myocardial oxygen demand could be considered as a reflection of the systemic hypotension and hypoperfusion. Since coronary blood flow occurs predominantly during diastole, low diastolic pressures, in particular, would reduce coronary blood flow and since diastolic pressure depends on systemic vascular resistance, perturbations of this in addition to total intravascular volume could have a detrimental effect on myocardial oxygen delivery.

SO, SHOULD I GIVE SHOCK DOSES OF CRYSTALLOIDS?

In summary, there is good experimental evidence that gastric dilation reduces venous return to the heart and that this effect is progressive over time. Also, reduced myocardial blood flow occurs at a time when myocardial oxygen demand is high creating the risk of heart muscle compromise. In addition, some of these experiments demonstrate that simply reducing intragastric pressure alone does not restore the circulation back to normal; this can only be achieved by additional fluid therapy. Good documentation of how compromised the circulation of clinical patients with GDV actually is lacking but serum lactate levels in affected patients suggests that hypoperfusion can be severe. In emergency practice, the clinician must rely on subjective indicators of perfusion such as mucous membrane colour, capillary refill time and pulse rate and quality. It would be an error to ignore these basic physiologic parameters when assessing the circulatory status of any patient. The clinician must, however, accept that such parameters are subjective, not "exact," and a mental "risk:benefit" calculation is needed when considering therapy. Among a population of dogs that have the potential to be severely hypovolemic, which option do we currently believe is the safest: 1) to "overdo" the fluid therapy in a dog that was only mildly compromised or 2) to "underdo" the fluid therapy in a dog that was severely compromised? This is bearing in mind that "shock" fluid doses (90 mL/kg/hr) should only be administered for one hour and progress of the patient during this period should be carefully monitored. The author would argue that it is generally safer to "overdo" fluid therapy for a short period of time, in a patient that didn't need it, rather than "underdo" fluid therapy in an animal that was severely compromised. Ultimately, the skill and experience of the clinician making the initial and subsequent clinical assessment of the animal will determine how much fluid is given.

REFERENCES/FURTHER READING

1. de Papp E, Drobatz KJ, Hughes D. Plasma lactate concentration as a predictor of gastric necrosis and survival among dogs with gastric dilatation-volvulus: 102 cases (1995-1998). J Am Vet Med Assoc. 1999;215(1):49-52.
2. Lantz GC, Bottoms GD, Carlton WW, Newman S, Cantwell HD. The effect of 360° gastric volvulus on the blood supply of the nondistended normal dog stomach. Vet Surg. 1984;13:189-196.
3. Passi RB, Kraft AR, Vasko JS. Pathophysiologic mechanisms of shock in acute gastric dilatation. Surgery 1969;65(2):298-303.
4. Merkley DF, Howard DR Eyster GE. Experimentally induced acute gastric dilatation in the dog: Cardiopulmonary effects. J Am Anim Hosp Assoc. 1976;12:143-148.
5. Orton EC, Muir WW. Hemodynamics during experimental gastric dilatation-volvulus in dogs. Am J Vet Res. 1983;44(8):1512-1515.
6. Orton EC, Muir WW. Isovolumetric indices and humoral cardioactive substance bioassay during clinical and experimentally induced gastric dilatation-volvulus in dogs. Am J Vet Res. 1983;44:1516-1520.
7. Badylak SF, Lantz GC, Jeffries M. Prevention of reperfusion injury in surgically induced gastric dilatation-volvulus in dogs. Am J Vet Res. 1990;51(2):294-299.

8. Davidson JR, Lantz GC, Salisbury SK, Kazacos EA, Bottoms GD. Effects of flunixin meglumine on dogs with experimental gastric dilatation-volvulus. Vet Surg. 1992;21(2):113-120.

9. Wingfield WE, Betts CW, Rawlings CA. Pathophysiology associated with gastric dilatation-volvulus in the dog. J Am Anim Hosp Assoc. 1976;12:136-141.

10. Barnes GE, Laine GA, Giam PY, Smith EE, Granger HJ. Cardiovascular responses to elevation of intra-abdominal hydrostatic pressure. Am J Physiol. 1985;248(2 Pt 2):R208-213.

11. Horn WA, Gilmore DR, Dietz AE, Freden GO. Effects of gastric distention-volvulus on coronary blood flow and myocardial oxygen consumption in the dog. Am J Vet Res. 1985;46(1):98-104.

12. Schober KE, Cornand C, Kirbach B, Aupperle H, Oechtering G. Serum cardiac troponin I and cardiac troponin T concentrations in dogs with gastric dilatation-volvulus. J Am Vet Med Assoc. 2002;221(3):381-388.

13. Lantz GC, Badylak SF, Hiles MC, Arkin TE. Treatment of reperfusion injury in dogs with experimentally induced gastric dilatation-volvulus. Am J Vet Res. 1992;53(9):1594-1598.

BEYOND LIGATING A PDA: SURGERY THAT CARRIES A HEALTH WARNING

Daniel J. Brockman, BVSc, CVR, CSAO,
Diplomate ACVS and ECVS, FHEA, MRCVS
Royal Veterinary College, University of London
Hatfield, Hertfordshire, United Kingdom

Although many trained surgeons are comfortable performing closed cardiac procedures such as ligation of a patent ductus arteriosus (PDA) and subtotal pericardectomy, only a few veterinary surgeons the world over perform open heart surgery regularly and perhaps even fewer can boast reliable long-term results for the therapy they perform. The reasons for this include the prevalence of surgically correctable cardiac disease in veterinary patients, the apparent success of non-surgical treatment (eg, balloon dilation for pulmonic stenosis), the risk surgical treatment poses to the patient, the techniques currently available, and the cost of such treatments. For these reasons, cardiac surgery in animals has fallen massively behind when compared with the repertoire of procedures currently offered to human patients with heart disease. Ironically, the techniques used in human patients to facilitate open heart surgery today are largely the same as the techniques developed by pioneers such as Gibbon, Lillehei, Taussig and others, as a result of experiments with dogs and cats. More recently, open heart surgery programs have been or are being developed at different centers throughout the world, increasing the availability, safety, and success of open heart surgical therapies in the dog.

Traditionally, open heart surgery was performed under total venous inflow occlusion (TVIO), placing time constraints on the duration of procedures. The trade-off for increasing the "safe" occlusion time for a patient was a reduction in the likelihood of successfully reviving the patient at the end of the procedure.

VENOUS INFLOW OCCLUSION

Normothermic	3–5 minutes*
	*(8 minutes – Hunt)
Mild hypothermia (30°C)	9 minutes
Moderate hypothermia (25°C)	15 minutes
Deep hypothermia (20°C)	45 minutes

This time constraint often meant that procedures were designed to be fast rather than accurate and that some procedures needed to be aborted before the surgical goals were achieved. These techniques did, however, allow resection of fibromuscular atrial bands (as in cor triatriatum dexter), resection of pulmonic valve leaflets, or placement of a pulmonary outflow patch to treat pulmonic stenosis, and the resection of right ventricular outflow tract tumors. Studies demonstrating the long-term results of, for example, pulmonary outflow patching under TVIO, do not exist. Although short-term survival for patients undergoing such procedures is high at some institutions, the evidence, via personal communication, is that long-term results are either poor or at least very inconsistent.

The ability to open the heart without the time constraint that TVIO creates would allow the surgeon to perform a more accurate operation for even the relatively simple congenital cardiac diseases such as pulmonic stenosis. This should result in better long-term results. Theoretically, such techniques would open the way not only for treatment of congenital heart diseases but also offer some hope for all dogs that develop progressive acquired valvular disease. Longer duration open heart surgery can be achieved in two ways, as discussed below.

CARDIOPULMONARY BYPASS
- Controlled cross circulation
- Heart-lung machine
- Unlimited time

The use of a large dog as the "oxygenator," as in controlled cross circulation, is considered unethical in many countries, leaving the heart-lung machine as the best means to perform prolonged open-heart surgery in dogs.

Equipment
In addition to standard surgical and anesthetic equipment, an artificial pump (roller head pump) and an artificial lung (oxygenator) are required to perform open heart surgery (Figure 1).

Personnel
A dedicated coordinated team effort is required to perform operations under cardiopulmonary bypass. This team includes: two surgeons, two scrub nurses, one anesthetist, and an anesthesia nurse or technician, a perfusionist to run the heart-lung machine, and critical care specialists to perform the postoperative care for these animals. In addition, cardiologists need to be prepared to offer surgical therapy to their patients and need to coordinate the medical heart therapy prior to and following surgical therapy.

Reinventing the Wheel
Unfortunately, over the last few years, those involved in such programs have to a large extent had to relearn the lessons learned by early workers in the human field of cardiac surgery many years ago. The author of this article has been involved in an open heart surgery program over the last 8 years and has concluded, as other workers have, that:

1. All members of the team (cardiologists, surgeons, anesthetist, perfusionist, critical care clinicians) have to be dedicated to the program, understand their roles, and be coordinated by a single leader.
2. Size matters: The insult associated with being on a heart-lung machine using current protocols is magnified in small dogs. This means that small dogs often die of bypass-related complications using protocols that are well tolerated by larger (>15 kg) dogs.

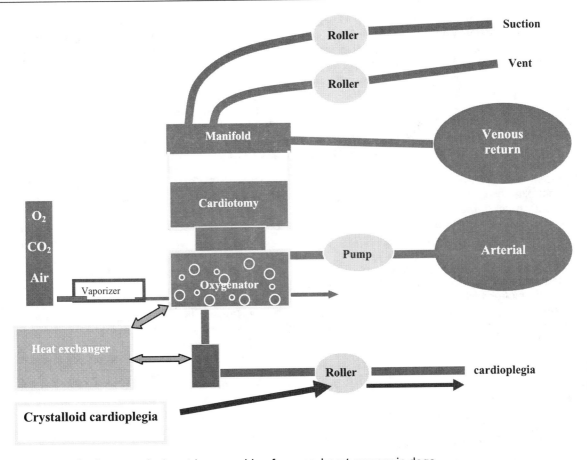

Figure 1. Schematic diagram of a heart-lung machine for open-heart surgery in dogs.

3. At the start of a program, attempt relatively simple operations in dogs that have not exhausted their myocardial reserve, preferably animals with congenital disease.

4. Dogs with end-stage heart disease are not good candidates for surgical therapy performed by an inexperienced team.

5. Because of problems associated with long-term patient anticoagulation, mechanical valve replacement is fraught with long-term problems; tissue valves that do not require patient anticoagulation may be a better valve option for small animals.

6. This is an expensive, high-risk endeavor that will be a drain on hospital resources. In order to survive within a hospital, it must be successful—that is, the patients must at least survive.

The Future

As centers around the world gain experience and expertise in the field of open heart surgery, the repertoire of procedures will be extended to include congenital and acquired valve defects, along with other congenital heart diseases. In addition, as skill levels increase, it will become possible for workers in this field to offer therapies to dogs of all sizes, along with cats and perhaps even horses.

OPEN RESECTION OF PULMONIC STENOSIS

Congenital stenosis of the pulmonary outflow tract is, along with patent ductus arteriosus and subaortic stenosis, one of the three most common congenital cardiac conditions seen in dogs. It is rare in cats. Pulmonic stenosis (PS) is characterized as being subvalvular, valvular, or supravalvular according to the anatomic location of the constriction. In the most common form of PS (valvular), valve pathology varies from fusion of otherwise normal valve leaflets within a normal valve annulus, to fibrotic deformed valve leaflets in a pathologically narrowed valve annulus. Secondary cardiac changes such as right ventricular hypertrophy can add a dynamic component to the stenosis that may influence treatment options and choice. In addition, concurrent anomalies of the coronary artery exist in some breeds, making treatment even more problematic.

Commonly, the severity of pulmonic stenosis is graded as mild, moderate, or severe, based on the pressure gradient estimated, by calculation, from the velocity of blood flow across the stenosis, derived by Doppler ultrasound interrogation. Such ultrasound examinations are typically performed in the conscious animal. Interestingly, historically, pressure gradients to classify the severity of a lesion were taken from pressure traces derived from catheter "pull-out" procedures that were performed in anesthetized animals. However, the severity of the pressure gradient, the presence of clinical signs and the degree of secondary cardiac changes (right ventricular hypertrophy) are all taken into consideration when determining a treatment plan for an affected animal. Generally, animals affected clinically or those with "severe" disease on the basis of their pressure gradient, are considered as candidates for intervention.

Treatment options include procedures directed at the valve alone and procedures that have been designed to treat the valvular deformity, valve annulus narrowing, and subvalvular muscular hypertrophy simultaneously. No single treatment option is endorsed by a report of a carefully controlled clinical trial, with long-term outcome, in "significant" numbers of animals. Treatments that carry the least risk to the patient like balloon valvuloplasty (BV) have, therefore, gained popularity despite the lack of evidence documenting long-term efficacy in small animals, largely because of the well-documented effect of similar techniques in human patients. The "higher risk" surgical procedures have been reserved for dogs that have failed nonsurgical treatments or dogs that are not considered "good" candidates for nonsurgical treatment.

TREATMENT OPTIONS
Valve Alone
- **Balloon valvuloplasty:** Often the first-choice for clinicians treating valvular PS in a breed that doesn't suffer from aberrant coronary artery anatomy (even if subvalvular infundibular muscular hypertrophy exists) where the pulmonic valve annulus is a normal size
- **Closed valvulotomy:** Using a mechanical valve dilator. Largely superseded by BV.
- **Open valvectomy via pulmonary arteriotomy:** Performed under total venous inflow occlusion (TVIO). Used in dogs/cats when valvular disease alone is present and in patients that have failed BV or in patients in which BV was not possible or considered inappropriate

Valve, Valve Annulus, and Muscular Hypertrophy
- **Closed patch grafting:** Six dogs reported in the literature
- **Modified open patch grafting:**
  - **Orton – Partial ventriculostomy under TVIO.** Four dogs reported
  - **Hunt – "quick sew" under TVIO.** Eight dogs reported in the literature
  - **Sackman – incised patch under TVIO.** In book chapter
- **Open patch grafting (Ccrdiopulmonary bypass):** None reported in literature. Success described by several workers. Perhaps gives the best opportunity to examine the valve leaflets and excise hypertrophied muscle. Most accurate placement of a "patch". Not appropriate for small patients!!
- **Conduits:** Only failed conduits reported in clinical cases in the literature. Success has been described by some workers

For many patients with severe or symptomatic PS, balloon valvuloplasty represents the safest first line of treatment even if infundibular muscular hypertrophy exists. For patients with predominantly valvular disease (ie, normal valve annulus), in which BV is not possible or fails, the best view of the right ventricular outflow tract is achieved under cardiopulmonary bypass. Although this approach is associated with the highest short-term risk to the patient, it probably offers the best chance at long-term palliation or improvement.

ATRIOVENTRICULAR VALVE REPLACEMENT
Pathoanatomy
The mitral and tricuspid valve can suffer from both congenital and acquired (endocardiosis) deformity that creates predominantly valvular incompetence and occasionally stenosis. Replacement of such valves in people is commonly performed and typically is done before secondary myocardial changes are advanced.

Valve Replacement in Dogs
Experience with replacement valves in dogs is in its infancy. Mechanical valves have been placed in the mitral position in dogs but, although dramatic results were obtained in the short term, difficulty in maintaining life-long anticoagulation resulted in devastating failure of the valve in many patients. Tissue valves (valves made from bovine pericardium or porcine valves) obviate the need for life-long anticoagulation in people and should be similar in dogs. Early results of tricuspid valve replacement using both bovine pericardial and porcine aortic valves suggest that inability to manage anticoagulation even in the short term can prove devastating in the long term for dogs undergoing valve replacement.

SURGICAL MANAGEMENT OF TETRALOGY OF FALLOT
Pathoanatomy
The primary pathoanatomy seen in dogs with Tetralogy of Fallot (ventricular septal defect, pulmonic stenosis, and overriding aorta) can all be explained by embryologic developmental defects of the endocardial cushions comprising the conotruncal septum.

Pathophysiology
Right to left shunting of blood results in underperfusion of the lungs, leading to systemic hypoxia and cyanosis. Compensatory polycythemia may be seen. The contribution of infundibular muscle to the right ventricular outflow tract obstruction can create both a dynamic and progressive component to this disease, accounting for worsening of signs with exercise and progression of disease despite fixed valvular and septal abnormalities.

Therapeutic Options
- **Medical/conservative:** Some mildly affected animals do not require any treatment and will enjoy a good lifestyle; others will require medical therapy (beta-blockers) to give an acceptable quality of life.

It has been suggested that approximately 25% of affected animals will not be controlled by conservative/medical means (Eyster et al. 1976).

- **Surgical**: Surgical treatments fall into two main categories: primary repair and palliative procedures.
  - o **Primary repair** of Tetralogy of Fallot has been described several times in the veterinary literature (Herrtage et al, 1983; Lew et al, 1989); this requires cardiopulmonary bypass, advanced surgical expertise, and currently carries a high mortality rate.
  - o **Palliative surgical procedures**: These were used extensively in human medicine prior to the advent of cardiopulmonary bypass and primary repair. Currently, some are used in infants as a "bridge" to primary repair, in severely affected individuals.
    - o **Potts anastomosis.** Side to side anastomosis of the aorta to the left main pulmonary artery
    - o **Blalock anastomosis.** Anastomosis of the left subclavian artery to the left main pulmonary artery
    - o **Modified Blalock-Taussig anastomosis.** The development of synthetic materials such as polytetrafluorethylene (PTFE) (Gore-Tex) that are relatively non-thrombogenic and can be created in tube form has allowed surgeons to modify existing techniques.
    - o **Others:** Microvasular anastomosis of the left internal thoracic artery to the pulmonary artery has been described in a cat that had a failed "Fontan" procedure (anastomosis of the right atrium to the pulmonary artery).

INTESTINAL ANASTOMOSES – IMPROVING YOUR RESULTS

Gary W. Ellison, DVM, MS, Diplomate ACVS
College of Veterinary Medicine
University of Florida, Gainesville, FL

Wound dehiscence of an intestinal anastomosis often leads to generalized bacterial peritonitis and subsequent death. Therefore, factors which negatively affect visceral healing are potentially of great clinical significance to the surgeon. Factors that cause intestinal anastomoses to leak include etiology of obstruction, failure to adequately identify ischemic tissue, improper suturing or stapling technique, and factors that negatively affect wound healing such as sepsis, malnutrition, and antineoplastic therapy.

IMPORTANCE OF TISSUE APPOSITION

Direct approximation of the wound edge allows for optimum rapid healing characterized by primary intestinal wound healing. With good apposition rapid mucosal re-epithelialization, and early formation of young well-vascularized collagen between the submucosa, muscularis, and serosa occurs. Other advantages of approximating patterns for intestinal anastomosis are 1) lumen diameter is not compromised, 2) wound strength meets or exceeds everting or inverting wound strengths, and 3) adhesions are minimal. The crushing suture has been shown to cause more tissue ischemia directly at the suture line and its use is discouraged.

Mucosal eversion or tissue overlap retards healing and should be avoided. Delayed fibrin seal formation, delayed mucosal re-epithelialization, increased mucocele formation, prolonged inflammatory response, and marked adhesion formation all characterize everted healing. Eversion may initially widen the lumen diameter, but the prolonged inflammatory response usually narrows the lumen sometimes resulting in stenosis. Everting anastomoses also have an increased tendency for leakage especially in the face of a septic abdomen and should never be used in the colon.

Inversion of the wound edge creates an internal cuff of tissue that reduces lumen diameter. Hemodynamic compromise of the inverted submucosa occurs resulting in mucosal edema and necrosis. After 5 days the internal cuff usually sloughs. Inverting anastomoses are characterized by a rapid serosa to serosa seal and minimal adhesion formation. Because of their safety against leakage, inverting patterns may be the preferred technique for the colon.

The GIA and TA autostaplers lay a double row of staples for security and when used in combination create a functional "end to end anastomosis." The GIA portion of the anastomosis is inverted whereas the TA portion of the anastomosis is everted. Recent studies have shown that leakage rates are similar to hand sewn techniques but autostapler usage significantly reduces surgical time.

A rapid alterative to sutured anastomosis is the use of an AutoSuture 35 skin stapler with stainless skin staples (United States Surgical Corp., Norwalk, CT). After triangulating the intestine with three stay sutures, the skin stapler is used to place staples every 2 to 3 mm around the perimeter of the wound. These closures are more rapidly done than hand-sewn anastomosis and have similar bursting strengths but mucosal eversion may occur between staples.

SELECTION OF SUTURE MATERIAL, NEEDLE TYPE, AND NUMBER OF SUTURES

Both absorbable and nonabsorbable suture materials have been used successfully for anastomosis. The braided nonabsorbable suture materials such as silk or Dacron may harbor bacteria, creating a granulomatous inflammatory reaction or draining suture sinus. Monofilament nonabsorbable sutures such as Nylon and polypropylene are safe in contaminated environments. However, polypropylene has been associated with foreign body adherence in one case series. Absorbable suture materials are usually used since the GI tract heals very rapidly and suture tensile strength is only needed for 2 to 3 weeks. Absorbable suture materials reported in the literature include **chromic gut, polyglycolic acid** (Dexon), **polygalactin 910** (Vicryl), **polydioxanone** (PDS), **polyglyconate** (Maxon), and **poliglecaprone** (Monocryl). Of these, surgical gut is not recommended for anastomosis because it is rapidly broken down by collagenase. Polygalactin 910 and polyglycolic acid are multifilament derivations of glycolic acid which retain good tensile strength for up to 28 days. Both sutures have good knot tying and handling characteristics with the exception of significant tissue drag. Vicryl is commonly used for intestinal anastomosis in Europe with good published success. Polydioxanone (PDS) and polyglyconate (Maxon) are polyester monofilament suture materials which are also absorbed by hydrolysis and therefore are unaffected by contaminated environment. They maintain up to 40% of their original tensile strength after 3 weeks. Many surgeons are starting to use shorter-acting monofilaments such as Monocryl or Biosyn for intestinal anastomosis. They have similar handling properties to PDS but its tensile strength are resorbed by within 10 to 21 days. The newer "Plus" sutures are impregnated with the antibacterial agent Tryclosan. Their efficacy in reducing infection in contaminated dermal wounds may foster an increased use in intestinal anastomosis.

Suture size, needle type and number of sutures are also important factors to consider. For cats, I use 4-0 suture on an RB1 needle. Usually 12 to 16 sutures are needed to complete the anastomosis. For dogs I typically use 3-0 suture on an SH needle and 18 to 20 sutures are needed to complete the anastomosis. Alternatively skin staples can be used to construct the anastomosis.

Small intestinal resection is limited to 70% of its length in adult dogs and 80% in puppies. Beyond that short bowel syndrome with malabsorption, maldigestion and chronic diarrhea will result. After transection, the wound edges are trimmed to remove everted mucosa and suturing is begun at the mesenteric border. Sutures are then placed on the anti mesenteric border, then at the 3 and 9 o'clock position before filling in the gaps.

All anastomoses should be covered with a vascularized omental flap which is tacked in place. Omentum is useful in 1) restoring blood supply to a devascularized area, 2) facilitating lymphatic drainage, and 3) minimizing mucosal leakage and secondary peritonitis. The role of omentum is significant when one considers that in one study 90% mortality rates were seen with intestinal anastomoses after omental resection was performed in dogs. Free omental flaps are not as effective as pedicle omental flaps and may in fact lead to anastomosis failure.

OTHER FACTORS EFFECTING DEHISCENCE

Healing of visceral wounds is negatively affected by a number of factors. **Chronic weight loss of 15% to 20%** due to cancer cachexia or other reasons has a negative effect on visceral wound healing. Correction of cachexia as well as early postoperative enteral feeding appears to increase collagen deposition and bursting wound strength. **Glucocorticoids** have a negative effect on wound healing when given in large doses prior to the third day after wounding. **NSAIDs** appear to affect the early inflammatory phase of wound healing, but do not appear to interfere with the proliferative phase of wound healing or have a significant negative effect on visceral healing strength. **Radiation** therapy interferes with fibroblast mobilization, replication, and collagen synthesis as well as causing sclerosis of microvasculature, thereby reducing oxygenation at the wound site. Whenever possible, radiation therapy should be initiated after visceral wound healing is complete. The negative effects of cancer on wound healing appear to be secondary to nutritional deficiencies rather than direct tumor impairment on wound healing. Visceral wound healing may actually be mildly augmented owing to release growth factors by the neoplasm. **Effects of chemotherapeutic agents on visceral wound healing are variable.** Drugs such as vincristine, vinblastine, and azathioprine seem to be safe when used in therapeutic doses. Drugs such as cyclophosphamide, methotrexate, 5-FU, and doxorubicin have been shown to delay wound healing in both experimental and clinical studies. Cisplatin appears to significantly impair intestinal wound healing in rats and should be used with caution after intestinal surgery.

NUTRITIONAL DEPLETION

Tissue trauma, sepsis, burns, and major surgery induce major metabolic changes in small animal patients. With each of these stresses the animal's basic metabolic rate is accelerated and protein metabolism occurs, leading to a potential state of negative nitrogen balance. Protein-calorie malnutrition (PCM) occurs because of starvation, when a metabolic response to injury becomes prolonged, or with hypermetabolism secondary to sepsis. It takes only 5 to 10 days of anorexia to compromise the immune system and deplete the body's muscular and hepatic glycogen stores. When PCM is present cell mediated immunity is impaired, there is a high risk of infection, anemia and hypoproteinemia and impaired wound healing.

Caloric and protein depletion in animals has been shown to inhibit visceral healing, but only after a loss of 15% to 20% of body weight. Decreases in wound breaking strength are directly proportional to the carcass weight loss. It is estimated that 75% of animals with elective surgical wounds attain functional wound union during the period of negative nitrogen balance; however, extended PCM from muscle, visceral, or plasma tissue losses increases the risk for visceral wound disruption. Impaired visceral wound healing is due to both a prolonged lag phase of healing and diminished capacity for fibroplasia within the logarithmic phase.

EFFECT OF EARLY POSTOPERATIVE ENTERAL FEEDING ON VISCERAL HEALING

Malnutrition induces intestinal mucosal atrophy, reduced motility, increased incidence of ileus and the potential for bacterial translocation through the bowel wall, with resultant sepsis. Impaired wound healing due to nutritional causes may be ameliorated by feeding an enteral or parenteral diet that supplies energy needs in the form of fatty acids and sugars and provides essential amino acids. Feedings of high protein meals after injury can optimize conditions for normal visceral wound healing. Amino acids provided through enteral nutrition are utilized for the synthesis of structural proteins such as actin, myosin, collagen, and elastin.

Early if not immediate postoperative enteral feeding has been shown to have a positive influence on the healing rate of intestinal anastomosis in dogs. Bursting pressures and collagen levels of ileal and colorectal anastomosis were compared in Beagles fed elemental diets versus those fed only electrolyte and water for 4 days. The dogs fed elemental diets had nearly twice the bursting strengths of the control group and nearly double the amount of both immature and mature collagen at the wound site. Total parenteral nutrition (TPN) does not appear to ameliorate the mucosal atrophy or increase collagen deposition as does enteral nutrition. In human studies, the incidence of septic complications was significantly lower in people fed between eight to 24 hours after surgery versus those maintained on TPN. In addition, early fed patients had a reduced incidence of postoperative ileus and reduced hospital stay.

REFERENCES

1. Braga M. Early postoperative enteral nutrition improves oxygenation and reduces costs compares with total parenteral nutrition. Clin Nutr. 2001; 29:242-248.
2. Chatworthy HW, Saleby R, Lovingood C. Extensive small bowel resection in young dogs: its effect on

growth and development. Surgery. 1952; 32:341.

3. Coolman BR, Ehrhart N, Pijanowski G, et al. Comparison of skin staples with sutures for anastomosis of the small intestine of dogs. Vet Surg. 2000; 29:392.

4. Ellison GW: Wound healing in the gastrointestinal tract. Sem Vet Med Surg. 1989; 4:287.

5. Erikoglu M, Kaynak A, Beyatli EA, et al. Intraoperative determination of intestinal viability: a comparison with transserosal pulse oximetry and histopathological examination. J Surg Res. 2005; 128(1):66.

6. McCaw DL. The effects of cancer and cancer therapies on wound healing. Sem Vet Med Surg. 1989; 4: 281.

7. Ralphs SC, Jessen CR, Lipowitz AJ. Risk factors for leakage following intestinal anastomosis in dogs and cats: 115 cases (1991-2000). J Am Vet Med Assoc. 2003; 223(1):73.

8. Weisman DL, Smeak DD, Birchard SJ, et al. Comparison of a continuous suture pattern with a simple interrupted pattern for enteric closure in dogs and cats: 83 cases (1991-1997). J Am Vet Med Assoc. 1999; 214(10):1507.

GASTROPEXIES AND COLOPEXIES

Gary W. Ellison, DVM, MS, Diplomate ACVS
College of Veterinary Medicine
University of Florida, Gainesville, FL

GASTROPEXY

Rationale

By definition, gastropexy describes the fixation of the stomach to nearby structures or body wall as a means of preventing recurrence of gastric dilatation-volvulus (GDV). Although gastropexy procedures reportedly diminish the recurrence rate of GDV, their reliability in producing permanent adhesions between the stomach and abdominal wall is not well documented.

Most North American surgeons use an antral gastropexy procedure to fix the gastric antrum to the right abdominal wall. The three major categories of "permanent" antral gastropexies used in North America are the **tube gastrostomy** described by Parks (1976); the **incisional gastropexy** described by MacCoy (1982) and the **circumcostal gastropexy** described by Fallah (1982). In addition, two modifications of muscle flap techniques, one using a "muscular flap" from the abdominal wall (Shulman) and another using a "belt-loop" from the gastric muscularis (Whitney), have been described.

Clinical Results

Potential advantages of the **tube gastropexy** are that 1) the surgery is rapid and easy, 2) that the tube not only creates a permanent adhesion of the gastric antrum to the abdominal wall preventing recurrence of volvulus but also 3) allows for continued gastric decompression in the early postoperative period. In addition, 4) slurried food or medications can be offered through the tube. The main disadvantages of the technique are the 1) nursing care and long hospital period required for tube management and 2) the potential for fatal peritonitis secondary to leakage around the tube or early removal by the dog.

Clinical studies of the tube gastrostomy have yielded encouraging results. Flanders (1984) reported recurrence of volvulus in only 1 of 29 dogs treated with tube gastrostomy for a follow-up time ranging from 14 to 40 months. However, there was a mortality rate of 31% during the first week after surgery. Johnson (1984) reported on 76 cases where this technique was used with only a 5% recurrence rate. Older studies describe a recurrence rate as high as 29% (Walshaw 1976) as well as a 17% complication rate (Fox 1985) including premature dislodging of a tube, peritonitis, subcutaneous cellulites, or persistent stoma drainage.

Advantages of the **incisional gastropexy** are that 1) the procedure is rapidly done, 2) the stomach lumen is not entered, and 3) fibrous connective tissue enters the abdominal rectus muscle and stomach wall to form a strong mature adhesion. The potential disadvantage is that the gaseous decompression is not provided in the postoperative period. The incisional gastropexy is popular among many North American surgeons but unfortunately no good retrospective studies are available to determine its clinical efficacy.

The **circumcostal technique** has become popular for use in academic medicine because it probably forms a stronger adhesion. It is reported to be more difficult to perform than the other techniques but the author disagrees with this statement. Potential advantages include 1) a viable muscle flap adhesion as well as 2) a more proper anatomic placement of the stomach. Potential disadvantages include a prolonged surgical time, potential for rib fracture, and potential for pneumothorax because of the close proximity to the diaphragm. Lieb (1984) reported on 39 dogs with circumcostal gastropexies to have a slightly lower recurrent rate (2.6% at 13.7 months) than dogs with tube gastrostomy.

Belt loop gastropexy offers similar advantages to the circumcostal and incisional gastropexies in that the gastric lumen is not entered and the risk of peritonitis is minimal. The technique is easily performed by an unassisted surgeon. Although the belt loop gastropexy has not been evaluated biomechanically one would suspect that breaking strengths would be superior to incisional or tube gastrostomy techniques but not quite as secure as circumcostal techniques since the base of the flap is narrower than in the latter technique.

Ventral midline gastropexy was described in the mid 1990s as a method of rapid gastropexy which simply put involves inclusion of wall of the stomach in the ventral midline closure. Over 170 dogs were successfully treated in this manner. The serosa of the stomach is abraded with a dry sponge immediately prior to closure. The original article described using Vicryl but we choose to use 0 or #1 monofilament polypropylene in a simple continuous pattern including the linea alba and the gastric muscularis. Obviously the veterinarian must be cautious if future exploratory laparotomy is needed.

Laparoscopic-assisted gastropexy is a relatively new noninvasive method of fixing the gastric antrum to the right gastric wall using a laparoscope. It is used as a prophylactic procedure for those animals who have previously bloated or those which are at risk for developing GDV. After insufflating the abdominal cavity and introducing the camera a second portal is made in immediately caudal to the floating rib. The gastric antrum is grasped with a Babcock tissue forceps and exteriorized thru a 2- to 3-cm incision. The muscularis is then incised and opposed on both sides to the external oblique muscle. Routine subcutaneous and skin closure are performed.

Postoperative Management

Diligent postoperative care is mandatory for successful outcome of the gastric dilatation volvulus patient. Most dogs that die in the postoperative period will do so within the first 3 to 4 days after surgery. After major gastric resection the animal receives nothing by mouth (NPO) for a period of 24 to 48 hours. Maintenance fluid, electrolyte, and acid-base status is critical during this period. Maintenance fluid should be given at a rate of 40-60 mL/kg per day. Although many dogs maintain normal serum potassium levels following GDV, a total body potassium deficit may exist because of the NPO status, vomiting, oral gastric innervation and removal of gastric secretions. Supplementation of 20 mEq of potassium chloride therefore is usually added to each liter of fluids to help maintain total body potassium. Hypokalemia can also contribute to the development of cardiac arrhythmias, and gastrointestinal ileus.

COLOPEXY

Rectal or anorectal prolapse is a double-layer evagination of the rectum (sometimes including the anorectal junction) through the anal canal. It is seen most commonly in kittens with severe endoparasitism, enteritis, and associated tenesmus. In older cats, rectal prolapse most commonly occurs secondarily to dystocia in queens. It has also been reported secondary to urethral obstruction in male cats.

Diagnosis

Diagnosis is made by visual examination of a tube-like mass of varying length which protrudes from the anal orifice. It is important to distinguish a true rectal prolapse from a prolapsed ileocolic intussusception. A well-lubricated thermometer is gently passed between the anus and the prolapsed mass. With a rectal prolapse the fornix is located within a cm or less of the anus whereas with a prolapsed intussusception, the probe can be easily passed for a distance of 5 to 6 cm past the mass. Occasionally only the mucosal portion of the rectal wall will be exposed. **Rectal mucosal eversion** may occur secondarily to some of the previously mentioned conditions but usually reduces spontaneously following treatment of the primary disease.

Treatment

Management of rectal prolapse depends on 1) degree of tissue viability and 2) number of recurrences. If the rectal mucosa is viable (red oxygenated blood oozes from its surface) and it is the cats first occurrence, reduction and an **anal purse-string suture** is initially attempted. Under general anesthesia or epidural analgesia, the edematous mucosa is lubricated with K-Y jelly and gently massaged to reduce swelling. Cold hypertonic solutions such as 50% dextrose have been advocated to reduce edema by vascular constriction and osmosis; however, warm isotonic solutions may serve to dilate the blood vessels and better allow interstitial edema to be removed by gentle manipulation. After reduction of the prolapse, a pursestring suture of 2-0 nylon is preplaced at the anocutaneous line immediately cranial to the anal sac duct orifices. A well-lubricated EDTA blood collection tube or similar sized tube is then placed into the rectum and the purse-string is tied tight enough to gently appose the rectal mucosa against the tube. The tube is then removed, leaving a purse-string, which is tight enough to prevent recurrence but loose enough to allow defecation of softened stool. The suture can be left in for a week or more without deleterious effects.

If the rectal prolapse is viable but not digitally reducible or if there is a history of multiple recurrences, then a **colopexy** procedure is performed. Colopexy has been especially effective in cats in which purse-string management is ineffective and the risks of suture line dehiscence or rectal stricture after amputation are high. After performing a midline laparotomy, gentle traction is placed on the descending colon and reduction of the prolapse is confirmed by an assistant under the drape. The colopexy is performed to the left abdominal wall with the colon in slight traction. A 5 mm x 1 cm elliptical section of peritoneum is removed from the abdominal wall 2 cm lateral to the midline. A similarly shaped area of colonic serosa is removed with a No.15 blade. The raw bleeding surfaces are then apposed with five or six simple interrupted sutures of 3-0 nylon or polypropylene taking care not to penetrate into the lumen of the colon. Usually three or four colopexy sites are created along the length of the colon.

When the prolapsed segment is devitalized an **amputation** and **rectal anastomosis** is performed. A devitalized prolapse is usually dark purple or black in appearance and exudes cyanotic blood from its often ulcerated surface. Amputation of the prolapse can be carried out in one of two methods. A lubricated blood collection tube can often be passed through the apex and into the lumen of the prolapse. This allows three or four full-thickness mattress retention sutures to be passed immediately caudal to the anocutaneous line. The prolapse is then sharply resected 1.0 cm from the anus and the tube is removed. The outer and inner walls of the rectum are then apposed with full-thickness simple interrupted sutures of 3-0 synthetic absorbable suture. The stay sutures are removed and the anastomosis retracts back through the anus. An alternate technique is to make a dorsal 180 degree incision through both layers of the rectum at the base of the prolapse. The dorsal rectal wall is apposed with two rows of simple interrupted sutures, the first engaging the muscularis and the submucosa and the second apposing the submucosa and mucosa. The remainder of the prolapse is then incised around the perimeter and anastomosed in similar fashion. Potential complications after amputation and anastomosis of rectal prolapse include dehiscence of the anastomosis or formation of postoperative strictures. Suture line dehiscence is often fatal unless detected early. Rectal strictures are initially managed by dilating the constricting ring with a rectal or vaginal speculum under general anesthesia followed by 2 weeks of prednisolone therapy. If the stricture recurs, excision of the fibrous ring must be attempted surgically.

Postoperative Care

Elimination of postoperative tenesmus is often necessary for successful case outcome. Local anesthetic ointments instilled rectally or epidural analgesia may be effective for the short-term period. Stool softeners such as dioctyl sodium sulfosuccinate or Metamucil are advisable in addition to dry cat food, which is higher in fiber. For kittens symptomatic treatment in the form of intestinal antibiotics, protectants, or anticholinergics is advisable if diarrhea is present. It is most important to identify primary causes and treat accordingly.

REFERENCES

1. Glickman LT, Glickman NW, Shellenburg DB, et al. Multiple risk factors for the gastric dilatation volvulus syndrome in dogs: A practitioner/owner case control study. J Am Anim Hosp Assoc. 1997; 33:197-204.
2. Glickman LT, Glickman NW, Shellenburg DB, et al. Epidemiologic studies of bloat in dogs. Purina Veterinary Previews 1997; 2:10-15.
3. Badylak SF, Lantz GC, Jeffries M. Prevention of reperfusion injury in surgically induced gastric dilatation volvulus in dogs. Am J Vet Res. 1990; 51:294-299.
4. Ellison GW. Gastric dilatation volvulus: Surgical prevention. Vet Clin North Am: Sm Anim Pract. 1993; 27:513-521.
5. Glickman LT. Epidemiology of gastric dilatation-volvulus in dogs. Waltham Focus. 1997; 7:9-11.
6. Engen MH. Management of rectal prolapse. In Bojrab MJ (ed): Current Techniques in Small Animal Surgery, 3rd ed.. Philadelphia, Lea & Febiger, 1990.

Additional references available from the author upon request.

HOW I USE VACUUM-ASSISTED WOUND CLOSURE: AKA THE VAC

Gary W. Ellison, DVM, MS, Diplomate ACVS
College of Veterinary Medicine
University of Florida, Gainesville, FL

Vacuum-assisted wound closure (VAC) is a noninvasive, active wound management therapy exposing the wound bed to local subatmospheric negative pressure through a closed system in order to facilitate wound healing. Initially introduced in human medicine for the treatment of chronic wounds, VAC removes fluid from the extravascular space, improving circulation and enhancing the proliferation of granulation tissue.

A VAC system consists of several elements. Sterile polyurethane open-cell foam is cut to conform to the surface of the wound. The foam is placed within the wound making sure the foam is in contact with the entire wound surface. An egress tube runs from within the foam to another tube, which is connected to a reservoir and a vacuum pump. A plastic sheet with adhesive on one side is placed over the sponge and around the tubing creating an airtight seal with the skin around the wound margin. Subatmospheric pressure then applies a controlled suction force uniformly to all tissues on the surface of the wound.

Beneficial effects on wound healing have been documented in several animal models. Reported benefits include increases in tissue blood flow, granulation tissue formation, and skin flap survival when compared with conventional bandaging techniques. VAC wound dressings also demonstrate a significant increase in the rate of bacterial clearance in experimentally infected.

Based on promising results in animal models, VAC has become a mainstay in human wound management. The successful treatment of acute, sub-acute, and chronic wounds is well documented throughout human medical literature. Vacuum-assisted closure has been used to treat degloving injuries, compartment syndrome, dehiscence of surgical wounds with or without exposed orthopedic implants, bones, ligaments, or tendons, and to prevent postoperative seroma formation. VAC dressings have gained wide acceptance as a bolster dressing for full- and split-thickness skin grafts and to enhance re-epithelialization of skin graft donor sites. The utility of VAC has also been recognized in human emergency medicine for the treatment of abdominal compartment syndrome, damage control laparotomy, open drainage of both the abdominal and thoracic cavities and nonsurgical treatment of enterocutaneous fistulas.

EQUIPMENT AND APPLICATION OF VACUUM-ASSISTED CLOSURE DRESSINGS

It is essential that basic wound care principles be applied to all wounds prior to the application of VAC therapy. Proper debridement of devitalized tissues is essential for successful would closure and to eliminate any potential nidus for bacterial growth. Inability to thoroughly debride wounds prior to the application of VAC may result in the proliferation of granulation tissue over necrotic tissues resulting in delayed wound healing and abscess formation.

The vacuum-assisted wound closure device and methodology are subject to US and foreign patents, and applications assigned to Wake Forest University. A worldwide license for VAC has been assigned to Kinetic Concepts, Inc. (KCI), San Antonio, TX, and the VAC is a trademark of KCI. A VAC system has several essential elements. Sterile open cell polyurethane foam, plastic egress tubes, collection reservoirs and an adjustable suction pump capable of intermittent or continuous negatives pressures ranging from –50 mmHg to –200 mmHg are all available through KCI.

The open cell polyurethane foam is available in three sizes. Each foam dressing comes in a sterile package with two transparent plastic self-adhesive sheets. The foam can be cut to conform to the shape of the wound. The foam should be placed within the wound so that it is in contact with the entire wound surface, especially the deep margins of the wound. Foam should be placed within the wound fully expanded and care should be taken to avoid tightly packing foam into wounds. Foam bandages available through KCI are often too large for dogs and cats. The foam can be cut to shape and excess foam utilized in future VAC bandages.

A plastic fenestrated egress tube is inserted into a hole cut into the foam or placed between two pieces of foam. Placement of the tube fenestrations directly on the wound should be avoided as this may cause pressure necrosis in tissues around the fenestration sites and result in clogging of the vacuum system. Once the foam and plastic tubing are in place the two are then covered with an adhesive plastic sheet that extends several centimeters beyond the wound margins. In veterinary patients it is helpful to cleanly shave all hair surrounding the wound in order to facilitate adherence of the plastic sheet and establish an airtight seal. In areas with difficult bandage conformation, we have also found it helpful to apply stoma paste to the skin around the wound to aid in adherence of the skin to the plastic adhesive sheet. It is essential that an airtight seal be established in order to maintain constant negative pressure and prevent desiccation of the underlying tissues. The egress suction tube is then attached to a collection reservoir and to the vacuum pump. When the bandage is properly placed, a closed system is created consisting of the wound, foam, suction tube, collection reservoir, and suction pump.

A continuous negative pressure setting of 125 mmHg is most commonly used. Initial animal studies showed improved blood flow and granulation tissue formation with intermittent suction; however, when intermittent suction was performed in the clinical setting on human patients, increased wound discomfort was noted. For weeping wounds and postoperative prevention of seroma and edema formation, a lower negative pressure setting of 50 mm Hg is used.

The frequency of VAC bandage changes depends on the characteristics of the individual wound. Vacuum-assisted closure bandage dressings are typically changed every 2 to 3 days. If VAC bandages are left in place over 4 to 5 days, granulation tissue may grow into the open cell foam requiring surgical removal of the foam bandage. Highly contaminated and infected wounds may require daily bandage changes and copious lavage. If a foul odor is noted while changing VAC bandages, bandage changes should be performed more frequently and hydrotherapy initiated. In veterinary patients, bandage changes can usually be performed under heavy sedation. If extended VAC therapy is to be performed, the foam can be cut out through the plastic adhesive sheets while leaving the portion of the sheet adhered to the skin in place. This reduces skin irritation and minimizes discomfort experienced during bandage changes. New adhesive sheets are placed over the previously applied bandage to avoid pulling the adhesive sheet away from the skin.

APPLICABLE HUMAN LITERATURE REVIEW
Nonhealing Wounds

Vacuum-assisted closure was initially developed for the nonsurgical treatment of chronic nonhealing wounds in human patients. A report of 175 human patients suffering from chronic nonhealing wounds attributed to pressure ulcers, dehisced wounds, venous stasis ulcers, radiation ulcers, vasculitic ulcers, and diabetic ulcers. Of the 175 patients treated with VAC therapy 171 responded favorably resulting in complete closure or closure following a less-invasive skin graft or skin flap. In a study comparing VAC versus traditional wet-to-dry bandages for the treatment of 36 chronic nonhealing wounds, VAC treated wounds decreased in size by 78% compared with a 30% size reduction in wounds treated with wet-to-dry bandages. Histologic evaluation of VAC treated wounds also showed marked granulation tissue formation and angiogenesis while the wet to dry treatment group showed inflammation and fibrosis.

Surgical Dehiscence

Vacuum-assisted closure has been used extensively in human surgery for the closure of surgical dehiscences. Closure of median sternotomies and various spinal and orthopedic procedures have all been reported. The use of VAC therapy has been shown to decrease the wound management time required before a delayed secondary closure could be performed as well as speed closure by nonsurgical means when second intention healing is relied on alone. The human literature also supports the use of VAC therapy in cases of surgical dehiscence with exposed orthopedic hardware, bone or tendons. The VAC system maintains these wounds in a closed environment preventing further contamination and enhances the rate of granulation tissue formation over exposed bone, tendon, or orthopedic implant.

Degloving Injuries and Skin Grafting

The ability of VAC to produce granulation tissue over exposed bone and tendon has made it an ideal form of wound therapy for appendicular degloving injuries and several human studies support such claims. In human patients, degloving injuries are treated with VAC therapy in a number of ways. Reports of appendicular degloving injuries treated with surgical reattachment of the skin and an overlying VAC bandage has resulted in skin survival rates between 60 and 100%. When skin reattachment is not a surgical option, degloving injuries are often treated with VAC dressing until a healthy granulation bed is formed. A split-thickness skin graft with an overlying VAC bandage can then be used as a bolster dressing. Human split-thickness skin graft survival is reported to be between 95% and 100% using this technique. The reported benefits of VAC bandages used as a bolster for human split-thickness skin grafting include evacuation of excessive fluid and removal of degradation products, immobilization of the skin graft to the recipient bed, bandage conformation to irregular surfaces, enhanced neovascularization. In addition, VAC bandage application to graft donor site wounds re-epithelialized significantly faster than donor sites managed with traditional bandaging techniques.

Skin Avulsions

Increased survival of skin flaps and skin avulsions injuries have been reported in both human patients as well as various animal models. In veterinary patients, these injuries can be difficult to manage since any attempt to stabilize the orthopedic injuries often results in further vascular compromise of skin, which is relying primarily on the subdermal plexus for survival. The increased anatomic dead space and avascular tissue created by these physiologic degloving injuries also create a favorable environment for bacterial growth.

Prevention of Postoperative Swelling and Seroma Formation

The VAC system has been used in humans as a dressing for fasciotomy wounds after compartment syndrome. In a retrospective study comparing, VAC to simple saline soaked dressings for fasciotomies, patients treated with VAC dressings had more rapid resolution of edema fluid from the tissue, allowing earlier definitive closure. In addition, a greater proportion of VAC treated wounds underwent primary closure rather than skin grafting for wound coverage. In human surgical wounds associated with a high risk of seroma formation or post-operative weeping, VAC dressings placed over the surgical incision at a low negative pressure (50 mmHg) have resulted in the prevention of seroma formation and the successful transition to a dry wound that healed uneventfully with one 24-hour application.

Abdominal and Thoracic Uses

The VAC system has been used in human thoraces for the treatment of surgical dehiscence following median sternotomy and abdominal cavities after damage control laparotomy and for the treatment of abdominal compartment syndrome. Separation of the open celled foam from the abdominal and thoracic viscera was performed in some cases with fenestrated sheets of silicon. Enterocutaneous fistula formation has been

1533

reported as a result of foam eroding through the serosal surface of the intestines. These enterocutaneous fistulas were treated nonsurgically with VAC using a series of progressively smaller foam pieces with finer pore size until the fistulous tracts were sealed and healed by second intention.

Complications and Contraindications

Few complications exist in the human literature regarding VAC therapy. The most common is mild skin irritation from contact with the foam. The manufacturer has proposed several contraindications to VAC therapy. Though the VAC system will debride wounds to some extent, it will not remove grossly necrotic or devitalized tissue and should not be used in place of proper surgical debridement. The treatment of osteomyelitis with the VAC system alone is also contraindicated. Though VAC can be used over infected bone, resolution of osteomyelitis may be dependent on sequestrectomy where indicated and appropriate antibiotic therapy. VAC bandages are not recommended for the treatment of fistulas tracts to organs or body cavities in cases were the cause of the fistula is unknown, although reports exist in the human literature describing such techniques. The VAC system should not be used in wounds associated with known malignancies, since the application of the VAC bandage will likely increase blood flow and stimulate cellular proliferation within the wound bed. Finally, care should be taken when placing VAC dressings near exposed arteries and veins. It is possible for the foam to erode through vasculature resulting in extensive blood loss. Similarly, VAC dressings should be used with caution in patients with coagulation abnormalities or patients with active bleeding.

LARYNGEAL PARALYSIS

Eric Monnet, DVM, PhD, FAHA,
Diplomate ACVS and ECVS
College of Veterinary Medicine and Biomedical Sciences
Colorado State University, Fort Collins, CO

The laryngeal functions are to regulate airflow, voice production, and prevent inhalation of food. If the intrinsic muscles and/or the nerve supply of the larynx are not normal, laryngeal function is not normal.

The cricoarytenoideus dorsalis muscle abducts the arytenoid cartilages at each inspiration. The laryngeal recurrent nerve innervates this muscle. Lesions to the laryngeal recurrent nerve or to the cricoarytenoideus dorsalis muscle result in laryngeal paralysis in dogs and cats. Laryngeal paralysis can be unilateral or bilateral

ETIOLOGY

Congenital and acquired forms of laryngeal paralysis have been recognized in dogs and cats.

Congenital Laryngeal Paralysis

Congenital laryngeal paralysis has been reported in Bouvier des Flandres, bull terrier, Dalmatian, Rottweiller and Huskies. Bouvier des Flandres and bull terrier cases have mostly been reported from Europe while the Dalmatian and Huskies cases are mostly from the United States. Laryngeal paralysis has a hereditary transmission in Bouvier des Flandres with an autosomal dominant trait. Wallerian degeneration of the laryngeal recurrent nerves and abnormalities of the nucleus ambiguus are both present. Dogs with congenital laryngeal paralysis are clinical at an early age (before one year old) than dogs with acquired laryngeal paralysis.

Acquired Laryngeal Paralysis

Acquired laryngeal paralysis is most commonly reported in Labrador retrievers, Golden retrievers, St. Bernards, and Irish Setters at an age of 9 years old. It has been reported in cats. Acquired laryngeal paralysis is more frequently idiopathic; however, other causes should be ruled out. Diseases and conditions may contribute to laryngeal paralysis. A cranial mediastinal or neck mass stretching or compressing the laryngeal recurrent nerve can induce a laryngeal paralysis. Trauma to the laryngeal recurrent nerve during dogfights or during surgery in the neck is a cause of laryngeal paralysis. Laryngeal paralysis in the cat has been diagnosed after bilateral thyroidectomy. Finally, neuropathy involving the laryngeal recurrent nerve or myopathy involving the intrinsic muscle of the larynx, and endocrine insufficiency (hypothyroidism) that can induce a polyneuropathy or a polymyopathy are other causes of laryngeal paralysis in the adult dog.

CLINICAL FINDINGS
History

The presenting signs are similar for the congenital and acquired forms. Progression of signs is often slow; months to years may pass before an animal develops severe respiratory distress. Early signs include change in voice, followed by gagging and coughing, especially during eating or drinking. Endurance decreases and laryngeal stridor (especially inspiratory) increases as the airway occlusion worsens. Episodes of severe dyspnea, cyanosis, or syncope occur in severely affected patients. Male dogs are approximately three times more affected than females. Laryngeal paralysis can be accompanied with various degrees of dysphagia which significantly enhances the probability of aspiration after surgical correction of the laryngeal paralysis.

Physical Examination

The physical examination of dogs with laryngeal paralysis is fairly unremarkable. Dogs have an inspiratory dyspnea that is not alleviated with open mouth breathing. Mild lateral compression of the larynx significantly increases inspiratory dyspnea. Referred upper airway sounds are present during auscultation of the thoracic cavity. Auscultation of the thoracic cavity and the lung field may reveal the presence of pneumonia in the cranial lung lobe due to aspiration. Palpation of the muscle mass may reveal skeletal muscle atrophy in cases of polyneuropathy. The tibial cranial muscle is very commonly atrophied in dogs with endocrine polyneuropathy. A complete neurologic examination is required to evaluate the animal for a polyneuropathy.

Laboratory Findings

Complete blood count and chemistry profile are usually within normal limits. Hypercholesterolemia, hyperlipidemia, and augmentation of liver enzymes activity are present on the chemistry profile for dogs with hypothyroidism. A thyroid profile with endogenous TSH and free T4 is then required to further define the diagnosis. Laryngeal paralysis has inconsistent correlation with hypothyroidism.

Radiographic Examination

It is necessary to perform a radiographic examination of the thoracic cavity for the evaluation of the lung parenchyma and the esophagus. Aspiration pneumonia is common finding preoperatively in dogs with laryngeal paralysis. If aspiration pneumonia is present the surgical intervention should be delayed until the aspiration pneumonia resolved. Megaesophagus might be present in dogs with laryngeal paralysis especially if the paralysis is due to polyneuropathy or polymyopathy. Megaesophagus places the animal at more risk for aspiration pneumonia after surgery. Radiographic examination of the larynx is unremarkable.

Laryngeal Examination

A laryngeal examination under general anesthesia is required for the diagnosis of laryngeal paralysis. A light plane of anesthesia is required to be able to evaluate the laryngeal function during each inspiration. Thiopental or propofol is used intravenously as needed for the anesthesia. The animal should be anesthetized to the point at which the mouth can be opened easily and a laryngeal reflex is still present. If the animal is too deeply anesthetized the larynx looks paralyzed even in the normal animal. If the plane is too deep it is important to let the animal approach consciousness and examine the laryngeal function during this time. During the laryngeal examination, motion of the arytenoid cartilage is observed during inspiration. Dopram intravenously can be used to stimulate the central respiratory center and have a better laryngeal examination. The animal should be placed in sternal recumbency and the head elevated to the level that it is normally carried. In the normal animal the vocal fold and the arytenoids should abduct during inspiration and passively relax during expiration. The arytenoid cartilages and the vocal cords are immobile and drawn toward midline during inspiration if the animal has laryngeal paralysis. If the paralysis is unilateral only one cartilage is not moving. Edema and erythema of the mucosa of the arytenoid cartilages is present on the dorsal part of the larynx and appear to be due to repeat trauma of the arytenoid touching each other at each inspiration.

TREATMENT

Medical Treatment: Emergency Treatment

Animals are usually presented with acute cyanosis or collapse as a result of upper airway obstruction. Most animals in a cyanotic crisis precipitated by upper airway obstruction recover initially with medical therapy. Excitement or increase in the ambient temperature can trigger an acute onset of inspiratory dyspnea. Excitement or increase in the ambient temperature increases the respiratory rate, which results in trauma to the mucosa of the arytenoid cartilage. Inflammation and acute swelling of the mucosa of the arytenoid cartilages can exacerbate the chronic airway obstruction and induce an acute onset of inspiratory dyspnea. A vicious circle is then initiated.

Corticosteroids are given intravenously (dexamethasone, 0.2 to 1.0 mg/kg BID) to reduce laryngeal inflammation and edema. At the same time, oxygen is administered by mask or oxygen cage to alleviate hypoxia. Hyperventilating hyperthermic animals (temperature >105°F) must be cooled with an alcohol or ice-water bath. Sedation with acepromazine intravenously is indicated (0.1 mg/kg with a maximum dose of 3 mg) if the animal is still stressed. Fluid therapy is administered with caution, because some animals with severe upper respiratory tract obstruction develop pulmonary edema. Diuretics are indicated in these patients. If the patient condition is deteriorating, an emergency tracheostomy is recommended to bypass the upper airway.

Surgical Treatment

Laryngeal surgery is directed at removing or repositioning laryngeal cartilages that obstruct the rima glottidis. The four currently recognized surgical procedures used to correct laryngeal paralysis are (1) unilateral or bilateral arytenoid cartilage lateralization, (2) ventricular cordectomy and partial arytenoidectomy via the oral or ventral laryngotomy approach, (3) modified castellated laryngofissure, and (4) permanent tracheostomy. Arytenoid cartilage lateralization is currently the most common surgical treatment.

Arytenoid Cartilage Lateralization

This procedure has been used successfully to treat laryngeal paralysis in cats and dogs. Arytenoid lateralization has been performed bilaterally or unilaterally. Unilateral arytenoid lateralization is sufficient to reduce clinical signs of laryngeal paralysis. A unilateral lateralization can be performed through a ventral or a lateral incision. It is our preference to perform lateralization through a lateral incision.

The animal is positioned in lateral recumbency for a unilateral lateralization, and a skin incision is made over the larynx just ventral to the jugular groove. The sternohyoid muscle is retracted ventrally to expose the lateral aspect of the thyroid and cricoid cartilages. The larynx is rotated to expose the thyropharyngeal muscle, which is transected at the dorsocaudal edge of the thyroid cartilage. The wing of the thyroid cartilage is retracted laterally, and the cricothyroid junction may be incised. Incision of the cricothyroid joint gives a better exposure but it is not always needed. Its transection might reduce the diameter of the rima glottidis after arytenoid abduction. The cricoarytenoideus dorsalis muscle or the fibrous tissue left is dissected and transected. The cricoarytenoid articulation is detached from caudal to cranial with Metzembaum scissors. The sesamoid band connecting the arytenoid cartilages dorsally is left intact. However, dorsal displacement of the arytenoid results and creates distortion of the rima glottidis. The disarticulated arytenoid cartilage is only attached to the vocal cord, aryepiglottic fold, and laryngeal mucosa. Invasion through the laryngeal mucosa is avoided.

The arytenoid cartilage is sutured to the caudo-dorsal part of the cricoid cartilage. This provides an adequate laryngeal airway with only a unilateral tieback. Placement of the suture on the caudo-dorsal part of the cricoid provides a physiologic position of the suture. One 2-0 nonabsorbable suture is placed in a simple interrupted suture pattern from the muscular process of the arytenoid cartilage to the caudo-dorsal edge of the cricoid cartilage and tightened to maintain the arytenoid in position. An interrupted mattress sutures can be used in large breed dogs. In cats, it is recommended to use small suture material 3-0 or 4-0 mounted on a pledget to prevent tearing through the cartilage. The arytenoid cartilage does not need to be displaced caudally. It is the author's impression that the arytenoid cartilage needs only to be maintained in position and stabilized at inspiration.

An assistant should be available to observe per os the size of the laryngeal opening achieved to ensure that adequate abduction of the laryngeal cartilages has been obtained. Excessive abduction may lead to aspiration of food or fluid. The wound is closed by suturing the thyropharyngeal muscle and routinely closing the subcutaneous tissue and skin.

Complications associated with laryngeal lateralization include aspiration pneumonia, persistent cough exacerbated after drinking, seroma, breaking of the suture and fragmentation of the arytenoid cartilage. Breaking of the suture or fragmentation of the cartilage induce recurrence of the clinical signs of laryngeal paralysis. Laryngeal lateralization should then be performed on the other side. If the procedure has been performed bilaterally a partial laryngectomy needs to be performed. Seroma formation is very common and is self-limited. The incidence of aspiration pneumonia is more common in bilateral laryngeal lateralization compared to unilateral. In a study, 42% of the dogs with bilateral lateralization experienced an episode of aspiration pneumonia. Water and food should be completely withdrawn after surgery for 24 hours. Two or three meatballs should be delivered 24 hours after surgery under constant direct supervision. If the animal can handle meatballs with aspirating, ice cube and then water can be delivered. The animal should be closely watched for the next 2 weeks. The animal is at risk for aspiration pneumonia for its entire life after surgery.

Permanent Tracheostomy

Permanent tracheostomy is a surgical option for the treatment of dogs with laryngeal paralysis. The permanent tracheostomy bypasses the upper airway obstruction without inducing any modification in the size of the rima glottidis. This surgical technique is therefore more valuable for dogs at high risk of aspiration pneumonia (myopathy, megaesophagus, hiatal hernia, gastrointestinal disorder). Animals responded well to the treatment and owners were satisfied. Permanent tracheostomy requires attention and maintenance from the owners.

HOW I TREAT LARYNGEAL PARALYSIS

Eric Monnet, DVM, PhD, FAHA
Diplomate ACVS and ECVS
College of Veterinary Medicine and Biomedical Sciences
Colorado State University, Fort Collins, CO

The laryngeal functions are to regulate airflow, voice production and prevent inhalation of food. If the intrinsic muscles and/or the nerve supply of the larynx are not normal laryngeal function is not normal.

The cricoarytenoideus dorsalis muscle abducts the arytenoid cartilages at each inspiration. The laryngeal recurrent nerve innervates this muscle. Lesions to the laryngeal recurrent nerve or to the cricoarytenoideus dorsalis muscle result in laryngeal paralysis in dogs and cats. Laryngeal paralysis can be unilateral or bilateral.

Medical treatment is necessary in an emergency situation; however, the surgical treatment is the definitive treatment. Laryngeal surgery is directed at removing or repositioning laryngeal cartilages that obstruct the rima glottidis. The four currently recognized surgical procedures used to correct laryngeal paralysis are (1) unilateral or bilateral arytenoid cartilage lateralization, (2) ventricular cordectomy and partial arytenoidectomy via the oral or ventral laryngotomy approach, (3) modified castellated laryngofissure, and (4) permanent tracheostomy. Arytenoid cartilage lateralization is currently the most common surgical treatment.

ARYTENOID CARTILAGE LATERALIZATION

This procedure has been used successfully to treat laryngeal paralysis in cats and dogs. Arytenoid lateralization has been performed bilaterally or unilaterally. Unilateral arytenoid lateralization is sufficient to reduce clinical signs of laryngeal paralysis. A unilateral lateralization can be performed through a ventral or a lateral incision. It is our preference to perform lateralization through a lateral incision.

The animal is positioned in lateral recumbency for a unilateral lateralization, and a skin incision is made over the larynx just ventral to the jugular groove. The sternohyoid muscle is retracted ventrally to expose the lateral aspect of the thyroid and cricoid cartilages. The larynx is rotated to expose the thyropharyngeal muscle, which is transected at the dorsocaudal edge of the thyroid cartilage. The wing of the thyroid cartilage is retracted laterally, and the cricothyroid junction may be incised. Incision of the cricothyroid joint gives a better exposure but it is not always needed. Its transection might reduce the diameter of the rima glottidis after arytenoid abduction. The cricoarytenoideus dorsalis muscle or the fibrous tissue left is dissected and transected. The cricoarytenoid articulation is detached from caudal to cranial with Metzembaum scissors. The sesamoid band connecting the arytenoid cartilages dorsally is left intact. However, dorsal displacement of the arytenoid results and creates distortion of the rima glottidis. The disarticulated arytenoid cartilage is only attached to the vocal cord, aryepiglottic fold, and

laryngeal mucosa. Invasion through the laryngeal mucosa is avoided.

The arytenoid cartilage is sutured to the caudo-dorsal part of the cricoid cartilage. This provides an adequate laryngeal airway with only a unilateral tieback. Placement of the suture on the caudo-dorsal part of the cricoid provides a physiologic position of the suture. One 2-0 nonabsorbable suture is placed in a simple interrupted suture pattern from the muscular process of the arytenoid cartilage to the caudo-dorsal edge of the cricoid cartilage and tightened to maintain the arytenoid in position. An interrupted mattress sutures can be used in large breed dogs. In cats, it is recommended to use small suture material 3-0 or 4-0 mounted on a pledget to prevent tearing through the cartilage. The arytenoid cartilage does not need to be displaced caudally. It is the author's impression that the arytenoid cartilage needs only to be maintained in position and stabilized at inspiration.

An assistant should be available to observe per os the size of the laryngeal opening achieved to ensure that adequate abduction of the laryngeal cartilages has been obtained. Excessive abduction may lead to aspiration of food or fluid. The wound is closed by suturing the thyropharyngeal muscle and routinely closing the subcutaneous tissue and skin.

Complications associated with laryngeal lateralization include aspiration pneumonia, persistent cough exacerbated after drinking, seroma, breaking of the suture and fragmentation of the arytenoid cartilage. Breaking of the suture or fragmentation of the cartilage induce recurrence of the clinical signs of laryngeal paralysis. Laryngeal lateralization should then be performed on the other side. If the procedure has been performed bilaterally a partial laryngectomy needs to be performed. Seroma formation is very common and is self-limited. The incidence of aspiration pneumonia is more common in bilateral laryngeal lateralization compared to unilateral. In a study, 42% of the dogs with bilateral lateralization experienced an episode of aspiration pneumonia. Water and food should be completely withdrawn after surgery for 24 hours. Two or three meatballs should be delivered 24 hours after surgery under constant direct supervision. If the animal can handle meatballs with aspirating, ice cubes and then water can be delivered. The animal should be closely watched for the next 2 weeks. The animal is at risk for aspiration pneumonia for its entire life after surgery.

PERMANENT TRACHEOSTOMY

Permanent tracheostomy is a surgical option for the treatment of dogs with laryngeal paralysis. The permanent tracheostomy bypasses the upper airway obstruction without inducing any modification in the size of the rima glottidis. This surgical technique is therefore more valuable for dogs at high risk of aspiration pneumonia (myopathy, megaesophagus, hiatal hernia, gastrointestinal disorder). Animals responded well to the treatment and owners were satisfied. Permanent tracheostomy requires attention and maintenance from the owners.

HOW DO I TREAT A PORTOSYSTEMIC SHUNT?

Eric Monnet, DVM, PhD, FAHA
Diplomate ACVS and ECVS
College of Veterinary Medicine and Biomedical Sciences
Colorado State University, Fort Collins, CO

Portosystemic shunt (PSS) is an abnormal vessel that shunts portal blood from the splanchnic circulation to flow directly to the systemic circulation by passing the liver. Toxins, hormones, nutrients, escaping bacteria, and exogenous drugs also bypass the liver resulting in hepatic encephalopathy (HE). Hepatic growth and size are maintained by normal portal blood flow (80% of the total liver blood flow) and hepatotrophic hormones (insulin, glucagon). Diversion of portal blood flow results in atrophy of the liver inducing further deterioration of liver function. Dogs or cats with congenital portosystemic shunt present with multiple clinical signs related to HE. Differentiation between single congenital and multiple acquired shunts is important, as their treatment and prognosis differ greatly. Treatment of choice for congenital shunt is partial or complete surgical ligation of the anomalous vessel; this may result in fatal portal hypertension in patients with acquired shunt. Portal hypertension secondary to primary liver disease (ie, hepatic cirrhosis) result generally in the development of acquired shunts.

Congenital portosystemic shunts may be classified as single or multiple and intrahepatic or extrahepatic. Five types of PSS have been described. Eighty percent of the PSS are single, 72% are extrahepatic, and 95% are between the portal vein and the caudal vena cava.

Surgery is recognized as the treatment of choice for PSS. Because liver needs hepatotrophic substances from portal blood flow, deterioration of liver function can be expected if the shunted blood flow is not surgically corrected in a physiologic direction. Medical treatment will not correct this alteration; therefore long-term survival is not expected. In one study, only 2 of 8 dogs with medical treatment were still alive at 6 months. Life expectancy of 2 months to 2 years is generally reported; the actual time presumably being dependent on the amount of portal blood flow. Restoring the flow of hepatotrophic substances to sinusoidal milieu results in substantial hepatic regeneration and reversal of functional impairment.

Patients with PSS experience a reduction in absorption, metabolism, and clearance of drugs due to liver impairment. Fentanyl can be used for sedation. Mask induction with isoflurane followed by endotracheal intubation is the method of choice. Dextrose (2.5%) is important during surgery and the immediate postoperative period to maintain blood glucose. Cephalosporin perioperatively is recommended. Ischemic episode can occur in the bowel during manipulation of the PSS that will may result in bacterial embolization .

A standard ventral midline celiotomy is performed from the xiphoid to pubis to explore the portal system. The portal vein and caudal vena cava are located by retracting the duodenum medially. The portal vein is identified ventral to the caudal vena cava at the most dorsal aspect of the mesoduodenum. The caudal vena cava is examine for identification of any abnormal blood vessels. Normally, from the renal and phrenico-abdominal veins to the hile of the liver there should be no blood vessels entering the caudal vena cava ventrally. Any blood vessel in this area should be suspect as an extrahepatic shunting blood vessel. Turbulence in this portion of the vena cava is another important clue for locating a possible shunt. If nothing abnormal is noticed the left omental bursa is entered and all tributaries from the portal vein are identified. Most often, shunting vessels come from the gastrosplenic vein in dogs and left gastric vein in cats. If no shunting vessel can be located, investigation for an intrahepatic shunt is started. Inspection of the hepatic veins cranial to the liver and inspection of liver lobes for dilation are the first steps in identification of an intrahepatic shunt.

Complete occlusion of the shunt at the time of surgery is associated with a better prognosis. However, complete occlusion may not be possible at the time of surgery because the liver parenchyma cannot accommodate the augmentation in blood flow. It then results in portal hypertension. Occlusion of a PSS has been performed traditionally with a suture placed around the shunt and tight while the portal pressure was measured. This technique resulted in acute or chronic portal hypertension in 15% to 20% of the cases. Acute portal hypertension resulted in death in most of the cases. Chronic portal hypertension induced ascites and the opening of acquired shunts.

To palliate to these problems and achieve complete occlusion of the PSS gradual occlusion has been performed with ameroid constrictor or cellophane band. Both of these devices induce a slow and complete occlusion of the PSS over 4 to 8 weeks. The liver parenchyma can then accommodate the augmentation in blood flow without inducing portal hypertension.

A strip of cellophane 1 cm wide is folded three times on itself. It is then placed around the shunt vessels without inducing any occlusion of the shunt. The cellophane is stabilized with a vascular clip.

Postoperatively, patients are examined for signs of portal hypertension: sepsis, abdominal pain, bloody diarrhea, and ascites. If signs of portal hypertension occur, the patient is taken back to surgery and the suture released. Failure to remove the ligature will result in septic shock and death. Hypothermia during surgery and postoperatively should be corrected aggressively. Dextrose (2.5%) intravenously is maintained. Thrombosis of the portal vein has been reported as complication of a partial ligation of intrahepatic PSS. Postoperative seizures have been reported as a complication of ligation of PSS and they carry a poor prognosis. Seizures may occur immediately or up to 3 days postoperatively.

Surgical mortality associated with treatment of PSS can be as high as 20%. The intraoperative and immediate postoperative periods are most critical.

Hypothermia and hypoglycemia should be anticipated and treated promptly. With the devices for gradual occlusion the incidence of complications seems significantly reduced.

Postoperatively the animal should be maintained on a low-protein diet, amoxicillin or neomycin, and lactulose. Bile acids should be monitored at 1, 3, and 6 months after surgery. Lactulose should be interrupted one month after surgery. The antibiotics should then be removed from the treatment. Three months after surgery the diet can be progressively returned to normal. If the animal is showing signs of hepatic encephalopathy then the low protein diet is re-instituted.

With cellophane bile acids do not come to within normal limits before 3 to 6 months after surgery. The cellophane is inducing a slow and progressive occlusion of the shunt.

LAPAROSCOPIC GASTROPEXY

Eric Monnet, DVM, PhD, FAHA
Diplomate ACVS and ECVS
College of Veterinary Medicine and Biomedical Sciences
Colorado State University, Fort Collins, CO

A preventive gastropexy can be performed using the laparoscope simply by exteriorizing the pyloric antrum region of the stomach through the right abdominal wall. The animal is placed in dorsal recumbency and the telescope portal is placed on the midline at the level of the umbilicus.

The instrument portal receives grasping forceps that are used to localize and grasp the pyloric antrum. The cannula entry site for the grasping forceps is placed 2 cm behind the last rib on the right side and at the junction of distal and proximal third of the last rib. A 5-mm atraumatic grasping forceps with multiple teeth is used to grasp the pyloric antrum mid-distance between the lesser and the greater curvature. The stomach is then pulled close to the cannula. If there is too much tension to bring the pyloric antrum to the body wall the pyloric antrum should be grasp again closer to the body of the stomach. Deflation of the pneumoperitoneum is also helpful to reduce the tension on the stomach wall. The incision for the cannula is extended through the abdominal wall. One should watch the scalpel blade internally as a scalpel blade enters parallel to the cannula shaft and then cuts away from the cannula increasing the incision to approximately 5 mm in length in a direction parallel to the last rib. Electrocautery can be used to perform the dissection through the abdominal wall. It is important not to touch the cannula with the cautery during the dissection because it can cauterize the stomach wall. An incision length of approximately 5 cm is made. Once the stomach is firmly seated against the cannula, the stomach, the grasping forceps and cannula are pulled through the abdominal wall simultaneously thus exteriorizing a section of the stomach wall.

Two stay sutures are then placed in the stomach wall to prevent it from falling back into the abdominal cavity. An incisional gastropexy is then performed using a No. 15 scalpel blade to incise the serosa and the muscularis layer over a 5-cm length. Metzembaum scissors are next used to develop the seroso-muscularis flap. Cruciate suture pattern (3-0 monofilament absorbable suture material) is used to pexy the seroso-muscularis flap to the transverse abdominal muscle. The external and internal oblique muscles are closed with a continuous suture pattern. Subcutaneous tissue and skin are closed in a routine fashion. The telescope is then removed and the incision closed.

PRINCIPLES OF GASTROINTESTINAL SURGERY

Eric Monnet, DVM, PhD
Diplomate ACVS and ECVS
College of Veterinary Medicine and Biomedical Sciences
Colorado State University, Fort Collins, CO

Gastrointestinal surgery is performed very commonly in small animals for biopsy, removal of a foreign body, upper gastrointestinal bleeding, resection of a necrotic segment of intestine, resection of necrotic portion of the stomach, and resection of a neoplasia. Approximately 10% of dogs with gastric dilatation-volvulus have a devitalized gastric wall requiring gastrectomy. Ischemic injury occurs most commonly in the fundic area along the greater curvature. Upper gastrointestinal bleeding results from chronic renal and liver disease, mast cell tumor, gastrin producing neoplasia of the pancreas, gastric neoplasia and non steroidal anti-inflammatory drugs. Gastrotomy, gastrectomy, enterotomy, and enterectomy are the procedures routinely performed. General principles common to all of these procedures have to be followed.

FLUID THERAPY

Animals with gastrointestinal disease require fluid replacement for rehydration and correction of acid–base deficit. Dogs and cats with vomiting and diarrhea might be hypovolemic which can result in hypotension at the time of anesthesia. Acid–base imbalance can also result in severe hypotension and arrhythmias at the time of surgery.

Incidence of gastric foreign bodies is high in dog and cat. The most characteristic sign is vomiting, which could be intermittent because vomiting reflex is trigger when the foreign body is located in the pyloric antrum. Metabolic acidosis is the most common modification with gastric foreign body. Hypokalemic alkalosis can occur if obstruction of the pylorus is present.

Vomiting animal from intestinal foreign materials may have a normal pH or be in metabolic acidosis. Metabolic acidosis results from loss of duodenal, pancreatic, and bile secretions more than gastric fluid.

ANTIBIOTIC PROPHYLAXIS

Gastrointestinal surgery is considered as a clean-contaminated surgery. Therefore antibiotics are required during the procedures. Most common bacteria encountered during gastrointestinal surgery are: *Escherichia coli, Enterococcus* spp, *Streptococcus, Staphylococccus aureus, Proteus,* and *Bacteroides fragilis.* In the stomach the bacteria population is more limited than in the rest of the intestine because of the acid environment. In the colon the population of anaerobic bacteria is elevated. Before surgery the patient is placed on prophylactic intravenous antibiotic. For the surgery of the stomach, ampicillin or first generation cephalosporin (20 mg/kg IV every 60 min) can be used. For the rest of the intestine, second generation antibiotics are preferable because they a have a broad spectrum against gram-positive and gram-negative bacteria. Cefoxitin (20 mg / kg IV every 90 min) is the antibiotic of choice. A combination of ampicillin enrofloxacin can be used also. Antibiotics are interrupted at the end of the procedure unless the animal has peritonitis. The animals need to be watch closely for signs of infection.

TIMING OF SURGERY

Gastric foreign bodies need to be removed when diagnosed because they can induce inflammation of the gastric wall and pyloric or intestinal obstruction. Bleeding gastric ulceration or bleeding mass of the stomach need to be removed surgically as soon as possible. The patient needs to be stabilized as best as possible before surgery with blood transfusion. Dogs with bleeding ulcer may exsanguinate in their stomach.

Intestinal perforation and peritonitis requires immediate surgical attention. Surgery for mechanical obstruction of the intestines is performed as soon as possible. The risk of ischemic necrosis caused by vascular obstruction increases with time. Necrosis of the mucosa results in translocation of bacteria and sepsis. Strangulation of a loop of intestine is suspected when acute and severe abdominal pain is present. It requires immediate surgical attention. Septic shock with a poor response to medical treatment is commonly associated with strangulation. Distention of the intestinal lumen with gas and fluid results from air ingested, gas due decomposition of intestinal content, gas diffusion from blood, decreased fluid absorption, and increased fluid production.

ASSESSMENT OF VIABLITY
Stomach

No objective criteria exist to evaluate the gastric wall viability. Absence of peristaltic wave, pale greenish to gray serosal color, thin gastric wall, and lack of bleeding after partial thickness incision are signs of gastric wall devitalization.

Intestine

Viability is assessed by coloration of the serosa, peristalsism, pulse in the jejunal arteries, and utilization of intravenous fluorescein. Fluorescein at the dose of 15 mg/kg is injected intravenously. Fluorescein emits a gold green fluorescence when exposed to ultraviolet light. Viable intestine has a smooth uniform green gold fluorescence. Hyperemic intestine has a brighter color than normal. Nonviable intestine has patchy fluorescence or no fluorescence. The fluorescence can also be located around blood vessel.

CHOICE OF SUTURE MATERIAL AND NEEDLES

A wide range of suture materials has been used during gastrointestinal surgery. It is recommended to use synthetic absorbable monofilament suture materials. Synthetic sutures are stronger sutures than gut and more resistant to infection. Synthetic absorbable sutures are absorbed primarily by hydrolysis, which is more predictable than enzymatic digestion. Monofilament cannot harbor bacteria and do not have a wick effect like braided suture therefore they are resistant to infection. Polydioxanone (PDS) or polyglyconate (Maxon) size 4.0 or 3.0 are the recommended sutures for gastrointestinal surgery. A taper needle is recommended for placement sutures in the stomach wall and the intestine.

ASEPSIS

Every effort should be made to prevent contamination of the abdominal cavity during gastrointestinal surgery. The stomach or the loop of intestine are "packed off" the rest of the abdominal cavity. Layers of moist laparotomy sponges are used. Intestinal content is moved away for the surgical site with gentle manipulation and atraumatic clamps are placed to prevent the intestinal content to come back. Stay sutures are placed in the stomach to elevate the stomach wall and prevent spillage of stomach content into the peritoneal cavity.

After completion of the surgery, the peritoneal cavity is lavaged with warm sterile saline solution to removed gastrointestinal spillage and blood clots. Usually 1 liter of saline is used for a 10-kg dog. The entire fluid is eliminated with surgical suction to get the peritoneal cavity as dry as possible.

Gloves and instruments are then changed. New surgical towels are placed on the edges of the laparotomy. The abdominal cavity is then closed routinely.

SURGICAL TECHNIQUES

A midline celiotomy is required for any surgery on the gastrointestinal tract. The surgery should start with a complete abdominal exploration to evaluate the entire length of the gastrointestinal tract, the liver, the pancreas, the lymph nodes, the urinary system and the adrenal glands.

SURGERY OF THE STOMACH
Gastrotomy

Gastrotomy incision is performed in a relatively avascular area, midway between the lesser and the greater curvature of the stomach. One stay suture is placed at each end of the planed gastrotomy incision. Stay sutures are used to manipulate the stomach and bring the stomach wall to the edge of the abdominal incision. The stomach is walled off with moist laparotomy sponges to prevent contamination of the abdominal cavity with gastric content. A No. 11 blade is used to stab the gastric wall next to one stay suture. Then, a Metzenbaum scissors is used to extend the gastrotomy incision. The incision should be long enough to remove the foreign body without tearing the stomach wall. Hemorrhage occurs mainly in the seromuscular layer and can be controlled by ligation with fine absorbable sutures. The foreign body is extracted and the gastrotomy closed. Gastrotomy is closed with one layer simple apposition pattern with 3-0 monofilament absorbable suture. The abdominal cavity is lavage with warm saline prior to closure. Surgical gloves are

changed and a new pack of instruments is then used to complete the abdominal closure.

Electrolyte and acid-base imbalances are corrected by intravenous electrolyte solution. Fluid therapy is maintained until oral fluid intake is adequate. Water is offered 12 to 24 hours after recovery from anesthesia. If the patient is not vomiting, then small amount of bland diet can be offered. The amount of food is gradually increased over the next four days. Peritonitis after gastrotomy is a rare complication. Gastritis requires treatment with cimetidine or ranitidine and sulcralfate.

Gastrectomy

Gastrectomy is required to resect the necrotic stomach wall during GDV. Stomach wall resection after rupture of a gastric ulcer requires wide margin since gastric ulceration could be associated with gastric adenocarcinoma or gastric lymphoma.

Two options are available: gastrectomy with either traditional suture technique or stapling suture. Gastrectomy with automatic stapling equipment is associated with the best post surgical outcome during GDV. This is the recommended technique.

Gastrectomy during GDV

Branches of the short gastric arteries and left gastro-epiploic artery supplying the area to be resected are ligated. Necrotic gastric wall is resected with Metzenbaum scissors to the level of healthy gastric tissue. A two-layer closure with inverting pattern using 3-0 absorbable monofilament suture is necessary to close the stomach. This technique is associated with 60% mortality. If autostapling equipment is available a Thoraco-Abdominal device (TA 55 or 90) can be used to perform the gastrectomy (Figure 1). The TA 55 or 90 placed two staggered row of staples respectively 55 or 90 mm long. The length of staples for stomach wall resection should be 4.8 mm. The TA 55 or 90 is first clamped on healthy stomach wall. The two row of staples are then fired and a 15 blade is used to resect the devitalized stomach wall. The TA is then released.

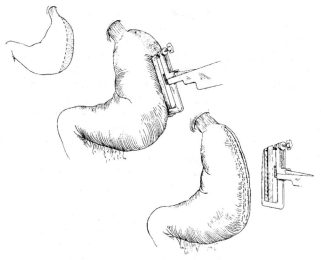

Figure 1.

The suture line is then inspected to be sure that all the staples are in correct position and then a simple inverting suture line is applied. The advantages of this technique include decrease surgical time and decreased abdominal contamination from gastric spillage. Mortality rate with the autostapling equipment is close to 10%. Stomach rupture at the time of surgery is associated with severe peritonitis.

Gastrectomy for Ulcer or Mass

After identification of the stomach ulcer or tumor, the healthy stomach is retracted with stay sutures to prevent gastric spillage. The stomach wall is then resected around the lesion. The stomach wall is highly vascular. Bleeding blood vessels on the line of incision are ligated with 4.0 monofilament absorbable sutures. Staples can be used to close the gastrectomy. Hand suture can be performed if stapling equipment is not available. Two inverting continuous sutures are used to close the stomach after gastrectomy. A Cushing suture followed by a Lembert is the traditional technique. However, one simple continuous apposition suture can be used to close the stomach.

Electrolyte and acid-base imbalances are corrected by intravenous electrolyte solution. Fluid therapy is maintained until oral fluid intake is adequate. Water is offered 12 to 24 hours after recovery from anesthesia. If the patient is not vomiting, then small amount of bland diet can be offered. The amount of food is gradually increased over the next four days. Peritonitis after gastrotomy is a rare complication. Gastritis requires treatment with cimetidine or ranitidine and sucralfate.

SURGERY OF THE INTESTINE
Enterotomy

A variety of foreign bodies can be ingested by young animals. Linear foreign bodies are more common in cats. Once, an object has passed through the pylorus, the next smallest lumen are the distal duodenum and the proximal jejunum.

Plication of the intestinal indicates the presence of a linear foreign body. Usually one end of the linear body is still located in the stomach and need to be released first. Particular attention is paid to mesenteric border especially with a linear foreign material. Linear foreign body can cut through the mesenteric border and induce leakage of intestinal content. Multiple enterotomy may be required to remove the entire linear foreign body. Enterectomy is required if the mesenteric border has been damaged.

Enterotomy is performed immediately distal to the foreign material. Intestine is walled off the abdominal cavity to prevent leakage of intestinal content inside the abdominal cavity. The incision on the antimesenteric border should be long enough to extract the foreign body without tearing the intestine.

The enterotomy is then closed with a simple interrupted appositional pattern with 4-0 monofilament absorbable suture. Since the submucosa is the only holding layer, it needs to be incorporated in the suture.

The submucosa tends to retract away from the edge of the incision. The everted mucosa can be trimmed away to allow better exposure of the submucosa.

A serosal patch can be performed to improve blood supply to the enterotomy site and increase its tensile strength. The abdominal cavity is lavage with warm saline prior to closure. Surgical gloves are changed and a new pack of instruments is then used to complete the abdominal closure.

Enterectomy

An enterectomy is indicated if the intestine is not viable (intussusception, volvulus) perforated by a linear foreign material at the mesenteric border, or if a intestinal neoplasia is present. End to end anastomosis is the preferred technique to perform an enterectomy. Intestine is walled off the abdominal cavity to prevent leakage of intestinal content inside the abdominal cavity. Enterectomy requires double ligation of the branches of the arterio-venous supply of the portion of intestine to resect (Figure 2).

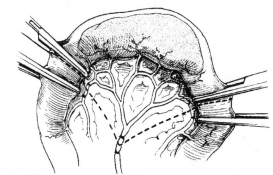

Figure 2.

The terminal arcade is also double ligated. Transection is performed between the double ligations. Crushing clamps are then placed on the portion of intestine that is going to be resected. The clamps are either placed perpendicular or at a slight angle toward the normal intestine. Non-crushing clamps are placed on the normal intestine 4 to 5 cm away from the enterectomy site after milking away the intestinal content. The intestine is transected with a scalpel blade using the crushing clamps as guide. Since the submucosa is the only holding layer, it needs to be incorporated in the suture. The submucosa tends to retract away from the edge of the incision. The everted mucosa can be trimmed away to allow better exposure of the submucosa (Figure 3) Anastomosis is performed with simple interrupted or continuous appositional pattern with 4-0 monofilament absorbable suture (Figure 4).

If the two extremities of the intestine are not of equivalent diameter the smaller diameter segment can is incised on the antimesenteric border to create a larger spatulated edge (Figure 4). A serosal patch can be placed around the enterectomy site to improve blood supply and tensile strength.

The abdominal cavity is lavage with warm saline prior to closure. Surgical gloves are changed and a new pack

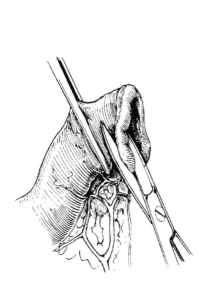

Figure 3.

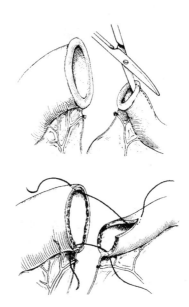

Figure 4.

of instruments is then used to complete the abdominal closure.

Electrolyte and acid-base imbalances are corrected by intravenous electrolyte solution. Fluid therapy is maintained until oral fluid intake is adequate. Water is offered 24 to 48 hours after recovery from anesthesia. If the patient is not vomiting, then small amount of bland diet can be offered. The amount of food is gradually increased over the next 4 days. Peritonitis after intestinal surgery is possible especially after removal of linear foreign body. Patients should be closely monitored for signs of peritonitis for at least 3 days after surgery. Dehiscence of the intestinal anastomosis is the most common 3 days after surgery.

POSTOPERATIVE MONITORING

Postoperatively the patients should be monitored for signs of peritonitis, hypotension, disseminated intravascular coagulation, and pain. Leakage after gastrointestinal surgery can happen within 24 hours of surgery if the suture technique was not correct or 3 to 4 days after surgery at the peak of the debridement phase. Clinical signs of peritonitis will be tachycardia, tachypnea, acute abdominal pain, hypoglycemia, and hyperthermia. An abdominocentesis is then required to confirm the presence of bacteria in the abdomen. If bacteria are presented pass 8 hours after surgery, the anastomosis is leaking and a second surgery is required.

GASTROSTOMY FEEDING TUBE

Eric Monnet, DVM, PhD, FAHA
Diplomate ACVS and ECVS
College of Veterinary Medicine and Biomedical Sciences
Colorado State University, Fort Collins, CO

Nutritional support is required for anorexic patients, debilitated patients, patients in a high catabolic stage (peritonitis, sepsis, burns), or stressed patients (surgical patient). Nutritional support allows a faster soft tissue healing, a better immune system response and a faster recovery from the patient. Nutritional support can be performed with food intake stimulation, force feeding, and feeding tubes. Vitamin B, valium (0.2 mg/kg IV), and ciproheptadine (2 mg/cat 2 to 3 times a day) have been used to stimulate food intake in dogs and cats with variable results. Force feeding with a syringe or tube is possible for one day or two. Force feeding places lot of stress on the animal and may induce aspiration pneumonia. Feeding tube placed either surgically or under endoscopy is the most efficient technique to provide nutritional support to a patient. Feeding tubes can be easily placed at the end of an abdominal surgery and may avoid lot of complications and troubles after surgery. Gastrostomy and jejunostomy tubes are the two most commonly used feeding tube in small animal.

Gastrostomy tubes are more commonly placed during abdominal exploration. However, they can be placed with a limited flank approach or percutaneously with an endoscope.

SURGICAL TECHNIQUE DURING ABDOMINAL EXPLORATION

The greater curvature of the body of the stomach is identified. The greater curvature of the body of the stomach is manipulated to identify the are with e least amount of tension after placement against the left abdominal wall behind the last rib. A purse-string suture with 3-0 monofilament absorbable suture is placed in the gastric fundus in the identified area (Figure 1 B).

A Foley catheter (18 to 20 French) is inserted first through the left abdominal wall just behind the last rib (Figure 1 A). A stab incision is made in the middle of the purse-string suture and the tip of the Foley introduced in

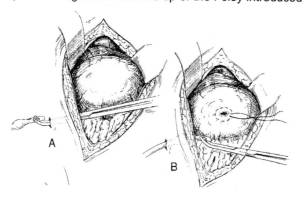

Figure 1.

the stomach (Figure 2 C). The balloon of the Foley catheter is inflated with appropriate amount of saline and the purse-string suture tied. Four gastropexy sutures (3-0 monofilament absorbable material) are placed between the stomach wall and the abdominal wall (Figure 2 D and E). The sutures are evenly distributed around the Foley catheter. A Chinese finger trap suture is placed around the Foley catheter on the skin.

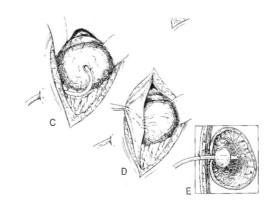

Figure 2.

FLANK APPROACH

After surgical preparation of the left flank, a rigid stomach tube is inserted through the mouth into the stomach. The stomach tube is rotated to tent up the skin of the left flank. With the tube maintained in place a skin incision is performed over the tube. Blunt dissection of the abdominal wall is performed over the tube. When the peritoneum is opened, the stomach wall is identified on the top of the tube. The stomach wall is then pexied to the abdominal wall with four mattress sutures. The stomach can then be removed. A purse-string is placed in the stomach wall and a Foley catheter is introduced after puncture with a No. 11 blade in the middle of the purse-string. The purse-string is tight and the skin closed. The Foley catheter can be tunneled under the skin before it penetrates in the stomach.

PERCUTANEOUS ENDOSCOPIC GASTROSTOMY TUBE PLACEMENT

Percutaneous endoscopic gastrostomy (PEG) tubes are inserted with the aid of general anesthesia. The animal is placed in right lateral recumbency and the flank area behind the last rib is surgically prepared. The endoscope is introduced in the stomach through the mouth. The stomach is insufflated with carbon dioxide. The stomach wall is then getting in contact with the abdominal wall. The lighted tip of the endoscope is turned to visualize the wall of the body of the stomach. A large needle is inserted into the stomach under the control of the endoscope. A nylon suture is inserted in the needle and grabbed in the stomach with a grasper inserted through the endoscope. The suture is pulled through the mouth while the endoscope is withdrawn. A mushroom tip catheter is then attached to the nylon suture coming out through the mouth. The lubricated catheter is pulled into the stomach by the suture exiting the body wall. Resistance will be encountered when the tip of the catheter hit the stomach/body wall. Firm traction is applied o the suture and counter-traction is applied to body wall to be able to pull the catheter through. A rubber flinge is fitted down the tube to prevent slippage of the tube. The flinge is glued to the catheter.

The tube can be removed by applying firm traction of the tube that will collapse the mushroom. In large breed dog the mushroom can be cut and pass through the feces.

The gastrostomy tube is removed by cutting the Chinese finger trap, deflating the balloon and pulling the catheter. Very often, the balloon is ruptured after 2 weeks because of the acid content of the stomach. If the tube needs to be maintained for more than 2 weeks a mushroom tip catheter is preferred to a Foley catheter

The fistula between the stomach and the skin is going to close quickly. Usually there is no leakage of stomach content through the fistula.

Feeding is started 24 hours after placement of the gastrostomy tube. Leaks of food can occur around the tube if the feeding is started to early. The correct amount of gruel for the patient is administered through the catheter. The catheter needs to be flushed every 4 hours to prevent its obstruction. The tube needs to stay in place for at least 7 days before its removal to allow appropriate sealing of the pexy. The gastrostomy tube can be kept for several weeks. It is recommended to start feeding with 1/4 maintenance and to increase the caloric intake by 1/4 every day. If animal shows abdominal discomfort, vomiting or diarrhea the caloric intake is decreased by a 1/4. The amount of food required daily is divided in four feedings.

SELECTED LARYNGEAL PROBLEMS: VOCAL FOLD GRANULOMAS

Gerhard U. Oechtering, Prof.Dr.med.vet., Dipl. ECVAA
Johanna P. Hueber, DVM
Claudia Noeller, Dr.med.vet.
Department of Small Animal Medicine
University of Leipzig, Germany

During the last few years we have diagnosed intra-laryngeal masses in dogs on a regular basis. Most of these masses were associated with the vocal folds and were predominantly located at the vocal process. Histopathology revealed vocal fold granuloma.

In the literature, vocal fold granulomas (VFG) are described in great detail in humans and also in horses. Analyzing our data, we can summarize the following findings. All dogs with vocal fold granulomas belonged to a brachycephalic breed; the majority were French Bulldogs. Altogether nearly one third of our brachycephalic dogs had these laryngeal masses. Specific clinical signs were very difficult to separate from those of brachycephalic airway syndrome (BAS) because all these dogs were referred for surgical therapy of BAS. Except for a very few animals with large masses obstructing more than one third of the laryngeal inlet, we had the impression that these masses did not cause any additional problems other than the brachycephalic symptoms. With the exception of those masses having a colliculus shape, we removed all of the masses surgically, either with a carbon dioxide laser or with high-frequency surgery. Recurrence therapy included topic application of either mitomycin or corticosteroids or anti-acid therapy. Recurrence rate after topical administration of drugs as the sole therapy was 100%. Unfortunately, we started using the anti-acid therapy comparatively late, but there is some incidence of therapeutic success, in concordance with findings in humans.

Currently we can only speculate on possible reasons for this disease in brachycephalic dogs: (1) We know that in the course of upper airway obstruction the larynx is exposed to continuous micro-trauma due to stridor and stertor. (2) We also know that most brachycephalic breeds suffer from gastrointestinal alterations including esophageal problems. In many of our cases, we diagnosed a typical widening of the esophagus immediately cranial to the base of the heart. This cavity was filled with gastric fluid very often. A continuous contact of the glottis with gastric acids possibly causes a chemical traumatism und consecutive inflammation.

At present we can say that surgical removal together with antiproliferative therapy does not seem to prevent recurrence of vocal fold granulomas, and that there are first hints that anti-acid therapy is beneficial.

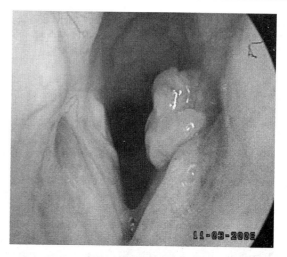
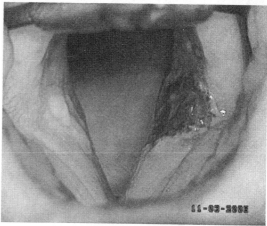

Figure 1. Vocal fold granuloma in a French Bulldog, before (*top*) and after (*bottom*) surgical removal.

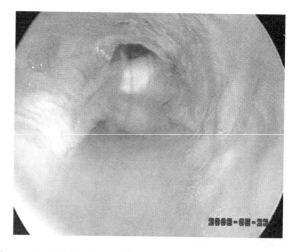

Figure 2. Widening of the oesophagus cranial to the base of the heart with accumulated gastric fluids

TRACHEOSTOMY

Michael Tillson, DVM, MS, Diplomate ACVS
College of Veterinary Medicine
Auburn University, Auburn, AL

A tracheostomy is an artificial opening between the skin and the tracheal lumen. It is created to allow the entrance of air into the respiratory tract while bypassing the nasal cavity, the nasopharynx, and the upper airway. In veterinary surgery, a tracheostomy can be placed as a emergency technique or as a adjunct to other surgical intervention.

Tracheostomy is an important surgical procedure. Indications for performing a tracheostomy can be broadly grouped into emergent and planned categories. Emergent tracheostomy is used in situations where there is a severe upper respiratory tract obstruction. Situations demanding an emergent tracheostomy typically occur with little advance warning and may, in some situations, be performed under less than optimal conditions; for example, in an unstable patient in severe respiratory distress, at the cage-side or in the critical care unit, and with inadequate patient preparation. Planned tracheostomies are performed to provide an airway for patients prior to diagnostic or surgical procedures of the upper airway or oral cavity where there is the potential for severe airway obstruction or where orotracheal intubation compromises the surgical field. Planned tracheostomies are performed under aseptic and controlled conditions. They offer the clinician an excellent opportunity to become familiar with the steps of performing a tracheostomy in a calm, minimally stressful environment.

INDICATIONS

The primary indication for a tracheostomy is life-threatening upper airway obstruction; either current or anticipated. Other indications include prolonged ventilatory assistance in conscious or semi-conscious patients, removal of aspirated materials, and maintenance of a patent airway for oxygen delivery (with or without anesthetic gases) during surgeries of the upper airway or oral cavity.

Tracheostomy tubes are helpful in a wide variety of surgical procedures. These include upper respiratory surgeries (soft palate resections, ventriculo-cordectomies, laryngectomies, modified castellated laryngeofissures, etc), tracheal surgeries, and surgeries involving the oral cavity when a) there is significant risk of postoperative airway obstruction or b) an endotracheal tube increases the difficulty of the surgical procedure. Tracheostomy tubes should be considered in any case where a patient is placed under general anesthesia for evaluation of respiratory distress or in those patients with upper respiratory compromise. Since recovery from anesthesia is always a high risk period in animals with upper airway disease, prophylactic tracheostomy tube placement allows a smoother and less anxious recovery for both patient and surgeon.

The placement of a tracheostomy tube can be considered an emergency or an elective procedure However, tracheostomy tube placement is rarely a "crash" procedure—that is, a procedure done on the spur of the moment, required to prevent death from anoxia. In most cases, patients requiring tracheostomy tubes can be oxygenated after inducing anesthesia with a small endotracheal tube or a red rubber catheter. This allows for the immediate oxygen delivery to the patient. In those rare cases where intubation is not possible, the insertion of a large-gauge (14-gauge) catheter or needle placed into the tracheal lumen to allow for oxygen delivery may be the difference between success and failure.

PROCEDURE

The patient is placed in dorsal recumbency with the head extended and the neck supported/arched. The ventral midline of the neck is clipped from the cranial aspect of the glottis to the sternum and halfway around the sides. The skin is incised from the larynx extending 5 to 6 rings caudally. The subcutaneous tissue is dissected and the sternohyoideus muscle is identified. The sternohyoideus is split on the midline and the trachea is exposed. A few moments should be taken to clear the tracheal surface and recheck the position of the proposed tracheal incision. The trachea is cleared approximately ½ the distance around, taking care to identify and preserve the major vessels and nerves in the area (jugular vein, carotid artery, cranial thyroid artery, recurrent laryngeal nerve, vago-sympathetic trunk).

Once the proposed insertion point is identified, stay sutures (2/0 nylon) are placed around a tracheal ring cranial and caudal to the proposed incision (make sure the endotracheal tube cuff is not incorporated with these sutures). These stay sutures will be left in place to provide the surgeon with the ability to manipulate the trachea without instrumentation. Once the site is prepared and the tube is ready, the endotracheal tube is removed and an incision is made into the tracheal lumen. Hemorrhage into the lumen is gently removed. While applying gentle traction to the distal stay suture, the proximal portion of the trachea is gently depressed and the tracheostomy tube is inserted. One or two simple interrupted sutures (2/0 nylon) are used to close the extremes of the skin incision. A nonadherent pad is covered with a topical antibiotic and placed around the tracheostomy tube. The tube is secured around the neck using umbilical tape. The tube and pad are secured with a light wrap, taking care to avoid occluding the tube.

The most common incision technique is a horizontal incision between tracheal rings. This incision encompasses 50% to 60% of the circumference of the trachea. Care should be taken to prevent injury to the neurovascular structures laying lateral to the trachea. A second technique involves a longitudinal (vertical) incision across several tracheal rings. Although this technique decreases the risk of injury to other structures, it does incise multiple tracheal rings.

The third technique (transverse flap tracheostomy) involves the formation of a flap from the ventral wall of the trachea. The flap is created as a "lazy U" incision beginning 3 to 5 rings below the cricoid cartilage and extending 2 to 3 rings toward the thoracic inlet. The primary advantage of a transverse flap tracheostomy is the ease of changing the tracheostomy tube. With this procedure, the tube can be quickly changed by a single individual. No increase in stricture formation was reported when the flap method was compared to standard tracheostomy incisions. Before placing the tracheostomy tube, the transverse flap technique elevates the trachea toward the skin incision by relocating the paired sternohyoideus muscle dorsally to the trachea. This action, raising the trachea closer to the skin, makes tracheostomy tube insertion less complicated and can also be performed with other incision techniques.

Since an incision into the tracheal lumen cannot be considered sterile, temporary tracheostomies are allowed to close by second intention healing. Stay sutures around the tracheal rings are removed, the site gently cleaned and an occluding bandage applied over the wound site. The bandage must be changed and the incision monitored for signs of infection. The site should close in 3 to 4 days. If this is not the case, the patient should be placed under general anesthesia and the site inspected, cultured and débrided.

In most cases, antibiotics are not required for patients with a tracheostomy. A temporary tracheostomy is not an automatic indication for systemic antibiotics. With proper tube management, anything other than a minor superficial infection should be uncommon. Furthermore, systemic antibiotic usage may contribute to the overgrowth of antibiotic resistant strains of bacteria. However, if the patient requires antibiotics for their pre-existing disease, then appropriate therapy should be provided. Patients requiring long-term tracheostomy tube placement may benefit from regular bacterial culturing of the tracheostomy tube or from routine bronchoalveolar lavage to monitor the bacterial flora within the respiratory system.

TRACHEOSTOMY TUBE SELECTION

Characteristics of tracheostomy tubes are important for in the management of the patient with a tracheostomy. As has been shown on TV "doctor shows," any hollow tube (pens, drinking straws, etc) can be placed as a temporary tracheostomy tube. However, tracheostomy tubes actually have certain desirable characteristics; large enough to allow adequate air exchange, rigid enough to maintain shape but flexible enough to prevent damage to the trachea. In veterinary medicine, it is helpful if the tubes can be cleaned and re-sterilized to help defray costs.

Double-lumen tracheostomy tubes (Shiley, Irvine, CA) are preferred for tracheostomy tube placement. A double-lumen tracheostomy tube allows the inner cannula to be unlocked and removed for cleaning and then replaced. The outer cannula remains in place providing a patent airway for the patient. The use of a double-lumen tube decreases the stress created by the routine removal of tracheostomy tubes for cleaning. The disadvantage of double-lumen tubes is the structure; two tubes, one inside the other, results in a larger outside diameter are a proportionally smaller inner diameter. This means a double-lumen tube provides the patient with a smaller airway when it is compared with a single-lumen tube with the same outside diameter. In practice, this is not a major concern in most patients and is more than compensated by the easier tracheostomy tube management double-lumen tubes offer. In smaller patients, double-lumen tubes become impractical since the diameter of the inner lumen is too small. In these patients, single-lumen tubes are used but, extra care is required to prevent obstruction.

Many tracheostomy tubes come with low pressure, high volume cuffs. The cuff should only be inflated on a tracheostomy tubes when it is being used for ventilation (anesthesia or mechanical ventilation). Keeping the cuff inflated at other times increases irritation to the tracheal mucosa and could prevent the movement of air around the tube in the event the lumen becomes occluded.

CONSIDERATIONS AND COMPLICATIONS

Respiratory tract drying results from air by-passing humidification and warming normally provided by the nasal passages. Oxygen supplementation (O_2 cage or intra-tracheal oxygen) increases the drying effect as the dry gases are inhaled. These factors and a decreased effectiveness of the mucociliary mechanism result in thickened, inspissated respiratory secretions (mucus) which are poorly cleared from the respiratory tract. This accumulated material can quickly and effectively cause tracheostomy tube occlusion. Drying can not be prevented—rather, it is managed. The key is continuous humidification of inspired air. The best method involves humidification of oxygen flowing to a patient. Environmental humidification can be accomplished using a nebulizer or a home-made steam generator (microwave a bottle of saline and place the end of the in-flow oxygen line in it to create that "steamy bathroom" effect). Any oxygen source used for supplementation must be humidified before exposure to the patient. Intermittently infusing sterile saline into the tracheostomy tube and trachea is another method used in maintaining the health and hydration of the respiratory tract. Sterile saline (0.1 mL/kg) is infused every 2 hours, up to maximum 5 mL.

Daily wound management includes bandage changes, cleaning the area around the tracheostomy stoma and the application of a topical antibiotic ointment. Tracheal damage is minimized by using a tracheostomy tube less than 2/3 the tracheal diameter and repositioning the tracheostomy tube at each bandage change. Tracheal aspiration is performed using low levels of suction and gentle technique. Subcutaneous emphysema can result from a disparity between tracheostomy stoma size and size of the skin incision. When the skin is closed over the stoma opening, air expelled from around the tracheostomy tube migrates into the subcutaneous tissues. Subcutaneous emphysema is generally self-limiting but could create a life-threatening situation or indicate other complications (tracheal laceration or necrosis).

Incision into the tracheal lumen and placement of a tracheostomy tube results in significant changes in the normal function of the trachea. There is disruption of the mucociliary apparatus (resulting in retained respiratory secretions), cilia loss, epithelial ulceration and inflammation of the submucosal layer. The disruption of the respiratory clearing mechanism predisposes the patient to bronchopneumonia or bronchi obstruction with resulting lung atelectasis. Management techniques used with tracheostomy tubes are, in part, designed to help compensate for these changes.

When properly performed, elective placement of a tracheostomy tube should have a low rate of associated morbidity and mortality. Other situations requiring a tracheostomy tube (positive-pressure ventilation, severe respiratory disease) may have significant morbidity or mortality associated with the underlying disease. Complications attributed to tracheostomy tube placement include: tracheal stenosis, asphyxiation from tube kinking, displacement or occlusion, selective bronchial intubation and local infection.

The primary complication is the occlusion of the tracheostomy tube and patient death from asphyxiation. For this reason, the tracheostomy tube must be cleaned on a routine basis and the patient maintained in a facility with 24-hour monitoring. Obstruction is prevented by routine removal and cleaning of the tracheostomy tube and periodic suctioning of the trachea and tracheostomy tube to remove accumulated material. Regular cleansing of the tracheostomy tube is important to remove build-up within the lumen. This maintenance is easier with a double lumen tracheostomy tube. Endotracheal tubes should not be used as tracheostomy tubes in the postoperative patient. Their length predisposes them to selective intubation of a bronchus, increased secretion accumulations and they can more easily kink when improperly secured. It is vital that correct placement of the tracheostomy tube be confirmed when removal and replacement of the entire tube is required for cleaning. Inexperienced personnel can inadvertently lodge the tube in subcutaneous (SQ) tissues instead of the tracheal lumen, especially if the patient is struggling or becomes anxious during tube manipulations.

Properly performed, tracheal stenosis should be minimal and generally any stenosis should be sub-clinical. The type of tracheal incision (horizontal, vertical and flap) have not been shown to have a significant difference in percentage of stenosis after healing. However, additional trauma to the trachea (from over-inflated cuffs, excessively rigid tubes, poor tube management or overly aggressive tissue handling) can result in a clinically significant tracheal stenosis. In some patients, resection of the affected area is required. Stenosis has been described in three locations within the tracheal lumen: the incision site, the area of the tracheostomy tube cuff or the tip of the tracheostomy tube.

PERMANENT TRACHEOSTOMY

A permanent tracheostomy is a definitive treatment for specific diseases. It creates a permanent opening (stoma) for the tracheal lumen on the ventral surface of the neck; bypassing the nasal and pharyngeal portions of the respiratory system.

For the creation of a permanent tracheostomy, a portion of overlying skin is removed from the proposed stoma site. The trachea is elevated by separating the sternohyoideus muscles and suturing them together dorsal to the trachea. A stoma is created by removing the ventral aspect of 3 to 4 rings including the associated annular ligaments. The trachea is then sutured to the subcutaneous tissues to secure it in position. The tracheal mucosa is elevated and suture to the skin edge to form a mucocutaneous junction.

If a permanent tracheostomy is created after the surgical resection of the proximal trachea or the laryngeal area, the trachea can be curved to allow the tracheal stump to become the stoma. While this appears convenient, modification of the tracheal stump, by incising the trachea on a bevel, creates a more effective opening and decreases the chances of the trachea kinking during movement of the neck.

The formation of a mucocutaneous junction is the most important step in the formation of a permanent tracheostomy. Accurate apposition of tracheal mucosa to skin edge is vital to prevent postoperative stricture of the stoma.

The postoperative care of a patient with permanent tracheostomy is vital. Since the surgical procedure creates a direct communication between the environment and the tracheal lumen, care must be taken to prevent aspiration of foreign materials (grasses, excessive dust, leaves, water, etc). Covering the opening with a mesh material has been discussed as a method of avoiding gross contamination. Grooming and daily care is important. Hair must be kept trimmed short and the stoma site cleaned daily. Obviously care is taken in bathing animals with permanent tracheostomy and swimming is out. A petroleum-based ointment may be applied around the stoma to help prevent drying and irritation.

Obese patients need to lose weight. Animals with excessive skin folds on the neck require additional attention to prevent skin-fold dermatitis and occlusion of the stoma by the folds. In some cases, surgical removal of excessive skin may be required.

A permanent tracheostomy involves a great deal of commitment by the owner and is not a procedure to be undertaken lightly.

ADDITIONAL READINGS
1. Tillson DM. Tracheostomy. Veterinary Surgical Secrets, ed 2. Philadelphia: Hanley & Belfus, Medical Publishers. 2004, chap. 23, pp. 85-88.
2. Fingland RB. Temporary tracheostomy. Kirks' Current Veterinary Therapy XII Small Animal Practice. Philadelphia: WB Saunders, 1995, pp179-183.

3. Hedlund CS, Tangner CH, Waldron DR, Hobson HP. Permanent tracheostomy: perioperative and long-term data from 34 cases. J Am Anim Hosp Assoc. 1988;24:585-591.

4. Macintire DK, Henderson RA, Wilson ER, Huber ML. Transverse flap tracheostomy: a technique for temporary tracheostomy of intermediate duration. J Vet Emerg Crit Care. 1995;5:25-31.

5. Smith MM, Saunders GK, Leib MS, Simmons EJ. Evaluation of horizontal and vertical tracheotomy healing following short duration tracheostomy in dogs (Abstract). Vet Surg. 1994;23:416-417.

SURGERY AND BIOPSY OF THE KIDNEY

Michael Tillson, DVM, MS, Diplomate ACVS
College of Veterinary Medicine
Auburn University, Auburn, AL

ANATOMY

The kidney is secured in a protected position within the abdominal cavity and technically it lies in the retroperitoneal space. Complete examination of the kidney requires careful dissection of the kidney from its retroperitoneal attachments. This will result in hemorrhage from vessels entering the capsule. These vessels are relatively few in the normal kidney but may increase in the diseased kidney. Ligation or fine electrocautery will allow for a relatively blood-free surgical field. Some procedures are possible without completely freeing up the kidney from its normal attachments, but if you do have to free the kidney completely, it is important to secure it back into position. Failure to secure the kidney could result in torsion of the renal vascular and subsequent loss of the kidney.

The renal artery branches off the aorta and feeds the kidney directly. Renal arteries frequently branch before entering the hilus of the kidney. The right renal artery is reported to branch more frequently than the left. In a few cases, there can be multiple braches off the aorta to the kidney but I have infrequently encountered these. You may encounter multiple braches from a single renal trunk, but these branches arise very close to the aorta. The renal arteries enter the hilus and branch to form the arcuate arteries at the corticomedullary junction. Damage to the arcuate arteries will cause substantial bleeding during renal surgery or biopsy. When encountered during surgery, these should be avoided, ligated, or cauterized to limit hemorrhage. The renal veins drain into the gonadal vessels on the left and into the vena cava on the right.

SURGICAL CONSIDERATIONS

Most urinary surgery can be performed with a good, basic soft tissue instrument pack. However, there is some equipment and specific instrumentation which will make your procedures much easier. Surgical suction is important. This can be a free-standing unit or a built-in system. It will allow the aspiration of fluids and permits complete abdominal lavage whenever there has been leakage or possible contamination. Electrocautery should be a standard instrument in every surgical suite where soft tissue surgery is performed. Abdominal retractors, such as Balfour retractors, are extremely important for visualization and access to the kidney and the ureters. Right-angle forceps, in several sizes, are helpful during dissection around the renal pedicle. Small instrumentation, such as tenotomy scissor and fine tissue forceps help with manipulating small vessels and the proximal ureter. I find various types of vascular clamps are valuable. Small "bulldog" type clamps can be used to occlude the vascular pedicle of the kidney and can be used to temporarily occlude the ureter. Vascular loops (soft elastic bands) can be used to occlude renal vessels and ureters. These can be placed through a large bore (8–12 Fr) red-rubber catheter to form a Rumel tourniquet. Moistened umbilical tape can be used for the same purpose. Large, curved, "Satinsky" type clamps can be used to obtain vascular occlusion in abnormal kidneys which may be difficult to elevate to permit vessel visualization. Malleable retractors and laparotomy sponges are helpful for urinary surgical procedures. Hemostatic agents, such as Gel-foam, improve hemostasis and help decrease the risk of post-operative bleeding. The caveat about hemostatic agents is that they will generally not stop brisk hemorrhage and may be much less effective in animals with low (or ineffective) platelets or other coagulation abnormalities. Thus, it is vital to control hemorrhage by other means (digital pressure, cautery, ligation or hemostatic clips) and rely on hemostatic agents for supplemental control.

The final "instrument" that is helpful for most renal and ureteral surgery is an assistant. Whether this person is another veterinarian or a veterinary technician (or a student), the availability of an extra set of hands makes renal surgery much easier, faster and safer for the patient. It is worth the investment and the cost to the owners to have additional help scrubbed in during these procedures.

Most suture materials have been used in the urinary system but with the variety available at this time, small (4/0–7/0), monofilament, absorbable sutures should represent the mainstay of the materials needed for urinary surgery. I tend to prefer PDSII and Monocryl sutures for most procedures. In a few rare situations, I have used a nonabsorbable material (polypropylene) for urinary surgery. As important as your selection of suture material is the choice of needles for renal surgery. Having a fine suture on a huge needle does not promote the atraumatic tissue handling important in renal surgery. Fine, taper-point needles should be available for urinary procedures.

While a flank approach can be used for renal surgery, especially biopsy, a ventral midline approach is more common. Adequate incision length is important to help with visualization of the entire urinary system.

No matter the type of renal surgery, active diuresis of the patient after the procedure is indicated. In addition to fluid support, opioid analgesics should be considered. I avoid the use of nonsteroidal anti-inflammatory drugs (NSAIDs) or alpha-2 agonists for postoperative analgesia after renal procedures.

RENAL BIOPSY

Renal biopsies are important for both diagnostic and prognostic information relating to kidney disease. The cause of renal disease, its duration, and potential reversibility can be determined from an adequate, appropriate renal biopsy. Persistent proteinuria requires a renal biopsy to differentiate glomerulonephritis from renal amyloidosis. Renal biopsy is vital in prognosticating causes of acute renal failure. Biopsies showing tubular damage without damage to the basement membrane should carry a more favorable prognosis and may encourage owners to seek aggressive, supportive therapies, such as hemodialysis. In a few circumstances, such as suspected renal lymphoma, a renal aspirate might provide the needed diagnostic information.

Considerations

Renal biopsies can be problematic. Pre-biopsy concerns include complete evaluation of renal parameters and assessment of the patient's clotting ability (ie, buccal mucosal bleeding time, platelet counts). The renal cortex should be biopsied to avoid the major vessels, nerves, and ureter in the renal hilus. This is accomplished by directing the biopsy needle along the long axis of the kidney. Furthermore, biopsy of the renal medulla may result in significant hematuria if the biopsy needle advances into the renal pelvis.

The technique used for obtaining a kidney biopsy is normally determined by the size of the sample needed. Needle biopsies can provide some information using ultrasound guidance or a key-hole technique; however, many clinicians prefer small needles (18-gauge) for "blind" biopsy samples and this may result in too few glomeruli for a confident histopathologic diagnosis. Larger needle biopsies (14-gauge) can be taken under direct or laproscopic visualization allowing the surgeon to evaluate and control any post-biopsy hemorrhage. Incisional biopsies can be obtained if large samples are needed; however, I seldom use incisional biopsies unless a nephrotomy has already been performed. If a renal biopsy is needed, I simply incise a thin slice off the incision edge and close.

The most common type of biopsy uses a "Tru-cut" biopsy needle. It is important to avoid directing the biopsy needle toward the central area of the kidney as it is possible to create a tract that will permit hemorrhage into the renal pelvis. This can result in substantial hemorrhage into the urinary tract and could possibly lead to urinary obstruction. Tru-cut biopsies can be obtained 1) as a blind, percutaneous procedure, 2) percutaneously under ultrasound guidance, 3) through a "key hole incision" 4) under laproscopic guidance and 5) under direct visualization at the time of exploratory surgery.

RENAL SURGERY
Nephrotomy

Indications for performing a nephrotomy include removal of urinary calculi (nephroliths), renal biopsy and occasionally partial resection of the kidney for trauma or neoplasia. It should be remembered that nephrotomy will reduce renal function by 20% to 50% in the postoperative period.

After dissecting the kidney free from its peritoneal attachments, the decision is made about the scope of the incision to be made. Hemorrhage is controlled with temporary vascular occlusion of the renal artery and vein. This can be accomplished with the placement of vascular clamps ("bulldog" clamps or curved vascular clamps) or by digital occlusion. I frequently place the kidney in the palm of my hand with the vascular pedicle between my fingers allowing me to effectively occlude

and release the vascular pedicle. When removing a small nephrolith, a small "key hole" incision into the renal pelvis may suffice. A 23- or 25-gauge hypodermic needle can be used to probe for the calculi and then an 11 blade passed along the needle to create the nephrotomy. The incision is expanded as required to allow the insertion of forceps into the pelvis for stone extraction. Direct pressure across the incision site will generally control the hemorrhage, but I always place a few mattress sutures (4/0 PDS II) in the renal capsule for additional support. If a large nephrolith is removed, a bisectional nephrectomy is performed. The nephrolith is removed and the recesses of the renal pelvis are gently probed and flushed to remove any remaining fragments. I also pass a urinary catheter into the ureter to ensure no stones or stone fragments have become lodged in the proximal ureter. If you need a renal biopsy, this is the time to take a thin slice from the edge of the incision. Nephrotomy closure is accomplished by applying direct, digital pressure to appose the incised renal tissue and then suturing the renal capsule with a fine, absorbable suture using a continuous pattern. The renal capsule is frequently friable in a diseased kidney and may not hold sutures well. Gentle technique must be used to avoid pulling the suture material through the capsule. Additional sutures (mattress sutures) may be placed as required to control hemorrhage. Re-secure the kidney to prevent torsion.

Pyelolithotomy

This procedure is used if urinary calculi have moved from the renal pelvis into the proximal ureter. Incision into the proximal ureter results in much less hemorrhage and minimal compromise of renal function. Access to the renal pelvis requires some dissection of fat from the ventral surface of the kidney. I normally do not dissect the kidney free of its attachments but rather retract the renal vein out of the way. A small, longitudinal incision is made into the proximal ureter/renal pelvis. Pinpoint cautery helps control hemorrhage and vascular clamps can be used to occlude the ureter if required. Care is needed to avoid incising the opposite wall of the ureter, as this will result in urine leakage. Once the stone is removed, the renal pelvis can be palpated and flushed to help dislodge any additional fragments. I also pass a catheter distally to ensure patency of the ureter going to the bladder. Closure is performed with fine sutures (5/0, monofilament suture) placed in a simple continuous or simple interrupted pattern. It is also possible to close some longitudinal pyelolithotomy incisions in a transverse manner. This will decrease the risk of ureteral stenosis secondary to the incision closure. Injection of saline into the renal pelvis will allow you check for a water-tight closure. If, as part of your dissection, you freed up the kidney from its peritoneal attachments, it should be secured to prevent torsion.

Nephrectomy

Removal of a kidney is indicated for severe trauma, uncontrollable hematuria, severe pyelonephritis, hydronephrosis, renal neoplasia, neoplasia of adjacent structures, some cystic conditions and severe, non-functional kidneys secondary to renal calculi. Nephrectomy is relatively straight forward, but there area several important points to consider. The first is to have confirmation that renal function can be maintained by the remaining kidney. Renal size alone is not a good indicator of which kidney is normal and which kidney is abnormal. Optimally, glomerular filtration rate (GFR) determination is performed before surgery, if nephrectomy is being considered. Scintigraphic GFR determination provides the total GFR for each kidney and for the kidneys combined. In some cases, the normal and the abnormal kidney may be combing to maintain a low normal GFR which keeps the renal function within normal limits. However, in this case, the removal of the abnormal kidney could result in enough of a reduction in GFR that the animal would be compromised. In this situation, the surgeon may attempt to save the "abnormal" kidney if feasible. Personally, I find this to be the toughest decision to make in many cases involving abnormal kidneys and ureters.

To remove the kidney, it should first be freed from its peritoneal attachments. Once the kidney can be manipulated, isolate the renal vein (which is more ventrally located) and then isolate the renal artery. I like to clear the artery to the level of the aorta to check for early branching. Normally, I try to pre-place my ligatures. This way I can rapidly ligate the artery and then the vein. In cases of neoplasia, some recommend ligating the venous side first, but this will result in significant congestion of the kidney. (Practically speaking, the manipulation during the dissection has probably already resulted in the shedding of any tumor emboli.) The renal artery can be ligated on the arterial side with a circumferential suture and a transfixation suture, circumferential suture and hemostatic clips or any combination that makes you sleep well at night. I also double ligate the renal vein. Remove the kidney and check the renal fossa for any persistent bleeding. Use ligation or cautery to staunch any hemorrhage.

After completing the dissection of the kidney, the ureter is removed. Ligation and transection of the ureter at the urinary bladder is the preferred technique in small animals. This minimizes the risk of the ureter harboring bacteria in a "blind sac." It does require an extension of the abdominal incision caudally to permit visualization and transection of the ureter. Care is taken not to damage other nearby structures during this process.

ADDITIONAL READING

1. Rawlings CA, Diamond H, Howerth EW, Neuwirth L, Canalis C. Diagnostic quality of percutaneous kidney biopsy specimens obtained with laproscopic vs ultrasound guidance in dogs. J Am Vet Med Assoc. 2003:223:317-321.
2. Rawlings CA, Howerth EW. Obtaining quality biopsies of the liver & kidney. J Am Anim Hosp Assoc. 2004;40:352-358.
3. Rawlings CA, Bjoring DE. Christie BA. Principles of urinary surgery. In: Slattter D (ed.): Textbook of Small Animal Surgery, 3rd ed. Philadelphia: WB Saunders. 2002, pp. 1594-606.
4. Rawlings CA, Bjoring DE. Christie BA. Kidneys. In: Slattter D (ed.): Textbook of Small Animal Surgery; 3rd ed. Philadelphia: WB Saunders, 2002, pp. 1606-1618.

HOW I TREAT AURAL HEMATOMA

Michael Tillson, DVM, MS, DIplomate ACVS
College of Veterinary Medicine
Auburn University, Auburn, AL

Aural hematomas are common and sometimes frustrating to treat. There are numerous techniques for managing aural hematomas. We'll review those in this discussion.

ANATOMY

Let us begin with a few quick reminders about the ear. The pinna of the ear is comprised of skin covering a sheet of cartilage. Normally, the skin is tightly attached to the cartilage by the perichrondrium. The cartilage is perforated with foramina which allow for the passage of blood vessels. Trauma to the ear causes disruption of these vessels and the accumulation of blood between the cartilage and the skin. This results in the formation of an aural hematoma. Normally, the hematoma forms on the medial aspect of the pinna. It can be limited in scope or cover the entire medial surface.

ETIOLOGY

The underlying etiology for hematoma formation is not clear; mite infection, otitis externa, trauma, immune-mediated processes and allergic hypersensitivity have all been implicated. The pathogenesis is not clear either. Head shaking, external trauma from scratching and other traumatic events have been suggested as contributing factors. One group of investigators found degeneration of the pinna cartilage suggesting that hematoma formation may be a "chronic/acute" process. If the ear is left untreated, the resulting scar tissue will distort the pinna into a "cauliflower-type" ear.

ANESTHESIA/SEDATION

Although many hematomas appear simply, the pinna is very sensitive and most dogs poorly tolerate manipulation of an aural hematoma without sedation or general anesthesia. In the academic setting, we normally use general anesthesia for hematoma repair; but, in a more efficient practice setting, heavy sedation might be practical. Remember, however, that sedatives such as medetomidine may create the illusion of light anesthesia but dogs under sedation with alpha-2 agonists can still respond violently and unexpectedly to simulation of the ear canal or the pinna. Since your face and hands are going to be rather close to the teeth during this time, extra care is warranted.

SURGICAL TECHNIQUES

Drainage. In an acute aural hematoma, management can occasionally involve simple drainage of the accumulated blood. This can be done using a large gauge needle and gentle suction. Placement of modified suction drains (such as described by Swaim) can also be used and can prolong drainage in the event there is further bleeding into the space. Drainage is normally ineffective if the hematoma has been present for an extended period of time (allowing for the formation of a fibrin clot). In this case, some of the distention might be removed and the dog may be more comfortable but significant alteration in the appearance of the ear will probably still occur.

Incision. Most surgical texts describe techniques for incising the pinna and expressing the hematoma, and associated clot, through the incision site. Longitudinal incisions or "S" incisions are made on the ventral aspect of the pinna. The incision is opened and the fibrous clot is removed. The resultant cavity is gently lavaged with warm saline until all material is removed. At this point, sutures are placed to obliterate the dead-space while healing occurs. A gap of 3 to 7 mm is left between the wound edges to prevent premature healing of the incision site and to allow for continued drainage of the pinna. Sutures are normally placed in a "through and through" manner.

Punctate Hematoma Management. Currently, my preferred technique involves using a dermal biopsy punch to make multiple circular holes in the ventral surface of the pinna. Although I keep trying to use a smaller size, I have found a 6 or 8 dermal biopsy punch works the best for me. The smaller sizes don't make a substantial hole for drainage and these holes may close before the healing is complete. Formation of granulation tissue in the holes left by the punch should help eliminate dead space and minimize the potential for a reoccurrence of the hematoma.

In cases where there is a large fibrous clot within the hematoma, it may be necessary to combine an incision with several punctate holes in order to extract the fibrous material. Make the incision no larger than necessary to remove the clot and then fenestrate the remaining area of the hematoma with the biopsy punch. Suture the ear using a fine, monofilament suture material. I place a single suture on the edge of each hole with a bite into the underlying cartilage.

BANDAGING

I like to bandage the ear after aural hematoma repair. In dogs with floppy ears, I normally bandage the ear over the top of the head. In prick ear dogs, place a Telfa pad on the inner surface and then use additional bandage material to create a "form" for the ear. Using gauze and then adhesive tape, secure the pinna around the form. Additional bandage material is needed to secure the ear in a stable position on top of the head. The result may result in the appearance of a lop-sided unicorn but will help keep the ear in an erect position during the initial stages of healing. This decreases the chances of permanent disfigurement and maximizes the potential for a cosmetic outcome.

OTHER COMMENTS

The reason for the development of the aural hematoma should be investigated. Cytology, culture and sensitivity, a thorough cleansing of the ear canal, and a complete aural examination should be performed while the dog is under anesthesia. This should be done before dealing with the hematoma since blood contamination might alter visualization or culture results.

ADDITIONAL READING

1. Harvey RG, Harari J, Delauche AJ. Ear Diseases of the Dog and Cat. London: Manson Publishing, 2005.
2. Fossum TW. Surgery of the Ear. Small Animal Surgery 2nd ed. St. Louis, MO: Mosby, 2002, pp 246-249.

ABDOMINAL BIOPSY PROCEDURES: INTESTINES AND LIVER

Michael Tillson, DVM, MS, Diplomate ACVS
College of Veterinary Medicine
Auburn University, Auburn, AL

INDICATIONS

One of the primary indications for performing abdominal exploratory surgery is to make or confirm a working diagnosis. To accomplish this, surgeons use their knowledge and surgical skills to evaluate the organs exposed during a laparotomy. However, even the most skilled surgeon can not discern microscopic pathologies within organs. For this reason, it is critical that the surgeon be comfortable with a number of different biopsy techniques that can be used to gain samples from organs, whether they appear grossly normal or abnormal.

Biopsies are the essence of the exploratory surgery. Leaving an abdomen after exploratory surgery without obtaining biopsies is unforgivable. It generally represents a wasted diagnostic effort, wasted money, and an unwarranted risk to the patient. ***The bottom line - when you complete an abdominal exploratory, you should have either 1) fixed the problem or 2) have a specimen for a pathologist to evaluate.***

This article discusses various biopsy techniques. The goal will be to make you more comfortable with obtaining those biopsy samples. Many surgeons are uncomfortable with the potential for causing more harm, by trying to biopsy an organ, than they are of not getting the diagnostic information that they need. You should practice these techniques on a cadaver. This will give you additional confidence about the biopsy procedure and make you more comfortable with any special equipment needed for biopsy sampling. Consider these methods—some tried and true, some (hopefully) a novel approach. And make sure you have plenty of formalin!

INTESTINAL BIOPSIES

Intestinal biopsies are the most common request for surgical biopsies. Endoscopic biopsies are often not deep enough to be diagnostic and full-thickness biopsies are needed for histopathologic evaluation. For all intestinal biopsies, a few rules are applicable.

1. Samples need to come from various portions of the intestinal tract. I normally obtain a duodenal, two to three jejunal, and an ileal biopsy. A gastric biopsy is not routinely obtained unless requested or unless the stomach appears abnormal during exploration. I also avoid biopsies of the colon due to the higher bacterial content and the less forgiving nature of colonic healing.

2. Before incising the intestine for the biopsy, make sure you have isolated the segment to be biopsied with moistened laparotomy sponges. The lumen of the intestines needs to be occluded before incision to prevent expulsion of intestinal contents. This can be accomplished using 1) an assistant's fingers, 2) vascular clamps (such as a ductus clamp) or a 3) Penrose drain placed around the intestine through a small fenestration in the mesentery). Other techniques may also be use but I avoid intestinal clamps and certainly don't recommend rubber sheathing on any clamp used to occlude the intestines.

3. Moistened gauze sponges are used to remove any ingesta that leaks from the incision and are discarded off the table.

4. Surgeons should take care to avoid damaging or distorting biopsy samples. They should use needles or very gentle pressure with tissue forceps. They should go directly into a formalin container to avoid dehydrate or being inadvertently discarded.

5. You should obtain intestinal biopsies from the antimesenteric surface, unless there is a specific lesion located in another area. Most GI diseases are generalized. Taking a biopsy on the antimesenteric surface is easier and has a lower risk of compromising the local vascular supply.

Several different techniques are available for taking intestinal biopsies; these are described below. The first technique is to incise the antimesenteric surface with an 11 blade and take a small elliptical portion of the bowel. The second technique is to make a 6- to 8-mm longitudinal incision along the antimesenteric surface and then close the incision in a transverse fashion. This creates "dog-ears" at either end of the incision that are trimmed away with Metzenbaum scissors. This technique gives you two small, full-thickness biopsies.

Another technique uses a 4- to 6-mm dermal biopsy punch to create a circular biopsy in the antimesenteric surface. I have grown to prefer this technique and have encountered relatively few complications with it. The primary complication occurs if the surgeon presses too hard and the punch incises the mesenteric surface. This breech may not be noticed and could lead to subsequent intestinal leakage. A second "issue" is the punch may force the sample into the intestinal lumen. In most cases, a little gentle pressure in either side of the biopsy site pushed the sample back through the site and it can be lifted with your suture needle or tissue forceps. The final issue concerns the re-use of the biopsy punch. While dermal biopsy punches can be cleaned and re-sterilized, a punch that is re-used (and re-used and re-used) can become quite dull. Steam sterilization will dull the instrument faster than EtO sterilization. A dull punch means less cutting and more pressure to force through the tissues. However, this problem is easily resolved; throw out the dull punch and getting a new one!

Once the biopsy is complete, trim away any everted mucosa (additional specimen?) and close the biopsy site with several simple interrupted sutures. My preference is a absorbable, monofilament (ie, 4/0 PDS) on a taper needle. I close the central portion first and then place additional sutures on either side until the incision is closed. We routinely check biopsy site closures by inserting a 25-gauge needle into the intestinal lumen, occluding the intestines on each side of the incision and injecting saline into the lumen. Fill the lumen until it is gently distended. If there is no leakage, you can feel comfortable about the closure. If an area leaks, place another suture or remove and replace all the sutures are required. Placing an omental wrap or using a sersoal patch should be considered when additional sutures are impractical or significant support is needed.

Complications and concerns associated with intestinal biopsies include biopsy site dehiscence, peritoneal contamination and standard concerns associated with any abdominal surgical procedure. Biopsy site dehiscence should be a rare complication and is generally associated with inadequate closure of the biopsy site, failure to engage the submucosa in sutures apposing the biopsy incision, or the presence of severe intestinal disease. Hypoproteinemia and hypoalbuminemia have not been associated with increase risk of intestinal dehiscence after biopsy, although extra care is warranted in animals suffering from these conditions. Other factors, such as pre-existing intestinal or peritoneal disease, may create a higher risk for any individual animal.

LIVER BIOPSY

The liver is the second most commonly requested organ for biopsy. You can encounter generalized disease of the entire hepatic parenchyma or specific and focal lesions within a specific liver lobe. For either of these situations, you need to be able to take biopsies which are representative of the disease process.

Liver biopsy is indicated when a patient demonstrates persistent elevation in hepatic enzymes, has abnormalities identified on imaging studies or abnormal results on liver function tests. While needle or "Tru-cut" biopsies can be performed in a less invasive manner (blind, ultrasound guided, key-hole or laparoscopic), they have been associated with excessive hemorrhage and inadvertent trauma to biliary structures or other organs. Furthermore, needle biopsies are contraindicated in patients with microhepatica, severe, uncorrectable coagulation abnormalities, serve ascites, suspected hepatic cysts or abscesses, or vascular masses. Surgical biopsy at the time of laparotomy is preferred for these patients.

SURGICAL BIOPSY

Advantages of surgical biopsy include visualization of the entire abdomen, close inspection and the ability to palpate the individual liver lobes, direct control of associated hemorrhage and the ability to collect of additional samples (ie, bile culture) of diagnostic importance. It also allows the surgeon to perform other diagnostic procedures (ie, portography or manography) for evaluation of portal pressures) or to attempt surgical correction of the underlying condition. Surgical biopsies Liver biopsies are normally taken as a "guillotine" or ligature biopsy, a wedge biopsy or a punch biopsy.

Guillotine biopsy is my preferred technique for obtaining liver biopsies. It is best used for generalized liver conditions. The biopsy is performed on a portion of the liver, generally the tip of a liver lobe that can be encircled with a strand of suture material. Once the area to be biopsied has been identified, a suture (small, monofilament, absorbable) is passed around the target. The suture is tightened and it cuts through the liver parenchyma separating the biopsy specimen and simultaneously ligating any vessels which might bleed after the specimen is removed. A couple of particulars for consideration:

1. Take advantage of naturally occurring fissures in the liver lobes to help determine the biopsy specimen.
2. Make small, "nick" incisions, along the sides of the liver lobe if natural fissures are not present. Use your Metzenbaum scissors for this task. This will prevent the suture from sliding off the tip as it is tightened down.
3. Use this for generalized disease or routine biopsy. Guillotine biopsy (aka "ligation biopsy") is less effective for focal lesions that are away from the tips of the liver lobe.
4. Large tissue samples can be obtained using the guillotine biopsy. These are often needed for determination of elemental toxicities (eg, copper).

Wedge biopsy works well for masses or lesions near an edge that cannot be taken with the guillotine technique. Simply isolate the target lesion and incise a wedge from the tissue. Sutures are placed to control hemorrhage and to appose tissues. You can place horizontal mattress sutures on the ventral and dorsal surface to close the wedge or you can place "through and through" mattress sutures parallel to the edges of the wedge to stop hemorrhage.

Punch biopsy can be taken using a dermal biopsy punch on the surface of the liver. The target tissue is isolated and supported with the surgeon's left (non-dominant) hand. A sharp punch is placed at the edge of the lesion and gently rotated until it cuts into the liver to the desired depth. Sharp scissors (Metzenbaum) are inserted along the incised tissue and dissect the plug of liver tissue away from its bed. Direct pressure, a mattress suture or hemostasis aids (eg, Gelfoam [Pfizer], Surgicel [Ethicon] or VetSpon [Novartis]) can be placed in the defect, and are used to control any hemorrhage. Remember, obtaining a biopsy sample with some adjacent "normal" tissue may help the pathologist in the interpretation. Care must be taken with the punch technique to avoid damaging large vessels or biliary ducts. The risk of inadvertent damage to these structures increases as the punch in driven deeper into the liver parenchyma and as the lesion to be biopsied moves away from the edge and towards the liver hilus.

Needle biopsy uses an automatic or a manual needle to obtain a core sample of the target tissue. Often called a "Tru-cut" biopsy, the biopsy needle has an internal obturator/stylet with a tissue capture chamber that slides through a hollow outer sheath. The obturator is sharpened and the hollow sheath has a cutting edge. As the needle is fired, the obturator moves forward, allowing a tissue specimen to fall into the "specimen chamber". The external sheath then moves forward, cutting the tissue and securing the tissue within the specimen chamber. Now the needle can be withdrawn from the tissue with the tissue sample protected inside the sheath. The obturator is advanced and the tissue specimen is gently teased from the chamber. Now, cytologic impressions can be made or the sample can be placed directly into formalin. The needle can be re-used for the next biopsy sample.

Advantages of the needle biopsy include ease of operation (with a minimal amount of instruction), rapid action and the ability to take samples from areas that might be difficult to biopsy otherwise. A needle biopsy can also be used to obtain ultrasound guided biopsies. Disadvantages include variable sample size (based on needle size, lesion size and tissue type), a "blind" component to the biopsy (trying to estimate exactly where the needle is heading) and the potential to sample/injure tissues beyond the intended lesion (another organ, the operator's fingers). However, the sampling speed and easy operation, especially when combined with the visualization provided by a laparotomy, make a biopsy needle a favorite biopsy tool.

FINAL COMMENT

For all biopsy specimens, care must be taken to avoid crushing or distorting the specimen. Prompt placement into an adequate volume of formalin also helps to minimize artifacts.

URETHRAL SURGERY: ANASTOMOSIS, OTOMY and OSTOMY

Michael Tillson, DVM, MS, Diplomate ACVS
College of Veterinary Medicine
Auburn University, Auburn, AL

URETHRAL PROCEDURES

To begin, the following are some general comments about urethral surgery in dogs and cats. There is a significant amount of hemorrhage during urethral surgery. Persistent irrigation is the best way to maintain a clear surgical field since the use of electrocautery and excessive blotting of blood with surgical gauze creates urethral trauma that could impact the final results of the procedure.

After surgery, it is important that the surgical site not be disturbed. A natural clot forms over the surgical site and the tendency is to wipe this off and clean the wound. With very few exceptions, I leave this natural bandage in place and avoid further irritation to the surgical site. It is also important that your patient recovers from anesthesia wearing an Elizabethan collar (or a similar device) to prevent self-mutilation of the surgical site. Finally, most urethral procedures will result in substantial post-surgical hemorrhage when the animal urinates. This is to be expected. Urethrotomy incisions, especially those healing by second intension, will bleed every time the animal urinates for 2 to 10 days after the procedure. This degree of postoperative hemorrhage may necessitate patient hospitalization during this time to minimize client concerns. Careful monitoring of the packed cell volume (or HCT) should be done in these patients, especially if they were anemic prior to surgery.

Urethral Retropulsion

Retropulsion is accomplished with the patient under general anesthesia. Additional anesthesia can be accomplished using local anesthetics infused up the urethra or by an epidural with a short-acting anesthetic. Next, a well-lubricated catheter is placed in the urethra to the level of the obstruction. The type of catheter is left to the individual, but I find that a large bore, red rubber catheter works well although a stiffer, polypropylene catheter might work well in some cases. I find that a Foley-type catheter is not stiff enough to help dislodge the obstruction and the use of Foley balloon impairs my ability to advance the catheter.

An assistant dons a glove and places their finger in the rectum. Placing ventral pressure on the urethra will permit the urethra to be distended. The primary clinician infuses saline into the urethra (through the catheter), distending it. Ideally, this will result in some loosening of the obstructed stones. In a coordinated manner, the urethral pressure through the rectum is released and the catheter advanced. At this point, some of the stones should be retropulsed back up the urethra. It is seldom that a single effort at retropulsion relieves the obstruction. In fact, it may require several attempts to free up the obstruction (if it is going to be relieved).

One important consideration is the volume of fluid infused during the retropulsion procedure. You can inadvertently infuse a great deal of saline during retropulsion and you must be careful to not over-distend the bladder; especially, if there was already a substantial amount of urine in the bladder. I always drain the urinary bladder after relieving the obstruction and leave the catheter in place to prevent the retropulsed stones from returning to the urethra. If this works, then a urethrotomy incision can be avoided.

Urethrotomy

Most urethrotomy procedures in dogs are related to urinary obstruction from calculi that passed into the urethral but became obstructed at the os penis. If a single stone is involved, urine may pass around it but as multiple stones begin to accumulate behind the primary stone, the flow becomes more and more diminished until obstruction is complete. Before committing to a urethrotomy incision to remove the obstruction, attempts should be made to retropulse the stones into the urinary bladder (see previous section)

If a urethrotomy incision is needed to remove an obstruction, it is normally performed over the proximal base of the os penis in the dog. Care must be taken to stay on the midline or excessive hemorrhage may be encountered if the incision strays into the cavernous tissues. Small, Gelpi-type retractors can be used to maintain the incision. The retractor penis muscle is identified and dissected free from the penis. It can be moved to the side. The presence of a urinary catheter in the urethra makes accurate identification of the urethra much easier.

Urethrotomy closure can be accomplished through primary suture closure or by letting the urethrotomy incision heal by second intension. Primary suture closure requires meticulous apposition of the mucosal edges to minimize stricture formation. A fine (5/0 or smaller), monofilament, nonabsorbable suture is my preference. Poor apposition will result in granulation tissue formation and this can lead to stricture. I normally allow urethrotomy incisions to heal by second intention. The dog will urinate from the distal urethra and the urethrotomy incision for several days but I have never experienced urethral stricture after letting a dog heal by second intension.

Surgical Considerations for Canine Scrotal Urethrostomy

Urethrostomy in the dog is normally performed as a scrotal urethrostomy. In this location, the urethra is relatively superficial and curves from a perineal position to the ventral abdomen allowing gravity to help prevent urine scald or urine migration into the subcutaneous tissues. Accurate apposition the urethral mucosa to the skin, creating a "muco-cutaneous" junction, is essential to creating a permanent urethrostomy. Intact dogs undergoing permanent urethrostomy should be castrated and a scrotal ablation performed. Intact dogs also bleed more from the surgical site, especially when they are stimulated. Care is needed with the ablation to ensure there is enough skin to permit the creation of a tension-free muco-cutaneous junction.

Surgical Considerations for Feline Perineal Urethrostomy

Accurately apposing the urethral mucosa to the skin (thereby creating a "muco-cutaneous" junction) is essential to creating a permanent urethrostomy. Perineal is the accepted, standard location in cats. Castration is performed in intact cats. The penis and scrotum are dissected free and the surrounding tissues are bluntly and sharply dissected. The ischiocavernosus muscle is transected at the pelvic attachment and the urethra should be freed to the level of the bulbourethral glands. This may require further sharp and blunt dissection. This degree of dissection is important since inadequate dissection promotes stricture of the urethrostomy in the post-operative period. The penis is amputated and the urethra incised longitudinally up to the bulbourethral glands. I still use the recommendation that you should be able to insert a pair of Kelly hemostats to the box-lock; if not, need further dissection is needed. Careful suture placement is required to accurately appose the urethral mucosa to the skin edge without tension. Creating a muco-cutaneous junction is essential since granulation tissue promotes stricture formation.

Urethral Resection and Anastomosis

This is a relatively uncommon surgery in veterinary medicine. Indications include urethral trauma, neoplasia (eg, prostatic adenocarcinoma, transitional cell carcinoma), and iatrogenic injury. If urethral resection is being planned, it is essential to review the pertinent anatomy for nerves and vascular supply to the urethra and bladder. The surgical plan should include some mechanism for urinary diversion during healing. A cystostomy tube or a urethral catheter can be used.

This is a challenging surgery and good visualization is a must. Fine, monofilament suture, in a simple interrupted appositional pattern is best for the anastomosis. It is important there not be any tension across the anastomosis site. The resected edges are apposed with full-thickness bites. Suture the dorsal side first - knots on the outside of the lumen. A single layer closure is adequate in most cases and will minimize lumen diameter compromise. Care must be taken to avoid inadvertently catching the far wall with your suture. Having a urethral catheter in place at the time of suturing may help this. A Foley catheter can be used to pull the bladder caudally toward the urethra. A contrast study can be used to evaluate the procedure and to check for healing. In most cases, I pull the catheters in 7 to 10 days. It is a good idea to re-check the urethra in 30 to 45 days to evaluate for stricture formation

Temporary or Permanent Cystostomy

A cystostomy catheter is placed when temporary or long-term urinary diversion is required. This may be secondary to acute or chronic urethral obstruction (from neoplasia or calculi) or severe urethral trauma and is considered to be a "salvage procedure." It may be the best method of urinary diversion after urethral surgery, particularly when urethral catheterization might damage or disrupt the surgical site or the healing process. I have place temporary cystosotmy catheters using human nephrostomy catheters in a few cases where urinary diversion was needed. This can be useful in animals requiring additional stabilization before a lengthy anesthesia and surgical episode.

Placing a cystostomy catheter is similar to performing a cystopexy. The site is determined and a Foley catheter is passed into the abdominal cavity at that site. Place either an interlocking box or a double purse-string suture in the bladder wall. Make a stab incision into the bladder and insert the catheter into the lumen. Temporarily inflate the catheter bulb and again check the location of the pexy. Tighten the interlocking box and secure the bladder against the body wall. If additional sutures are to be placed, advance the catheter into the center of the bladder to avoid puncturing the bulb when passing sutures. Secure the catheter with a "finger-trap' suture on the outside and connect it to a closed collection system.

When removing a temporary cystostomy catheter, the catheter can simply be pulled after deflation of the balloon and the site bandaged. The wound will rapidly contract and granulate closed. While this is useful when we want to remove the catheter, it also means that if the catheter is prematurely dislodged, it must be replaced immediately or an additional surgery may be required to re-insert the catheter.

An alternative to a cystostomy tube might be insertion of an urethral stent. These stents have been placed for specific urethral obstruction secondary to neoplasia or trauma.

SPECIAL CONSIDERATIONS
Suture Materials

Many options exist for suturing the urinary system. My preference is a fine, monofilament, absorbable suture. This would include PDS II and Maxon. Monocryl is very strong but has a rapid absorption rate in tissue and therefore I only use it in normal bladders where I expect rapid and complete healing in a short period of time.

Monofilament, nonabsorbable sutures (polypropylene >> nylon) can be used in situations where the healing is expected to be delayed. In general, this is not a suture recommended for urinary closure. Braided, absorbable sutures have mixed reviews for use in the urinary bladder. Vicryl is considered acceptable but Dexon is not recommended for use in the acidic environment of the bladder. Chromic gut has been used as well but is not currently recommended. This is in spite of a recent study that showed that gut had the least change in suture strength after being soaked in urine inoculated with *E. coli* bacteria. The reason for this is related to the mechanism of degradation for chromic gut sutures. The inflammatory reaction, specifically the response of the macrophages, is responsible for the break-down of chromic gut. The absence of macrophages from the test systems in this report would account for the minimal change in the strength of the suture material - even in inoculated urine. Braided, nonabsorbable sutures can be used for external ligatures but should not be placed where they could enter a lumen or cause obstruction secondary to an inflammatory reaction.

You can consider urinary surgery to be "plumbing", meaning that non-leak apposition is required for the best results. Therefore, careful tissue handling, accurate tissue apposition and careful suture placement is required for the best results. Remember that while the urethra will heal quickly and completely when properly handled and apposed, it is also true that the wound can fall apart if the tissues have been excessively traumatized or made avascular by the inciting injury or poor surgical technique.

Catheters After Urinary Surgery?

The need to place a urinary catheter after urethral surgery is controversial. I do not place indwelling urinary catheters if 1) the patient is otherwise healthy and able to get up to urinate on a regular basis, 2) the bladder closure was secure, 3) the hospitalization facility can assist frequent urination (24-hour care) and 4) there is no medical need to document the amount of urine being produced by the patient.

If a catheter is placed, then two important items must be addressed: 1) the urinary catheter must be placed using aseptic technique and secured to the patient and 2) a closed collection system for collection of the urine. It is important to remember urinary catheters have been shown to increase the risk of stricture formation if the catheter creates too much irritation.

GENERAL CONSIDERATIONS OR "ODDS AND ENDS"

Handle the urinary tract gently. It is easily inflamed and rough handling results in greater postsurgical irritation (prompting clients to call frequently to report "'Fluffy' is always squatting and straining). Use gentle lavage to remove hemorrhage, don't wipe the mucosal surface. Be conservative with suction and avoid or minimize incisional manipulation with forceps or hemostats. Avoid excessive electrocautery along bladder incisions. "Pin-point" application can be accomplished using forceps and the cautery wand. Excessive carbonization from electrocautery delays healing and may promote granulation tissue formation.

It is not unusual for patients to have postsurgical hematuria. Normally, the hemorrhage is short lived, with the majority occurring immediately after surgery. Some hematuria will occur, especially at the end of micturation, but the frequency and the amount should steadily decrease. Severe postsurgical hemorrhage can occur if hemostasis was incomplete and a vessel is hemorrhaging into the bladder lumen. In rare situations, transfusion or reoperation may be required to control blood loss.

ADDITIONAL READINGS

1. Stone EA, Barsanti JA. Urologic Surgery of the Dog and Cat. Philadelphia: Lea & Febiger, 1992.
2. Smeak DD, Newton JD. Canine scrotal urethrostomy. In: Bojrab MJ, Ellison GS, Slocum B (eds.): Current Technique of Small Animal Surgery (4th). Baltimore: Williams & Wilkins, 1998, pp 465-468.
3. Bojrab MJ, Constantinescu GM. Perineal urethrostomy in the cat. In: Bojrab MJ, Ellison GS, Slocum B (eds.): Current Technique of Small Animal Surgery (4th). Baltimore: Williams & Wilkins, 1998, pp 468-474.

EVIDENCE-BASED DIAGNOSIS, TREATMENT, AND PREVENTION OF CANINE INFECTIOUS RESPIRATORY DISEASE

Brad Fenwick, DVM, PhD, Diplomate ACVM
College of Veterinary Medicine
University of Tennessee, Knoxville, TN

While there are a number of medical conditions that occur more frequently than respiratory diseases in pet dogs, infectious respiratory disease is second to none in group-housed dogs and is second only to musculoskeletal conditions in racing and sporting dogs. The environmental and epidemiologic circumstances, etiology, prevention, and medical management of respiratory infections in these populations of dogs requires approaches that are similar but not identical to those used in individual cases. Beyond the initial benefits provided by the development of vaccines against select viruses, disturbingly little progress has been made in the reliable prevention and treatment of canine infectious tracheobronchitis (kennel cough) specifically, and more generally, in the canine infectious respiratory disease complex. Progress requires a new degree of cooperation and information sharing between dog owners, trainers, kennel managers, practicing veterinarians, and scientists. With that background, the topic of canine infectious respiratory disease is an excellent candidate for the strategic application of the principles of evidence-based medicine.

EVIDENCE-BASED MEDICINE (EBM)

At its roots, medicine of all types has been based on the informed application of current knowledge as measured against the specific characteristics of the individual case. In veterinary medicine, advancements in our understanding of best practices in the diagnosis and treatment of disease are strongly based on shared clinical observations and experience. Such an informal and opinion-based approach can be an effective but painfully slow and incremental approach to improving medical services. The fact is that many clinical decisions are not based on valid scientific evidence. Research has repeatedly found that "informal group discussions have the lowest validity and greatest potential for bias." In response to profound increases in medical knowledge, rapid growth in open-source communication systems, better informed and engaged clients, and increases in practice liability, EBM emerged as a rational strategy to address these pressures and to enhance clinical practice.

As first defined by Sackett et. al. over 10 years ago, "Evidence-based medicine is the conscientious, explicit and judicious use of current best evidence in making decisions about the care of individual patients. The practice of evidence-based medicine means integrating individual clinical experience with the best external clinical evidence from systemic research." Since then numerous articles and books have been published, a number of conferences have been held, databases and journals established, and working groups established across a diverse array of disciplines, including more recently veterinary medicine. As a complement to problem-based learning, increasing numbers of medical schools have added an "evidence" class to their curriculums.

EBM is based on combining clinical experience, the unique characteristics of a specific case, and the best scientific evidence available in order to make an informed medical decision. It provides a problem-based structure that critically accounts for and causes one to recognize the ignorance, uncertainty, and the reliability of current knowledge upon which prevention, diagnosis, and treatment strategies are based. When incorporated as a standard for establishing routine clinical protocols, EBM becomes the foundation for continuous learning and improvement. It also provides clarity as to the gaps in our knowledge and in so doing serves to focus the efforts of both basic and clinical research.

As is the case with formal research, the value of EBM flows from the formation of a well-crafted question that relates to a specific clinical problem. Such a question drives the process of finding and evaluating what is known and what is not known. The process of "just-in-time-learning" is both more satisfying and the retention greater than reviewing the contents of dozens of journals or relying on textbooks. The process is now possible because of the availability of searchable Internet-based public databases and open-source publications, the results of which can made available online or even downloaded to a hand-held personal digital assistance (PDA).

The evidence that EBM has a positive impact on clinical practice is strong and growing. While studies specific to veterinary medicine are limited, there is reason to believe that the findings of how physicians find and use data would be similar. Sackett found that only about 50% of the time was the initial clinical plan supported by the latest literature and that 25% of the time a review of the literature caused the plan to be modified and that 25% of the time a completely new plan was used. This data was later reproduced in a second study, which found that a review of the medical literature changed the medication, diagnostic test, or prognostic outlook in 47% of the cases.

The application of EBM to infectious respiratory disease can be a particularly productive approach because of 1) the complexity of the respiratory system, 2) the number and variety of etiologic agents involved and the fact that they often act in consort to produce clinical disease, 3) difficulties with arriving at a confirmed diagnosis, 4) the consequences of treatment failures, and 5) the ongoing frustrations in reliably preventing disease outbreaks. The difference with the standard application of EBM to an individual patient is that when applied to a contagious disease the approach also requires a population-based prospective.

While not specific to infectious diseases of the respiratory system, a powerful benefit of EBM is that it motivates clinicians to sharpen their skills in critically evaluating the validity and clinical application of published research while at the same time encourages scientists to design research projects that produce data upon which the best medical decisions can be based. The challenge in veterinary medicine is that there is not enough scientifically sound information to address many of the most significant clinical questions. To address this knowledge gap requires a greater level of cooperation, which is of particular value in veterinary medicine because of the disproportionate relationship between the availability of funds to conduct well-controlled clinical research and the vast amount of readily available case-based clinical experience. The full utilization of clinical experience and data is becoming increasingly important as research costs increase and acceptance of experimentally re-created disease in healthy animals declines.

APPLYING EBM TO CANINE INFECTIOUS RESPIRATORY DISEASE COMPLEX

The goal of this presentation is to provide an evidence-based approach to the diagnosis, treatment, and prevention of infectious respiratory disease in group-housed dogs with special attention to racing Greyhounds. The guideline is intended for private and track/regulatory veterinarians, as well as trainers. It is not intended to replace clinical judgments based on local or unique circumstances and should not be viewed as a comprehensive or used as a sole source of guidance information. Given the scope and complexity of the subject, the following is provided as an example focused on the most common etiology of kennel cough, *Bordetella bronchiseptica*.

Diagnosis

Descriptions of the clinical characteristics associated with confirmed causes of infectious respiratory disease show that there is considerable variability among dogs infected with the same organism and that regardless of the cause; all have clinical presentations that include coughing and nasal discharge. Clinical and research evidence makes it clear that it is not possible to arrive at a reliable etiologic diagnosis based on clinical presentations and routine laboratory data alone. It is also important to remember that "not all dogs that are infected cough and not all dogs that cough are infected."

General hints as to etiology can be gained from the epidemiologic characteristics of a disease outbreak when measured against the characteristics of the population involved. Classically, viral infectious (distemper, influenza) are characterized by a high percentage of susceptible dogs developing some signs of disease. On the other hand, under the correct circumstances outbreaks of *B. bronchiseptica* have the same disease occurrence and severity pattern of a viral infection. In addition, while incubation period is of lesser value, the duration of disease symptoms can be helpful in that duration of virus-induced disease is generally shorter. Response to treatment is also not a reliable indicator of the etiology. Regardless of cause, the clinical symptoms will continue until the respiratory track has healed.

A confirmed diagnosis requires the isolation/ identification of a respiratory pathogen in several typical cases. There is reasonable research and clinical data to suggest that the sampling methods, timing and location, as well as the laboratory involved are important factors in arriving at an etiological diagnosis with confidence. This is a particular concern with *B. bronchiseptica*. The applications of molecular diagnostic methods (polymerase chain reaction [PCR] and others) have been very helpful and are quickly becoming more widely available for respiratory pathogens, including *B. bronchiseptica*. However, because of the great sensitivity of these methods, the fact that some respiratory pathogens induce a chronic asymptomatic carrier state, and multiple infections are not uncommon, finding a respiratory pathogen is not a foolproof indication that it was the causative microorganism.

Secondary bacterial pneumonia is the most serious consequence following infection with a primary respiratory pathogen. Fortunately, these complicated cases occur in a small percentage of the dogs with primary infections (generally 3% to 5%), but at the same time such cases require significantly greater medical interventions and have much greater mortality rates if not treated promptly, including the use of an effective antimicrobial agent. A sudden onset and rather straightforward clinical signs and laboratory findings generally characterize a diagnosis of secondary bacterial pneumonia.

Treatment

While there are a number of publications concerning the use of various medications in the treatment of canine infectious respiratory disease, well-designed appropriately controlled clinical research is rare. Except in cases of secondary bacterial pneumonia or chronic disease, the value of using antibiotics even in known cases of *B. bronchiseptica* has not been confirmed. Evidence in support of the use of antibiotics rests primarily with preventing secondary bacterial pneumonia, reducing the transmission rate, and their use as prophylaxis in preventing disease following exposure. Current evidence indicates there is no value in the use of antitussives, expectorants, or anti-inflammatory drugs in terms of significantly reducing the clinical course of primary uncomplicated respiratory infections.

Given the nature of infectious respiratory disease, and particularly in complicated cases, treatment is often initiated prior to etiologic confirmation and the susceptibilities determined. *B. bronchiseptica* is uniformly resistant to cephalexin. Regardless of the primary cause, antimicrobial selection in the treatment of clinical cases is aimed primarily at the goal of preventing secondary infections and as such single broad-spectrum or combinations of microbial agents are appropriate. Clinical evidence supports the use of combinations as the preferred approach as treatment failures in individual cases are most often associated with a rare resistance pattern. When used to prevent infection and to control outbreaks of kennel cough on a population basis, the use of a single antibiotic (see below) is supported by clinical experience as well as by data involving control of *B. pertussis* outbreaks in humans.

Prevention

The success of vaccines in controlling infectious diseases in dogs, including in particular respiratory viruses, has been profound. Many diseases that were once commonplace are now rare. While we fight infectious disease everyday, vaccines have given us an upper hand against major respiratory diseases such as canine distemper and adenovirus type 2. If warranted by appropriate risk analysis, it is reasonable to predict that vaccines against more recently recognized viral causes of kennel cough such as canine influenza and corona virus will be equally successful. Intranasal kennel cough vaccines evaluated in an animal shelter only reduced coughing by approximately 25% in comparison to a placebo vaccine.

In contrast, while *B. bronchiseptica* vaccines are used with the same or greater frequency of the virus vaccines, *B. bronchiseptica* has been confirmed to be involved in a majority of kennel cough outbreak. In contrast, current vaccines have a more reliable benefit in reducing the occurrence and severity of experimentally induced disease. As is the case with pertussis vaccine failures and more frequent outbreaks of whooping cough, the nature of this apparent contradictory data concerning *B. bronchiseptica* relates to the critical difference in the antigenic characteristic between vaccine and disease causing field strains. Until a new generation of antigenically correct *B. bronchiseptica* vaccine becomes available, the experimental data supports alternating between intranasal with injectable vaccines.

The disease prevention value of environmental condition control, hygiene, isolation, quarantines, and post-exposure antimicrobial prophylaxis are based primarily on theoretical rationale as well as logical extensions of information concerning *B. pertussis* infections in humans because reliable *B. bronchiseptica* specific scientifically valid clinical evidence is generally not available. In the case of pertussis, the scientific and clinical evidence is strong that the use of a macrolide (particularly erythromycin) as post-exposure prophylaxis in direct and environmental contacts is an effective means of preventing symptomatic infection in susceptible individuals. The dosing level and schedule is the same used in the treatment of whooping cough (four divided doses per day, 40–50 mg/kg/day total for 14 days). Sensitivity patterns for canine strains of *B. bronchiseptica* support the use of doxycycline (2.5–5.0 mg/kg PO q12h) and enrofloxacin (15 mg/kg/day PO).

CONCLUSION

While it is necessary and appropriate for individuals to exercise professional judgment in the prevention, diagnosis, and treatment of canine infectious respiratory disease on a population basis, the cooperative application of EBM in the crafting and evaluation of clinical practice guidelines presents the opportunity to achieve a number of important goals. Goals and outcomes under current practices have not and are unlikely to be achieved. These include advancing the reliability of disease prevention, diagnosis, and treatment strategies; defining the circumstances where professional judgment is applied such that this highlights critical gaps in our understanding and serves to set a research agenda; and ultimately enhancing the effectiveness of the veterinary care provided to dogs that are group housed or periodically exposed to a larger population.

REFERENCES

1. Sackett D, Rosenberg WMC, Gray JAM, Haynes RB, Richardson WS. Evidence based medicine: what it is and what it isn't. Br Med J. 1996;312:71-72.
2. Evidence-based Veterinary Medicine Association. http://www.ebvma.org/index.html
3. Sackett DL, Straus SE, Richardson WS, Rosenberg W, Haynes RB. Evidence-Based Medicine. How to Practice and Teach EBM, 2nd ed. Edinburgh: Churchill Livingstone, 2000.
4. Geyman JP, Deyo RA (eds.): Evidence-Based Clinical Practice: Concepts and Approaches. Boston: Butterworth Heinemann, 2000.
5. Cockcroft PD, Holmes MA. Handbook of Evidence-Based Veterinary Medicine. Oxford, UK: Blackwell Publishing, 2003.
6. Dawes M. Evidence-based practice: a primer of health care professionals, 2nd ed. Edinburgh, UK: Churchill Livingstone, 2005.
7. Buonavoglia C, Martella V. Canine respiratory viruses. Vet Res. 2007;38:355-373.
8. Brownlie SE. A retrospective study of diagnosis of 109 cases of canine lower respiratory disease. J Small Anim Pract. 1990;31:371-376.
9. McKiernan BC. Diagnosis and treatment of canine chronic bronchitis. Twenty years of experience. Vet Clin North Am Small Anim Pract. 2000:30(6):1267-78.
10. Radharkrishnan A, Dorbatz KJ, Culp WTM, King LG. Community-acquired infectious pneumonia in puppies: 65 cases (1993-2002). J Am Vet Med Assoc. 2007:230(10):1493-1497.

Additional references available from author upon request.

REGENERATIVE MEDICINE: A NEW SOLUTION FOR OUR OLD ENEMY, PAIN

James S. Gaynor, DVM, MS, Diplomate ACVA & AAPM
Animal Anesthesia and Pain Management Center
Colorado Springs, CO

The concept of using stem cell therapy as a form of regenerative medicine was born out of a lack of satisfactory therapy for degenerative diseases, such as osteoarthritis. Regenerative medicine also came to the forefront due to a lack of adequate healing of traumatic ailments. These include non-union fractures and tendon and ligament injuries. The goal of stem cell therapy is to initiate tissue regeneration and homeostasis, not just healing. In this way, strength, range of motion and performance are enhanced while minimizing scars, pain, and potentially future related disease.

Stem cells are primitive cells which are present in virtually every tissue. They are capable of differentiating many different tissue types (Figure 1). They are self-renewing and act as trophic factories. This allows these adult stem cells to treat traumatic and degenerative diseases, including bowed tendons, ligament injuries, osteoarthritis, and osteochondral defects in horses and dogs.

A key concept is that this type of regenerative medicine utilizes ADULT stem cells. These adult stem cells are derived from adipose tissue from inguinal, caudal scapular or intra-abdominal areas, making them a readily available source, much easier to collect and much more plentiful than those derived from bone marrow. As mentioned above, these cells are able to differentiate into multiple lineages implicating their potential in bone, cartilage, and cardiac repair. Fractions isolated from adipose tissue contain a heterogeneous mixture of regenerative cells, including:

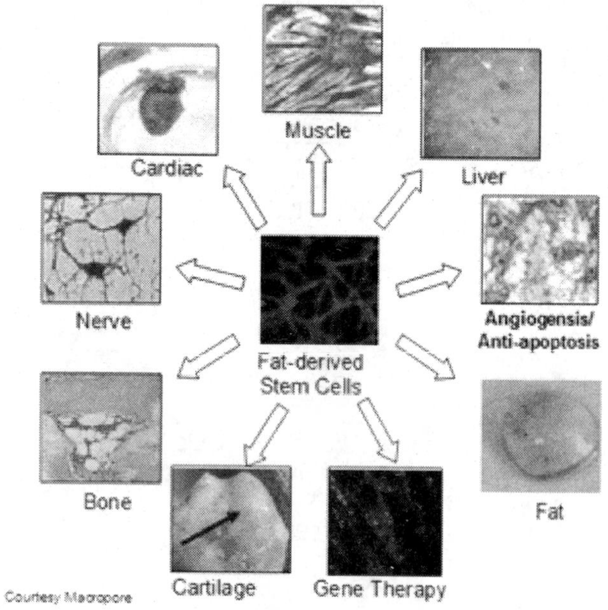

- Mesenchymal stem cells
- Endothelial progenitor cells
- Pericytes
- Immune cells
- Fibroblasts
- Other growth factor-secreting bioactive cells

There are multiple advantages of using stem cell regenerative medicine over a more traditional approach. The first is that stem cells do not rely on a single target receptor or a single pathway for their action. They can have very global effects. In addition, the regenerative cell mixture is delivered either directly to the traumatic wound (eg, tendonitis, desmitis, fracture) or is delivered systemically (eg, liver disease, renal disease). In the case of arthritis, stem cells are injected directly into two to four affected joints, or intra-articularly and intravenously to induce a more global effect. Once again the regenerative cells can differentiate into many tissue types, induce repair, and stimulate regeneration. They can also "communicate" with the cells of their local environment through paracrine and autocrine modalities, creating the optimal environment for natural healing. They also produce a variety of both secreted and cell surface substances that regulate tissue growth, integrity, and function.

Currently, over 200 dogs have been treated for osteoarthritis and orthopedic procedures. Most patients had elbow, hip, or knee problems. Initial studies demonstrate that intra-articular administration of regenerative stem cells significantly decreases pain and improves comfort in the majority of cases. Duration of the benefit from a single injection varies from several months to more than one year (Figures 2, 3, and 4). The current indications for regenerative stem cell therapy in dogs include osteoarthritis and tendon and ligament injuries.

As more research is conducted, the likelihood of expanding the indications for stem therapy increases. Besides the overwhelming scientific data demonstrating the clinical efficacy of regenerative cellular therapy in animal models of osteoarthritis, osteochondral defects, tendon repair, and fractures, many additional studies demonstrate success in treating systemic disorders such as cerebral and myocardial infarction, muscular dystrophy, and immune-mediated disorders.

Figure 1. Differentiation of Adipose into Various Tissues

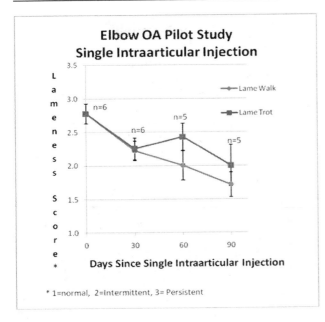

Figure 2. The effect of a single intra-articular injection of stem cells on walking and trotting lameness scores in dogs with elbow osteoarthritis.

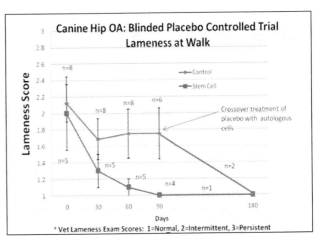

Figure 3. The effect of intra-articular stem cells on a walking lameness score in dogs with hip osteoarthritis

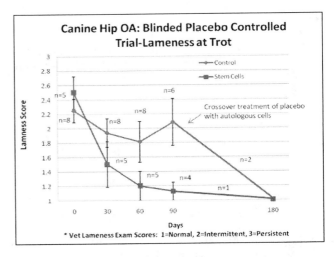

Figure 4. The effect of intra-articular stem cells on a trotting lameness score in dogs with hip osteoarthritis.

STATE OF THE RACING GREYHOUND INDUSTRY

Gary Guccione
Executive Director, National Greyhound Association and
American Greyhound Council
Abilene, KS

One of the biggest news items to come out of 2007 with respect to the sport of Greyhound racing was the passage of legislation that will permit the installation of slot machines in racetracks in Kansas—the state recognized as the very cradle of the Greyhound industry in the United States. It is in Kansas that the National Greyhound Association—the sport's official registry—and the Greyhound Hall of Fame are headquartered. In addition, Abilene (hometown of these two institutions) has long been recognized as the capital of the Greyhound world. More Greyhounds are raised in Dickinson County (where Abilene is the county seat) than any other county in the United States.

After years of frustration and effort, the Greyhound and horse racing industries combined to finally persuade legislators that such a bill was beneficial to the state of Kansas, as well as to the racing industry and the ancillary businesses that service the sport, particularly those that are agriculturally related. The racetracks in Kansas have been on the verge of closing for years, due largely to the competition from casinos in neighboring states and even on Indian reservations within the state. The legislation—endorsed and signed by Gov. Kathleen Sebelius in April—should put the racetracks on a more level playing field with their competitors, breathing new life into the tracks, as well as the race-breed industries in the state.

In addition, the legislation calls for the development of four destination casinos in the areas of Kansas City, Wichita, Dodge City, and Pittsburg (Southeastern Kansas). However, the bill requires approval of voters by referendum for both the racetrack slots and the destination casinos for either plan to move forward. Voters in Wyandotte County (the Kansas City area, where the Woodlands dual-purpose racing facility is located) approved the racetrack measure by an 82% margin in June. In a shocker (despite polls showing the issue as much as 18 percentage points ahead on election day), voters in Sedgwick County voters (the Wichita area) turned down the racetrack slots proposal in a very tight vote (less than 250-vote difference among 100,000 votes cast) on August 7—which tempered to a considerable degree the enthusiasm generated by the new legislation. (Incidentally, approval of the destination casino in that county failed by a wide margin.) A third track, Camptown, in the Southeast corner of the state, will reopen its live racing program (which has been dormant for a number of years) and also offer slot-machine gaming.

The bill is facing some legal challenges, but those close to the issues expect the tracks to be up and running with slots by the spring of 2008. The destination casinos will not likely be in operation for several more years, giving the racetracks a head start in building up a loyal clientele.

Kansas thus joins other states that offer additional casino-type games to their Greyhound racing menu: Rhode Island, Iowa, and West Virginia. In addition, similar games are offered at Mardi Gras Racetrack (formerly Hollywood) in Broward County in Florida; Southland Park in W. Memphis, Arkansas, and VictoryLand in Shorter, Alabama. Meanwhile, racetracks (Greyhound and horse) in other states continue to lobby for legislation that will permit them to also expand their gaming operations, offering a wider variety of games at their venues. Tracks in Miami-Dade County in Florida are anxious for a vote later in January 2008 that might allow them to offer the same games as those facilities in its neighboring county (Broward).

Despite making vast strides in addressing animal welfare issues in the last couple of decades, Greyhound racing still faces criticism from the animal rights world, particularly from the Massachusetts-based organization Grey2K USA. In 2007, Grey2K USA made a bold effort to ban the sport in the state of New Hampshire. Convinced that the sport was indeed humane and that it placed high priority on the welfare of its athletes, the New Hampshire legislature easily defeated the measure. Later in the year, Grey2K USA announced it would make a third stab at trying to ban Greyhound racing in Massachusetts. (Two previous efforts failed—one in 2000 by a close referendum vote, and again in 2006 when the referendum question was muddied because it had been tied to two unrelated issues, rendering it void in the eyes of the state's high court; the question never went to a vote of the people.)

Another noteworthy event in 2007 was the second annual running of the sport's only million-dollar stake—the Derby Lane Million (DLM) at the sport's historic facility, in St. Petersburg, Florida. For the second straight year, a Greyhound bred in Abilene, Kansas (Flying Stanley) captured the event, worth a half-million dollars to his ownership team. (The first Derby Lane Million was won by Greys Calibrator in 2006.) Flying Stanley has already become the sport's all-time leading money winner with more than $600,000 in earnings thus far. Derby Lane has announced that a third DLM will be staged in February and March of 2008.

A growing concern among Greyhound owners in 2007 was the apparent trend of a number of racetracks cutting back on their live-racing programs. Numerous tracks that were once year-round operations have shaved their racing programs down to seasonal operations, while continuing to offer simulcast wagering year-round to their customers. Wonderland Park (Boston) and Seabrook (NH) were examples of this in New England. In 2007, such tracks as Melbourne (FL), Sarasota (FL), and Hinsdale (NH) joined these ranks, with Corpus Christi (TX) announcing its intentions of racing just 2 weeks of live racing in 2008, then simulcasting the rest of the year. In Colorado, the Cloverleaf track near Loveland announced that it would not run a live meet in 2007 (but would only simulcast). The Mile High Track near Denver picked up those dates, assuring there'd be year-round racing in Colorado for 2007—but Cloverleaf did not apply for any live dates in 2008, and Mile High applied only for dates running from March through October. That leaves two 2-month gaps with no racing for the year—something Greyhound kennels and breeders in the state will have a difficult time sustaining.

Not surprisingly, in Kansas—following the slots defeat in Sedgwick County—Wichita Greyhound Park announced it would be closing its doors permanently later in the year.

Florida underwent some legislative changes in 2007 that helped lead to the cutbacks of live-racing dates by Melbourne and Sarasota. For years, tracks in Florida were required to stage live racing on whatever days they also chose to offer poker. That law was amended in 2007, allowing some tracks to shorten their live racing season, but keep their poker tables in operation on their dark days. For the first time ever, Tampa tried running a year-round season at the same time nearby Derby Lane was running its live meet. The plan failed, and on August 9, Tampa announced it would close its live-race program in 10 days, making a deal with Derby Lane to run the rest of its dates at its competitor's track across the bay. This left most of the kennels that had anticipated a lengthy season at Tampa in a bind.

While racetracks that offer other types of gaming have been able to supplement their purses with profits from slots and gaming revenue, most other tracks continue to experience declines or stagnation in business—not unlike the trend in other types of pari-mutuel racing, such as Thoroughbreds, Quarterhorses, Standardbreds. While millions continue to enjoy racing, many younger Americans have been turning their entertainment interests toward the quick-play, instantaneous gratification games of chance. This has negatively affected racing purses—and, consequently, the number of people willing to participate in Greyhound breeding and ownership.

The inability of purses to keep pace with expenses has naturally led to a steady reduction in the number of Greyhounds bred in the past decade and a half. The National Greyhound Association reports that breeding registrations have taken another major nosedive in the last four years. This is pursuant to a 35% drop from 1992 to 1999, followed by a leveling off period early on in the 2000s. The new, major decline began in 2004 when breedings were down 10%, followed by a 14% decline in 2005 and another 10% drop in 2006. News of Kansas' passage of a slots bill spurred some new enthusiasm in the game, especially among breeders in the state of Kansas itself. As a result, the decline in the first half of 2007 dropped to just 7%. Still, the overall decline the past 4 years already exceeds the downsizing that took

place in the 1990s. Projections for 2007 showed the probable individual registration of less than 20,000 new Greyhounds for the year 2007—a far cry from the more than 39,000 new pups registered in 1993. There is no reason to believe that the declines will not continue into 2008 and beyond.

Meanwhile, the industry's vigilant attention to animal welfare continues on a very steady and positive path. More than 20,000 Greyhounds each year are being placed into homes as pets, mostly through the more than 300 adoption agencies on the continent that deal almost exclusively in retired Greyhounds. That means that well more than 90% of all Greyhounds are either being retired into homes as pets or going on to a second career as broods or sires back on the farm. The industry spends millions each year on the adoption effort, with the work of the American Greyhound Council (a joint effort begun in 1987 by the NGA and the American Greyhound Track Operators Association) leading the way. Today, Greyhound pets in America easily outnumber the Greyhounds still linked to the racing industry, and the gap grows wider with each passing year.

The AGC's milestone event in 2007 was the release of its second major textbook, *Care of the Racing & Retired Greyhound*—written by Drs. Linda Blythe and A. Morrie Craig of Oregon State University and Drs. James Gannon and Des Fegan of Australia. (The first three authors had written the original text, *Care of the Racing Greyhound*, in 1994.) The new book promises to follow in the footsteps of its predecessor and become one of the most popular books in the Greyhound world. Its appeal is primarily to breeders, trainers, and all veterinarians who treat Greyhounds—whether young pups, racing Greyhounds or Greyhounds that have been retired as pets.

The AGC also continues with its efforts, in conjunction with Dr. Brad Fenwick of the University of Tennessee, to develop a vaccine to combat the outbreaks of kennel cough and secondary infections caused by *Bordetella bronchiseptica*. It is hoped that 2008 will be the breakthrough year. Other AGC projects, aimed at improving the care administered to Greyhounds, include: continuation of the Greyhound Health Research & Information Network (GHRIN) program, which monitors the day-to-day health status of racing Greyhounds at all tracks across the country (GHRIN, which went on-line midway through 2005, can be viewed at www.ghrin.org); farm inspections; support of canine educational programs; funding assistance to local and national adoption agencies; and research grants (including one, through the Morris Animal Foundation, to help improvement of pain management in association with treating osteosarcoma).

TENDON, LIGAMENT, & MUSCLE INJURIES – LOCATION, SEVERITY, TREATMENT, & RECOVERY

Ian G. Holsworth, BSc, BVSc (Hons), MACVSc (Surgery), Diplomate ACVS
Veterinary Medical and Surgical Group, Ventura, CA

Soft tissue injuries to the musculoskeletal system are common among canine athletes and comprise the majority of lameness-inducing and poor performance conditions. Classification of the connective tissue injuries into specific anatomic locations with determination of the tissue type involved is crucial in the initial investigation of an injury. Once localized the severity of the tissue compromise can be assessed and graded according to an accepted scheme. Specific treatment regimes, whether medical or surgical, will be dictated by the grade of injury and recovery guidelines can be determined.

Two mechanisms for trauma to the muscle, tendon, and ligament are possible. The first is direct trauma from external contact resulting in laceration or contusion to the soft tissue structure. In the event of bone fracture the fractured bone ends may also be responsible for soft tissue damage as the fracture ends displace through surrounding tissue planes. The second mechanism is strain. Every tissue has a load-deformation relationship which dictates the amount of energy that can be absorbed by a tissue until the yield point is reached. Below the yield point the tissue deforms in an elastic fashion with return to its original form when the load is removed. Further load on the tissue beyond the yield point results in permanent deformation in the structural character of the tissue which results in permanent damage in many cases. If load continues to the failure point complete rupture or separation of the tissue occurs which is a catastrophic event. Strains in the ligament, tendon and muscle have been classified into grades to allow the severity of the injury to be assessed and a treatment plan formulated. Muscle injuries are classified in a four-grade system:

- Grade 1 muscle strains are characterized by pain, spasm of the affected muscle, mild muscle fibre tearing, an intact fascial sheath and no obvious hemorrhage.
- Grade 2 strains have an intact fascial sheath but have a hematoma present within the muscle belly.
- Grade 3 strains have significant muscle fibre tearing, a torn fascial sheath and diffuse hemorrhage into the adjoining tissues.
- Grade 4 strains are complete ruptures of the muscle belly with separation of the muscle into two or more distinct portions.

Ligaments and tendons strains may also be graded in a similar fashion with three grades. Mild disruption of their constituent Type 1 collagen fibers with hemorrhage, stretching, and tearing is Grade 1. Grade 2 are partial ruptures of the tendon or ligament with moderate fiber damage and Grade 3 are severe rupture with complete disruption of all collagen fibers.

Localization and grading of connective tissue injuries requires a thorough history from the presenting owner to establish cause, chronicity, progression and historical severity. A gait exam allows lameness grading and observation of conformational abnormalities. A thorough orthopedic and neurological examination of the complete musculoskeletal system completes the initial evaluation of the patient. Once localized, palpation of the affected muscle, tendon or joint allows some assessment of severity. Soft tissue imaging of the affected area by diagnostic ultrasound or magnetic resonance imaging (MRI) allows more complete visualization of connective tissue structural abnormalities and radiography and computer tomography (CT) may be utilized to determine any bony involvement. The combined findings of these examinations should allow accurate tissue localization and grading of injury severity.

In canine athletes there are certain connective tissues that are more commonly injured than others. This predisposition to injury varies according to breed and athletic endeavour and risk factors increase with age and amount of training and competitive exposure each individual undergoes. Of great significance in older and heavily worked athletes is a gradual decrease in the yield point of connective tissue with cumulative loading of the tissue. The occurrence of microtrauma and the progressive accumulation of repair tissue within structures results in a loss of elasticity and the presence of poorly organised collagen tissue that is prone to re-injury. Also demonstrated in human studies on chronic Achilles tendinosus patients is the presence of new blood vessel (neovascularisation) and accompanying nerve fibers at the site of tendon degeneration and damage. These neovessels and nerves have been demonstrated as the source of pain sensations in the damaged Achilles area and obliteration of these structures during physical therapy or interventional treatments results in a significant improvement in patient comfort and function. In dog models of tendon damage the same neovessels and nerves are present and are derived from fibrovascular adhesions between the damaged tendon and the tendon sheath. Techniques to limit the formation and decrease the post-traumatic persistence of the neovessels and nerves may improve functional recovery from connective tissue trauma in our patients.

The treatment of Grade 1–2 muscle, tendon, and ligament strains is commonly conservative with initial analgesia, cold therapy and passive rehabilitation. Transition to active rehabilitation and heat therapy is determined on clinical response to initial therapy and the structure injured and to what degree. Results are optimised if supervision is close and rehabilitation limits are closely observed. With significant lacerations (>40% of structure transected), some Grade 3 and all Grade 4 muscle strains and Grade 3 tendon and ligament ruptures surgical therapy is indicated. The critical role of repair technique is to provide a stiff and strong repair with avoidance of repair-site elongation (gap formation).

Gap formation greater than 3 mm delays the development of repair site strength and must be avoided. Use of external coaptation (splint, casts, external fixators) is recommended to prevent early active mobilization which increases gap formation. Passive-motion rehabilitation in the early postoperative period allows moderate amounts of tendon excursion (2 mm) at low levels of tendon force which inhibits adhesion formation and promotes healing. With many ligament ruptures primary repair is challenging, incomplete or not possible and augmentation of joint stability with autologous tissue grafting or synthetic replacement material is utilized. Healing ligaments are weak and only regain about 60% of normal tensile strength after one year. Persistent joint instability due to ligamentous elongation during the healing period is an issue that must be assessed, as chronic joint subluxation/instability may be the sequulae. Excellent postoperative care of external limb supports, judicious use of pain medication, appropriate initiation of physical therapy and meticulous restriction of moderate and high impact activity is essential for treatment success.

REFERENCES

1. Roe SC. Injury and diseases of tendons (Chap. 16). In: Bloomberg MS, Dee JF, Taylor RA (eds.): Canine Sports Medicine and Surgery. Philadelphia: WB Saunders, 1998.
2. Eaton-Wells RD. Muscle injuries in the racing greyhound (Chap. 15). In: Bloomberg MS, Dee JF, Taylor RA (eds.): Canine Sports Medicine and Surgery. Philadelphia: WB Saunders, 1998.
3. Johnson KA Carpal injuries (Chap. 17). In: Bloomberg MS, Dee JF, Taylor RA (eds.): Canine Sports Medicine and Surgery. Philadelphia: WB Saunders, 1998.
4. Boemo CM, Eaton-Wells RD. Medial displacement of the tendon of origin of the biceps brachii muscle in 10 greyhounds. J Small Anim Pract. 1995; 36(2):69-73.
5. Ohberg L, Alfredson H. Effects on neovascularisation behind the good results with eccentric training in chronic mid-portion Achilles tendinosis. Knee Surg Sports Traumatol Arthrosc. 2004;12(5):465-470.
6. Alfredson H, Ohberg L, Forsgren S. Is vasculo-neural ingrowth the cause of pain in chronic Achilles tendinosis: An investigation using ultrasonography and colour Doppler, immunohistochemistry, and diagnostic injections. Knee Surg Sports Traumatol Arthrosc. 2003;11(5):334-338.
7. Ditsios K, Leversedge FJ, Gelberman RH. Neovascularization of the flexor digitorum profundus tendon after avulsion injury: an in vivo canine study. J Hand Surg [Am]. 2003;28(2):231-236.
8. Silva MJ, Boyer MI, Gelberman RH. Recent progress in flexor tendon healing. J Orthop Sci. 2002;7(4):508-514.
9. Grewal R, Chan Saw SS, Varitimidus S. Evaluation of passive and active rehabilitation and of tendon repair for partial tendon lacerations after three weeks of healing in canines. Clin Biomech. 2006;21(8):804-809.

TRAUMATIC JOINT INSTABILITY - ASSESSMENT, TREATMENT & RECOVERY

Ian G. Holsworth, BSc, BVSc (Hons), MACVSc
(Surgery), Diplomate ACVS
Veterinary Medical and Surgical Group, Ventura, CA

Traumatic injuries to the articular joints of the canine athlete are commonplace and vary in their severity from mild sprain to catastrophic failure of the joint's support system. Localization of injury to a specific joint, physical and diagnostic imaging examination of the soft tissue and bony support structures, and grading of the injury severity are the initial diagnostic steps that are followed. Once localized and graded, a treatment plan can be formulated which will dictate the duration of recovery and allow some speculation on the ability of the patient to resume athletic activity and to what functional level the patient may eventually return.

Normal joint anatomy is structured to facilitate predictable, energy-efficient and pain-free movement. The joint capsule, ligaments, bone-cartilage contour, and surrounding tendons and muscles provide mechanical stability by restricting translational movement, excessive rotational movement and controlling the degree of flexion and extension, abduction, and adduction to a physiological acceptable range. A second major function of the joint is to support the musculoskeletal system and transmit load.

The relationship between joint use, joint injury, and joint degeneration is a complex one. In humans, participation in sports that subject joints to high levels of impact and torsional loading increases the risk of joint injury and subsequent trauma-initiated joint degeneration. Individuals with abnormal joint anatomy or alignment, previous significant joint injury, osteoarthritis, joint surgery, joint instability, disturbances of joint or muscle innervation, or inadequate muscle strength have increased risk of joint damage during participation in high-impact athletics.

Primary and secondary stabilizers support joints; a loss of primary stabilizers results in joint instability. Normal loading of the joint is well tolerated by the cartilage bed, underlying bone, support ligaments, and muscle-tendon units; however, with excessive loading progressive failure of the stabilizers occurs, leading to instability. The degree of excessive loading or the frequency with which it occurs will dictate the amount of damage to the joint, a high velocity impact in an accident situation may render a joint unusable in terms of force transmission due to failure of multiple anatomic structures. Chronic overloading of a joint's load tolerance may result in equally debilitating injury albeit from a more insidious breakdown and incomplete repair process.

When assessing acute damage to a joint structure it is crucial that the patient is well restrained (physically and/or chemically), effective analgesia has been administered, and the patient is relaxed. The joint is stability tested through a full range of motion with force applied in multiple directions against the primary stabilizers and the examination is repeated until a complete understanding is obtained of the degree of laxity present. Once the examiner is satisfied with the palpation findings diagnostic imaging should be employed to more fully evaluate the degree of damage to affected structures. The simplest imaging step is radiographic exam of the affected joint. Two views should always be obtained at a minimum; obtaining stressed views to further evaluate abnormal joint movement can be beneficial. Definitive evaluation of bony damage in the joint (intra-articular) or adjacent to the joint (peri-articular) may be very challenging in the elbow and small multi-bone joints of the canine carpus and tarsus. In these cases multi-slice computer tomography increases diagnostic accuracy and improves treatment decision-making. In joints with a large degree of soft-tissue stabilizers (shoulder, hip, knee) magnetic resonance imaging is becoming more popular in an attempt to increase diagnostic accuracy.

Treatment of joint instability may be conservative or surgical. Conservative treatment consists of supporting the unstable joint in a set position with external splintage or casting, restricting the patients exercise to prevent further damage to the joint and initiating a physical therapy and mobilization program at an appropriate time to allow progressive rehabilitation of joint movement, force transmission and avoid excessive stiffening and loss of range of motion. Surgical treatment consists of open or arthroscopic approach to the joint if intra-articular damage is suspected, visual assessment of the damaged support structures, primary repair or secondary augmentation of the primary joint stabilizers and introduction of postoperative external splintage or coaptation. Following surgical repair, temporary joint immobilization by external coaptation, patient exercise restriction, staged return of joint movement and load through development of a physical therapy plan and routine re-assessment of progress is recommended. The decision to perform either a conservative or surgical plan for the patient depends on the joint that is injured, the severity of the laxity and the primary stabilizers damaged, the time delay between instability recognition and presentation to a veterinary care facility and the goals of the client and patient regarding mobility and movement of the affected limb in the long term.

The prognosis for high-end athletes and performance return are often difficult to predict with joint instability. With moderate to severe damage to joint support systems a loss of the joint's range of motion is not unusual and even with surgical reconstruction, meticulous aftercare and well-supervised, staged return to activity a decrease in performance may often occur.

REFERENCES

1. Todhunter RJ, Johnston SA. Osteoarthritis (Chap. 154). In: Slatter DH (ed.): Textbook of Small Animal Surgery, 3rd ed. Philadelphia: WB Saunders, 2003.
2. Buckwalter JA. Sports, joint injury, and post-traumatic osteoarthritis. J Orthop Sports Phys Ther. 2003;33(10):578-588.

LINKING PUPPY TRAINABILITY AND NUTRIENT STATUS

Russ Kelley, MS
P&G Pet Care,Lewisburg Innovation Center
Lewisburg, OH

Genetics and environment are key contributors to the development of the puppy and ultimately determine the characteristics that will be expressed as an adult. Environment can be continually modified (for better or worse) throughout growth and development; however, an animal's genetic potential is, to a degree, fixed at the time of conception. Traditionally, nutrition has been characterized as the supply of necessary building blocks for organ and system growth. Clearly, this remains vitally important; however, it is becoming increasingly evident that nutrition can also significantly impact the achievement of genetic potential in the puppy in ways not previously appreciated.

Trainability may be considered a combination of willingness to learn/please (attitude/motivation), ability to understand what the trainer wants (intelligence), and ability to remember the tasks being taught (memory). Expectations of a puppy's ability to learn vary immensely among owners, ranging from the very basics like coming when called or sitting to multiple sets of more complex skills as required by dogs serving the Military or individuals with disabilities. Given enough time and the proper stimuli, all puppies possess the ability to learn a given task. However, how well the task is performed will vary greatly from dog to dog and be influenced by an array of factors such as the puppy's genetic makeup, how the puppy is raised and trained (environment), and its health status, which is itself a reflection of genetics and environmental influence. Nutrient status is seldom directly included in discussions regarding an animal's trainability. However, when one considers that nutrition is a major environmental factor that also has an enormous impact on health status, it is a factor that will likely receive greater attention in the future.

MATERNAL INFLUENCES

A series of past efforts have demonstrated that a bitch's nutrient status is influenced by several key factors including diet, stage of her reproductive cycle, and her reproductive history. This occurrence is not unique to the dog with similar results observed in other mammalian species, including humans. Reductions in maternal nutrient status have been reported for several nutrients including essential fatty acids (EFA), select minerals and vitamins. While all of these nutrient classes are critical for optimal health, the major focus of this report will be how a puppy's trainability is linked to EFA status and how the puppy's EFA status is influence by nutrition.

A bitch's EFA status, particularly DHA (docosahexaenoic acid – 22:6n-3) status, has been shown to be influenced by the composition and content of the dietary lipids, her reproductive history, and litter size, although the latter had less influence than the previous factors.[1-4] In addition, it was found that a puppy's DHA status was strongly influenced by maternal status as well the bitch's reproductive history. It remains unclear if the decline in a puppy's DHA status from later litters is a response to repeated reproductive activity or an aging response, but puppies from subsequent litters have consistently been found to have significant reductions (up to 50%) in DHA status when compared with puppies born earlier to the same bitch. This occurrence would be expected in cases where bitches have been maintained on diets that contain only minimum levels of DHA; however, this has also been observed in bitches that have been maintained on diets with sufficient DHA levels to maintain maternal DHA status.

Currently, there is little to no prospective data available that examines the interaction of nutrition, parity (reproductive history) and a puppy's learning performance. However, a study by Mundell does provide substantial retrospective data that strongly suggest the existence of such an interaction.[5] Mundell examined the effect of parity on reproductive performance and puppy outcome of some 5500 puppies in terms of successively becoming a Service Dog. Mundell reported a significant impact on both reproductive performance and graduation rate. Although Mundell did not discuss in detail exact behaviors, the study did report the number of behavior related releases were significantly affected by parity, increasing approximately 25% in 5th parity puppies compared to 1st parity. Interesting, Mundell reported that the number of medical releases were not affected by parity number, suggesting that health status was not compromised.

DIETARY INFLUENCES OF DHA

Numerous studies in several species have demonstrated the benefits of DHA regarding the development and function of neurological tissues.[6] The impact of dietary DHA on puppy status and trainability has also been previously reported.[3,4] Puppies were produced from bitches fed various levels of DHA with puppies weaned onto and maintained on their respective maternal diet for a period 16 weeks. During weeks 9 to 16 of the study, puppies were evaluated for their performance in a 2-arm maze to assess their trainability. A significant ($P < 0.05$) effect of dietary DHA level was observed with the greatest percentage of puppies (68%) achieving at least 1 success criterion when fed the High DHA diet compared with the Low DHA group, which produced the fewest successes (30%). While success rate increased in a dose-dependant manner, puppies from the Medium DHA group (42%) did not differ from the High or Low DHA group (Figure 1).

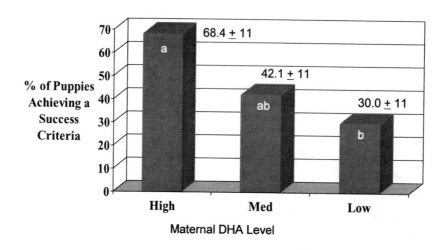

Figure 1. Effect of dietary DHA on puppy trainability. Different superscript denotes significant difference at $P < 0.05$.

CONCLUSION

As mentioned earlier, genetics and environment are key contributors to the development of the puppy and ultimately determine the characteristics that will be expressed as an adult. Admittedly, numerous questions remain unanswered in terms of the mechanisms impacting nutrient status and nutrient–genetic interaction, but clearly a relationship between nutrient status and trainability exist and while improved nutrient status alone cannot overcome inferior genetics and/or training programs, it certainly should not be a puppy's limiting factor.

REFERENCES

1. Kelley RL. Canine reproduction: What should we expect? In: Reinhart GA, Carey DP (eds.): Recent Advances in Canine and Feline Nutrition, Volume III. Wilmington, OH: Orange Frazier Press, 2000, pp 225-242.
2. Kelley, RL, Lepine AJ, Burr JR, Shyan-Norwalt M, Reinhart GA. Effect of dietary fish oil on puppy trainability. Proceeding from the 6th Congress of the International Society for the Study of Fatty Acids and Lipids, Maternal & Infant Nutrition Workshop, 2004.
3. Kelley RL, Lepine AJ, Ruffing J, Vennard T, Reinhart GA. Impact of maternal dietary DHA and reproductive activity on DHA status in the canine. Proceeding from 6th Congress of the International Society for the Study of Fatty Acids and Lipids, 2004, p 149.
4. Kelley RL, Lepine AJ, Shyan-Norwalt MR, Burr JR, Reinhart GA. Impact of Maternal and Post-Weaning Nutrition on Puppy Trainability. Proceedings from the 4th International Working Dog Breeding Association Conference, 2005, pp 113-116.
5. Mundell PE. The effect of parity number on litter size, health and performance in working dogs. Proceedings from the 4th International Working Dog Breeding Association Conference, 2005, p 141.
6. Lauritzen L, Hansen HS, Jorgensen MH, Michaelson KF. The essentiality of long chain n-3 fatty acids in relation to development and function of the brain and retina. Progr Lipid Res. 2001; 40:1-94.

INTEGRATIVE MEDICINE AS IT APPLIES TO THE CANINE ATHLETE

Laurie McCauley, DVM
TOPS Veterinary Rehabilitation
Grayslake, IL
Canine Rehabilitation Institute
Aspen, CO and Wellington, FL

Canine athletes, whether they do recreational sports (agility, lure coursing, Frisbee) or functional sports (fieldwork, sled pulling, herding), push their bodies to the limits and in doing so increase their risk of an injury over pet dogs. Many of the injuries we see are also related to the individual sport in which they participate. On the other hand, some injuries, for instance cranial cruciate ruptures, can be seen in recreational and functional sporting dogs. Integrative medicine is not a silver bullet and will not heal all injuries, but there are many times integrative medicine can be utilized to speed the recovery or prevent the injury from occurring. Acupuncture, Manual Therapy (a combination of different hands on techniques), Homotoxicology, and Essential Oils will be discussed to aid your athletic canine patient to a life of reduced injuries and speedier healing when injuries do occur.

PREVENTING INJURIES

The first and foremost thought is to prevent injuries if at all possible. Stretching and warming the muscle tissue before working has been shown to decrease the rate of injuries. Flexion, extension, and rotation of the joints of all four limbs and the spine can be done standing and in under 10 minutes. Care must be taken not to put abnormal stress on any of the joints. Warming up the muscles is easily done by having the dog perform a slow trot for about 5 minutes. This should be gentle and easy, not tearing out after a toy as this will deplete some of their stored energy. After the dog has finished their competition or job, they should be walked again for 5 minutes to cool down. This increases blood flow through the muscles preventing the lactic acid from settling into the muscle tissue and creating stiffness or soreness which would otherwise slow them down for their next feat.

Stretching starts with the dog standing and the handler either kneeling next to the dog or if the dog is a small breed, the handler can stand and the dog can on a table. Distal joints cannot be fully flexed or extended until the proximal joints are flexed or extended; therefore, we always start with the proximal joints. When we start we need to be cognizant of where the dog is shifting their weight. If they are shifting their weight onto the limb we want to stretch, it will be more difficult for the handler and unbalancing for the dog. The easiest thing to do is to shift their weight towards your body and reach across their body to work on the opposite limb. By having them lean into you they are more stable and more comfortable. Keep the limb perpendicular to the ground as you bring the elbow to the chest, then the carpus to the shoulder, and then the foot to the forearm, flexing the toes as you do so. Hold for 10 seconds applying only as much pressure as you can comfortably apply as you pull your own pointer finger back (this will be explained in lecture). By placing the dog's elbow in your palm you can guide their limb forward into full extension (shoulder, elbow, and carpus). Place your other hand on their chest to aid their balance. Do not let the limb rotate. If full range of motion is not achieved, massage the triceps and deltoid muscles as one of these two muscles is usually the cause for this restriction. This position should only be held for 10 seconds. Then, by placing your palm at carpus, the limb can be moved into shoulder flexion with elbow and carpus extension. This stretches the biceps brachii, pectoral, serratus ventralis, rhomboideus, trapezius, and supraspinatus muscles. If full motion is not achieved, these muscles should be checked and massaged if they are not lengthening fully. This should be held for 10 seconds. This whole process should be repeated 2 to 4 more times. The shoulder, as with the hip, is a rotary joint. Lean the dog into your body, support the limb and hold it at or above the elbow with one arm and with the other arm hold the dog across the chest and place your hand over the shoulder to monitor for pops and grinding. Rotate the limb at the shoulder 5-10 times (this should encompass full abduction and adduction).

The rear limb is very similar to the forelimb as we use the same amount of pressure, start proximal and work distal, the 10-second rule applies, and the limb should stay perpendicular to the floor. Shift the dog's weight into you slightly and lift the opposite limb bringing the stifle to the chest. Make sure you do not torque the joint by adding any rotation. Then bring the hock to the hip, flex the hock and then the toes. Hold for 10 seconds. Cup the hock with one hand and bring the limb forward while the other hand prevents the stifle from rising (rotation and torque of the hip) or going under the ribcage. Hold this stretch for 10 seconds. Then place the hand that was on the hock, on the stifle and guide the limb back so the hip, stifle, and hock are all in extension. Hold this for 10 seconds. Repeat this sequence 2 to 4 times. To rotate the hip, place one hand over the hip joint and the other supporting the limb at or above the stifle. The hip should be rotated, resulting in full abduction and adduction 5 to 10 times.

The spine can be stretched in lateral flexion, flexion, and extension. The easiest way to do this is with cookie stretches. Using tasty treats, ask the dog to bring their nose to their shoulder. There should be no rotation of the head. Holding the cookie close to the body wall at the level of the shoulder, bring the cookie to the hip and then down to the rear toes giving nibbles to the dog as you move the cookie. If they do not get any treats as they do this, they lose interest rather quickly. After repeating this on the other side, take the cookie to the chest, down to the floor, and between the front legs until they are in a headstand position. This is lateral flexion and then straight flexion. To obtain full extension of the spine, ask the dog to bring their front feet on to an elevated surface and take the cookie toward the sky. If the dog is standing with all four feet on the ground, the only thing that will extend will be their lower cervical spine. By having the feet elevated, the cervical, thoracic, and lumbar spine are all extended. Each stretch only needs to be held for 3 to 5 seconds.

To flex the whole thoracolumbar spine, cat stretches are useful. By placing your pointer fingers together at the first rib and applying moderate pressure up and at a 45° angle back and slowly moving your fingers back until meeting the thigh, each of the dog's facet joints are opened and then closed. Three repetitions are all that are needed. If the dog has lordosis, this often visually improves by the time the third stretch is completed.

If any of these stretches are painful to the dog, this may indicate an injury and further diagnostics may be needed.

TREATING COMMON INJURIES

There are many injuries common to canine athletes. We can not go through all of them, but will start with the head and work our way down covering some of injuries that are most easily treated with integrative medicine.

If when doing cookie stretches the dog has trouble laterally flexing his head to his shoulder without rotating it, or if the cookie isn't worth the discomfort of turning, then the neck musculature is examined for muscle knots/trigger points (capitus rectus muscles or brachiocephalicus muscle). If an obvious knot is present this can be manually worked out with ischemic compression, longitudinal strokes, circles, or cross fiber massage. Traction of the neck is often very helpful (be careful of your hand placement). There are acupuncture points on the sides of the neck, palpated as depressions, which can be injected with the homotoxicology remedy Traumeel. Traumeel is indicated for bruising, muscle stiffness or soreness, and inflammation. Inject 0.2 to 0.5 mL into the subcutaneous tissue at each point.

If there is restriction of motion along the thoracic spine or pain is palpated anywhere along the spine, depressions can usually be found and injected. Depressions are found by running your fingers along the Spinalis muscle. Any depressions found are acupuncture points. The dog will usually improve relatively quickly. Massage, laser (4–8 Joules/cm²), and ischemic compression can be used on any trigger points along the Spinalis muscle as well. For any dogs that are prone to back injuries or have chronic carpal hyper-extension, the Ligaplex supplements from Standard Process or Ligatone may beneficial. Ligaplex I and Ligaplex II support the ligaments and tendons. Ligaplex II is may also be utilized as a preventive supplement to protect against tendon and ligament injuries.

Teres major strain (aka "agility pit") is seen when a dog does a plant and twist when the muscles are not stretched beforehand. There can be lameness, slowing down over jumps, or trouble wrapping after a jump in one direction. It is diagnosed by placing two fingers up into the armpit to stroke the teres major muscle and finding discomfort when wiggling your fingers. Relief can be brought about by gentle massage and stretching. Flex the shoulder, place two fingers in to the armpit and gently massage the muscle as you bring the shoulder

into extension. If discomfort is felt, immediately return the shoulder to flexion and start again. This therapy can be done from twice a day to twice a week and is usually resolved within 1 to 2 weeks if treated correctly. As with any muscle injury, Traumeel tablets can be given as well to reduce inflammation and muscle tenderness. The dose for a 5- to 30-pound dog is ½ tablet two to three times daily; the dose for dogs over 30 pounds would be 1 tablet two to three times daily. A dog under 5 pounds could receive ¼ tablet two to three times daily or two to three drops of the liquid preparation two to three times daily. This remedy, as with all homotoxicology and homeopathy, is best given away from food. Arnica, in a tablet or cream form, can be used as well for these injuries.

Strains in the triceps muscle can be seen in field, freestyle, agility, Frisbee and lure coursing dogs. A thickening of the long and lateral head of the triceps is palpated and there may be restrictions in full shoulder extension. As in most muscle strains (others commonly affected are sartorius, tensor fascia lata, gracilis, gluteal, and flexor carpi ulnaris muscles), oral Traumeel, MSM (at 750–1500 mg/50 pounds), TID cryotherapy (10 minutes on, 10 minutes off, 10 minutes on), Laser therapy of 2–4 Joules/cm², therapeutic Ultrasound (72 hours post injury), and massage (gentle the first 4–7 days and then with more pressure to break up the fibrous tissue and increase circulation) can be utilized. Most muscle strains are palpated as a thickening with heat and tenderness on digital palpation. The injury to the sartorius is usually at the proximal aspect of the muscle just below the wing of the ileum. Tensor fascia lata injuries are located just caudal to where the sartorius injuries are felt. Sometimes both muscles are equally affected. The gracilis muscle is on the medial aspect of the thigh and should be palpated (with the semimembranosus and semitendinosus as the hip is flexed and the stifle is extended). Gracilis injuries are commonly seen with agility and racing dogs. Gluteal muscle strains are palpated between the wing of the ileum and the greater trochanter. The Flexor Carpi Ulnaris muscle is palpated easily as it attaches to the accessory carpal bone. When strained it may be two to three times its normal thickness and hot. All muscles need to be palpated while the limb is non-weight bearing.

Essential oils can be rubbed into injured muscles to relive discomfort and speed healing. Commonly used oils include:

- Lavender, the universal oil, which can be used topically to help relax dogs; can be applied to a wound, insect bite, or burn to decrease pain and speed healing; and relieve discomfort from osteoarthritis when applied topically (diluted in oil).
- Birch, related to willow, contains methyl salicylates, which has analgesic, antispasmodic, and anti-inflammatory properties, and can be applied topically to relieve pain and inflammation associated with tendonitis, muscle stiffness, and osteoarthritis.

- German Chamomile also has a calming effect as well as antispasmodic and anti-inflammatory properties.
- Cypress improves circulation and supports the neurological system. It is also antibacterial and repels insects. It can be used topically on wounds, to lessen scar formation, and over joints with osteoarthritis.

Other muscles commonly injured with working dogs include the iliocostalis and iliopsoas muscles. The iliocostalis muscle along with the Gluteal muscle affect motion of the sacroiliac (SI) joint. The SI joint is palpated at a 20° medial to lateral angle. Palpating straight dorsal to ventral can jam the joint and is contraindicated. If the joint doesn't move, palpate the iliocostalis and gluteal muscles. The Iliocostalis may have twine-like fibers coming from the wing of the ileum toward the ribs if it is causing the problem. If the gluteal muscle is the problem, it will feel like there is a finger in the middle of the muscle perpendicular to the muscle fibers, or the whole muscle may be rock hard. Massage, laser, therapeutic ultrasound, phonophoresis, and topical heat all can be useful. Again, Traumeel or Arnica may help as well. The typical Iliopsoas injury is seen when an agility dog crashes into a tire and hyper extends the SI joint. The iliopsoas, made up of the psoas major and the Iliacus muscles, can be strained. It is common for there to be lameness for a short while and then no lameness, but the dog doesn't put full weight on the limb when standing. To test for this injury, the rear limb is placed in full extension and then internally rotated. As the Iliopsoas attaches to the lesser trochanter, this creates a full stretch. This should be done very slowly as when the muscle is strained, it is very painful. Massage and stretching are the way to heal this injury, but care must be taken as the femoral artery runs across this muscle and an unskilled person may occlude blood flow to the limb. This is not a muscle for you to teach your average client how to massage. Laser and ultrasound are not recommended, as they may affect the femoral artery as well. When stretching, bring the hip into full flexion, massage the muscle (found by following the body wall and pushing the intestines out of the way) and slowly extend the hip. If too much pressure is placed on the muscle or if the hip is extended too quickly, the dog may try to bite you. This should only be massaged and stretched for 5 to 7 minutes, two to seven times a week as too much too fast may do more harm then good. Traumeel can be injected into two acupuncture points for immediate relief of pain. Those points are Bladder 28, located 1.5 cun lateral to the caudal border of the spinous process of the 7th lumbar vertebrae (a cun is the width of the 3rd rib) and Gall Bladder 28, cranial and ventral to the cranial dorsal iliac spine.

With all muscle strains, restricted activity for 2 to 3 weeks is needed to allow time for the muscle to heal followed by a slow return to normal activity over another 3 to 4 weeks depending on the degree of the injury. Leash walks are always the first activity to be re-instated.

Bleeding of any kind (cuts, worn pads, nails that have been broken or torn off) can be treated with the Chinese Herb formula Yunnan Bai Yao. It comes in capsules that can be opened up and the herb applied directly to the wound, it can also be taken orally if a dog has trouble clotting and a wound or injury is likely. The Yunnan Bai Yao package comes with little red pills as well. These are to be ingested if there is excessive bleeding or shock. For those vets who do surgery and have nicked a spleen, this is a very handy, inexpensive tool to have in the clinic. It can also be applied to nails that have been cut to the quick.

Toe injuries are also very common. Jammed toes, fractured toes, torn medial or lateral collateral toe ligaments, fractured sesamoids. First determine what the injury is. If it is a hot swollen joint, a radiograph is needed to determine if there is a fracture. If a fracture is present, restrict activity for at least 4r weeks. If no fracture is found, cryotherapy, traction +/- rotation, and oral and topical Traumeel or topical Arnica are indicated. Cryotherapy slows nerve conduction reducing pain and degradation enzyme activity. When the ice is removed there is rebound vasodilatation with increased blood flow to speed healing. Traction and rotation stimulate the nociceptive receptors in the synovial capsule decreasing pain as well as stretching the capsule to break up fibrous adhesions, which would otherwise restrict motion. Partially torn ligaments can be repaired with a technique called Prolotherapy. The injection of dextrose, procaine, plus or minus other ingredients at the insertion of the ligament triggers the body to produce fibrous tissue where it is needed to increase stability of the joint and relieve pain. This may need to be done several times a week to every 3 weeks for two to five treatments. Laser therapy of an injured collateral ligament can also speed healing. Dosing of 4 to 8 Joules/cm² daily to twice weekly is advantageous. Cross friction massage can be started gently at 2 weeks post injury and more aggressively at 3 to 4 weeks to help the collagen fibers lay more parallel enhancing the tensile strength.

Many injuries are common in working dogs. I have chosen those that do not require surgery that I see most commonly. Ministering to canine athletes is thrilling to me. To prevent injuries, and to hasten the recovery of those that do occur, allows these dogs to continue to do what they were bred to do, well into their geriatric years.

CHONDROPROTECTIVE AGENTS: FACT OR FICTION?

Ron McLaughlin. DVM, DVSc, Diplomate ACVS
College of Veterinary Medicine
Mississippi State University, Mississippi State, MS

In recent years, efforts have been made to identify alternative treatments for the medical management of osteoarthritis (OA). Research has focused on slowing the progression of cartilage degradation and promoting cartilage matrix synthesis. Products are now available that may have a positive effect on cartilage matrix, enhance hyaluronic acid production, inhibit catabolic enzymes in osteoarthritic joints, and encourage normalization of the synovial fluid and cartilage matrix. These agents reportedly enhance cartilage health by providing the necessary precursors to maintain and repair cartilage.

Chondroprotective agents are defined as compounds that (1) support or enhance macromolecular synthesis by chondrocytes, (2) support or enhance synthesis of hyaluronan by synoviocytes, (3) inhibit degradative enzymes or inflammatory mediators, and (4) remove or prevent formation of fibrin, thrombi, or plaque in synovium and/or subchondral blood vessels. There are currently numerous products available that claim to be "chondroprotective"; however, at the present time, no known agent has been scientifically proven to fulfill all of these requirements. Fortunately, some products currently on the market do to fulfill some of the requirements of a "chondroprotective" agent. The term *disease modifying osteoarthritis agent* is preferred over the term *chondroprotective agent* in most literature. Since many of the products act by gradually becoming incorporated into the cartilage matrix, the term *slow-acting disease modifying osteoarthritis agent* is often used. These products can be further divided into parentrally or orally administered products.

INJECTABLE DISEASE-MODIFYING OA AGENTS:
Adequan
Adequan® (Luitpold Pharamceuticals) is a polysulfated glycosaminoglycan (PSGAG). Known as Arteparon in Europe, this agent been used to treat OA for many years and is approved for use in horses and dogs. It appears to be very safe at recommended doses. Studies have shown that injected Adequan does reach therapeutic levels in serum, synovial fluid, cartilage and tendons. Although experimental evidence of Adequan's positive anabolic effect on cartilage is conflicting, its ability to decreases cartilage catabolism has been shown in numerous studies on both horses and dogs. The effects of intramuscular administration of PSGAG was evaluated in growing pups with hip dysplasia. Treatment from 6 weeks to 8 months of age resulted in less subluxation (as determined by radiography) and improved coxofemoral congruity at 8 months of age. Joint pathology scores obtained at necropsy indicated a trend toward more normal synovial fluid volume and lower ligament volume in treated puppies, although the improvements were not statistically significant. These findings suggest Adequan may be useful if administered early in the disease process. In another study, DeHann evaluated the effects of Adequan as a treatment for hip dysplasia in 84 adult dogs. Lameness, range of motion (ROM), and pain on manipulation of the hip joints were evaluated. The results indicated that dogs given Adequan had a greater improvement in orthopedic scores compared to a placebo group; however, the differences were not statistically significant. Unfortunately, the absence of a control group in this study may have caused a type II statistical error and prevented the identification of a positive effect.

Other studies evaluating the effect of PSGAG on joint health after transection of the cranial cruciate ligament in dogs have been equivocal. Treatment did not preserve cartilage biochemical and biomechanical properties in one study, but did improve joint health in another. However, a study evaluating the effects of systemic administration of Arteparon found it provided partial protection to the articular cartilage from damage caused by meniscetomy in the canine. This was demonstrated histologically by reduced surface fibrillation, diminished chondrocyte cloning, and maintenance of alcianophilia. Another study in 8 horses found that intra-articular PSGAG protected cartilage during a chemical insult to the joint but had no effect in a physical articular cartilage-defect model. However, in an experiment where postoperative exercise and intra-articular PSGAG were used in 18 ponies with osteochondral defects, the combination of exercise and PSGAG in individual joints resulted in a significant decreased bone remodeling.

Although numerous dose recommendations have been reported for the use of Adequan in dogs, a dosage of 5 mg/kg IM twice weekly is common. Complications associated with Adequan administration are rare. PSGAG is a heparin analog and when injected in cats has produced a transient, dose-dependent increase in activated partial thromboplastin time. Therefore, its use in animals with bleeding disorders should be avoided. Concurrent use with NSAIDs that exhibit strong anti-thromboxane activity should also be avoided.

Hyaluronic Acid (HA)
HA (hyaluronic acid, sodium hyaluronate) is a non-sulfated GAG that is a major component of synovial fluid. It is administered primarily by intra-articular injection, though a form of HA for intravenous administration is available for use in horses (Legend®, Bayer). HA is postulated to enhance joint health by increasing the viscosity of the joint fluid, reducing inflammation, and scavenging free radicals. In a research study of HA used to treat dogs with transected cranial cruciate ligaments, a positive effect on cartilage biochemical parameters was noted. Based on experience and scientific evidence from its use in humans and in horses, HA may be beneficial in treating OA in dogs. However, HA has not been commonly used to treat OA in dogs.

ORAL DISEASE-MODIFYING OA AGENTS

Many oral disease-modifying osteoarthritis agents are marketed as nutritional supplements. Currently, there are few regulations to ensure the products actually contain the agents listed on the label or that the agents, if present, are available in adequate quantities. As a result, variation among available products is significant and the results obtained from scientific evaluation of one product may not apply to other seemingly similar products.

Many of the oral disease modifying agents contain glucosamine and chondroitin sulfate in various forms. It is reported that they are absorbed by the GI tract, become incorporated into joint tissues, and provide the necessary precursors to maintain cartilage health and perhaps even promote cartilage repair. Anecdotal reports, in vitro studies, and published clinical trials indicate that these agents are effective in treating OA.

Glucosamine is an amino-monosaccharide nutrient that has exhibited no toxicity even at high oral doses. It is a precursor to the disaccharide unit of glycosaminoglycans, which comprise the proteoglycan ground substance of articular cartilage. Studies using radiolabeled compounds in man and animals have shown that 87% of orally administered glucosamine is absorbed and is eventually incorporated into the cartilage matrix. Excretion of glucosamine is primarily via urine and feces. Glucosamine reportedly acts by providing the regulatory stimulus and raw materials for synthesis of glycosaminoglycans. Since chondrocytes obtain preformed glucosamine from the circulation (or synthesizes it from glucose and amino acids), adequate glucosamine levels in the body are essential for synthesis of glycosaminoglycans in cartilage. Glucosamine is also used directly for the production of hyaluronic acid by synoviocytes.

In vitro biochemical and pharmacological studies indicate that the administration of glucosamine may normalize cartilage metabolism and stimulates the synthesis of proteoglycans. In one study, glucosamine stimulated synthesis of glycosaminolgycans, prostaglandin and collagen by chondrocytes and fibroblasts, suggesting it not only provides raw material for their production, but may actually up-regulate synthesis. The effects of glucosamine sulfate on human chondrocyte gene expression was also evaluated, assessing its effects on type II collagen, fibronectin, stromelysin and proteoglycans in normal adult chondrocytes. Glucosamine modulated the expression of cartilage proteoglycans, decreased stromelysin mRNA levels in osteoarthritic chondrocytes, and preserved the constitutive expression of type II collagen and fibronectin in both normal and osteoarthritic chondrocytes.

Clinical trials have also been performed to evaluate the effects of glucosamine on OA in humans. A double-blind, randomized, placebo-controlled study evaluating the effects of glucosamine sulfate in 252 patients with knee OA found oral glucosamine was significantly more effective than placebo in improving pain and joint motion. Another study evaluated glucosamine sulfate in 80 patients with OA by scoring articular pain, joint tenderness, swelling, and restriction of active and passive movements. Treated patients experienced a reduction in overall symptoms nearly two times greater and more rapidly than those given a placebo, and samples of articular cartilage analyzed by scanning electron microscopy appeared more normal in patients treated with glucosamine. A study using semi-quantitative scoring of pain at rest and during passive movements, restricted function, and walking-time over 20 meters found OA patients treated with glucosamine sulfate were significantly improved compared with those given a placebo. And, in a randomized, double-blind, parallel-group study of 200 patients with active knee OA, glucosamine was found to be as effective as ibuprofen in controlling symptoms. These studies indicate that glucosamine may have a positive effect on cartilage health and helps control symptoms associated with OA in humans.

Chondroitin Sulfate (CS) is a long chain polymer of a repeating disaccharide units (galactosamine sulfate and glucuronic acid). It is the predominant glycosaminolycan found in articular cartilage and can be purified from bovine, whale, and shark cartilage sources. Bioavailability studies in rats, dogs and humans have shown 70% absorption of CS following oral administration. Studies in rats and humans using radiolabeled CS (^{99m}Tc-CS) have shown that CS does reach synovial fluid and articular cartilage.

The effect of CS on cartilage has been investigated in several in vitro studies. When human articular chondrocytes were cultivated in clusters in the presence CS, prostaglandin levels were significantly increased and collagenolytic activity was decreased. A similar study indicted that CS competitively inhibited degradative enzymes of prostaglandins in cartilage and synovium by its long chain length. In a study of rabbits with chymopapain-induced stifle arthritis, prostaglandin depletion was reduced by the administration of CS.

Clinical trials in humans have also found CS to be effective in reducing the symptoms of OA. In a placebo-controlled, double-blinded study of 120 patients with OA of the knees and hips, treatment with CS resulted in significant improvements in pain-scale scores and pain-function index. In another study of 42 patients with knee OA, CS treatment significantly reduced pain and increased joint mobility. Bone and joint metabolism (as assessed by various biochemical markers) also stabilized in the patients treated with CS while remaining abnormal in patients receiving a placebo. Hyaluronate concentrations and viscosity were increased, and collagenolytic activity was decreased, in the synovial fluid of OA patients treated with CS for 10 days. These clinical trials indicate that CS has a positive effect in controlling the symptoms associated with osteoarthritis in humans.

Combinations of glucosamine and chondroitin sulfate are commonly used together as a disease modifying osteoarthritis agent. It is reported that these agents work synergistically. One of the most popular products available for use in animals, Cosequin® (Nutramax Laboratories), is derived from bovine trachea and contains purified glucosamine hydrochloride, chondroitin sulfate, manganese and ascorbate. Cosequin has been used in numerous studies evaluating its efficacy in the treatment of OA.

In a survey of small animal practitioners on the perceived efficacy and safety of Cosequin, the percentage of practitioners that rated the clinical efficacy of the compound to be "good" or "excellent" relative to improved mobility, alleviating pain, and improved attitude in animals were 89%, 83%, and 85%, respectively. A study evaluating the effects of Cosequin on hematologic variables in clinically normal dogs found significant decreases in hematocrit, hemoglobin, WBC, and segmented neutrophil variables on days 3 and 14 of treatment. A significant decrease in platelet count was reported on days 14 and 30. However, no changes were seen in prothrombin time, activated partial thromboplastin time, mucosal bleeding time, or biochemical variables and the conclusion was that Cosequin causes only minor changes in hemostatic variables.

In an in vivo study of the effects of Cosequin on cartilage metabolism in dogs, serum samples were collected after treatment with Cosequin and tested for circulating glycosaminoglycan content. Median serum glycosaminoglycan levels were significantly increased in treated dogs. When normal calf cartilage segments were exposed to the serum from the treated dogs, the biosynthetic activity of chondrocytes was significantly increased and proteolytic degradation of the cartilage segments cultured in serum was reduced. In a similar study, cartilage stimulatory and antiproteolytic activity were evaluated using sera of 30 dogs treated with Cosequin for 1 month. Serum glycosaminoglycan levels were increased by 42% after 1 month. Radiolabeling techniques were then used to study the biosynthetic and degradative responses of bovine cartilage exposed to the canine serum. Cartilage segments cultured in canine serum had a 50% increase in glycosaminoglycan biosynthesis and a 59% reduction in median proteolytic degradation. These in vitro studies suggest that Cosequin promotes glycosaminoglycan synthesis and suppresses proteolytic enzymes.

Several in vivo studies have also investigated the use of Cosequin for treatment of OA. In a study of 16 dogs with experimental cranial cruciate ligament injury (with and without surgical stabilization) dogs receiving Cosequin treatment had subjectively less osteoarthritis and a more normal joint translation than control dogs. In a study of acute synovitis in dogs, those pretreated with Cosequin showed a reduction in joint inflammation (as measured by nuclear scintigraphy) and improved clinical lameness scores over controls.

Cosamin®, the version of Cosequin used in humans, was evaluated in a study assessing the progression of cartilage lesions in rabbits using a joint instability model. Rabbits treated with Cosamin had less severe cartilage lesions as measured using the modified Mankin grading system. In a recent double-blind study sponsored by the National Institutes of Health (NIH) and published in the New England Journal of Medicine, over 1,500 patients of 40 years of age and suffering from knee osteoarthritis were treated with a placebo, celecoxib, or a combination of glucosamine and chondroitin sulfate (found in Coasmin). The study found that the combination of glucosamine and chondroitin sulfate was effective in managing moderate to severe knee pain, and that this combination was superior to either agent used alone. These in vivo studies suggest that treatment with Cosequin has a positive clinical effect in osteoarthritic patients.

Dasuquin™ (Nutramax Laboratories) is the latest joint supplement marketed for management of OA in dogs. It is a combination of glucosamine, chondroitin sulfate, decaffeinated tea polyphenols, and avocdado/soybean unsoponifiables (ASU). Tea polyphenols may have a positive effect on cartilage health and provide oxidative balance in the body. ASU has been shown to be more effective than chondroitin sulfate in inhibiting the expression of certain OA mediators responsible for cartilage breakdown. In in vitro studies, ASU has been shown to decrease the expression of COX-2 enzyme, TNF-α, IL-1, and PGE_2 in chondrocytes. The combination of ASU with glucosamine and chondroitin sulfate decreased the expression of numerous pro-inflammatory mediators, including TNF-α, IL-1β, and iNOS. Dasuguin is also available with MSM (methylsulfonylmethane), a source of organic sulfur also used to support joint health.

SUMMARY

Although no agent has been shown to provide all of the beneficial effects required of a "chondroprotective agent," many products have been shown, through in vitro studies and controlled clinical trials, to be useful in the treatment of OA. Additional prospective clinical trials (random, double-blind, placebo controlled studies) are needed to confirm the efficacy of disease-modifying agents in the treatment of OA; and additional laboratory research is needed to better understand the mechanisms by which these products may enhance cartilage health.

Reference are available from the author upon request.

REHABILITATION CONSIDERATIONS IN DOGS WITH PERFORMANCE-INDUCED INJURIES

Darryl L. Millis, MS, DVM, Diplomate ACVS, CCRP
College of Veterinary Medicine
University of Tennessee, Knoxville, TN

Performance events for dogs are increasing in popularity. Canine agility sport activities are the most rapidly growing events for dogs. Other canine sporting events continue to be of interest, including sled dog racing, flyball, hunting, Frisbee events, and coursing. Regardless of the sporting event, there are a number of injuries that occur in dogs, some of which are minor, and others which may end a dog's competitive career. There are a number of factors which may reduce the chances of injuries. Rehabilitation may improve the chances of a dog returning to activity.

PREVENTION

While some injuries are unavoidable, prevention of injuries is preferable to having a major injury. The optimal prevention program involves proper selection of a dog for a particular event, initiating training at the proper age, having an appropriate conditioning and training program, educating owners regarding evaluation of their dog after each workout, and regular evaluations to be certain that overuse injuries are not occurring.

Proper Selection: Some dogs are more suited for certain sports than others. Many physical attributes important to sporting dogs are inherited, including size, speed, strength, endurance, and agility. Tall dogs with long legs are more suited for running and endurance events, while those with a shorter build may be better suited for power activities. Conformation may affect the forces that are placed on the limbs during activity. For example, dogs with less angulation to the joints had higher forces placed on the forelimbs while jumping than dogs with greater angulation to the joints.

Training Programs: A proper training program is essential to prevent injuries. Cardiovascular conditioning is essential to prevent fatigue. As animals tire, their coordination becomes compromised, rendering them more susceptible to injury. Training programs should be as sport-specific as possible. For example, it is essential that sled dogs undergo conditioning in the snow to strengthen shoulder and hip muscles for pulling the sled through snow. To increase strength (or endurance), a load that exceeds muscle and/or cardiopulmonary metabolic capacity must be achieved during exercise. The systems must also be exercised to fatigue to promote improvement. Dogs involved in speed events must develop muscle strength to allow rapid contraction velocity of muscles to cause joint motion to drive the body forward. Dogs involved in flyball must accelerate as quickly as possible in a straight line for just a few seconds, jump four times, decelerate very rapidly, turn, and accelerate as quickly as possible, and jump over the hurdles again. In designing a strengthening program, there is a need to focus on strengthening pelvic limbs, for acceleration and jumping, and on the forelimbs for braking and turning.

Conditioning begins early in life, but caution should be exercised regarding training programs in skeletally immature dogs. Most people involved with agility training do not recommend intense training over jumps until 12 to 18 months of age. These guidelines are prudent because the concussive forces associated with jumping may damage developing cartilage. For example, large dogs jumping over a 25-inch jump place the equivalent of 310% of their body weight on their forelimbs when landing, while those jumping over a 37" obstacle place the equivalent of 430% of their body weight on their forelimbs.

It is also important to consider changes in fitness and conditioning following injury or a period of rest. In one study, endurance decreased by 41% in dogs whose activity was restricted for 8 weeks. These changes were reversible with 8 weeks of retraining.

Early Detection: Early detection of problems may result in reduced recovery time and may prevent career-threatening injuries. Early detection of overwork may allow the dog to recuperate prior to permanent damage. Owners should be taught to palpate their dog's limbs, joints, back, and neck for any problems before and after each training session. They should also be counseled regarding subtle changes in performance, such as resisting turning at speed, or approaching a jump in an awkward fashion. In particular, any forelimb lameness that becomes visibly apparent is likely a significant injury because the ability to detect forelimb lameness while subjective forms of gait analysis is relatively poor. Often, there may be a difference in weight bearing of 20% to 30% between the lame forelimb and the ipsilateral forelimb before becoming visible during normal gait evaluation.

SPORTING INJURIES

Osteoarthritis is the most common condition of sporting dogs. It is more common in dogs with abnormal joint biomechanics, either as a result of conformation abnormalities or injury. The majority of orthopedic problems encountered in sporting dogs appear to result from developmental orthopedic diseases, such as hip dysplasia, elbow dysplasia, patellar luxation, and osteochondritis dissecans. These diseases may remain undiagnosed for months to years until intense activity promotes the development of clinical signs. In most instances, changes such as osteoarthritis are present in the affected joints when the problem is diagnosed, confirming the chronicity of the problem. Rehabilitation can have a profound effect on osteoarthritis in the sporting dog.

Rupture of the cranial cruciate ligament is probably the most devastating injury in sporting dogs. In addition to the ruptured ligament, dogs develop osteoarthritis. Sprains and strains occur relatively commonly, but they are frequently undiagnosed. Dogs with mild injuries may be rested and treated conservatively. Carpal hyperextension syndrome is a serious sprain involving the carpal ligaments and palmar fibrocartilage, usually requiring fusion of the joints. Strains of the biceps and supraspinatus muscles may occur, especially in dogs that frequently jump or are trained in muddy conditions. Muscle injuries are graded according to the severity, with the gracilis, tensor fascia latae, triceps, iliopsoas, gastrocnemius, and biceps femoris muscles most commonly affected. Infraspinatus muscle contracture is a well-recognized condition.

The level of competition has rapidly increased over the past several years, with competitive events stressing increased speed and efficiency of performance. For example, high level agility competitors often approach a jump at a diagonal and literally begin turning when over the jump and while landing. This puts a great amount of strain on the forelimb, particularly the shoulder joint and may, over time, result in damage to supporting structures of the glenohumeral joint.

Treatment of Acute Injuries

The earlier an acute injury is treated, the better the prognosis and the less likely that there will be permanent damage. Frequent and thorough evaluation is the key to early detection. In some instances, a dog may compensate for an underlying injury, resulting in a problem in another joint or limb. For example, dogs alter their spinal motion when they have a hind limb lameness. With a unilateral rear limb lameness, the back goes from a normally relatively passive connector of the front and rear limbs, to an active motion part to help advance the affected rear limb forward. Essentially, dogs flex the back laterally to the side that is lame to help pull the limb forward. This presumably aids excess stress and strain to the back and may contribute to muscle soreness or spondylosis in some cases.

The goals of early rehabilitation following injury or immediately after surgery are to control inflammation and edema, preserve joint range of motion, and decrease deconditioning effects, such as loss of cardiovascular conditioning and muscle mass. Modalities that have some ability to increase the healing process may also be applied, such as therapeutic ultrasound and low level laser therapy. The therapist must also be aware of the strength profile of healing tissues and resist the temptation to overstress healing tissues. For example, muscle healing requires more than 6 weeks for adequate strength to develop. Healing tendons have 56% tensile strength at 6 weeks and 79% tensile strength at 1 year. Healing ligaments attain 50 to 70% tensile strength at 1 year. Healing and recovery rates, however, vary with the patient's age, the severity of injury, and the specific tissue damage.

Cryotherapy is applied during acute tissue injury to reduce tissue injury and secondary inflammatory responses. The primary effects of cryotherapy include vasoconstriction, reduced blood flow, reduced cellular metabolism and permeability, decreased nerve conduction velocity, analgesia, reduction of edema, and decreased muscle spasm. Several methods may be used to apply superficial cold. The simplest method of ice application is to wrap a plastic bag containing crushed ice in a thin damp cloth and apply directly over the affected area. To prevent skin damage, prevent direct contact of the ice pack with the animal's skin. Apply for 20 to 30 minutes at a time. Unfortunately, cryotherapy may not be effective for tissues at depths greater than 3 cm.

Range of Motion and Stretching Exercises

Active range of motion (ROM) is necessary for a successful outcome. Some patients not receiving early ROM exercises after surgery for cranial cruciate ligament rupture have reduced stifle extension, which is permanent in some dogs if they do not receive appropriate rehabilitation.

Although it may be necessary to immobilize a limb, the consequences should be realized. Reduced ROM occurs after joint immobilization and it may take 8 to 12 weeks of remobilization for improvement. Rehabilitation may help shorten this time. To perform ROM, the patient should be placed in lateral recumbency with the affected limb up. Slowly flex the treated joint, while maintaining the other joints in a neutral position, until the patient shows initial discomfort, then slowly extend the joint until initial discomfort. A number of joints may be simultaneously placed through a functional ROM. Flexing and extending all of the joints of a limb in a pattern that mimics a normal gait pattern is also beneficial. For most conditions, 15 to 20 repetitions, performed 2 to 4 times per day are likely adequate. As the ROM returns to normal, the frequency may be reduced. Patients may benefit by performing activities which encourage a greater ROM, such as swimming or walking in water. Other activities include walking in snow, sand, or tall grass, crawling through a play tunnel, climbing stairs, and walking over cavaletti rails.

Stretching techniques are often performed in conjunction with ROM exercises to improve flexibility of the joints and extensibility of periarticular tissues, muscles, and tendons. Stretching is performed to elongate pathologically shortened tissues, and to increase flexibility and joint motion. Stretching takes tissues beyond the normal ROM. Overstretching should be avoided to make certain that tissues are not damaged. Scar tissue adhesions between normal tissues tie down the tissues and prevent normal gliding motion. Scar tissue adhesions may be prevented with appropriate stretching and perhaps deep tissue massage.

Muscles, ligaments, tendons, joint capsule, and skin, respond differently to stretching. The therapist must consider which tissues are limiting mobility and choose the appropriate techniques to help achieve more normal function. The acute effect of stretching is immediate elongation of the elastic component of the musculotendinous unit. A chronic stretch over time with the target tissues of the limb immobilized in an elongated position may result in sarcomeres being added to lengthen muscle tissue.

As tissue is stretched to the end of a ROM, the tissue remains elastic, and release results in return to its normal resting position. If the stress continues, there may be plastic deformation. Caution should be used to avoid stretching too rapidly, which may cause tissue damage or stimulation of the muscle spindle and an increase in muscle contraction. Static stretching involves placing the joint(s) in a position so that the muscles and connective tissues are stretched while held with the tissues at their greatest length for 15 to 30 seconds. After stretching, the tissues are allowed to return to a neutral position, and then the stretch is re-applied for up to 20 times in a session. A stretching program performed 3 to 5 times per week may increase flexibility. Heating tendons prior to stretching may result in less tissue damage and greater elongation. Therapeutic ultrasound is frequently used to warm tissues for stretching.

Proprioception and Balance Activities

Sporting dogs need to have well-developed balance and proprioception to adjust to the specific challenges of their activities, and injury often affects proprioception and joint position awareness. Proprioception decreases with fatigue, injury, and age in people. Proprioceptive training includes activities that may be performed at low or high speed that require an awareness of limb position in space. They include walking in circles or figure-of-eight, and walking across obstacles of various shape, height, and spacing. Balance exercises are exercises requiring rapid responses to changes in slopes, such as walking on a trampoline, balance or wobble board, or standing on a physioroll.

Other Modalities

Reconditioning activities are initiated after early rehabilitation activities have been initiated. Reconditioning may be initiated in a dog that is walking and trotting with minimal lameness following a cranial cruciate ligament injury, or in a dog with a fracture that has a mature bridging callus. Walking, trotting, and light running will help to provide adequate stress to the cardiovascular and musculoskeletal system conditioning.

The emphasis then shifts from protection of the injured area to aggressively loading the area in preparation for return to activity. The entire body must be considered in rehabilitation and prepared for the sport, not just the injured joint or body part. Strengthening and endurance activities should be gradually introduced during rehabilitation, being certain that the condition is not exacerbated. Power-building activities, such as jumping, sprinting, and pulling weights, should be closely monitored. Judicious use of nonsteroidal anti-inflammatory drugs should be considered to help achieve goals of increased performance while helping to control inflammation. Aquatic activities are very useful in patients with osteoarthritis to help with active ROM, muscle development, and cardiovascular fitness. They do not help to build bone mass, however. Therefore, rehabilitation should include some sport-specific activities.

REFERENCES

1. Loonam JE, Millis DL, Evans M, Moyer TL, Hamilton S. The effect of therapeutic ultrasound on tendon heating and extensibility. Proc Vet Orthop Soc, Steamboat Springs, CO, 2003.
2. Marcellin-Little DJ, Levine D, Taylor R. Rehabilitation and Conditioning of Sporting Dogs. Vet Clin North Am Small Anim Pract. Nov-Dec, 2005.
3. McMaster W. A literary review on ice therapy in injuries. Am J Sports Med. 1977; 5:124-126.
4. Millis DL, Levine D, Taylor RA. Canine Rehabilitation and Physical Therapy. 1st ed. Elsevier, 2004.
5. Olson J, Stravino V. A review of cryotherapy. Physical Ther. 1972;62:840-853.
6. Olson VL. Evaluation of joint mobilization treatment. A method. Physical Ther. 1987;67:351-56.
7. Schollmeier,G, Sarkar,K, Fukuhara,K, Uhthoff, HK. Structural and functional changes in the canine shoulder after cessation of immobilization. Clin Orthop. 1996;(323):310-15.
8. Yanoff SR, Hulse DA, Hogan HA, Slater MR, Longnecker MT. Measurements of vertical ground reaction force in jumping dogs. Vet Comp Orthop Traumatol. 1992;5:44-50,

ANESTHESIA AND ANALGESIA IN GREYHOUNDS

Luisito S. Pablo, DVM, MS, Diplomate ACVA
College of Veterinary Medicine
University of Florida, Gainesville, FL

Anesthesia and acute pain management in Greyhounds has evolved over the years spurred by a better understanding of the physiological and pharmacological peculiarities of this breed and the introduction of new anesthetic and analgesic drugs. However, it is interesting to note that over the last 8 years publications dealing with anesthesia and analgesia in Greyhounds are few. It appears that interest in Greyhound anesthesia has waned, producing a lack of information that might change how we handle anesthesia and analgesia in this breed. The purpose of this presentation is to review anesthesia and analgesia in the Greyhound. The anesthesia records of all the Greyhounds anesthetized at the University of Florida Veterinary Medical Center in the last 6 years (2002–2007) were also reviewed to supplement the available literature.

WHAT MAKE GREYHOUNDS DIFFERENT

Greyhounds possess certain characteristics that make them different from other dog breeds. In general, they appear to be nervous and agitated in unfamiliar surroundings. Gentle handling and sedation prior to inducing anesthesia are important. Their body-surface-to-volume ratio is greater compared to other breeds. This fact in addition to having very short hair and low body fat make them susceptible to hypothermia during anesthesia.

Greyhounds also have some clinicopathological values that are different compared to other breeds of dog. They have a higher packed cell volume (PCV) and lower serum total protein and albumin concentrations. Higher PCVs increase blood viscosity and can result in mucous membranes appearing "cyanotic" despite normal hemoglobin oxygen saturation. Increased blood viscosity due to a higher PCV may be counterbalanced by lower serum total protein leading to inconsequential effects during anesthesia. Other reported differences include lower white blood cell counts and higher red blood cell indices. Lower platelet counts (150,000–170,000 platelets/µL) have been reported, although other reports have found platelet counts similar to other dog breeds. Greyhounds also have higher creatinine levels despite higher glomerular filtration rates compared with non-Greyhound dogs. Higher serum creatinine levels have been attributed to the high muscle mass in this breed.

Postanesthetic hyperthermia has been reported in the Greyhound breed. Many feel that this is related to stress during the postanesthetic period because they are very muscular and can generate heat easily. Researchers have investigated the susceptibility of Greyhounds to malignant hyperthermia and although it has been reported in this breed (Bagshaw et al, 1978;

Kirmayer et al, 1984), more conclusive evidence demonstrating increased predilection to malignant hyperthermia is needed (Cosgrove et al, 1992). It may be that the hyperthermia noted in some Greyhounds during anesthesia and postanesthesia is a different form of malignant hyperthermia.

Different pharmacokinetic and pharmacodynamic studies have led to the conclusion that some drugs have longer duration of action in Greyhounds because of impaired liver drug metabolism. This has been attributed to the reduced activity of a specific hepatic cytochrome P_{450} enzyme (Court M, 1999). Others believe that the lean body conformation (fat 15% of body weight) of Greyhounds may contribute to the slowed recovery from some intravenous (IV) anesthetics.

When preparing Greyhounds for anesthesia it is important to note if they are trained or completely untrained. It has been shown that trained Greyhounds have significantly lower systemic vascular resistance and increased cardiac index and stroke volume compared with life-long untrained Greyhounds and mongrels. The systemic arterial pressure tended to be higher in Greyhounds (Pape LA, 1986). These hemodynamic changes should be considered when monitoring Greyhounds during anesthesia.

PREANESTHETIC EVALUATION

A thorough physical examination before anesthetizing these animals is important. The choice of drugs and the anesthetic protocol should be tailored to the condition of the patient. Based on the age and condition of the patient, a complete blood count (CBC) and serum biochemical analysis may be required. For young and healthy patients, hematocrit, plasma protein level, BUN, and blood glucose level should be determined. In compromised or old patients, a CBC and serum biochemical analysis will be very helpful. Some drugs are best avoided in Greyhounds with hepatic and/or renal compromise. In some instances, urinalysis will aid in defining problems that may complicate anesthesia.

PREMEDICATION
Anticholinergics

Atropine and glycopyrrolate are the most common anticholinergics used in veterinary practice. They are indicated as premedicants to control salivation and airway secretion and prevent sinus bradycardia. In our practice, only 7.0% of Greyhounds were given an anticholinergic prior to anesthesia. The limited use of anticholinergics in our practice is based on the finding that these drugs are potentially arrhythmogenic. In addition, a dry mouth caused by anticholinergics is considered unpleasant based on human experience and a strong vagal stimulation during anesthesia cannot be prevented by premedicating with an anticholinergic. The concentration of the anticholinergic (given as a premedicant) during anesthesia will not be high enough to counteract strong vagal effects. It is our practice to treat sinus bradyarrhythmias on an as needed basis. In those patients with preexisting bradycardia an anticholinergic will be included in the premedication. The inclusion of an opioid in our practice does not warrant the routine use of an anticholinergic. If salivation is profuse upon presentation, an anticholinergic is also considered. Glycopyrrolate is considered a better antisialogogue. Atropine is given IM at 0.02 to 0.04 mg/kg while glycopyrrolate is given IM at 0.01 mg/kg. Glycopyrrolate has a longer duration of action than atropine.

Acepromazine

Acepromazine is a tranquilizer/sedative agent with alpha blocking properties. It is also known to have antiemetic and weak antihistaminic effects. It reduces afterload leading to a decrease in the workload of the heart during anesthesia. Arterial hypotension occurs in a dose-dependent fashion because of peripheral vasodilation. Administration of acepromazine results in a longer duration of sedation compared with other commonly used sedatives like the alpha$_2$ agonists. Arterial hypotension and long duration of action are the two major reasons why some practitioners avoid acepromazine.

Most Greyhounds appear nervous and agitated when presented for anesthesia. Very nervous Greyhounds will benefit from a dose of acepromazine. In fact, acepromazine is the most common sedative we use. The majority of our Greyhound patients (78%) received acepromazine as part of their preanesthetic medication. Acepromazine is given IM at 0.05 mg/kg. The dose is reduced by one half in older patients. It is best to leave the patient in a quiet room, undisturbed to get the maximum effect from acepromazine.

Acepromazine lowers the PCV, which is useful in Greyhounds because of their higher PCV. Decreasing the PCV will reduce the viscosity of the blood and in turn decrease the workload of the heart.

Benzodiazepines

Diazepam and midazolam are the two most common benzodiazepines used in veterinary practice. When administered by themselves, profound sedation cannot be expected in healthy patients. Some degree of agitation and restlessness can be seen in healthy dogs. There is no specific study looking at the sedative effect of midazolam alone in Greyhounds. However, there is a study (Platt SR, 2000) that compared intranasal and IV diazepam in Greyhounds given at 0.5 mg/kg. In this study, the Greyhounds became sedated and ataxic following IV administration although the sedative effect only lasted for up to 15 minutes. These drugs may be best utilized in depressed and medically compromised Greyhounds. These drugs provide stable cardiopulmonary function in sick patients. In our practice, only 6.0 % of Greyhounds received a benzodiazepine as part of premedication.

When used as premedicant, diazepam and midazolam can be given at 0.1 to 0.3 mg/kg IM or IV. Midazolam is water-soluble making absorption following IM injection more predictable. Diazepam is not water-soluble and is preferably given IV.

In Greyhounds, diazepam or midazolam can be used as part of the induction process together with ketamine. This combination is discussed more in the section on induction.

Opioids

An opioid is administered as a premedicant to provide analgesia. Some of the opioids also provide mild to moderate sedation. When given with acepromazine, the sedation is generally more profound. When a Greyhound is in pain or the surgical procedure will be painful, an opioid should be part of the preanesthetic medication. There are three main types of opioids used for analgesia: full agonist, partial agonist, and agonist-antagonist. Full agonists include morphine, meperidine, hydromorphone, oxymorphone, fentanyl, and methadone. An example of a partial agonist is buprenorphine. Butorphanol is classified as an agonist-antagonist. The full agonists are more efficacious in relieving pain than the partial agonists and the agonist-antagonists. As a rule, Greyhounds that have or will have severe pain following a surgical procedure require a full agonist opioid. In cases involving moderate to mild pain, a partial agonist or agonist-antagonist may be chosen.

The adverse effects of opioids include vomiting, sinus bradycardia, defecation, panting, dysphoria, excitement, urinary retention, respiratory depression, and histamine release. Dogs appear to be less sensitive than humans to the respiratory depressant effect of opioids. The adverse effects of opioids are manageable and some can be prevented by following the necessary precautions. For example, morphine and meperidine should be given IV slowly to prevent massive histamine release. Excitement and dysphoria can be minimized by the concomitant administration of a sedative like acepromazine.

In our practice, the most common opioids used were hydromorphone (58.4%), morphine (20.3%), butorphanol (7.1%), and buprenorphine (4.4%). Some Greyhounds did not receive an opioid because of the non-painful nature of the procedure.

Alpha$_2$ Agonists

The alpha$_2$ agonists that can be used in dogs include xylazine, medetomidine, and romifidine. These drugs will provide sedation, analgesia, and muscle relaxation. In our practice, we reserve these drugs for sedating dogs that will require minor procedures like taking radiographs, bandage changes, and skin testing. Experience indicates that alpha$_2$ agonists are very useful drugs in Greyhounds. However, there are no specific studies of the pharmacokinetics and pharmacodynamics of alpha$_2$ agonists in this breed.

When used for sedation, combining an opioid with an alpha$_2$ agonist is useful. By combining the two, a lower dose of the alpha$_2$ agonist is needed. Opioids and alpha$_2$ agonists can also be reversed making it easier to manage outpatients. Medetomidine can be used as premedicant in healthy patients at 10 to 20 µg/kg IM.

INDUCTION

Anesthetic induction can be accomplished by the use of injectable or inhalant agents. The use of an injectable agent is more common because it minimizes stress and the induction process is much quicker. A recent study looking at perioperative fatalities in anesthetized small animals showed that mask induction is associated with a higher probability of mortality. All of our Greyhound patients in the last 6 years were induced with an injectable agent or a combination of injectable agents.

Barbiturates

The studies that showed that Greyhounds have impaired liver drug metabolism involved the IV induction agents. It has been shown that Greyhounds recover slower from thiopental and thiamylal (both thiobarbiturates) compared with mixed-breed dogs. Delayed recovery was associated with higher blood concentrations of the thiobarbiturates and lasted more than 8 hours (Robinson et al, 1986). In addition to slow recovery, the Greyhound also recovered poorly. This is characterized by vocalization, delirium, and struggling. Initially, it was postulated that delayed recovery was mainly due to delayed drug redistribution secondary to the lean body conformation of Greyhounds. However, a pharmacokinetic study later revealed nonlinear drug disposition in the Greyhound dog indicating the involvement of metabolism. It is now believed that the impaired liver drug metabolism of thiobarbiturates is due to the reduced activity of a specific hepatic cytochrome P_{450} enzyme (Court, 1999). Presently, the use of thiopental is strongly discouraged in Greyhounds because of prolonged and rough recoveries.

Methohexital is an ultrashort-acting oxybarbiturate, which can be used in Greyhound dogs because its administration results in the shortest duration of anesthesia compared with the other barbiturates (Sams et al, 1985). However, recovery in mixed-breed dogs given methohexital was still shorter than in Greyhounds. It can also cause myoclonic activity and excitement during anesthetic induction. With the introduction of propofol in veterinary practice, methohexital use in Greyhound dogs has stopped. If available, it is given at 3.0 to 5.0 mg/kg IV with the initial calculated dose given more rapidly than when using propofol to minimize excitement and the rest of the dose given to effect.

Propofol

Propofol is the most common IV induction agent (76%) we use in Greyhounds. It has a quick onset of action and is known not to accumulate in the body following a constant rate infusion. Recoveries in Greyhounds following propofol are generally better than those seen with thiopental. However, one study has shown that Greyhounds still recover slowly following propofol anesthesia. In this study, the non-Greyhounds stood in about 28 minutes after stopping the propofol infusion while the Greyhounds stood in about 63 minutes (Robertson, 1992). These observations are supported by a pharmacokinetic study showing that Greyhounds eliminated propofol at a rate about half that found in mixed-breeds (Zoran, 1993).

The common side effects of propofol seen in Greyhounds are similar to those seen in other breeds of dogs and include apnea, hypotension, hypoventilation, and myoclonus (muscle tremors). In one study with a limited number of Greyhounds used, 50% showed muscle tremors during anesthetic induction and maintenance using propofol (Robertson, 1992).

Following premedication with a sedative, propofol can be given IV using a calculated dose of 4.0 mg/kg. Half of this dose should be given slowly and the rest given to effect. Without premedication, the calculated dose is increased to 6.0 to 8.0 mg/kg.

In some cases, IV diazepam or midazolam can be given with propofol during induction. Preferably, ¼ of the calculated propofol dose is given first followed by IV diazepam or midazolam at 0.2 mg/kg. The remainder of the propofol is given to effect. By incorporating diazepam or midazolam, the cardiopulmonary depressant effects of propofol are reduced.

Benzodiazepine-Dissociative combinations

The benzodiazepine-dissociative combinations that can be used in Greyhounds include: 1) midazolam and ketamine, 2) diazepam and ketamine, 3) zolazepam and tiletamine (Telazol®). Anesthetic induction using these combinations in Greyhounds is considered good. The induction is characterized by an easy transition to unconsciousness. There is an absence of struggling, vocalizing, and paddling. However, excessive chewing and licking may be observed in Greyhounds not given any sedative before induction (Hellyer, 1991). We prefer to give a sedative before administering a benzodiazepine-dissociative combination. In the series of Greyhound anesthesia performed at UF, 17.6% received diazepam and ketamine as induction agents. All of these patients were premedicated with acepromazine and/or an opioid. The doses of diazepam (midazolam) and ketamine are 0.25 mg/kg and 5.0 mg/kg, respectively. For Telazol, the IV dose is 2.0 to 4.0 mg/kg. It is advisable to maintain anesthesia using an inhalant agent to reduce the incidence of rough recoveries associated with these combinations. When a single IV injection of diazepam-ketamine and propofol were compared in Greyhounds, it was observed that the recovery from diazepam-ketamine was inferior (Mansager, 1990). This observation is explained by the persistence of the effect of the dissociative agent.

Alpha$_2$ Agonist-Ketamine Combination

Following profound sedation with an alpha$_2$ agonist given either IM or IV, ketamine can be administered IM or IV. Medetomidine is given at 40 µg/kg while xylazine can be given at 1.0 to 2.2 mg/kg IM. Following an IM dose of 40 µg/kg of medetomidine, ketamine at 5.0 mg/kg IM resulted in an anesthetic state that allowed endotracheal intubation. A combination of IM xylazine at 1.0 mg/kg and IM ketamine at 15.0 mg/kg also will result in an anesthetic state (Moens, 1990). However, it is important to note these dosages are based on non-

Greyhound dogs. The author prefers this combination in young and healthy Greyhounds. These combinations can be used as induction agents as well as for short-term anesthesia. If an inhalant agent is used for maintenance, the requirement for anesthesia is much less when compared to other anesthetic protocols. The patient should be monitored very closely with special attention given to the depth of anesthesia.

MAINTENANCE

Anesthesia in Greyhounds can be maintained using either inhalant or injectable agents. The use of inhalant agents is preferred in Greyhounds primarily because the duration of action of inhalant agents is not dependent on liver metabolism. In addition, the depth of anesthesia can be changed much quicker with inhalant anesthesia. The use of IV anesthetic agents is reserved for special cases when an inhalant agent cannot be delivered via an endotracheal tube such as bronchoscopy, airway examination and airway surgical procedures. It is important to remember that propofol, the agent of choice for total IV anesthesia, results in relatively longer recovery times in Greyhounds.

Isoflurane and sevoflurane are the two most common inhalant agents used in small animal practice. The main advantage of sevoflurane is the quicker recovery because of its lower blood solubility. Because of this property, the depth of anesthesia can also be changed quicker when compared with isoflurane. Both inhalant agents will cause cardiopulmonary depression in a dose-dependent manner. Presently, sevoflurane is still more expensive than isoflurane. For the 6-year period from 2002 to 2007, 96% of anesthetized Greyhounds received isoflurane for maintenance and only 1.7% were maintained with sevoflurane. The rest were given propofol for maintenance because the procedures prevented the insertion of an endotracheal tube. For anesthetic maintenance, the isoflurane vaporizer can be set at 1.5% to 2.0% while sevoflurane, having a higher MAC in dogs, is set at 2.5% to 3.5%. These settings are based on the assumption that premedicants are given to the patients. Higher settings may be needed in very painful procedures and in those patients without premedicants or given low dosages of premedicants.

COMPLICATIONS

There was no mortality associated with anesthesia in the 113 Greyhounds we anesthetized from 2002 to 2007. One was euthanized because of the primary disease. During anesthesia, the most common complications in Greyhounds we observed included sinus bradycardia (26.5%), arterial hypotension (23.9%), hypoventilation (22.1%), hypothermia (13.3%), sinus tachycardia (9.7%), apnea (8.8%), and dysrrhythmia (7.0%). About 33.0% of our Greyhound patients had anesthesia without any complications. Even though complications were encountered in this series of patients, appropriate actions were taken to prevent morbidity and mortality. Close monitoring is essential in recognizing these complications and should always be part of appropriate anesthetic management.

RECOVERY

The postanesthetic management of Greyhounds is similar to other dogs. Postanesthesia care should include continuous monitoring, pain management, cardiovascular and respiratory support, body temperature maintenance, minimizing distress, and providing comfort. Some Greyhounds will recover in a dysphoric state, which should be managed by administering a sedative (acepromazine, 0.02 mg/kg IV). Only 6% of our Greyhound patients had dysphoria, restlessness, and agitation immediately after tracheal extubation. Those that are in pain should be given an opioid immediately. As a general rule, an opioid should be administered to a patient that had a surgical procedure before it regains full consciousness. The opioid can be administered during the surgical procedure, right before tracheal extubation or immediately after extubation. Acute pain management will be discussed in the following section. As a result of stress, Greyhounds can develop hyperthermia in recovery. There are reports of mortality in Greyhounds because of profound hyperthermia. Hyperthermia should be managed by administering a sedative and cold IV fluids. Additional measures include spraying the patient with tap water and directing an electric fan to the patient. Cold packs can be applied to the body where the major vessels are located. In extreme cases, a cold enema and gastric lavage can be performed.

ACUTE PAIN MANAGEMENT

Acute pain management is an integral component of anesthesia in Greyhounds. Any Greyhound that is in pain and will be painful during the surgical procedure needs to be managed appropriately. Effective pain control will prevent central sensitization while uncontrolled pain can interfere with wound healing and function of the immune system and reduce caloric intake. It is also possible that acute pain, if not controlled, can result in chronic pain syndromes. In human studies, it has been shown that effective pain control improves morbidity following surgery.

There are general principles that apply to acute pain management. Administration of systemic analgesic(s) and/or performance of local anesthetic technique(s) before the pain occurs should be the goal during anesthesia. By doing this, postoperative pain can be controlled easily. Trauma patients should have analgesics once their conditions are stabilized. This is important to reduce the nociceptive facilitation caused by the injury. In Greyhounds with severe pain, a multi-modal approach to pain control should be instituted.

Acute pain management in Greyhounds should include the different pain modalities depending upon the severity of pain. There are many options currently available to veterinary practitioners including opioids, nonsteriodal anti-inflammatory drugs, local anesthetic techniques, NMDA receptor antagonist (ketamine), IV lidocaine, alpha$_2$ agonists and other miscellaneous modalities that can improve pain control in Greyhounds.

Opioids

All Greyhounds that will undergo painful procedures should be given an opioid. It is important to remember that there are no absolute contraindications for the use of opioids. It is given as a part of preanesthetic medication, during surgery (depending upon the length of the procedure and severity of pain), and postoperatively. There are cases that will require an opioid CRI for consistent pain control. The opioids and corresponding dosages that we have used in Greyhounds are listed in Table 1. The full agonists (morphine, hydromorphone, oxymorphone, and fentanyl) are more efficacious in controlling severe pain. All of the opioids can be used in cases with mild to moderate pain. The choice is then influenced by the duration of action, frequency of side effects, cost, and controlled substance designation. In our practice, hydromorphone (58.4%) and morphine (20.3%) are the two most common opioids used for controlling perioperative pain.

It is disappointing to note that studies specifically looking at the pharmacokinetics and pharmacodynamics of the different analgesics in Greyhound are very scarce. The dosages here are mainly extrapolated from dosages used for the general population of dogs. There was a study done which compared the side effects of morphine (0.5 mg/kg IM) and butorphanol (0.1 mg/kg IM) in halothane-anesthetized Greyhounds. The study concluded that morphine resulted in lower heart rates and lower body temperature (Carter, 1987). However, the reduction in heart rate and body temperature caused by morphine is considered mild and clinically acceptable.

Nonsteroidal Anti-inflammatory Drugs (NSAIDs)

NSAIDs have become an important component of multi-modal pain therapy because they possess both anti-inflammatory and analgesic properties. Any surgical procedure will result in inflammation. NSAIDs inhibit the primary enzymes (COX-2) involved in the inflammatory process. By inhibiting the prostanoids, the development and transmission of pain after tissue injury are also controlled. The addition of an NSAID to the anesthetic protocol also reduces the reliance on opioids to control pain. NSAIDs can be administered preoperatively, intraoperatively or postoperatively. It is ideal to administer an NSAID preoperatively to ensure good concentration in the potential area of inflammation before the injury happens. However, concerns about its toxicity have forced some practitioners to give it postoperatively especially if cardiovascular monitoring is inadequate during anesthesia. The NSAID is given postoperatively when the patient has recovered from the cardiovascular depressant effects of the anesthetics.

Adverse effects of NSAIDS include gastrointestinal ulceration, impaired platelet function, and renal ischemia. Patient selection is very important when making the decision to give an NSAID. Patients with known hepatic disease, gastrointestinal disease, coagulopathies, renal disease and hypovolemia are not good candidates for NSAID administration. Those patients receiving corticosteroids should not be given an NSAID. It is also important to wait for at least 4 to 5 days before switching NSAIDs (Robertson S, 2003).

For perioperative pain management, we prefer NSAIDs with injectable forms. Since some of the premedicants we use can cause vomiting, an injectable form is better than the oral preparation. Presently, carprofen and meloxicam have injectable forms. In our practice, carprofen is the most commonly used NSAID. A possible explanation for this choice is the availability of carprofen in tablet form making dosing in bigger dogs easier (average weight of Greyhounds in the case series, 31.5 kg). The duration of administration of an NSAID following surgery differs among practitioners. The duration of administration will depend on the surgery performed and the comfort level of the patient.

Table 1. Dose and Duration of Action of the Opioids

Opioids	Dose	Duration
Morphine	0.3–1.0 mg/kg IM, SC 0.05–1.0 mg/kg slow IV 0.1–0.5 mg/kg/hour CRI	2–6 hours 1–2 hours duration of CRI plus 30–60 mins
Hydromorphone	0.05–0.2 mg/kg IV, IM, SC 0.01–0.04 mg/kg/hour CRI	2–6 hours Duration of CRI plus 30–60 mins
Oxymorphone	Same as hydromorphone	Same as hydromorphone
Fentanyl	1.0–2.0 µg/kg IV 0.3–2.0 µg/kg/min IV Given intraop 2.0–5.0 µg/kg/hour IV Given postop	15–18 minutes Duration of CRI plus 30–60 mins Duration of CRI plus 30–60 mins
Buprenorphine	0.01–0.03 mg/kg IV, IM	4–8 hours
Butorphanol	0.2–0.5 mg/kg IV, IM	1–2 hours

Table 2. Dose, Route and Frequency of Administration of the NSAIDs Used Perioperatively

NSAIDS	Dose and Route	Frequency
Carprofen	≤ 4.0 mg/kg SC ≤ 2.0 mg/kg SC, PO	On induction, intraoperatively, or immediately after surgery. Repeat every 12 hours
Meloxicam	≤ 0.2 mg/kg IV, SC ≤ 0.1 mg/kg IV, SC, PO	On induction, intraoperatively, or immediately after surgery Repeat every 24 hours

There is no study on the use of the above-mentioned NSAIDs in Greyhounds. It is interesting to note that the pharmacokinetics of celecoxib was studied in Greyhounds. In this study, celecoxib was given daily for ten days. The maximum concentration of celecoxib was lower after the 10th day (Hunter, 2005). There is no available data on the chronic use of carprofen and meloxicam in Greyhounds and we cannot extrapolate the findings from the celecoxib study. As such, close observation is needed when Greyhounds are taking NSAIDs for long periods of time.

Local Anesthetics and Peripheral Neural Blockade

Regional anesthesia can be used as an adjunct to general anesthesia. These local anesthetic techniques should be performed when the Greyhound is under general anesthesia and before the surgery starts. The local anesthetic technique that is needed depends on the surgical procedure involved. For abdominal procedures, thoracotomies, and hindleg procedures, a lumbar epidural block using bupivacaine can be performed. For the legs and head, specific nerve blocks can be performed. For example, a mandibular nerve block can be performed before performing mandibulectomy. Repair of radial and ulnar fractures will benefit from a brachial plexus block. Line infiltration using local anesthetic can also be performed before an abdominal incision. Likewise, local anesthetic can be administered via a soaker catheter tunneled into a surgical wound. This is useful in total ear can ablation and leg amputation.

Bupivacaine, which has a long duration of action, is the preferred local anesthetic used for these techniques. Sometimes, lidocaine is mixed with bupivacaine in a 1:1 volume ratio to take advantage of lidocaine's quicker onset of action.

NMDA Receptor Antagonist (Ketamine)

Activation of the NMDA receptors results in wind-up (central sensitization). Microdosages of ketamine have been shown to block the NMDA receptors decreasing wind-up. These microdosages of ketamine are not associated with the adverse CNS signs (hallucination, increased muscular movement, or seizure) typically seen with higher doses of ketamine. If a ketamine CRI will be used during surgery, ketamine is used as the induction agent together with a benzodiazepine. During surgery, ketamine is given at 0.6 mg/kg/hour. Postoperatively, the rate is reduced to 0.12 to 0.18 mg/kg/hour. The use of ketamine appears to reduce the tolerance of patients to opioids. By itself, a ketamine CRI will not be able to completely control pain and an opioid should be included in the analgesic plan.

Lidocaine (IV Infusion)

IV lidocaine has been shown to be effective in neuropathic pain. In humans, perioperative lidocaine infusions have preventive effects on postoperative pain. It also reduces the morphine consumption following a major abdominal surgery. Lidocaine also reduces the MAC of isoflurane in a dose-dependent manner in dogs. The loading dose for lidocaine is 1.0 to 2.0 mg/kg IV. It is then followed by a CRI of 3.0 mg/kg/hour. Lidocaine can be given together with an opioid and ketamine for better pain control in Greyhounds that are suffering from severe pain.

Alpha₂ Agonists

Alpha$_2$ agonists provide analgesia through the alpha$_2$ receptors in the dorsal horn of the spinal cord. Medetomidine is the alpha$_2$ agonist most commonly used for perioperative pain management. It is known to be synergistic with opioids in providing analgesia. We use medetomidine when the patient continues to whine and vocalize despite repeated administration of sedatives like acepromazine and an opioid. It is not usually used by itself because of the profound sedation and the notable cardiovascular effects. Medetomidine is given initially at a dose of 1 to 2 µg/kg IV. Then, a CRI of 1 to 5 µg/kg/hour is started. The rate of infusion should be adjusted according to the sedation shown by the dog. Sinus bradycardia is expected during a CRI of medetomidine (40 to 60 beats per minute).

Miscellaneous Steps

Good nursing care should be part of perioperative pain management. Anxiety and distress should be minimized in patients recovering from anesthesia. Sometimes, a patient simply needs a reassuring voice and caring personnel who spend time with the dog. Application of cold packs on the surgical site will reduce the degree of inflammation and pain. A patient recovering from surgery should be in a quiet environment and provided with good bedding. The urinary bladder should be checked, as a full bladder will result in discomfort. Maintaining normal body temperature will also help to produce uneventful and restful recovery.

References are available from the author upon request.

LOCAL AND SYSTEMIC CONSEQUENCES OF PERIODONTAL DISEASE AND ITS MANAGEMENT

R. Michael Peak, DVM, Diplomate, AVDC
Tampa Bay Veterinary Specialists
Largo, FL

Periodontal disease is defined as the inflammation, active or inactive destruction of the periodontal tissues: gingiva, periodontal ligament, cementum or alveolar bone. The incidence has been reported and remains one of the most common disease processes seen in animals and humans. Since this is such a widespread problem in humans, much research has been focused over the last 30 years investigating the cause and effect of periodontal disease in humans. There has not been as much research directly related to companion animals, but in many cases, dogs are used as the periodontal model for human research and that information can be extrapolated for veterinary use. While most all dogs develop some level of periodontal disease by the age of 4 years, some breeds, such as smaller dogs, are predisposed. Furthermore, periodontal disease tends to increase with age, complicating preventative and treatment measures involving anesthesia. Also, some breeds, such as Greyhounds and miniature Schnauzers, can show an aggressive form of periodontal disease at a young age, called localized juvenile periodontitis, which results in rapid loss of bone support around the roots of teeth, chronic infection, and ultimately the loss of these teeth.

Due to the innate nature of periodontal disease in dogs, the fact that bacteria are a part of the normal flora of the oral cavity, and the lack of owner/pet compliance with oral hygiene, periodontal disease will likely develop in many if not most veterinary patients. This chronic source of infection could have other potential systemic and overall health implications. One of the few studies in veterinary medicine directed at the systemic effects of periodontal disease in canines found there was an association between advanced periodontal disease and microscopic changes in the heart, liver and kidney tissues. There are other studies in humans that concur with these findings and study the effects of periodontal disease with the frequency of cardiovascular disease/stroke, diabetes, pulmonary disease, osteoporosis, inflammatory bowel disease, and pre-term, low-birth-weight babies. What may be more difficult to measure are the effects of all the chronic inflammatory mediators associated with periodontal disease such as C-reactive protein, interleukins, as well as tumor necrosis factor and how these inflammatory mediators impact other distant organs. C-reactive protein has been shown to be elevated in humans with extensive periodontal disease and is associated with an increased risk of atherosclerosis. The effects of chronic infection may have far reaching consequences.

In the early 1960s, Socransky is given credit for identifying bacteria within plaque and subsequently, several human periodontal researchers reported that bacteria associated with the development of plaque were intimately and directly involved with the formation of periodontal disease. Since that time, studies have been directed toward identifying the bacteria contained within plaque and those that may be associated with periodontal disease in both dogs and humans. The conclusion has been that although there are slight differences in the species of bacteria, in general, the disease process is very similar. In fact, these early studies in many instances were performed on Beagle dogs. We now know that within minutes of the teeth being cleaned a pellicle of glycoproteins form on the tooth surface providing the substrate for bacterial colonization. We also know the initial colonization will be predominately by gram-positive bacteria and that as the disease progresses to more advanced stages of periodontal tissue loss and periodontal pocket formation, the bacterial flora changes from gram-positive cocci to predominately gram-negative rods. These gram-negative rods flourish in the anaerobic environment of the periodontal pocket and along with the host inflammatory mediators result in significant periodontal tissue destruction. Locally within the periodontal pocket, the result is the loss of alveolar bone support surrounding the tooth root—periodontitis. As this progresses, the chronic infection continues deeper into the alveolar bone creating a localized area of osteomyelitis and eventually complete loss of periodontal attachment and if not prevented, tooth loss.

Harvey et al in a study of 49 dogs with moderate to severe gingivitis found the subgingival bacteria to be 58% aerobic and 42% anaerobic.[17] The study went on to categorize these bacteria into species. The primary gram-negative species that was cultured at that time was called *Porphyromonas gingivalis*. *Porphyromonas gingivalis*, a black-pigmented anaerobic bacteria (BPAB), is considered to be one of the primary etiologic agents responsible for periodontal bone loss in humans and has garnered much attention in the search to control periodontitis. A recent study has more precisely identified the pathogenic black-pigmented anaerobic bacteria associated with advanced periodontal disease in dogs. Hardham et al found *Porphyromonas gingivalis* was not, in fact, associated with periodontal disease in dogs,[19] but a very similar strain (catalase positive, unlike *P. gingivalis*) was found, *Porphyromonas gulae*. In this study, the most prominent BPAB were *Porphyromonas salivosa*, *Porphyromonas denticanis*, and *Porphyromonas gulae*. One of these types of bacteria was recovered in 76% of the 33 dogs tested. Furthermore, to prove the pathogenicity of these bacteria an additional study was performed in mice. These same three bacteria were found to be responsible for the most net alveolar bone loss when placed in the gingival sulcus of otherwise healthy mice. If the studies in humans are accurate in that *Prophyromonas gingivalis* is a major periodontopathogen and a significant cause of periodontal bone loss in people, a similar conclusion can be drawn that these very similar bacteria can be considered major causes of periodontitis in dogs. The studies by Hardham et al support this theory.

Porphyromonas gulae has also been isolated in a number of other animals with signs of periodontal bone loss. Ultimately, the prevention and/or control of these bacteria may be the key to preventing alveolar bone infection, alveolar bone loss, tooth loss, and prevention of pro-inflammatory mediators associated with periodontitis in dogs.

In the late 1990s, with the association made between *Porphyromonas gingivalis* and periodontitis in humans, various modalities of control of these bacteria were proposed. One such hypothesis was the advent of a periodontopathogen vaccine directed at *P. gingivalis*. Page et al proposed creating a bacterin for P.gingivalis and tested such a vaccine in non-human primates.[21] Using suture/ligature-induced periodontitis, in comparison with a control group, immunization with *P. gingivalis* bacterin induced protection. Following the isolation of the primary agents located in the periodontal pockets of advanced periodontal disease in dogs, a study was undertaken in mice to investigate the possibility of developing a vaccine for these bacteria. Hardham et al proposed a monovalent *Porphyromonas gulae* vaccine and tested this bacterin in mice challenged with this bacteria. The research confirmed that the administration of a *P. gulae* vaccine could elicit an immune response that could provide protection against alveolar bone loss. Further, when the gingival sulcus of these test subjects were cultured, *Porphyromonas gulae* was found in large quantities in the control, but only in minimal levels in those vaccinated. This gave strong evidence that the vaccinated group not only were protected against bone loss, but also had less of the periodontopathogen burden. This monovalent vaccine also gave cross protection when challenged with other *Porphyromonas* strains, *P. salivosa* and *P. denticanis*. The systemic inflammatory mediators were not measured in this study, but could be decreased due to the lower bacterial load and reduced alveolar bone loss.

The mode of action of this vaccine is still under investigation, but it is proposed that IgG is stimulated as a response of immunization and responsible for the protective effects. There is normally a continuous flow of serum-derived fluid in the normal gingival sulcus called the gingival crevicular fluid. As inflammation, gingivitis, and periodontitis ensue, this gingival crevicular fluid flow increases. IgG is found in the gingival crevicular fluid and could attach to the targeted bacteria preventing further penetration into the periodontal attachment. This may allow neutrophils and macrophages to more easily detect, attach, and destroy these pathogenic organisms, thus preventing advancing alveolar bone loss.

These studies supported the rationale of the vaccine and measures were taken to seek approval for use by the USDA in canines. A provisional license was granted based on these studies and another showing a reduction of periapical bone loss in dogs immunized and challenged with *Porphyromonas* bacteria endodontically. For the provisional license to be granted, there had to be a need for the product that no other product could provide, there needed to be scientific data of a "reasonable expectation of efficacy," and safety studies equal to those for full licensure had to be performed and the product shown to be safe. Those studies have been done and a provisional license has been granted. Long-term studies to evaluate the efficacy of the prevention of periodontitis have been proposed and are under investigation.

Clinically, this vaccine could be a significant tool against the loss of periodontal tissues and chronic periodontal infection. As with any medication or immunization, the clinician must take into consideration the chance his patient may develop this disease and the reward of providing protection with respect to the risk involved. This is one of the very few modalities that does not rely heavily on client compliance on a regular basis to be effective, which is one of the major reasons we see such advanced periodontal disease in veterinary patients. It is important to recognize what the vaccine is geared to do and equally important to educate your staff and clients what the vaccine is not intended to do.

As the research has shown, this vaccine is directed toward one group of bacteria, the BPAB, *Porphyromonas*. The vaccine theoretically should not alter other plaque bacteria. As such, one would still expect to see plaque and eventually calculus to develop. Immunized patients will still need to have other home care regimens in place for a complete oral hygiene program. Owners should be instructed to continue brushing efforts, use dietary therapy where appropriate, continue to use plaque retardants, oral rinses, and anything else deemed effective for plaque and calculus control. The overall result of the vaccine should be a decreased incidence of periodontitis, periodontal bone loss, and ultimately less tooth loss due to advanced periodontal disease. Hopefully, when periodontitis results in bone loss, the effects will be less significant and take longer to develop, giving an earlier warning and potentially more options for treatment instead of simply extraction. It is important to also note that dental examinations, scaling, and periodontal probing will continue to be relevant and important to detect the true disease below the gingival margin. The research has shown 76% of the studied dogs had one of the major *Porphyromonas* bacteria present when there was periodontitis. Conversely, 24% had periodontitis, yet yielded none of the *Porphyromonas* bacteria targeted by the vaccine. This means there could still be a few cases of advanced periodontal disease even in vaccinated animals. This further emphasizes the fact that there will continue to be a need for thorough oral examination under anesthesia. Overall, the expectation is that there will be less "unforeseen extractions" due to periodontal disease not noted on physical examination.

As mentioned earlier, one of the difficult parameters to measure is the systemic ramifications of the prevention of periodontitis and chronic alveolar osteomyelitis. We have long recognized the potential for bacteremia during dental procedures and some of the distant organ effects of advanced periodontal disease have been studied, but there could be potentially many more significant benefits of preventing the chronic infection, chronic immune stimulation, and chronic release of inflammatory mediators.

Early vaccination of those patients prone by either signalment or familial history could result in not only prevention of periodontitis and tooth loss, but other systemic consequences as well. In certain breeds such as Poodles, Schnauzers, Yorkshire terriers, and Greyhounds, especially those with familial histories of periodontal disease, vaccination should afford some protection against the development of Localized Juvenile Periodontitis. Also, since periodontal disease tends to develop as pets get older, this may help reduce the need for anesthesia in the geriatric patient as well as helping to reduce anesthetic needs in breeds with idiosyncrasies to anesthesia such as the Greyhound.[25, 26] Furthermore, since the incidence of periodontal disease is so high in veterinary patients, this could potentially be beneficial in all pets. In older patients, or those who have shown a propensity for periodontal disease, vaccination after the teeth have been cleaned and any existing periodontal disease treated should help prevent further pathology. Ideally, prevention of periodontal disease before it has the chance to develop is the best course of action, because in many instances, once the alveolar bone is lost, it is difficult if not impossible to regain.

In a perfect world, clients would have all the time necessary to perform home oral hygiene for their pets and every pet would be compliant. Unfortunately, in the busy and hectic schedules of most people's lives, this is not the case. As a result, we will continue to see the high incidence and ramifications of poor pet oral hygiene and the systemic consequences. Luckily, studies in human and veterinary medicine have underscored the importance of periodontal disease and identified of some of the pathogenic bacteria responsible for much of the periodontal tissue infection and alveolar osteomyelitis. This information has led to a breakthrough in the management of these periodontopathogens and may ultimately have far reaching benefits for all pets...and one day possibly humans. When we consider the incidence of periodontal disease in the veterinary patient population, the result of the constant infection and release of inflammatory mediators, and the eventual bone/tooth loss associated with periodontitis coupled with the lack of owner compliance and the safety shown with this vaccination, the protection via vaccination is well warranted.

REFERENCES

1. Lund, EM, Armstrong, PJ, et al. Health status and population characteristics of dogs and cats examined at private veterinary practices in the United States. J Am Vet Med Assoc. 1999; 214(9): 1336-41.
2. Harvey CE. Periodontal disease in dogs. Etiopathogenesis, prevalence, and significance. Vet Clin North Am Small Anim Pract. 1998; 28(5): 1111-28.
3. Hoffman T, Gaengler P. Epidemiology of periodontal disease in poodles. J Small Anim Pract. 1996;37(7): 309-16.
4. Harvey CE, Shofer FS, et al. Association of age and body weight with periodontal disease in North American dogs. J Vet Dent. 1994;11(3): 94-105.
5. DeBowes, LJ, Mosier, D, et al. Association of periodontal disease and histologic lesions in multiple organs from 45 dogs. J Vet Dent. 1996;13(2): 57-60.
6. Xiaojing, LI, Koltveitt, KM, et al. Systemic diseases caused by oral infections. Clin Microbio Rev 2000; 13(4):547-558.
7. Scannapieco FA. Systemic effects of periodontal diseases. Dent Clin North Am. 2005;49: 533-550.
8. Van Dyke TE, Dowell, DR, et al. Potential role of microorganisms isolated from periodontal lesions in the pathogenesis of inflammatory bowel disease. Infect Immun. 1986: 671-677.
9. Genco R, Offenbacher S. Periodontal disease and cardiovascular disease, epidemiology and possible mechanisms. J Am Dent Assoc. 2002;133: 14s-22s.
10. Paquette DW. The periodontal infection-systemic disease link: a review of the truth or myth. J Int Acad Periodontol. 2002;4(3): 101-109.
11. Elter JR, Offenbacher S. Relationship of periodontal disease and edentulism to stroke/TIA. J Dent Res. 2003; 82(12): 998-1001.
12. Slade GD, Ghezzi EM, et al. Relationship between periodontal disease and C-reactive protein among adults in the atherosclerosis risk in communities study. Arch Intern Med. 2003;163:1172-79.
13. Listgarten MA. Dental plaque: Its structure and prevention, J Dent Children. 1972: 347-351.
14. Linde J, Hamp S, et al. Plaque induced periodontal disease in beagle dogs. J Periodont Res. 10:243-255.
15. Rateitschak, KH, Rateitschak, EM, et al, Color Atlas of Dental Medicine: Periodontology, 2nd ed, Thieme Publishing, 1989, pp 19-31.
16. DeBowes LJ. Effects of dental disease on systemic health. Vet Clin North Am Small Anim Pract. 1998; 28(5):1057-1062.
17. Harvey CE, Thornsberry C, et al. Subgingival bacteria—comparison of culture results in dogs and cats with gingivitis. J Vet Dent. 1995;12(4): 147-150.
18. Kumagai Y, Yagishita H, et al. Molecular mechanisms for connective tissue destruction by dipeptidyl aminopeptidase IV produced by the periodontal pathogen Porphyromonas gingivalis. Infect Immun. 2005;73(5), 2655-2664.
19. Hardham J, Dreier K, et al. Pigmented-anaerobic bacteria associated with canine periodontitis. Vet Microbiol. 2005;106: 119-128.
20. Fournier D, Mouton, et al. Porphyromonas gulae sp. Nov., an anaerobic, gram-negative coccobacillus from the gingival sulcus of various animal hosts. Int J Sys Evol Microbiol. 2001; 51: 1179-1189.
21. Page RC. Vaccination and periodontitis: myth or reality. J Int Acad Periodontol. 2000; 2(2): 31-43.
22. Hardham J, Reed M, et al. Evaluation of a monovalent companion animal periodontal disease vaccine in an experimental mouse periodontitis model. Vaccine. 2005; 23: 3148-3156.

23. Nieves MA, Hartwig P. Bacterial isolates from plaque and fromblood during and after routine dental procedures in dogs. Vet Surg. 1997; 26(1): 26-32.

24. Tou SP, Adin DB. Mitral valve endocarditis after dental prophylaxis in a dog. J Vet Intern Med. 2005; 19:268-270.

25. Freeman WE. Idiosyncrasies in greyhounds that can affect their medical care. Vet Med. 2005; 592-600.

26. McKelvey D, Hollingshead KW. Small Animal Anesthesia & Analgesia, 2nd ed. St. Louis, MO: Mosby, 2000, p 220.

CURRENT PERSPECTIVES ON CRANIAL CRUCIATE LIGAMENT INSUFFICIENCY IN DOGS

Antonio Pozzi, DMV, MS, Diplomate ACVS
College of Veterinary Medicine
University of Florida, Gainesville, FL

Cranial cruciate ligament (CCL) rupture is one of the most common causes of hind lameness in dogs. The CCL maintains stability of the stifle joint, thus injury to the CCL will result in joint instability and predispose the joint to degenerative changes. In dogs, the majority of CCL ruptures occur under normal activity, likely due to structural deterioration of the ligament and not because of a traumatic injury. Rupture of the CCL due to degeneration can present acutely even in young dogs and eventually becomes bilateral. Osteoarthritis, meniscal injury, and persistent lameness commonly occur with CCL rupture. Therefore, the pathologic condition related to CCL rupture is often referred to as "cruciate disease." Cranial cruciate ligament rupture is particularly common in large and giant breed dogs; however, any breed, size, or age of dog may be affected. Although clinical features and treatment options have been well discussed in the veterinary literature, the disease mechanisms for CCL rupture are poorly understood.

MECHANISMS OF CCL RUPTURE

Exact causes and disease mechanisms of CCL ruptures are undefined and remain controversial. Rupture of the CCL associated with major traumatic injury is rare. It is usually unilateral involving multiple ligamentous injuries of the stifle and is more common in puppies and typically associated with avulsion of the ligament at the tibial attachment site distally. In contrast, most pathologic cranial cruciate ligament ruptures are bilateral midsubstance incomplete or complete tears associated with degenerative changes that may be primary or secondary, or a combination of multiple factors. Several risk factors have been proposed for CCL rupture. Rupture of the CCL has significant association with breed, body weight, and neutering. Other factors, such as aging, gender, conformational variation, medial patellar luxation, inactivity, and obesity have also been associated with CCL rupture. The effect of TPA on CCL rupture in dogs has yet to be established. The risk of CCL rupture is higher in certain breeds, such as the Rottweiler, Labrador and Chesapeake Bay retriever, Newfoundland, Akita, Neapolitan mastiff, Saint Bernard, and Staffordshire bull terrier. Larger dogs weighing >22 kg are at greater risk of cruciate disease and tend to develop CCL rupture at younger ages. Conformational variation such as straight stifle, narrow intercondylar notch, steep tibial plateau slope, MPL, valgus and varus deformities of the stifle, and repeated stress and microinjury can result in progressive degenerative joint disease and CCL rupture. Straight stifle and narrow intercondylar notch, together with excessive rotation of the tibia and extension of the stifle, may cause constant impingement and abnormal compression of CCL against cranial aspect of intercondylar notch. Medial patellar luxation, genu varum and excessive internal rotation of tibia, or steep tibial plateau slope may cause increased stress on CCL and predispose it to rupture. Although anatomic differences in the shape of the proximal tibia have been documented in dogs with cruciate disease, its role in cruciate disease is unclear because many dogs with a steep tibial plateau angle do not develop cruciate disease.

TREATMENT OPTIONS

Treatment of CCL insufficiency aims to resolve lameness caused by joint instability and provide good long-term function of the affected hindlimb. Conservative management of dogs weighing less than 15 kg typically results in acceptable limb function, with reported success rates ranging from 84% to 90%. Surgical intervention is, however, advocated for the majority of dogs with CCL insufficiency in order to re-establish joint stability, mitigate secondary degenerative joint disease, and address any concurrent meniscal injury. Over the past 50 years, a plethora of surgical techniques has been described to treat this condition. This evolution of surgical procedures reflects the controversy that exists regarding the optimal management of CCL insufficiency, and to date, no one procedure has consistently demonstrated superior clinical efficacy.

Traditional methods of repair attempt to impart stability by utilizing an autogenous, allogenic, or synthetic structure placed within or about the stifle that mimics the function of the normal CCL. Extra-articular techniques utilize peri-articular heavy gauge suture or wires, or the transposition of soft tissues to reduce stifle laxity, whereas intra-articular techniques attempt to anatomically reconstruct the CCL using autogenous tissues, allografts or synthetic materials. Most authors cite good to excellent limb function in the majority of dogs that have undergone extra- or intra-articular procedures.

As surgical techniques continue to evolve, the current stem of innovations has focused on the concept of creating functional stability in the CCL deficient stifle by altering bone geometry. In 1984, Slocum described the cranial tibial wedge osteotomy (CTWO), a surgical procedure that attempts to eliminate cranial subluxation of the tibia during weight-bearing by reducing the caudally directed slope of the tibial plateau. By establishing dynamic stability of the CCL-deficient stifle, passive restraint against laxity is not required. Recognition that stabilization could be achieved in this manner led to the development of several proximal tibial osteotomy procedures, such as the tibial plateau leveling osteotomy (TPLO), and the proximal tibial intra-articular osteotomy (PTIO). The more recently described tibial tuberosity advancement (TTA) procedure attempts to dynamically neutralize cranio-caudal instability by altering the relative alignment of the patella tendon to the tibial plateau. Though there are few studies evaluating long-term function of any of these tibial osteotomy techniques, most have been associated with favorable clinical results.

The optimal treatment for cranial cruciate insufficiency is yet to be defined, partly because depends on several factors. The following factors should be considered when choosing the surgical treatment for CCL insufficiency:

1. Experience of the surgeon on the CCL repair technique
2. Differences in conformation (ie, steep tibial plateau angle, femoral or tibial deformities...) between subjects and breeds
3. Size of the dog
4. Degree of instability/chronicity
5. Level of activity of the dog
6. Concurrent medial patella luxation

The following recommendations (originating from clinical experience) may be helpful in the decision-making of CCL repair.

1. Optimize one or two techniques for CCL repair. Any technique may be successful if performed accurately.
2. Improve the meniscal evaluation and treatment. Failure of CCL repair is often due to poor management of the concurrent meniscal pathology.
3. Select the best cases for yourself, and refer the rest (it sounds funny, but it is not):
   a. Ideal patients for ANY techniques are thin, well muscled, small to large breed dogs with unilateral CCL insufficiency, without specific conformation abnormalities (ie, steep tibial plateau) and with compliant owners.

b. An obese large breed dog with a long history of lameness and severe muscle atrophy is NOT an easy case for anyone.

4. Select the candidate based on the technique. This is a controversial topic, but the following are some guidelines:
   a. Non-overweight, well muscled, small to large dogs, with unilateral CCL insufficiency, without specific conformation abnormalities may be good candidates for lateral suture stabilization.
   b. Very active large dogs may be candidates for a tibial leveling procedure.
   c. Any dog with steep tibial plateau (>30–35 degrees) may be a candidate for a tibial plateau leveling procedure.
   d. Medium size dogs with small bone or any dogs with tibial deformities may be good candidates for CTWO rather than TPLO.
   e. Dogs with tibial deformities, severe muscle atrophy and steep tibial plateau angles may not be good candidates for TTA.
   f. Giant breed dogs are challenging cases with any technique and may not have the same prognosis as medium-large dog.
5. Treat concurrent medial patella luxation.
6. Educate your clients to the postoperative management. Many failures of CCL repair are due to poor client compliance.
7. Use appropriate instrumentation and assistants.
8. Charge for your time and the quality of work that you are doing.
9. Ask advice about more complex cases.

MODERN KENNEL CONCEPTS

Terry L. Terlep, DVM
Emergency Veterinary Clinic
Ft. Meyers, FL

Modern kennel concepts encompass the newest designs and the latest construction materials and methods. Our goal is to develop the ultimate in kennels. Construction considerations should include a facility that is both functional and efficient while considering the needs and safety of both dogs and people. Other considerations include the demands of the site, desires of the owners, owner's financial means, community zoning laws, and construction codes.

The more time you spend planning your kennel, the better the results will be. It is acceptable to challenge the traditional designs of the past and create your own concepts. The designs will vary widely depending on the use of the facility (for example, a commercial boarding kennel verses a private breeding or training facility).

Regardless of the intended use of the facility, you want to avoid the appearance of a prison by using light, bright colors, skylights where possible, colorful flooring materials, live hanging flower baskets both inside and outside the kennel and tasteful planting of trees and shrubs. The safety of animals and employees is a primary concern of any kennel operation. Safety factors for animals include air quality, surface temperatures, and humidity control. Human safety factors include such considerations as noise protection, slip proof floors, air quality, air exchanges, and ambient temperatures.

Exhaust systems are a must to prevent diseases. Twelve to fifteen air exchanges per hour should be adequate with a 50% fresh air make up. Acceptable temperatures range from 60°F to 80°F. Ceiling fans move a lot of air which allows you to dry floors and set air conditioners at a higher temperature. HEPA filters (high efficiency particulate air filters) are useful to filter air and clean it thoroughly. They are 99.97% efficient and can filter 0.3 micron particles from the air. Desiccate units remove moisture from the air and are capable of reducing temperatures of 95°F to 80°F. Heat recovery ventilators (HRV) are very efficient at conserving heat from the air before it is exhausted to the outside, thereby saving energy costs. Heating the facility and its associated costs is a very important consideration due to the ever increasing costs of fuel and energy. Hot water radiant floor heating works well and when combined with other heating systems allows you to conserve energy and money.

Confinement areas vary widely from cages to inside runs to inside house/outside house runs. Inside the building runs should be a minimum of 15 to 30 square feet with a 3-foot minimum width. Provide a resting bench which is hinged to the wall and covers the cleaning trough at the rear of the kennel run. Water supply can be via water pans, buckets, lick its, or automatic waters. This water is supplied either up from the slab or from overhead. Only galvanized metal piping should be used as a supply line for water inside the run.

It is imperative that the floor of the run have adequate slope for proper drainage. Floors should slope from one-fourth inch to one inch per lineal foot. Privacy panels between the runs are helpful to stop cross kennel contamination with stool and urine, prevent urine spray, reduce noise and help reduce fence fighting. Materials used commonly are of concrete block, stainless steel, aluminum, galvanized metal and fiberglass reinforced plastic (FRP). Outside runs can be any desired size depending on the breed size and intended use of the facility.

Standard kennel run sizes are 3 feet to 8 feet wide and 8 feet to 20 feet in length. Privacy walls which are 24 inches tall, or curbs which are 4 inches wide and 4 inches tall, should be constructed to prevent urine and stool contamination. The pipe and wire used to construct the runs is a very important factor with respect to cost and durability. Pipe choices are stainless steel, aluminum, and galvanized steel. Stainless steel and aluminum do not rust and are not adversely affected by urine, moisture, and chemicals used for cleaning.

The pipe should be one inch outside diameter (OD) or larger, and schedule forty or greater. If galvanized pipe is to be used, it should be galvanized inside and outside with a smooth coat spray on the outside. Galvanized paint should be used on all welds. All runs should be covered and a perimeter fence installed to prevent escape. A swimming pool screen enclosure around the outside runs will prevent insect problems and can be used to provide some shade. It is very important that a portion of the outside runs be fully shaded in the summer months.

Chain link fencing is the most popular enclosure material and is available in many sizes and of various quality. Chain link is attractive and in most cases long lasting. Wire of nine, eleven, or thirteen gauge is the commonly used sizes and openings of one to two inches are normally used. Eleven-gauge wire with a one and one-half inch opening is the most popular size used today.

It is important that the ends of the wire are knuckled over to prevent injury to dogs. The wire should be attached to the bottom rail by either hand lacing the wire with 13-gauge wire or with the use of a tension bar. Random placed wire clips are not used as they are not secure enough for most kennel runs.

When choosing wire for the runs it should be electro-galvanized before weaving (GBW). Hot dip galvanizing after weaving leaves some sharp edges and often times if not thoroughly galvanized. Aluminum grills are also used for enclosures because they are attractive and rust free and easy to maintain although costly. Runs, whether inside or outside, require a trough to carry urine, water and feces away for disposal. Troughs should be a minimum of 6 inches wide, 2 to 12 inches deep, and slope one-half to one inch per foot to a drain which should be located at one end of the trough. Troughs on the inside kennel runs are located at the back of the run and should be covered with a hinged resting bench. Outside runs should have a trough located just beyond the far end of the run and the installation of a 24-inch splash wall will help make cleaning much easier.

Kennel flooring and finishing is a very important consideration which should be completed prior to using the new facility. The degree of slope from the front of the run to the back of the run should be from one fourth inch to one inch per linear foot. The greater the slope the faster it dries and urine pooling is eliminated.

Concrete is the most popular flooring used and has many advantages over other types of flooring. Concrete can be sealed, color stained, painted or covered with various materials. Concrete should be reinforced with the use of rebar and fiber mesh which prevents cracking. Polypropylene filaments should be added at one and one-half pounds per cubic yard of concrete to add strength. A magnesium zinc flusilicate liquid concrete hardener can be used and the use of a penetrating sealer/hardener is recommended. Avoid the use of non-penetrating sealers. They are not recommended because they sit on top of the floor and will quickly peel. Concrete stains that are mixed with the wet material before it is poured come in any desired color and are an inexpensive alternative to other flooring choices.

Other materials that are used as kennel flooring include MMA (methyl methacrylate) poured flooring, poured epoxy, ceramic tile, terrazzo, brick pavers, quarry tile and stone. A popular flooring choice in many boarding facilities is an elevated plastic or plastic coated expanded metal. These floors are normally 18 inches to 24 inches off the floor. The size of the openings is an important consideration and should be a minimum of one-half inch by one and one-half inches. These floors are easy to clean and allow dogs to stay dry and clean. PVC (poly vinyl chloride) coated expanded metal floors should be nine gauge metal with one-eighth inch coatings and a minimum of one-half inch openings. The disadvantage of this type of flooring is that it is very heavy and difficult to remove to clean. Plastic (one hundred percent polypropylene) raised flooring is lightweight, durable and easy to clean and comes with various size openings. This flooring has stood the test of time in the swine industry and is both indestructible and inexpensive.

Gate latches should be sturdy, easy to operate, escape proof and capable of opening from outside or inside the run. Popular choices are the never fail and two way latch. Kennel doors are available in various styles for different uses. Pickwick doors are designed for the frame to swing out and the panel to swing in. Five sixteenths inch aluminum frames are best and come with 13 by 19-inch or 17 by 29-inch openings. Guillotine doors are popular and should have aluminum channel door guides with acrylic or aluminum, used for the door material. Rubber flap dog doors consist of a hanging rubber flap with a magnet at the bottom of the flap which contacts the metal frame to allow self closure.

Ceilings in the inside kennel should be nine feet in height. An aluminum frame grid with USG Kapok-Armstrong ceiling tile that is a vinyl faced fiberglass ceiling with random fissures and has a .75 NRC (noise reduction coefficient). Ceilings in the outside run area are optional although the use of metal roofing attached to the bottom of the trusses improve the appearance of the area and prevents insect webs and bird nests in the rafters. Concrete block walls, whether they are privacy walls between runs or structural walls, should be painted or covered and the use of two part epoxy paint gives a beautiful appearance and is very easy to maintain. Ceramic tile can also be used to cover these walls.

Other considerations in kennel concepts include:

1. Ceiling-mounted retractable hose reels
2. Hot water heater
3. Rodent proof feed room
4. Feeding cart
5. Insect misting system
6. Automatic dishwasher
7. Grooming/bathing area with dryer system
8. Heated whelping room with attached puppy run
9. Leaf blower to dry floors and runs
10. Wet/dry vacuum
11. Pressure washer
12. Washer and dryer in laundry room
13. Electric walk-on scale

FELINE WOUND HEALING — IT'S NOT A SMALL DOG

Mark Bohling, DVM
College of Veterinary Medicine
University of Tennessee
Knoxville, TN

Cats comprise the second largest patient group overall in small animal practice; some practices see a majority of feline patients and a few specialize exclusively in feline medicine and surgery. Cats differ from dogs in many important areas of their anatomy and physiology, and we are continually adding more areas to the list of ways in which the cat is not a small dog. Wound healing is yet another aspect of feline physiology in which the cat differs significantly from the dog, and those practitioners who deal with cat wounds can benefit from an understanding of these differences and how they can affect clinical feline practice.

OPEN WOUND HEALING: FELINE COMPARED WITH CANINE

Differences in closed wound healing between cats and dogs begin to be noted within 24 hours after creation of identical experimental wounds. The first difference to be seen is in the gross appearance of the wound. At 24 hours post-wounding in the dog, the skin at the wound margin is typically moderately swollen and red. The wound bed is moist, and a moderate amount of wound fluid will be noted in the bandage when it is removed. In contrast, an open wound in the cat is usually much less "disturbed" in appearance, with little if any swelling and redness at the skin margins. Much less wound fluid will also be seen in the bandage material. The next differences are noted at post-wounding day 4 or 5, when the first visible granulation tissue is starting to appear in the wounds of dogs; this granulation tissue is typically first seen in the bottom or base of the defect. In cats, no granulation tissue is visible until 1 to 2 days later, and when it does appear, it is usually seen at the cut skin margin rather than on the base of the wound. Granulation tissue proliferation also proceeds more slowly in cat wounds; a 2-cm-square wound is filled with granulation tissue to the level of the surrounding skin in an average of about 7 days in dogs, but this takes between two and three times as long in cats.

CLOSED WOUND HEALING: FELINE COMPARED WITH CANINE

The gain in wound tensile strength is directly proportional to fibroblast recruitment, proliferation, and collagen secretion. The slower onset of the proliferative phase in cat wound healing translates to a slower gain in sutured wound strength compared with the dog. Cat wounds were on average only half as strong as dog wounds when tested via tensiometry at 7 days post wounding. In addition, problematic healing of closed wounds appears to be more frequent in feline patients than in canine patients (see below).

ROLE OF THE SUBCUTIS IN WOUND HEALING

The subcutaneous tissues serve as an adipose storage depot, cushion, and conduit for the passage of cutaneous nerve, vascular, and lymphatic supply. In addition, more recent investigation has shown that the subcutis appears to serve as a major contributor to normal cutaneous wound healing, and that removal of large portions of subcutis has a profound negative impact on wound healing. The contribution of the subcutis to wound healing (and the resultant delay in healing when it is removed) is not the same for all species. Experimental data has demonstrated that removal of the subcutis has a much greater negative impact on wound healing in the cat than in the dog. This is exemplified by the fact that 2 x 2 cm open wounds in cats, with subcutis removed, failed to heal in 3 weeks, while corresponding wounds in dogs were healed in about 2.5 weeks on average.

SPECIAL FELINE WOUND HEALING PROBLEMS

Cats also appear to be different from dogs in that certain types of problem wounds are seen exclusively or at least predominantly in cats. One such wound is the indolent pocket wound. This wound is typically a large defect of the skin and subcutis and is usually located in the axillary region. The etiology is thought to be related to the presence of a foreign body; the assumed scenario is that one of the cat's forelimbs becomes entrapped by its collar. Similar collar, rope, and chain-related injuries are frequently seen in dogs, and after removal of the foreign material and cleansing of the wound, such wounds have a high rate of rapid uncomplicated healing. In contrast, when seen in cats, these wounds are often chronic nonhealing wounds characterized by the formation of an indolent pocket. An indolent pocket wound is defined as an open wound, completely lined with granulation tissue, in which there is overlying non-adherent skin at the wound margin. The deep aspect of this overlying skin is also lined with granulation tissue, so that granulation tissue from the deeper wound bed is in contact with granulation tissue from the skin, but the two areas never adhere or heal together, nor does the pocket thus formed ever completely fill in. Rather, it remains as a blind cul-de-sac around the wound margin. Indolent pocket wounds are also seen in dogs and other species including man; however, they do appear to form more readily in cats in situations that would have resulted in normal uncomplicated healing in other species, and also seem to be particularly resistant to treatment when seen in cats.

Another special wound healing problem seen in cats is the phenomenon of the so-called "pseudohealing" wound. Pseudohealing wounds are closed wounds; in this scenario, an apparently routine closure and uncomplicated healing is the first event. The patient is rechecked for suture removal at the usual interval around 14 days post op and the wound appears to be healed and quiescent. After the sutures are removed, however, the wound completely dehisces when the patient puts the least amount of normal stress on the wound, for example, by jumping up onto a chair. The dehisced wound edges are typically noted to have very little if any bleeding. Pseudohealing wounds have usually been associated with large subcutaneous defects such as seen after resection of a large neoplasm, or closure of a ruptured abscess.

CLINICAL APPLICATION TO FELINE WOUNDS

Knowing about the uniqueness of cats is of no particular value unless we can translate that information into better patient care. In the case of differences in wound healing, there are several practical recommendations that can help improve surgical outcomes and reduce complication rates, particularly with challenging, more invasive procedures such as major mass resection:

1. Gain of strength in sutured wounds in cats occurs more slowly than in dogs; therefore, leave skin sutures in place for a longer period (10–14 days for cats versus 7–10 days for dogs). If the closure is "challenged" (eg, large resection, radiation therapy) leave in place 21 days or more.

2. The subcutaneous tissues make a major contribution to wound healing, and loss of subcutis seems to be particularly damaging to wound healing in the cat; therefore, subcutis should be debrided somewhat conservatively rather than aggressively. When subcutis must be resected, the defect in the subcutis should be closed by apposition if this can be accomplished without excessive tension. If much subcutis has been removed, appositional closure of the subcutaneous defect may not be possible. In these cases other measures such as tacking sutures should be used to bring skin in better direct contact with underlying blood supply.

3. Wound healing stimulants, particularly stimulants of granulation tissue, may be of particular use in large open wounds in cats and should be considered. They may be contraindicated, however, in closures after resection of fibrosarcoma or other mesenchymal neoplasms, since many wound healing stimulants function by promotion of fibroplasia. More research in this area is needed before an evidence-based recommendation can be made.

THE PULLEY SUTURE

Mark Bohling, DVM
College of Veterinary Medicine
University of Tennessee
Knoxville, TN

Management of tension is an important goal of primary wound closure, particularly when a large defect has been created via trauma or tumor resection. A certain amount of wound tension is expected in normal wound closures. In fact, mild wound tension can even be beneficial to wound healing. Although healing has been classically described in terms of discrete phases, in reality the events of wound healing occur in an overlapping fashion. This means that even during the proliferative phase of healing, remodeling is already beginning to occur. Remodeling during skin healing allows collagen fibers in the scar to orient along lines of tension. In bone, this property of tissue remodeling has been formalized as Wolff's law and allows remodeling bone to develop greatest strength where most needed. Although not formalized into a "law," the same property has been described for skin. Therefore, a mild amount of tension in the healing skin wound actually contributes to the more rapid development of scar strength and a secure closure when compared to a completely tension-free closure. Therefore, the goal in most wound closures should be the management or reduction of excess tension, not the elimination of all tension.

A variety of suture patterns and other techniques have been developed to control this tension. The properties of an ideal tension management technique are that it should be:

1. Easily executed
2. Secure – does not easily unravel or become untied, even with patient movement or manipulation
3. Versatile – able to be used in a variety of tissues and surgical applications
4. Able to be used for high or low tension closures
5. Compact – minimizes the amount of foreign material implanted into the wound
6. Flexible – able to withstand the shocks and tension changes associated with patient activity
7. Non-elongating – does not stretch, or if it does, stretches at a slower rate than biological creep so that the skin does not end up becoming the principal channel for tension again
8. Implantable and absorbable, or readily removable and well tolerated.

Many suture patterns and techniques meet some or most of these ideals; none meets all of them. One simple suture technique, developed by Henderson a number of years ago, but reported only recently (Austin and Henderson, Vet Surg 2006), is the modified "pulley" suture. This suture pattern works on the same principle as the block and tackle. The block and tackle is a simple piece of equipment for lifting and pulling loads. It works by the principle of force–distance tradeoff: by suspending a load between multiple pulleys, the force required to lift or pull the load is spread out over a greater length. The pulling force is decreased but the distance (amount of rope pulled in) is increased in proportion, that is, a reduction in force to 1/2 requires a 2X increase in length of rope pulled to move the load. The pulley suture works on the same principle. The suture is passed through the tissues twice instead of once; twice as much suture passes through the "pulleys" (ie, tissues) and the load (pulling tension) is reduced by half. In this author's opinion, the major benefit of this suture pattern, however, is not the reduction in effort required to close a defect. The major benefit is that the reduction in pulling tension also translates to a continuous tension reduction after closure. This again follows from the pulley principle—the reduction in load is experienced as the load is being lifted, and also as it remains in the static lifted position. From a wound-healing standpoint, this means reduction in the crushing force applied to the tissues enclosed within the suture bites, and thus reduced risk of ischemic necrosis of those tissues. Since most dehiscences are the result of ischemic necrosis of the sutured tissues rather than mechanical failure of the suture material, the major benefit of the pulley suture is the ability to close wounds under tension with a reduced risk of dehiscence.

The pulley suture can be used in many applications in which tension and/or risk of dehiscence are concerns. It has been used very effectively in closure of large defects following tumor removal, and in abdominal closures of large animals (up to 400+ lb tigers), and hernia repair. One caution regarding the pulley suture is that because it works so well at reducing tensile load at closure, it is possible to pull tissues together when that would not have ordinarily have been possible. The tension on such closures may be so great that dehiscence still occurs. A good rule of thumb with the pulley suture is that if the closure still feels rather tight as one is bringing the tissue into apposition, it is better to employ either a different technique or an additional technique to manage the tension.

TIPS ON PREVENTING WOUND HEALING PROBLEMS

Steven F. Swaim, DVM, MS
College of Veterinary Medicine
Auburn University, Auburn, AL

Over the years, the author has seen and experienced some practices that are helpful in managing wounds. These include some "do's" and "don'ts" that may prevent wound healing problems.

GENERAL PRACTICES
Wound Closure, Bandages, Bedding and Clients

Closure. In the presence of chronic wound infection, eg, chronic fibrosing interdigital pyoderma, on which surgical debridement will be done, use preoperative systemic antibiotics. These should be based on culture and sensitivity tests, and are used to prevent septicemia.

When dealing with an infection by an unusual organism, eg, *Nocardia* or atypical *Mycobacterium*, do not try to close the wound until *all* infection is under control; otherwise it will disrupt.

For wounds that are in areas that will be difficult to bandage or immobilize, consider using punch skin grafts placed in pockets.

Bandages. To immobilize wound repair sites in the axillary or inguinal area of cats, place a box with a hole in the side or a large paper sack in the cage. Cats get in these and sit with all joints flexed; thus, immobilizing them. Similarly, "cage" (dog and cat) or "aquarium" (snake) bandages can be used when it will be difficult to bandage large body areas. Medication is placed on the wound(s) and the animal is placed in the cage/aquarium with no bedding. Medication will get on the container sides as the animal moves about and it serves as a "bandage" to keep medication on the wound(s).

To remove the last layer of a bandage that is adhered to a wound, wet it with some warm 2% lidocaine shortly before removal.

Bedding. To prevent decubital ulcers on large dogs that are unable to move, bed them on *thick* foam rubber padding covered with vinyl. Cover any bedding that is used with an artificial sheep skin covering to wick urine away from the skin. At least daily part the hair and check over boney prominences for hyperemia— a sign of early decubital wounds.

Owner involvement and help. When owners are to be involved in wound care, as with all home care, always give all written and oral instructions to the owners before the pet is given to them. Owners hear little if any instruction given after they receive their pet.

If an owner will be treating an open wound at home, they often do not appreciate the wound contraction process when they see the wound daily. However, progress can be monitored and shown to the owner at weekly checks. The veterinarian can trace the wound on clear acetate, date it, and place it in the animal's record. When laid out over the wound a week later, progress of healing is seen.

If you are going to have owners change bandages at home, it is best to give them instructions on removing and replacing bandages, let them watch you change a bandage, and then have them do a bandage change under your supervision. It is especially helpful to do this with leg and paw bandages to help ensure that they do not get them on too tight. Related to this is instruction on taping: The author always uses adhesive tape on limb and paw bandages and has clients do likewise. The owner should always pretear tape strips before applying them to help avoid getting them too tight.

HEAD AND EAR
Lips

When dealing with wounds or surgery around the lips and nares, it is important to prevent licking of the area. This can be done by placing some simple interrupted sutures of stainless steel in the area, leaving short sharp tags on the sutures.

Tongue

Do not place an anesthetized dog on a grill or grate type surface to recover from anesthesia, or if it is placed on a grill or grate, have a towel under the head. It is possible for the animal's tongue to drop from the mouth between grate or grill openings. The result is tongue swelling, and when the dog recovers from anesthesia, severe self-inflicted trauma occurs.

Head Bandages

Head and ear bandages require some special attention. If adhesive tape is used for a head bandage, the rostral-most piece of tape is important because it keeps the bandage from slipping caudally. It should be applied carefully with half the tape width on the bandage and the other half on the hair of the head. Use the heat of your hand and the dog's body to ensure adhesion of the tape.

When an ear is taped over the top of the dog's head and it is necessary to medicate the ear canal, a hole can be cut through the bandage over the external auditory opening for medication application. When this is done, it is obvious the ear is taped over the top of the head. When it is not done, the ear could be over or under the head. In such cases, the ear should be drawn and labeled on the bandage to help avoid it being cut at bandage removal. If elastic tape is used on a head bandage and is placed while the animal is still anesthetized, it should be observed carefully after extubation to be sure taping was not too tight causing respiratory obstruction.

PERINEAL
Surgical Positioning

During perineal surgery when the animal's hind quarters are elevated with the pelvic limbs hanging over the table edge, the edge of the table should be well padded. This will help prevent bilateral compression of the femoral nerves and having a dog that cannot extend the stifles to walk following surgery.

Suture Reminder

If a purse-string suture is used in the anus to prevent fecal contamination of the surgical site, leave long tags or even marked tags. These are reminders for postoperative removal as well as cotton ball removal if they have been used in the anus and rectum.

Cautery of Anal Sacs

Chemical cauterization can be used to remove/destroy the anal sacs. Silver nitrate swabs can be used for this. DO NOT place formalin in the anal sac as a means of chemical cauterization. Severe damage to the surrounding soft tissues may occur.

LIMB AND PAW
Early Precautions

If an animal has had trauma to a distal limb, there are no open wounds, but there is orthopedic damage (ie, fractures), do not place a fully encasing cast on the limb. Such a cast placed early following trauma does not accommodate the swelling that will occur. Swelling within the cast places pressure on tissues, to include blood vessels. The result is tissue ischemia and slough. Use bivalved casts in such instances.

When a pouch flap is considered for reconstructing a limb wound, it is wise to bandage the dog's or cat's limb along its side prior to performing the surgery. If the animal will not tolerate its leg bandaged in this position, it is better to learn this before the surgery and select an alternate reconstruction technique, rather than have the animal destroy a pouch flap following surgery.

Surgical Preparations

With paw wounds on the dorsum of the paw, the *entire* paw should be clipped and scrubbed. Hair left in the interdigital area and on the palmar/plantar surface of the paw provides a good area for bacterial growth to complicate wound management. Pledgets of cotton placed in these areas help keep them dry during wound management. In addition, nails should be clipped as part of wound management, and if there is a groove remaining on the palmar/plantar nail surface, an 18-gauge needle should be used clean it out prior to scrubbing the paw. A chloxhexidine scrub and solution should be used for preparation rather than povidone iodine for better residual activity.

Following aseptic preparation of the paw/limb, it can be protected during transport to the surgical area by sterile aluminum foil wrapped around the limb. It is moldable, water resistant, and easily removed in the surgery room.

Bandaging

Bandaging a forelimb and/or paw is made easier if the elbow and carpus are extended during the procedure. This is easily accomplished when the animal is in lateral recumbency with the affected limb uppermost. The person restraining the animal simply pushes on the animal's elbow. This extends all joints, making bandage changing easier.

To enhance healing of wounds over the point of the elbow, pressure on the wound and movement (elbow flexion) must be prevented. These can be prevented by incorporating splinting material in the elbow-limb bandage to keep the joint immobilized in extension. Such splinting could be a lateral limb and shoulder splint, cranial aluminum rod loop splint, or pipe insulation "donut" pad.

Three techniques can be used to help keep pressure off paw pad wounds to enhance healing. A foam sponge pad (intermediate compressible, Comforfoam, HiTech Foam, Lincoln, NE) with a "donut" hole to go over the metacarpal/metatarsal pad can be incorporated in the bandage for pressure relief on these pads. Second, a triangular piece of foam the size of the metacarpal/metatarsal pad is incorporated in the bandage under this pad to elevate the digits and relieve pressure on digital pad wounds. Third, a "clam shell" splint can be placed on the limb to put it in a toe dancing posture and relieve pressure on all pads.

Pressure can be relieved over convex surfaces where taping might put pressure on the skin over such areas (eg, point of the hock carpal pad). "Donut" pads made from cast padding (Specialist Cast Padding, Johnson & Johnson Orthopedics, Raynham, MA) can be placed with the "donut" hole over the convex surface.

When using porous adhesive tape to hold a limb/paw bandage in place, the adherence of the proximal-most piece of tape can be enhanced by placing a hexamethyldisiloxane acrylate (Cavilon No Sting Barrier Film, 3M Health Care, St. Paul, MN) on the skin near the top of the bandage. It also helps prevent epidermal stripping when tape is removed.

To help protect a paw bandage from water when a dog is in a wet environment, duct tape can be used. However, if it is not completely water-tight, any water that gets in stays in. Also, duct tape does not allow the bandage to "breathe". It does have the advantage of helping deter bandage molestation. Other means for clients to keep bandages dry include placing a bread sack or self-adherent plastic food wrap over the bandage. However, these should not be held in place with rubber bands and should not be left on when the dog is not in a wet area. They do not allow the bandage to "breathe."

At the time of bandage removal it is much more comfortable for the bandager and "bandagee" (dog or cat) if the bandage is removed in layers, rather than trying to cut through the full-thickness of the bandage. Carefully, cut the tape only with a razor blade, and snip with bandage scissors between the tape and secondary layer. Find an end to the secondary layer, and unwrap it. Do not try to cut through all bandage layers. This is uncomfortable for the animal. Moisten the primary layer with warm 2% lidocaine prior to removal.

When major surgery has been done on a paw, especially the plantar or palmar surface, and it is time to discontinue bandages, booties can be used as the transition between bandages and no bandages.

Personal experience is a good teacher, and learning from the experiences of others is also a good teacher!

SKIN GRAFTING: PRACTICAL PATCHES FOR PROBLEM WOUNDS

Steven F. Swaim, DVM, MS
College of Veterinary Medicine
Auburn University, Auburn, AL

Autogenous skin grafts are segments of skin that are separated from the body and placed on another area of the body where they heal in place. Grafts have been defined as a piece of skin that is dead when it is put in place, but it may come to life later (Gilles and Millard). Grafts are used on areas of the body where there is insufficient skin to move or create flaps for wound closure, usually on the distal limbs. Four forms of grafts are practical for small animal practice: mesh, strip, paw pad, and punch grafts.

MESH SKIN GRAFTS

A proper wound bed is necessary to place a graft. This is either a bed of healthy granulation tissue or a wound that is vascular enough to produce a bed of granulation tissue. Wound management to obtain such graft beds may require removal of abnormal tissue (eg, tumors), staged debridement, and application of topical medications, including wound healing stimulants, with bandages.

Three reasons grafts do not heal are infection, hemorrhage, and movement. Meshing a graft allows blood or exudate to drain from under the graft, thus allowing the graft to contact the graft bed securely. Tacking sutures can be used between mesh holes of the graft to immobilize it on the wound. These sutures also help pull the graft into concavities on the wound surface for adequate graft-wound contact.

If the graft bed is composed of granulation tissue, the surface should be scraped with a number 10 scalpel blade the day before grafting to help remove any coagulum and surface flora on the wound. Neurolept-analgesia may be necessary to do this. The wound is then bandaged with a gauze sponge coated with 0.1% gentamicin sulfate ointment.

On the day of surgery the area around the wound is prepared for aseptic surgery, not doing anything to the wound itself. The lower cranio-lateral thoracic graft donor area is also prepared for aseptic surgery. After draping the wound and donor area, a number 15 scalpel blade is used to remove epithelium from the wound edge if a granulation tissue bed is present. A pattern is made of the wound by laying a piece of sterile towel over the wound to obtain a blood imprint of the wound. The pattern is then cut to the shape of the wound.

The pattern is laid over the lower cranio-lateral thoracic area *being careful not to turn the pattern over* during the transfer. The pattern is placed such that the direction of hair growth will be the same as the hair around the wound. Methylene blue or a skin marking pen is used to trace around the pattern, and a scalpel blade is used to cut around the traced line. The graft is removed from the body, and the donor site is closed with

"walking" sutures, subcuticular sutures, and skin staples or sutures.

The graft is fixed dermal-side up to a piece of sterilized cardboard (back of a writing tablet) by stay sutures of silk placed through the edge of the graft and pulled through slits cut in the cardboard edge. A faster alternative is to fix the graft to a piece of sterile corrugated cardboard with hypodermic needles. *All* subcutaneous tissue is removed from the dermis using sharp-sharp scissors and thumb forceps. A number 11 scalpel blade is used to cut staggered parallel rows of slits in the graft. The slits are about 1 cm long and 0.5 cm apart.

The graft is removed from the cardboard; it is placed on the defect and sutured along one edge. If the mesh holes are not open to allow drainage when the remaining edge of the graft is opposed to the remaining wound edge, 2 to 3 mm of skin are trimmed from the free graft edge before suturing/stapling it to the remaining wound edge. After the graft edges are affixed in place, simple interrupted tacking sutures are placed between some of the mesh openings to fix the graft to the wound, especially where the graft is over a wound concavity.

The wound is then bandaged with a semiocclusive nonadherent pad that has a *thin* coating of a 0.1% gentamicin sulfate ointment on it, an absorbent wrap, and adhesive tape. A metal splint (eg, Mason metasplint) is incorporated in the bandage to add stability, especially if the wound is over a joint. Generally, bandages are changed daily during the first postoperative week, every other day during the second week, and once or twice the third week postoperatively. Sutures are removed 10 days after grafting. Bandaging is generally discontinued after the third week.

Graft survival depends on plasmatic imbibition, inosculation, and capillary ingrowth. During plasmatic imbibition, a graft absorbs fluid and cells from the wound surface. The graft may appear cyanotic and edematous for the first 1 to 3 days. With inosculation and ingrowth of capillaries, the graft's circulation is further increased. As circulation increases the graft becomes less edematous and regains a more natural color.

The adherence of a graft to the wound is initially by a weak fibrin attachment. The fibrin is invaded by fibroblasts that produce ground substance followed by their production of collagen for a stronger graft adherence. As inter- and intramolecular collagen bonding occurs, the graft adherence becomes progressively stronger.

The use of a wound healing stimulant to enhance graft healing can have positive and negative effects. They can be used to enhance early formation of granulation tissue over exposed bone or tendons for early graft placement. However, if they are used after a mesh graft is placed they can be "too much of a good thing." Although the graft revascularizes nicely, granulation tissue may become exuberant in the mesh holes. This can result in mechanical obstruction of contractual healing of the mesh holes, ie, delayed healing until the granulation tissue regresses. Thus, if a wound healing stimulant is used after grafting, it should be used judiciously, eg, every second or third day with discontinuance when granulation tissue is at the level of the skin graft surface.

STRIP SKIN GRAFTS

Strip skin grafting is a simple procedure and requires no special equipment. After a bed of healthy granulation tissue has formed, which could be enhanced by wound healing stimulants, parallel grooves are cut in the granulation tissue. The grooves are approximately 5 mm wide, 2 to 3 mm deep, and 3 to 4 mm apart. After the grooves are prepared, full-thickness strips of skin approximately 5 mm wide are cut from the skin on the lower cranio-lateral thoracic region. After removing subcutaneous tissue from each strip, they are laid in the grooves in the granulation tissue and anchored at each end with a simple interrupted nonabsorbable suture. Where indicated, the strips can be further immobilized to the sides of the grooves by simple interrupted sutures. Bandaging is like that for mesh grafts.

As the grafts heal, epithelial tissue grows from the grafts' edges to cover the remaining granulation tissue and the grafts tend to widen to some degree. Those grafts usually do not have a good hair regrowth, and thus, they are not as cosmetic as other types of reconstruction. They lend themselves best to longitudinal limb wounds.

PAW PAD GRAFTS

Paw pad grafts can be considered for reconstruction or salvage when all of the metacarpal or metatarsal pad has been lost from a limb and it is not feasible or possible to use a digital pad for replacement by phalangeal fillet (eg, all digits have been lost). Paw pad grafts can be considered for reconstruction or salvage. A healthy bed of granulation tissue can be enhanced by using wound healing stimulants on the wound. After a bed of healthy granulation tissue has developed in the area of the missing pad, a piece of sterile developed x-ray film with a 6 x 8 mm rectangular hole in its center is used to trace recipient sites around the edge of the granulation tissue bed using methylene blue or a skin marking pen. These sites are excised to create recessed beds for digital pad grafts.

The same x-ray film pattern is used to trace grafts in the center of digital pads. All subcutaneous tissue is removed from these grafts after they are excised. The grafts are placed in the previously created recipient sites. They are sutured in place with simple interrupted 5-0 polypropylene sutures at each corner of each graft. Donor sites are bandaged and allowed to heal as open wounds.

A paw bandage is applied as previously described for mesh grafts, and metal splints (Mason metasplints) in the form of a "clam shell" splint are incorporated in the bandage. Bandages are changed every 1 to 2 days.

Sutures are removed from the grafts at 10 to 14 days after grafting and the hard darkened stratum corneum is removed from the grafts. This should reveal an underlying viable pad graft.

As the grafts heal, dense keratinized epithelium will advance from the grafts to cover the wound center, and the wound will contract to coalesce the grafts to provide a suitable weight-bearing tissue. Although there is no fibroadipose cushioning tissue under the grafts, they compensate for this by becoming very hard to withstand the stress placed on them.

PUNCH SKIN GRAFTS

Punch skin grafts are small segments of skin that are placed in incised pockets. These grafts are used on wounds that are located in areas where it will be difficult to bandage and where there will be movement.

After a bed of granulation tissue has formed, which could be enhanced by wound healing stimulants, a number 15 scalpel blade is used to make parallel rows of pockets 2- to 4-mm-deep and 5- to 7-mm apart in the granulation tissue. The blade is inserted almost parallel to the wound surface with the opening of the created pocket dorsally.

The punch grafts are harvested with a 6-mm-diameter dermal biopsy punch from the lower cranio-lateral thoracic area. The punch is inserted at an angle parallel to the direction of hair growth to obtain as many intact hair follicles as possible. All subcutaneous tissue is removed from each graft.

It is important to place a graft in each pocket as the pocket is made. Do not make all the pockets and then try to remember which ones you have placed grafts in.

The granulation tissue of the pocket serves as a bandage to immobilize the graft in place and protect it. In areas where a scab can form over the grafted area, the scab acts as an additional bandage over the wound. A restraint device may be indicated to protect the area if it cannot be bandaged.

As the grafts heal, the overlying granulation tissue pockets recede. Epithelial tissue spreads from the grafts' edges to cover intervening granulation tissue, wound contraction coalesces the grafts together, and some hair grows back on the grafts. Although they may not be as cosmetic as a mesh graft, these grafts provide skin coverage over areas that are difficult to bandage and where there will be movement.

REFERENCES

1. Paveletic MM. Atlas of Small Animal Reconstructive Surgery, 2nd ed. Philadelphia: WB Saunders, 1999, pp 365-379.
2. Swaim SF, Henderson RA. Small Animal Wound Management, 2nd ed. Baltimore: Williams & Wilkins, 1997, pp 295-370.

USE OF WOUND HEALING STIMULANTS IN AN ALTERNATING REGIMEN

Steven F. Swaim, DVM, MS
College of Veterinary Medicine
Auburn University, Auburn, AL

Veterinarians are called on to treat problem wounds. These wounds present a challenge either from their size or their chronicity. A seven-day alternating clinical regimen for wound management has been used to treat such wounds. Three topical wound healing stimulant medications are used in the regimen.

A hydrophilic Acemannan-containing medication (CarraSorb, Carrington Laboratories, Irving, TX) enhances the early inflammatory stage of healing by stimulating macrophages to produce interleukin-1 and tumor necrosis factor alpha, which results in fibroblast proliferation, neovascularization, and collagen deposition (granulation tissue). Epidermal growth and motility are also enhanced. The hydrophilic property pulls fluid through the wound tissue to bathe it and reduce edema. In addition, if the animal is on systemic antibiotics, the wound is bathed from the inside-out with antibiotic-laden fluids.

A D-Glucose polysaccharide Maltodextrin N.F. (IntraCell, Macleod Pharmaceuticals, Ft. Collins, CO) is hydrophilic, chemotactic for macrophages, and it has some antibacterial properties. It reportedly provides energy for wound healing cells for their continuance of the wound healing process.

A tripeptide–copper complex (Iamin Hydrating Gel, Procyte Labs, Redmond, WA) is a macrophage chemoattractant and stimulant of collagen systhesis and angiogenesis, and results in reduced levels of matrix metalloproteases associated with chronic wounds.

It has been noted in preclinical research and on clinical cases that when something has an effect on wound healing, it has its greatest effect during the first 7 days of application. Thus, these three wound healing stimulants have been used in an alternating 7-day regimen to treat challenging acute (eg, large wounds and wounds with exposed bone) and chronic wounds in dogs and cats. This report is based on objective observations in various preclinical wound management studies and subjective observations of clinical cases.

FELINE SKIN FOLD FLAPS

Don R. Waldron, DVM, Diplomate ACVS and ABVP
Virginia-Maryland Regional College of Veterinary
Medicine, Virginia Tech
Blacksburg, VA

Skin flaps are excellent sources for reconstructing wounds in dogs and cats. Skin flaps in dogs are based either on the subdermal plexus, which is the generalized microcirculation that exists in the dermis of animals, or in some cases on specific large perforating arteries. The latter have been termed "axillary pattern flaps" (APF) and are discussed and described in most veterinary surgical texts.

Several types of advancement flaps are available for reconstruction of defects. Dr. G.B. Hunt described the use of elbow and flank fold advancement flaps for use in the dog and cat in 1995. The amount of skin available for reconstruction following mobilization of the elbow or flank folds is substantial. These folds are most useful for closing large wounds in the pectoral or inguinal areas of the feline. Cats usually have well-developed skin folds; however, their presence in dogs is less predictable.

CLINICAL USE

The skin and subcutaneous tissue of the ventral abdomen and thorax may be affected by disease that requires large areas of tissue excision. Pyogranulomatous panniculitis caused by *Mycobacterium* spp, neoplasia of the skin or subcutaneous tissue, trauma, burns, and abscesses may be indications for reconstructive techniques in this area. Options for reconstruction of large defects especially if the defect crosses midline may be limited due to excess tension in the area. APFs may be used in some cases but if the lesion extends across midline in the inguinal area the caudal superficial epigastric artery may be compromised bilaterally.

Both the flank fold and elbow folds consist of laterally (outer) or medially (inner) layers of skin separated by loose connective tissue. Division of the fold distal attachments to the limb creates in both cases large U-shaped flaps of skin which can be advanced locally to cover sternal or inguinal defects without decreasing limb mobility.

SURGICAL TECHNIQUE

The animal is placed in dorsal recumbency and hair is clipped around the defect that is to be closed/covered with the skin fold(s). The axial and abaxial aspects of either the forelimbs or rear limbs is clipped to the midantebrachial or midcrural levels and prepared for aseptic surgery.

The lesion is excised or if a defect is already present epithelial edges are excised in preparation for receiving the donor flap. Flaps can be created on one or both sides by retracting the elbow fold caudally from the forelimb or the flank fold cranially from the rear limb.

Medial and lateral skin incisions are created along the border of the limb and the incision is carried to the area where the limb is attached to the trunk. Use of the "pinch test" is recommended to assess how large the defect can be and still permit closure. The flap is dissected below the level of the subcutaneous tissue from distal to proximal resulting in a generous U-shaped flap that can be advanced over the wound. The elbow or flank fold flaps can be positioned one in front of the other to cover large defects. It is possible to access by celiotomy the omentum, which can be used in conjunction with the flank folds for reconstructing large inguinal defects. Generally, we prefer to use "active" closed suction drains such as a Jackson-Pratt or Snyder drains rather than Penrose drains to create effective drainage at the recipient site.

It is possible in theory to create flaps from all four limb sites and use them concurrently to close extremely large defects. In theory, these flaps can also be constructed so they can be used to cover defects on the lateral body wall.

The donor site wounds on the forelimb and rear limb are closed with a continuous pattern in the subcutaneous tissue and interrupted sutures in the skin.

REFERENCES

1. Hedlund CS. Principles of plastic and reconstructive surgery. In Fossum TW (ed.): Small Animal Surgery, 3rd ed. St. Louis, MO: Mosby-Elsevier, 2007, pp 211-215.
2. Pavletic M. Pedicle grafts. In Slatter DH (ed.): Textbook of Small Animal Surgery, 3rd ed. Philadelphia: Saunders, 2003, pp 292-321.
3. Hunt GB. Skin fold advancement flaps for closing large sternal and inguinal wounds in dogs and cats. Vet Surg. 1996;24:172-175.

FELINE AXILLARY PATTERN SKIN FLAPS

Don R. Waldron, DVM, Diplomate ACVS and ABVP
Virginia-Maryland Regional College of Veterinary
Medicine, Virginia Tech
Blacksburg, VA

Axial pattern flaps (APF) are a type of pedicle flap that includes a large direct cutaneous artery and vein. The inclusion of a direct cutaneous artery allows movement of a large skin segment that is predictably robust with a large percentage of the flap surviving.

APFs were first reported by Pavletic in the 1980s. Subsequently, many APFs have been described in the canine and feline by various authors. In general, the direct cutaneous vessels of the dog and cat are similar, thus landmarks for construction of the flaps are similar but do have minor variation in regards to lengths of the specific flaps. Some flaps in cats are capable of covering larger defects when compared to the dog especially on the extremities.

General guidelines for construction of axial pattern flaps include the following:

- Carefully consider the appropriate anatomic landmarks for development of each flap.
- Position the animal and use the "pinch test" to assess the size of the donor flap that may be constructed and allow closure of the donor site without excessive tension.
- Use of a sterile marking pen is recommended to "map" out the flap to ensure Inclusion of the intended artery. Flaps are usually constructed in a "peninsular" design and rotated into adjacent or more distant defects.
- A "bridge incision" is made to join the donor and recipient sites allowing the flap to be positioned in the created defect. Alternatively, if the flap is to be used more distally, the flap can be "tubed" rather than making a long bridge incision.

The most commonly used APFs, their landmarks in cats, and clinical uses are described here.

CAUDAL SUPERFICIAL EPIGASTRIC APF

The caudal superficial epigastric APF is an extremely versatile flap that is used for closure of defects of the flank, inguinal area, perineum, thigh, and importantly, the rear limbs. This flap when used for reconstruction of the rear limb can extend as far as the tarsus in the cat. In comparison, the flap reaches only to the level of the stifle in the dog.

Landmarks
- Mammary teats, ventral midline,

Incisions/Surgery
- Medial incision caudal ventral midline to include the skin and teats #2, 3, 4.
- Lateral incision two times the distance from nipples to midline ("pinch test")

The flap is dissected from the abdominal wall in the same fashion as performing a mastectomy and rotated into the defect using a "bridge incision" in most cases. The flap is sutured with 3/0 or 4/0 nylon and a padded bandage applied to the recipient site.

THORACODORSAL APF

The thoracodorsal flap is utilized to cover defects of the axilla, thorax, and forelimb. This flap can reach as far as the carpus in the cat but is limited to the olecranon in the dog.

Landmarks
- Spine of the scapula
- Caudal edge of the scapula (shoulder depression)
- Vessel originates in caudal shoulder depression

Incisions/Surgery
- Cranial incision based on acromion and runs parallel and over the spine of the scapula to the midline if necessary.
- Caudal incision two times the distance from the acromion to the shoulder depression and the same distance caudal to the depression and the incision parallel to the original incision. Either a bridge incision or "tubing" is utilized to place the flap on the forelimb or other locations.
- Ventral limit from acromion through axilla.

CAUDAL AURICULAR APF

This flap is based on the caudal auricular artery, which originates in the depression just caudal to the ear and supplies the lateral cervical skin. The flap is useful for reconstruction of the lateral and dorsal (temporal) facial areas.

Landmarks
- Caudal auricular depression
- Dorsal midline
- Ventral midline
- Rostral edge of scapula caudally

Incisions/Surgery
The flap is based rostrally at the caudal edge of the ear. Take care to do the "pinch test" to assure closure of the donor site. Sometimes the donor site is closed as a "Y" on each end and linearly in the middle.

SUPERFICIAL TEMPORAL APF

This flap is useful for facial reconstruction especially defects involving the orbit and rostral facial area.

Landmarks
- Zygomatic arch
- Caudal orbit
- Rostral pinnal area

Incisions/Surgery
The flap is based on the zygomatic arch ipsilaterally and may extend across the temporal area to the

contralateral arch. Use the "pinch test" to determine the width of the flap that may be constructed.

CAUDAL ARTERY APF

This flap consists of the skin from the tail that is preserved after "deboning" the tail by amputation. The skin of the tail is supplied by two arteries that course in the lateral skin. The flap may be used for defects in the perineal area, tail head area, or caudal rear limb.

Landmarks/Surgery
- Base of the tail

A linear incision is made on EITHER the dorsal or ventral midline over the length of the tail. The incision is made dorsally for dorsal defects and ventrally for ventral defects. The skin flap is then dissected free of the caudal vertebrae and the tail amputated at the base preserving the skin flap. The flap is moved into the recipient defect and sutured with 3/0 or 4/0 nylon.

NASAL PLANUM RESECTION IN THE CAT

Don R. Waldron, DVM, Diplomate ACVS
Virginia-Maryland Regional
College of Veterinary Medicine
Blacksburg, VA

Neoplasia of the nasal planum in cats is relatively common. Although various timors including fibrosarcoma affect the nasal planum the most common tumor is squamous cell carcinoma (SCC). This disease is most common in cats with lightly pigmented skin and may affect the pinna of the ears in addition to the nasal planum. Non-neoplastic disease of the nasal planum, such as eosinophilic granuloma complex also occurs so an appropriate incisional deep biopsy of the suspected lesion for histologic diagnosis is indicated prior to definitive surgery.

BIOLOGY, CLINICAL SIGNS, AND CLINICAL ASSESSMENT OF FELINE SCC

Nasal planum SCC typically begin as erythematous, crusty erosions or ulcerations on the nasal planum. These erosions typically are present for weeks to months as the disease develops. The median age for the disease was reported as 12.5 years in one study involving 61 cases.

Once SCC is present, the lesion may be carcinoma in situ, superficial SCC, or deeply invasive SCC. The disease is locally invasive but rarely metastasizes to lymph nodes or lungs.

General anesthesia is necessary for incisional biopsy of the suspected lesion. Prior to anesthesia, thoracic radiographs are taken although pulmonary metastasis is regarded as rare. Routine blood work including FeLV status is appropriate during the clinical workup. In the study cited above, 13 of 61 cases had other disease processes such as diabetes, hyperthyroidism, cardiomyopathy, or renal disease.

Computed tomography (CT) and magnetic resonance imaging (MRI) may be useful imaging techniques for determining the depth of tumor invasion of the nasal planum.

TREATMENT OPTIONS

Several modalities including radiation, photodynamic therapy, intralesional chemotherapy, laser surgery, and conventional surgery have been used with varying success in treating nasal planum SCC. Many cats will respond positively to some of the above therapeutic modes but cure of the disease is most likely with surgical resection of the nasal planum and rostral conchal cartilage as needed.

A 360-degree incision is made around the nasal planum and into the nasal cavity and skin. Bleeding is typically profuse and suction and local blotting are used to allow visualization of the surgical field. A 360-degree purse-string type of nylon or polyprolene suture may be placed in the skin around the periphery of the lesion. The purse-string should not be tied too tightly or stricture of the surgical site may result. Alternatively, simple interrupted sutures may be placed around the periphery of the lesion.

I have no experience with laser excision of the nasal planum but likely its use would result in decreased hemorrhage during resection.

SURGICAL RESULTS

The suture (s) is removed in 14 days and any scab/crust also removed while the cat is sedated. Complications such as stricture of the newly created nares seem uncommon. If stricture occurs, reoperation, placement of silastic stents and placement of metallic stents have been reported.

Median survival times of cats with SCC of the nasal planum undergoing surgery are approximately 673 days and days. Interestingly, it seems that "dirty margins" may not necessarily be significant. Nevertheless, attaining clean surgical margins continues to be the goal of surgical resection.

MARINE MAMMALS AS SENTINELS FOR OCEANS AND HUMAN HEALTH

Gregory D. Bossart, VMD, PhD
Center for Coastal Research–Marine Mammal Research and Conservation Program
Harbor Branch Oceanographic Institution, Ft. Pierce, FL

As the effects of global climate change become better understood, concern is being raised about the health of the Earth's aquatic ecosystems. This concern is particularly prevalent in the United States, where more than half the human population now inhabits coastal freshwater or marine ecosystems. The concept of marine sentinel organisms may provide one way of evaluating aquatic ecosystem health. Such sentinels are used to gain early warnings about current or potential negative trends and impacts. In turn, such indicators and warnings will permit us to better characterize and potentially manage negative impacts on human and animal health associated with our oceans.

Marine mammals are sentinels for oceans and human health because many species have long life spans, are typically long-term coastal residents, feed at a high trophic level and have unique fat stores that can serve as depots for anthropogenic toxins. In addition, marine mammals are charismatic megafauna that typically stimulate a human behavioral response and are thus more likely to be observed. Similarly, diseases that impact these species may make humans more likely to pay attention to ocean health issues. The threats to marine mammals are ultimately related to the size, growth rate, consumption patterns and behaviors of humans. Therefore, it is in our own best interest to determine marine mammal health patterns that could potentially impact our own well being.

Marine mammal sentinel species include the Californian sea lion (*Zalophus californianus*), Atlantic bottlenose dolphin (*Tursiops truncatus*), southern sea otter *(Enhydra lutris nereis)*, bowhead whale (*Balaena mysticetus*), polar bear (*Ursus maritimus*), and the endangered West Indian manatee (*Trichechus manatus latirostris*).

INFECTIOUS DISEASE

Newly documented complex diseases involving emerging infectious and neoplastic components are being reported in some marine mammal species. In turn, these diseases may provide important information on aquatic ecosystem health. For example, approximately 20% of sexually mature stranded California sea lions have an unusually high incidence of a newly described urogenital cancer, which is associated with a novel herpesvirus, as well as exposure to anthropogenic contaminants such as PCBs and DDTs that persist in the sea lion's feeding grounds. Genetically inbred sea lions, and those with a specific MHC genotype, are more likely to develop urogenital cancer. In addition, orogenital neoplasia associated with another novel herpesvirus and papillomavirus recently was reported in coastal Atlantic bottlenose dolphins in Florida (Figure 1). It is suspected that this latter disease may be associated with environmentally associated immunologic suppression. These data suggest that interactions occur among genes, anthropogenic toxins, immunologic factors and/or viruses in these common marine mammals that share a coastal environment with humans.

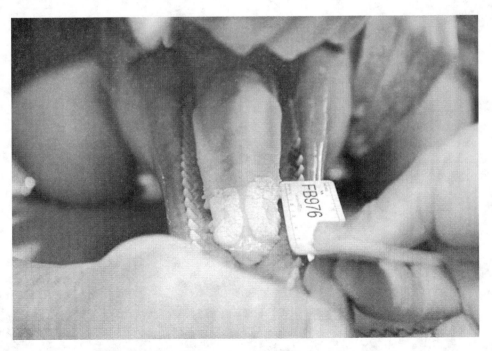

Figure 1. A novel oral sessile papilloma in a free-ranging Atlantic bottlenose dolphin discovered as part of a dolphin health assessment program in Florida.

. Toxoplasmosis is a major cause of mortality among southern sea otters and is potentially fatal to humans. A recent seroprevalence analysis to *Toxoplasma gondii* showed infection in 52% of beachcast sea otters, and 38% in live sea otters, sampled along the California coast. As coastal predators, otters serve as sentinels of marine ecosystem pathogenic protozoans since they share the same environment and consume some of the same foods as humans. Investigations of the pathogenesis of sea otter *T. gondii* infections provide crucial information of terrestrial parasite flow and the emergence of disease at the interface between wildlife, domestic animals and humans.

We recently reported the emergence lobomycosis in epidemic proportions in a free-ranging Florida bottlenose dolphin health assessment study along Florida's Atlantic coast (Figure 2). Lobomycosis is a rare chronic mycotic disease of the skin and subcutaneous tissues caused by a yeast-like organism known as *Lacazia loboi* (formerly *Loboa loboi*). The organism has not been cultured to date in vitro; therefore, diagnosis depends on identification of the characteristic yeast-like cells in tissue or exudates. Dolphins and humans are the only species known to be naturally susceptible to infection with *Lacazia loboi*. The reasons for the emergence of this rare disorder are unclear, but data indicate that the disease may be associated with an immunosuppressive co-factor of environmental origin. Emerging diseases of marine mammals are particularly sensitive to environmental perturbations, whether of anthropogenic or natural origins. Thus, these dolphins may serve as a sentinel species for a public health hazard. Limited evidence exists to suggest that lobomycosis may be transferred from infected animals to people. However, the high prevalence of lobomycosis in the dolphin population of this Florida coastal region, which is used extensively for recreational purposes, raises concerns for zoonotic or common source transmission.

ANTHROPOGENIC TOXINS

Polar bears, bowhead whales, and bottlenose dolphins can serve as direct sentinels for coastal ecosystem pollution. Organohalogens and heavy metal contaminant bioaccumulation among polar bears and bowhead whales may reflect Arctic Ocean health. In turn, many Alaska residents are dependent upon marine resources and a distinct human relationship exists with polar bear health since both species feed on similar prey and the polar bear itself is consumed.

Bottlenose dolphins reside in ocean, coastal, and estuarine communities, and are exposed to a variety of persistent pollutants. Bottlenose dolphins from the eastern US coast and the Gulf of Mexico have a coastal habitat and many are year-round residents in waters surrounded by human activity. Elevated organohalogen compounds have been found in dolphins from this region including PCBs and organochlorine pesticides and polybrominated diphenyl ethers (PBDEs) in blubber and perfluoro alkyl compounds (PFCs) in liver. Interestingly, an increase in dolphin tissue PFCs concentrations was found in a free-ranging health assessment study to occur within a 2-year period from 2003 to 2005 with mean concentrations increasing 1.3-fold in plasma from dolphins inhabiting coastal waters of Charleston, South Carolina and 2.3-fold in plasma from dolphins inhabiting the coastal waters of east-central Florida. As apex

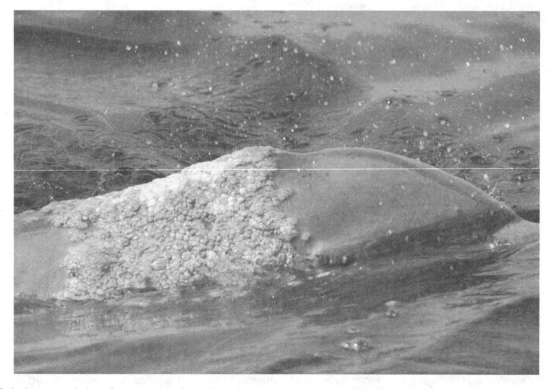

Figure 2. Lobomycosis in a free-ranging Atlantic bottlenose dolphin from Florida.

predators, marine mammals, such as dolphins, have extensive fat stores and have been known to accumulate high levels of persistent organic lipophilic pollutants. During periods of fasting, starvation, lactation, or other physiological demands, stored blubber lipids may be mobilized which may not only potentially redistribute known chemicals such as PCBs but now also the PFCs. This increase in PFCs is of concern in these dolphin populations as well as the coastal human population that are exposed to the same toxins.

HARMFUL ALGAL BLOOMS

Harmful algal blooms (HABs), and the potent neurotoxins they produce, are associated with mass mortalities of dolphins, sea lions and manatees. The range of biotoxins produced by HABs is extensive and these toxins directly or indirectly impact human health. Biotoxins associated with HABs includes: brevetoxins, the cause of neurotoxic shellfish poisoning; saxitoxins, the cause of paralytic shellfish poisoning; okadaic acid, the cause of diarrhetic shellfish poisoning; and others. The HAB problem is significant, growing worldwide and poses a major threat to human and ecosystem health and marine mammals appear to be good sentinels for the ecosystem and public health effects of HABs.

Recent often unprecedented endangered Florida manatee and Atlantic bottlenose dolphin epizootics have been associated with potent marine neurotoxins known as brevetoxins, which are produced by the 'red tide' dinoflagellate *Karenia brevis*. Brevetoxins are known to kill large numbers of fish and cause illness in humans who ingest toxic filter-feeding shellfish (neurotoxic shellfish poisoning) or inhale toxic aerosols. The pathogenesis of brevetoxicosis is suspected to involve direct inhalation of toxins (in manatees) or ingestion of toxins in food sources (in manatees and dolphins). Important new data indicate that brevetoxin vectors such as seagrasses can result in delayed or remote manatee exposure causing intoxication in the absence of toxin-producing dinoflagelates. Thus, unexpected toxin vectors may account for manatee deaths long after or remote from a dinoflagellate bloom. Diagnosis of brevetoxicosis is typically by exclusion and may be based on pathologic findings and postmortem demonstration of the toxins in fluids and tissues. Immunohistochemical staining is used to determine the presence, abundance and distribution of brevetoxins in tissues. The present data suggest that manatee mortality resulting from brevetoxicosis may not necessarily be acute but occur after chronic inhalation and/or ingestion and involve the release of inflammatory mediators that result in fatal toxic shock. The inhalational route of brevetoxin exposure appears to be unique in marine mammals but shared with humans. Increases in human pulmonary emergency room diagnoses are temporally related to 'red tide' occurrences, which may be increasing in frequency along Florida coastlines.

Marine mammals are proving to be good sentinels for oceans and human health due to their many unique natural attributes. New opportunities for interdisciplinary and multi-institutional studies are emerging for utilizing marine mammal sentinel species and this approach will undoubtedly expand as new species are evaluated. As well, this approach provides a new avenue for better understanding the interface between intriguing ecosystem and public health issues.

REFERENCES

1. Bossart GD. Marine mammals as sentinel species for oceans and human health. Oceanography. 2006; 19(2): 44-47.
2. Bossart GD. The Florida manatee: on the verge of extinction? J Am Vet Med Assoc. 1999; 214:10-15.
3. King DP, Hure MC, Goldstein T, et al. Otarine herpesvirus-1: a novel gammaherpesvirus associated with urogenital carcinoma in California sea lions (*Zalophus californianus*). Vet Microbiol. 2002; 2277:1-7.
4. Ylitalo GM, Stein JE, Hom T, et al. The role of organochlorines in cancer-associated mortality in California sea lions (*Zalophus californianus*). Marine Pollution Bull. 2005; 50: 30-39.
5. Bossart GD, Ghim S, Rehtanz M, et al. Orogenital neoplasia in Atlantic bottlenose dolphins (*Tursiops truncatus*). Aquatic Mammals. 2005; 31(4): 473-480.
6. Acevedo-Whitehouse K, Gulland FMD, Greig D, Amos W. Disease susceptibility in California sea lions. Nature. 2003; 422:35.
7. Conrad P, Kreuder C, Mazet J, et al. Linkages between cats, run-off and brain disease in sea otters. Symposium, Marine Mammals on the Frontline: Indicators for Ocean and Human Health. American Association for the Advancement of Science, St. Louis, Missouri, February 18, 2006.
8. Reif JS, Mazzoil M, McCulloch SD, et al. Lobomycosis in Atlantic bottlenose dolphins (*Tursiops truncatus*) from the Indian River Lagoon, Florida. J Am Vet Med Assoc. 2006; 228: 104-108.
9. O'Hara TM, Hoekstra PF, Hanns C, et al. Concentrations of selected persistent organochlorine contaminants in store-bought foods from northern Alaska. Int J Circumpolar Health. 2005; 64:303-313.
10. Bossart GD, Baden DG, Ewing RY, Roberts B, Wright SD. Brevetoxicosis in manatees (*Trichechus manatus latirostris*) from the 1996 epizootic: gross, histologic and immunohistochemical features. Toxicol Pathol. 1998; 26:276-282.
11. Flewelling LJ, Naar JP, Abbott JP, et al. Red tides and marine mammal mortalities. Nature. 2005; 435:755-756.

SWIM WITH THE FISHES: GETTING STARTED WITH PET FISH IN PONDS

Helen E. Roberts, DVM
Aquatic Veterinary Services of Western New York, PC
Orchard Park, NY

The practice of companion animal aquatic practice (pet fish) is a growing segment in today's private practice sector. According to the APPMA (American Pet Products Manufacturers Association) 2005-2006 National Pet Owners Survey, Americans own 139 million freshwater fish and 9.6 million saltwater fish. These owners are all potential clients! Most patients presented to a private practice are pond fish, goldfish and koi, averaging 70% in most fish practices.

Building a pond fish practice requires an understanding of the potential clients and their needs; increasing the public awareness of aquatic veterinary services that can be offered through marketing and networking; a small investment in some additional equipment; and continuing education of the interested practitioner.

CLIENT DEMOGRAPHICS AND NEEDS

The average small animal hospital dog and cat client probably has fish in aquariums, and may have ornamental ponds with fish (Figure 1). Most veterinary hospitals are unaware of these "unlisted" patients simply because they have never inquired. Most fish owners still seek advice for their fish health concerns from the original source of their fish including pond supply and water garden centers, pet stores, and their pond-owning neighbor.

Similar to other exotic pet owners, most pond fish hobbyists are very Internet savvy. In fact, a majority of their husbandry information may derive from online sources such as hobbyist message boards, live chats, and forums. Examples of Koi and goldfish hobbyist message boards include:

- www.koiphen.com
- http://www.koivetforums.com/forums/index.php
- http://members4.boardhost.com/koimag/
- http://www.thegab.org

A small percentage of pond fish owners, particularly koi owners, belong to a koi and pond club. The Associated Koi Clubs of America has a complete list of all member clubs on its Web site, www.akca.org. A club typically meets once monthly. At a meeting members share their experience, listen to speaker lecture on a pond related topic, and exchange ideas, livestock, and plants. The Goldfish Society of America fills a similar niche for goldfish owners. Their website is www.goldfish society.org.

Pond fish owners thirst for information that helps them maintain healthy pets and prevent disease outbreaks. Unfortunately, many receive inaccurate or incomplete information from their current sources. An aquatic veterinarian can offer these services and much more. Education, as with other exotic pet owners, is an integral part of the diagnosis and treatment of sick fish. Once owners are educated in the advantages of working with a veterinarian for their fish health issues, these owners often become long-term clients.

MARKETING

Development of a fish practice will require marketing. Many fish owners, and some veterinarians, are unaware that aquatic animal veterinary practitioners exist. Although some practitioners may be reluctant or apprehensive to market themselves, marketing yourself locally in the community can be critical to the success or failure of your new niche practice. The most efficient way to begin treating pet fish is to add this service to an existing exotic or small and exotic animal practice. A simple way to show your interest is with an aquarium (or several) and/or a small pond in the waiting room (Figure 2). A display or sign describing your willingness to treat pet fish, the names and ages of the fish in the tank or

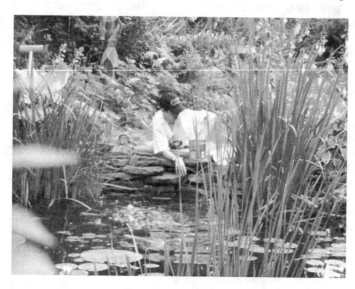

Figure 1. The author's son hand feeding fish in their backyard pond.

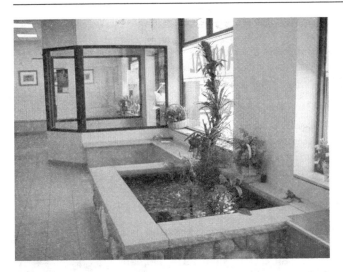

Figure 2. Waiting room pond at the author's practice, 5 Corners Animal Hospital in Orchard Park, NY.

pond, and a description of the equipment can be used to market this service to existing clientele. In our practice, we have a naming contest for any new fish added to the pond. We have found that feeding the fish is something the clients' children look forward to doing. We even have clients and their children stop by just to feed the fish!

Clients do notice changes in the tank or pond. It is very important that the pond or tank be aesthetically pleasing and appears healthy. Sick fish should be removed, if possible, or an explanation of their illness should be given to the receptionist detailing the problem and treatment efforts for the invariable client questions. Our practice has found clients will often call to see how "Spot" is doing! It is an advantage to purchase fish that are not unique in appearance. This helps when the need arises to replace them due to disease or other mishap. Although the pretty white goldfish with the heart shaped mark becomes a favorite with clients and staff, it is hard to duplicate. Quarantine of new additions is essential to reduce the incidence of disease and prevent widespread mortalities in your population. The water should be clear and free of algae. I have visited several practices that display filthy tanks with sick fish. Some clients may wonder about the quality of health care given to their own pets if the veterinarians' "pets" do not appear healthy.

Announcing your services to local veterinarians is another effective way to market your new practice or new interest. Many practitioners are unwilling, either through lack of time, knowledge or desire, to practice veterinary medicine on fish. Start by sending a letter out to all your colleagues and include referral forms and history questionnaires that can be completed by the client. I send referral forms to most practices in my area, particularly the ones who offer exotic animal services. It is not unusual for the veterinarians in the area to ask your advice for their own fish!

In order to be able to practice aquatic medicine, it is important to reach your target audience. Water garden centers, niche koi dealers, and pet stores are the most common sources of fish health advice for the public. This is where the client originally purchased the pet(s). It is a good idea to try and develop a relationship with these businesses. Many stores will be relieved to refer these people to you, particularly after a few over the counter remedies have failed. Do not underestimate the experience some employees and owners of these businesses have. They can be a great resource on the most current equipment available, trends in the industry, husbandry information, and unique information on certain species. In many cases, they may become clients themselves. Through diplomatic interactions, referrals will usually increase. Acknowledge the referral by sending the client back to the same retail center to purchase any over the counter needs and equipment if relevant. Develop a professionally appearing clinic brochure with your logo that can be given to their customers. Many of the locally owned businesses offer seminars to their customers. This is very common with koi dealers and water garden centers. Offer to give a seminar on fish health and how veterinarians can be an integral part of their fish keeping experience.

Joining the tropical fish club or local pond club in your area is a great way to meet fish enthusiasts. The Associated Koi Clubs of America (AKCA) has a complete listing of pond clubs on their Web site (www.akca.org). The AKCA will also list veterinarians who treat fish (specifically koi) on their site. Pond and tropical fish clubs are a great way to meet potential clients and learn more about this interesting hobby. Fish hobbyists are very knowledgeable about their pets and related accessories or equipment so be sure to take the time to listen and learn from them. The clubs have regular seminars and speakers at their meetings, this is a great opportunity to talk about your practice and what you can offer them.

The widespread establishment of the Internet in our society can help the beginning pet fish veterinarian. Web sites, message boards, and forums by the hundreds exist for pond fish, especially koi. Site may also have listings for fish veterinarians, such as www.fishdoc.net and www.akca.org. You can "lurk" or post on some message boards to get an idea of the common problems fish owners are dealing with.

The aquatic veterinarian and diagnostic lab database (www.aquavets.com) is another excellent resource. The database allows users to perform searches that pools information on aquatic veterinarians and diagnostic laboratories. Users can easily search by species, disease, location and other categories to quickly scan the 2,300 veterinarians and 110 diagnostic laboratories in the system. The database was developed in response to the growing demand by pet fish owners, aquaculture stakeholders and industry, and veterinarians for access to aquatic animal practitioners. The URL may change soon but users should have ample advance warning and be directed to the new site.

Finally, develop a "fishy" logo for the aquatic portion of your practice or add fish to your existing logo. Once you have a few fish clients, you will be amazed at the word of mouth referrals you may get.

NETWORKING AND CONTINUING EDUCATION

A new organization that hopes to serve and advocate for veterinarians in aquatic animal medicine has been recently incorporated. More information can be found at www.aquavets.org.

With interest in pet fish medicine increasing, many national and regional veterinary conferences are now including lecture sessions on aquatic animal medicine. Several veterinary schools and other universities also offer short week or weekend courses. Online education courses are available through Veterinary Information Network (VIN) and a few universities including Kentucky State University, www.kyvu.org. Due to the unique nature of fish health, educational opportunities also exist outside traditional veterinary venues. The American Fisheries Society Fish Health Section (AFS FHS) lists many fish health related meetings on their Web site, http://web.fisheries.org/units/fhs/.

SPECIAL EQUIPMENT NEEDS

Pond fish practice requires ambulatory visits. Some cases may need to be hospitalized or examined in the hospital but the best assessment of pond fish health is seeing the fish and the environment they live in. Most equipment required is already present in small animal hospitals such as glass slides, coverslips, syringes, needles, and surgical instruments. Ambulatory equipment should be fairly sturdy (or packed well) and easily transported pondside. A wheeled tool box (for example, Husky®, available from Home Depot; Figure 3) with two drawers and a removable top section makes an ideal mobile equipment carrier. The tool box will fit in most SUVs or trucks and keeps equipment from getting lost or damaged in a moving vehicle. The tool box should be strapped down to prevent mishaps.

Because a majority of fish disease situations involve poor water quality; reliable, accurate water testing kits are required for ambulatory calls. Some recommended choices are: Hach Fish Farmers Water Quality Test Kit (a freshwater kit that tests ammonia, nitrite, pH, dissolved oxygen, alkalinity, total hardness and carbon dioxide-FF-1A, www.hach.com), a hydrogen sulfide test kit, a chlorine test kit, a copper test kit and an electronic salinity meter (0.1–10.00 ppt). For some marine water chemistry parameters, additional test kits may be required. Initial purchasing can be quite confusing so be sure to contact customer support. Most of the author's water testing kits are from Hach or LaMotte (www.lamotte.com) and she has found their customer support to be very good.

Most external parasites found on skin and gill scrapes will not survive on the slide for a trip back to the office, a microscope that can be easily transported is essential for onsite diagnostic cytology. An example of a good scope to have for pond calls is the Field Microscope (FM31 series) by Swift. Several size capture nets and bowls should be on hand, including a sock net for koi capture. These nets and bowls must be able to be cleaned and disinfected between pond calls. Plastic containers of various sizes with lids can be used for examining, sedating, and treating fish on site (Figure 4). They can also double as equipment storage between calls. A field surgery "pack" should include sterile instruments, sterile gloves, biopsy specimen jars, anesthesia (MS-222, Finquel®, www.argent-labs.com) and an anesthesia holding chamber with a fluid delivery system. Dermal masses, lacerations, and fin tears are the most common surgical procedures that can easily be treated pondside with a portable surgery kit.

Starting a pond fish practice can be challenging but the rewards of treating these animals are great. The need is growing and more practitioners will be asked to care for "wet pets" in the future. With a few small changes and a moderate investment in equipment, it is easy to get started.

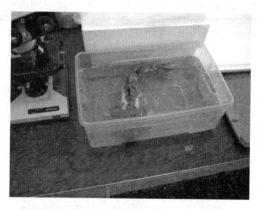

Figure 4. A koi ready to undergo anesthesia for a dermal mass removal performed pond side.

REFERENCES

1. American Pet Products Manufacturers Association (APPMA) 2005-2006 National Pet Owners Survey (NPOS).
2. Roberts HE. Aquatic medicine for the exotic practitioner. Exotic DVM. 2005;7(3):87-91.
3. Francis-Floyd, R. Incorporating Pet Fish Into Your Small Animal Practice. University of Florida, Institute of Food and Agricultural Sciences, Gainesville. Fact Sheet VM 147. Available: http://edis.ifas. ufl.edu/VM108 (August 2007).
4. Lewbart, GA. Emergency and critical care of fish. Vet Clin North Am Exot Anim Pract, 1998;1:233-250.

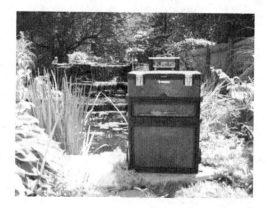

Figure 3. A portable toolbox easily holds equipment for pond calls.

LIFE SUPPORT SYSTEMS FOR POND FISH

Helen E. Roberts, DVM
Aquatic Veterinary Services of Western New York, PC
Orchard Park, NY

Pond keeping, and subsequently the keeping of pond fish, is on the rise nationwide. A backyard pond can be anything from a simple liner filled hole with a crude filter to an investment of several hundred thousand dollars involved an intricate network of PVC, water, waterfalls, and faux rocks. As with other areas involving the combination of art and technology, life support equipment for ponds is a constantly evolving market. In addition to being able to assess the health of the pond inhabitants, it is important to recognize key elements in a pond's design. Not only does equipment knowledge lend you credibility in the eye of the client, this knowledge allows the clinician to make educated evaluation of the adequacy of the equipment. Life support system evaluation involves assessing the pond location, construction materials, volume and size of the pond for current population, and filtration and other equipment present.

LOCATION, LOCATION, LOCATION

Typically, ponds are placed where the homeowner can enjoy them the most. Ponds are usually constructed close to the house, near a viewing window or next to (or incorporated into) a deck design. The site should be assessed for potential rainwater runoff, predator access, amount of sunlight and shade, possibility for falling debris, leaves, etc. into pond. The author has seen cases where ornamental copper flashing on a roof created copper toxicity after a period of heavy rains. Rain ran over the copper flashing and accumulated to toxic levels in the water, causing fish deaths. Long-term rated (25–50 year) roofing shingles can contain a copper based algaecide which may also contribute to water toxicity. Ponds constructed near fences can have potential for future problems. Treated lumber and paint or stain may contain toxic additives that can leach into the water. The pond owner should be advised to use extreme caution when repainting or restaining a fence adjacent to the pond.

Trees near a pond can provide excessive amounts of shade in northern climates preventing full growth of the aquatic plants. Leaf debris and pine needles will easily clog a mechanical filter if not removed by the pond owner on a regular basis during the fall.

Electric supply for the pumps, filters, and air hoses should be safe and not an obstruction to traffic. Long extension cords and non GFI based outlets can pose a hazard to both the fish and the owner.

An area to easily do water changes or drain the pond without excessive flooding issues is invaluable. Most pond designs do not account for water changes, drainage and full cleaning, and capture of the fish. Hiding areas of rock, PVC, and other materials can be useful to the fish when evading predators but also serve well to "protect" them from the fish veterinarian.

The margins of the pond should be evaluated for ease of predator access. Ornamental ponds are seen as an easily accessible buffet by many predators. Stone "beaches" are very appealing but make the pond inhabitants an easy meal for wading birds of prey such as herons. Mink, raccoons, domestic cats, and predatory birds are a few examples of pond predators. Heron decoys, pond netting, motion-activated water sprinklers, and low voltage electric fencing may reduce or eliminate predator access.

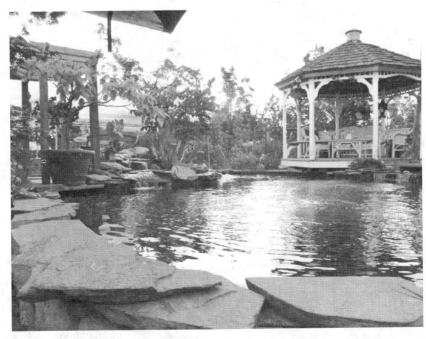

Figure 1. Pond built incorporating existing deck and gazebo. Photo courtesy of Walt Oldenberg.

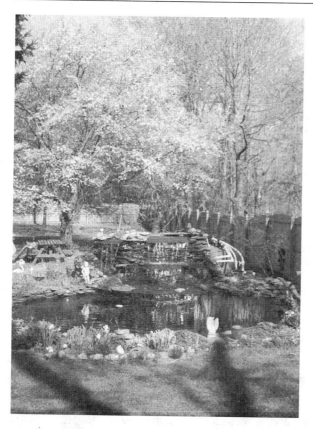

Figure 2. The author's 11, 000 gallon backyard pond

POND CONSTRUCTION MATERIALS

Modern ornamental ponds are constructed using plastic, high density polyethylene (HDPE), rubber or PVC liners; concrete or Gunnite; spray on polyurea liners; preformed ponds of UV treated PVC or plastic; and fiberglass. Each material has its own advantages and disadvantages. Construction materials may have tendencies to leak (especially liners), be easily chewed or gnawed on by rodents, crack (concrete, Gunnite) with earth movement, and generally deteriorate over time due to constant exposure to the elements.

SIZE AND VOLUME

Most pond owners will, over time, develop high stocking densities. The owners either acquire too many fish or purchase fish that grow larger than they anticipated. Some strains or lines of koi can get over three feet in length. Zoos, aquariums, and pet stores often receive requests to take or trade in fish that are too large. Goldfish tend to breed frequently and have a high fecundity. It is not unusual to start with half a dozen goldfish and end up with several hundred in a year or less. Fish <u>can</u> be kept at high densities for short times, such as in commercial aquaculture systems but most owners do not adapt their equipment to meet the high demands. Many pond owners who build a small pond initially go on to build a larger pond or two. In fact, there is a cautionary saying among hobbyists, "Build your last pond first."

Large fish, such as koi, seem to be healthier in ponds with larger volumes and depth. A rule of thumb such as an inch per gallon, does not apply well to large fish, assuming it was accurate for smaller fish. The author recommends a conservative 500 to 1000 gallons per koi to pond owners. One of the reasons for the conservative number is that pond owners will often push any volume given to the limit!

The required depth of the pond varies with geographical location and climate. In northern climates where freezing occurs and fish are to be left to over winter in a pond, it must be of a minimum depth determined by the frost line. In the author's region, Western New York, the recommended minimum pond depth is three feet. For ponds with fish that winter indoors, the depth may be less.

Minimum depth is a consideration in warmer climates also. Ponds that are too shallow in any region can experience severe and rapid temperature fluctuations that can adversely affect fish health. Minimum depth requirements should be used to prevent heat stress.

FILTRATION

Filters, regardless of type or style, mainly perform the same functions. Filters are used for mechanical filtration (removal of large particulate matter, settled waste products or solids and suspended solids from the water); biological filtration (by provide a high density surface area for colonization by nitrifying bacteria for nitrogenous waste removal); and chemical filtration (ultraviolet sterilization, carbon pads, zeolites).

Filters are usually an external flow through system although some internal filters may be found designed to operate on the same principle as an under gravel filter in home aquariums. Filters receive water from the pond by a gravity fed design or pump-fed design. Pond water is removed from the pond via gravity, a submersible pump, or an external pump and flows into pipes (typically made of PVC). The water may first enter a settling chamber or Vortex chamber (to allow solid waste particles to settle on the bottom and be removed later via a bottom drain) or be channeled through a large filter mat to remove particles (suspended and large). The water may pass through one or more areas containing brushes, and mats designed to remove particles in decreasing size and finally enter a chamber containing biological media. Many companies have designed products for colonization of nitrifying bacteria. These products may look very different and be constructed of different materials but all have a high surface area per volume for bacterial colonization. It is important to realize this is not the only site of biological filtration. Bacteria colonization all surfaces of the pond and equipment including pipes, waterfalls, filter containers, etc.

The owner should be questioned on maintenance of the filters including cleaning, backwashing, and rinsing practices. Evaluate filters for lack of power, leakage, and evidence of poor maintenance including odor and debris accumulation. The water exiting the filters to return to the pond should be examined for heavy particulate accumulation, clarity, and odor. It is not uncommon for poorly maintained filters to be the initiating cause of fish health problems.

Pumps should appear to be in good working order (Figure 3). Leaking pumps can contribute to gas supersaturation and stray voltage issues. Flow rates and retention time (within the filter) should be assessed also. Most ponds turn over one to two times an hour. A pump's listed gph (gallons per hour) may be higher than actual due to the plumbing. A vertical rise ("vertical discharge pressure head") in the flow of pumped water, sharp bends in the pipes, and small diameter pipes may all contribute to lower flow rates. There are several methods a home owner can use to measure the flow rate at different sampling sites in the pond plumbing design. Submersible pumps may contain oil and leak into the pond when seals are damaged.

OTHER EQUIPMENT

The aquatic practitioner should always make a point of observing the area surrounding the pond and the pond equipment storage area for various pieces of equipment, medications, and water treatments. Most koi keepers keep several nets including a large, circular catch net and a sock net. Large air pumps may be used to supply additional aeration to ponds, especially in hot weather.

Ultraviolet lamps ("filters") may be seen in the plumbing design or as a part of a filter unit. Depending on the wattage and water flow rate, they can be used for disinfection, algae control, or microscopic parasite control. Bulbs need to be changed often as with UV bulbs for some reptiles. The owner should know the flow rate and wattage depending on the filter's use and when the UV bulb was last changed. Ozone generators are

sometimes used for disinfection in ponds although its use is not as commonly seen as in indoor aquariums.

Assessment of fish health involves a critical evaluation of the environment and the equipment used to maintain that environment. Without this evaluation, the diagnosis may be incomplete and health problems may not resolve or resolve only to reappear.

REFERENCES

1. Atkinson S (ed.). Garden Pool, Fountains and Waterfalls. Sunset Books, 1997.
2. Wildgoose WH. BSAVA Manual of Ornamental Fish, 2nd ed. British Small Animal Veterinary Association, 2001.

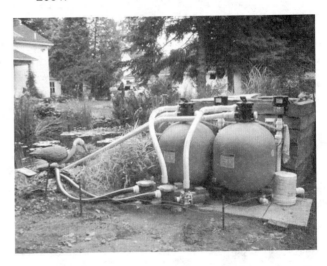

Figure 3. Bubble bead filters and attached pumps on the author's pond.

TREATING NEMO: THERAPEUTIC APPROACHES FOR POND FISH

Helen E. Roberts, DVM
Aquatic Veterinary Services of Western New York, PC
Orchard Park, NY USA

A multimodal, systemic approach should always be used when treating pet fish. Fish health problems are usually multifactorial. Treatment and management of disease may include the use of pharmaceuticals, water additives, pesticides, nutritional support and other management changes, and equipment modification. It is important to identify all the potential causes (stressors) that may have contributed to disease outbreaks.

ENVIRONMENTAL PROBLEMS
Water Quality

Water quality problems, identified by diagnostic water chemistry testing, are corrected with multiple measures. The source water should always be tested in addition to the pond water before pond construction begins. Municipal water should always be dechlorinated or "aged" before use. Well water may be very low in dissolved oxygen concentration, highly alkaline, or contain toxic levels of heavy metals, etc. The author has seen clients use diverted streams as a source for pond water. The possibility of infectious diseases and parasites is very high. Likewise, the effluent discharge from the ornamental pond may contain medications and additives that can harm native fish, invertebrates and plants.

For severe water quality issues, fish may need to be removed and temporarily housed in another pond or large tank. A temporary pond can be made from an inflatable outdoor swimming pool or plastic vats (Figure 1). The temporary facility needs to be monitored for water quality problems and netted to prevent jumping accidents. For accumulations of nitrogenous wastes, such as ammonia and nitrite, water changes are the core to treatment. Additional management changes include: increasing the size and capacity of biofiltration; adding additional aeration; the addition of salt to reduce osmotic stress (Figure 2); reducing or stopping feeding; reducing stocking density; and instruction in proper filter maintenance.

Low dissolved oxygen levels may be seen for a variety of reasons. Corrective measures include: adding aeration; removal of severely affected fish to tanks that can be oxygenated; reducing the water temperature if possible; reduction of feeding and stocking densities; delaying fish movement and additional capture stresses; and repair of faulty equipment if needed.

When toxins are detected in the water, steps should be taken to remove the source of contamination, such as pond ornaments and copper tubing, in addition to the contaminated water. Serial water changes should also be employed.

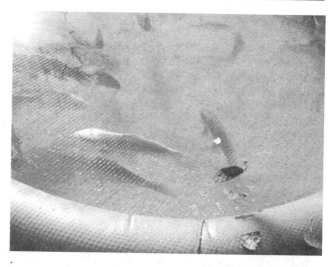

Figure 1. Fish temporarily housed in an inflatable swimming pool during a pond cleaning

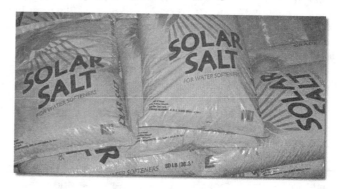

Figure 2. Salt, sodium chloride, is a commonly used additive in the treatment of many fish health problems.

Traumatic Injuries

Most pond owners will have fish that experience traumatic injuries. Traumatic injuries can be traced to poor pond design, predators, careless fish handling, secondary to fish behaviors (flashing and spawning), and inter- or intra-species aggression.

Treatment should include management of the injury, mitigation of risk factors, and medications. Ulcers and other wounds should be debrided under anesthesia. Gentle cleaning of the wound can be done using sterile saline, a dilute povidone-iodine or dilute chlorhexidine solution. Topical medications such as silver sulfadiazine, povidone-iodine ointment and other antibiotic ointments can be applied. The area should be dried with a gauze sponge to increase adherence of the topical treatment. Tricide-Neo® (Molecular Therapeutics, LLC, Athens, GA) solution can be used as a topical spray on infected wounds on a daily or intermittent basis (treatment interval based on severity of the wound and potential capture stress to the patient). Parenteral antibiotics are used if the wound is deep, infected, or involves a wide expanse of tissue. Enrofloxacin 10 mg/kg IM or ICe (Baytril®, Bayer) or ceftazidime 20 mg/kg IM (Fortaz®, GlaxoSmithKline) are good initial choices when indicated. The author also gives a one time injection of carprofen 2.2 to 4.4 mg/kg IM (Rimadyl®, Pfizer Animal Health) for pain management and inflammation when appropriate.

Predator-related injuries indicate the need for changes to the pond layout or surrounding area (Figure 3). Nets can be placed over the pond to prevent easy access to herons (Figure 4). It is best to try to anchor the edges of the net off the ground as snakes and other small pond inhabitants can get tangled in the fabric. Small birds may also get tangled in the netting. Remind the clients that large invertebrates such as dragon flies may not be able to access the pond or leave from under the net once hatched. Alternatively, a low voltage electric fence can be placed around the pond. Herons typically land near the ponds'edge and wade into the pond. A jolt of electricity may deter them and other predators.

Owners may not fully understand the trauma and stress that can be induced by netting and handling. It is important to include client education on proper handling and netting techniques as a part of a treatment plan. Most koi can be gently maneuvered into a capture bowl rather than being suspended in a net. Netting has the potential to damage fins, tails, and remove necessary skin mucus from the fish. Seine nets may be more effective and less stressful than long poled nets for certain species of "nervous" fish such as "Orfe." If a long time has been spent chasing the fish, this will result in additional stress and possible compromise to the fish' health.

The environment needs to be searched for potential harmful objects and ornamentation. "Spitter" statues may be plumbed with copper tubing; decorative rocks and floating ornaments may have sharp edges. Most pond fish are curious and like to explore their surroundings. "Normal" equipment and plumbing such as filter intake pipes can be hazardous. The author has treated traumatized fish that became wedged in intake pipes, trapped in skimmer boxes, and had taken a "ride" through the bottom drain pipe to end up lodged in the pre-filter straining basket!

INFECTIOUS DISEASES

In order to control or limit infections, it is important to discuss quarantine procedures and biosecurity measures with the pond owner (Figure 5). All new livestock or pets (fish, amphibians, and invertebrates) need to be quarantined for a minimum period. Remind the owner never to add the shipping or transport water to the new pond or quarantine system. The author recommends one year quarantine for new koi, although this is very conservative. Most fish can be adequately quarantined for 30 to 90 days. Two approaches are used in quarantine: observation alone and treatment on an as needed basis or observation and the use of a protocol involving prophylactic treatments for parasites and other common problems. New plants need to be dipped in a solution and rinsed before placing in the pond. Potassium permanganate is often used as a dip to remove infectious stages of parasites and other pathogens. Nets and other equipment that can act as

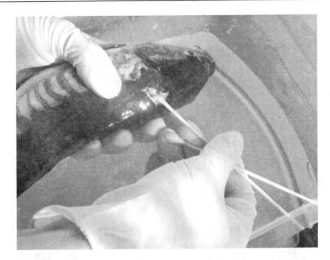

Figure 3. The author debriding and cleaning a heron induced puncture wound on an anesthetized koi.

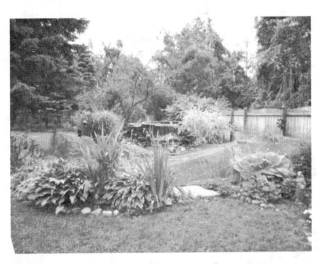

Figure 4. Netting over a pond that has experienced predation by herons.

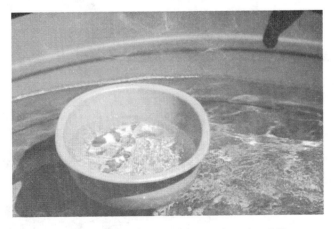

Figure 5. Koi (Kohaku) placed in capture bowl for pre-purchase examination.

fomites should not be shared between ponds. Equipment should be disinfected after use and dried whenever possible.

Both parasites and people can serve as disease vectors. Infestation with some parasites can result in spread of bacterial disease and, possibly, some viral diseases. The owner should be encouraged not to allow people to put their hands in the water if they have visited other ponds, such as on a pond tour day.

The client will often call for treatment advice of a bacterial disease. This frequently occurs after several unsuccessful attempts themselves. Questioning the client on previous medications used is very important. Clients often use a "poly-pharmacy" approach to problems. This practice may actually make the disease situation worse. Most clients do not understand all the possible factors that can predispose fish to disease. What resembles a primary bacterial problem to them may actually be primarily an ectoparasite infestation and poor water quality. For this reason, a physical exam and a site visit should always be part of fish disease treatments.

In general, strict adherence to good water quality management practices and the addition of salt to reduce stress is applied to most disease situations. Specific treatments based on the diagnosis of the problem can be more effective with these practices.

Parasites

Once a parasitic cause of disease has been identified, management changes and medical treatment can be instituted. For example, trichodinosis is often seen on debilitated fish due to other causes such as poor water quality, overcrowding, and other infectious diseases. These stressors need correction if the infestation is to resolve properly. In stressed fish, parasites can be fatal, the "last straw".

It is important to know the life cycle of the parasite in order to effectively treat. Live bearing flukes need multiple treatments to be effective and egg laying flukes need both multiple treatments and a longer duration of treatment. It is also important to know the effects of treatment on the biological filter. Some treatments may adversely affect the filter, killing essential bacteria. On the other hand, some parasite life stages may be located in the filter and treatment would not be complete unless the medication enters the filter. Maintaining excellent water quality remains an integral part of the treatment process.

Bacterial and Viral Diseases

Koi keepers may experience outbreaks of cutaneous ulcer disease. Goldfish and other fish can appear to be "suddenly" septic. Most infections are secondary although primary bacterial pathogens do exist. Stressors that precipitate disease outbreaks include poor water quality, shipping, careless handling, overcrowding and overfeeding, ectoparasites, concurrent viral and other bacterial diseases, hypoxia, predation, and temperature stress. Management of the disease may include drastic husbandry changes in addition to appropriate systemic (and possibly topical) antimicrobials, and other medications. The most common problems the author sees in pet pond fish practice are poor water quality, overcrowding, overfeeding, and ectoparasites. Again, quarantine and biosecurity practices need to be discussed in addition to other management changes.

Although it may be simple to try (and tempting) to dispense the "magic bullet" pharmaceutical for fish disease outbreaks, treatment must include necessary management changes. Treatment failures are common when common stressors are not identified and corrected.

REFERENCES
1. Noga, EJ. Fish Disease: Diagnosis and Treatment. St Louis, MO: Mosby, 1996.
2. Wildgoose, WH. BSAVA Manual of Ornamental Fish, 2nd ed. British Small Animal Veterinary Association, 2001.

TENPUKU: IT'S NOT JUST SUSHI

Helen E. Roberts, DVM
Aquatic Veterinary Services of Western New York, PC
Orchard Park, NY

One of the most frequent client complaints in a pet fish practice is of a buoyancy disorder in fish, primarily fat bodied goldfish. The fish either presents positively buoyant (a "floater") or negatively buoyant (a "sinker"). Most cases can be traced to swim bladder (gas organ, air bladder) disorders but other diseases can have a similar presentation.

ANATOMY

The swim bladder is a retroperitoneal organ derived from gastrointestinal tissue. It is located dorsally, immediately ventral to the posterior kidney in most cyprinid fish. There can be a direct connection from the swim bladder, via the pneumatic duct, to the esophagus (physostomous fish) or no connection (physoclistous fish). Physoclistous fish maintain the appropriate amount of gas in the swim bladder by one or more retia mirabilia. Physostomous fish may also possess a rete mirabile counter current system. The swim bladder can have one (trout), two (goldfish, koi) or three (codfish) lobes. The entire purpose of the swim bladder remains unknown. It does function to maintain proper buoyancy but may also function in detection of pressure fluctuations, detection of sound, production of sound, and respiration.

CLINICAL PRESENTATION

Buoyancy disorders can present with a variety of nonspecific clinical signs including permanent, intermittent, or partially abnormal buoyancy. Fish may be anorectic or have normal appetites, lethargic or active, have evidence of systemic disease, or have mucoid stools. Fat-bodied goldfish such as Ryukins, Orandas, Ranchus, Lionhead, Moors, and Pearlscale varieties are most commonly affected (Figure 1).

ETIOLOGIES

Buoyancy disorders can have multiple etiologies. In a recent retrospective study, necropsy and histopathology on 35 affected goldfish revealed systemic granulomatous disease (23%), fluid in swim bladder (23%), polycystic kidney disease (17%), and other internal diseases (20%). No discernable pathology was found in 17% of the goldfish examined. In addition, poor water quality, low water temperatures, neoplasia, improper diet, pneumatic duct torsion, and congenital abnormalities have also been incriminated.

DIAGNOSTIC APPROACH

All fish with health problems should be evaluated with a standard minimum database including a comprehensive history, indirect and direct physical examination, water quality testing, a direct fecal exam, and exfoliative cytology of the skin and gills. Physical examination may reveal firm or fluctuant abdominal distention.

Additional diagnostics for buoyancy disorders include a neurologic examination, radiography, and ultrasonography. Contrast radiography can be utilized to differentiate the gastrointestinal tract from coelomic organs or masses. It is not unusual to see a missing lobe, hyperinflation or under inflation of a lobe on radiographs. (Figures 2, 3, and 4) Fluid in the swim bladder may also be visible on radiographs. Alternately, the swim bladder may appear normal and other causes such as intestinal gas, ileus, and enteritis may be noted. Polycystic kidney disease may be detected either by ultrasonography or radiographs.

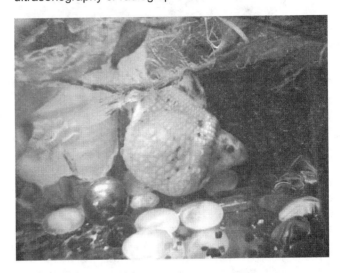

Figure 1. Calico Pearlscale goldfish with typical round bodied appearance.

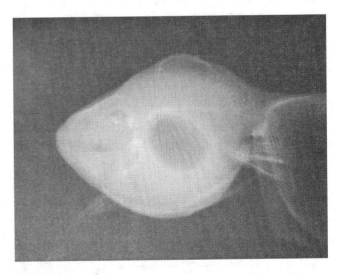

Figure 2. Lack of cranial swim bladder lobe and hyperinflation of remaining lobe in a Ryukin.

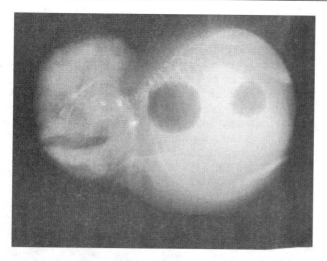

Figure 3. Polycystic kidney disease in an Oranda with secondary displacement of the caudal swim bladder lobe.

Pneumocystocentesis should be performed if fluid accumulation is suspected or visible radiographically or on ultrasound. Any fluid collected should be submitted for cytology, including acid fast staining, and culture.

THERAPEUTIC APPROACH

Underlying water quality issues need to be addressed. Chronic exposure to high nitrate levels has been implicated in some cases of swim bladder abnormalities. Elevated nitrate levels are easy to prevent with monitoring and frequent water changes. Salt can be added at a level of 0.1% to reduce the osmotic gradient and as an aid in stress reduction. The author treated one case where the buoyancy disorder appeared to be idiopathic by slowing raising the water temperature to 75°F. Normal buoyancy was achieved and maintained as long as the water temperature remained stable.

The dietary history should be evaluated, including any supplements and fresh foods given by the client. Intermittent buoyancy has been observed in some fish with the practice of feeding flake food formulations. A change to a sinking pellet may correct the problem. Goldfish can be fed a variety of fresh foods including green vegetables, a small amount of fruit, and shrimp. A commercial herbivorous or omnivorous gel food (Mazuri®, PMI Nutrition International, St. Louis, MO) can be used as base and supplemental food can be mixed in. Fasting for 48 to 72 hours followed by offering a shelled green pea has also been effective in some cases that don't initially respond to dietary management.

Metronidazole, fed at rate of 1% body weight, can be mixed into a gel food and fed exclusively for 14 days. This may be particularly effective in cases of enteritis, even if no parasites were observed in the fecal flotation.

Parenteral antibiotics may be administered if infectious pneumocystitis is suspected or pending aspirated fluid culture results. The author's initial choices are enrofloxacin 10 mg/kg IM or ICe (Baytril®, Bayer) or ceftazidime 20 mg/kg IM (Fortaz®, GlaxoSmithKline).

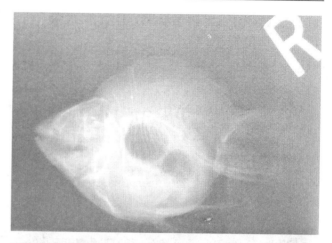

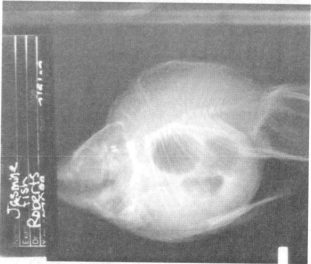

Figure 4. Right (*top*) and left (*bottom*) lateral views of a Ryukin with enteritis and secondary displacement of caudal lobe of the swim bladder.

Various mechanical and surgical methods have been utilized in an attempt to correct abnormal buoyancy including flotation devices, surgically implanted sterile weights, percutaneous pneumocystocentesis, slings, and surgical partial pneumocystectomy.

Buoyancy disorders remain, for the most part, a frustrating, complex disorder. Clients should be aware that full resolution, and even a diagnosis, may not be possible. When a cause can be identified, proper treatment can sometimes to resolution of the abnormal buoyancy.

REFERENCES

1. Lewbart GA. Green Peas for Buoyancy Disorders. Exotic DVM. 2000, 2(2):7.
2. Palmeiro BS. Sink, float or swim: Battling Tenpuku disease (buoyancy disorder) in goldfish. Proceedings AVMA, July 2007.
3. Stoskopf MK. Fish Medicine. Philadelphia: WB Saunders, 1993.
4. Wildgoose WH, Buoyancy disorders of ornamental fish: a review of cases seen in veterinary practice. Fish Vet J. 2007;(9):22-37.

SURGICAL COELOMIC EXPLORATION

Helen E. Roberts, DVM
Aquatic Veterinary Services of Western New York, PC
Orchard Park, NY

Surgical exploration of the coelomic cavity of pet fish is an essential part of any companion aquatic animal practice. Indications include traumatic, penetrating injuries; elective gonadectomy; exploration of the coelomic cavity; coelomic mass removal; and as a method to acquire biopsy samples.

PATIENT SELECTION

Koi and goldfish are relatively hardy fish and make good surgical candidates. As with any species, care should be taken to thoroughly evaluate each patient prior to surgery to maximize survivability and surgical success.

A minimum database (MDB) should be completed in all fish cases. In addition to an extensive verbal history (including questions on appetite, weight loss if applicable, behavior in the pond, duration of presenting problem and prior medical conditions) and a thorough physical examination of the patient, the clinician should also perform water chemistry testing and wet mount cytologic exam for external parasites of the skin and gills. Other diagnostic techniques such as radiography and ultrasonography may help to give further information prior to surgical exploration. Preoperative blood testing can be performed as in other species. In house testing using the Abaxis VetScan® for plasma biochemical values has recently been explored. A packed cell volume (PCV) and total protein should also be evaluated preoperatively. Septic, cachectic, anemic, or lethargic patients do not make good surgical candidates. Stabilization should be attempted whenever possible to reduce the risk of perioperative complications, including death.

The surgeon should be familiar with the normal internal anatomy of the patient. In the event the species presenting is a novel one, anatomy reference texts should be consulted if available.

PREOPERATIVE AND PERIOPERATIVE MEDICATIONS

There is a great deal of debate regarding the ability of fish to perceive pain. It is commonly agreed among fish practitioners that aquatic patients should receive adequate analgesia. Butorphanol 0.4 mg/kg IM (Equanol®, Vedco) is commonly given perioperatively, prior to recovery. Depending on the indication for surgery and anticipated length of surgery, preoperative antibiotics may be used. The author gives 10 mg/kg enrofloxacin IM (Baytril®, Bayer Health Care) or ceftazidime 20 mg/kg IM (Fortaz®, GlaxoSmithKline) when indicated.

ANESTHESIA

Tricaine methanesulfonate or MS-222 (Finquel®, Argent Chemical Laboratories, Redmond, WA and Tricaine-S® (Western Chemical, Ferndale, WA) is currently the only FDA-approved anesthetic for use in finfish. Using a gram scale, weigh the MS-222 powder and sodium bicarbonate (baking soda, Arm and Hammer®) prior to use. A ratio of one part MS-222 is added to two parts sodium bicarbonate to buffer against the acidic effects of MS-222 when used in freshwater. Clients should be advised to bring several one gallon jugs containing water from the patient's pond or tank for use in induction, anesthesia maintenance, anesthesia recovery, and transport home.

Most koi and goldfish can be induced at 100 to 150 mg/L (ppm). The dose should be reduced for debilitated patients. Monitor opercular movements and fish behavior until the desired plane and stage of anesthesia is reached. A surgical plane of anesthesia is usually readily maintained at 50 to 100 mg/L (ppm).

The author's anesthetic "table" with positioning device is shown in Figure 1.

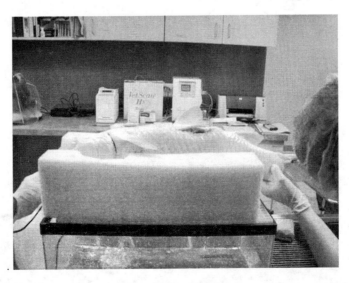

Figure 1. Koi anesthetized and in dorsal recumbency for surgical exploration of the coelomic cavity.

SURGICAL PREPARATION AND APPROACH

A ventral midline approach is the most common technique used for exploration of the fish coelomic cavity. The patient is placed in dorsal recumbency and held using a positioning device or table. In large fish, scales can be gently removed to allow for easier entry. The incision site can be gently cleaned with sterile gauze or a dilute surgical prep solution (povidone-iodine or chlorhexidine). Use of a sterile, clear plastic drape allows the surgeon to better monitor the patient, reduces moisture loss, and helps to prevent contamination of the coelomic cavity. The initial incision is usually made just caudal to the pectoral fins and extending just cranial to the pelvic fins. Care should be taken to not damage the delicate, underlying intestinal tract. The incision can be extended if needed but may require cutting the pelvic girdle. Retractors can provide better visibility as the skin of fish is rigid, unlike most mammals.

SUTURE SELECTION

Results from a suture study in koi show monofilament suture material, such as PDS® (Ethicon) and Maxon® (Tyco Healthcare Group), and nylon cause less tissue reactivity than braided sutures. Closure is generally done in one layer for small fish but may be done in two layers in larger fish, such as mature koi. Fish do not absorb sutures so external sutures need to be removed in 2 to 4 weeks, depending on healing status of the incision.

RECOVERY

The patient should be monitored in a recovery tank until swimming movements have resumed and the fish is ventilating well. Prolonged salt (sodium chloride) immersion at 1 to 3 g/L in the recovery tank may help reduce osmotic stress and potentially aid in healing of the surgical incision. The water should be heated to optimize wound healing. For pond fish, this is generally 20 to 23°C. Water quality should be monitored daily and water changes done as indicated to maintain optimal conditions for healing. A cover or net should be placed over the tank to prevent jumping and further injury. Some practitioners advise the use of a "buddy" fish from the patient's tank to reduce stress and provide companionship.

REFERENCES

1. Fontenot DK, Neiffer DL. Wound management in teleost fish: Biology of the healing process, evaluation and treatment. Vet Clin North Am Exotic Anim Pract. 2004;(7):57-86.
2. Hurty C, et al. Histological evaluation of the tissue reaction to five suture materials in the body wall of koi (Cyprinus carpio). Proc Am Assoc Zoo Vet and Intl Assoc Aquatic Anim Med, 2000.
3. Lewbart GA, et al. Surgical removal of an undifferentiated abdominal sarcoma from a koi carp (Cyprinus carpio). Vet Rec, 1998;(143):556-558.
4. Lewbart GA. Surgical techniques in the Koi patient. Exotic DVM. 2001;(3.3):43-47.
5. Palmeiro BS. Utilizing the Abaxis VetScan® as a Diagnostic Tool in Koi (Cyprinus carpio). Proceedings AVMA Convention, July 2007.
6. Wildgoose WH. BSAVA Manual of Ornamental Fish, 2nd ed. British Small Animal Veterinary Association, 2001.

DIAGNOSTIC EXAMINATION IN PET FISH MEDICINE

Stephen A. Smith, MS, DVM, PhD
Virginia-Maryland Regional College
of Veterinary Medicine
Virginia Polytechnic Institute and State University
Blacksburg, VA

As more time and money are invested into aquarium and ornamental fish, the demand for providing veterinary services for these species has become more widespread. As a result, a number of clinical techniques have been developed for fish that can yield valuable diagnostic information. Most of these techniques are easy to accomplish, relatively inexpensive, and do not require any specialized equipment other than would normally be available in a general veterinary practice. The non-lethal techniques include the skin, fin and gill biopsies, fecal analysis, blood sampling, injection and aspiration techniques, and radiology. Most of the biopsy, bleeding, injection, and aspiration techniques can be performed on fish without the use of anesthesia, although light sedation of the fish often simplifies the task, making the procedure less stressful on both the fish and diagnostician. The lethal technique, or necropsy, can be performed on fish and can either include collection of individual tissues for large fish or preservation of the whole fish for small fish.

FISH SEDATION/ANESTHESIA

Fish should be sedated or anesthetized for any procedure that is painful or stressful on the animal. Depending on the species of fish, the type of procedure, and the desired length of sedation/anesthesia required, fish can be administered a variety of anesthetic agents by a variety of routes including intraperitoneally, intramuscularly, orall,y or via the water. However, the most common method for minor non-lethal procedures is to directly immerse the fish in an aerated, sodium bicarbonate (v/v) buffered anesthetic solution. Tricaine methanesulfonate (MS-222, Finquel®) is the most widely utilized anesthetic agent for this type of administration. As a general rule, sedation is reached in 3 to 5 minutes at 20 to 50 mg MS-222 per liter of water, while surgical anesthesia is reached in 5 to 8 minutes at 50 to 150 mg MS-222 per liter of water. Onset and duration of sedation or anesthesia in a fish is dependent upon on a number of factors including water temperature and the species, size, and general health of the fish. By continuously monitoring the fish for changes in behavior and respiratory activity, the fish can be removed from the anesthetic solution when the desired depth of sedation or anesthesia is reached. When the procedure is finished or in case of anesthetic overdose, the fish can be immediately placed in a separate container of fresh aquarium water for recovery.

FISH HANDLING

To avoid abrasion to the skin and gill tissues, fish should always be handled with latex or vinyl gloves that have been rinsed of all powder or other contaminants. Fish should never be handled with bare hands, or placed on a cloth or paper towel that might absorb moisture from the mucus and skin of the fish.

SKIN BIOPSY

The skin is a primary target organ for many of the infectious pathogens of fish. Therefore, a skin biopsy (or mucus smear) is one of the most useful and commonly acquired samples for diagnosing problems in a fish. A skin biopsy is performed by gently scraping, in a cranial to caudal direction, a small area of the surface of the fish with the edge of a microscope slide coverslip. Care should be taken to use only a minimal amount of pressure to obtain this scraping, since removal of the epithelium or deeper scales damages the skin and can result in osmoregulatory imbalance or secondary bacterial and fungal infections in the fish. The sample should be immediately transferred to a drop of aquarium water (either fresh or salt water depending on the species of fish) on a glass microscope slide and a coverslip carefully applied. This wet mount should then be examined under the compound microscope for the presence of free-swimming, attached, or encysted protozoa, metazoan parasites, fungal hyphae, or bacteria.

FIN BIOPSY

A fin biopsy (or fin snip) is obtained by cutting a small piece of tissue from the edge or tip of one of the fins or tail. The fin snip should be immediately transferred to a drop of aquarium water on a glass microscope slide, the tissue sample spread to its full extent and a coverslip carefully applied. This wet mount should then be examined under the microscope for the presence of protozoan or metazoan parasites, fungal hyphae, or bacterial colonies.

GILL BIOPSY

A gill biopsy (or gill snip) is obtained by inserting the tip of a fine pair of scissors into the branchial (gill) cavity behind the operculum (or gill cover) and cutting off the distal tips of several of the gill lamellae. As only the tips of the lamellae are removed, only a minimal amount of bleeding should occur. The excised gill tissue should be immediately transferred to a drop of aquarium water on a glass microscope slide, the individual elements of the gill tissue separated by teasing the lamellae apart and a cover slip carefully applied. This wet mount should then be examined under the microscope for the presence of protozoan or metazoan parasites, fungal hyphae, or bacterial colonies.

FECAL EXAMINATION

Evaluation of fecal material from fish for the presence of internal parasites is accomplished with techniques similar to those used in terrestrial animals. A fresh fecal sample can be collected with a pipette from either the bottom of the aquarium or hanging from the vent of the fish. If an appropriate sample cannot be acquired from the environment or if examination of a specific individual is desired, the application of gentle pressure on the sides of a netted fish often produces a fecal sample near the vent of the fish. A fecal specimen is generally best examined by placing the material on a glass microscope slide, covering the sample with a coverslip, and observing the material directly with a compound microscope. The fecal specimen can also be processed by standard floatation or sedimentation techniques and evaluated for parasite (coccidia, nematodes, trematodes, cestodes, and acanthocephalans) eggs and larvae.

BLOOD SAMPLING

A non-lethal blood sample can be obtained from fish from the heart, dorsal aorta, or tail using a syringe and needle. Venipuncture of the caudal vessels of the caudal peduncle (tail) can be accomplished via a ventral midline or lateral approach. Fish blood coagulates rapidly and, thus, the use of heparinized syringes and needles and avoidance of tissue fluid contamination are necessary for proper blood sampling. Hematology and serum chemistry can be determined by standard hematologic methodology, but interpretation of values in most species of fish may be difficult at the present time and are of limited value. Some hemoprotozoans may also be identified in the blood of fish.

TISSUE AND FLUID SAMPLING

Celoemic or tissue aspirates can be obtained in fish using techniques similar to those used in terrestrial animals. Sedation or anesthesia facilitates the acquisition of proper samples using these standard techniques and greatly reduces the potential for injury to the fish. Samples can then be evaluated by cytologic, bacteriologic, viral, and/or parasitologic techniques.

IMAGING TECHNIQUES

Radiography has been used in fisheries biology to facilitate the non-destructive examination of the vertebrae, fin rays, and other skeletal elements of fish for morphological description. The use of radiography as a diagnostic tool in aquatic medicine can also provide useful information on the morphology of abnormal or injured fish. Radiography is accomplished by lightly sedating the fish, removing the fish from the anesthetic solution and positioning the fish on a piece of plexiglass, plastic, or Saran wrap covering a film cassette. After the radiographic film is exposed using a high-detail tabletop technique, the fish is immediately returned to a container of fresh aquarium water for recovery from sedation. Alternatively, a fish can be radiographed directly in water using a modified plexiglass restraining box. This technique can reduce the amount of stress on the fish; however, the technique requires a higher dose of x-rays due to the depth of water in the box and generally produces a lower quality image. Digital radiography and special imaging techniques, including xeroradiography, ultrasound, computed tomography (CT), and magnetic resonance imaging (MRI), have also been rapidly gaining acceptance as diagnostic techniques in fish medicine.

FISH EUTHANASIA

Fish can be humanely euthanized with an overdose or prolonged exposure to tricaine methanesulfonate (150 to 200 mg buffered MS-222 per liter of water). Depending on the temperature and concentration of MS-222, this may take as long as 15 minutes for cessation of respiratory and cardio activity. Other compounds that can be used to euthanize fish include benzocaine hydrochloride, 2-phenoxyethanol, carbon dioxide, but not clove oil. Cervical separation behind the head area after sedation/anesthesia is also an acceptable method of euthanasia.

NECROPSY

A necropsy starts with a complete external examination of the fish including skin, fins, eyes, oral and opercular cavities, gills and vent. After collection of external samples (lesions, parasites, and representative gill arch) the internal coelomic cavity and visceral organs can be examined. A small incision is made in the ventral surface of the fish just in front of the pectoral fins and the cut continued caudally along the entire length of the ventrum to the vent. Care should be taken to not cut into the vent or intestinal tract of the fish to avoid contamination of the coelomic cavity. After viewing the visceral organs *in situ*, the organs can be removed from the coelomic cavity by cutting through the anterior end of the esophagus just in front of the liver. Then, the entire gastrointestinal tract and other visceral organs can be removed from the coelomic cavity by pulling the visceral mass caudally toward the tail. This will often include both the swimbladder and the gonads. A bacterial culture of the posterior kidney can be obtained using a sterile culturette, cotton swab, or plastic loop. Slight pressure while rotating the swab may be needed to penetrate through the thin membrane covering the surface of the kidney. Then, tissues may be taken for impression smears, viral isolation, or histopathology. To obtain brain tissue for bacteriologic, histologic, or toxicologic evaluation, an incision is made on both sides of the head to each eye from the incision previously made just behind the head to sever the spinal cord. Tissue is bluntly removed from the head of the fish to expose the underlying cartilaginous tissue of the skull. Removing the cranium of the skull exposes the underlying brain tissue that may be collected for various assays.

REFERENCES

1. Andrews C, Exell A., Carrington N. The Manual of Fish Health. Morris Plains, NJ: Tetra Press, 1988.
2. AVMA Guidelines on Euthanasia. Schaumburg, IL: American Veterinary Medical Association, 2007, pp 20-21.
3. Gratzek JB. Aquariology: The Science of Fish Health Management. Morris Plains, NJ: Tetra Press, 1992.
4. Hrubec T, Smith SA. Fish hematology. In: Feldman B, Zinkl J, Jain (eds.): Scham's Veterinary Hematology. Philadelphia: Lippincott, Williams & Wilkins, 2000, pp 1120-1125.
5. Longshaw M, Feist SW. Parasitic diseases. In:

BSAVA Manual of Ornamental Fish. Gloucester, England: British Small Animal Veterinary Association, 2001, pp 167-184.

6. Post GW. Textbook of Fish Health. Neptune, NJ: TFH Publications, 1983.

7. Smith SA. Non-lethal clinical techniques used in the diagnosis of fish diseases. J Am Vet Med Assoc.. 2002.;220:1203-1206.

8. Smith SA. Parasites of Fish. In: Zajac A (ed.): Veterinary Clinical Parasitology, 7th ed. Ames, IA: Blackwell, 2006, pp 265-279.

9. Stoskopf MK. Tropical fish medicine. Vet Clin North Am. 1988; 18.

10. Stoskopf MK. Fish Medicine. Philadelphia: WB Saunders, 1993.

ITCHY FISHY AND OTHER PARASITIC DISEASES OF PET FISH

Stephen A. Smith, MS, DVM, PhD
Virginia-Maryland Regional College
of Veterinary Medicine
Virginia Polytechnic Institute and State University
Blacksburg, VA

Parasites are the most common pathogen of tropical and ornamental fish. Some parasites are very host-specific, while others are cosmopolitan in the wide range of fish hosts they can affect. Fish may serve as an intermediate, paratenic, or definitive host, and the parasites can inhabit the skin, gill, lumen, or parenchyma of almost any tissue of the fish. There is an immense diversity of parasites in fish and these include protozoans, trematodes, cestodes, nematodes, acanthocephalans, crustaceans, and arthropods.

PROTOZOAN PARASITES

Probably the most universally recognized parasite of pet fish is *Ichthyophthirius multifiliis*, commonly called "Ich" or "white spot disease." This parasite affects all species of freshwater fish worldwide, and is an important pathogen of warm water tropical fishes. This holotrich ciliate is an extremely large parasite (up to 1000 µm) with a prominent horseshoe-shaped or C-shaped nucleus. Infection usually results in clinical signs of multiple, small, raised white lesions on the skin and fins of the fish. The life cycle includes a trophozoite stage, which is embedded in and feeds on the epithelial tissues of the fish, a cyst stage in the water, which undergoes multiple divisions producing numerous smaller, free-swimming ciliated stages, and the cilitated tomite stage, which is released into the water column and is infective to the fish. The complete life cycle can be completed in as short a time period as a few days to weeks depending on environmental temperature. The equivalent organism in marine species of fish is *Cryptocaryon irritans*. This parasite is similar to *I. multifiliis* in almost all aspects of its life cycle, clinical signs and pathogenisis, except that the organism is only found in marine waters and the nucleus is not horseshoe-shaped or C-shaped.

Chilodonella spp. is a dorsoventrally flattened, oval parasite with cilia located in distinct bands along the body of the protozoan. This is an external parasite of freshwater tropical and pond-reared fishes. Although this parasite does not generally penetrate the epithelial tissue of the host, the parasite causes irritation of the gills and fins resulting in hyperplasia and fusion of gill lamellae and hyperplasia of fin tissue.

A multitude of species of *Trichodina* spp. and *Trichodinella* spp. infest freshwater, brackish, and marine species of fishes. These ciliated, circular protozoans have a prominent internal denticular ring. Most species of these parasites infest the gills and skin of fish, but a few species also infest the urinary bladder and oviducts of freshwater and marine tropical fish. Gill-inhabiting species are generally most pathogenic where the parasite causes irritation to the gill tissue and respiratory problems

Several parasites are sessile on the fish host and include *Scyphidia* spp., a small urn-shaped protozoan with oral cilia, and *Trichophyra* spp., a pin cushion-like ciliate parasite. Both parasites can inhabit the skin and gills of the fish, and can cause problems in ornamental species and pond-reared goldfish. These parasites can cause clinical disease if found in large numbers on the gills where the parasite causes irritation to the gills with resulting respiratory distress. Another sessile parasite of fish is *Epistylis* spp., a colonial, stalked ciliated protozoan. This is primarily a parasite of goldfish and bottom-dwelling, pond-reared fish, where the parasite attaches to the skin and sometimes produces superficial lesions.

Tetrahymena spp., the cause of "guppy disease" or "tet" in tropical aquarium fishes (especially guppies and mollies), is a small, cylindrical to pyriform-shaped facultative ciliate. The parasite can invade the skin, and progress to the deeper musculature and internal organs of the fish.

Ichthyobodo spp. (older name *Costia* spp.) is a very small, pyriform-shaped flagellate of freshwater and occasionally marine fishes. This pathogenic parasite can be found either attached to the skin or gills, or motile in wet mounts. This parasite is approximately the size of a red blood cell and is often overlooked. Other flagellates that infect the intestinal tract or skin of freshwater fish include *Spironucleus* spp. and *Hexamita* spp. In general, these small, oval to pyriform-shaped parasites cause poor body condition, inappetence, weight loss, unthriftiness, emaciation and sometimes death. *Spironucleus* sp. is an endoparasite of the intestinal tract of angelfish, with clinical signs ranging from nonpathogenic to severely pathogenic. Large numbers of the protozoan in the intestine can cause sloughing and necrosis of epithelium resulting in emaciation and mortality. *Hexamita* sp. has historically been associated with a disease syndrome known as "hole-in-the-head" of cichlids, which involved discus, oscars, angelfish, and other Central American and African cichlids. However, the protozoan etiology has not been definitively proven for this disease.

There are a number of species of parasitic dinoflagellates infesting either marine or freshwater fish worldwide. *Amyloodinium* spp. infests numerous marine species and causes a disease syndrome commonly called "velvet disease" or "rust disease," while *Piscinoodinium* spp. infest freshwater species of fish. These parasites have a trophozoite stage that may be found attached to gills, fins or skin of the fish. The feeding stage then detaches from the host and encysts in the environment where it produces numerous free-swimming, infective dinospore stages. The attached trophozoites may cause hyperplasia and fusion of gill lamellae, and can be extremely pathogenic to captive fish where parasite numbers often expand rapidly.

Many different species of sporozoan (microsporidean) parasites have been reported from fishes. *Plistophora* spp. causes a disease called "neon tetra disease," which is usually progressively fatal in neon tetras; and also affects other tropical fish species such as angelfish, rasboras, and swordtails. The parasite produces a whitish cyst (xenoma) within tissues of the host, which contains numerous intracellular spores. After the cyst ruptures, infective spores are released into the water where they are ingested by fish. Other species of sporozoans parasitic in tropical and ornamental fish included *Glugea* spp. and *Heterosporis* spp.

As with many species of domestic animals, coccidiosis can be a significant parasitic problem in fish, especially in younger animals. Several species of *Eimeria* and *Goussia* have been recorded from various ornamental fishes. The parasites follow the typical coccidian life cycle with oocysts being passed in the feces. Heavy infections can result in poor growth, emaciation, and death.

HELMINTH PARASITES

Numerous species of myxosporidean parasites infect freshwater or marine species of tropical and ornamental fishes. These parasites (*Kudoa* spp., *Myxidium* spp., and *Myxobolus* spp., etc.) commonly cause boil-like cysts in the musculature and internal organs of a fish. *Hoferellus* spp. causes significant renal pathology in goldfish and carp. Transmission to other fish is through rupture of the cyst and release of infective spores into the water.

Almost all species of cold to warm, fresh to brackish to marine fish may be infested by monogeneans. There are numerous species of monogeneans, including the more common *Gyrodactylus* spp., *Dactylogyrus* spp., and *Benedenia* spp, and most are host specific. These parasitic flatworms have a direct, one-host life cycle and cause pathology by attachment to tissues with hooks, hooklets, clamps, or other clasping device and by their abrasive feeding activity. This attachment and feeding activity causes irritation to the gills and skin, increased mucus production and hyperplasia of epithelial tissues, and allows the entrance of secondary bacterial infections through the resulting lesions.

Larval and adult digenetic trematodes, cestodes and nematodes infect many species of fish. Larval forms use fish as an intermediate host for development and generally cause minimal pathology in the host fish, but heavy infections can result in chronic emaciation and stunted growth. Migration of the larval parasites can also cause pathology and leave fish susceptible to secondary bacterial and fungal infections. Examples of larval digenetic trematodes of fish include *Clinostomum* sp. (yellow grub), *Posthodiplostomulum* sp. (white grub), *Neascus* sp. (black spot), and *Diplostomulum* sp. (eye fluke). Adult forms of the various helminth parasites use fish as a definitive host for completion of their life cycle. Adult digenetic trematodes, cestodes, nematodes, and acanthocephalan parasites mainly inhabit the lumen of the intestinal tract and generally cause minimal pathology in the host fish, however heavy infestation can cause emaciation and poor growth.

CRUSTACEAN PARASITES

There are a number of important crustacean parasites that infest fish. These include *Learnea* spp. (anchor worm), *Ergasilus* sp. (copepods), and *Argulus* sp. (fish louse). *Learnea* spp. commonly occurs on goldfish, carp, Koi, and other pond-reared fishes. As its name implies, the anterior end of the adult parasite is deeply embedded into the musculature of host while the posterior end and eggs sacs hangs free from the host. There is often an intense, focal inflammatory response and epithelial hyperplasia around the site of parasite attachment. *Ergasilus* sp. is another form of copepod parasite that only attaches externally to the gills of many species of pond-reared tropical and ornamental fish. *Argulus* sp. is a dorsoventrally flatten copepod parasite with two prominent sucking disks, two dark-colored eyespots, and a piercing stylet. Damage to the fish is caused by penetration of the stylet into host tissue and the removal of blood and cellular material from the cell. There is often a severe local reaction at the site of stylet penetration suggesting a toxic substance is released by the parasite to facilitate feeding. All of these parasites produce lesions on the external surface fish and may also serve as mechanical vectors for certain bacterial, viral and protozoal diseases.

MISCELLANEOUS PARASITES

Several species of freshwater (*Piscicola* spp.) and marine (*Myzobdella* spp.) leeches infest various species of fish, and larval stages (glochidia) of freshwater clams and mussels also infect the tissues of various species of freshwater fish.

REFERENCES

1. Gratzek JB. Parasites associated with ornamental fish. Vet Clin North Am. 1988;18:375-400.
2. Hoffman GL. Parasites of North American Freshwater Fishes. Ithaca, NY: Cornell University Press, 1999, pp 1-548.
3. Longshaw M, Feist SW. Parasitic diseases. In: BSAVA Manual of Ornamental Fish. Gloucester, England: British Small Animal Veterinary Association, 2001, pp 167-184.
4. Smith SA. Parasites of fish. In: Zajac A (ed.): Veterinary Clinical Parasitology, 7th ed. Ames, IA: Blackwell, 2006, pp 265-279.
5. Smith SA, Noga EJ. General parasitology of fish. In: Stoskopf MK (ed.):. Clinical Fish Medicine. Philadelphia: WB Saunders, 1992, pp 131-148.

BACTERIAL LESIONS AND SEPSIS OF PET FISH

Stephen A. Smith, MS, DVM, PhD
Virginia-Maryland Regional College
of Veterinary Medicine
Virginia Polytechnic Institute and State University
Blacksburg, VA

The majority of the bacterial pathogens of fish are opportunistic pathogens, and generally occur secondary to suboptimal water quality (low oxygen content, high ammonia concentration, high organic content, or elevated temperature), poor husbandry (overcrowding, handling), or trauma. Thus, stress or a stressful event can be a predisposing factor for an outbreak of a bacterial disease in fishes. Most fish bacteria are gram-negative aerobes or facultative anaerobes, but there are also a few gram-positive organisms that are significant pathogens. Although a bacterial outbreak can occur at any time of the year, most bacterial infections of fish have a distinct seasonal occurrence due to the bacteria's dependence on an optimal temperature range of 18–25°C. As a result, incubation of bacterial cultures at room temperature is more appropriate for most fish pathogens than the typical mammalian incubation temperature.

Aeromonas hydrophila is one of the most common bacterial pathogens of freshwater fishes. The bacterium is a motile, gram-negative bacilli with a single flagellum, and belongs to a group of organisms, along with *A. sobria*, that cause a clinical syndrome commonly called "motile aeromonas septicemia." The organism is ubiquitous in freshwater habitats worldwide, and can also be found as part of the normal intestinal flora of fish. The organism primarily causes disease in warm and cool water fish such as tropical fish, goldfish, koi, and baitfish, and most epizootics occur in the spring or early summer. Clinical signs of an *A. hydrophila* or *A. sobria* infection in fish include exophthalmia, external hemorrhages, dermal ulcerations, abdominal distention, and raised scales. Infections can present as a rapidly fatal septicemia with few gross lesions or a chronic ulcerative skin disease with focal hemorrhage, ulceration, and inflammation. Convalescent fish may serve as a reservoir for this organism.

Aeromonas salmonicida is a non-motile, gram-negative bacilli that belongs to the "non-motile aeromonad group" of bacteria. This bacteria is an obligate fish pathogen and has limited ability to survive long-term outside the fish host. This pathogen is probably best known for causing "furunculosis" in coldwater salmonids, but atypical strains of this organism (*A. salmonicida* subsp. *achromogenes* may cause "goldfish ulcer disease" in goldfish and "erythrodermatitis" of carp. Clinical signs in these fish include hemorrhagic ulcerative dermatitis often without septicemia.

Vibrio spp. are gram-negative motile organisms that primarily occur in marine and estuarine fish, waters and sediments. Although predominantly pathogens of marine and estuarine fishes, these organisms also can cause disease in freshwater fishes. Infections produce skin ulcers with erythema of the skin and oral cavity, and hemorrhages of the tail and fins. There may also be hemorrhages of the gills and skeletal muscle, and most infections ultimately progress to septicemia. Vibriosis is sometimes called "red pest," "red boil," or "red plague" due to the erythema and petechial hemorrhages of the skin. Predominant pathogens in this group include *V. anguillarum*, *V. ordalii*, *V. alginolyticus*, *V. damsela*, and *V. vulnificus*. While *Vibrio damsela* appears to be a specific pathogen of damselfish, *V. anguillarum*, *V. alginolyticus,* and *V. vulnificus* appear to indiscriminately infect fish.[1] As these organisms are typically marine organisms, culture media may need to be supplemented with 2%–3% NaCl for optimal growth.

Flavobacterium (older generic names *Cytophaga* and *Flexibacter*) *columnaris* causes a disease commonly known as "columnaris" or "columnaris disease." This motile (flexing or gliding) gram-negative bacteria often has a "haystack" or "column" type of colonial appearance on fish. This yellow-pigmented, filamentous bacterium infects most species of freshwater fish, especially pond-raised carp, goldfish and tropical fish.[1,4] In scaleless fish, the infections generally appears as small circular lesions with a necrotic center, that may have inflamed hyperemic margins. In scaled fish, the infection often starts with frayed fins and spreads toward the trunk of body. Lesions of the skin frequently begin with little or no hemorrhage, and progress to superficial erosion and ulceration of the body. Infected gills appear hemorrhagic and necrotic, with infection then becoming systemic. The organism does not grow well on typical culture media such as TSA, BHI, or blood agar, and is best isolated on a selective media such as Cytophaga agar (Table 1), where it produces a cream to yellow colored, spreading colony. A presumptive diagnosis may be based on the observation of typical bacterial columns on wet mounts of the skin or gills, but a definitive diagnosis is based on culture and identification. Though fish probably serve as a primary reservoir of infection, the organism can survive for long periods of time in the water and sediment. Another *Flavobacterium* species, *F. branchiophilia* is the cause of "bacterial gill disease (BGD)" of pond-raised and ornamental fishes. This bacterium primarily affects the gill tissue where the infection produces hypertrophy of gill epithelium, followed by proliferation of gill tissue with clubbing and fusion of the gill lamellae. Clinical signs include

Table 1. Cytophaga Agar (Anacker and Ordal, 1959)

Tryptone	0.5 g
Yeast extract	0.5 g
Sodium acetate	0.2 g
Beef extract	0.2 g
Agar	11.0 g
Distilled water	1000 mL

Adjust to pH 7.2, autoclave, and pour plates.

anorexia, surface swimming, orientation of fish against the water current, and mortality due to impaired respiration, impaired excretion, and impaired osmotic balance.

Two species of *Edwardsiella* are important pathogens of the commercial catfish industry; however, both gram-negative organisms can also affect a wide range of fish species. *Edwardsiella ictaluri*, the cause of enteric septicemia of catfish, can cause disease in non-ictalurid fishes where an infection presents as either an ulcerative skin disease or a gastrointestinal septicemia. *Edwardsiella tarda*, the etiologic agent for "emphysematous putrefactive disease" of catfish, is not as pathogenic as *E. ictaluri* but affects a wider range of warm water fish species.[2] Clinical signs include lethargy, abdominal distention, abnormal swimming behavior, and superficial skin lesions to necrotic ulcerations that may lead to deep muscle abscesses. This bacteria produces hydrogen sulfide and necrotic material in the deeper abscesses may have a foul odor.

Yersina ruckeri, which causes a disease known primarily as enteric redmouth disease (ERM) of salmonids, has also been reported to occur in freshwater minnows and goldfish and some marine species of fish. This motile, gram-negative bacterium is transmitted by direct contact of fish and/or contaminated water. Clinical signs may include lethargy, anorexia, exophthalmia, hemorrhage of the eye, subcutaneous hemorrhages of the fins and gill filaments.

Pseudomonas fluorescens, another gram-negative bacterium, has been reported as causing disease in aquarium fish. Although generally a secondary pathogen due to elevated temperatures and/or poor husbandry, this organism may also be a primary pathogen. Infections generally result in a bacterial hemorrhagic septicemia where the clinical signs include petechial hemorrhages of the oral cavity, opercula and ventral body surfaces.

Streptococcus spp., a group of gram-positive spherical or oval bacteria, have been reported from both freshwater and marine ornamental fish. Three specific groups of pathogens have been isolated from fish and include alpha-hemolytic, beta-hemolytic, and non-hemolytic strains. This is a major disease of cultured striped bass and tilapia, and ornamental cichlids and marine butterflyfish.[7] Clinical signs are typical of general bacterial infections in fish and include exophthalmia, hemorrhages of the fins and body surfaces, abnormal swimming behavior, and skin ulcerations. Transmission is most likely via direct contact with infected fish or water, or through the feeding of contaminated fish foods.

Numerous species of acid-fast, gram-positive *Mycobacterium* can cause pathology in fishes, including *M. marinum*, *M. fortuitum* and *M. piscium*. Infections have been reported in marine, brackish and freshwater where the organism most commonly causes a chronic, systemic, granulomatous disease (piscine tuberculosis). Although considered to infect all species of fish, a number of species of fish appear to be more susceptible to infection including goldfish, rainbow fish, neon tetras, swordtails, betas, groumais and zebra danios.[5,6] Clinical signs may include anorexia, listless, lethargy, emaciation, exophthalmia, generalized "fin rot", deformities of the vertebral column and head, loss of normal coloration and chronic, non-healing, skin ulcerations. The clinical signs and progression of disease is dependent on the species of fish infected, the route of exposure, stress factors and water temperature. Internal pathology may include small nodules (granulomas or tubercles) in the kidney, spleen, liver, gastrointestinal tract, muscle, and gills. Fish probably serve as the primary reservoir of infectious material, but the organism can survive in the water column and biofilm of aquatic systems. Transmission is probably by oral ingestion of the organism in tissues or feces from infected fish and ingestion of contaminated feed, but also by direct infection of the organism from the water through existing skin abrasions. Transovarial transmission has also been reported in Mexican platyfish.[5] These organisms are typically slow growers and often need to be cultured on special medias such as Lowenstein-Jensen and Middlebrook 7H10 media. Importantly, all of these organisms have a significant zoonotic potential for humans where the disease is called "fish handlers disease." Human infection with any of the aquatic *Mycobacterium* spp. most commonly occurs as localized cutaneous granulomas on the extremities.

Nocardia aesteroides is another acid-fast gram-positive organism that causes a chronic granulomatous disease in tropical ornamental fish such as neon tetras and groumais. Clinical signs of nocardiosis in fish are similar to those described for mycobacteriosis. Therefore, typical clinical signs include skin ulcers, exopthalhamia, anorexia, and emaciation. Importantly, the clinical signs and pathology are often so similar that misdiagnosis of the disease with mycobacteriosis commonly occurs if bacterial samples are not cultured and identified.

A *Chlamydia*-like organism has been reported as the etiological agent for epitheliocystis. The intracellular organism produces small white nodules on the gill and sometimes the skin of freshwater and marine fish species. The disease is generally an incidental finding, but heavy infections can cause dyspnea and impaired respiration. Definitive diagnosis of this disease is by histological examination where large granular basophilic inclusions occur in cysts within the gill or skin tissue.

Definitive diagnosis of bacterial diseases in fish must be based on culture and identification of the organism as clinical signs and pathology are similar for many of the fish bacterial pathogens. Samples for bacterial culture may be obtained from the skin, gills or external lesions, but it should be remembered that these exterior sites are exposed to the water and may grow multiple non-pathogenic and pathogenic species that are representative of the environment. Bacterial samples from fish with systemic disease are most commonly obtained aseptically from the posterior kidney, but may also be acquired from the anterior kidney, spleen, liver, brain or other specific tissue depending on the clinical signs and pathology observed. Piscine bacterial cultures should be incubated at room temperature and may take several days to grow detectable colonies. In addition, some bacterial species may also need selective or modified media to grow particular fish isolates.

REFERENCES

1. Austin B, Austin DA. Bacterial Fish Pathogens: Disease in Farmed and Wild Fish. New York: John Wiley & Sons, 1987, pp 1-364.
2. Barker G. Bacterial diseases. In: Wildgoose WH (ed.): BSAVA Manual of Ornamental Fish. Gloucester, England: British Small Animal Veterinary Association, 2001, pp 185-193.
3. Guzman E, Shotts EB. Bacterial culture and evaluation of diseases in fish. Vet Clin North Am. 1988;18:365-374.
4. Inglis V, Roberts RJ, Bromage NR. Bacterial Diseases of Fish. New York: John Wiley & Sons, 1993, pp 1-312.
5. Smith SA. Mycobacterial infections in pet fish. Semin Avian Exotic Pet Med. 1997; 6:40-45.
6. Stoskopf MK. Bacterial diseases of freshwater tropical fishes. In: Stoskopf MK (ed.): Clinical Fish Medicine. Philadelphia: WB Saunders, 1992, pp 559-563.
7. Stoskopf MK. Bacterial diseases of marine tropical fishes. In: In: Stoskopf MK (ed.): Clinical Fish Medicine. Philadelphia: WB Saunders, 1992, pp 635-639.

DIAGNOSTIC DIFFERENTIALS FOR WEIGHT LOSS IN ANGELFISH

Stephen A. Smith, MS, DVM, PhD
Virginia-Maryland Regional College
of Veterinary Medicine
Virginia Polytechnic Institute and State University
Blacksburg, VA

A commercial producer of freshwater angelfish (*Pterophyllum scalare*) was experiencing significant mortality of both juvenile and adult broodstock fish. Water quality parameters were evaluated for the facility and specimens of both juvenile and adult fish were sampled for diagnostic evaluation. The history included the addition of new broodstock approximately one year ago, chronic increasing mortality in all stocks over the last 6 months, and several unsuccessful chemotherapeutic treatments (oxytetracycline, copper, etc.) in the past 2 months. The juvenile angelfish were fed mainly live brine shrimp napulii and a commercial flake diet, while the adult angelfish were fed mainly the same commercial flake diet and frozen bloodworms. Water quality parameters for the recirculation system housing the juvenile angelfish were temperature 68°F, pH 7.3, hardness 171 mg/L, ammonia 0.4 mg/L, nitrite 0.1 mg/L, nitrate 0.2 mg/L; water quality parameters for the recirculation system housing the adult angelfish were temperature 75°F, pH 7.6, hardness 183 mg/L, ammonia 0.1 mg/L, nitrite 0.1 mg/L, nitrate 0.0 mg/L.

Clinical signs in the juvenile angelfish included lethargy, anorexia, stunted growth, "wasting syndrome," and unacceptable mortality (35%–85%) for all spawns in the past 6 months. Clinical signs in the adult angelfish included anorexia, stunted growth, abdominal distention, superficial to deep ulcerative skin lesions, tumor-like growth on the lips of several individuals, missing eyes on several individuals, reduced spawning activity, reduced fecundity, and reduced hatch success.

At necropsy, the majority of the juvenile angelfish appeared emaciated with no body fat observed in the coelomic cavity. Several of the fish had distended intestinal tracts with material that appeared to be food. The majority of the adult angelfish also appeared emaciated with no body fat in the coelomic cavity. The abdominal distention noted in several individuals was the result of fluid accumulation in the coelomic cavity. The intestinal tract of most of the examined fish had only a small amount of food material, and the liver, posterior kidney and intestinal tracts of several fish had numerous small, cream-colored, raised nodules on the surface of each tissue.

Histopathology of the juvenile angelfish revealed moderate to severe gill hyperplasia, but no protozoan or metazoan parasites. The intestinal tract was filled with food material and included plant material and numerous brine shrimp eggs shells. The intestinal tract also had a few nematodes migrating through the epithelium of the intestinal wall. The remainder of the tissues was unremarkable. Histopathology of the adult angelfish revealed moderate to severe gill hyperplasia, and numerous small, biflagellated parasites, some of which were attached to the gill epithelium. The ulcerative skin lesions penetrated through the epidermal and dermal layers of the skin into the deeper musculature and contained several granulomas. The intestinal tract had a small amount of food material, numerous flagellates in the lumen of the tract, and a few nematodes migrating through the epithelium of the intestinal wall. These nematodes were considered to be adult stages as there were numerous eggs within the worms. The liver, spleen, anterior and posterior kidneys, intestinal tract and gonads of all fish examined had multiple granulomas within the parenchyma of each organ. A modified Fites stain showed that these granulomas contained abundant small, rod-shaped bacteria that stained acid-fast positive.

What is your diagnosis, and what are your health management and/or therapeutic recommendations?

DIAGNOSIS

Juvenile angelfish diagnosis – Poor water quality of low temp, elevated ammonia, and hard water; gill pathology from water quality; nutritional problem with brine shrimp egg shells occluding intestinal tract, severe *Spironucleus* sp., and larval *Capillaria* sp.

Adult angelfish diagnosis – Poor water quality of hard water, high pH; gill pathology due to *Costia* sp.; lip fibroma causing nutritional deficiency in some individuals; mild *Spironucleus* sp.; adult *Capillaria* sp. with eggs, and disseminated systemic mycobacteriosis.

RECOMMENDATIONS

The suboptimal water quality issues (low temperature, elevated ammonia, high pH, and hard water) are generally easy to modify and make appropriate for inducing spawning behavior in angelfish. The nutritional problem facing the juvenile angelfish (brine shrimp shell occlusion) can be corrected with changes in management protocols (decapsulation of brine shrimp eggs, and careful collection of only napulii stages). The nutritional problem facing the adult angelfish (lip fibroma) may be more difficult to manage as this tumor-like syndrome is reported to be caused by a retrovirus-like particle. Infected individuals should be culled from the population, but subclinical individuals (both adults and juveniles) may still exist in the population and go undetected until the fish reach an older age. The parasitic issues (*Costia* sp. on the gills, *Spironucleus* sp. in the intestine, and larval and adult *Capillaria* sp. in the intestine) are manageable with proper management and antiparasitic compounds.

Unfortunately, the most significant diagnosis (disseminated systemic mycobacteriosis) is a serious problem from both a therapeutic and management perspective. There are no therapeutics proven efficacious for piscine mycobacteriosis, and the bacterial disease in the fish and system (water and biofilm) presents a zoonotic hazard. Thus, the final recommendation would be to depopulate and disinfect the entire facility.

REFERENCES

1. Floyd RF. Health management of angelfish. Florida Cooperative Extension Service, University of Florida, Gainesville, FL. Circular 882, 1991, pp 1-15.
2. Francis-Floyd R, Bolon B, Fraser W, Reed P. Lip fibromas associated with retrovirus-like particles in angelfish. J Am Vet Med Assoc. 1993; 202:427–429.
3. Longshaw M, Feist SW. Parasitic diseases. In: BSAVA Manual of Ornamental Fish. Gloucester, England: British Small Animal Veterinary Association, 2001, pp 167-184.
4. Lowry T, Smith SA. Aquatic zoonoses associated with food, bait, ornamental and tropical fish. JAVMA 2007; 231:876-880.
5. Smith S.A. Culture and maintenance of angelfish in the laboratory. In: Stolen JS, Fletcher TC, Rowley AF, Zelikoff JT, Kaattari SL, Smith SA (eds.): Techniques in Fish Immunology, Volume 3. Fair Haven, NJ: SOS Publications, 1994, pp A9-A10.
6. Smith SA. Mycobacterial infections in pet fish. Semin Avian Exotic Pet Med. 1997; 6:40-45.
7. Smith SA. Non-lethal clinical techniques used in the diagnosis of fish diseases. J Am Vet Med Assoc. 2002;220:1203-1206.

PET, ORNAMENTAL, AND FOOD FISH ZOONOSES

Stephen A. Smith, MS, DVM, PhD
Virginia-Maryland Regional College
of Veterinary Medicine
Virginia Polytechnic Institute and State University
Blacksburg, VA

As veterinary medicine expands into the pet and ornamental industry, veterinarians will increasingly come into contact with potential zoonotic diseases specific to aquatic species. These pathogens have generally been of little concern to veterinarians dealing primarily with terrestrial animals. In additional to the variety of pathogens that are transmissible to humans from aquatic species via consumption, a number of specific pathogens can also be encountered during examination, handling, and treatment of aquatic species. Therefore, it is important for veterinarians to be aware of these potential zoonotic pathogens and be familiar with ways to minimize risk of exposure. In addition, like terrestrial veterinary medicine, it is also important for veterinarians to inform clients of the potential risks of maintaining aquatic species.

The interaction of pathogens between humans and aquatic species is complicated because of the aqueous medium essential to the aquatic organism and the various potential routes of transmission. Many of the potential zoonotic pathogens are commensal organisms in the aquatic species and do not cause disease in the animal; thus an apparently healthy fish may have the potential to transmit a particular pathogen to humans. In addition, many of the clinical signs of a potential zoonotic disease in an aquatic species have little relevance to the clinical signs that may develop in humans affected with the pathogen.

As there are no reported parasitic, viral, or fungal zoonoses acquired from contact with aquatic species, bacteria are the only agents of concern for zoonotic infections from fish. However, the variety of bacterial species associated with aquatic organisms is vast and includes both gram-negative and gram-positive bacteria that are potential zoonotic pathogens. Aquatic animals live in a wide range of aqueous conditions, which directly influence the types and diversity of bacterial species that are associated with certain aquatic species. For example, *Aeromonas* spp. are more commonly associated with freshwater species, whereas *Vibrio* spp. are more commonly associated with marine species.

GRAM-NEGATIVE BACTERIA
Aeromonas Species
Aeromonas spp. are gram-negative bacteria that are ubiquitous in both the aquatic and terrestrial environments. These bacteria compose a large portion of the bacterial population found in most freshwater aquatic organisms and can be found in fish from a wide range of water temperatures from warm to cool to cold water. *Aeromonas hydrophila, A. caviae, A. sobria,* and *A. schubertii* frequently cause disease in ornamental and food fish, and have all been implicated in human disease.[1] Interestingly, *Aeromonas salmonicida,* the cause of furunculosis in salmonids, goldfish ulcer disease in goldfish and erythrodermatitis in carp, does not appear to present a zoonotic potential.

Clinical signs of *Aeromonas* spp. infections in fish are seldom specific and include ulcerative lesions of the skin, lesions around the base of the fins, exophthalmia, abdominal distention, and raised scales, all of which are general, nonspecific clinical signs of bacterial infections in fish. Anemia, hepatomegaly and ascites may also develop in affected fish depending on the severity of the infection. Aeromonad infections in fish are often secondary to other stressors such as suboptimal water quality and/or poor husbandry practices.

The primary route of transmission to a veterinarian or other persons handling fish is contact with mucus or tissues from infected fish. Abrasions that are already present on the hands of the veterinarian or fish handler, as well as, cuts or puncture wounds caused by directly handling fish are common routes of entry. In healthy individuals, the most common signs of an *Aeromonas* spp. infection include localized wound swelling; however, *Aeromonas* spp. infections in immunocompromised individuals can prove life threatening.

Vibrio Species
Vibrio spp. are gram-negative bacteria that are often associated with marine and brackish water fishes because of the preference for these bacteria for waters of high salinity. Despite being more prevalent in saltwater environments, *Vibrio* spp. can also be occasionally isolated from freshwater fish. These bacteria proliferate at warmer temperatures and more commonly cause disease during the warmer months.

Clinical signs in fish infected with *Vibrio* spp. are similar to those of other bacterial infections and include anorexia, lethargy, skin ulcers, exophthalmia, and erythema around the anus and bases of fins. *Vibrio* spp. can also be cultured from the skin and gastrointestinal tracts of fish that appear clinically normal. In humans, *Vibrio vulnificus* infection is the most common fish-derived *Vibrio* spp. infection with the major route of exposure being through puncture wounds. Clinical signs of such infections in humans are necrotizing fasciitis, edema and swelling in the immediate area of the puncture wound.

Edwardsiella, Escherichia, Salmonella, and Klebsiella Species
Another group of bacterial organisms that are associated with fish species or freshwater aquatic environments belong to the *Enterobacteriaceae*. These gram-negative bacteria include *Edwardsiella spp., Escherichia spp., Salmonella spp.,* and *Klebsiella spp.,* all of which have a zoonotic potential. Of these, *Edwardsiella ictaluri* and *Edwardsiella tarda* are important primary pathogens of fish that can cause major losses in the commercial catfish and ornamental industry. *Edwardsiella ictaluri,* the etiologic agent of enteric septicemia of catfish, causes circular areas of

hyperemic skin, hemorrhage at the base of fins, raised hemorrhagic lesions on the top of the head that often ulcerate, exophthalmia, abdominal distention, anorexia, and abnormal swimming behavior. *Edwardsiella tarda*, or emphysematous putrefactive disease of catfish, causes typical nonspecific clinical signs of a bacterial infection with hemorrhage and ulcerations of the skin. This particular pathogen can progress to develop large gas-filled abscesses in the muscles and skin of the fish.

The greatest potential for a human infection with any of these pathogens is through puncture wounds received during handling or examination of fish, or by contamination of existing cuts and abrasions. Infections can remain localized at the point of entry or can become systemic and result in meningitis.

GRAM-POSITIVE SPECIES
Mycobacterium Species

There are also a number of gram-positive species of bacteria associated with aquatic organisms that are considered potential pathogens of humans. A number of *Mycobacterium* spp. (*M. marinum, M fortuitum, M chelonei, M ulcerans, M chesapaeki,* and *M shottsii*) have been isolated from fish. These gram-positive, acid-fast bacteria have been cultured from a variety of freshwater, brackish, and marine species of ornamental, bait, and food fish. All of the aquatic *Mycobacterium* spp. can produce acute to chronic disease in fish with varying clinical signs of exophthalmia, lethargy, scale loss, abdominal distention, pigment changes, poor body condition, and skin ulcers. Infected fish may transmit the infection to other fish in an aquarium or tank by ingestion of infected feces or tissues, or contamination of the water. In people who handle or work with fish, *Mycobacterium* spp. infections, called "fish handlers' disease" or "fish tank granuloma," typically result in granulomatous nodules or ulcerative lesions on the extremities due to the bacteria's preference for lower body temperatures. However, a few rare cases of systemic mycobacteriosis in humans have been reported.

Streptococcus iniae

Streptococcus iniae is another gram-positive bacteria that causes multiple clinical signs, including abdominal distention, petechial hemorrhage of the dermis, exophthalmia, and death, in various species of freshwater and marine fish.[30-32] Several species of fish (tilapia, striped bass, and their respective hybrids) appear to be predisposed to infection with *S. iniae* and may be chronic carriers of the bacterium. Most human infections are a result of contamination of an existing wound or a puncture wound during handling of live or dead fish. Humans infected with *S. inae* develop cellulites, systemic arthritis, endocarditis, and meningitis.

Erysipelothrix rhusiopathiae

Erysipelothrix rhusiopathiae is also a gram-positive bacteria that is ubiquitous in freshwater and marine environments. Although the bacterium has no apparent effect on fish, it is often associated with fish skin and mucus. Human infections with *E. rhusiopathiae* are typically a result of contact or handling of animal tissues. Disease in humans has several forms, ranging from a localized skin infection to a diffuse cutaneous form to a systemic form which may affect the heart and heart valves of the infected individual.

PREVENTION OF ZOONOTIC DISEASES

Similar to other disciplines of veterinary medicine, prevention is a much more effective way of avoiding zoonotic diseases than responding to existing infections. Discussion of biosecurity principles with clients and implementation of appropriate biosecurity plans for aquaculture facilities are important in reducing the introduction and minimizing the spread of a pathogen in an animal population. It is also advisable to have clients seek veterinary guidance prior to purchasing fish and arrange pre-purchase examinations of fish, especially when large numbers or expensive fish are involved.

Establishment of a quarantine area or tanks that are separate from existing populations is one way of reducing zoonotic pathogens and also other disease agents from entering the clients' fish populations. New fish should be held in quarantine for 30 to 45 days to allow adequate observation of behavior, feeding, and development of clinical signs. This period of time is generally sufficient to allow the detection of most active pathogens in new fish, although chronic, subclinical infections such as *Mycobacterium* spp. may not be apparent. The quarantine area or facility should be treated as a separate area and should be equipped with separate nets, feed, and tank cleaning supplies to prevent contamination to existing populations of fish.

In production facilities, large numbers of food, bait, or ornamental fish may be entering and leaving a facility throughout a production cycle. Any one of these incoming fish has the potential to introduce a new disease that may or may not have zoonotic potential. Recommendations to clients to implement an all-in, all-out production cycle can decrease the quarantine requirements and help prevent the spread of some infections within a facility. The period between production cycles should also allow a thorough disinfection of the facilities, removing bacterial and viral pathogens, and interrupting the life cycles of parasites.

Avoidance of contact with the fish and water is the single most effective way to prevent human infection, thus basic hygiene and thorough hand washing after contact with fish or water that contains fish is a good preventative protocol. This contact can be further decreased by the use of gloves when working with fish or aquatic systems, thereby reducing exposure to previous cuts or abrasions. Clients should also be cautioned that immunocompromised individuals may be at increased risk for infection with a zoonotic pathogen and their contact with aquarium water and fish should be limited. Finally, clients seeking advice regarding zoonotic diseases should also be advised to talk with their personal physicians.

References available from the author upon request.

REPRODUCTIVE TRACT DISEASES: GETTING OUT OF THE BIND

M. Scott Echols, DVM, Diplomate ABVP
Westgate Pet and Bird Hospital
Austin, TX

Reproductive tract disease is commonplace in avian medicine, especially among female birds. The unique anatomy and physiology of the avian reproductive tract results in a highly productive, but poorly accessible organ system. This is commonly represented as a hen producing numerous eggs and subsequently becoming "egg bound" or developing egg yolk peritonitis. Although many reproductive tract diseases can be managed medically, there is a definite need for surgical intervention in some cases. Surgical approaches to the coelom and management of some reproductive tract diseases are discussed in the following article in this proceedings. Management, whether surgical or medical, will be discussed for most male and female avian reproductive tract diseases. *The remainder of this article has been adapted from Echols MS. Surgery of the avian reproductive tract. Seminars in Avian and Exotic Pet Medicine, V11(4):177-195, 2002 with permission from Elsevier.*

Primarily due to highly productive laying hens, avian reproductive tract disease is very common in pet and even commercial avian practice. With the advancements in diagnostics and therapeutics available to birds, many reproductive tract diseases can be medically managed. However, several diseases can only be treated surgically. Because of past literature describing procedures such as salpingohysterectomy as "difficult and risky," many practitioners are rightfully cautious about performing avian reproductive tract surgery. Just as with diagnostics and therapeutics, anesthetic techniques, instrumentation, a better understanding of respiratory physiology and surgical techniques have also advanced in birds. Now with the progression and public awareness of these 'advancements', avian practitioners are being called upon to perform more difficult surgical procedures in birds. Again, avian coelomic surgery will be discussed at another presentation during this conference.

BASIC STABILIZATION OF BIRDS WITH REPRODUCTIVE TRACT DISEASES

Common presenting complaints in female birds with reproductive tract disease include abdominal swelling, broken bones, cloacal prolapse, anorexia, depression and behavior changes. In all cases, stable birds should be thoroughly evaluated (history, physical examination, complete blood count, chemistry panel and radiographs) to determine the extent of the problems present. Critically ill birds should first be stabilized (oxygen, fluid therapy, antibiotics, etc) as deemed appropriate by the attending clinician. As a note, many reproductively active females have varying degrees of medullary (polyostotic) hyperostosis preventing the placement and use of intraosseous catheters. Up to three fourths of the medullary cavity's hematopoetic tissue can be replaced by medullary bone during polyostotic hyperostosis. Fractures present should be bandaged until surgical options are available (severe medullary hyperostosis may also preclude surgical fracture repair).

DISEASES OF THE AVIAN OVARY
Cystic Ovarian Disease

Although the cause is often unknown, cystic ovarian disease has been reported in numerous bird species. Cystic ovaries are sometimes secondary to neoplasia. Depending on their size, ovarian cysts may be found incidentally if small or may cause abdominal distension when large and/or numerous and can be associated with ascites. Large or numerous cysts can often be diagnosed non-invasively using ultrasound. Cysts can be treated by ultrasound guided transabdominal aspiration or more directly via celiotomy or endoscopy. If collected, evaluate the fluid for evidence of infection or other abnormalities. Severe cystic disease may require partial or complete ovariectomy and should include biopsy for histopathologic evaluation. Leuprolide acetate has also been suggested to reduce or resolve ovarian cysts in birds and offers a noninvasive treatment option.

Oophoritis

Ovarian infections can be life-threatening and are often associated with septicemia. Salmonella *pullorum* is the etiologic agent of pullorum disease of poultry and most frequently affects the ovary. Clinically affected birds usually show more severe, but general signs of illness and if not treated quickly, peritonitis and death may result. Abnormally shaped, colored or partially ruptured follicles identified during celiotomy or endoscopy should be carefully aspirated for cytologic and microbiologic analysis and broad spectrum antibiotics pending culture results initiated. The Storz injection needle with Teflon guide (Karl Storz Veterinary Endoscopy America, Goleta, CA) is particularly useful as an endoscopic means to aspirate ovarian follicles. If possible, completely drain the abscessed follicle(s) being careful to not contaminate the abdomen. Partial or complete ovariectomy may be required for chronically infected and caseated follicles.

Reproductive Tract Neoplasia (Ovary and Oviduct)

Ovarian cancer is reported with some frequency in birds and can be associated with egg retention, ascites, cystic ovarian disease, medullary hyperostosis, abdominal hernias, oviductal impaction and general malaise. One study noted that 38% of USDA Inspection Service mature fowl condemnation is the result of neoplastic disease, most of which are from the genital tract. Fredrickson states "there is indeed a unique propensity for hens (poultry) to develop cancer of the reproductive system in the almost total absence of tumors at other sites." Granulosa cell tumors and ovarian adenocarcinomas are most frequently reported but carcinomas, leiomyosarcomas/leiomyomas, adenomas, teratomas, dysgerminomas, fibrosarcomas, lipomas and lymphomatosis have all been identified in bird ovaries.

Oviductal tumors are less common than ovarian neoplasia and include adenocarcinomas/adenomas, adenomatous hyperplasia, carcinoma and carcinomatosis.

Granulosa cell tumors and possibly other reproductive tract neoplasms may be functional and cause increased plasma hormone levels. Granulosa cell tumors have been cited as common in older female budgerigars (*Melopsittacus undulatus*) and may be functional resulting in hyperestrogenism. Polyostotic (medullary) hyperostosis may also result as a paraneoplastic syndrome with functional ovarian and oviductal neoplasms. Interestingly, one study found that hyperestrogenism did not cause polyosostic hyperostosis in several species of birds with various neoplastic and non-neoplastic reproductive tract diseases.

Clinical signs vary and are non-specific for most reproductive tract diseases and include abdominal swelling, dyspnea ascites, poor or altered reproductive performance and lethargy. If the mass compresses the overlying lumbar or sacral nerve plexus, lameness (usually left sided) may be seen. Diagnosis can be further supported using radiography, ultrasonography, exploratory celiotomy, endoscopy and biopsy. Once a definitive diagnosis is made, options for therapy include chemotherapy, radiation therapy and partial or complete ovariectomy, but all carry a guarded prognosis at best.

DISEASES OF THE AVIAN OVIDUCT
Congenital Defects

Congenital defects have been identified in birds and include large cysts on a rudimentary oviduct of a budgerigar and discontinous or atretic oviducts in domestic fowl. Persistence of the right ovary and/or oviduct has been reported in numerous species and are often found incidentally. Cystic dilatation is common with persistent right oviducts in poultry species. Each defect should be evaluated on a case-by-case basis and may require surgical modification or removal based on the associated clinical signs.

Ectopic Ovulation, Ectopic Eggs and Egg Yolk Peritonitis

Ectopic ovulation occurs when the infundibulum fails to engulf an ovum or fails to retain the ovum because of oviductal rupture or reverse peristalsis. The ectopic ovum is not developed. Potential causes include infundibulum failure from oviductal fat, trauma or disease, exuberant reverse peristalsis and oviductal disease. Ectopic ovulation is thought to occur frequently and has been reported in 28.6% of necropsied birds from nine orders in one study. The author has also seen ectopic ovulation associated with a persistent right oviduct in a chicken. Ectopic ovulation usually results in mild, self-resolving, sterile yolk coelomitis and usually requires no or minimal supportive therapy (fluid therapy, anti-inflammatories, etc).

Partially and completely shelled ectopic eggs result when a developing egg goes into the ceolomic cavity through an oviductal rupture or via reverse peristalsis from oviductal or even cloacal disease. Anything affecting the oviduct function such as cloacal or oviductal masses (including egg binding, impactions and neoplasia), salpingitis, cystic hyperplasia and oddly shaped or large eggs can result in ectopic eggs. A large ectopic egg can cause a penguin-like stance and is often associated with ascites and varying degrees of depression in many birds. Diagnosis can often be suspected using radiography, ultrasonography and sometimes endoscopy (depending on how much debris is in the coelom), but celiotomy is often required for definitive diagnosis. Ectopic eggs should always be considered when conservative therapy for egg binding fails. Partially and fully formed ectopic eggs should be surgically removed after stabilizing the patient and determining the underlying cause(s).

Severe sterile and life threatening septic egg yolk peritonitis may also result from ectopic ovulation or eggs. Acute egg yolk peritonitis may result in significant depression, anorexia and ascites and rarely, respiratory distress and death. Secondary diseases resulting from sterile and septic yolk peritonitis include pancreatitis, splenitis, yolk-thromboembolic disease, hepatitis, nephritis and coelomic adhesions. Septic yolk peritonitis may obviously result in or from septicemia and has been most commonly noted with coliforms such as *E. coli*, *Yersinia pseudotuberculosis* and *Staphylococcus* spp. Abdominocentesis and cytologic fluid analysis and culture are used to definitively diagnose yolk peritonitis. If needed, celiotomy and endoscopy can be used to assess the associated internal pathology. Severe egg yolk peritonitis, especially when associated with bacteria, includes aggressive supportive care, antimicrobials, identifying and resolving causative factors if possible and occasionally may require surgical removal, irrigation of the caudal coelomic cavity and placing a drain tube. If irrigation is used, be careful to prevent fluid from entering the lung tissue.

Egg Binding and Dystocia

Egg binding, dystocia and other reproductive tract diseases (egg yolk peritonitits, cystic ovary, etc) are common problems in pet bird medicine. Oviposition is the expulsion of the egg from the oviduct and is conducted by vigorous contraction of the uterine muscles and peristalsis of the vagina. Egg binding is simply defined as prolonged oviposition (egg is arrested in oviduct longer than normal for the given species) while dystocia implies the developing egg is within the distal oviduct either obstructing the cloaca or prolapsed through the oviduct-cloacal opening. Dystocia is often more advanced than egg binding alone, has many potential causes and is commonly associated with functional (malformed eggs, cloacal masses and obesity), metabolic (calcium imbalance and nutritional deficiencies), environmental (temperature changes, lack of exercise and other stressors) and hereditary diseases. Because this topic is frequently described in the current avian literature, egg binding and its management will only briefly be described here.

Oviduct Cystic Hyperplasia

Cystic oviductal hyperplasia or dilatation has been reported in budgerigars, other psittacines and poultry. Although little etiologic information is forwarded, cysts may occur secondary to improper formation of the oviduct. Affected oviducts are often thickened with white to beige masses and distended with brown or white mucoid fluid. Affected birds may show no signs (and the oviductal hyperplasia is discovered incidentally) or signs typical of reproductive tract disease. Antimicrobials may be tried if organisms are recovered from aspirated samples, otherwise salpingohysterectomy is indicated.

Oviduct Impaction

An impacted oviduct is usually distended and simply contains caseated material and misshapen, ruptured, soft-shelled, partially or fully formed eggs. Potential causes include excess mucin and albumin secretion secondary to inspissated egg material and cystic hyperplasia. Salpingitis is often found concomitantly, especially in older birds. Metritis, salpingitis, egg binding, dystocia and neoplasia commonly precede oviductal impactions.

Typical of most reproductive tract diseases, vague clinical signs with or without abdominal swelling and ascites are common with oviductal impaction. Some birds may show persistent 'broodiness' with recent cessation of egg laying. Oviductal impactions have been reported in Budgerigars, cockatiels, canaries, African grey parrots (Psittacus erithacus) and poultry. Definitive diagnosis is made at celiotomy or sometimes via ultrasound and endoscopy with aspiration of the oviductal contents. Chronic oviductal impactions may be found incidentally during exploratory celiotomy and are often associated with a history of sudden cessation of egg laying several months or years prior to presentation. Acute impactions may be treated by salpingotomy, culture and appropriate antibiotic use and oviductal flushing while severe or chronic disease are best treated with salpingohysterectomy.

Oviduct Prolapse

Powerful abdominal contractions combined with the process of oviposition can result in oviductal prolapse which is often secondary to dystocia. Predisposing factors may include large or abnormally shaped eggs, malnutrition, general debilitation and systemic illness, disease of the oviduct and sometimes, normal egg laying. In turkeys selected for high meat yield, decreased vaginal collagen has been associated with uterine prolapse. The uterus is most commonly prolapsed but the vagina and other portions of the oviduct may also prolapse. The cloaca may also prolapse and should be distinguished from the oviduct.

Because the exposed tissue can rapidly become devitalized and infected, aggressive treatment with warm saline flushes, antibiotics and replacement of the prolapsed oviduct is warranted. If the prolapsed oviduct is edematous, topical dextrose, dimethyl sulfoxide (DMSO) and/or steroids may be needed to reduce the swelling. If an egg is present in the prolapsed or coelomic oviductal tissue, ovocentesis and digital crushing is often needed to reduce associated pressure and aid in eggshell removal. After stabilizing the bird, remove the egg medically if possible and replace the prolapsed tissue. Two transcloacal sutures may be required to prevent the immediate recurrence of prolapsed tissue.

Surgical removal is indicated when the oviduct is necrotic and/or the egg (or its fragmented shell) cannot be removed medically or pass on its own. If an oviductal torsion is present distal to the egg (within the oviduct), attempting to force deliver the egg will often result in further damage. Oviductal torsion, neoplasia, adhesions, and other anatomic disorders should be considered if a bound egg cannot be delivered without forceful techniques and surgical options should be pursued.

Oviduct Torsion

Oviductal torsion has been reported infrequently as a cause of egg binding. Torsion of the oviduct may occur following a tear of the dorsal, and possibly ventral, oviductal ligament(s). In four reported cases, all birds presented with signs of egg binding and/or general lethargy and had a history of previously laying 'many eggs' prior the oviductal torsion. One cockatiel presented thin with lethargy, depression and abdominal distension and died despite emergency therapy. Of the three birds presented live, two cockatiels were treated with salpingohysterectomy and one eclectus parrot (Eclectus roratus vosmaeri) was treated with a hysterotomy (salpingotomy), egg removal, torsion correction and subsequent closure of the oviductal ligament tear. All birds recovered uneventfully from surgery. The eclectus successfully laid normal clutches after surgery.

Salpingitis and Metritis

Salpingitis, inflammation of the oviduct or salpinx, is common in birds. In poultry, salpingitis has been listed as the most prevalent form of reproductive tract disease. E. coli infections are fairly common in poultry and can cause salpingitis, but Streptococcus sp, Mycoplasma gallisepticum, Acinetobacter sp, Corynebacterium sp, Salmonella sp and Pasteurella multocida have all been implicated from various species. Some ground-nesting species, such as Anseriformes and emus, may develop non-lactose fermenting, gram-negative (Pseudomonas aeruginosa, Proteus mirabilis, P. vulgaris) salpingitis. Non-infectious salpingitis can also be seen, especially with chronic, sterile oviductal impactions. Metritis is inflammation within the uterine portion of the oviduct and may result from or cause egg binding, chronic oviductal impaction and rupture, peritonitis and septicemia. Prosthogonimus ovatus and other related trematodes (flukes) can inhabit the oviduct of Anseriformes and Galliformes and result in salpingitis with heavy infestations. Other infectious agents ascending from the vagina or cloaca or descending from air sacculitis, pneumonia and septicemia can also cause salpingitis. Specifically in poultry, vent cannibalism has been implicated as a precursor to salpingitis.

Birds with nonseptic salpingitis or metritis often show vague signs of illness, while septic birds are usually clinically very ill. One distinctive feature is that egg shell deformities and embryonic and neonatal infections are often secondary to metritis. Definitive diagnosis is made at celiotomy or endoscopy with aspiration of oviductal fluid for cytologic and microbiologic analysis or if the oviduct has no liquid contents, biopsy with culture. Base antibiotic use on culture and sensitivity results. If trying to spare the oviduct, repeated endoscopic evaluation, direct and indirect oviductal flushing and long-term antimicrobials are recommended. Salpingohysterectomy is indicated for severe cases or those non-responsive to appropriate antimicrobials.

DISEASES OF THE MALE AVIAN REPRODUCTIVE TRACT SYSTEM
Orchitis

Ochitis, or inflammation of the testicle, is usually due to bacterial infections and may originate from septicemia, renal obstruction, cloacitis, or even prolapsed or ulcerated phalli. Affected birds may show signs of septicemia, but the author has seen cases of focal orchitis with no associated clinical signs or, reduced fertility only. Orchitis may be diagnosed with aspiration and cytologic and microbiologic analysis via endoscopy or celiotomy when the whole testicle appears abnormal or, biopsy when focal lesions are seen. Initial treatment for bacterial orchitis should be antibiotics based on culture and sensitivity results. If a focal granulomatous lesion is seen and appropriate antimicrobials have proven ineffective, the testicle can be partially ablated by removing only the affected tissue. Clamp with hemostats or hemoclip the testicular tissue dorsal (towards the blood supply) to the lesion(s) and remove using cold excision, electrocautery or laser. Avian testicular tissue seems to have great regenerative capabilities and may redevelop following partial ablation. En bloc surgical removal of the affected testicle is indicated for diffuse, non-medically-responsive orchitis.

Testicular Neoplasia

Testicular neoplasia has been reported in numerous bird species and includes sertoli and interstitial cell tumors, seminomas, teratomas and lymphoproliferative diseases. Although most are benign, sertoli cell tumors seem to be the more prevalent testicular neoplasm in birds. Reported neoplasms of the epididymis and ductus deferens include leiomyosarcoma and carcinoma. Chronic weight loss, abdominal swelling and unilateral paresis are most commonly associated with testicular cancer in birds. Specifically, budgerigars may become feminized and change cere color from blue to brown. Surgical removal of the affected testicle is the treatment of choice and carries a good prognosis as long as metastasis is not present. As noted in the literature and in the author's experience, many testicular tumors are cystic. Cystic testicular masses can be aspirated and drained during surgery to reduce their mass and facilitate removal.

Cystic Testicular Disease

Non-neoplastic cystic testicular disease is very infrequently reported and its significance is not clear. Cystic dilatation of the seminiferous tubules, and subsequently the testes, has been consistently produced in fowl fed a diet high in sodium. Cystic testicles have also been noted in chickens fed egg albumen as a source of protein. Dilatation of the seminiferous tubules, but not gross cystic testicular change, has been noted in (chicken) roosters affected with epididymal cysts and stones of unknown origin. As mentioned above, cystic testicles may be neoplastic and cancer should be considered. Due to the potential for neoplastic disease, cystic testicles should be drained and biopsied, if not removed.

Disorders of the Phallus

Partial and complete phallic prolapses are possible in birds with large phalli and are usually secondary to local infection, trauma and extreme weather fluctuations. Over exuberant vent sexing and mating, fecal contamination and *Neisseria* spp (suspected sexually transmitted in geese) have all been implicated causes of phallic infections. A prolapsed phallus may become enlarged and ulcerated and compound the problem. Frostbite and resultant necrotizing dermatitis of a prolapsed phallus has been discussed in ostriches. Birds with severe prolapse and infection may be significantly depressed and often lose interest in copulation. Clean exposed phalli and carefully debride abnormal tissue prior to replacement. Topical antibiotic creams, DMSO and systemic antibiotics may be beneficial and their use is based on clinical findings. The cloaca may need partial closure (via a mattress or transcloacal suture) to prevent recurring prolapses. Severely necrotic phalli may need surgical debridement.

References are available from the author upon request.

SURGERY OF THE COELOM

M. Scott Echols, DVM, Diplomate ABVP
Westgate Pet and Bird Hospital
Austin, TX

A basic understanding of general surgical principles should be understood prior to avian surgery. Although there are many anatomic and physiologic differences between birds and mammals, surgical techniques are very similar. Due to small patient size and anatomic differences (avian air sacs, for example), microsurgical instrumentation and magnification with focused light is often necessary for efficient bird surgery. Because of physiologic variations (compared with mammals, birds exchange oxygen on inspiration and expiration and can frequently go into cardiac arrest following relatively brief apnea), anesthetic techniques in avian species are very different and are discussed elsewhere.

Doolen listed several principles that hold very true to maximize avian surgical success. First is to minimize hemorrhage. The second is to minimize tissue trauma. Third is to minimize anesthetic time. Fourth is to minimize anesthetic and metabolic complications. Last, provide postsurgical support and analgesia. These seem simple enough, but are very important to understand and practice during all avian surgical procedures.

Prior to considering avian surgery, familiarize yourself with the numerous potential surgical "tools." These tools include radiosurgery, microsurgical instruments, endoscopes, high-powered microsurgical loops with light, operating microscopes, laser units, and other items that have become commonplace with avian surgery. Consult with surgical instrument companies, colleagues, and the continuing education resources widely available.

The author's most commonly used instruments and "tools" used with avian surgeries are discussed in this article. Although little information exists on suture material in birds, chromic catgut, polyglactin 910, polydioxanone (PDS), monofilament nylon and monofilament stainless steel have been evaluated in rock doves (*Columba livia*). In a separate study of polygalactin-910, chromic catgut and polydioxanone used in cloacopexy surgery in pigeons, the authors concluded that inflammation and fibrosis were most prominent with polygalactin-910. From this information and the author's experience, PDS is slowly absorbed and causes minimal tissue reaction making it suitable for both internal and skin closure use. For the purposes of this discussion, PDS will be used for all monofilament, absorbable sutures in bird surgeries.

CELIOTOMY

The left lateral celiotomy provides good exposure to the female reproductive tract, left testes, proventriculus/ventriculus, spleen and left kidney and ureter. Place the anesthetized patient in right lateral recumbency with the wings pulled dorsally, the right leg caudally and the left leg cranially. In some cases, the left leg is best pulled caudally, especially when a more cranial approach to the lateral abdomen is required. Tape the extremities in place with masking tape (or any other tape that is easily removed). Make a longitudinal incision from cranial to caudal in the left paralumbar area. The incision may extend from the cranial extent of the pubis to the uncinate process of the last rib. If needed, the incision can be further extended cranially by incising through the last rib(s) at the costocondral junction(s). Use radiosurgery, laser, sutures or simple hemostasis to control hemorrhage. Once through the skin, bluntly dissect through the lateral abdominal muscles (external oblique, internal oblique and transverses abdominus mm.) to expose the underlying ventriculus (cranial) and intestines (caudal). At this point, the abdominal air sac is visible dorsally. Palpebral or similar retractors are very useful to better expose the underlying structures.

A ventral midline, transverse or combination celiotomy is used to expose the middle and/or both sides of the abdominal (coelomic) cavity gaining access to the liver, intestines, pancreas, cloaca and the oviduct (when enlarged). The incision is made on the ventral midline from just caudal to the sternum extending caudally to the interpubic space. The supraduodenal loop (ileum) lies relatively ventral along the midline of the caudal abdomen and can be easily transected if not careful. For this reason, the midline incision should be made as cranial as possible unless the caudal ventral abdomen must be explored as with some cloacal surgeries. After the skin incision is made, the linea alba is tented upward and carefully transected being careful not to damage underlying organs.

The transverse and combination ventral celiotomy can be used to increase exposure to the abdominal cavity in birds. A transverse incision is made midway between the vent and sternum. If needed, a ventral midline incision is used in conjunction with the transverse incision to increase exposure. As discussed above, underlying structures should be carefully avoided when incising through the underlying abdominal wall.

LIVER BIOPSY

Liver biopsy is a fairly common procedure and is very useful in determining hepatic pathologic change. Liver biopsy is obviously indicated when hepatic disease is suspected, but is also useful in determining response to therapy. Ideally, a thrombocyte estimate and capillary clot time (normal is less than 5 minutes) should be performed prior to surgery. With that stated, avian platelets can only be estimated, as they tend to clump in birds. If a coagulopathy is suspected, give vitamin K_1 (0.2–2.5 mg/kg IM) 24 to 48 hours preoperatively. If ascites is present, as much fluid as possible should be drained via coelomocentesis prior to surgery. A cranial ventral midline abdominal (just caudal to the sternum) approach works well for most hepatic biopsies.

Incise through the midline skin and linea alba to gain access to the cranial abdomen and ventral hepatic peritoneal cavities. With hepatomegaly, the liver is readily visible and the right lobe is usually larger. With microhepatica, the liver is tucked under the sternum. Use cup-end biopsy forceps or curved hemostats to collect a small piece of liver. Typically the edge of the liver is biopsied using either instrument while the cup-end forceps are more appropriate for selecting specific lesions and with microhepatica. When biopsying the liver's edge, bleeding is often minimal and sutures are rarely required. If hemorrhage is persistent, use hemostats to clamp on the bleeding area until hemostasis is established. If possible, collect extra tissue for culture and electron microscopy. Close the muscle and skin layers as with other abdominal surgeries.

Although complications such as uncontrolled hemorrhage, perforation of intestines and other underlying organs and introduction of ascitic fluid into the air sacs are reported, these problems are fairly uncommon with the abdominal approach discussed above. Even with severe liver disease, complications such as clinically evident coagulopathies are uncommon in the author's experience.

Selected laboratory values will likely change following a liver biopsy. In pigeons and quails undergoing ultrasound guided tru-cut liver biopsies, AST, CK, LDH, AP, TP and albumin were measured before and 1 week after surgery. In pigeons the AST and albumin both significantly increased post-surgically while only AST increased in the quails. In a study of mixed wild raptors, 'liver and kidney' values increased within 5 days after liver biopsy.

PROVENTRICULOTOMY/VENTRICULOTOMY

Proventriculotomy and ventriculotomy are reserved for the removal of foreign bodies not eliminated via conservative therapy or non-retrievable using endoscopy or other less invasive techniques. Most reported cases involve gastrointestinal impactions in ratites, but have also been described in kiwis (*Apteryx australis*), sarus cranes (*Grus antigone*) and umbrella cockatoos (*Cacatua alba*). This same approach is also used to obtain biopsies for suspected proventricular dilatation disease and cancer, address perforating ulcers and to explore the serosal surface of the proventriculus, isthmus and ventriculus. Prior to surgery, conservative therapy using bulking agents, fluid therapy and basic support should be attempted.

For adult birds undergoing proventriculotomy/ventriculotomy, fast the patient for at least 12 hours to help 'clean' the gastrointestinal tract. If possible, use hand feeding formula 1-2 days prior to surgery as these easily digestible foods tend to leave little residue in the ventriculus. (Also discontinue feeding formulas 6-12 hours prior to surgery.) Pre- and post-operative antibiotics should be considered as with other animals undergoing enterotomies.

A midline combined with transverse ventral or left lateral celiotomy may be used. If the ventriculus is displaced medially (as supported by contrast study radiographs), the ventral midline approach is more appropriate. Otherwise, the left lateral approach is more commonly used.

Once located, place stay sutures in the white tendinous portion of the ventriculus to help retract the organ(s) out of the coelomic cavity and improve exposure. Due to its location, the proventriculus cannot be exteriorized but visualization is improved with ventriculus retraction. It is best to pack moist sponges around the retracted organs to help prevent coelomic contamination. Incise into the relatively avascular isthmus and extend the incision cranial into the proventriculus or caudal into the ventriculus as needed. At this point, both the proventriculus and ventriculus can be explored. Due to the massive mobile muscular tunic and high tensile strain on the tendinous centers, the ventriculus does not have a good site for incisional entry. Additionally, an endoscope may be introduced to improve visualization and help retrieve foreign bodies when present. Irrigation and suction are often needed-be careful not to contaminate the coelomic cavity. Use fine monofilament, absorbable suture in a simple continuous pattern to close the wound. Oversew with a continuous inverting pattern. Meticulous closure is required to help prevent dehiscence.

The ventriculus may also be approached via the caudoventral sac. The ventriculus has two blind sacs (craniodorsal and caudoventral) covered with relatively thin muscles. Incise through the muscle fibers to enter the ventricular lumen. Again, use meticulous closure. This tissue does not invert, so use interrupted sutures placed close together. In a study of Coturnix quail undergoing caudoventral sac ventriculotomy, ventricular mucosal healing was not complete until 21 days post-surgery.

LOWER INTESTINAL SURGERY

Lower intestinal surgery is rarely reported in avian medicine. Both metallic and non-metallic intestinal foreign bodies are described in multiple bird species. Non-metallic lower gastrointestinal foreign bodies are rarely described in avian medicine and are most frequently linear, occasionally form a nidus or enterolith and diagnosed based on palpation or necropsy. Radiographs, with or without barium or iodine (especially if gastrointestinal perforation is suspected), and ultrasound may also aid in diagnosis. One case report describes a 14-month-old female Eclectus parrot (*Eclectus roratus*) with a mineralized intestinal foreign body. The foreign body and proximal part of the duodenum were removed and the bird recovered uneventfully. The details of the actual surgery were not included other than the foreign body was brittle upon removal and had a central fiber like structure. One paper briefly notes that an ostrich died of complications associated with small intestinal resection and anastomosis performed because of a perforating intestinal foreign body. The same ostrich underwent a proventriculotomy 2 months previously.

Intestinal resection, repair, and anastomosis are delicate procedures in birds. Use microsurgical instruments to remove necrotic or damaged bowel and spare healthy tissue and the surrounding vascular supply. Use 6-0 to 10-0 absorbable monofilament suture on ¼ circle atraumatic needles for intestinal anastomosis and enterotomy closures. Six to eight simple interrupted sutures are often necessary for end-to-end anastomosis. Enterotomy closures should be performed so as to limit intestinal stricture.

The following and last section on Avian Reproductive Tract Surgery has been adapted from Echols MS. Surgery of the avian reproductive tract. Seminars in Avian and Exotic Pet Medicine 2002; 11:177-195, with permission from Elsevier.

SURGERY OF THE FEMALE REPRODUCTIVE TRACT
Anatomy of the Avian Oviduct

The oviduct is suspended within the coelomic cavity via a dorsal and ventral ligament. The cranial, middle and caudal oviductal arteries running in the dorsal mesentery, supply blood to the oviduct. The origins of each vessel vary between species but some generalization can be made. The cranial oviductal artery arises from the left cranial renal artery, aorta or external iliac artery. The middle oviductal artery comes from the left ischiadic artery or its branch, the medial renal artery. Finally, the caudal oviductal artery arises from the left internal iliac artery or the pudendal artery. The veins draining the cranial oviduct empty into the caudal vena cava (via the common iliac vein), while those draining the caudal oviduct enter the renal portal or hepatic systems.

Salpingohysterectomy

Salpingohysterectomy is the surgical removal of the oviduct, infundibulum to uterus, is indicated for chronic egg laying and any oviduct disease that cannot be medically managed and is reported as the "therapy of choice for overproduction of eggs." Every attempt should be made to understand the bird's overall health status prior to surgery, as the patient should ideally be stable. Birds with septic yolk peritonitis generally carry a poor prognosis. Patients with underlying health problems such as various lung, liver and kidney diseases can also complicate surgery. Otherwise healthy salpingo-hysterectomy candidates typically do well and surgery is often straightforward especially when the oviduct is small and inactive. Oviductal hypertrophy occurs secondary to elevated estrogen levels during sexual activity and can take up most of the left side of the intestinal-peritoneal portion of the coelomic cavivity. This oviductal hypertrophy includes increased vascularity and risk of bleeding during surgery. If the patient is stable, time permits, and increased reproductive tract vascularity is suspected, the author will "condition" the bird prior to surgery. "Conditioning" includes improving nutritional status (if necessary) and attempting to turn off the bird's sexual cycle. This process may take weeks to months and often results in decreased vasularity and lower patient morbidity.

In the author's experience, a left lateral approach offers the best exposure to the female avian reproductive tract, but a ventral midline approach can also be used. Perform a left lateral celiotomy. After incising through the left abdominal air sac, the ovary and oviduct are readily visible. Gently retract the cranial oviduct (infundibulum area) out the incision and hemoclip or cauterize suspensory ligament vessels as needed. The closer the bird is to laying, the larger the vessels present. Depending on the size, the cranial, middle and/or caudal oviductal artery (ies) may need to be hemoclipped or cauterized. Once visualized, hemoclip the base of the oviduct just proximal to its junction with the cloaca. Excise the oviduct.

Cystic follicles should either be aspirated (drained) or removed. If the follicle is accidentally incised, yolk will leak into the abdomen. Simply "mop up" excess yolk and other fluid if present. Collect culture and samples for histopathologic evaluation as needed.

Cesarean Section and Reproductive Tract Sparing

Cesarean section is indicated when the bird's reproductive capabilities need to be spared and is typically limited to egg binding with an otherwise normal, or minimally diseased oviduct. Depending on the location of the egg, a caudal left lateral or ventral midline approach is used. The oviduct should be incised directly over the bound egg and away from prominent blood vessels. After removing the egg, inspect the oviduct for other abnormalities and collect biopsies and cultures as needed. Close the oviduct in a single simple interrupted or continuous layer using fine (4-0 or smaller) absorbable suture material. Abdominal closure is standard. The author recommends resting the hen from reproductive stimuli for two to four weeks or longer as dictated by culture and/or histopathologic results.

SURGERY OF THE MALE AVIAN REPRODUCTIVE SYSTEM
Anatomy of the Avian Testicle

Avian male reproductive anatomy consists of three main gross structures, the testes, epididymis and ductus deferens. The paired testes are located ventral to their respective left or right cranial renal division. The mesorchium connects the testes to the dorsal body wall. The left testicle is typically larger than the right in most young birds, but this relationship can change as the bird ages. In seasonal breeders, such as some passerines, the testes can increase 300 to 500 times in size and should not be interpreted as neoplasia. In addition to size, the color of the testicles can also change with fluctuating hormone levels ranging from black in the sexually immature or inactive cockatoos to white or yellow in the chicken.

The epididymis is located at the testicular hilus, or dorsomedial aspect of the testes. The ductus deferens continue from the epididymis as highly convoluted tubes running lateral to and alongside the ureters and then terminate at the urodeum as a papillae ventral to the ureteral ostium. Budgerigars and passerines have a 'ball of tissue' (seminal glomus) at the distal end of the ductus deferens that serves as sperm storage and forms a prominent projection (cloacal promontory) that can be used to sex some birds.

The testicular artery arises from the cranial renal artery and provides most of the arterial blood supply to the testes. An accessory testicular artery may arise directly from the aorta. The venous drainage is returned either directly to the caudal vena cava or forms a common stem with the adrenal veins. Kremer and Budras found that two testicular veins empty directly into the caudal vena cava of Peking drakes (*Anas platyrhynchos*). Given the diversity within the class Aves, it is likely that multiple variations of the testicular vasculature exist.

Castration

Avian castration is infrequently discussed, especially in comparison to salpingohysterectomy, suggesting that male reproductive tract diseases are relatively uncommon. Although caponization is common in the poultry industry (performed between 1 and 2 weeks of age), routine castration is rare in pet birds, especially psittacines. As a result, there is little information regarding the behavior altering effects of castration in pet birds. Until further studies are available, castration should be used judiciously to alter avian behaviors, especially in adult birds and should always be considered secondary to more conservative methods of behavior management. However, castration has real benefit with testicular cancer, abscesses/granulomas, cysts and other conditions that may not respond to medical management alone.

Several methods of castration have been forwarded and include simple extraction (caponization), laser ablation, intracapsular suction, and en bloc surgical excision. Even with early age caponization, testicular regrowth is well documented. This supports the need for complete testicular removal, which is why the author prefers en bloc surgical excision.

Use a cranial left lateral approach or ventral midline incision with transverse flap to evaluate the testes. Due to the cranial location, the lateral celiotomy is often extended cranially by cutting the last two ribs to improve exposure to the testes. Depending on the species, puncture through the caudal thoracic and/or the abdominal air sac(s) to expose the left testis. The right testis may be exposed through the same incision by cutting through the midline junction of the corresponding air sacs or the process may be repeated with a right lateral celiotomy. With gentle traction, pull the testis ventrally and hemoclip the dorsal blood supply. If two can be placed, then incise between the hemoclips and remove the testis. Otherwise, use electrocautery to carefully free the testis from the hemoclip and vascular cord. The cautery should destroy any remaining testicular cells attached to the hemoclip but be careful to not damage the overlying blood vessels, kidney or adrenal gland. Alternatively, if the testicular blood supply is small, a hemostat can be temporarily used in place of a hemoclip and the testis pulled free. Leave the hemostat on the vascular stump for 1 to 2 minutes prior to release. Use direct pressure hemostasis as needed. Diode laser excision can also be used through this approach and may be performed without the need for direct hemostasis. Closure is routine.

References are available from the author upon request.

GETTING JUICED ABOUT PANCREATIC DISEASE

M. Scott Echols, DVM, Diplomate ABVP
Westgate Pet and Bird Hospital
Austin, TX

AVIAN PANCREAS

In most avian species, the pancreas is trilobed with the third, or splenic, lobe sometimes being detached from the other two. The duodenal loop encircles most of the avian pancreas. In most species, each lobe has a separate draining duct. In general, the ducts all drain into the duodenum often at the distal duodenal loop.

The functions of the pancreas can be divided into exocrine and endocrine. The avian exocrine pancreatic enzymes such as amylase, carboxypeptidases, deoxyribonucleases, elastases, ribonucleases, trypsin, chymotrypsin and lipases are similar to those found in mammals. Also of note, the intestinal wall mucosa can produce amylase, lipases and other enzymes that aid in digestion. Amylase levels are highest in the jejunum of birds.

The primary endocrine function of the pancreas is glucose metabolism. Following feeding, plasma glucose and amino acids stimulate the release of insulin from pancreatic B cells. The insulin aids the liver in glycogenesis. With low blood glucose concentration, glucagon (pancreatic A cells) increases and insulin decreases. Elevated glucagon (catabolic) stimulates glycogenolysis, gluconeogenesis, and lipolysis in the liver. Somatostatin (pancreatic D cells) controls the ratio of insulin to glucagon released from the pancreas. Pancreatic peptides (F cells) are stimulated by cholecystokinin, secretin, absorbed amino acids and gastrin and are glycogenolytic without producing hyperglycemia. The interactions of the endocrine pancreatic components with other body systems and diabetes mellitus are very complex and will not be further covered here.

PANCREATITIS

When digestive enzymes such as protease, phospholipidase, and trypsin are activated within the pancreas, pancreatitis can result. Subsequent damage results in further release and activation of these enzymes into ducts and extracellular tissue. Resultant free radical production can produce further damage.

The actual initiating cause of pancreatitis is sometimes difficult to identify; however, several factors have been noted. Viral diseases including Paramyxovirus type 3 (especially in *Neophema* spp), adenovirus, herpesvirus, polyomavirus and avian influenza A can all cause variable pancreatic inflammation and necrosis. Bacterial invasion (presumably through the intestinal tract or systemically) can also cause pancreatitis. Obesity-related pancreatitis, especially those psittacine species on all-seed diets, is commonly discussed. Some species such as quaker parakeets (*Myiopsitta monachus*) are especially prone to acute pancreatic necrosis and death. The author has also observed this syndrome in macaws (*Ara* spp). Zinc toxicosis results in pancreatic vacuolization and acinar cell degeneration. Secondary damage from egg yolk peritonitis (coelomitis) may also cause pancreatitis. Birds with exocrine pancreatic insufficiency often have pale voluminous feces and may exhibit chronic weight loss. Primary and metastatic pancreatic cancer may also be encountered.

DIAGNOSING PANCREATIC DISEASE

As with mammals, diagnosing pancreatitis in birds can be difficult. Gastrointestinal dysfunction (vomiting, diarrhea, ileus, polyuria, polydipsia, and coelomic distension) and pain (anorexia, lethargy, aggression, wide-based stance, kicking, coelomic feather damaging and obsessive chewing) are some of the nonspecific signs associated with pancreatitis. Blood amylase is probably the best noninvasive method used to diagnose pancreatitis. However, blood amylase may also increase with proventricular, ventricular and small intestinal disease, renal disease, glucocorticoid administration and coelomic inflammation and is therefore not specific to pancreatic disease. Pancreatic biopsy is the method of choice for diagnosing pancreatic diseases.

TREATING PANCREATIC DISEASE

Strategies for treating pancreatic diseases have been adapted from the mammalian literature. Immediate care often consists of fluid therapy to correct fluid deficits and promote tissue perfusion, analgesics (butorphanol), intestinal motility stimulants (metaclopramide and cisapride) to counteract intestinal ileus and parenteral antibiotic therapy. Zinc and other toxicoses should also be treated. Omega-3 fatty acids may also be used for their anti-inflammatory and lipid stabilizing effects. Converting birds on an all seed diet to a lower fat diet is also appropriate. Plasma transfusions may help by replacing protease inhibitors and slowing or stopping further pancreatic damage in cases of life threatening pancreatitis. Contributing gastrointestinal foreign bodies should be addressed ideally with conservative means or surgical removal if needed. Pancreatic enzymes can be added to food to 'pre-digest' a meal for birds with exocrine pancreatic insufficiency. Surgical debulking and chemotherapy may be considered in cases of pancreatic neoplasia.

PANCREATIC BIOPSY AND DUODENAL ASPIRATION

Pancreatic biopsy is indicated when pancreatic disease, such as pancreatitis and neoplasia, is suspected and accurate diagnosis is needed for individual case management. A cranial ventral midline approach is used similar as with liver biopsy. The dorsal and ventral pancreatic lobes rest between the ascending and descending duodenal loop. The duodenum is located to the right of midline and is often covered by a thin peritoneal membrane. Incise through the thin membrane and gently retract the duodenal loop. After examining the pancreas and duodenum for gross abnormalities, select the distal (free) end of the dorsal pancreatic lobe (unless another site is clearly abnormal). Using hemostats, clamp the pancreas just distal to its distal-most vessel coming off the duodenum. Remove the distal pancreatic fragment and submit for pathologic evaluation. Usually, a 3- to 8-mm section of pancreas is harvested. Remove the hemostats, but re-apply if bleeding occurs. Sutures to control hemostasis are rarely indicated. Close the abdomen in standard fashion.

Pancreatic duct ligation results in severe damage to the pancreas. Most of the pancreas lies within the duodenal loop and has one to three draining ducts that enter the terminal duodenum in close proximity to the bile and hepatic ducts. The potential complications of bile duct ligation are listed below. Pancreatic duct ligation results in atrophic pancreatic acini and interstitial fibrosis in chicks (similar to what is noted with the same procedure in mammals). Pancreatic duct obstruction has been a proposed cause of stunting syndrome in chickens.

If both bile ducts are ligated (chickens), severe fibrosing cholehepatitis results within 28 days. The typical lesions that result from extrahepatic bile duct ligation in poultry include cholestasis, fibrosis, proliferated biliary ductules and increased Ito (fat storing) cells within the liver. While not jaundiced, chickens with both bile ducts ligated also developed intensely yellow stained droppings 6 to 7 days post surgery. Bile duct ligation results in atrophic and sclerotic testes 10 weeks post surgery in 1-year-old chickens likely as a result of the hepatic fibrosis and obstructive cholestasis the procedure causes.

A high-grade pancreatic exocrine adenocarcinoma was removed from a 5-year-old male cockatiel via celiotomy. The report describes a "large, firm, white multinodular pedunculated mass (2.5 cm in diameter) that originated between the distal portion of the pancreas and ascending loop of the duodenum." The authors also reported they removed the distal tip of the pancreas adjacent to the mass at the same time. Neoplastic cells were surgically evident at the biopsy margins. Six weeks after surgery, the bird was doing well and celecoxib (10 mg/kg PO SID) was administered for 3 months. One hundred forty-two days post surgery the bird presented with dyspnea and died during diagnostic sample collection. The bird had diffuse metastatic pancreatic adenocarcinoma. Of note, the bird had acute diffuse renal tubular necrosis (possibly due to the celecoxib).

The birds and their pancreas seem to tolerate pancreatic surgery well. Following 99% pancreatectomy in chickens, the splenic pancreatic lobe undergoes a rapid enlargement (400% increase) over 16 days. Partially depancreatomized chickens, with splenic lobe intact, also seem to maintain metabolic parameters remarkably well although a post-surgical transitory hyperglycemia may be noted. One conclusion drawn is that the avian splenic lobe appears to be "extremely competent following removal of the major avian pancreatic lobes in adjusting to the demands placed on it for adequate nutrient absorption and distribution." Total

pancreatectomy is fatal, but subtotal pancreatectomy (leaving the splenic lobe intact) results in transient "diabetes" that resolves in 12 days in Peking ducks

Duodenal aspiration may be helpful in identifying occult parasitic (Giardia spp and other protozoa) and Mycobacteria spp infections and small intestinal bacterial overgrowth. Via a ventral midline surgical approach, the duodenal loop is isolated (see above). Using a 25-gauge or smaller needle, aspirate the duodenal contents for culture and cytology. Additionally, use another needle with the bevel side up to aspirate the mucosal surface of the duodenum. Oftentimes, occult mycobacterial organisms can be recovered cytologically by aspirating affected thickened duodenal mucosa. Closure is standard and the collected samples should be processed/evaluated as soon as possible.

REFERENCES:

1. Gelis S. Evaluating and treating the gastrointestinal system. In: Harrison GJ, Lightfoot TL (eds): Clinical Avian Medicine Volume I. Palm Beach, FL: Spix Publishing, 2006, pp 411-440.
2. Hudelson S, Hudelson PM. Endocrine considerations. In: Harrison GJ, Lightfoot TL (eds): Clinical Avian Medicine Volume I. Palm Beach, FL: Spix Publishing, 2006, pp 541-557.
3. Martland MF. Histopathology of the chick pancreas following pancreatic duct ligation. Vet Rec. 1986;118:526-530
4. Onderka DK, Langevin CC, Hanson JA. Fibrosing cholehepatitis in broiler chickens induced by bile duct ligations or inoculation of Clostridium perfringens. Can J Vet Res. 1990;54:285-290
5. Handharyani E, et al. Immunohistochemical and ultrastructural study of Ito cells (fat-storing cells) in response to extrahepatic bile duct ligation in broiler chickens. J Vet Med Sci. 2001;63:547-552
6. Yoshioka K, et al. Testicular atrophy after bile duct ligation in chickens. Vet Pathol. 2004;41:68-72
7. Chen S, Bartrick T. Resection and use of a cyclooxygenase-2 inhibitor for treatment of pancreatic adenocarcinoma in a cockatiel. J Am Vet Med Assoc. 2006;228:69-73
8. Hazelwood RL, Cieslak SR. In vitro release of pancreatic hormones following 99% pancreatectomy in the chicken. Gen Comp Endocrinol. 1989;73:308-317
9. Laurent F, Karmann H, Mialhe P. Insulin, glucagon and somatostatin content in normal and diabetic duck pancreas. Horm Metabol Res. 1987;19:134-135
10. Baron EJ, Finegold SM: Microorganisms encountered in the gastrointestinal tract. In: Baron EJ, Finegold SM (eds): Diagnostic Microbiology, ed 8. St. Louis: The CV Mosby Company, 1990, p 246
11. Speer BL. A clinical look at the avian pancreas in health and disease. In: Proceedings Association Avian Veterinarians Annual Conference, St Paul, MN, 1998, p 57.

RESPIRATORY DISTRESS AND THERAPEUTICS

M. Scott Echols, DVM, Diplomate ABVP
Westgate Pet and Bird Hospital
Austin, TX

Respiratory distress is common in avian practice. By classifying the type of respiratory disease, clinicians are better able to determine a cause and resolution. This article attempts to help practitioners classify and treat various forms of respiratory disease in awake and anesthetized birds.

ACUTE RESPIRATORY DISTRESS

Acute respiratory distress is a potentially life-threatening emergency condition seen in birds. Its causes can be divided into large airway disease, parenchymal disease, coelom space disease, and small airway disease. Prior to differentiation, all avian patients experiencing acute respiratory distress should be gently handled to minimize stress and provided with supplemental oxygen in preparation for more aggressive diagnostics.

LARGE AIRWAY DISEASE

Causes of large airway disease include tracheal obstruction (foreign body, fungal or bacterial granuloma, intratracheal neoplasia, stricture, and others) or oropharyngeal masses, granulomas, swelling, or other disorders that obstruct airflow in and out of the trachea. These birds often require rapid anesthetic induction, intubation to get past oropharyngeal masses or an air sac tube if the trachea is obstructed. Diagnostics (eg, tracheal endoscopy, tracheal wash, radiographs) follow once the patient is more stable.

Air Sac Breathing Tube

If the oral cavity or trachea is occluded preventing proper induction or maintenance of anesthesia or the air sacs need to be medicated, an air sac tube can be used. Patients with oral masses, tracheal obstructions, etc should be mask (if possible) or box induced. Anesthesia delivered via air sac breathing tubes has been successfully used in patients as small as zebra finches.

When anesthetized, place the patient in lateral recumbency and quickly, surgically prepare the paralumbar fossa (just behind the last rib). A small skin incision is made over the paralumbar fossa (same site as for surgical sexing) exposing a relatively thin layer of lateral abdominal wall muscles. Use right angle forceps to "punch" through the muscle layer and into the underlying air sac. Place a sterilized endotracheal, red rubber feeding or other tube into the air sac (either caudal thoracic or abdominal air sac, depending on the bird species and placement) and suture (the tube) to the skin. When properly placed, one can hold a down feather over the tube opening to watch for air movement or place a slide and watch for condensation. The tube diameter should be approximately the same size as the patient's tracheal lumen. Due to progressive micro-organism infection and air sacculitis, air sac breathing tubes should not be left in avian patients more than 5 days. In addition to infection, air sac breathing tubes can result in coelomic organ damage, life-threatening blood loss (from vessel laceration/trauma), air sac damage, and subcutaneous emphysema (which is usually self-limiting).

In studied sulfur-crested cockatoos (*Cacatua galerita*), delivering isoflourane and oxygen via caudal thoracic air sac intubation provided a reliable method of maintaining anesthesia and resulted in minimal alteration in respiratory function similar to endotracheal tube administration. In the same study, clavicular air sac intubation did not provide adequate ventilation or maintenance of anesthesia.

PARENCHYMAL DISEASE

Causes of parenchymal disease include smoke inhalation; fungal, viral, bacterial and parasitic pneumonia; and cardiogenic pulmonary edema. Bronchodilators (parental or via nebulization) and antibiotics may benefit birds with parenchymal disease. An air sac tube may also improve respiration in these birds, but is often a less dramatic improvement as is seen in birds with large airway disease. If a murmur, arrhythmia or muffled heart sounds are auscultated, cardiogenic edema or pericardial effusion may be present. Furosemide (2–4 mg/kg IV) and nitroglycerine ointment on the tongue may help stabilize the patient for additional diagnostics. Broncodilators, antibiotics, and antifungals should be considered with pneumonia.

COELOM SPACE DISEASE

Coelom space disease includes those causes of coelomic distension such as liver disease, egg-related and other peritonitis, heart disease, hypoalbuminemia and organomegaly. If fluid is present, coelomocentesis and standard fluid evaluation are recommended. Depending on fluid analysis, antibiotics may be indicated. Ultrasound and radiographs can be beneficial in differentiating coelomic masses, eggs, and fluid from each other. If present, egg binding is treated (eg, ovocentesis, fluid therapy, warmth). Organomegaly often requires a full medical work up to identify the problem and guide therapy.

Coelomocentesis

Coelomocentesis is indicated for birds with free coelomic fluid of unknown type or origin. Due to the coelomic, intestinal-peritoneal and dorsal and ventral hepatic-peritoneal cavities in normal birds, a single free "cavity" does not exist. Attempts at 'abdominal washes' are difficult and can result in fluid infusion into the abdominal or caudal thoracic air sacs potentially causing or contributing to respiratory distress. With increasing coelomic fluid, the avian air sacs become compressed, the coelom distends and the patient may develop varying degrees of dyspnea. An affected bird should be restrained with the long axis of its body oriented vertically, or slightly tilted forward, and head up. Use of anesthesia may be contraindicated due to potential respiratory compromise.

The ventral coelom is aseptically prepared and a small gauge needle (21- to 27-gauge) is inserted on the midline just caudal to the sternum (keel). As is needed to avoid the ventriculus (gizzard), the needle is directed to the right side of the body and any fluid present is aspirated. As with other avian fluids, the aspirated sample should be processed quickly and may be used for microbiological, cytologic, and biochemical analysis.

SMALL AIRWAY DISEASE

Small airway disease is often the most difficult to manage and may be due to inhalation of respiratory irritants such as Teflon fumes, aerosols, smoke, and candle suet. These respiratory irritants cause acute bronchoconstriction leading to cough and acute respiratory disease. This series of events creates a need for immediate therapy and bronchodilators are often the first line drugs. Because of a faster onset of action, nebulized bronchodilators are the first choice. Bronchodilators that stimulate beta-adrenergic receptors in bronchial smooth muscle (causing smooth muscle relaxation) are considered the most effective for treating acute bronchoconstriction and respiratory distress. Lichtenberger recommends the beta-agonist terbutiline first given as an aerosol or second, given IM (0.01 mg/kg).

Several nebulization options exist. Jet nebulizers are inexpensive; the most common and create a gas stream that draws drug solution up a tube and then pulverizes the mixture to form an aerosol spray. Ultrasonic nebulizers are more expensive and generate an aerosol using an ultra-high frequency vibrating piezoelectric crystal at the bottom of the drug solution. While ultrasonic nebulizers have faster nebulization time, smaller particle size, quieter operation and longer product life than jet nebulizers, studies in humans have shown little difference between the two types. Metered dose inhalers (MDI) can be used for rapid local administration of bronchodilators (such as albuterol). However, the actual dose of drug deposited in the lower airway is unknown using a MDI. Some MDI come with a soft facemask that can be used with larger psittacine birds.

Oxygen Administration

Facial or environmentally increased (cage) oxygen is essential for many critical avian patients. The indications for supplemental oxygen may include any type of respiratory or cardiac disease, shock, postsurgical recovery, and patient stress. Oxygen delivered by facial mask may not be well tolerated in some fractious, disoriented, and wild patients. If a specifically designed "oxygen cage" is not available, most incubators, cages and aquariums can be modified so that supplemental oxygen can be provided in a closed environment. For most critical avian patients kept in a closed chamber, a 40% oxygen saturation level is recommended. Pure oxygen is acceptable for short-term use when given via a facemask or in an enclosed environment.

It should be noted that oxygen "toxicity" in the form of pulmonary oxidative stress and toxicity with histologic changes in the lungs has been noted in budgerigars. The studied birds were kept in a high oxygen environment (95% O_2) for as little as 3 hours and developed signs of oxidative stress, perivascular edema, bronchial pneumonia and depletion of body antioxidants (carotenoids, alpha tocopherol) that worsened with prolonged oxygen exposure. This recent information further supports limiting the exposure to pure supplemental oxygen in avian patients.

RESPIRATORY DISTRESS WHILE UNDER ANESTHESIA

Birds in respiratory distress are frequently encountered in avian practice. Not only are birds brought in for emergency evaluation, but respiratory disease may develop during anesthesia. It is important for the attending clinician to recognize normal and abnormal respiratory patterns for birds undergoing anesthetic procedures and how to deal with problems when they arise.

Abnormal Breathing Patterns Should Be Identified and Resolved as Soon as Possible

Pathologic conditions such as pain (surgical manipulation), lung hemorrhage, and overheating can induce rapid breathing (**tachypnea**). With painful conditions, tachypnea usually resolves by inducing a deeper plane of anesthesia. Tachypnea associated with blood-filled lungs (hemorrhage) responds poorly to increasing the anesthetic dose. If lung hemorrhage is suspected or identified (visualized via endoscopy or laparoscopy), anesthesia should be stopped or continued only with great caution. In birds, lung hemorrhage can be fatal, especially if progressive; its cause is poorly understood and no treatments are currently described. Increased respiration due to overheating is most commonly noted when the avian patient is "light" or upon recovery, but sometimes hyperthermia contributes to mild tachypnea during deeper anesthetic planes.

Dyspnea, or difficult and labored breathing, often indicates poor ventilation. Tachypnea and dyspnea can be very similar, are often difficult to distinguish and share some common causes. Underlying diseases (heart, lung, and air sac disorders), as opposed to human induced overheating and pain, are more frequently associated with dyspnea in birds. Dyspnea may occur due to an obstruction (such as a mucus plug) in the trachea or endotracheal tube, poor cardiovascular perfusion (heart disease and anemia), fluid or blood-filled lungs (pulmonary edema, inflammation and hemorrhage) and decreased or diseased air sac space resulting from improper restraint/positioning, ascites, bleeding, organomegaly, other abdominal masses and air sacculitis. Correction of dyspnea is aimed at identifying and addressing the underlying cause.

Apnea, or cessation of breathing, is common in anesthetized birds and can be associated with multiple conditions. If apneic birds are not restored (artificially or naturally) to breathing, death may soon follow and faster than is noted in cats and dogs. Apnea is commonly due to poor ventilation, taping the beak closed (diving birds), excessive anesthetic, and hypothermia, but may also be associated with hypoglycemia, hypovolemia (blood or other fluid loss), and other underlying metabolic and systemic disturbances. Apnea is frequently preceded by decreased respiration. Identifying and correcting the causes of decreased respiration will help the monitoring nurse prevent apnea or respond more quickly, should it (apnea) occur.

When a bird's respiration begins to drop, first evaluate the patient's anesthetic dose, surgical conditions (eg, disrupting air sacs/lungs, excessive blood loss), and monitoring tools (eg, body temperature, heart rate). Correct obvious deficits as best as possible by lowering anesthetic dose, providing fluid support, maintaining patient body heat, and so on as needed. If decreased respiration is progressive, auscultate the lungs and trachea and determine if the passages are clear. Tracheal mucus plugs will often produce a "gurgling" sound that may only be heard with the aid of a stethoscope. Lung hemorrhage and edema may also result in abnormal respiratory sounds and should be considered as well. Remove the endotracheal tube (if present) and check for blood or mucus plugs that may be contributing to poor ventilation. In general, endotracheal tubes may need to be replaced every 30 minutes to decrease plug formation. Air sac tubes are an exception, as they rarely occlude with mucus and can be left in for days without problems. However, air sac tubes can become plugged with blood, other fluids and organ tissue and should be checked for patency as needed. The surgeon should be notified when the patient is becoming apneic so he or she can identify and resolve any surgical conditions that may be interfering with respiration.

If respiration decreases to the point of apnea, several steps should be taken to restore breathing. Quickly evaluate the patient as discussed in the above paragraph. If breathing cannot be restored, turn off all anesthetic gas, maintain oxygen flow, and manually ventilate the patient. When manually ventilating birds, provide enough pressure (8–12 cm H_2O) to create normal inspiratory depth and 10–12 respirations per minute. Some feel that artificial ventilation should be routinely provided to all anesthetized birds. To prevent trauma to the air sacs when providing positive pressure ventilation, limit the pressures to 15–20 cm H_2O.

In birds, decreased ventilation results in increased $PaCO_2$ which directly affects pH and acid-base balance. The expected response in an awake, healthy bird is to increase ventilation, which decreases $PaCO_2$ and increases pH. Birds must adequately ventilate to maintain proper acid-base balance. Anesthetized birds may not properly ventilate themselves and often require artificial ventilation. In ducks, the common parameters such as respiratory frequency and tidal volume alone cannot be used to monitor acid-base balance. Studies in Amazon parrots have clearly shown that intermittent positive pressure ventilation will decrease $PaCO_2$, which

subsequently affects pH and acid–base balance. Even birds that are self-ventilating while under anesthesia should be assisted with 4 to 6 respirations per minute.

The sternum may be moved ventrally and dorsally to provide ventilation if no endotracheal tube or sealed face mask is being used. If the air sacs have been exposed as part of surgery, the surgeon may need to temporarily "close" the surgical site with a finger to help permit more normal ventilation. If the patient is apneic, the surgeon must attempt to limit overall surgical time while the attending nurse increases the oxygen flow rate and continues assisted ventilation. Sometimes continued tissue manipulation will help the patient respond and begin breathing. Patients that become apneic and are restored should be maintained on a very light plane of anesthesia for the remainder of the procedure.

Cardiac Arrest Often Follows Prolonged Apnea or Dyspnea

Maintaining normal fluid volume, proper oxygenation, ventilation and monitoring, minimal use of cardiodepressive drugs, and appropriate anesthetic depth are all needed to help prevent cardiac arrest. Certainly, some underlying conditions may adversely affect the heart and may be precipitated by anesthesia. If cardiac arrest occurs, begin cardiopulmonary resuscitation. If possible, place an endotracheal tube (if not already present) and restore ventilation. Doxapram, a positive inotrope, can be given (to help stimulate respiration. Also consider Hetastarch at 5 mL/kg intravenously (IV) or intaosseously (IO) to increase blood pressure and improve organ perfusion. Manipulate the sternum, as described above, to assist circulation and ventilation. Due to anatomy, direct cardiac massage is very difficult. Intravenous, intratracheal, or intracardiac epinephrine (0.5–1.0 mL/ kg of 1:1,000) can be tried to stimulate the heart. Unfortunately, birds are very difficult to resuscitate once cardiac arrest occurs.

REFERENCES
1. Lichtenberger M. Emergency case approach to hypotension, hypertension, and acute respiratory distress. In: Association of Avian Veterinarians Annual Conference, San Antonio, TX, 2006, pp 281-290.
2. Ludders JW. Respiratory physiology of birds: considerations for anesthetic management. Semin Avian Exotic Pet Med. 1998;7(1):3-9.
3. Curro TG. Anesthesia of pet birds. Semin Avian Exotic Pet Med. 1998;7(1):10-21.
4. Jenkins JR. Hospital techniques and supportive care. In: Altman RB, Clubb SL, Dorrestein GM, et al (eds): Avian Medicine and Surgery. Philadelphia: WB Saunders, 1997, pp 232-252.
5. Brown C, Pilny A. Air sac cannula placement in birds. Lab Animal. 2006;35:23-24.
6. Mitchell J, Bennett RA, Spalding M. Air sacculitis associated with the placement of an air breathing tube. In Association of Avian Veterinarian Annual Conference, New Orleans, LA, 1999, pp 145-146.

7. Jaensch SM, Cullen L, Raidal SR. Comparison of endotracheal, caudal thoracic air sac, and clavicular air sac administration of isoflourane in sulphur-crested cockatoos (*Cacatua galerita*). JAMS. 2001;15(3):170-177.

8. Campbell TW: Cytology of abdominal effusions. In: Avian Hematology and Cytology. Ames, IA: Iowa State University Press, 1988, p 41.

9. Campbell TW: Cytology. In: Ritchie BW, Harrison GJ, Harrison LR (eds): Avian Medicine: Principles and Application. Lake Worth, FL: Wingers Publishing, 1994, pp 199-222.

10. Jenkins JR. Avian critical care and emergency medicine. In: Altman RB, Clubb SL, Dorrestein GM, Quesenberry K (eds): Avian Medicine and Surgery. Philadelphia: WB Saunders, 1997, pp 839-863.

11. Jaensch S, Cullen L, Raidal S. The pathology of normobaric oxygen toxicity in budgerigars (*Melopsittacus undulatus*). Avian Pathol. 2001;30:135-142.

12. Phalen DN. Principles of avian anesthesia. *In* TAMU Annual Exotic Pets Conference, College Station, TX, 2000, pp 19-22.

13. Edling TM. Anesthesia and Monitoring. In: Harrison GJ, Lightfoot TL (eds): Clinical Avian Medicine Volume 1. Palm Beach, FL: Spix Publishing, 2006, pp 747-760.

14. Edling TM. The effects of intermittent positive pressure ventilation on African Grey Parrots. In: Association of Avian Veterinarian Annual Conference, Portland, OR, 2000, pp 223-225.

15. Rupley AE. Emergency procedures: recovering from disaster. In: Association of Avian Veterinarians Annual Conference, Reno, NV, 1997, pp 249-257.

WOUND CARE AND MANAGEMENT

M. Scott Echols, DVM, Diplomate ABVP
Westgate Pet and Bird Hospital
Austin, TX

GENERAL WOUND ASSESSMENT

Avian wounds come in many forms and result from many causes. The general principles of wound management used in small animal practice are similar with bird medicine. Some anatomic and physiologic differences do exist with birds which may change some treatment strategies.

As a general rule, all wounded avian patients deserve a complete history and physical examination prior to setting a treatment plan. Antibiotics are considered with bite wounds, necrotic and infected tissue, and any time infection is a concern. When possible, culture and sensitivity should direct antibiotic choice; otherwise safe broad-spectrum antibiotics are recommended. Birds should be stabilized as much as possible prior to anesthetic events and provided with cardiorespiratory, dietary, and fluid support, pain management ,and hemorrhage control as needed.

Open wounds should be protected with bandages, surgical closure and/or semi-occlusive bandages. Necrotic wounds should be debrided prior to closure. Consider primary closure for clean wounds less than 24 hours old. Give burn wounds 3 to 7 days post injury to better delineate normal and dead tissue prior to surgical wound closure. Because avian skin is so thin and is rapidly revasularized, free skin grafts work better in birds than most other animals. When cleaning the injured site, create a 2- to 3-cm circumferential featherless zone around the wound.

Although little information exists on suture material in birds, chromic catgut, polyglactin 910, polydioxanone (PDS), monofilament nylon and monofilament stainless steel have been evaluated in rock doves (*Columba livia*). From this information and the author's experience, PDS is slowly absorbed and causes minimal tissue reaction making it suitable for both internal and skin closure use.

The function of the bird and how the injury will affect the avian patient should be considered. With some exceptions, injured wild birds should be managed with the intent to release the patient back to the wild. Many wounds may not be initially life-threatening but may result in long-term injuries that preclude normal flying, hunting or escape techniques. Some of these birds may need to be humanely euthanized.

General principles are provided. Addressing each type of possible avian wound goes beyond the scope of this article.

AVIAN SKIN

Avian skin is quite different from that in mammals. While birds have epidermal, dermal and subcutaneous layers, the epidermis is extremely thin with typically only three to five cell layers (except over thicker nonfeathered areas such as the feet, beak, legs and face). With the exception of the uropygial gland, avian skin typically lacks glands and is dry and inelastic over much of the body. However, individual keratinocytes act as holocrine glands and can produce oils.

Avian wound healing has been described in three phases including inflammatory, collagen and maturation. Wound healing in birds begins with a clot and inflammatory response much as with mammals. Heterophils and monocytes, later followed by lymphocytes, infiltrate the avian wound (inflammatory phase). Next fibroblasts and then capillaries proliferate (collagen phase). Last collagen fibers organize and ultimately orient themselves in relation to the tension placed on the edges of the wound (maturation phase). In this last phase, the wound contracts attempting to bring epithelial margins back together closing the wound and can take weeks to months to complete.

As another notable avian feature, normal bruising results in a greenish discoloration in the bird. After hemoglobin is broken down, biliverdin pigment accumulates giving the greenish color within 2 to 3 days post injury.

SKIN PROTECTIVE DEVICES

Aside from instances of self-mutilation, most birds will not continue to traumatize their wounds (surgical, injury, etc). Surprisingly, birds rarely pull at sutures after surgery. If birds do self-mutilate their wounds, this may suggest pain and the cause should be investigated and dealt with as needed (pain medications, evaluate the surgery site, etc.). Birds that have primary wounds from self-mutilation deserve a full medical and behavioral workup. Regardless, neck collars and bandages can be useful when birds self-traumatize their wounds or when open wound management is needed.

As a general rule, adherent bandages are used during the initial inflammatory stage of healing. Nonadherant bandages are reserved for the proliferative and remodeling stages of healing.

Nonstick (Tegaderm, 3M Company, St Paul, MN) or minimally adhesive (VetWrap, 3M Company Animal Care Products) bandaging material can be used to protect a tissue bed and prevent serum leakage from a wound. Semi-occlusive dressings (Tegaderm) may be poorly adhesive but can be laid over a cleaned wound and then covered with a bandage. Cyanoacrylic products or tissue glue (Nexaband, Veterinary Product Laboratories, Phoeniz, AZ) can be used to repair minor incisions or lacerations. Aseptically applied VET BIOSIST (Cook Veterinary Products, Spencer, IN), a protein matrix bandage consisting primarily of porcine collagen, is hydrated and sutured to a wound and acts as an epithelial framework. If the patient does not reject the VET BIOSIST, the bandage material is incorporated into the host tissue. The use of this product requires a light bandage covering.

Wet to dry bandages are beneficial in large wounds that are not amenable to primary closure. Clean the defect. Soak gauze bandages with an antiseptic solution or sterile isotonic fluid and lay over the wound. Apply a thicker layer of dry gauze sponges on top of the wet sponges and use a bandage to hold everything together.

Change the bandages frequently as removal debrides and keeps the wound clean and helps stimulate granulation tissue. Once a healthy granulation tissue bed is present, nonadherent bandages can be used. The wound will either contract and eventually close or surgical assistance may be required.

Create a fast, hard fixative using super glue and baking soda. Dr Pat Redig reported mixing cyanoacrylate adhesive (also known as 'super glue') or other thin modeling cyanoacrylate with baking soda. Simply apply baking soda over a desired area and then add a drop of cyanoacrylate. The combination rapidly forms a firm adhesive that can be shaped with a grinding tool and colored as needed. Additional layers can also be added as needed. This works great for filling in beak defects and building beak prostheses.

The simplest distracting device is to place a tape tag over a bandage that the bird can otherwise reach and damage. Butterfly the central portion of a tape strip leaving two sticky ends. The sticky ends are then applied to the bird's bandage leaving a tape tag sticking out. Until the birds get use to the bandage, they often only chew on the tag if at all.

Neck collars should be reserved for birds that insist on self-traumatizing their wounds. As mentioned above, the cause of the self-mutilation should be identified and corrected if possible. Neck collars should be temporary. There are a variety of neck collars available from homemade (plastic and radiographic film 'E-collars', foam pipe insulation, etc.) and manufactured (plastic clamshell, plastic circular disks, etc.) models. The author primarily uses foam pipe insulation because it is inexpensive, effective, easily placed and because it is soft it tends to not cause pressure wounds.

SKIN DISINFECTANTS

Oftentimes skin wounds should be cleaned prior to surgical closure or bandaging. While sterile saline and other isotonic solutions can safely be used to clean and irrigate superficial wounds, bacterial contamination is common requiring chemical disinfectants. Povidone iodine (1%) and chlorhexidine diacetate (0.05%) have both been found to be equally effective at cleaning skin (in mammals). However, povidine iodine has been associated with skin reactions in some dogs. Also, povidone iodine has been shown to be toxic to fibroblasts in concentrations as low as 1-5%. Chlorhexidine at 0.05% is considered very effective and safe as a wound irrigating solution. Hydrogen peroxide (3%) is minimally effective against most bacterial organisms but is sporacidal and should be used to clean wounds that may be contaminated with clostridial organisms. Hydrogen peroxide is also toxic to fibroblasts and other tissues and is used best as a single lavage treatment.

In birds, water-miscible ointments are optimal can be applied to the skin over wounds. Oil-based ointments should be avoided or used minimally because they inhibit normal thermoregulatory function of the feathers. Silver sulfadiazine cream (Silvadene Crème, Boots Pharmaceuticals, Lincolnshire, IL) is effective against most bacteria and fungi, promotes epithelialization, penetrates necrotic and eschar tissue (good for burn wounds) but can damage fibroblasts and impeded wound contraction. Use caution with topical steroid products as these compounds may be absorbed systemically from the skin in birds.

BANDAGING TECHNIQUES

Bandaging techniques are useful in stabilizing fractures, traumatic injuries and intravenous and intraosseous catheters. The avian leg is anatomically similar to the mammalian leg except for the tarsometatarsus and distal. It is difficult to immobilize femoral fractures with external fixation alone in birds. The cardinal rule of splinting (immobilize the joint above and below the fracture) should be followed. Bandaging material should be soft and pliable as cast padding for the initial layer followed by a self-adherent bandage (VetWrap) for the outer layer. Reinforce the bandage, when necessary, with wooden splints, aluminum rods or human orthopedic products such as Orthoplast (Johnson & Johnson Products, New Brunswick, NJ) or Hexcelite (Hexcel Medical Co, Dublin, CA). At room temperature Orthoplast and Hexcelite are firm, but after placing in hot water, can be made to conform to the shape of a bird's limb. Semi-occlusive bandages (Tegaderm) are useful for self-induced traumatic lesions and abrasions. Rectangular sheets are cut into strips before removing the opposite backing material.

Most simple mid-shaft fractures heal within 3 weeks in otherwise healthy avian patients. Other fractures may require 4 to 6 weeks to heal. Regardless, most fracture stabilizing bandages are left on for 4 to 6 weeks. Open fractures and comminuted fractures should be given a guarded prognosis. Open fractures should be treated with antibiotics based on culture and sensitivity results. Advise the patient's owner to use smooth-sided cages without perches (aquarium or plastic carrier) to prevent climbing during the healing period. Joints bound too long with a bandage may develop decreased range of motion. Splinted, or otherwise bandaged, birds should be regularly evaluated by an avian veterinarian and given physical therapy as needed.

Tape Splint

Tarsometatarsal and tibiotarsal fractures are easily diagnosed by palpation and can be supported with the use of a tape splint in small birds (< 300 g). Under anesthesia, the bird's leg is plucked and inspected for signs of a compound fracture. Some compound fractures are best stabilized surgically. Otherwise, the fracture is manually reduced and overlying skin is sutured or otherwise closed as needed. Once stable, run a thin strip of overlapping lightly adhesive bandage such as VetWrap from the foot to the distal femur (tibiotarsal fracture) or mid proximal tibiotarsus (tarsometatarsal fracture). Next, place overlapping butterfly tape strips up and down the bandage. Use hemostats to crimp both ends of the butterfly tape strips. Cut the free tape ends (leaving enough for the "crimp." Most uncomplicated tarsometatarsal and tibiotarsal fractures heal within 4 to 6 weeks.

"Football-type" Bandage

The "football-type" bandage is used to immobilize toes and as a temporary bandage for bumblefoot. A large ball of soft gauze is placed within the grasp of the foot. The toes are then bound to this ball by wrapping more gauze over and around them. The whole ball may be taped to the foot and the bird may be able to bear weight on it.

Plastic Spica Bandage

Plastic splints can be used for simple, aligned fractures of the femur in small birds (< 300 g). A splint can be molded from heat activated dental and other products or padded aluminum finger splints. This is a modification of a Robert Jones bandage discussed below, except that the padded molded splint extends from the tibiotarsus proximally and over the bird's pelvis in an inverted U-shape to immobilize the femur against the body of the bird.

Modified Robert Jones Bandage

The Robert Jones bandage should be limited to any fracture of the tibiotarsus, or soft tissue injuries of the hock joint and distal structures. This bandage is most useful in birds under 500 g. Use Thermoplast or similar material and cut in an L-shape. Adjust the size of the arms of the L based on the bird. Make the vertical portion of the L as long as the tibiotarsus and the horizontal portion as long as the tarsometatarsus. Next, place a layer of padding material around the leg from the foot up to the proximal femur. Add a layer of cling or cotton gauze, tightening gently while wrapping. Heat the thermoplastic splint in hot water until it becomes clear and malleable. Position and mold the splint along the lateral aspect of the leg. Wrap the final layer of VetWrap around the material before the splint hardens.

Schroeder-Thomas Splint

A Schroeder-Thomas splint is used to stabilize fractures of the tarsometatarsus and distal one third of the tibiotarsus. Indications for these splints include fractures of the tarsometatarsus in small psittacine birds and fractures close to the hock. Wire material used in the splint and should be made with two right-angle bends next to the ring at the top so that the splint is parallel to the long axis of the leg. Position the leg so with some flexion at the hock joint. Apply a light bandage to the leg with gauze and tape. Suspend the leg within the splint by alternating strips of tape placed cranially and caudally with the toes extended to the end of the splint. Cover the splint with bandage material.

Ehmer-type Bandage

Place the leg in an Ehmer sling like as used in a dog or cat. Fold the tarsometatarsus against the tibia, and wrap gauze around both. If necessary, bind the leg to the body. Use for a dislocated hip or for temporary stabilization of fractures involving the leg.

Figure of 8 Bandage

Birds with wing fractures commonly presents with a dropped wing. Some fractures heal well with external coaptation only, with return to full function. However, bandages should be reserved for wing fractures in birds not required to return to full flight (aviary and cage birds). The wing is especially amendable to splinting as it can be splinted in the normal physiological position. A figure-of-8 bandage provides adequate stabilization for fractures of the radius and ulna, carpometacarpus, and digits and when used in conjunction with a body wrap, some fractures of the pectoral girdle and humerus. This bandage is easily placed in anesthetized patients.

Hold the wing in a normal flexed position away from the body with primary and secondary wing feathers parallel to each other as the carpus is flexed. Incorporate all scapular (shoulder) feathers into the bandage. Apply a layer of light gauze wrap or cast padding beginning as high in the axilla as possible on the medial aspect of the humerus. Continue the wrap on the dorsal surface of the wing up to the carpus, and then circle the carpus from lateral to medial ending on the ventral portion of the carpus. Pass the bandage along the ventral wing surface from the carpus and back to the axillary region. Repeat until the wing is held lightly but securely in a flexed position. Excessive layering will cause a bulky and uncomfortable bandage. Cover the gauze or cast padding with a layer of VetWrap or similar material.

To form a body wrap, use the padding material to hold the wrapped wing next to the body in a natural position. The padding is placed around the body and caudal to the opposite wing at the axillary region. Repeat the body wrap going cranial to the opposite wing, forming a vest. Add a thin layer of VetWrap or similar material. Use caution such that the caudal extent of the ventral portion of the body wrap does not interfere with leg movement.

REFERENCES

1. Riggs SM, Tully TN. Wound management in nonpsittacine birds. Vet Clin Exotic Anim Pract. 2004;7:19-36.
2. Ritzman TK. Wound healing and management in psittacine birds. Vet Clin Exotic Anim Pract. 2004; 7:87-104.
3. Bennett RA, Yaeger MJ, Trapp A, Cambre RC. Histologic evaluation of the tissue reaction to five suture materials in the body wall of rock doves (*Columba livia*). JAMS 1997; 11(3):175-182.
4. Redig PT. Raptors: practical information every avian practitioner can use. Proc Annu Conf AAV 2006, San Antonio, Texas, pp 203-212.
5. Bowles HL, Odberg E, Harrison GJ, Kottwitz JJ. Surgical resolution of soft tissue disorders. In: Harrison GJ, Lightfoot TL (eds) Clinical Avian Medicine Volume II. Palm Beach, FL: Spix Publishing, 2006, pp. 775-829.
6. Chavez W, Echols MS. Bandaging, endoscopy, and surgery in the emergency avian patient. Vet Clin Exotic Anim Pract. 2007;10:419-436.

EMERGENCIES "DOWN THERE"

M. Scott Echols, DVM, Diplomate ABVP
Westgate Pet and Bird Hospital
Austin, TX

CLOACAL ANATOMY

The avian cloaca is the common endpoint of the digestive, urinary, and reproductive tracts. As a result, disease of any of the three systems may manifest as a cloacal problem.

The cloaca is a three-chambered structure starting proximally with the coprodeum which receives contents from the rectum. The coprodeal fold is an encircling sphincter-like ridge that separates the coprodeum and urodeum. The coprodeal fold can completely close off the coprodeum from the other cloacal chambers preventing contamination of semen and eggs during ejaculation and laying, respectively.

The second and more distal chamber is the urodeum and receives the ureters and oviduct (females) and ductus deferens (males). The urodeum is typically the smallest chamber in many birds. The urodeal mucosa is physically smoother and less vascular than the in the coprodeum. Urodeal retroperistalsis pushes urine and urates aborad into the coprodeum and rectum for water and solute resorption accounting for difference in ureteral urine and the urine found in droppings. The uroproctodeal fold separates the urodeum from the more distal proctodeum.

The most distal chamber is the proctodeum which is slightly larger than the urodeum in most species. The Bursa of Fabricius is located on the proctodeal dorsal midline. The bursa is the site of B-lymphocyte production and is most prominent in juveniles. The bursa is also a site frequently affected by viral diseases such as psittacine beak and feather disease virus. The opening into the bursa and its chamber can be seen during endoscopic cloacoscopy even in some mature birds. The bursa usually involutes between 2 and 6 months of age (but this is variable).

The distal most external structure of the gastrointestinal system is the vent. The vent has a dorsal and ventral lip and is surrounded by a sphincter of voluntary muscles. The partial eversion of the vent lips results in defecation.

INFECTIOUS DISEASES OF THE CLOACA

Several infectious agents may result in cloacitis. Bacterial cloacitis is reported as rare in birds; however, the author has seen numerous cases in psittacine birds. The most common presentation is fresh blood (microscopic or gross) in the droppings and bright red cloacal mucosa. Multiple bacterial organisms may be responsible and culture and sensitivity are useful. As a note, the avian coccygeomesenteric vein drains the lower intestines and, because of the renal portal system, may drain directly into the kidneys. Inflammatory products and infectious agents may be carried directly to the kidneys contributing to or causing renal disease. As a result, the author recommends antibiotic therapy with bacterial cloacitis.

Internal papillomatous disease related to avian herpes virus is sometimes responsible for irregular, cobblestone lesions in the cloacal mucosa of (primarily South American) psittacines. Severe lesions may result in proctodeal obstruction. Affected birds may have bloody droppings, tenesmus, flatulence, malodorous feces and vent staining. Acetic acid applied to the lesions usually causes a blanching response and herpes virus PCR can be used to give supporting diagnosis. Biopsy is required for definitive diagnosis. Multiple treatments have been reported and include sharp surgical excision, mucosal stripping, electrocautery, radiosurgery, silver nitrate cautery and laser surgery.

NONINFECTIOUS DISEASES OF THE CLOACA
Cloacaliths

Cloacoliths are firm urate aggregates that sometimes form in birds. While some occur spontaneously, others are induced iatrogenically after intervention for other cloacal disease (forceful cloacal sampling, manipulation or surgery). The cloacaliths may collect feces and result in varying degrees of obstruction, inflammation and infection. Gentle removal with anti-inflammatories, antibiotics, and frequent monitoring are often required. Chronic cases may heal slowly after cloacalith removal and may still result in recurring cloacaliths.

Cloacal Prolapse

Cloacal prolapse may include the cloaca, the oviduct and/or the intestines. Idiopathic cloacal prolapse is most frequently reported in male cockatoos. These birds are often physically normal otherwise and this is believed to be behavioral in origin. The cloacal prolapse is gently replaced and temporary transcloacal sutures are used to prevent recurrence. Oftentimes, birds have prolapsed their cloaca so long that all cloacal muscles and supporting structures are permanently stretched and non-functional. In these cases, ventplasty can be performed reduce the vent size such that cloacal prolapse does not recur. It should be understood that ventplasty will likely fail if the underlying cause of the prolapse is not resolved and the bird continues to strain postoperatively. These birds and their owners often need behavioral counseling as the primary mode of treatment.

Oviductal prolapse is most commonly seen in egg-laying birds that strain excessively. If the tissue is viable, gently replace it. Apply transcloacal sutures if the prolapsed material will not remain reduced. Radiographs help confirm that no other eggs are still present prior to applying transcloacal sutures. Perform a salpingo-hysterectomy if the tissue is necrotic or severely damaged. Supportive therapy is provided as needed.

Intestinal prolapse suggests that a fistula is present in the cloaca. Gently replace the tissue and provide supportive care (eg, antibiotics, fluid therapy). Transcloacal sutures can be used to reduce the risk of further prolapse. A full medical workup is often necessary to rule out underlying disease. Rarely, an exploratory coeliotomy is needed to stabilize the prolapse.

Neoplasia

Several cancer types can be found in the cloaca and usually arise from either epithelial tissue (carcinomas, adenocarcinomas), lymphoid (lymposarcoma) or smooth muscle (leiomyomas and leiomyosarcomas). The masses may appear to bulge externally and usually only cause problems when they ulcerate and become infected, grow to be so large as to be a physical problem, or metastasize. However, neoplastic masses that form within the cloaca may be externally unapparent and obstruct the ureter (causing renal disease), distal colon (causing fecal retention and obstruction) and/or oviduct (resulting in egg binding). All invasive neoplasias and specifically cloacal carcinomas carry a poor prognosis. Biopsy is required for definitive diagnosis. If possible, resect the mass. Treatment options may exist for some non-resectable neoplasia and the author recommends consulting with an oncologist.

Phallic Prolapse

Partial and complete phallic prolapses are possible in birds with large phalli and are usually secondary to local infection, trauma and extreme weather fluctuations. Over exuberant vent sexing and mating, fecal contamination and *Neisseria* spp. (suspected sexually transmitted in geese) have all been implicated causes of phallic infections. A prolapsed phallus may become enlarged and ulcerated and compound the problem. Frostbite and resultant necrotizing dermatitis of a prolapsed phallus has been discussed in ostriches. Birds with severe prolapse and infection may be significantly depressed and often lose interest in copulation. Clean exposed phalli and carefully debride abnormal tissue prior to replacement. Topical antibiotic creams, DMSO (dimethyl sulfoxide), and systemic antibiotics may be beneficial and their use is based on clinical findings. The cloaca may need partial closure (via a mattress or transcloacal suture) to prevent recurring prolapses. Severely necrotic phalli may need surgical debridement.

REFERENCES

1. Gelis S. Evaluating and treating the gastrointestinal system. In: Harrison GJ, Lightfoot TL (eds): Clinical Avian Medicine Volume I. Palm Beach, FL: Spix Publishing, 2006, pp 411-440.
2. Echols MS. Evaluating and treating the kidneys. In: Harrison GJ, Lightfoot TL (eds): Clinical Avian Medicine Volume I. Palm Beach, FL: Spix Publishing, 2006, pp 452-491.
3. Garner MM, Phalen D. Cloacal carcinomas in psittacines: is it herpes all over again? Proc AAV 2006 Annu Conf, San Antonio, Texas, pp 21-24.
4. Echols MS. Surgery of the avian reproductive tract. Semin Avian Exotic Pet Med. 2002;V11(4):177-195.

BLOOD MATTERS

Neil A. Forbes, BVetMed, FRCVS, Diplomate ECAMS
Great Western Exotics
Swindon, Wilts, UK

A SPECIFIC DIAGNOSIS
Why

As we all know, birds are ostensibly wild creatures: they have developed in the knowledge that "if I look sick today, some one is going to come and eat me." Moreover, they have a faster metabolic rate than mammals, so that once ill, they get sick and die quicker than mammals. It is therefore essential that the "sick bird" is presented immediately. In turn the veterinarian must not simply reach for the bottle of enrofloxacin, but instead make every effort to achieve a specific diagnosis such that the most appropriate therapeutic plan can be developed.

How

In order to reach that diagnosis, the clinician must put aside sufficient "quality time," outside a regular consulting period, to work up the case. While "blood" is indeed important, even that remains just "part of the picture." All too often, when a clinician is unfamiliar with the species he is presented with, the reaction is to rely on laboratory results to hang a diagnosis on. Such an approach (although we have all been guilty of it) is inappropriate. For each sick bird, the following diagnostic tools should be applied: full history taking, visual examination of the bird and its environment, physical examination, clinical pathology sample collection (blood, faeces, swabs, aspirates, etc.), radiography (at least two views at right angles, preferably additional exposures with varying exposure levels). Only at this stage will one decide if further more specialist techniques are required, eg, endoscopy, ultrasound, electrocardiography.

SAMPLE COLLECTION

A 23- or 25-gauge needle is used. If the sample is slow to draw due to vein collapse as suction is applied, clotting of the sample can result. For novices sampling smaller species, the syringe and needle maybe flushed with dilute (1:100) heparin to prevent clotting. The average blood volume of a bird can be taken as 10%. Ten percent of this can be removed from circulation for testing, that is, 1% of the bird's body weight. For a 300-g parrot, up to 3 mL of blood can be collected; for a 65-g parakeet, 0.65 mL, but one should consider the volume lost from circulation (eg, as a hematoma) as well as that collected in the syringe. Some species are easily restrained for blood collection; in others stress to the patient may be reduced by application of isoflorane. For hematology a smear should be prepared, as well as an EDTA sample (also required for lead and fibrinogen analysis). For biochemistry, heparin samples are suitable (including glucose). Avian blood may be collected from the following sites:

- **Basilic** (brachial, or superficial ulnar) vein, distal to the elbow on ventral aspect. This is easily performed in all species > 150 g unless the patient is anemic or has a collapsed circulation.
- **Medial metatarsal** (caudal tibial) vein, located on the medial aspect of the proximal metatarsus. It is not as readily seen as the basilic vein but is easily accessed in larger species, without need to cast the bird; it is not prone to hematoma formation. This site is especially useful in larger waterfowl.
- **Right jugular**, with or without anesthesia, depending on species. This is the easiest route for small birds. The neck is extended, the vein is readily visualized, and the feathers are parted to locate the apteria which is moved over the jugular. Hematoma can be an occasional problem in small species.
- **Toenail** clip can only be used for collection of samples for DNA sexing, as contamination can lead to clinical pathology inaccuracies.

SAMPLE QUALITY

Although we accept that blood samples should be collected, we first need to consider factors that will alter the value of our results. As birds deteriorate so fast, there is an advantage in processing samples in-house, but will your equipment give you results of a suitable consistency, accuracy, and usefulness? It is sad that commercially driven companies and clinicians will often conduct a barrage of tests that are inappropriate for the species that they are testing; there is no excuse for this practice. If tests are to be conducted in-house, there must be appropriate quality control, the test parameters must be of value, and the clinician must know how to correctly interpret them. The time of day the sample is taken, postprandial effects, sample-handling artefacts, delay in testing, and transportation artefacts should all be considered. Whether the sample is tested in-house or at a quality controlled commercial laboratory, the availability of normal values is mandatory. If using an external laboratory, use one that is accustomed to the species with which you are dealing, check that they have normal parameters, and seek advice on sample collection, handling, and transportation ideals.

INTERPRETATION

Normal values should be specific to the laboratory in question; even so a wide variation in "normality" can be anticipated, dependent on age, sex, caged/aviary living, breeding/non-breeding, diet, exercised or not, and so on. There is great benefit to be gained by sampling patients on a routine annual basis, first in the search for subclinical disease, but also so that the patient's normal blood values can be recorded on file. An inappropriate test or poor quality sample is bad. A wrongly interpreted sample is worse than not testing the bird in the first place.

WHAT DO WE WANT FROM OUR BLOOD SAMPLE

We are searching for the hidden (so many bird diseases present as "a fluffed sick bird"), confirming our anticipations and monitoring for responses to therapy.

Hematology

Most if not all hematology can be readily conducted in-house, and is the most beneficial and useful part of clinical pathology. Speed is of the essence and being able to differentiate as to whether the condition is infectious/noninfectious, if anemia is present, and if so is the bone marrow responding to it, is invaluable. The complete blood count (CBC) will reveal the following information:

- The number and character of red blood cells
- The total number, percentages, and characteristics of white blood cells
- The concentrations of solids in the plasma
- The number of thrombocytes in circulation, as an indication of bone marrow response
- The presence of blood parasites, or other morphologic changes which could lead to anemia.

Avian and mammalian blood cells do differ. Avian red cells are nucleated (which is why mechanical white cell counts are typically not possible). Regenerative anemia is represented by increased polychromasia of red blood cells (RBC). White blood cells (WBC) are similar to mammalian lines, except that mammalian Europhiles are replaced with heterophils and mammalian platlets are replaced with thromobocytes. There are significant variations in normal blood pictures between species, in particular the total WBC and the heterophil/lymphocyte ratios.

The following interpretations can be made:

- **Leukocytosis** – infections, noninfectious inflammation, necrosis, neoplasia, stress (macaws in particular – although no toxic changes in cells), heavy metal toxicosis
- **Moderate heterophilia** – infections, cellular necrosis
- **Severe heterophila** – chlamydophilosis, aspergillosis, tuberculosis (often with toxic changes in WBC)
- **Leukopenia** – extreme viral (in particular Circovirus) or overwhelming bacterial infections. Leukopenia can be associated with increased use of WBC (demonstrated by immature/toxic WBC), as opposed to reduced production (no immature or toxic WBC)
- **Lymphocytosis** – viral infections or certain stages of chlamydophilosis
- **Monocytosis** – indicates chronicity of an infection, with extensive necrosis and phagocyte activity (typically aspergillosis, chlamydophilosis and tuberculosis).
- **Eosinophilia** – is of inconsistent and unproven significance
- **Basophilia** – these are uncommon and most often associated with respiratory infections, resolving tissue damage, parasitism and some stages of chlamydophilosis.

Protein Electrophoresis

The division of plasma protein into separate groups, by the use of an electric current, gives a percentage of the total protein represented by different fractions. The ratios of the different fraction, yields information regarding the patient's physiological and immunological status. Plasma protein is divided into pre-albumin, albumin and globulin components. Globulins are subdivided into alpha, beta, and gamma fractions. The first assessment to be made should be the A:G ratio (albumin/globulin). A depressed A/G ratio (ie, less albumin, but increased globulin), which may be caused by reduced albumin production, or loss of albumin via gut or kidney, is a grave sign, which is compounded by an increased globulin level (associated with immunological reaction against infection, inflammation or neoplasia). An increased A/G ratio is consistent with an increasing albumin level (rare), or a decreasing globulin level (failure to produce or mount an immune response).

Pre-albumin and Albumin Fractions

The significance of pre-albumin fractions in birds is unknown. It may function as a transport protein, similar to albumin in other species. Pre-albumin may comprise 40% of total plasma protein, a reduction in pre-albumin appears to be synonymous with a reduced albumin fraction in other species. The albumin fraction represents 45% to 70% of total plasma proteins. In cases where pre-albumin is low, albumin tends to be low also. Albumin is responsible for maintaining osmotic pressure and as a transport protein as in mammals.

Globulin Fraction

The globulin fraction consists of alpha, beta, and gamma fractions. Alpha is subdivided into alpha1 and alpha2. Parasitism causes an elevation of alpha proteins. Other causes are as yet unidentified; elevations of alpha proteins are unusual. Beta proteins comprise other acute phase proteins and are represented by β2-macroglobulin, fibronectin, transferring and B-lipoprotein. Increases in B proteins tend to associated with chronic liver or renal disease, or chronic inflammatory diseases such as aspergillosis or chlamydophilosis; however, the most common reason for elevated B proteins is the transferring component, which is associated with egg production. A 1.5 to 2x elevation in B globulins, together with an elevation in blood calcium level is almost path gnomonic for an egg-laying female bird. Gamma globulins only appear as one peak in birds (compared with two peaks in mammals); elevation is associated with antibody production.

BIOCHEMISTRIES

Alkaline Phosphotase (AP) has no specific significance and is not applicable in birds.

Alanine Aminotransferease (ALT, SGPT) has no value in birds

Albumin. See the discussion above of electrophoresis. Dry chemistry analysis is very rarely of any value due to artifactual errors. Albumin may be useful (wet chemistry) as an indication of response following disease and if very low, a warning regarding the chance of ascites developing.

Amylase is difficult to interpret. A mild elevation is typically associated with gastrointestinal disease; marked elevations (>4x maximum range) are typically associated with pancreatic disease.

Aspartate Aminotransferase (AST, SGOT). The primary source is muscle, liver, and kidney. If CK, AST, LDH are all elevated it is likely to indicate muscle damage; if AST and/or LDH are elevated in the absence of CK elevation, this is typically indicative of liver damage. However, relative half-lives of different enzymes should also be considered. CK has a short half-life compared with AST, so after a muscle insult, the CK may have returned to normal but the AST is still raised, which might be interpreted as being liver derived while in fact it was muscle related. Intramuscular injections will cause elevations. It is the last enzyme to rise after muscle or liver damage (72 hours post damage), but also the last to normalize.

Bile Acid is the only indicator of liver function. Pre sampling starvation is required in birds with no gall bladder (e.g. pigeons and parrots). If a high level is detected, the sample should be repeated. After two high results liver biopsy is indicated, in order to determine the cause of the liver dysfunction.

Bilirubin has an inconsistent elevation in liver disease. High levels of bilirubin are usually indicative of obstructive jaundice. Yellow colouration of serum is often caused by food derived carotenoids

Calcium (Total) is linked to plasma protein. Ionized calcium levels are vastly more useful, as elevations or declines in total calcium may or may not affect functionally available calcium (ionised). Hypocalcaemia is a common cause of fitting in African greys. Calcium levels are controlled by parathyroid hormone, vitamin D3 levels and calcitonin. In psittacines, hypercalcaemia often occurs as an effect of vit D3 toxicity (the commonest vitamin toxicosis) but elevated blood calcium levels will also be seen just before egg laying. In such cases, polyostotic hyperostosis (increased medullary bone density) may be seen in the shafts of the long bones. Haemolysis of samples can cause false elevation, as can lipaemia. Hypoalbuminaemia, hypoparathyroidism, secondary nutritional or renal hypoparathyroidism and hypovitaminosis D may also cause hypocalceamia.

Cholesterol. The inconsistent significance may be associated with starvation, liver disease, hypothyroidism or excessive fatty diet.

Creatinine is not useful in birds.

Creatine kinase (CK) is associated with muscle damage, post intramuscular injections, or catabolism (weight loss due to inanition or disease). Its half-life is approximately 16 hours.

Glucose is elevated due to stress, starvation after eating, or persistently in diabetes.

Glutamate Dehydrogenase is the most consistently useful tissue enzyme for liver cell damage. Elevations can also be consistent with damage to kidney and brain.

Lactate dehydrogenase is present in muscle and liver (see AST above).

Lipase may be elevated with acute pancreatitis.

Phosphorus is inconsistent, and is elevated in chronic renal failure.

Protein (Total) should be measured by the biuret method to be accurate, although a temperature compensated refractometer is acceptable if the same is not lipemic. Reduced levels in malnutrition, malabsorption, renal disease, liver disease, elevated in dehydration, immune stimulation, best to assess with A/G ratio.

Urea is of limited value, elevated if dehydrated (4-5x), but not an indication of renal function..

Uric Acid is elevated with impaired renal function, dehydration, or physiological elevation within 12 hours of feeding in raptors. The kidney removes 90% of the blood uric acid, and 50% of the kidney must be destroyed to effect the blood uric acid level. Normal levels are not an indication of no renal damage.

Chloride is inconsistent

Potassium is elevated in renal disease, acidosis, adrenal disease, and hemolysis; and is decreased with diarrhea and alkylosis.

Sodium is elevated in salt poisoning and decreased in over hydration.

Bicarbonate is increased in alkalosis and decreased with acidosis.

SEROLOGY

A range of serologic and polymerase chain reaction (PCR) tests are now available for avian disease identification. Availability and interpretation varies in different areas and is rapidly developing.

FURTHER READING

1. Altman RB, Clubb S, Dorrestein G, Quesenberry K. Avian Medicine and Surgery. Philadelphia: WB Saunders. 1997.
2. Campbell TW. Avian Hematology and Cytology. Ames, IA: State University Press, 2nd ed., 1995.
3. Fudge AM. Laboratory Medicine: Avian and Exotic Pets. Philadelphia: WB Saunders, 2000.
4. Lumeij JT. Avian clinical biochemistry, In Kaneko JJ, Harvey JW, Bruss ML (eds.): Clinical Biochemistry of Domestic Animals. New York: Academic Press, 1997, pp 857-883.

IMAGING THE POSSIBILITIES

Neil A. Forbes, BVetMed, FRCVS, Diplomate ECAMS,
Great Western Exotics
Swindon, Wilts, UK

RADIOGRAPHY IN BIRDS

Radiography is a noninvasive, safe, and informative diagnostic tool to be used alongside other diagnostic information. A specific diagnosis is rarely made with one element of information alone. Radiographic appearance of ascites, gastrointestinal tract (GIT) obstruction, and cardiomegaly, for example, in birds resembles that of mammals. Radiology (at least two views at right angles, preferably with two different exposure levels) should be performed on all sick patients. Sick birds are often suffering from concurrent diseases; without a comprehensive workup, some diagnoses are likely to be missed. A parrot presented off color and weak with polyuria/polydipsia. and discolored cloacal excrement with an abnormal fecal gram stain, might be considered to have a bacterial GIT infection, while a radiograph might reveal heavy metal toxicity.

GETTING THE MOST OUT OF YOUR RADIOGRAPHS

All birds to be radiographed should be anesthetized. Consistent positioning is vital; a restraint device may be useful. High detail (mammography) film (ie, a slow speed film with small crystal size and hence high detail), together with appropriate single screen is essential. A short exposure time (<1/60 sec), light beam diaphragm with a minimized focal area, and a standard focal film distance of 1.05 m should be applied. Avian body radiographs have good natural contrast, so KV should be higher and mAs lower. However, using low exposure, minor inaccuracies become significant. If you increase KV by 10, you must halve the mAs. If your contrast is too great (very black and white), increase your kV and decrease your mAs. If your image is too 'gray' (eg, in an ascites case, where the air sacs are lost), then reduce your kV and increase your mAs. As our patients are generally less than 9 cm deep, grids (to reduce scatter) are generally contraindicated, as the benefit achieved is outweighed by the loss of definition created by the grid.

Film Faults
- **Overexposure** – film too black
  - KV, mA, time too high
  - Film focal distance too small
- **Underexposure** – film too pale
  - KV, mA, time too low
  - Film focal distance too high
- **Fogging**
  - Darkroom not light-tight
  - Safelight filter inappropriate for sensitivity of the film
  - Safelight strength/proximity to film
  - Radiation – keep unexposed cassettes away from radiation

Processing Faults
- **Overdevelopment** – Film too dark, contrast low
  - Developer too hot
  - Developer too concentrated
  - Developer time too long
- **Underdevelopment** – Film pale, especially the background
  - Developer too cold
  - Developer exhausted or weak
  - Insufficient time (commonest manual processing fault)

Automatic Processor Faults
- Roller marks, scratches
- Underdevelopment – not warming up
- Overdevelopment – malfunction
- Incorrect chemical concentrations
- Poor dying
- Lost films

Optimizing Results
- Reduce scatter – grids, collimation, lead
- Faster film – screen combinations (although this may cause a loss of resolution, due to larger crystal size)
- Reduce movement blur (use adequate restraint/GA)
- Use of 'Exposure Charts' (utilising the lowest KV, the highest MA and the shortest exposure time possible)

While radiographic texts are useful, a file of normal radiographic anatomy should be maintained. When dealing with >9000 species, even the most experienced clinician will not be familiar with the finer points of all species. With the advent of digital photography and e mail veterinary special interest groups and referral centres, it is now possible to seek a second opinion and seek assistance in interpretation without any delay in interpretation.

POSITIONING
Ventrodorsal (VD) View
The bird is placed in dorsal recumbency, with the keel directed 90 degrees from the cassette. The wings should be extended bilaterally 90 degrees from the body and the legs extended caudally. If wings and legs are each abducted equally, then there is every chance that the radiograph will be level. Position the carina (keel) of the sternum is over lying the spinal vertebrae.

Lateral View
The bird is placed in right lateral recumbency, with superimposition of the acetabula. The wings are both extended dorsally and maintained in place with sand bags or tape. The legs are retracted caudally, with the dependant (lower, ie, right) limb slightly cranial to the non-dependent limb. If positioned correctly, the acetabula, ribs, coracoid, and kidneys are all superimposed contralaterally.

INTERPRETING AVIAN RADIOGRAPHS
Skull
The cranium is fused. There are numerous interconnecting sinuses, the largest of which is the infra-orbital sinus, which is rostro-ventral to the eyes. The upper beak forms a synovial joint with the frontal bone via the articular and quadrate bones. The scleral ossicles form a boney ring, which is visible radiographically (shape shows major inter species variations).

Spine
The avian spine shows major variation from mammals. It may be divided into cervical (parrots 12, swans 25), **notarium** (fused thoracic, lumbar 1-3), free lumbar (lumbar 4) and **synsacrum** (fused caudal lumbar and pelvic), plus **pygostyle** (free caudal). The region of the one free lumbar (typically lumbar 4) vertebrae, is a natural hinging point and the most common area to suffer bruising (which can subsequently lead to an anaerobic environment which may facilitate anaerobic abscess formation), trauma, or spondylosis. So, in conclusion, only the neck, L4 and the tail (pygostyle) are susceptible to damage.

Thoracic Vertebrae
Birds have eight (in parrots) complete ribs.

Thoracic Girdle
The thoracic girdle consists of the **clavicle** (which fuse bilaterally to form the **furcula** - wish bone), the **coracoid,** and the **scapula.** These three bones form the **triosseum,** onto which the proximal humerus articulates. The tendon of the **supracoracoideus** passes through the **triosseal canal** (created at the pyramidal junction of the three bones). The sternum meets to form the carina (or keel) in the ventral midline. On the wing, the humerus articulates with the **ulna and radius.** The secondary feathers of the wing insert on the caudal periosteum of the ulna. The ulna and radius articulate with ulna and radius carpal bones at the **carpus,** which lead to the **carpo-metacarpus.** The manus has three digits (I - the alula, II - the major metacarpal, III - the minor metacarpal).

When radiographing extremities, always image and compare normal and abnormal limbs. There is so much inter species variation, that even experienced clinicians can be misled by normal structures.

Pelvic Girdle
The pelvic girdle consists of the **fused ilium and ischium and the unfused pubis.**

The femur has a small but recognizable femoral head, which sits neatly in an acetabulum. Most birds have four digits. The most medial caudal digit is numbered first, then the cranial medial toe etc. Digit 1 has 1 phalanx, digit 2 has 2, digit 3 has 3 and digit 4 has 4. Many hand-reared parrots (eg, >50% of African grey parrots) have suffered from metabolic bone disease. Survey radiographs of birds should always be thoroughly checked (especially limbs and ribs).

Hyperostosis / Polyostosis
This is increased medullary bone density of the long bones. Minor changes occur in egg-laying females. Major changes are seen in birds suffering from hyper-estrogenism, a frequent clinical problem in single 'frustrated breeder' pet owned parrots.

Trachea
Complete tracheal rings can be seen. There is marked species variation is position, length, and syringeal (voice box situated at the base of the heart) shape.

Lungs
On the lateral view the normal avian lung shows a honeycomb appearance. Loss of honeycomb, or focal densities indicate likely pulmonary pathology.

Air Sacs
Most birds have two cranial thoracic, two caudal thoracic, two abdominal, two cervical, and one clavicular air sac. Dark air-filled areas represent parts of each air sac and are visible in VD and lateral body views. None of the lines between air sacs should not be evident radiographically. The presence of air sac lines is indicative of air sacculitis (past or present), in which case endoscopy is indicated.

Heart
On the VD view, the avian heart should be seen lying between the 2nd and 6th thoracic ribs. In psittacines the heart base is best measured at the level of the 5th thoracic vertebrae, should not exceed 50% of the width of the thoracic cavity. On the lateral view the heart length should not (in psittacines), exceed 47% of the length of the sternum. On the VD view the heart - liver silhouette should resemble an 'hour glass' or figure of 8, shape. Macaws have a relatively smaller liver than other psittacines. The liver (coeliomic) outline should lie on or medial to a vertical line (on VD view) from the scapula to the acetabula. If the coeliomic silhouette is greater this is indicative of 'organomegaly' within the coeliomic cavity (liver, gonad, oviduct, adrenal gland, ascites, etc.).

Atherosclerosis may be apparent by the presence of mineralization in the great vessels cranial to the heart. If not hepatomegally is indicated.

Digestive System Radiography
The crop lies to the right of the midline on the VD view, cranial to the thoracic inlet. The proventriculus is left of the crop on the VD, and dorsal to the liver on the lateral view. The ventriculus often contains grit and is situated caudo-ventral to the proventriculus (except in ostriches in which it is anterior). The intestines occupy the dorso-caudal portion of the abdominal cavity. If the bird is positioned symmetrically and the liver shadow does not appear symmetrical, then a further extension on the left side is indicative for a **proventricular dilation**. Dilation of any part of the GIT is abnormal (unless the bird is a raptor and the dilation is due to the

presence of a 'casting,' ie, undigested fibrous matter prior to producing a pellet).

Dilation of the proventriculus indicates physical or functional gut dysfunction, (proventricular dilation syndrome [PDS], heavy metal poisoning, any form of infection (bacterial, viral, fungal) of the ventriculus or proventriculus or any form of GIT blockage or obstruction, eg, heavy nematode burdens, foreign bodies, torsions, strictures, or neoplasia.

Kidney

The kidney is seen most readily on the lateral view. The cranial lobe of the kidney is apparent below the lumbar spine, just cranial to the acetabulum. The other two lobes of the kidneys are placed sequentially caudal to this one. Just cranial and ventral to the cranial lobe of the lies the gonads. Gonad swelling may be confused with renomegally. Dehydration cause deposition of radio-opaque urates in the kidneys, which can be confused with renal calculi or renal mineralization consequent to hypervitaminosis D. If this is suspected the patient should be given copious fluid therapy and re-radiographed the following day.

Spleen

The spleen may on occasion be seen on the lateral view as a spherical object, cranial to the femur, at mid abdominal cavity height, just above the level of the proventriculus. The spleen should not be larger than 1.5x the diameter of the femur. When the spleen is visible, it is typically an indication of splenomegally, the commonest cause being chronic antigenic stimulation, most commonly psitticosis.

Loss of abdominal space will be seen as a loss of the hourglass shape on the VD, and may be seen as a loss of the radiolucent space between the proventriculus and the kidney. Such a finding is synonymous with any abdominal space-occupying lesion, which may be physiological (eg, prior to egg laying with distended oviduct and ovarian follicles), or pathological (eg, egg bound, organomegaly, egg peritonitis, neoplasia).[4] Any space-occupying lesion will expand at the expense of the air sacs.

In any such case GIT barium contrast, will delineate the position of the GIT, in relation to other organs. If plain radiographs show organomegally of unknown cause (while the patient is still anesthetized), a male dog urinary catheter should be measured and marked for appropriate distance (at which the proventriculus should be reached). The catheter is passed per os, via esophagus, crop, distal esophagus to the proventriculus. 6 mL/kg of barium is expressed into the proventriculus, continuing as one gradually removes the catheter. This technique will highlight proventriculus, distal oesophagus and crop, with no risk of aspiration, as would be anticipated if the barium where only placed into the crop.

HIGH-DEFINITION DIGITAL RADIOGRAPHY (HDDR)

This technique represents a major enhancement in imaging capability, which has been proven to achieve increased diagnostic abilities in both human and veterinary fields. In this system, image creation (generation of an x-ray beam), is identical to conventional radiography, but the creation of the image, and the manner in which this digital image can be manipulated, so as to maximize the diagnostic possibilities varies greatly. In HDDR, film is replaced with 'x-ray sensitive optical sensors, containing several million pixels. The photo electric converter (pixel), converts the reaction to an electrical impulse which is instantly digitalised. Pixel size will vary with equipment, but is likely to be approximately 100 microns in diameter, which compares with 200 to 400 microns with the highest quality CT scanner. The HDDR system uses a scintillator in place of intensifying screens. The greatest benefit of digital radiology is the opportunity to manipulate the image after initial processing, creating an ability to compensate for exposure errors, or simply to alter the exposure, to enable the detection of different anatomic structures with variable radio density. While a traditional screen/film system only permits a 20-fold change in x-ray exposure (from nothing to totally black), a digital system will permit a 10,000-fold change in exposure, with the ability to manipulate any one image, to see the effect of any exposure within that range, there by allowing one exposure to 'see all.'[2]

FLUOROSCOPY

Fluoroscopy is a valuable additional diagnostic tool that enables real-time radiography to be visualized on a screen. This technique is particularly valuable for assessing GIT motility (in suspect PDS cases), and also for assessing respiratory function in dyspneic birds that one does not wish to anesthetize.

ULTRASOUND

Ultrasound (US) is limited in birds (compared with mammals), due to the inability to penetrate air or bone. The most available access point is immediately caudal to the sternum. A scanner probe with a small foot print and high (10–14) MHz is most valuable. Despite these limitations US can be most useful diagnostic tool for noninvasive investigation of heart, liver, gastrointestinal tract, and urogenital system. The information gained by ultrasound, in contrast to radiography, is greatly superior, as indications of texture, consistency, dynamic movements, and functionality can be derived as opposed to simply the size and shape.

MICRO PET/CT SCAN, COMPUTED TOMOGRAPHY (CT) AND SPIRAL CT

These techniques are all now of increasing value in referral practices. They are of great value but time constraints prevent inclusion in this talk.

REFERENCES AND FURTHER READING

1. Brix G, Nosske D, Glattingi, et al. A survey of PET activity in Germany during 1999. European J Nucl Med Mol Imaging 2002;29;1091-1097.
2. Canon. CXDI Series Technical Guide [Physics], 2001.

3. Jones MP, Souza NJ, Avenell JS, Greenacre CB, Daniel GB. Clinical Use of Micro PET/CT scan for advanced diagnostic imaging in avian species. In: Proceedings 9th European AAV Conference. Zurich. 2007, pp 282-287.

4. Krautwald ME, Tellhelm B, et al. Atlas of Radiographic Anatomy and Diagnosis of Cage Birds. Verlag Paul Bracey. Berlin, 1992.

5. Paul-Murphy JP, Mccutcheon RA, Standing B, Steebeba EE, Converse AK. Using Positron Emission Tomography Imaging of the Parrot Brain to Study Response to Clinical Pain. . In: Proceedings 9th European AAV Conference. Zurich. 2007, pp 293-297.

SURGERY/ENDOSCOPY: THE PROS AND CONS

Neil A. Forbes, BVetMed, FRCVS, Diplomate ECAMS
Great Western Exotics
Swindon, Wilts, UK

WHAT ARE THE DETERMINING FACTORS?

This is a regular conundrum, particularly for the less experienced clinician, but also one which 'longer toothed' clinicians should keep asking themselves. The main factors in consideration are discussed in this article.

Availability of Equipment

Avian surgery of any type does require certain instrumentation. For conventional surgery, microsurgical instrumentation is a great asset. The latter should have normal-sized handles with only the tips miniaturized. The handles should preferably be counter-weighted in order to minimize finger fatigue. Atraumatic tissue forceps are essential (eg, Harris ring tip forceps). Conversely, relatively few instruments are required in an avian surgical kit; fine pointed scissors, needle holders, 2x artery forceps, atraumatic grasping forceps, and a retractor are the essentials. Spring-loaded, locking instruments will also greatly assist in preventing finger fatigue. In addition, illumination and magnification is required, as well as some form of adequate retraction system (eg, Lone Star Retractor). Against this the endoscopy route, requires suitable endoscopes (0 degrees [look straight ahead] and 30 degrees [look around], obturators (to gain access and protect the scope to prevent bending and rod breakage). If endoscopic surgery is contemplated, one will need biopsy forceps, grasping forceps, scissors and potentially more sophisticated instruments such as endo cautery, insufflators, and aspirators, etc.

Experience of Clinician

All surgical training, whether conventional or endoscopic, is ideally gained at conference wet labs, then reinforced with practical training on the job. Endoscopic surgery probably requires more 'further training,' when compared with avian conventional surgery, for the typical experienced small animal clinician. A lack of training is not a long-term reason to use one technique over another, but it may be a reason for a choice in the short or immediate term.

Size of Patient

This decision takes one both ways in different situations. On occasion, in a very small bird (say 100 g), the tracheal lumen may be too small to get an endoscope safely down. When it comes to tracheal surgery, the bigger the patient the more endoscopic surgery one can achieve. Certainly for endoscopic beginners, performing on a larger patient is far easier and hence safer; as one gains in experience and confidence, small patients also become comfortable and there is even more reason to use endoscopy on these small patients, so the iatrogenic stress and trauma caused by conventional surgery can be minimized.

Size of Access and Location of Lesions

Lesions in certain locations, eg, anterior thoracic air sac, syrinx, and infra-orbital sinus, would be very difficult to access with a conventional surgical approach (if highly destructive access surgery is to be avoided), whilst other lesions (eg, cloacal papilloma), lend themselves much more readily to conventional techniques.

Purpose — Diagnosis or Surgery

In general terms, endoscopy is a far quicker, safer, minimally invasive technique if one is simply making a diagnosis. The air sac system (designed with the express purpose of making life easier for avian vets) facilitates the visual examination of all internal organs; it is then only a small step further to collect endoscopic diagnosic biopsies from suspect internal organs (eg, liver, kidney, lung, spleen, pancreas, bursa of fabricius). The only downsides of such endoscopic techniques are the reduction in size of biopsy harvested and on occasion a marginally reduced ability to ensure the biopsy is representative of the entire or suspect parts of the organ. Hemorrhage while collecting the biopsy is very rare, at least once a practitioner is experienced.

Potential Risks of Either Technique

Contamination of other structures on removal of infective material—for example, the removal of an aspergilloma lesion from the cranial thoracic air sac, which could well also have secondary bacterial infection, might be readily achieved, with minimal risk of spreading infection, if carried out by conventional methods (although such a lesion should not normally be removed until it is considered to be inert).

With regard to size limitations in relation to tissue or debris to be removed via obturator, the same applies as discussed above: if a lesion is larger than the diameter of the obturator through which it needs to be recovered, then the lesion will break up and the risk of contamination increases.

When comparing the ability to control hemostasis, serious intraoperative hemorrhage is rare, but the surgeon's ability to deal with it may be greater if increased access is available (ie, with conventional surgery), although the down side is that the procedure will take longer to complete. This is particularly relevant with liver biopsy, as by definition liver pathology, and hence effect on clotting factor production, is likely to be present at a time when liver biopsy is indicated.

As far as the potential for collateral damage to adjacent organs, the more visible the surrounding organs are, the less risk of collateral damage. However, conversely, the illumination and magnification provided by an endoscope is typically superior to that of conventional surgery.

With endoscopy, there may be inability to see 'the bigger picture,' whereas conventional surgery may allow the surgeon to see the totality of the clinical scenario, particularly where multiple organs are involved. With endoscopy, the surgeon (particularly the less experienced) may not be aware of some issues.

The spillage of ascitic fluid from the coelom into air sac can be a problem if the endoscopic surgeon is unaware prior to prior to the procedure that the patient has ascites. Entry may be achieved, via the air sac into the coelom, and leakage of ascites into the air sac and lung may occur before one is aware of what is happening. This is potentially life threatening.

Endoscopy can be problematic when organomegaly or neoplastic masses have deranged normal anatomic positioning.

The inability to cope if something 'goes wrong' with endoscopic surgery is a potential concern–although an endoscopic surgery can generally be converted into a conventional access, there may be some time delay. In the event that something goes wrong during endoscopic surgery, the ability to resolve that matter may be restricted or delayed.

There is no doubt that wounds created at conventional surgery do take longer to heal. The larger the wound and the longer healing takes, the greater the risk of wound break down prior to total healing. Conventional surgical procedures generally take longer, thereby leading to an increased risk of the procedure over all.

CONCLUSION

If endoscopy is to be utilized, the surgeon should be adequately equipped, trained, and experienced. This being so, endoscopy should be used in all situations where the overall 'risk-benefit' profile of endoscopy is superior to that of conventional surgery. Although there are no hard and fast rules, there are certain situations in which one would always use endoscopy, while there are others where one would always use conventional access, with residual gray areas in between where a choice will be made due to the surgeon's personal preferences, equipment, and experience. As equipment advances and surgeon's skills increase, it is likely that more and more procedures should be completed endoscopically. As such, clinicians should keep challenging themselves in relation to optimum techniques, rather than just repeating their previous 'comfortable' procedures.

Always Use Endoscopy for:
- Tracheoscopy and treatment if possible

- Coeliomic (including thoracic) diagnostics, including assessment of gonadal activity
- Renal biopsy
- Sinography
- Retrieval of enteric foreign bodies if possible
- Salpingohysterectomy, orchidectomy or in immature birds
- Vasectomy in birds of any age
- Ingluvioscopy and proventriculoscopy

Always Use Conventional Surgical Approach for:
- Where reproductive disease is anticipated, where egg coeliomitis, egg shell fragments or other retained egg material are likely to be present
- Where lower GIT blockage, intussusceptions, non viable sections of GIT, etc., are anticipated
- Any situations where an enterotomy is required
- Salpingohysterectomy, orchidectomy in mature sexually active patients

The Gray Areas – Use Whatever Seems Right at the Time
- Lung and liver biopsy
- Cloacal examination and surgery
- Complex situations, with multi organ involvement
- Removal or treatment of abscessated material, including aspergilloma.

FURTHER READING
1. Doneley B, Harrison GJ, Lightfoot T (2006). Maximising information from physical examination. In: Clinical Avian Medicine Vol 1. (Eds)~Harrison GJ, Lightfoot TL.Spix Publishing. Palm Beach. pp153-212
2. Lierz M (2006). Diagnostic value of Endoscopy and Biopsy. In: Clinical Avian Medicine Vol 1. (Eds)~Harrison GJ, Lightfoot TL.Spix Publishing. Palm Beach. pp631-652
3. Lennox AM, Nemetz L. (2006). Diagnostics: Endoscopy vs. Exploratory Surgery of the Coeliom in the Avian Patient. In Proceedings 27th Annual Conference Association of Avian Vets. AAV Publications Bedford Texas. pp 371-372.
4. Hernandez-Divers SJ, Blasier M, Wilson H, Christian M. (2006). Endosurgical Treatment of Severe Air Sac Aspergillosis. In: In Proceedings 27th Annual Conference Association of Avian Vets. AAV Publications Bedford Texas. pp 363-365.

IS IT INFECTIOUS?

Neil A. Forbes, BVetMed, FRCVS, Diplomate ECAMS
Great Western Exotics
Swindon, Wilts, UK

INFECTIOUS CONDITIONS

A patient may have an infectious condition without it being a disease. Such a condition only becomes a 'disease' if the patient suffers as a consequence of the infection; this is not always the case. The fact that a patient has an infection does not mean it is contagious, ie, it is only contagious if the patient has the ability to pass on the infectious agent.

Any avian patient should be considered infectious until proven otherwise. There are simply too many serious infectious diseases, which may be clinical or subclinical, for any case to be automatically considered safe until proven to be so. We can consider diseases such as avian influenza, Chlamydophila, psittacine beak and feather disease, and herpes virus, all of which can be present in an avian patient, without any overt signs and yet still present serious risks of 'infection' to other birds, either by direct contact, fomite spread, or most serious of all by air spread.

WHY DOES IT MATTER IF IT IS INFECTIOUS?

Not only is it essential to determine if it is infectious and if so what the pathogen is, in order to ensure the patient gets the very best treatment as soon as possible, but perhaps even more important is the need to protect other patients and the biosecurity status of your facilities against contamination.

HOW DO WE RECOGNIZE IF A BIRD IS SUFFERING FROM AN INFECTIOUS CONDITION?

All clinicians are familiar with the signs of a 'sick bird'—fluffed up, loss of condition or weight, change of appetite and water consumption, change of normal position, perching place or stance, change in level of activity, standing on two legs rather than one, possibly even hanging onto the bars of the cage with his beak, loss or change of voice, respiratory stridor, tail bobbing, faecal changes, abnormal discharges (mouth eyes, nares, ears, preen gland, cloaca), lying down more, CNS signs, etc. However the presence of 'sick bird' clinical signs does not imply the bird is suffering from an infectious disease.

History Collection

In any sick bird situation, a full detailed history should be collected. Changes of diet, the introduction of new birds, the mixing of captive birds with wild stock, and previous disease history are all factors which may well increase the suspicion of an infectious disease. As with any sick bird, the author would recommend a full diagnostic workup, to include history, optical observation, physical examination, collection of clinical pathology samples (eg, blood samples), radiography, and if necessary other specialized diagnostic tests such as ultrasound, endoscopy, electrocardiography, etc. In view of the fact that birds hide the signs of illness for as long as possible (if I look ill some one might eat me), and on account of their higher metabolic rate (get sick quicker), wherever possible (so long as quality assurance can be guaranteed), samples should be tested onsite, with results available as soon as possible.

Hematology

Most if not all hematology can be readily conducted in-house, and this is the most beneficial and useful aspect of clinical pathology. Speed is of an essence and being able to differentiate as to whether the condition is infectious or noninfectious, if anemia is present, and if so is the bone marrow responding to it, is invaluable. The complete blood count (CBC) will reveal the following information:

- The number and character of red blood cells
- The total number, percentages and characteristics of white blood cells
- The concentrations of solids in the plasma
- The number of thrombocytes in circulation – as an indication of bone marrow response
- The presence of blood parasites, or other morphological changes which could lead to anemia.

Avian and mammalian blood cells do differ. Avian red cells are nucleated (which is why mechanical white cell counts are typically not possible). Regenerative anemia is represented by increased polychromasia of red blood cells (RBC). White blood cells (WBC) are similar to mammalian lines, except that mammalian neutrophils are replaced with heterophils and mammalian platelets are replaced with thromobocytes. There are significant variations in normal blood pictures between species, in particular the total WBC and the heterophil/lymphocyte ratios. The following interpretations can be made

- **Leukocytosis – infectious**: Chlamydophila spp, Aspergillosis, Mycobacteria (given sufficient time all the previous three tend to cause severe leukocytosis with monocytosis, although in early stages a straight forward mild leukocytosis may be all that is evident). Intestinal or respiratory parasites, viral disease, bacterial or other parasitic infections
  - **Noninfectious:** Inflammation (including trauma), necrosis, neoplasia, stress (macaws in particular – although no toxic changes in cells), heavy metal toxicosis
  - **Inflammatory**: Elevated uric acid levels, arthritis, allergies, egg yolk peritonitis
- **Moderate heterophilia** – Infections, cellular necrosis
- **Severe heterophila** – Chlamydophilosis, aspergillosis, tuberculosis (often with toxic changes in WBC).
  - **Assessment of heterophilia:** As can be seen above, there are many conditions of dissimilar causes, which all result in a degree of leukocytosis. The further assessment of heterophils, the degree of toxicity and

degranulation, will further assist the clinician in determining the cause.

- **Leukopenia** – extreme viral (in particular Circovirus) or over whelming bacterial infections. **Leukopoenia** can be associated with increase use of WBC (demonstrated by immature/toxic WBC), as opposed to reduced production (no immature or toxic WBC)
- **Lymphocytosis** – Viral infections or certain stages of chlamydophilosis
- **Monocytosis** – Indicates chronicity of an infection, with extensive necrosis and phagocyte activity (typically aspergillosis, chlamydophilosis, and tuberculosis).
- **Eosinophilia** – Is of inconsistent and unproven significance
- **Basophilia** – These are uncommon and most often associated with respiratory infections, resolving tissue damage, parasitism and some stages of chlamydophilosis.

Protein Electrophoresis

The division of plasma protein into separate groups, by the use of an electric current, gives a percentage of the total protein represented by different fractions. The ratios of the different fraction, yields information regarding the patients physiological and immunological status. Plasma protein is divided into pre-albumin, albumin, and globulin components. Globulins are subdivided into alpha, beta, and gamma fractions. The first assessment to be made should be the A:G ratio (albumin / globulin). A depressed A/G ratio (ie, less albumin, but increased globulin), which may be caused by reduced albumin production, or loss of albumin via gut or kidney, is a grave sign, which is compounded by an increased globulin level (associated with immunological reaction against infection, inflammation, or neoplasia). An increased A/G ratio is consistent with an increasing albumin level (rare), or a decreasing globulin level (failure to produce or mount an immune response).

Pre-albumin and Albumin Fractions

The significance of pre-albumin fractions in birds is unknown. It may function as a transport protein, similar to albumin in other species. Pre-albumin may comprise 40% of total plasma protein; a reduction in pre-albumin appears to be synonymous with a reduced albumin fraction in other species. The albumin fraction represents 45% to 70% of total plasma proteins. In cases where pre-albumin is low, albumin tends to be low also. Albumin is responsible for maintaining osmotic pressure and as a transport protein as in mammals.

Globulin Fraction

The globulin fraction consists of the alpha, beta, and gamma fractions. Alpha is subdivided into alpha1 and alpha2. Parasitism causes an elevation of alpha proteins. Other causes are as yet unidentified; elevations of alpha proteins are unusual. Beta proteins comprise other acute phase proteins and are represented by β2-macroglobulin, fibronectin, transferring, and B-lipoprotein. Increases in B proteins tend to associated with chronic liver or renal disease, or chronic inflammatory diseases such as aspergillosis or chlamydophilosis; however, the most common reason for elevated B proteins is the transferring component, which is associated with egg production. A 1.5 to 2x elevation in B globulins, together with an elevation in blood calcium level, is almost pathognomonic for an egg laying female bird. Gamma globulins only appear as one peak in birds (compared with two peaks in mammals); elevation is associated with antibody production.

FURTHER READING

1. Doneley B, Harrison GJ, Lightfoot TL. Maximising information from the physical examination. In: Clinical Avian Medicine, Vol 1. GJ Harrison, Lightfoot TL (eds): Zoological Education. Spix Publishing. 2006, pp 153-212.
2. Harris DJ. Avian clinical pathology. In: Scientific Proceedings BSAVA Congress. BSAVA Gloucester. 2007, pp 408-410.
3. Harcourt-Brown N, Chitty J. BSAVA Manual of psittacine Birds, 2nd ed. BSAVA. Gloucester, 2005.
4. Olsen GH, Orosz SE. Manual of Avian Medicine. St. Louis, MO: Mosby. 2000.

WHAT THE HECK IS WRONG WITH THIS BIRD?

Neil A. Forbes, BVetMed, FRCVS, Diplomate ECAMS
Great Western Exotics
Swindon, Wilts, UK

A SPECIFIC DIAGNOSIS

Why: As we all know, birds are ostensibly wild creatures: they have developed with the knowledge, that "if I look sick today, someone is going to come and eat me." Moreover, they have a faster metabolic rate than mammals, so that once ill, they get sick and die quicker than mammals. It is therefore essential that the "sick bird" is presented immediately. In turn the veterinarian must not simply reach for the bottle of enrofloxacin, but instead make every effort to achieve a specific diagnosis such that the most appropriate therapeutic plan can be developed. If a client ever presents a bird stating that it is not normal, believe them—do not send it home without a diagnostic workup and appropriate therapy.

How. In order to reach that diagnosis, the clinician must put aside sufficient "quality time," outside a regular consulting period, to work up the case. While "blood" is indeed important, even that remains just part of the picture. All too often, when a clinician is unfamiliar with the species he or she is presented with, the reaction is to rely on laboratory results to hang a diagnosis on. Such an approach (although we have all been guilty of it) is inappropriate. For each sick bird, the following diagnostic tools should be applied (taking into account the species and specific susceptibilities of that species):

- Full history collection, while maintaining visual observation of the bird and its environment
- Physical examination in a through and systematic manner
- Collection of relevant clinical pathology samples (blood, feces, swabs, aspirates, etc.)
- Radiography (at least two views at right angles, preferably additional exposures with varying exposure levels)
- Additional specialized tests as may be dictated necessary in view of species, history or other findings (eg, endoscopy, ultrasound, ECG)

As long as quality control can be assured, there is great benefit in samples being tested in-house (for reasons of expediency). However, it is still essential that appropriate initial fluid therapy and nutritional support be provided, plus symptomatic therapy pending the availability of results. When teaching undergraduates and clinicians, the single most important point to get across, is that the vast majority of diagnosis can be made by companion animal clinicians, so long as they are prepared to apply their basic training, to their feathered patient.

FURTHER READING

1. Doneley B, Harrison GJ, Lightfoot TL. Maximising information from the physical examination. In Harrison GJ, Lightfoot TL (eds): Clinical Avian Medicine, vol 1. Palm Beach, FL: Spix Publishing, 2006, pp 153-212.
2. Harris DJ. Avian clinical pathology. In Scientific Proceedings, BSAVA Congress. Gloucester, UK: BSAVA. 2007, pp 408-410.
3. Harcourt-Brown N, Chitty J. BSAVA Manual of Psittacine Birds, 2nd ed. Gloucester, UK: BSAVA, 2005..
4. Olsen GH, Orosz SE Manual of Avian Medicine. St. Louis, MO: Mosby, 2000..
5. Samour JH, Naldo JL Anatomical and Clinical Radiology of Birds of Prey. Elsevier, 2007.

AVIAN ZOONOSES: BEYOND AVIAN FLU

Neil A. Forbes, BVetMed, Diplomate ECAMS, FRCVS
Great Western Exotics
Swindon, Wilts, UK

PSITTICOSIS

Also known as parrot fever and ornithosis, psittacosis is caused by *Chlamydophila psittaci*, an obligate intracellular bacterial infection of birds that can cause severe pneumonia and other serious disease in humans (on average 250 reported cases per year in the US). Most cases resulted from exposure to infected pet birds, (cockatiels, parakeets, parrots, and macaws). Infected birds shed bacteria through feces and ocular/nasal discharges. Disease in humans is called psitticosis, parrot fever, or ornithosis. In a survey conducted by this author of 100 households with infected birds, humans only suffered disease in two households. Apart from exposure to infected pet birds, other persons at risk include pigeon fanciers and employees in poultry slaughtering and processing plants; veterinarians and technicians; zoo, laboratory and avian quarantine employees; farmers; game-keepers; and wildlife rehabilitators. Humans can be infected from brief, passing exposure to infected birds or their excretions so infection can arise from brief contact with an infected bird, eg, in a shop, zoo, or restaurant, where contact was so short that the patient has forgotten it. This problem is compounded as patients are often 'confused.' Person-to-person transmission has been suggested but not proven. Onset of illness typically follows an incubation period of 5 to 14 days (longer periods have been reported). Disease ranges from subclinical to systemic illness with severe pneumonia. Disease is fatal in less than 1% of properly treated humans; however, where a diagnosis is not made and no appropriate antimicrobials are provided, fatality levels can reach 15% to 20%. Human patients demonstrate sudden onset fever, headache, malaise, and myalgia. They usually develop a non-productive cough that can be accompanied by breathing difficulty and chest tightness. Splenomegally, and a non-specific rash are sometimes observed and are suggestive of psittacosis in patients with community-acquired pneumonia. The differential diagnoses include *Coxiella burnetii*, *Mycoplasma pneumoniae*, *Legionella* spp, other *Chlamydiaceae*, and respiratory viruses, eg, influenza. *Chlamydophila psittaci* can also endocarditis, myocarditis, hepatitis, arthritis, keratoconjunctivitis, and encephalitis. Severe illness with respiratory failure, thrombocytopenia, hepatitis, and fetal death has been reported among pregnant women.

Avian Chlamydiosis Transmission

Chlamydophila psittaci is excreted in the feces and nasal discharges of infected birds. The organism is environmentally labile but remains infectious for months in organic debris. Latently infected birds appear healthy but shed the organism intermittently, for months to years. Shedding can be activated by stressors, such as relocation, shipping, crowding, chilling, owner absence (eg, vacation) and breeding.

Clinical Signs

Incubation ranges from 3 days to several weeks. However, a latently infected bird can present with active disease with no identifiable exposure. Whether the bird has acute or chronic signs of illness or dies, depends on the species of bird, virulence of the strain, infectious dose, stress factors, age, and extent of treatment or prophylaxis. Clinical signs include lethargy, anorexia, ruffled feathers, ocular or nasal discharge, diarrhoea, yellow-green urates, anorexia, emaciation, dehydration, and death.

Diagnosis

Confirmation is on the basis of at least one of four laboratory results, including isolation of *C psittaci*, identification of antigen by immunofluorescence of patient tissues, a ≥ 4-fold change in serologic titer in two samples, at least 2 weeks apart, assayed simultaneously at the same laboratory, or identification of *Chlamydiaceae* within macrophages in Gimenez or Macchiavello stained smears bird's tissues. A probable case is defined as compatible illness and at least one of two positive results, including a single high serologic titer in 1 or more samples obtained after the onset of signs or detection of *Chlamydiaceae* antigen (identified by use of ELISA, polymerase chain reaction [PCR], or fluorescent antibody) in feces, a cloacal swab specimen, or respiratory tract or ocular exudates.

Treatment

All birds with confirmed or probable avian chlamydiosis should be isolated and treated. Birds with suspected avian chlamydiosis or birds previously exposed to avian chlamydiosis (ie, have been housed in the same air space) should be isolated and retested or treated. As treated birds can be re-infected, they should not be exposed to untreated birds or other potential sources of infection. To prevent re-infection, contaminated aviaries should be thoroughly cleaned and disinfected several days before treatment ends. While birds are under treatment the following care should be provided. Treatment comprises a maintained minimum inhibitory concentration (MIC) with doxycycline for 45 days, by weekly injections or medication in food or water.

Responsibilities of Veterinarians to Bird Owners

All new bird owners seen at the clinic should be advised of the risks of *Chlamydophila* infection. All new birds should be tested and isolated pending results. Owners should be advised not to mix their tested birds, with other birds of unknown health status, or to go where other birds have been. In the event of a patient testing positive, a **'written client advice sheet, detailing clinical signs in birds, clinical signs in humans, and action to be taken by concerned humans – visit your physician – take this piece of paper with you.'** Humans exposed to birds with avian chlamydiosis should seek medical attention if they develop influenza-like symptoms or other respiratory tract illnesses. The physician should consider psittacosis in ill patients exposed to birds and collect specimens for laboratory analysis.

SALMONELLOSIS

Salmonellosis is the most common and most serious zoonosis of the developed world, with some 5 million Americans affected annually. Although *Salmonella* spp are sensitive to many disinfectants as well as cooking, they do survive for extended periods in stagnant water and even longer in soil. Salmonellosis is transmitted to humans by eating contaminated (incompletely cooked) food and drinks, although fomites (including poor personal hygiene), is also a major factor. Humans have been infected from poultry, but also free living birds. Feral birds living on and flying away from refuse tips can form a significant route of transmission. Salmonellosis in humans typically presents as a gastro enteritis, although any organ can become infected, eg, arthritis, bronchopneumonia, endocarditis, meningitis, osteomyelitis, and pyelonephritis. Antiobiosis is generally contraindicated in humans, as it increases the chances of patients becoming carriers.

CAMPYLOBACTERIOSIS

Campylobacteriosis is an acute enteritis illness (with severe abdominal cramps) in humans with an incubation period of 2 to 5 days. Human infection is typically self-resolving in 7 to 10 days. Many infected birds become carriers (eg, 35% of migrating waterfowl and galliformes, although a very low rate in pet psittacines), creating a particular risk to humans. In the UK, birds opening foil milk bottle tops of door-step-delivered milk bottles has lead to significant outbreaks of infection.

YERSINIOSIS (PSEUDOTUBERCULOSIS)

Yersiniosis is a common bacterial infection of many groups of birds, but is less common in mammals. Zoonotic infection is most common in Europe and occurs only sporadically in the US. Pigeons and doves are the most common avian reservoir, resulting in zoonotic infection. Epizootics can occur in birds, leading to major mortalities, on occasions approaching 100%, in such cases massive environmental contamination can occur, resulting in human infection. In humans, incubation is typically 7 to 21 days, with the most common form being an acute mesenteric lymphadenitis with or without erythema nodosum. Severe enteritis can occur, with half of sufferers having hepatomegaly and jaundice.

NEWCASTLE DISEASE

This is a common and highly infectious disease of most species of birds. Humans working in close contact with birds (poultry farmers, slaughterers and veterinarians) can become infected from stock, or live vaccine. The incubation period in humans is 1 to 2 days. The most common clinical signs are unilateral or bilateral conjunctivitis, although fever, headache, lethargy, pharyngitis, encephalitis, and hemolytic anaemia can occur. Recovery is spontaneous after an illness of 3 days to 3 weeks duration.

ALLERGIC ALVEOLOITIS

This is a serious and underestimated disease that often affects pet bird owners after years of exposure to low-grade levels of avian feather antigen. It is an allergic alveolitis, resulting in hypersensitivity pneumonia, bronchiolitis, and interstitial pneumonia, which is classified as acute, subacute, or chronic. The acute form demonstrates 4 to 8 hours after large-scale exposure, resulting in coughing, dyspnea, and fever. The subacute form occurs after years of moderate exposure and is characterized by a dry cough and progressive dyspnea. Diagnosis is achieved on intradermal skin testing. If further exposure to avian antigen can be prevented, prognosis is good. The chronic form results from years of low-grade exposure to feather dander and is most common in the owners of pet birds. The disease is irreversible, causing dyspnea, nonproductive cough, weight loss, and respiratory rales. The lungs undergo chronic pulmonary fibrosis. To prevent further deterioration, the client must prevent exposure.

WEST NILE VIRUS

West Nile virus (WNV) is a flavivirus ('arboviridae') and is transmitted by arthropods (insects). The virus was first isolated in 1937 from a woman with pyrexia in the West Nile district of Uganda. WNV was first recognized as a cause of a human illness known as meningoencephalitis in Israel in 1957 and as a cause of horse disease in Egypt and France in the early 1960s. WNV is predominantly an infection of birds and mosquitoes. The virus circulates in the blood of the bird, then when mosquitoes take a blood meal from an infected bird they take up the virus as well. Other species infected (horses or humans) are incidental victims. Incubation in humans is 3 to 15 days. West Nile virus is not transmitted from "person-to-person." Eighty percent of infected humans are asymptomatic, 20% show mild influenza-like illness. Less than 1% develop more severe disease (encephalitis, meningitis). Patients may suffer headaches, fever, stiff neck, sore eyes, disorientation, muscle weakness, convulsions and coma, with occasional fatalities. WNV has been identified in Africa, Europe, the Middle East, west and central Asia, and the Americas. WNV was found in US for the first time in 1999 and is considered endemic. In 2005, 3000 cases were reported in the US. In temperate zones WNV occurs in late summer or early autumn, while in the tropics the virus can be transmitted all year round. Most mosquitoes that carry the WNV are likely to bite around dusk and dawn.

AVIAN INFLUENZA

Avian influenza (AI) naturally circulates in wild waterfowl such as ducks and geese, often causing few or no signs. Many other bird species are susceptible to infection which may lead to severe disease and high mortality. Outbreaks associated with high bird mortality are called Highly Pathogenic Avian Influenza (HPAI) (typically caused by H5 or 7), and are described according to properties of two surface proteins: hemagglutinin (H) and neuraminidase (N). In January 2004, avian influenza (HPAI) was confirmed in poultry in Vietnam. Subsequently, numerous outbreaks have occurred in a number of countries, sweeping from Southeast Asia, across Central Asia, and into western Europe. Very infrequently, AI viruses are transmissible to humans. Some 300 persons have become infected, of whom more than 50% have died. The World Health Organization comments that while avian HPAI has been very prevalent, it is reassuring that human infection has been so rare. However, increased infection of humans and human-to-human transmission remains a real threat, subsequent to viral antigen changes through 'shift' and 'drift.' The more virus is actively replicating (ie, active infection in birds), the greater the chance of this occurring. Outbreaks of influenza affecting many thousands and sometimes millions of people with high mortality occurred in 1918 ('Spanish'), 1957 (Asian), 1968 (Hong Kong), and 1977 (Russian). New subtypes of influenza caused these pandemics. These were probably formed by combination of genes from both avian and human influenza viruses, this is most likely to occur when a mammal (eg, humans and pigs) is concurrently infected with mammalian and avian virus strains. Emergence of new highly pathogenic avian influenza with the capacity to infect humans is a concern because it may lead to circumstances where a new subtype of influenza can develop that both causes serious disease and can spread from person to person. Humans are usually infected through close contact with live infected birds. Birds shed influenza virus in their feces, so contact with feces (for example by visiting enclosures or markets where birds have been recently kept) is also a possible transmission route. Evidence to support limited human-to-human transmission has also been described; this presents the major concern for the future.

The Role of the Veterinarian in Controlling AI

As avian veterinarians, we are all in the front line. Clinicians should train staff in the recognition of clinical signs and actions to take when the public calls concerning possible cases. The factors to consider are national biosecurity; personal, staff and public health; and prevention of contamination of your business facilities. In the UK, DEFRA will only call out to investigate if more than 10 birds are found dead; during office hours, at other times, and in other situations, we are on the front line.

CRYPTOSPORIDIOSIS

Cryptosporidiosis is caused by a coccidian parasite that is commonly found in numerous bird species. In humans, clinical signs comprise persistent diarrhea, malabsorption, abdominal pain, fever, and vomiting. Although no avian strains have been incriminated as yet the cause of human disease, because birds can become infected by mammalian strains, which could then contaminate human water supplies, it seems only a matter of time.

CRYPTOCOCCOSIS

Cryptococcus is typically caused by *Cryptococcus neoformans*, a saprophytic fungus, commonly found in soil contaminated by bird (especially pigeon) feces. Disease is rare in birds, but has been reported as disseminated disease in a number of psittacine species. Disease may affect the respiratory, gastrointestinal, or nervous systems, causing necrotic, granulomatous lesions with characteristic pale gelatinous exudates. Sinusitis (even with beak deviations), blindness, or paralysis can occur. Diagnosis is based on histopathology combined with culture. Culture alone is insignificant as the infection can be carried asymptomatically. Human infection generally occurs through contact with or handling or exudates or other infective material and can affect healthy as well as immunocompromised individuals. Clinicians must always be aware of this disease when treating atypical upper respiratory infections in birds.

MYCOBACTERIUM spp

This is worthy of note only in so far as human tuberculosis is commonly contracted by immuno-compromised individuals from contaminated soil. Infection from infected birds is extremely rare.

Other rare zoonotic pathogens include erysipelas, listeria, rabies, toxoplasmosis, and Giardia.

FURTHER READING
1. CDC. Division of Public Health Surveillance and Informatics. Available at: www.cdc.gov/epo/dphsi/casedef/psittacossiscurrent.htm.
2. Resources available from the World Health Organization.

TRIAGE: ASSESSMENT AND SUPPORT

Marla Lichtenberger, DVM, Diplomate ACVECC
Thousand Oaks Pet Emergency Clinic
Thousand Oaks, CA

Increasing numbers of birds are being kept as pets, and owners want to receive high quality medical care for these pets. Treatment of hypovolemic shock and critical care monitoring in birds are complicated by small patient size, physiological diversity and lack of research and clinical data on their response to therapy. Despite these impediments, the same principles and techniques of monitoring used in domestic animals can be applied to the avian patient. The goal of this and the following companion articles is to provide an in-depth presentation on the principles and pathophysiology of shock, types of fluids, monitoring techniques, and shock resuscitation methods for use in birds. Principles of cardiopulmonary-cerebral resuscitation will also be discussed. Arterial blood pressure measurement is an important tool in the management of the critically ill bird. The message of clinical importance is that fixed fluid regimens (eg, lactated Ringers), fixed volumes (eg, mL/kg) and rules of thumb are in most instances outdated, inappropriate and often times inadequate. Appropriate fluid therapy, combined with frequent patient evaluation and periodic blood pressure monitoring techniques, can produce astounding and at times miraculous results.

Most birds do not show signs of illness in the early stages of disease. Often, birds with chronic disease present as an emergency because of their ability to mask clinical signs of the disease until the condition is severe. In virtually all cases, I advise the receptionist to recommend the bird be brought in for an exam. If the owner is concerned enough to call, then the bird is probably very sick and needs to be seen. While all signs reported by the client can be of concern, sitting at the bottom of the cage, bleeding, respiratory distress, regurgitation and anorexia are considered true emergencies. The client should be instructed to bring the bird in a cage, if possible, otherwise instructs the owner about suitable alternatives (eg, box, cat carrier). The water dish should be emptied but the cage should not be cleaned prior to traveling to the hospital.

Once the bird has arrived, it is ideal to have a trained receptionist call for an immediate triage by a nurse. Prompt, accurate treatment is vital to a favorable outcome. The nurse should assess the condition of the bird in a room. In cases of bleeding, seizuring, head trauma and respiratory distress, the bird should be evaluated immediately by the veterinarian. If the bird is fluffed, weak or sitting at the bottom of the cage, they should be placed in a warmed incubator and oxygen is administered. The optimum temperatures for ill birds are 85 to 90°F (29–30°C).

PHYSICAL EXAMINATION

Initially the bird should be evaluated in its cage. Its posture, ability to ambulate and perch, respiratory status, interest in the environment, and fluffing of the feathers are assessed. The cage can be examined for discharges and vomit and sources of lead and zinc. Examine the feces (color, amount or blood), urates (normally is white to off white), and urine (an increase or change in color is abnormal) parts of the droppings. Following stress, birds frequently demonstrate polyuria.

Perform a complete physical exam as the condition of the bird allows. When handling a bird, it is best to work in a small room with low ceilings, closed window and no fans. Some birds, particularly finches and canaries, should be picked up in a darkened room. Prior to picking up the bird, you should determine if it is safe to restrain the bird. Weak birds and birds in respiratory distress could die during handling. Sudden death is no uncommon with restraint of obese budgies fed an inadequate diet. Efficiency is important when handling a bird. Setting up ahead of time for procedures to be performed will reduce the total restraint time. Proficiency in handling birds is an important factor in gaining client confidence. It is important to warn clients prior to picking up the bird what is going to happen. Most clients have never heard their bird scream or seen their bird struggle the way it does during restraint.

It may be better to postpone a complete physical exam in a weak bird or bird in respiratory distress. A quick one minute exam can be performed on a bird while taking the bird out of the cage and placing in the incubator. The head should be examined for oculonasal discharges and swellings. The oropharynx and choanal is examined for color mucous and presence of blunted papillae. The beak is examined for bleeding, symmetry, or fractures. Hydration is assessed by eyelid mobility, skin turgor, and dry mucous membranes.

The crop is palpated for presence of food or foreign bodies. Observation of refill time of the basilic (wing) vein will estimate perfusion status. Normal veins refill in 1 to 2 seconds after depression. The heart and lungs are auscultated. The respiratory rate and effort is evaluated. The pectoral muscle should be evaluated to judge the bird's body condition. The abdomen is palpated for signs of masses or fluid distention. In normal birds, it is difficult to palpate abdominal organs. An increase in the distance between the caudal end of the sternum and the pubis can suggest abdominal organomegaly, neoplasia or ascites. The vent should be examined for matting, redness or swelling. The grasp reflex of the feet will help determine weakness. The bird is also weighed on a gram scale.

SHOCK IN THE AVIAN PATIENT

Shock is defined as poor tissue perfusion from either low blood flow or unevenly distributed flow. This results in an inadequate delivery of oxygen to the tissues. This definition applies to all species of animals. Recent studies done by the author on shock in birds, has provided in-depth knowledge of a birds response to hypovolemic shock. Fluid resuscitation of the patient in hypovolemic shock can be a challenge and the clinician should understand the basic pathophysiology of shock, principles of perfusion, have knowledge of the different types of fluid and blood pressure monitoring techniques.

Appropriate fluid therapy, combined with frequent patient evaluation and blood pressure monitoring, can produce favorable outcomes.

Glucocorticoids

The use of glucocorticoids in the treatment of shock is controversial. These drugs have been extensively investigated in the shock syndrome. The side effects of immunosuppression, increased risk of infection (ie, aspergillosis, psittacosis), hyperglycemia, and gastric ulceration may outweigh their benefits. Their use in shock caused by hemorrhage and hypovolemia is not currently recommended.

Sodium Bicarbonate

The most important method of correction of severe metabolic acidosis is aimed at increasing the pH through increasing the extracellular fluid pH. Crystalloid fluids containing lactate, acetate, and gluconate (ie, Plasma-Lyte, Normasol R, LRS) are considered an important means of increasing the alkalinity of the extracellular fluid. Correction of acidemia initially begins with correction of the patient's perfusion and hydration status through the use of fluid therapy.

Blood gas parameters must be evaluated before considering the administration of sodium bicarbonate. Since this is rarely possible in the avian patient, use of sodium bicarbonate in shock is not recommended.

HYPOVOLEMIC SHOCK

Hypovolemic shock is caused by either an absolute or relative hypovolemia. Potential etiologies of absolute hypovolemia would be any cause of hemorrhage, including trauma, coagulopathy, gastrointestinal bleeding, surgical mishaps or a ruptured neoplasia. Examples of relative hypovolemia would include severe dehydration from gastrointestinal loss, or extensive loss of plasma as in a burn patient, or loss into a third-body space such as the coelomic cavity, uterus, or gastrointestinal tract.

The most common cause of hypovolemic shock is hemorrhage. When an animal begins hemorrhaging, there is a decrease in blood volume and decrease in venous return to the right side of the heart. This causes a decrease in return to the left side of the heart and therefore a decrease in cardiac output. With a substantial hypovolemia, blood pressure decreases below a mean arterial pressure of 60 mmHg or a systolic pressure of less than 90 mmHg. The carotid and aortic artery baroreceptors detect a decrease in stretch due to the decrease in cardiac output. This sends a neural signal to the vasomotor center in the medulla oblongata, which results in inhibition of vagal parasympathetic center and stimulation of the sympathetic center. This causes vasoconstriction of the veins and arterioles throughout the peripheral circulatory system and increases heart rate and strength of heart contraction. The humoral response is an increase in adrenal circulating catecholamines which in turn stimulates renin release via adrenergic receptors on cells of the juxtaglomerular apparatus (specialized smooth muscle cells in the afferent arterioles). Renin causes release of Angiotensin II, aldosterone, and antidiuretic hormone. There is a strong vasoconstriction and water retention, from their release causing an increase in extracellular fluid volume and an increase in blood pressure.

The pathophysiology of hemorrhagic shock is poorly understood in avian species. Acute blood loss of 30% to 40% of blood volume has been shown to result in 50% mortality (LD_{50}) in mammals. Blood loss is better tolerated in birds than in mammals. The LD_{50} for acute blood loss in ducks has been shown in a recent study to be 60% of the total blood volume.

A recent hemorrhagic shock study in mallard ducks (*Anas platyrhynchos*) documented an increase in heart rate and decrease in blood pressure following acute blood loss. That study may show that birds have a baroreceptor response to shock similar to that seen in mammals.

Isotonic replacement fluids are administered according to the patient's estimated dehydration, maintenance needs, and anticipated ongoing losses.

Red Blood Cell Regeneration After Acute Blood Loss

After acute blood loss, mammals are dependent on red blood cell (RBC) regeneration to maintain oxygen delivery to the tissues. In response to tissue hypoxia, erythropoietin stimulates RBC production by the bone marrow. Reticulocyte release from the bone marrow in mammals occurs rarely after 2 to 4 days and most commonly longer than 5 days after acute blood loss. Reticulocytosis, or polychromasia, is the hallmark of intensified erythropoiesis in mammals and birds, allowing classification of anemias into regenerative or nonregenerative types. A previous study done by the author, on acute blood loss in the duck documented an early regenerative response shown by presence of polychromasia starting at 12 hours after blood loss. The relatively short live span of the red blood cell (28–45 days) and presence of a nucleated red blood cell (RBC) may account for a birds' ability to mount a very early regenerative response. The use of early supportive care with fluid therapy in avian shock may help bridge the gap for the first 24 hours, after which birds can mount their own RBC regenerative response.

Fluid Selection

Individual characteristics of available fluids influence the dose, type, and volume of fluid administered. Crystalloids solutions can be used together with colloids during the resuscitation phase. Crystalloids are the mainstay of the rehydration and maintenance phases of fluid therapy. The three basic groups (ie, crystalloids, synthetic colloids, and hemoglobin-based oxygen carriers) of fluids will be discussed.

Fluid Therapy – Birds

Any sick, debilitated bird presenting for emergency care, should immediately be placed in a warm incubator (Temperature at 85–90°F [29.4–32.1°C]) with oxygen supplementation for 2 to 4 hours. When active external hemorrhage is present, this must be stopped immediately. Most birds benefit from the administration of warmed crystalloids at 3 mL/100 g BW IV, IO or SQ. Birds should be offered food and water during this time. When the bird appears stable (alert, responsive) and can be safely anesthetized with mask isoflurane or sevoflurane, diagnostics and treatment for hypovolemia and dehydration can be performed. Blood pressure monitoring using Doppler and an ECG can be used during these procedures.

The Doppler cuff can be placed on the distal humerus or femur and Doppler probe on the medial surface of the proximal ulna or tibiotarsus, respectively. The blood pressure of various avian species under isoflurane or sevoflurane anesthesia at the author's clinic is 90 to 140 mmHg systolic. When blood pressures are below 90 mmHg systolic, birds are treated for hypovolemia as given below. Bolus administration of crystalloids (10 mL/kg) and colloids (HES or Oxyglobin[®]

at 5 mL/kg) can be given IV or IO until blood pressure is greater than 90 mmHg systolic. In the author's experience one or two bolus infusions are usually required. In severely dehydrated birds that are not eating, IV or IO catheters are placed for replacement of dehydration losses with crystalloids. Estimation of the fluid deficit is based on estimated dehydration and body weight:

Estimated Dehydration (%) x Body Weight (g) = Fluid Deficit (mL)

Daily maintenance fluid requirements (2 mL/kg/hr) are added to the fluid deficit volume.

References are available from the author upon request.

AVIAN SHOCK: HOW TO KEEP THEM ALIVE

Marla Lichtenberger, DVM, Diplomate ACVECC
Thousand Oaks Pet Emergency Clinic
Thousand Oaks, CA

HYPOVOLEMIC SHOCK

Hypovolemic shock is caused by either an absolute or relative hypovolemia. Potential etiologies of absolute hypovolemia would be any cause of hemorrhage, including trauma, coagulopathy, gastrointestinal bleeding, surgical mishaps, or a ruptured neoplasia. Examples of relative hypovolemia would include severe dehydration from gastrointestinal loss, or extensive loss of plasma as in a burn patient, or loss into a third-body space such as the coelomic cavity, uterus or gastrointestinal tract.

The most common cause of hypovolemic shock is hemorrhage. When an animal begins hemorrhaging, there is a decrease in blood volume and decrease in venous return to the right side of the heart. This causes a decrease in return to the left side of the heart and therefore a decrease in cardiac output. With a substantial hypovolemia, blood pressure decreases below a mean arterial pressure of 60 mmHg or a systolic pressure of less than 90 mmHg. The carotid and aortic artery baroreceptors detect a decrease in stretch due to the decrease in cardiac output. This sends a neural signal to the vasomotor center in the medulla oblongata, which results in inhibition of vagal parasympathetic center and stimulation of the sympathetic center. This causes vasoconstriction of the veins and arterioles throughout the peripheral circulatory system and increases heart rate and strength of heart contraction. The humoral response is an increase in adrenal circulating catecholamines which in turn stimulates renin release via adrenergic receptors on cells of the juxataglomerular apparatus (specialized smooth muscle cells in the afferent arterioles). Renin causes release of angiotensin II, aldosterone, and antidiuretic hormone. There is a strong vasoconstriction and water retention, from their release causing an increase in extracellular fluid volume and an increase in blood pressure.

The pathophysiology of hemorrhagic shock is poorly understood in avian species. Acute blood loss of 30% to 40% of blood volume has been shown to result in 50% mortality (LD_{50}) in mammals. Blood loss is better tolerated in birds than in mammals. The LD_{50} for acute blood loss in ducks has been shown in a recent study to be 60% of the total blood volume.

A recent hemorrhagic shock study in mallard ducks (*Anas platyrhynchos*) documented an increase in heart rate and decrease in blood pressure following acute blood loss. That study may show that birds have a baroreceptor response to shock similar to that seen in mammals.

Isotonic replacement fluids are administered according to the patient's estimated dehydration, maintenance needs, and anticipated ongoing losses.

Fluid Selection

Individual characteristics of available fluids influence the dose, type, and volume of fluid administered. Crystalloids solutions can be used together with colloids during the resuscitation phase. Crystalloids are the mainstay of the rehydration and maintenance phases of fluid therapy. The three basic groups (ie, crystalloids, synthetic colloids, and hemoglobin-based oxygen carriers) of fluids will be discussed.

Fluid Therapy – Birds

Any sick, debilitated bird presenting for emergency care, should immediately be placed in a warm incubator (Temperature at 85–90°F [29.4–32.1°C]) with oxygen supplementation for 2 to 4 hours. When active external hemorrhage is present, this must be stopped immediately. Most birds benefit from the administration of warmed crystalloids at 3 mL/100 g BW IV, IO, or SQ. Birds should be offered food and water during this time. When the bird appears stable (alert, responsive) and can be safely anesthetized with mask isoflurane or sevoflurane, diagnostics and treatment for hypovolemia and dehydration can be performed. Blood pressure monitoring using Doppler and an ECG can be used during these procedures.

The Doppler cuff can be placed on the distal humerus or femur and Doppler probe on the medial surface of the proximal ulna or tibiotarsus, respectively. The blood pressure of various avian species under isoflurane or sevoflurane anesthesia at the author's clinic is 90 to 140 mmHg systolic. When blood pressures are below 90 mmHg systolic, birds are treated for hypovolemia as given below. Bolus administration of crystalloids (10 mL/kg) and colloids (HES or Oxyglobin® at 5 mL/kg) can be given IV or IO until blood pressure is greater than 90 mmHg systolic. In the author's experience one or two bolus infusions are usually required. In severely dehydrated birds that are not eating, IV or IO catheters are placed for replacement of dehydration losses with crystalloids. Estimation of the fluid deficit is based on estimated dehydration and body weight:

Estimated Dehydration (%) x Body Weight (g) = Fluid Deficit (mL)

Daily maintenance fluid requirements (2 ml/kg/hr) are added to the fluid deficit volume.

Cardiopulmonary-Cerebral Resuscitation

CPCR is a comprehensive term used to describe both the basic principles of cardiopulmonary resuscitation (CPR) as well as advanced life support and post-resuscitation care. The word *cerebral* resuscitation was added to cardiopulmonary resuscitation to identify the importance of being alive with complete neurologic function. The most recent International Heart Association guidelines for CPCR and emergency cardiac care in humans were published in 2000. The primary focus was use of evidence-based medicine. These guidelines were used to extrapolate the basic principles for mammals. I have taken this information and applied the same principles to the avian species.

The prognosis for respiratory arrest, especially when caused by isoflurane anesthesia overdose, is good. Cardiac arrest carries a poor prognosis, because direct compression of the heart is not possible because of the overlying sternum. Because birds do not have a diaphragm, closed-chest compressions in birds cannot utilize the thoracic pump mechanism to increase overall negative intrathoracic pressure.

Always monitor birds with a Doppler blood pressure and electrocardiogram when placing under gas anesthesia. The goal is to use these monitoring devices to identify cardiovascular instability early. Early recognition of cardiovascular instability is the key to success in avian medicine.

If the bird arrests on anesthesia, stop the anesthesia administration. Place an endotracheal tube and start positive-pressure ventilation with 100% oxygen. An alternative method for positive pressure ventilation is placement of an air-sac breathing tube. The bird is given an injection of naloxone (0.2 mL for a large bird and 0.1 mL for a small bird) IM (intramuscularly) to stimulate the respiratory centers. Epinephrine (0.01 mg/kg) and atropine (0.04 mg/kg) can be given IV (intravenous), IO (intraosseous), or via the endotracheal route (using a tom cat catheter inserted down the endotracheal tube and doubling the dose used for IV). Intracardiac injections should be avoided, because of risk for laceration of the coronary vessels. An electrocardiogram, Doppler blood pressure, and end-tidal CO_2 monitor can be used to evaluate the effectiveness of CPR resuscitation.

HYPERTENSION

The definition of hypertension in birds is somewhat vague. A study of normal conscious and anesthetized psittacine birds of different species reported mean systolic Doppler arterial pressures of 90 to 180 mmHg and 120 to 180 mmHg, respectively. In the authors' experience, systolic Doppler blood pressures greater than 200 mmHg (in conscious and anesthetized birds) are taken to indicate hypertension in birds.

Pathophysiology and Clinical Consequences

Signs of organ damage may be the presenting complaint in some patients with severe hypertension. The patients may present for ocular lesions (ie, retinal hemorrhages, detachments, and/or papilledema), neurologic signs (ie, confusion, seizures), cardiovascular signs (ie, ventricular hypertrophy and congestive heart failure) or renal system abnormalities (ie, glomerulonephritis).

Etiology of Hypertension

- Primary or essential hypertension
- Primary hypertension is common in people and has been documented in dogs, the prevalence is extremely low. Its presence in other animals and birds is unknown
- Renal disease

- Renal failure is relatively commonly associated with severe hypertension in dogs and cats (ie, 60% of renal failure patients), particularly in patients with protein-losing nephropathy (PLN). The presence of PLN and hypertension in birds is unknown. The author has treated a parakeet with hypertension secondary to a renal tumor.
- Atherosclerosis

Possible Risk Factors for Atherosclerosis

- Obesity and decreased exercise
- Obesity affects the function of many organ systems in the body and predisposes to a variety of diseases. These include coronary artery disease, myocardial infarction, heart failure, hypertension, and dyslipidemias (lower high-density lipoprotein [HDL], elevated low-density lipoprotein [LDL] and very low-density lipoprotein [VLDL], elevated triglycerides).
- The exact cause of hypertension in obese individuals is unclear. Most likely, it results from the additive effects of several organ derangements. As total body mass increases, blood flow also increases to the expanding adipose tissue. Body metabolic rate and oxygen consumption increase, stimulating an increase in cardiac output. Normally, the rise in cardiac output occurs with a reduction in systemic vascular resistance and maintenance of a normal blood pressure. However, as obesity becomes more severe, systemic vascular resistance and blood pressure increase.
- High-fat/cholesterol diet or hypertriglycerides/ cholesterol (hyperlipidemia)
- Hypothyroidism
- Exposure to stress factors as cold, cigarette smoke
- Hypertension

Treatment for Atherosclerosis

- Reduce fat and cholesterol in the diet
- Increase exercise
- Rule out hypothyroidism
- Decrease stress factors as exposure to cold, cigarette smoke
- Blood cholesterol reducing agents (e.g. Lipitor-not established in birds)
- Omega 3 fatty acids –may reduce serum cholesterol and triglyceride concentrations by decreasing the sybthesis of VLDL and LDL. 30 mg/kg PO q 24 hr
- Chitosan is a fiber supplement made from shellfish that reportedly binds (positive ion to negative lipoproteins) to lipids in the diet and decreases absortion of them. Give 30 min before meal and separate from omega 3 by several hours (increases break down of fatty acids) at 15 mg/kg
- Niacin reduces hepatic triglyceride synthesis and VLDL production; 50–300 mg/day/dog
- Arterial hypertension medications

Unless evidence for hypertension-related organ injury is seen (eg, retinal lesions, neurologic signs, renal disease), the decision to initiate antihypertensive therapy is not an emergency. The initial blood pressure should be taken and every effort should be made to minimize the risk that measured elevations in blood pressure represent a transient "white coat" effect, rather than a sustained elevation in blood pressure.

The optimum endpoint for antihypertensive therapy has not been established for dogs, cats, or birds with hypertension. In the absence of such information, treatment for arterial hypertension should be initiated cautiously with the goal of reducing blood pressure by 25% over weeks in patients without hypertension-related injury. In patients with acute, severe hypertension-related injury, rapid reduction in blood pressure may be necessary.

Angiotensin-Converting Enzyme (ACE) Inhibitors

ACE inhibitors inhibit the conversion of angiotensin I to angiotensin II, and thus attenuate angiotensin-mediated vasoconstriction and aldosterone release. These drugs also decrease glomerular efferent arteriolar vasoconstriction, and help reduce protein loss and inhibit the progression of glomerulosclerosis by lowering glomerular filtration pressure. ACE inhibitors, such as benazapril (0.5 mg/kg BID), have the potential renoprotective benefits and are therefore appropriate options for renal patients with hypertension. In the author's experience, ACE inhibitors generally produce a relatively small reduction in blood pressure in dogs and cats. However, because of their beneficial role in altering intraglomerular hemodynamics, proteinuria, and profibrotic effects of the intrarenal rennin-angiotensin system, ACE inhibitors may have renoprotective effects even in the absence of achieving adequate blood pressure control. In a recent study the ACE inhibitor, enalapril, reduced the severity of renal lesions that develop in dogs with surgically reduced renal mass. Further, in dogs with naturally occurring glomerulopathies, enalapril significantly reduced proteinuria and may have been beneficial in stabilizing renal function.

The author has measured a systolic blood pressure in a parakeet with a renal tumor that was greater than 300 mmHg. The bird was started on antihypertensive medication (Benazapril 0.5 mg/kg BID PO) and returned weekly for Doppler blood pressure measurements. Due to the stress level of the bird, he was anesthetized under sevaflurane anesthesia for weekly blood pressure measurements. The medication dose was adjusted with changes in these weekly blood pressure measurements.

Calcium Channel Blockers
- Cases:
  - Renal disease or tumor
  - Atherosclerosis or hyperlipidemia
  - Neurologic - confusion, dullness, weakness, seizures, ataxia, tremor (ischemia or atherosclerotic cerebellar/cerebral vessels)
  - Species - Amazon, cockatiel, cockatoo, or any older bird

References are available from the author upon request.

ANESTHESIA AND ANALGESIA: MONITORING THE DOWN AND OUT

Marla Lichtenberger, DVM, Diplomate ACVECC
Pet Emergency Clinic
Thousand Oaks, CA

Pain is present with many diseases as well as in association with surgical and traumatic conditions. The demonstration of pain is not always obvious; therefore, an animal should be assumed to be experiencing pain in any condition expected to produce pain in humans. The assessment and control of pain is an art as well as a science. Clinicians should keep in mind that the art of pain management is a continual learning experience requiring assessment and therapeutic adjustment for individual animals even when they are undergoing similar surgical procedures. Therefore, standard or rule-of-thumb analgesic and anesthetic protocols are not always appropriate.

If we accept that animals can experience pain, then how do we determine if a bird is or is not painful? It is likely that the tolerance of pain by birds varies greatly from individual, as it does in other species. This coupled with bird's innate ability to mask significant disease, and probably pain, make it difficult to assess pain. Compared to dogs and cats, very few investigations have been carried out on the assessment and alleviation of pain in birds. Most likely, as in cats the mainstay of pain assessment in birds appears to be behavioral.

There are certain behaviors that are commonly seen in birds suffering acute trauma or postoperative pain. Such birds are often depressed, immobile, silent, and appear and distanced from their environment. They do not respond normally to petting or attention; birds tend to hide when experiencing pain. They may also hyperventilate. In the author's clinic, birds appear to have a very similar response to pain as is seen in cats.

MULTIMODAL APPROACH

The process of nociception and pain involves many steps and pathways, so one analgesic agent is unlikely to alleviate pain completely. An effective management plan includes drugs of different classes, each acting at a different part of the pathway; this is termed *multimodal analgesia*. For example, a bird can be premedicated with an opioid, which will modulate pain; midazolam can be added to relieve anxiety; a local anesthetic block could be incorporated to inhibit transmission; and a nonsteroidal anti-inflammatory drug (NSAID) can be added pre- or postoperatively to alter transduction. This approach also allows smaller doses of each drug to be used as the effects are additive and may reduce any undesirable side effects from larger doses of individual drugs.

Constant rate infusions (CRIs) are delivered intravenously at a constant rate, frequently over a long period of time. Constant rate infusions have several advantages. They allow the drug to be titrated to effect resulting in a reduction in the total amount of drug used, frequently resulting in fewer side effects, less "rollercoaster" analgesia, fewer hemodynamic effects, and more cost-effectiveness. Disadvantages include a slow rise in plasma concentrations to therapeutic levels, which is why a loading dose of the drug is frequently given prior to starting the CRI. No published studies have been done in birds demonstrating the use of a CRI infusion of analgesia.

The easiest way to administer a CRI is via an automated mechanical pump system. In veterinary medicine, syringe pump systems are the most common delivery system and are mandatory for the small volumes used for birds. These are small pumps that can utilize 1 cc to 60 cc syringe for delivery of the drug through an intravenous extension line. The syringe pump is advantageous because it allows very small volumes of drug to be delivered at a constant rate infusion.

PAIN MANAGEMENT OPTIONS IN BIRDS

There is no doubt that in the bird, pain management in clinical practice is presently inadequate. The bird patient has an undeserved reputation for adverse respiratory depression after opiate treatment. In the authors' opinion, birds become very comfortable and sleep normally after administration of opioids postoperatively. Birds have mainly kappa pain receptors and therefore respond to kappa agonist drugs for pain relief. Fear of these adverse effects has resulted in many birds not receiving analgesics before or after surgery or trauma.

ANESTHETIC DRUGS USED IN BIRDS

The three major classes of analgesics employed for acute pain management are opioids, NSAIDs, and local anesthetics.

Opioids

Birds continue to have an undeserved reputation of having "respiratory depression" after administration of opioid drugs. Resting very quietly without pain is being interpreted as respiratory depression. When used appropriately, opioids can be administered to birds and are safe and effective for alleviating pain. Opioids in general have a very wide margin of safety and excellent analgesic properties. In veterinary medicine, the most commonly used opioid constant rate infusions (CRIs) are fentanyl, hydromorphone, morphine, and butorphanol. Some animals may respond better to one opioid over another depending on individual variability, species, and source of pain.

Butorphanol (Dolorex®, Intervet) continues to be the most commonly used opioid in ferrets despite recent questioning of its analgesic properties. Described as an agonist-antagonist agent, its agonist activity is exerted at the kappa receptors and its antagonist actions are demonstrated at the mu receptors. Opioid drugs in this class exert a ceiling effect, after which increasing doses do not produce any further analgesia. Butorphanol appears to be an effective visceral, but a poor somatic, analgesia. Butorphanol is a poor analgesic choice for surgery patients where there will be somatic and visceral pain, however. Its ceiling effects limits its use to minor procedures, and the frequent dosing required is inconvenient and expensive. When used in the author's clinic, for treatment of pain in the bird we prefer to use it as a CRI, instead of repeated dosing. Higher doses repeated throughout the day can also be used in avian medicine for pain relief. The drug is repeated every 2 to 3 hours.

Tramadol (opioid-type drug) is another possible drug to be used orally for postoperative pain control. Tramadol binds to opiate receptors and also inhibits reuptake of norepinephrine and serotonin. The agent thus stimulates two endogenous, antinociceptive mechanisms in the spinal cord and the brain stem. The doses that are currently used have been extrapolated from human medicine.

Nonsteroidal Anti-inflammatory Drugs (NSAIDs)

NSAIDs are excellent agents for alleviation of acute postoperative and traumatic pain. As in other species there are concerns about preoperative use of NSAIDs in birds. The main concern relate to inhibition of prostaglandin synthesis, which may lead to gastrointestinal erosion, impaired renal function, and bleeding. The limited ability for glucuronide conjugation in ferrets can prolong the duration of action of the NSAIDs, but with appropriate changes in dose and dosing intervals they can be used safely. The advantages of this category of drugs are their long duration of action and that no Drug Enforcement Administration (DEA) paperwork is required. In young birds with no evidence of renal disease, this group of drugs is a good choice.

Injectible carprofen has become available in the United States, but it is unlikely to be labeled for use in birds. Carprofen is not a potent inhibitor of prostaglandin synthetase and has proved to be a safe agent in ferrets. Ketoprofen (Ketofen, Fort Dodge Animal Health) is available as an injectable agent, but because of its COX-1 inhibition, should be reserved for postoperative administration. Meloxicam (Metacam®, Boehringer Ingelheim Vetmedica, Inc., St. Joseph, MO) is recently available as an injectable and oral form, and is the most commonly used NSAID in the bird. It has primary COX-2 inhibition. NSAIDs should not be used in animals with preexisting renal disease, hypovolemia, or bleeding disorders or if severe surgical hemorrhage is anticipated. Flunixin meglumine is an NSAID and is a very potent inhibitor of cyclo-oxygenase. The author warns against its use with pre-existing renal disease, hypovolemia, or bleeding disorders as with NSAIDs. Newer NSAIDs that are specifically COX-2 inhibitors may be safer to use in birds than flunixin.

Local Anesthetics

Local anesthetic agents can be employed successfully in birds. The two most commonly used agents are lidocaine (lidocaine HCl oral topical solution, USP 2%, Hi-Tech Pharmacal Co.) and bupivacaine (bupivacaine HCl, 0.5%, Abbott Laboratories).

An advantage of this group of drugs is their low cost and uncontrolled status. A complete sensory block prevents nerve transmission, making use of these agents one of the most potentially practical pre-emptive techniques. Local anesthetics can be infiltrated into the surgical skin site, or discrete nerve blocks can be preformed.

EQUIPMENT USED TO MONITOR ANESTHESIA IN BIRDS

The following equipment commonly used in small animals can also be used to monitor anesthesia in birds. The lecture will discuss how we use this equipment in practice and present case discussions commonly seen in avian practice.

- End-Tidal CO_2
- Pulse oximetry
- Indirect blood pressure monitoring
- Temperature monitoring
- Electrocardiogram
- Respiration rate

References are available from the author upon request.

DEALING WITH FLUFFLED, RUFFLED PATIENTS

Marla Lichtenberger, DVM, Diplomate ACVECC
Thousand Oaks Pet Emergency Clinic
Thousand Oaks, CA

Increasing numbers of birds are being kept as pets, and owners want to receive high quality medical care for these pets. Treatment of hypovolemic shock and critical care monitoring in birds are complicated by small patient size, physiological diversity, and lack of research and clinical data on their response to therapy. Despite these impediments, the same principles and techniques of monitoring used in domestic animals can be applied to the avian patient. The goal of this article is to provide an in-depth presentation on the principles and pathophysiology of shock, types of fluids, monitoring techniques, and shock resuscitation methods for use in birds. Principles of cardiopulmonary-cerebral resuscitation will also be discussed. Arterial blood pressure measurement is an important tool in the management of the critically ill bird. The message of clinical importance is that fixed fluid regimens (eg, lactated Ringer's), fixed volumes (eg, mL/kg), and rules of thumb are in most instances outdated, inappropriate, and oftentimes inadequate. Appropriate fluid therapy, combined with frequent patient evaluation and periodic blood pressure monitoring techniques, can produce astounding and at times miraculous results.

Most birds do not show signs of illness in the early stages of disease. Often, birds with chronic disease present as an emergency because of their ability to mask clinical signs of the disease until the condition is severe. In virtually all cases, I advise the receptionist to recommend the bird be brought in for an exam. If the owner is concerned enough to call, then the bird is probably very sick and needs to be seen. While all signs reported by the client can be of concern, sitting at the bottom of the cage, bleeding, respiratory distress, regurgitation, and anorexia are considered true emergencies. The client should be instructed to bring the bird in a cage, if possible; otherwise instruct the owner about suitable alternatives (eg, box, cat carrier). The water dish should be emptied but the cage should not be cleaned prior to traveling to the hospital.

Once the bird has arrived, it is ideal to have a trained receptionist call for an immediate triage by a nurse. Prompt, accurate treatment is vital to a favorable outcome. The nurse should assess the condition of the bird in a room. In cases of bleeding, seizuring, head trauma, and respiratory distress, the bird should be evaluated immediately by the veterinarian. If the bird is fluffled, weak, or sitting at the bottom of the cage, they should be placed in a warmed incubator and oxygen is administered. The optimum temperatures for ill birds are 85 to 90°F (29–30°C).

SHOCK IN THE AVIAN PATIENT

Shock is defined as poor tissue perfusion from either low blood flow or unevenly distributed flow. This results in an inadequate delivery of oxygen to the tissues. This definition applies to all species of animals. Recent studies done by the author on shock in birds have provided in-depth knowledge of a bird's response to hypovolemic shock. Fluid resuscitation of the patient in hypovolemic shock can be a challenge and the clinician should understand the basic pathophysiology of shock, principles of perfusion, and have knowledge of the different types of fluid and blood pressure monitoring techniques. Appropriate fluid therapy, combined with frequent patient evaluation and blood pressure monitoring can produce favorable outcomes.

A companion article in this proceedings, "Avian Shock: How to Keep Them Alive," discusses general principles of hypovolemic shock, blood pressure monitoring, and characteristics of fluids. These principles will then be applied to treatment of hypovolemic shock in the avian species. The importance of pain management and nutrition will also be discussed. IN a second companion article, The second part of this article discusses principles of CPCR (cardiopulmonary-cerebral resuscitation) and ARD (acute respiratory distress).

Glucocorticoids

The use of glucocorticoids in the treatment of shock is controversial. These drugs have been extensively investigated in the shock syndrome. The side effects of immunosuppression, increased risk of infection (eg, aspergillosis, psittacosis), hyperglycemia and gastric ulceration may outweigh their benefits. Their use in shock caused by hemorrhage and hypovolemia is not currently recommended.

Sodium Bicarbonate

The most important method of correction of severe metabolic acidosis is aimed at increasing the pH through increasing the extracellular fluid pH. Crystalloid fluids containing lactate, acetate, and gluconate (eg, Plasma-Lyte, Normasol R, LRS) are considered an important means of increasing the alkalinity of the extracellular fluid. Correction of acidemia initially begins with correction of the patient's perfusion and hydration status through the use of fluid therapy.

Blood gas parameters must be evaluated before considering the administration of sodium bicarbonate. Since this is rarely possible in the avian patient, use of sodium bicarbonate in shock is not recommended.

Fluid Selection

Individual characteristics of available fluids influence the dose, type, and volume of fluid administered. Crystalloids solutions can be used together with colloids during the resuscitation phase. Crystalloids are the mainstay of the rehydration and maintenance phases of fluid therapy. The three basic groups (ie, crystalloids, synthetic colloids, and hemoglobin-based oxygen carriers) of fluids are discussed.

Fluid Therapy in Birds

Any sick, debilitated bird presenting for emergency care, should immediately be placed in a warm incubator (temperature at 85–90°F [29.4–32.1°C]) with oxygen supplementation for 2 to 4 hours. When active external hemorrhage is present, this must be stopped immediately. Most birds benefit from the administration of warmed crystalloids at 3 mL/100 g BW IV, IO, or SQ. Birds should be offered food and water during this time. When the bird appears stable (alert, responsive) and can be safely anesthetized with mask isoflurane (Abbott Laboratories) or sevoflurane (Abbott Laboratories), diagnostics and treatment for hypovolemia and dehydration can be performed. Blood pressure monitoring using Doppler and an ECG can be used during these procedures.

The Doppler cuff can be placed on the distal humerus or femur and Doppler probe on the medial surface of the proximal ulna or tibiotarsus, respectively. The blood pressure of various avian species under isoflurane or sevoflurane anesthesia at the author's clinic is 90 to 140 mmHg systolic. When blood pressures are below 90 mmHg systolic, birds are treated for hypovolemia as given below. Bolus administration of crystalloids (10 mL/kg) and colloids (HES or Oxyglobin® at 5 mL/kg) can be given IV or IO until blood pressure is greater than 90 mmHg systolic. In the author's experience 1 or 2 bolus infusions are usually required. In severely dehydrated birds that are not eating, IV or IO catheters are placed for replacement of dehydration losses with crystalloids. Estimation of the fluid deficit is based on estimated dehydration and body weight:

Estimated Dehydration (%) x Body Weight (g) = Fluid Deficit (mL)

Daily maintenance fluid requirements (2 mL/kg/hr) are added to the fluid deficit volume.

References are available from the author upon request.

FEEDING THE STARVED BIRD

Susan Orosz, PhD, DVM, Dipl. ABPV-Avian & ECAMS
Bird and Exotic Pet Wellness Center
Toledo, OH

OVERVIEW

Malnutrition has been defined as a nutritional deficit associated with an increased risk of adverse clinical events such as morbidity or death. Malnutrition has been treated clinically in hospitalized human and animal patients through both enteral nutrition (EN) and total parenteral nutrition (TPN). A review of the evidence from a group of clinical trials in human patients examined a number of factors comparing EN and TPN administration. The researchers concluded that EN was associated with lower costs, improved nutritional outcomes, less mucosal permeability, and greater wound healing. There also appeared to be a decrease in septic morbidity of enterally fed, abdominal trauma patients. The review found that abdominal trauma patients benefited from EN preferentially over TPN. EN was the preferred method of supplying the metabolic needs for all critically ill patient types examined, except for head-injured patients. In those patients, either TPN or EN was acceptable, depending on the mental status of the patient. This has important ramifications to our avian patients that are critically ill as well.

Although the relationship between poor nutritional status and increased susceptibility to disease has been recognized clinically for a long time, mechanisms that modulate the immune system have been poorly understood, particularly with avian patients. While research in the past has focused on micronutrient deficiencies and their role in an altered immune system, newer studies are investigating the use of supraphysiologic levels of micronutrients as immune modulators.

One area that has been investigated is the role of energy in patients that are critically ill. These patients most often have decreased energy intake. However, studies that have investigated the effects of decreased energy intake on immune function have produced variable results. Studies of intracellular and viral pathogens suggest that mild to moderate undernutrition may be protective. These studies suggested that this undernutrition may affect pathogen growth more than host immunity. However, further review of these studies suggested that the altered immune function may have been the result of micronutrient deficiencies rather than from a pure decrease in energy. Fernandes and Venkatraman[3] found that a 60% to 70% decreased energy intake tended to have a biphasic effect on the immune system in mice. This decrease in energy primarily affected cell-mediated immunity both early and late in life. They also found that lowered energy intake slowed the aging of the immune system and significantly increased life expectancy.

Pharmacologic doses of arginine have been shown to promote wound healing at least by increasing the accumulation of hydroxyproline. It may be that arginine may be used as a precursor for proline in the formation of collagen. Additionally, arginine has been found to be immune stimulating by preventing thymic atrophy and by increasing the responsiveness of peripheral blood monocytes to T-cell mitogens. In brain-injured patients, the addition of glutamine and probiotics in their enteral formula decreased infection rates and days of ventilation. This data suggests that these patients have increased energy and protein needs and they improve with glutamine supplementation.

The polyunsaturated fatty acids (PUFA) of the n-6 and n-3 series are also implicated in affecting immunity and its response. The n-6 PUFA arachidonic acid is the precursor for prostaglandins, leukotrienes, and other related compounds that have specific roles in the inflammatory process. A number of studies have examined the anti-inflammatory role of the n-3 PUFA of fish oils, eicosapentaenoic acid (EPA), and docosahexaenoic acid (DHA) in cardiovascular and inflammatory/autoimmune diseases suggesting that they have a beneficial effect. Data from clinical and research studies suggest that the balance of n-6 to n-3 should be closer to 2:1 for parenteral nutrition with a markedly reduced immune system.

A dietary source of vitamin C is not normally required in many species of birds, as they are able to manufacture ascorbic acid. However, the rate of natural production may be insufficient during various stresses, physical trauma, and infection. In chickens, when ascorbic acid was increased above maintenance in the diet, there was improved resistance to a variety of infections and wound healing. This would suggest that with these types of conditions, as well as with liver and/or kidney failure, avian patients should be supplemented with vitamin C.

Malnutrition has been associated with an increased risk of wound-related complications. In addition to T cell impairment and alteration of granulocyte function, wound healing can also be delayed with malnutrition. Additionally, it has been observed in humans that increased levels of vitamin E interferes with healing and fibrosis and antagonize the promotion of wound healing with vitamin A.[11,12] This problem also occurs with birds. High levels of vitamin E (>1000 IU/kg) in pelicans resulted in them developing hemorrhagic problems because these levels of vitamin E produced a deficiency of vitamin K. This same problem can occur with other fat-soluble vitamins like vitamin A.

Malnutrition commonly occurs in hospitalized patients, in part from altered metabolism as a consequence of disease or surgery. Malnutrition can also result from a variety of causes including decreased intake and/or a reduced ability to digest, absorb, or metabolize nutrients. A number of disorders may increase the risk of malnutrition—those that alter the loss of protein and electrolytes and those that alter nutrient requirements. The first group (alteration of protein and electrolyte loss) includes vomiting, draining wounds, burns, ileus, diarrhea, abcesses, and malassimilation. The second group (alteration of nutrient requirements) includes trauma, blood loss, liver disease, sepsis, drug-nutrient interactions, burns, multiple surgical procedures, chronic renal diseases, fever, and cancer.

Enteral nutrition provided immediately post-operatively also has positive benefits for mammalian patients and presumably for birds. In a study in rats, the loss in total body water (TBW) was less in the early-fed group compared to the delayed group. This change in patient management also was shown to reduce catabolism while increasing the rate of wound healing.

STARVATION AND ILLNESS

In order to understand the nutritional requirements of birds during metabolic crises, it is important to understand basic principles of energy metabolism. Carbohydrates and protein produce the same amount of energy when metabolized in the living bird. However, fat yields twice as much energy as carbohydrates and protein. Clinically, this would suggest that when there is a significant energy deficit, fats should be considered as the primary energy source. For example, the energy of dry seeds contains 6 times the energy content of fresh fruit.

While these values represent the gross energy content, digestible energy represents the energy of the food that is absorbed from the GI tract. A small portion of the digestible energy is excreted as uric acid, and energy is also excreted in urine and feces. The energy retained in the body is the metabolizable energy. The energy available for use by the bird is the metabolizable energy less a loss resulting from an increase in the metabolic rate when food stuffs are absorbed by the gastrointestinal tract. Diets that are more elemental, with short carbon chains, may have a greater likelihood of improving birds that are debilitated, because less energy is needed to digest and transport short-chain nutrients across the intestinal tract.

When birds are deprived of food, their heat production diminishes as well as their metabolic rate. Glycogen reserves are usually depleted within 24 hours of a fast and gluconeogenesis begins within several days quickly. Gluconeogenesis is the metabolism of protein for glucose to supply needed energy during starvation or with increased metabolic demands with disease. Once glycogen is depleted, fat is preferentially metabolized as the source for energy. Liver and muscle incur the greatest losses in weight after adipose tissue when a bird is not eating. Muscle mass is often gauged by palpation of the pectoral muscles clinically. Understanding that glycogenolysis occurs rapidly, and that the liver loses its mass quickly, allows the clinician to predict and treat liver failure more effectively with cachexia.

Simple starvation differs from critical illness in a number of ways. With simple starvation, the metabolic activity decreases, resulting in hypometabolism. To maintain a normal blood glucose, the animal decreases its insulin concentration in the blood while increasing glucagon through increased hepatic glycogenolysis, increased gluconeogenesis, and use of glycogen stores. This combination of hormones increases lipolysis,

thereby increasing ketone bodies in the bloodstream while producing a mild acidosis. Once the hepatic glycogen stores are depleted, amino acids derived from skeletal muscle proteins and visceral proteins become the energy source for glucogenesis. Eventually, the liver uses immunoglobulins and lymphokines as a protein source for energy, complicating immune function.

Critical illness differs from simple starvation. One important difference is that critically ill patients are in a hypermetabolic state, due to local tissue injury or changes in homeostasis. Therefore, patients become hypoglycemic and acidemic quickly as a consequence of neuroendocrine activity. Activation of the neuroendocrine system by critical illness gears up the sympathetic nervous system in accordance with the degree of stress. This activation increases levels of cortisol in mammals, presumably corticosterone in avians. The neuroendocrine system results in an increase in glucagon, due to the increased metabolism associated with the illness. This can result in a rapid depletion of nitrogen and potassium, complicating healing and recovery. The increased concentration of the adrenal steroids results in glucose intolerance in the tissues, despite hyperinsulinemia.

Sepsis further complicates metabolic needs. Oxygen consumption, cardiac index, and metabolic rates increase in septic patients beyond that of nonseptic patients. Septic patients also tend to use fat as the primary source of energy. Sepsis in critically ill patients increases the risk of multiple organ failure.

NUTRITIONAL ASSESSMENT

Nutritional assessment should be performed as soon as possible upon admission to enhance patient outcome. The history should include a dietary history to help understand potential nutritional deficiencies or excesses, or if the patient is malnourished. Body weight has been determined to be one of the best assessors of mammalian nutritional status. In humans, if the patient has lost more than 10% of their body weight, nutritional support is indicated, even if the patient is obese.[13] These factors need to be taken into account with avian patients as well. Obese birds that suddenly stop eating have greater risk, especially if they have significant fat in their liver or have liver failure as they switch to ketone body formation as their energy source.

CONCLUSION

Therefore, enteral nutrition is indicated in alert patients, whether mammalian or avian, when they exhibit anorexia, have undergone a 5% to 10% weight loss, have a decreased level of serum albumin, or there are clinical indications of protein loss such as reduced pectoral mass (birds). Enteral nutrition should be used with caution and knowledge in its administration. Tube feeding should always be performed knowing and guarding against possible complications. Avian patients should be weighed at approximately the same time each day and prior to gavage feeding. After the diet has been tube fed, the patient should be returned immediately to its hospital cage without stress and, to avoid aspiration, without touching the crop. Tracking the bird's weight helps to determine if the type of enteral nutrition and the volume is appropriate to meet its metabolic demands.

The clinician needs to understand the types of products that can be used enterally and how to match the correct ingredients with the symptoms of the patient. Elemental diets that are calorically dense using fat are appropriate for use in debilitated patients. These patients need adequate levels of amino acids to meet the metabolic demands and to rebuild tissues after gluconeogenesis has reduced their mass. Those avian patients that appear to have liver failure and/or are hypoglycemic need simple carbohydrates as well to provide adequate levels of carbohydrates to meet the immediate need for glucose. Diets that are gavage-fed need to be tailored to the conditions of the patient to enhance overall success. It is hoped that this review of critical illness will provide the avian clinician with the information needed to provide appropriate nutritional support for the most important metabolic factors to enhance patient outcome.

REFERENCES

1. Smith LC, Mullen JL. Nutritional assessment and indications for nutritional support. Surg Clin North Am. 1991;71:449-457.
2. Heyland DK. Nutritional support in the critically ill patient. A critical review of the evidence. Crit Care Clin. 1998;14:423–440.
3. Fernandes G, Venkatraman JT. Dietary restriction: Effects on immunological function and aging. In: Klurfeld DM (ed.): Nutrition and Immunity. New York, NY: Plenum Press, 1993, pp 91-120.
4. Good RA, Lorenz E. Nutrition and cellular immunity. Int J Immunopharm. 1992;14:361.
5. Kirk JS, Barbul A. Role of arginine in trauma, sepsis, and immunity. J Parenter Enteral Nutr. 1990;14:226-229.
6. Barbul A, Lazarou SA, Efron DT, et al. Arginine wound healing and lymphocyte immune responses in humans. Surgery. 1990;108:331-337.
7. Falcao deArruda IS, de Aguilar-Nascimento JE, Benefits of early enteral nutrition with glutamine and probiotics in brain injury patients. Clin Sci (Lond). 2004;106:287-292.
8. Anderson M, Fritsche KL. (n-3) Fatty acids and infectious disease resistance. J Nutr. 2002;32:3566-3576.
9. Calder PC. N-3 polyunsaturated fatty acids and inflammation: from molecular biology to the clinic. Lipids. 2003;38:343-352.
10. Grimm H, Schott J, Schwemmle K. [Development of an immuno-neutral lipid emulsion for optimal postoperative management of intensive care patients]. [Article in German]. Langenbecks Arch Chir Supl Kongressbd. 1998;115:599-604.
11. Albina JG. Review: Nutrition and wound healing. J Parenter Enteral Nutr. 1994;18:367–376.
12. Bowers TL. Nutrition and immunity part 2: The role of selected micronutrients and clinical significance. Vet Clin Nutr. 1997;4:96-101.
13. Thatcher CD. Nutritional needs of critically ill patients. Compend Contin Educ Pract Vet. 1996;18:1303–1313.
14. Alverdy J, Aoys E, Moss G. TPN promotes bacterial translocation from the gut. Surgery. 1988;104:185–190.
15. Burkholder WJ, Swecker WS. Nutritional influences on immunity. Semin Vet Med Surg (Small Anim). 1990;5:154–166.
16. Maguid MM, Collier MD, Howard LJ. Uncomplicated and stressed starvation. Surg Clin North Am. 1981;61:532-543.
17. Aoki TT, Finley RJ. The metabolic response to fasting. In: Rombeau IL, Caldwell MD (eds.): Parenteral Nutrition. Philadelphia: WB Saunders; 1984, pp 9-28.
18. Long CD. Energy balance and carbohydrate metabolism in infection and sepsis. Am J Clin Nutr. 1977;30:301-310.
19. Hasselgren PO, Jagenburg, R, Karlstrom L, et al. Changes of protein metabolism in liver and skeletal muscle following trauma complicated by sepsis. J Traum. 1984;24:224-228.
20. Watters JM, Wilmore DW. The metabolic responses to trauma and sepsis. In: Degroot LJ (ed.): Endocrinology. Philadelphia: WB Saunders; 1989, pp 2367-2393.
21. Davis CL, Newman RJ, Molyneux SG, Grahme-Smith MB. The relationship between plasma catecholamines and severity of injury in man. J Traum. 1984;24:99-105.

THE SEIZURING BIRD

Susan Orosz, PhD, DVM, Dipl. ABVP-Avian & ECAMS
Bird and Exotic Pet Wellness Center
Toledo, OH

SEIZURES: WHAT ARE THEY?

What is a seizure in a bird? The common tonic clonic seizure is one where the bird starts out with a vague preictal phase where the bird has an abnormal behavior, tries to hide, or gets agitated. This phase is most often missed by the owner. The classic seizure is the one where the bird stands upright and becomes opisthotonic with the head stretched out and backward over the back. The wings extend and the bird starts shaking them. The beak is commonly open and closed in relation to the wings shaking and some birds may scream. The seizures are usually symmetrical and the tonic phase is when the muscle tone increases, followed by the clonic phase of relaxation in quick alternating successions. In the post ictal phase after the muscle exertion has ended, the bird is commonly sleepy, may act blind, appear ataxic or act disoriented.

Partial motor seizures are less common and are much more difficult to diagnose. They often affect a leg or wing. The bird is temporarily unable to control its shaking and the bird's attention is directed toward the affected limb.

STABILIZING THE PATIENT

While it is important to determine the etiology of the seizure, it is important to stabilize the avian patient first. The history will help discern the underlying cause but may be taken by the technician or as the clinician is working on the patient. Just like with dogs and cats, prolonged seizures can result in permanent deficits.

The first step is to administer diazepam (valium) to potentially control the seizure at 0.5 to 1.0 mg/kg. While it is commonly administered intravenously (IV) in small animals, it is difficult to hit a vein in birds that are actively seizuring, so the intramuscular (IM) or intraosseous route (IO) can be used. Since the drug can be absorbed across mucous membranes, it can be administered cloacally as well. The first dose is often administered by IM injection in the pectoral muscle and if the seizure continues then another dose or another route should be used. The calculated dose can be administered up to 3 times and if that does not control the seizure, a constant rate infusion of 1.0 mg/kg/hr in saline should be considered or the use of phenobarbital at an infusion rate of 2 to 10 mg/kg/hr.

From a simplistic view, most seizures result from intracranial swelling or from decreases in blood levels of calcium or glucose. If the seizure cannot be controlled with the use of diazepam or phenobarbital, then one must rapidly add other potentially life saving medications. In-house testing of blood levels of calcium and glucose are ideal and if low, help determine if either needs to be supplemented by IM or IV administration. Blood levels of glucose are much higher in birds normally than in mammals. The blood glucose levels in birds normally range from 250 to 350 mg/dL. While there is controversy over the role that glucose plays with seizures, blood glucose values less than 150 mg/dL should warrant intervention with 50% dextrose by IV or IO administration at 1 mg/kg. The author has administered 50% dextrose in the pectoral muscles of very small birds when access was limited. Dextrose can be administered IV over longer periods of time at 5% but remember that it is hypertonic at that dose. Dilution to 2.5% is preferred especially if it is used in subcutaneous fluids.

Low blood calcium values more often result in seizures in African grey parrots although other birds with low calcium levels may seizure as well. Calcium values in the blood may also be low with heavy metal toxicosis as there is a competitive absorption transport system and lead will impede calcium absorption, for example. Calcium is often administered intramuscularly at a dose of 50 to 100 mg/kg diluted or by slow IV administration. Birds with low calcium values need to be assessed nutritionally to determine if their vitamin D3 levels are low as the underlying cause. If that is the case, oral administration of calcium will not be effective for long-term management after the initial crisis has passed.

Intracranial pressure from brain swelling is a difficult medical problem to solve. Administration of a short-acting steroid may be of some benefit, but birds are exquisitely sensitive to steroids and their administration can result in adrenal crisis or severe immune suppression. Prednisolone sodium succinate may be considered at a dose of 10 to 20 mg/kg IV or IM. Dexamethasone sodium phosphate at 2 to 4 mg/kg may be used at 2 to 4 mg/kg IM or IV very 12 hours. Most avian clinicians will use steroids only once or at most twice in an emergency situation such as a seizure. Mannitol can be used when there is brain edema, due to its osmotic effect to draw fluid from the tissues. It can be administered at 0.5 to 1.0 mg/kg over a 20-minute IV infusion period.

THE ETIOLOGIES OF SEIZURES

There are a number of disorders that result in seizures and they are commonly divided into intracranial and extracranial causes. The intracranial causes result from increased pressure in a closed cranium. These causes include: congenital malformations such as hydrocephalus (cockatoos more commonly have hydrocephalus), neoplasia, inflammatory diseases that are often infectious, vascular disease from hemorrhage or infarcts, acquired epilepsy, trauma or degenerative conditions. Infectious diseases that are associated with seizures in birds include: avian paramyxoviruses such as exotic Newcastle's disease; psittacosis, particularly in cockatiels; West Nile virus; Western equine encephalomyelitis (WEE) virus; Eastern equine encephalomyelitis (EEE) virus; herpes virus or duck viral enteritis virus in waterfowl; picornavirus or duck viral hepatitis virus in ducklings; fungal granulomas such as with aspergillosis; and bacterial septicemia. Seizures may be observed in birds with proventricular dilitation disease, particularly cockatoos. Budgerigars more commonly develop tumors and the tumor type that results in seizures in young male budgies is the pituitary adenoma.

One of the more common problems that alter consciousness and potentially result is seizures in companion birds is concussive trauma to the head from hitting windows or doors and ceiling fan collisions. There will be a history of head trauma often with evidence of blood in the oropharynx, or ear, or the retina may be detached. The same treatments may be considered along with furosemide and oxygen therapy.

In addition to head trauma, there are a number of extracranial causes that are often labeled as metabolic causes. One common cause in companion birds is from heavy metal toxicosis with lead as the most frequently observed problem. Other intoxications that can result in seizures include organophosphates, carbamates and mercury toxicosis. Hypocalcemia causing seizures is more common in African grey parrots, although other birds can be hypocalcemic and not seizure. Hypoglycemia can uncommonly result is seizures, although this metabolic condition more often causes weakness and vague changes in mentation. Hepatic encephalopathy is associated with abnormal hepatic function that leads to depression, changes in behavior and seizures, particularly after eating a meal. Hypoxia, particularly hypoxia resulting from vascular accidents of the major vessels to the cranium, or atherosclerosis can lead to seizures. Thiamine deficiencies in fish-eating birds or raptors on a pure meat diet may lead to seizures that respond to thiamine or B complex injections. Idiopathic causes may occur but may just represent our lack of knowledge of certain disease processes.

NARROWING THE DIFFERENTIAL LIST

Susan Orosz, PhD, DVM, Dipl. ABPV-Avian & ECAMS
Bird and Exotic Pet Wellness Center
Toledo, OH

In human medicine, it has been determined that the history and physical exam accounts for 80% of the diagnosis. Diagnostic tests then are used to help the physician confirm if their different list is appropriate or if there needs to be a reevaluation of that list. This suggests that to narrow the list, the astute clinician needs to properly evaluate the patient in relation to the history.

The signalment of the avian patient is just as important as that of a dog or cat. Often I have had clinicians call and say that they have a sick parrot and ask what should they do for it. That would be unheard of when a clinician refers a small animal. For example, is it a hen blue-fronted Amazon parrot or a black-capped male conure? The presenting complaint may need to be narrowed or defined when examined. Is the bird on the bottom of the cage because it is a female wanting to lay an egg or a male that is weak and depressed from an infectious disease process? The 7-year-old female blue-fronted Amazon parrot on the bottom of the cage egg laying is very different than the 6-month-old male black capped conure on the bottom of the cage recently purchased at a bird show.

The history is a major component in narrowing the differential list. Part of the history is based on the physical appearance of the avian patient. If the bird is stable on observation, then there is time for a detailed history. In stable patients, the history should include information regarding husbandry, where and when purchased, and how the bird interacts with the people in its surroundings. What the bird eats is more important than what is offered. Knowing the diversity of foods provided is important for behavioral considerations. The cage and toys used are important from a behavioral perspective and for understanding the potential for heavy metal toxicosis.

When and where a bird was purchased is extremely valuable in determining its exposure to infectious diseases. The purchase of a new bird into the household and the type of bird is also important. The other caveat is the owner's exposure to other birds (eg, by visits to bird fairs, pet stores, and breeding facilities). If the bird is new or there has been an exposure within the past 6 months, this throws the bird into a "new bird" classification, suggesting infectious diseases are more important on the differential list. By knowing the period of incubation of serious bird diseases, the clinician will know if a particular disease is more likely to be ruled in or out of the differential list. This helps determine the diagnostic testing appropriate for the patient. For example, a cockatoo that has been in the house for 3 years but is now having feathering problems may be suggestive on a noninfectious disease until you find out that 6 months ago the owners purchased a lovebird that died 5 weeks later.

If the bird is unstable, the history needs to address the above concerns about infectious disease exposure, along with concerns about trauma and toxin exposure. When the event occurred and how the bird acted after the trauma is very important for the diagnostic and treatment plan. The physical exam will help gain clues as to the ability of the owner to relay reliable historical information. Sometimes the acute emergency was really a chronic problem that was not picked up by the owner soon enough.

Acute toxicosis can occur in free-ranging birds in the house or exposure from owners' lack of knowledge. Since the avian respiratory tree is much more sensitive to inhalants than the human respiratory system, birds are acutely sensitive to a number of toxins that are airborne. Examples include: nonstick cookware containing teflon or polytetrafluorethylene, self-cleaning ovens and drip pans; carbon monoxide and automobile exhaust; smoke from a variety of sources including tobacco, candles with scents, wood or kerosene burning fires; paint fumes; natural gas leaks, and cleaning products such as bleach or ammonia and aerosol sprays.

Birds may also ingest house plants or other plant-based toxins, including avocado. Avocado ingestion and inhalants lead to acute and severe respiratory signs. Plant toxicoses often lead to vomiting or regurgitation, leading rapidly to depression and then to neurologic signs. Lead and zinc ingestion may lead to acute signs particularly when the levels are high. A bird with lead toxicosis, depending on the amount ingested, is associated with signs of depression and/or seizures, regurgitation, and fecal droppings with frank or digested blood. The signs with zinc toxicosis are more vague and owners may not know if their bird has ingested this heavy metal. Signs on presentation include polyuria, polydipsia, diarrhea, regurgitation, and weight loss from anorexia; if toxicosis is severe, then seizures may also occur.

Trauma commonly results in an emergency presentation. The bird standing in the cage with blood on the cage floor or the walls near the cage should be examined for a blood feather. Birds caught on toys need to be freed and provided with supportive care as soon as possible. Birds flying into walls and windows, smashed by doors, hit by ceiling fans, grabbed by dogs or cats, or in other ways traumatized need emergency support. The bird that is bitten or at least been in the mouth of a cat needs to be seen as soon as possible. This is because the most important commensal organism, *Pasteurlla sp*, can kill the bird in the first 24 to 48 hours. Birds may act normal at first and so the owner is hesitant to bring in the bird. A bactericidal drug should be administered that shows therapeutic efficacy; appropriate care for the wound and the patient should be initiated and the prognosis should be conveyed as guarded.

CLINICAL EXAMINATION

The clinical examination has two main components—the physical examination and the behavioral exam. The physical examination includes observations of the patient and its interactions with its owner and palpation and auscultation of the patient. The second component associated with observations is the behavioral exam. To complete the behavioral exam, photos of the cage and the area where the bird lives are important, along with recordings of the behavior in its home environment. Observational skills often need to be sharpened, compared to those needed for a dog or cat. The signs of birds tend to be more subtle. This may result from their relationship in the food chain—psittacine birds are preyed upon by carnivorous species. They are also flock animals and to show signs suggestive of a problem would cause the flock to expel that bird, leading to its death.

Subtle Signs of Illness

Getting the avian patient to the veterinarian early on in the course of the disease improves the prognosis. Owners should be taught to recognize subtle sign illness on their first appointment. These signs can be communicated through a handout, as well, but should be explained by the tech staff with emphasis by the veterinarian. Subtle signs of illness may include subtle changes in their appearance and posture along with changes in the quality and color of their feathers. The nares or nostrils may have material in them or wetness on the feathers surrounding them. There may be swellings of the head, or changes in breathing including abnormal sounds or the bird stops vocalizing. Any changes to the color or volume of the droppings, increased amounts of urine or changes in the amounts of food consumed or water drunk should be investigated. Behavior changes are cause for concern. Changes in the legs, feet or beak, increased size of an organ, changes in breathing should also be considered.

Clinicians presented with a bird should watch for these, along with dullness to the eyes, eyes sunken into the skull, indicating dehydration; swellings around the head, suggesting an upper respiratory tract infection or tumor; nasal discharge resulting from an upper respiratory tract infection; fluid, clear or purulent, above the nares or on the cranial margin of the carpus or the wrist on the wing; the bird rubbing its head to "wipe its nose" to clear discharge or to relieve pressure exerted in the sinuses; scratching at the nares or the side of the head frequently; sneezing often, particularly with a discharge; or feather loss around any part of the head, particularly the area around the nares or nostrils

Serious Signs of Illness

Serious signs of illness include any of the following: eyes closed with long periods of sleepiness; drooping wing or wings; falling off the perch; noticeable and noisy breathing; vomiting/regurgitation; bird remaining on the bottom of the cage; fluffed and ruffled feathers; bird sitting horizontal posture on the perch; any abnormal posture; not vocalizing; not eating or drinking; tail bobbing with each breath; bleeding; soiled vent; standing on only one leg; open-mouthed breathing; or seizuring or any abnormal behavior.

EVALUATING CLINICAL SIGNS

After the physical examination is complete, the clinician needs to determine the number of systems affected, the part(s) affected, and the extent. It should be decided if the symptoms are compatible with an infectious disease, trauma, or organ failure or altered function. If the bird is presented for a behavioral problem, is it exclusively behavioral or is there an organ system problem that results in the condition observed?

Recognizing patterns of disease is an important part of determining the differential list. Acutely infected birds have a normal pectoral muscle mass and their signs usually develop rapidly and are more severe than chronically infected patients. Chronically infected birds commonly have reduced pectoral mass, as they are often partially anorexic or cannot meet the metabolic demand of their disease process over a period of time. This is because birds undergo body plundering of their pectoral muscle mass to meet their metabolic needs. The protein from the muscle is converted to energy through gluconeogenesis. That is why it is important to palpate the pectoral muscle mass. Smaller birds will use their muscle mass for energy faster than larger birds but all will use their muscle mass as the medical condition drains the body of energy.

An example of using the signalment in relation to the physical exam findings is the following. You perform a physical exam on a pigeon and you find that the bird has normal pectoral muscle mass and is bright and alert with torticollis or infrequent neurologic signs—the differential list should include Paramyxovirus-1. Then you do a physical exam on an adult Amazon with neurologic signs. This bird is not bright and alert but fluffed and depressed. It also has increased respiratory effort with increased bronchovesicular sounds and watery diarrhea. The big differential that needs to be addressed is exotic Newcastle disease—another Paramyxovirus that is velogenic and reportable to state and federal agencies. The seriousness of this disease and its possible transmission to other birds places it a special category requiring a definitive diagnosis.

When signs are localized to a system, the diagnostic workup should focus on the common diseases affecting the system. Diagnostic tests need to be performed in order of the most critical for ruling in or out a disease for determining the diagnosis. The shotgun technique of running multiple blood tests and diagnostics does not work—birds have a small blood volume and are easily stressed. The maximum blood to be withdrawn should not exceed 1% of the body weight. A diagnostic plan needs to be developed and thought out before taking any samples. This reduces the need to pick the bird up a second time further adding to stress and causing untoward results. Remember that diagnostic tests help to rule in or out differentials and help to arrive at a diagnosis. It is important to always remember to treat the bird and not the lab results. Owners want answers at the least cost. If you are stumped, remember to refer the bird to another clinician with more experience or expertise or to call a colleague for advice. They may be able to think of something that you may have missed.

The owner will think more highly of you for referring their beloved pet to a clinician with a greater expertise.

There are a greater number of diagnostic tests that are available to the clinician now compared with those 5 years ago. With all tests it is important to understand the sensitivity and the specificity of the test that you choose to help arrive at the diagnosis. Although there are a number of labs offering tests, it is important to choose a lab that has a long-term reputation for performing quality testing for companion birds. Sample size and turn around time are also important considerations. For example, fungal cultures take a considerable amount of time and the wise clinician will start the avian patient on appropriate antifungal drugs for its species and its clinical condition while waiting for the lab results. Fungal cultures of a nasal flush should be compared against the much faster turn around time for an *Aspergillus* sp polymerase chain reaction (PCR) test.

A minimum database for companion birds really is based on the differential diagnosis list. Radiographs represent an extension of out hands and eyes but ultrasound has helped understand organs in a very different way. A CBC helps determine if there may be an infectious or inflammatory response. A monocytosis is suggestive of a more chronic disease, fungal disease, avian mycobacteriosis, or psittacosis. The avian profile helps to determine if there may be liver or kidney involvement or if the concentration of the common inorganic ions are out of the normal range. Biopsies for histopathology or culture help to definitively diagnose the condition of the avian patient.

Gram stains of the choanal slit and the cloaca or fresh feces have been an old standard of avian medicine where more recently cultures have replaced these as the more definitive test. Those of us that have used Gram stains and know how to interpret them use them to rule in or out differentials with the advantage of their quick access to information. The gram stain of the choanal slit, for example, gives the clinician information regarding the nutritional status of the patient that impacts its immune function. Companion birds should not have any or just a few bacteria or fungal organisms on their choanal gram stain. Large numbers of gram-negative rods when the bird is sick would suggest a treatment plan that would differ from one with large numbers of gram-positive rods and/or cocci with large numbers of budding yeasts. A bird that is fluffed and depressed with few to no gram-negative rods or gram-positive rods suggests some other cause for the underlying problem. Gram stains are often used in combination with cultures.

Parasite exams using a number of techniques are becoming increasingly important in young birds that are raised in large commercial operations. Giardiasis and encephalitis are becoming problems in cockatiel and budgerigar flocks when infected birds pass the disease to other birds at pet stores, or when chicks are infected by their diseased parents. Fecal floats and direct smears can be performed in the clinician's office while electron microscopy, zinc sulfate and ELISA testing from reputable labs can be helpful in finding some of these elusive organisms.

All of these tests need to be used in relation to the clinical condition of the avian patient. There are increasing numbers of tests but they need to be used based on their level of reliability and appropriateness. There are a number of infectious diseases that companion birds acquire where there are no good diagnostic tests available. Clinical judgment and experience remains an important part of avian medicine.

RECOMMENDED READING

1. Orosz SE. Diagnostic workup plan. In: Olsen GH, Orosz SE (eds): Manual of Avian Medicine. St. Louis, MO: Mosby; 2000.

DIAGNOSING THE FUZZIES

Susan Orosz, PhD, DVM, Dipl. ABVP-Avian, DECAMS
Bird and Exotic Pet Wellness Center
Toledo, OH

Mycotic infections can be divided into two basic types based on the fungal phase that the organism is most commonly observed—the mycelial phase and the yeast phase. The mycelial phase most commonly observed is *Aspergillus* and most common species is *fumigatus*. It is this mycelial phase that is the "fuzzie." However, this article will focus on several fungal pathogens in birds—*Aspergillus* sp, *Candidia* sp, and *Macrorhabdus ornithogaster*—and how to diagnose these infections.

ASPERGILLOSIS
Pathogenesis
One of the most common or at least most difficult-to-treat respiratory infections is from *Aspergillus* sp. Free-living birds tend to be free of *Aspergillus* species, and serologic testing of antibodies in raptors has been negative. Turkeys infected with *Aspergillus* produce moderate to severe fibrino-heterophilic or granulomatous air sacculitis. The air sacs appeared thickened, opaque, and or filled with fibrinous to gelatinous material. Macrophages invade the area quickly along with heterophils. Edema and fibroplasia develop early on, which stiffens the air sac, reducing its functional capabilities. Around 7 days into the disease process, lymphoid hyperphasia develops. It is important to note that titer values (obtained from AGID and ELISA tests) were not helpful clinically at predicting mortality—only weight loss was helpful in these research studies using turkeys.

There is also concern that bacterial components including the lipopolysaccharide (LPS) portion of the cell wall in *Pasteurella mutocida* reduces pulmonary performance initially, setting up an *Aspergillus* infection. LPS may also interfere with the phagocytic role of the epithelial lining of the lung and air sacs. Gliotoxins produced by some strains of *Aspergillus* sp may be an important factor in the pathophysiology of aspergillosis, with direct cytotoxic effects and immunosuppression.

Diagnosis
Aspergillosis can be difficult to diagnose in companion psittacine species. These birds can present with a chronic or acute infection. The acute form results in clinical signs in a few days: dyspnea, lethargy, depression, anorexia, weight loss, emaciation, exaggerated respiratory effort, cyanosis, and sudden death. The chronic form is often referred to with respiratory tract signs through an immunocompromising event. Signs include a change in voice character or quality, loss of voice, respiratory stridor, ataxia, torticollis, and possible seizures.

No definitive test is available, producing black or white results. Instead the clinician must rely on multiple tests and experience in arriving at a diagnosis. Hematologic findings can include a heterophilic leucocytosis, monocytosis, lymphopenia, hyperproteinemia, and a nonregenerative anemia. The total WBC is often > 20,000/μL but may be in the normal range when the bird experiences immune suppression. The plasma biochemical analytes are nonspecific with AST and CK commonly elevated, but not consistently. Radiographs do not typically demonstrate visible lesions until the latter stages of disease when the patient decompensates. Radiographic observations include a prominent parabronchial pattern, loss of definition or asymmetry of the air sacs, hyperinflation of the abdominal air sacs, thickening of the air sac membranes, and soft tissue opacities within the respiratory tree.

Endoscopy allows for visual inspection of the respiratory tree and biopsy for cytology and culture. White, yellow, grey, or green plaques can be visualized lining the walls of the air sacs and within the lung parenchyma during the latter stages of the disease process.

The swab or biopsy should be cultured on Sabourad's dextrose agar. Culture of the organism in the absence of lesions, however, is not diagnostic. However, Gram stains and culture can help to identify the organisms obtained from the plaque. Usually, *Aspergillus* colonies form blue-green colonies at 48 hours.

Plasma or serum electrophoresis can be useful when monitoring disease progression and the response to therapy. Acute infections often demonstrate an increase in beta globulins, while chronic ones show an increase in beta or gamma fractions or both. However, birds with immune suppression may have hypoproteinemia.

There are several labs with ELISA tests developed for the detection and levels of *Aspergillus* antibody. These tests tend to perform better with chronically infected birds except for owls. However, false positives have been noted as well as false negatives, particularly with immune-suppressed birds or those with relatively walled-off granulomas. One lab provides an ELISA test of the detection of antigen and was adapted from human use. This test also requires clinical experience for interpretation as false positives and negatives occur.

CANDIDIASIS
Candida has been identified as an increasingly prevalent infectious agent in a variety of animals and has caused severe disease in humans. Gram-negative bacteria have been replaced with gram-positive bacteria and *Candida* as the most common bloodstream pathogens in humans in hospitals in the United States. Previously considered opportunistic diseases, particularly in neonates, they are increasingly difficult to cure. Normally the host defense system and the normal bacterial flora of the gastrointestinal tract keep yeasts like *Candida* under control. Although small numbers of non-budding organisms are considered normal flora in healthy florivores, in this author's experience, they are not present except when carried into the tract by food items, such as breads.

Candida affects the mucocutaneous surfaces that often include the GI tract and in particular the oropharynx, crop, and esophagus. Common signs included delayed crop emptying, crop stasis, regurgitation, anorexia, depression, and poor digestion of food. In chicks where the upper GI tract is affected, they do not grow properly and may appear stunted. The droppings of birds with GI tract involvement are abnormal and may be watery. Cockatiels, budgerigars, and cockatoos are considered higher risk psittacine species. Systemic infection has resulted in CNS signs in a flock of canaries, along with GI signs.

Candidiasis, when it affects the crop may be called thrush in raptors or sour crop in psittacines. It is most commonly caused from *Candida albicans* but may be from *C. parapsilosis*, *C. krusei*, and *C. tropicalis*. In young birds it is associated with improper handfeeding and a noncompetent immune system. These infections can often result from the administration of antimicrobials in adult and young birds. Antifungals specific for yeasts may need to be considered in the treatment plan of the avian patient.

The diagnosis of candidiasis may be difficult if the lesions are deep within the GI tract. Gram stains of swabs or biopsy specimens are important for identifying gram-positive budding yeasts or those with pseudohyphae. Flushes using pH balanced solutions of the nares and upper respiratory tract are helpful and examination are helpful in determining if these organisms are involved with the infection or complicating it. *Candida albicans* are basophilic gram positive oval shaped organisms measuring 3.5–6.0 x 6–10 µm. The presence of pseudohyphae suggests a more severe infection. Systemic candidiasis is currently rare in birds but may become more common, as it is in humans. In these cases, *Candida* sp. may be isolated from the blood, bone marrow, and/or parenchymatous organs.

MACRORHABDIASIS

Macrorhabdus ornithogaster has only been recently identified as a yeast, as it was previously thought to be a large rod-shaped bacteria, a "megabacterium." This organism was implicated in a syndrome of budgerigars that was described as "going light." It is a long straight rod 3 to 4 µm wide and 20 to 80 µm long. The organism may be longer as they often occur as long chains of cells where the separation between them are not visualized. On a gram stain, the thick cell wall may not stain with only the cytoplasm staining and they may not take up common cytology stains. For this reason, it is often difficult to visualize this organism, particularly the live bird.

Proventricular scrapings or a flush from the proventriculus is used for an antemortem diagnosis. Sick birds are more likely to shed organisms in their droppings. Wet mounts of unstained droppings examined under 40 and 100x and with a lowered diaphragm are more likely to be rewarding. Often multiple samples will need to be examined to find the organism. A new PCR test may be helpful at diagnosing this organism.

The implication of *Macrorhadus ornithogaster* producing disease remains unclear. Birds may shed organisms but appear normal on physical examination. Sick birds may shed a large number of organisms but may not shed any. It may be considered a pathogen while others believe it to be a commensal.

The organism appears to be prevalent in budgerigar aviaries with fecal shedding ranging from 27% to 64% based on fecal shedding. It has also been commonly observed in parrotlets, cockatiels, and lovebirds. Additionally the organism has been found in chickens, turkeys, geese, ducks, and ostriches.

In budgerigars, there may be an acute or a chronic presentation. Birds presenting with an acute presentation suddenly go off feed and regurgitate with or without bloodstaining. Death occurs within several days. The chronic form may be more common. Budgies appear hungry and are observed grinding food in their beak but not ingesting it. Regurgitation is common including birds presenting with matted feathers with regurgitated material around their heads. Undigested seeds may be found in the droppings. Other birds may have diarrhea with or without melena. These birds will have reduced pectoral muscle mass and appear to be "going light." These signs are not pathognomonic for this disease as candidiasis and other conditions may present similarly.

Parrotlets and lovebirds present with similar signs as with budgies. Parrotlets were observed to present acutely with regurgitation and melena. Lovebirds were observed to have significant numbers of organisms in their droppings but were also infected with pscittacine beak and feather disease (PBFD).

RECOMMENDED READING

1. Orosz SE. Antifungal drug therapy in avian species. Vet Clin North Am Exotic Anim Pract. 2003;6(2):337-350.
2. Orosz SE. Overview of aspergillosis: Pathogenesis and treatment options. Semin Avian Exotic Pet Med. 2000; 9:1-8.
3. Jones MP, Orosz SE. The diagnosis of aspergillosis in birds. Semin Avian Exotic Pet Med. 2000:9; 52.
4. Orosz SE. Itraconazole. Literature review. Aspergillosis in companion birds, dogs and cats: treatment with itraconazole. Informational brochure. Brussels, Belgium: Janssen Animal Health; 2005.
5. Phalen DN, Implications of *Macrorhabdus* in clinical disorders. In: Harrison GJ, Lightfoot TL (eds.): Clinical Avian Medicine, Vol II. Palm Beach, FL: Spix Publishing; 2006, pp 705-709.

DISTINGUISHING VIRAL DISEASES

Susan Orosz, PhD, DVM, Dipl. ABPV-Avian & ECAMS
Bird and Exotic Pet Wellness Center
Toledo, OH

AVIAN POLYOMAVIRUS

Avian polyomavirus (APV) is a nonenveloped DNA virus that is very stable in the environment. This virus is a significant problem for aviculturists and pet stores as it is associated with economic losses of chicks and young birds. When it manifests in adult birds, they are most likely concomitantly infected with psittacine beak and feather disease or are severely stressed. Macaws, conures, and ecletus parrots are the species more commonly associated with this disease. Birds that are exposed generally develop symptoms 10 to 14 days after exposure although the route of infection has not been verified; it is suggestive that it is through the respiratory tract. Once infected, viremia occurs about 7 to 10 days post exposure. The hallmark of this disease is hemorrhage—from petechial to ecchymotic in the skin to massive hemorrhage in the organs. There is often severe hepatic necrosis and immune complex glomerulopathy. Most birds die from this disease. Those birds that do not develop symptoms remain viremic for a period of time and shed virus in their fecal droppings and feather dander. Birds that maintain an antibody titer do not appear to be persistently infected but will clear the virus over time.

Clinical Presentation for Budgerigars

Budgie breeders should be suspicious of APV when they start losing chicks in the nest at approximately 10 to 20 days of age. Dead chicks have abnormal feather development; skin discoloration; abdominal distention with ascites and/or crop swelling; appear stunted; hepatomegaly with necrosis; and variable hemorrhages. Some chicks will show neurologic signs particularly head tremors preceding death as the virus has been shown to affect the cerebellum. Not all chicks die and those that live may present with abnormalities of the primary and secondary remiges or flight feathers. These birds have been described as runner or creepers as these alterations of the flight feathers ground them. This condition also occurs with another virus, PBFD virus, and so must be distinguished.

Clinical Presentation for Lovebirds

Clinical symptoms are similar to those in nestling budgies but the disease appears to be protracted to up to 1 year of age. These older birds are often infected with PBFD virus and may help to explain the delay in the development of symptoms. Inclusion bodies can be found in multiple organs as are found in the budgies.

Clinical Presentation in Nestling Cockatoos

Young cockatoos of approximately 4 to 8 weeks of age are presented stunted and/or with reduced pectoral muscle mass in acute respiratory distress. One important differential is of food aspiration but on necropsy birds have a generalized interstitial pneumonia. Histologically, there are large numbers of inclusion bodies that appear to be in type II pneumocytes. Data from Phalen suggest that this form of APV is a specific variant of the virus.

Clinical Presentation in Non-Budgerigar Species

The species most commonly observed include conures at less than 6 weeks of age, and macaws and ecletus parrots at 14 weeks of age or less. Most birds are being hand fed when they develop slowing of the crop and regurgitation with weakness, pallor and bruising under the skin. They may be found dead with no premonitory signs. Older birds may show bleeding from the nares and may occur when stressed.

Adult Parrots with APV

Adult psittacines most commonly do not show signs of disease with APV. They may or may not shed virus briefly and are asymptomatic. Those with symptoms are infected with PBFD or are highly stressed. The signs are similar to nestlings with bruising or hemorrhaging, crop stasis, and GI tract slowing. In cockatoos, there can be an atypical progressive encephalopathy.

PSITTACINE BEAK AND FEATHER DISEASE

Psittacine Beak and Feather Disease (PBFD) is a nonenveloped DNA virus and has a number of variants. There does not appear to be a relationship between the variant and the host or pathogenicity in work in Australia. In the United States, there appears to be a variant for lories and lorikeets. Because of the number of variants, PCR testing requires the DNA utilized to detect the virus has a conserved part of the DNA or multiple assays need to detect the variants.

Birds infected with the virus shed it in their feather and skin dander, crop secretions, and feces. Transmission is most likely from ingestion or inhalation. Vertical transmission is suspected. The virus replicates in a large number of tissues including the skin and feathers, crop, esophagus, intestine, thymus, and the cloacal bursa. Feather dysplasia is a hallmark of the disease and the feathers have a pinched appearance, appear abnormal, and/or have bleeding into the shaft. There is often hyperkeratosis of the feather sheath with thickening and retention. Growing feathers may be clubbed, appear to be bowed, or have dystrophic lines resulting in fractures along its length. Birds do not make their normal powder down.

Beak lesions are more commonly found in some of the cockatoo species, little corellas, and galahs. Early on there is hyperkeratosis of the beak and elongation and overgrowth. Longitudinal fissures can appear leading to fractures of the distal end of the beak. The beak then will separate from the underlying bone which is very painful and causes the bird not to eat.

Acute infection occurs more commonly in nestlings and is associated with depression and regurgitation. If they live long enough, they have abnormal feathers as in the chronic form that develops rapidly with annular constricting bands at the base of the feathers. This disease has often been described as birdie AIDS as it is associated with immune suppression leading to secondary bacterial and fungal infections that kill the affected bird.

Clinical Presentation in African Greys
Young birds from 7 weeks to 9 months presented with crop status, regurgitation, and weakness. Feather loss and changes may or may not be present. Acutely presenting young have massive liver necrosis.

Clinical Presentation in Lovebirds
Lovebirds from Texas are commonly affected with PBFD virus and may or may not show signs of the disease. There seems to be birds that are asymptomatic birds that are transiently affected and when presented with signs they are typically young birds. The birds may appear unthrifty, have areas where feathers do not regrow, or have a delayed molt. The lorry variant has been reported to be common to lovebirds.

Clinical Presentation in Budgerigars
Birds with PBFD are found in breeding flocks and present with feathering like those with APV- absence of the primary and secondary flight feathers, Dystrophic feather changes as in cockatoos are not common.

PSITTACID HERPESVIRUS (PsHvs)
The alpha herpesviruses are the causes of Pacheco's disease and internal papillomatosis of psittacines. There are three major serotypes of the PsHv1 and within those serotypes there are four genotypes. The relationship of pathogenicity and species affected between serotypes and genotypes is beginning to unfold. Genotypes 1, 2, and 3 are highly pathogenic to Amazon parrots. Genotype 4 is most common in macaws and conures. Pacific species such as cockatoos and cockatiels are relatively resistant to Pacheco's disease. Birds that become infected with PsHvs often are found positive by polymerase chain reaction (PCR) throughout life but may not shed presently. Those that are persistently infected may go on to develop internal papillomatosis.

Pacheco's Disease
This disease often manifests as an outbreak where multiple birds are housed. Initially a single bird is found dead with no promontory signs. Often Amazons are found dead where there are macaws and/ or conures in the collection as well. Breeding or recent changes signaling some type of stressor immediately precedes the death. Usually, a bird is acutely ill with profound lethargy, anorexia, and depression that precedes the passing of bright green feces or sulfur yellow urates. Often birds die within minutes to at most several days from the onset of signs.

Diagnosis is often at necropsy. The bird is well muscled with hepatomegaly, splenomgaly, and renal swelling. There may be epicardial or serosal hemorrhage. The liver is often pale yellow with diffuse mottling. Eosinophilic with possible basophilic intranuclear inclusions are apparent in hepatic cells and along bile ducts.

Internal Papillomatosis
Papillomatous lesions of the oropharynx and cloaca are most commonly observed in the affected species which include macaws, Amazons and hawk-headed parrots. Conures are infrequently affected. Lesion may extend from the oral cavity into the proximal portion of the GI tract. Birds often present because the owner observes frank blood on the cage papers and/ or a protrusion from the cloaca. In other birds that are affected at the proximal end of the GI tract, the bird may be wasting as food has a mechanical blockage from the presence of the lesions. A small number of birds that have internal papillomatosis will develop bile duct carcinoma.

PARAMYXOVIRUS 1 (PMV-1)
There are nine serogroups of paramyxoviruses and within each of the serogroups there are a number of strains. Within group 1 is a number of strains and those that are highly pathogenic to chickens or termed velogenic is exotic Newcastle disease (END). Those strains of virus that cause hemorrhagic lesions of the digestive tract are termed the viscerotropic velogenic Newcastle disease virus (VVND), while those that produce respiratory and neurologic signs are the neurotropic velogenic Newcastle disease virus (NVND). Mesogenic strains cause fewer symptoms and pigeon paramyxovirus is the most important disease for the exotic animal veterinarian.

END in parrots results in nonspecific signs and these include respiratory signs with weight loss, depression, and diarrhea. Birds that have neurologic signs that accompany these others should be considered suspicious. Ataxia, head bobbing, and opisthotonus and paralysis may occur. If these signs reflective of respiratory, GI, and CNS involvement occur in a bird, it is important to contact the regulatory veterinarian in your state.

PMV-1 in pigeons is associated with two differing presentations. In the CNS form, the bird is bright but has torticollis and/or ataxia. The other form is polyuria with or without neurologic signs.

RECOMMENDED READING
1. Phalen DN. Implications of viruses in clinical disorders. In: Harrison GJ, Lightfoot TL (eds.): Clinical Avian Medicine, Vol II. Palm Beach, FL: Spix Publishing; 2006, pp 721-746.

THE PATH TO HISTO RESULTS

Susan Orosz, PhD, DVM, Dipl. ABPV-Avian & ECAMS
Bird and Exotic Pet Wellness Center
Toledo, OH

Gross necropsy, coupled with appropriate diagnostic testing, is an important tool in avian medicine. It serves a number of functions including determining a final diagnosis—often not obtained until the necropsy. Clinical signs and antemortem diagnostics are often not truly understood until the necropsy is complete. Diagnosis at necropsy helps the clinician to develop an improved treatment plan for future animals with the same diagnosis or clinical signs. It often helps grieving owners alleviate their guilt with the death of their animal family member. Necropsy is a necessary and practical component of flock management. It forms part of the data base needed to provide improved husbandry for the management to enhance flock health. With legal considerations and/or dissatisfied clients, the necropsy should always be performed by a veterinary pathologist that routinely does avian necropsies and histopathology and a person that is recognized for their training and expertise in that area of pathology. A dog and cat lab will not suffice.

A significant misunderstanding can occur for clients when necropsies are suggested, but good communication can help alleviate their concerns. In certain situations, the owner has spent a considerable amount of money, yet their animal has died. The owner has just started to grieve when the clinician suggests a necropsy. I have had owners become angry and confused with the suggestion, thinking that you did not actually know what was wrong with their pet. "Why would you want to do that … I thought you knew what was wrong and were treating my pet correctly and now you don't know what was wrong?" they retort. That problem needs to be headed off at the pass in the beginning of the communication of their pet's condition. They need to understand that we know a certain amount but not all. An important part of the communication process is imparting the understanding that the necropsy will help us as avian clinicians understand more about this condition. The veterinarian needs to be sincere that it will help and then do the necropsy with skill and thought. The client should never construe the necropsy as a way for the clinician to make more money. It should be offered, particularly when a zoonotic disease like psittacosis is suspected.

The costs associated with the necropsy need to be determined on the front end. That is often a big problem as most owners will not pay a bill that arrives in the mail a month after their bird has died. Additionally, it sets up bad client perceptions when the bill is more than quoted. I think this is one of the most difficult problems from a costing perspective as most pathologists when performing the post will want to run a number of diagnostic tests when they observe certain conditions. Unfortunately, those costs get added on and the clinician ends up eating the bills. For this reason, it is important to think through the potential costs for ALL of the tests that are appropriate and estimate accordingly.

One way that we handle necropsies is to gently discuss with the client beforehand the possibility of a postmortem exam with those cases that have a unique problem and those that have a poor prognosis and are hospitalized patients. We often do the gross necropsy of those patients without an added cost to the client. After the gross necropsy is completed and then at that point, we might suggest further diagnostic tests that may help us further understand the condition for other birds in the future. Most often that would include histopath, so we take representative tissues while performing the necropsy.

As our society becomes more inclusive of others and their religions, it is also increasingly important that veterinarians become aware of other ways of thinking and how this might affect client response. For example, some religions require that the dead be buried before nightfall in a 24-hour period and the taking of tissues may not be appropriate from a religious perspective. The veterinarian should suggest and explain what the necropsy is all about so that the person can make decisions appropriately. We should not be so offended by the negative response some may give about the suggestion of a necropsy as it might be based on their religious perspective. The flip side is that the avian veterinarian is in a unique situation to provide support after the bird passes to help the owner be okay with their grief. Society is more accepting of the grief of a pet owner with a dog or cat family member, but avian owners often only hear the common response, "It is only a bird."

Like all components of veterinary medicine, it is important to proceed in a systematic manner. A detailed history is important, particularly when the bird and/or the owner's facilities are unknown. As with surgery, proper equipment is needed to protect you from potential infectious diseases. Mask and gloves are a minimum precaution and the carcass should be wetted down before invading the body cavity. Often water with a disinfectant is used as the wetting agent.

From the history and the physical examination, a differential list should be developed. This will help remind you of other diagnostic test specimens that may be needed as you proceed to inspect the organs and body cavity. These should be ready and available. The external body and organ should be examined including the feathers, beak, and uropygial gland. The infraorbital sinus can be inspected by making a coronal section through the head if that has been approved by the owner. If not, an incision can be made either above or below the jugal bone of the head and a swab can be used to obtain any samples required.

The coelomic cavity can be opened by making a longitudinal incision along the ventral midline. The ribs on either side of the sternum can be cut with a scissors and lifted towards the head as you inspect the air sacs. You should "be able to read a newspaper" through the air sacs. They may contain yellowed fat or be cloudy or have material on them from infection. Swabs for culture or polymerase chain reaction (PCR) should be taken of the air sacs at this point and then samples for histopath. The organs should be inspected and any abnormalities noted.

RECOMMENDED READING

1. Rae M. Diagnostic value of necropsy. In: Harrison GJ, Lightfoot TL (eds.): Clinical Avian Medicine, Vol II. Palm Beach, FL: Spix Publishing; 2006, pp 661-678.
2. Schmidt RE, Reavill DR, Phalen D (eds.): Pathology of Pet and Aviary Birds. Ames, IA: Iowa State Press; 2003.

DECIPHERING LIVER DISEASE

Laura Wade, DVM, Diplomate ABVP (Avian)
Specialized Care for Avian & Exotic Pets
Broadway Veterinary Clinic, PC, Lancaster, NY

Liver disease is commonly encountered in avian patients and the liver is often involved in systemic disease processes. In birds, liver disease is rarely due to a single cause and usually involves multiple pathologic processes. One of the diagnostic challenges is that there are many nonspecific physical and laboratory signs and some birds with liver disease show no signs of illness. In addition, there are often concurrent diseases present and often the bird is in critical condition by the time liver disease is evident to the owner. The diagnosis of liver disease requires a combination of evidence based on the history, physical examination, and laboratory and imaging diagnostics. Ultimately, histopathology is used to obtain a definitive diagnosis which is vital to optimizing a treatment plan. Understanding some of the unique aspects of avian liver anatomy and physiology will greatly aid in the deciphering of liver disease in birds.

LIVER ANATOMY AND PHYSIOLOGY

The liver is the largest gland in the body and is larger in birds than mammals compared to body size. The avian liver surrounds the heart and consists of two lobes (right and left) joined at midline. In many species, including parrots, the right lobe is larger and depending on the species, one of the lobes is divided (in passerines, the right lobe is divided). The gallbladder is present in most species (except pigeons, parrots, and ostriches) and lies along the visceral surface of the right lobe. In most species, two hepatic ducts drain into the ascending duodenum; in the pigeon and ostrich, it drains into the descending duodenum. Blood is supplied to the liver from a branch of the celiac artery via the right and left hepatic arteries. The liver also receives blood from the stomach and intestines via the portal vein. This blood supply may be supplemented by additional flow from the kidney via the renal portal vein. Blood flow out of the liver to the vena cava is via the hepatic portal veins.

The liver has numerous vital body functions, including digestion, metabolism of proteins, fats and carbohydrates, selective storage of vitamins and minerals, and detoxification. It is also important in the manufacture of blood clotting proteins, red blood cells and production of vitamins. The liver is also the major source of uric acid from protein metabolism. Because birds lack mesenteric lymph nodes, the liver is an important immune system filter for the intestines.

Biliverdin and Bile Acids

Biliverdin is the major avian bile pigment and biliverdinuria is responsible for the green discoloration of the urates of birds with liver disease. Birds lack bilirubin reductase and excrete unconjugated biliverdin into bile as the major end product of heme catabolism. Unlike unconjugated bilirubin in mammals, any biliverdin produced can be readily excreted into urine and does not accumulate to any extent in the plasma or tissues.

Bile acids are synthesized from cholesterol and are secreted, extracted and excreted by the liver. Bile acids are actively reabsorbed by the small intestine (jejunum and ileum) and transported back to the liver via portal circulation. Approximately 90% to 95% of the bile acids are extracted in the first pass through liver. During and immediately after meals, the bile acid pool recycles 2 to 5 times via the enterohepatic cycle. Plasma levels of bile acids therefore rely on the integrity of the enterohepatic cycle and hepatobiliary function. Abnormalities in hepatic uptake, storage, excretion or perfusion delay extraction of bile acids from circulation. Chronic hepatic disease leading to fibrosis, and hepatic atrophy/hypoplasia may lead to a decrease in bile acids.

DIAGNOSIS

History and Causes of Liver Disease

Liver diseases may have a primary infectious or noninfectious cause(s) or may be secondary to other conditions, such as obesity, malnutrition, trauma, cardiac disease, and air sacculitis. It is important to critically review the bird's history, especially regarding diet and nutritional supplementation, egg-laying history, exposure to toxins, exposure to other birds, and so forth. Birds that eat a high percentage of sunflower seeds and peanuts are prone to hepatic lipidosis. A diet that includes seeds and nuts may also contain mycotoxins that can be hepatotoxic, especially aflatoxin B_1. Over-supplementation of vitamin A and D_3 can cause hepatic toxicosis. Other hepatotoxins include zinc, lead and copper, some plants, pesticides and certain medications. Some species (toucans, mynahs, lories) are especially prone to abnormal hepatic iron storage (hemochromatosis). Female birds actively laying eggs can have problems with excessive fat mobilization to the liver.

Birds may develop liver disease from infectious diseases. Common bacterial causes are *E. coli*, *Salmonella* sp, *Chlamydophila psittaci*, and *Mycobacteria* sp. Viruses affecting the liver include polyomavirus, herpesvirus, adenovirus and circovirus (PBFD) among others. Other organisms, such as parasites and fungi are less common. Liver tumors (bile duct carcinoma, hepatocellular carcinoma, hemangiosarcoma, lymphosarcoma) are common in older birds and may originate from the liver, or migrate to the liver from other tissues. Birds with chronic cloacal papillomas may develop liver tumors due to herpesvirus infection.

Physical Examination and Clinical Signs

Clinical signs of liver disease in birds vary with the severity and duration of the disease process. Hepatic dysfunction occurs after severe injury or repeated significant insults. The liver has considerable functional reserve and regenerative capacity. Only lesions that affect the majority of hepatic parenchyma are likely to produce signs of hepatic failure. Birds with liver disease often have polyuric, yellow to bright green stools (biliverdinuria). Many also have subtle, nonspecific signs such as weight loss, lethargy, anorexia, polydipsia, and regurgitation. More liver-specific signs include abnormal feather quality and pigmentation and an overgrown upper beak and nails are especially in chronic cases. Birds with advanced liver disease often exhibit abdominal enlargement and dyspnea due to enlarged liver and coelomic fluid. In severe cases, neurologic signs (seizures) and bruising or hemorrhages may be observed. Unexpected death without apparent signs is possible, especially in acute or severe disease.

Laboratory Diagnostics

Diagnostic tests assess the presence and severity of hepatic damage, help determine prognosis and monitor progression of disease. Each test is limited by its particular sensitivity, specificity and degree of invasiveness. The biochemical evaluation of hepatic function in avian species is not as straightforward as it is in mammals. Because of the nonspecific nature of avian liver enzymes, levels outside the normal range do not always correlate with organ pathology.

Aspartate aminotransferase (AST) is probably the most sensitive indicator of liver disease in birds. AST is also found in heart and skeletal muscle, so increases must be interpreted with the help of other enzymes. Elevated AST indicates active damage to the liver or muscle. If CK is normal, it is more likely that AST is of liver origin. It is important to remember that AST is sometimes normal even in some cases of severe liver disease. Albumin, glucose, cholesterol, triglycerides and uric acid are either entirely or partly produced within the liver and decreased blood values may be associated with liver disease. In birds with fatty liver disease, however, cholesterol is usually elevated.

The complete blood count (CBC) often reveals an elevated white blood cell count, which is a nonspecific indication of inflammation or infection. Chronic liver disease usually causes anemia, which may or may not be regenerative. Plasma protein electrophoresis (EPH) provides the best estimate of protein levels in birds. Inflammatory proteins (globulins) may be increased with chronic hepatitis. Bile acids (BA) produced in the liver may be poorly removed from the blood, resulting in elevated BA in birds with liver dysfunction, especially fatty liver disease. Approximately 75% of birds with liver disease will have abnormal BA. Chronic hepatitis may result in decreased bile acids due to lack of BA production.

Diagnostic Imaging

Screening radiographs give an indication to liver size and shape. Proper positioning is important to prevent artifactual alterations of the hepatic shadow and in most situations; gas anesthesia is required to achieve this. Normally, the liver should not extend past the sternum on the lateral view. If the bird has microhepatica, the proventriculus will be displaced in a cranioventral location; hepatomegaly displaces it in a caudodorsal location. Loss of the "hourglass" cardio-hepatic silhouette can be seen on the ventrodorsal view. IN addition, extension of the hepatic shadow beyond a line drawn between the scapula and acetabulum is also suggestive of hepatomegaly. Barium contrast radiographs are sometimes helpful to visually separate the superimposed gastrointestinal tract from the liver.

Ultrasound imaging has proven useful in cases where the liver is severely enlarged or abdominal fluid is present and allows evaluation of the liver parenchyma, hepatic vessels and gallbladder, if present. Lesions may often be detected earlier than radiography or endoscopy and anesthesia is not usually needed. Also, other abdominal lesions may be observed. A 6.5- to 7.5-MHz probe is placed caudal to the sternum and directed cranially (ventro-median approach). A right lateral approach is possible and a short fasting time will empty the GI tract and make liver visualization easier. Ultrasound-guided, fine-needle aspiration of the liver, although safer than biopsy, is usually of low-yield. This technique is good for identifying hepatocyte hemosiderin and vacuolization. A 22-gauge 1-inch needle is used with 0.5 mL suction. Hemorrhage is not typically clinically significant.

If fluid is present around the liver, removing it via coelomic centesis may be helpful in relieving pressure on the gastrointestinal and respiratory tracts. In addition, the fluid may be analyzed for abnormal cells and proteins (see Table 1 in a subsequent article in this proceedings, "Tricks of the Non-coelom").

Coelomic Effusion and Hepatic-Associated Ascites

Ascites is an increase in the amount of coelomic fluid normally found in the peritoneal spaces. The coelomic cavities are considered potential spaces because air sacs invaginate into and occupy most of the available space with the coelomic cavity under normal circumstances. See a more detailed description in a subsequent article in this proceedings, "Medical Surprises in the Coelom." The intestinal peritoneal cavity is a single midline cavity that extends from the liver to the vent. The two ventral hepatic peritoneal cavities are large, blind pouches that extend lateroventrally from the liver to the caudal body wall. The two dorsal hepatic peritoneal cavities are smaller spaces located craniodorsally in the abdomen. The right dorsal cavity is blind, but the left dorsal hepatic peritoneal cavity communicates freely with the intestinal peritoneal cavity. The liver is encapsulated within the right and left dorsal and right and left ventral hepatic peritoneal cavities. Ascitic fluid may accumulate within one or more of these five peritoneal cavities, usually resulting in abdominal enlargement.

Most of the parenchyma of the left and right liver lobes protrudes into the blind-ending left and right ventral hepatic peritoneal cavities, respectively. The volume that accumulates in each peritoneal cavity is directly proportional to the surface area of the liver contained within that space. Large amounts collect in the right and left ventral hepatic peritoneal cavities with smaller amounts in the right dorsal hepatic peritoneal and intestinal cavities. As described above, the surface are of the liver contained in the left dorsal hepatic peritoneal cavity is smallest and this cavity also communicates with the intestinal peritoneal cavity. As a result, ascitic fluid drains caudally rather than accumulating in the left dorsal peritoneal cavity.

Liver Biopsy

When all signs point to liver disease and the definitive cause is not known, liver biopsy in stable patients offers the best diagnostic tool to obtain a definitive etiology. Histopathology is most likely to be useful for diagnosis of neoplasia, mycobacteriosis, hemochromatosis, and protozoal disease. The best time to biopsy is early as possible in the disease process so the liver can heal and to avoid the risk of anesthesia later when the bird is weaker. Biopsies may be obtained via percutaneous, laparoscopic ("key hole"), and endoscopic methods. Via a lateral approach, the liver can be visualized from the cranial and caudal thoracic air sacs.

A bird undergoing biopsy is fasted for 2 to 6 hours to empty the upper gastrointestinal tract. The bird is anesthetized and placed in dorsal recumbency (Figures 1 and 2). A small area of feathers is gently plucked over the lower half of the keel and abdomen and the skin is cleaned with a disinfectant solution. A clear Steri-drape is placed over the endoscopy site. A 5-mm incision is made in the skin just past the edge of the keel. The body wall is then carefully incised in similar fashion and a 2.7-mm rigid endoscope is inserted to view the liver structure. If the lesion appears to affect the whole liver, a 1- to 2-mm piece of the liver edge can be sampled with biopsy forceps. This piece is placed in formalin for histopathology. If possible, a second or third piece of liver is obtained for bacterial culture and in-hospital cytology. The biopsy site is observed for bleeding and the incision is closed with one or two small sutures. Complications are generally unusual and liver biopsy is not likely to be fatal unless performed too late in the disease process.

TREATMENT OF LIVER DISEASE

Treatment of liver disease focuses on decreasing clinical signs (loss of appetite, weight loss, bleeding), while addressing the pathologic changes present (inflammation, scarring, cancer). The most successful treatment plan is developed based on obtaining an accurate diagnosis. The liver is a strongly regenerative organ, and if not damaged too severely, will often be able to repair itself if the disease processes can be stopped. Concurrent treatment of other altered organ systems (cardiac, renal) that may be needed.

Acutely ill birds should receive supportive care, including environmental heat, oxygen, fluid therapy and administration of highly digestible food. Birds with anemia, low blood proteins or problems clotting benefit from vitamin K supplementation and may require blood transfusion. Chronically ill, overweight birds on poor diets may respond to diet improvement, vitamin and mineral supplementation and carefully supervised exercise. Antibiotics may be indicated, and should be administered based on culture and sensitivity results if possible. Several herbs that assist in liver detoxification and improve liver function may be used.

Prevention of many causes of liver disease is possible through administration of a well-balanced diet free of hepatotoxins. Healthy birds should be examined yearly and routine laboratory analysis should be performed periodically. Birds at risk for liver disease should be evaluated every 6 months, especially birds that are receiving any long-term liver metabolized medications. Frequent monitoring and follow-up is extremely important for all birds with active liver disease.

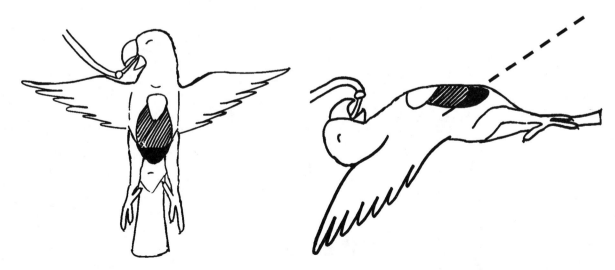

Figures 1 and 2. Dorosventral (Figure 1, left) and lateral (Figure 2, right) views of liver biopsy site in anesthetized parrot. The heart is surrounded by the liver with enlarged portion (black) projecting caudally past the edge of the keel. The white x (Figure 1) and the dashed black line (Figure 2) indicate location of entrance of endoscope.

REFERENCES

1. Hochleithner M, Hochleithner C, Harrison L. Evaluating and treating the liver. In: Harrison GJ, Lightfoot TL (eds): Clinical Avian Medicine, vol. 1. Palm Beach, FL: Spix Publishing, 2006, pp 441-449.
2. Lumeij JT. Hepatology. In: Ritchie BW, Harrison GJ, Harrison LR (eds): Avian Medicine: Principles and Application. Lake Worth, FL, Wingers Publishing. 1994, pp 522-537.
3. Schmidt RE. The avian liver in health and disease. Proc Annu Conf Assoc Avian Vet. 1999; 273-289.
4. Davies RR. Avian liver disease: etiology and pathogenesis. Semin Avian Exotic Pet Med. 2000; 9(3):115-125.
5. Jaensch S. Diagnosis of avian hepatic disease. Semin Avian Exotic Pet Med. 2000; 9(3):126-135.
6. Redrobe S. Treatment of avian liver disease. Semin Avian Exotic Pet Med. 2000; 9(3): 136-145.
7. Wheler Cl. Webber RA. Localized ascites in a cockatiel (Nymphicus hollandicus) with hepatic cirrhosis. J Av Med Surg. 2002; 16(4):300-305.
8. Krautwald-Junghanns, ME. Ultrasonography of the avian liver and gallbladder. Proc Annu Conf Assoc Avian Vet. 2006; 53-58.
9. Nordberg C, et al. Ultrasound examination and guided fine needle aspirate of the liver in Amazon parrots (Amazona species). J Avian Med Surg. 2000; 14(3):180-184.
10. Grizzle JM, et al. Use of milk thistle to reduce aflatoxin poisoning in pigeons (Columba livia). Proc Annu Conf Assoc Avian Vet. 2007; 373-375.

DISEASES ABOVE THE PYLORUS

Laura Wade, DVM, Diplomate ABVP (Avian)
Specialized Care for Avian & Exotic Pets
Broadway Veterinary Clinic, PC, Lancaster, NY

In this article, intracoelomic upper GI tract organs above the pylorus include the coelomic (thoracic) esophagus, and stomach (proventriculus and ventriculus). Discussion will focus on more common stomach diseases seen in clinical companion avian practice (Table 1).

CLINICAL EXAMINATION OF THE AVIAN PATIENT WITH INTRA-COELOMIC UPPER GI DISEASE
History and Clinical Signs

When evaluating a patient with upper gastrointestinal disease, because of the high incidence of infectious, obstructive and toxic causes, it is important to obtain detailed information about diet, other bird health history, and access to possibly ingested objects and toxins. Anorexia and regurgitation are the most consistent findings in birds with disorders of the upper gastrointestinal tract. Weight loss, polyphagia, maldigestion, melena, and seeds in the droppings also occur.

Diagnostics and Treatment

Sometimes organisms in the coelomic esophagus and stomach will be passed into the crop via vomiting or into the feces via the intestines. Therefore, basic microscopic examination is useful, including yeast/parasite analysis (crop/fecal wet mounts and fecal floats), and bacterial, fungal, protozoal cyst analysis (Gram's stain, Diff-Quik and Acid-fast cytology). Depending on these preliminary findings and patient status, additional testing may include complete blood count, plasma biochemistry profile and protein electrophoresis, toxicology (lead/zinc), microorganism polymerase chain reaction (PCR), coelomic radiography (including barium or iohexol contrast), fluoroscopy, GI endoscopy, and surgical biopsy/histopathology. Birds that die should have a complete necropsy evaluation, especially in flock situations. Depending on the clinical signs and results of diagnostic tests, appropriate medications may be administered (Table 2).

ANATOMY AND DISEASES OF THE COELOMIC (THORACIC) ESOPHAGUS

The avian esophagus is thin-walled and distensible with a relatively greater diameter than that of mammals. Esophageal fold development is large and extensive in birds that swallow whole food prey items. Parrots exhibit minimal esophageal fold development and possess a relatively narrow esophagus. Mucus-secreting glands are especially prevalent in the thoracic esophagus. Birds lack true upper and lower esophageal sphincters as found in mammals. The esophageal muscles contain an inner circular layer and an outer longitudinal layer. The thoracic esophagus innervated by the vagus nerve and the celiac plexus.

Lower Esophageal Diseases

Many diseases that affect the oropharynx, cervical esophagus and crop may on occasion manifest in lower esophageal diseases. In addition, some diseases affecting the proventriculus may extend into the distal esophagus. Infectious diseases include: primary and secondary bacterial infections, yeast infections, viral infections and flagellated protozoal and nematode parasites. Noninfectious diseases include foreign body penetration, hypovitiminosis A and neoplasia. Esophageal tumors may become large, necrotic and hemorrhagic and carcinomas may invade surrounding tissue.

Extra-GI causes should be considered as well, including thyroid enlargement (goiter), cardiac enlargement, lung mass, hepatic enlargement, renal failure and normal behavioral (courtship regurgitation).

ANATOMY, PHYSIOLOGY AND DISEASES OF THE STOMACH

The avian stomach lies in the left dorsal and left ventral regions of the coelomic cavity. It consists of two portions, a cranial proventriculus or glandular part and a caudal ventriculus (gizzard) or muscular part. The isthmus is the intermediate zone between the proventriculus and ventriculus. In birds, the proventricular chief cells secrete both hydrochloric acid and pepsin (pepsinogen), contrary to mammals. The ventriculus is the site of gastric proteolysis and in many species is also the organ of mechanical digestion. The stomach is innervated by the vagus nerve and the celiac and cranial mesenteric plexi (subvertebral ganglia from thoracolumbar paravertebral ganglia), which lie just under the serosa. Gastric motility appears to be under the influence of pace setting from the ileum and ceca, unlike gastroduodenal pacing as seen in mammals. The celiac artery supplies blood to the proventriculus and ventriculus.

Like the esophagus, the proventriculus also has an inner circular layer and outer longitudinal layer. The outer layer is poorly developed or absent in parrots. Resting on the surface of the epithelium in the highly muscular ventriculus is a hardened membrane, the cuticle (koilin layer) which is a carbohydrate-protein complex. The koilin acts as a grinding surface and protects the underlying mucosa from stomach acids. The ventriculus is thickened and biconvex in birds that feed on digestively resistant items. Most of the wall of the ventriculus consists of smooth muscle arranged in four semi-autonomous masses. Powerful asymmetrical contractions of these muscles allow for mixing and grinding of food. Food is propelled in alternate directions between the pylorus and ventriculus and occurs in three phases. During first phase, the isthmus closes. The thin muscles of the ventriculus contract and the pylorus relaxes, allowing food to be pushed into the duodenum. In the second phase, the isthmus relaxes while the duodenum and thick muscles of the ventriculus contract, refluxing food back into the proventriculus. The third phase is contraction of the proventriculus.

Proventricular and Ventricular Diseases

Bacterial infection can be primary but is usually secondary to immunosuppressive or other disease states. Usually gram-negative organisms, such as *E. coli, Klebsiella, Salmonella,* and *Enterobacter* sp are identified and typically also affect the intestine. *Mycobacteria* sp infection is occasionally seen, especially in the isthmus.

Common fungal diseases include *Macrorhabdus ornithogaster* (avian gastric yeast) and *Candida* sp, especially in finches. Proventricular dilatation disease (PDD) affects the myenteric plexi of the gastrointestinal tract, leading to segmental atrophy of smooth muscles (crop proventriculus, ventriculus, and small intestine) and subsequent delayed gastrointestinal motility and organ dilatation. Although *Cryptosporidia* sp usually infect the avian intestinal tract (especially in immunosuppressed individuals), proventricular cryptosporidiosis is seen in finches.

Noninfectious causes include impaction and/or perforation by foreign bodies, which are very common in ratites, anseriforms and galliforms and young psittacines. Ingested objects include wood, plant material, grit, metal, plastic other materials, including bedding in neonatal psittacines. Heavy and trace metal toxicosis (lead, zinc and copper) may cause mucosal irritation, erosion, epithelial necrosis, and koilin damage/sloughing. Proventricular neoplasia occurs in older birds, especially Grey-cheek and other *Brotogeris* sp and Amazon parrots with adenocarcinoma.

Recently, a retrospective review of cases submitted to two avian pathologists identified the five most common lesions identified in the proventriculus and ventriculus in companion birds: Proventriculuar dilatation disease (29%), avian gastric yeast (14%), gastric tumors (6%), endoventricular mycoses (3%), and cryptosporidiosis (2%). Lesions varied depending on the species (Table 1).

REFERENCES

1. Gelis S. Evaluating and treating the gastrointestinal system. In: Harrison GJ, Lightfoot TL (eds.): Clinical Avian Medicine, vol. 1. Palm Beach, FL: Spix Publishing, 2006, pp 411-440.
2. Hadley TL. Disorders of the psittacine gastrointestinal tract. Vet Clin Exotic Anim. 2005;8(2):329-349.
3. Morrisey JK. Gastrointestinal disease of psittacine birds. Semin Avian Exotic Pet Med. 1999;8(2):66-74.
4. Klasing KC. Avian gastrointestinal anatomy and physiology. Semin Avian Exotic Pet Med. 1999;8(2):42-50.
5. Rupley AE. Diagnostic techniques for gastrointestinal diseases of psittacine birds. Semin Avian Exotic Pet Med. 1999;8(2):51-65.
6. Schmidt RE. Pathology of gastrointestinal disease of psittacine birds. Semin Avian Exotic Pet Med. 1999;8(2):75-81.
7. Langlois I. The anatomy, physiology and diseases of the avian proventriculus and ventriculus. Vet Clin Exotic Anim. 2003;6(1):85-111.
8. Boutette JB, Taylor M. Proventricular dilatation disease: a review of research, literature, species differences, diagnostics, prognosis and treatment. Proc Assoc Avian Vet Conf. 2004;175-181.
9. Reavill D. Schmidt R. Lesions of the proventriculus/ventriculus of pet birds: 1640 Cases. Proc Annu Conf Assoc Avian Vet Conf. 2007;89-93.
10. Carpenter JW. Exotic Animal Formulary, 3rd ed. Philadelphia: WB Saunders;2005.

Table 1. Common Histopathologic Lesions of the Proventriculus (PV) and Ventriculus of Pet Birds

Bird Group	Common Findings	Pathologist Comments
African greys	PDD, 70%	
Amazons	Serositis/Peritonitis, 37% PV mineralization, 19% Gastric carcinoma (PV), 10%	Concurrent hepatitis and nephritis Underlying renal disease Older birds
Australo-Asian parakeets	*Macrorhabdus ornithogaster*, 27%	
Brotogeris sp.	Gastric carcinoma (PV), 47% Ulcerative proventriculitis, 33%	Older birds Systemic neoplasia, renal disease
Budgerigars	*Macrorhabdus ornithogaster*, 53% Gastric carcinoma (PV), 18% Idiopathic proventriculitis, 14% Mineralization PV, 4%	 *Chlamydophila*, bacterial enteritis, neoplasia Underlying renal disease
Caiques	Proventriculitis/Ventriculitis, 27/27%	Concurrent systemic disease, intraluminal foreign material
Cockatiels	PV gland mineralization, 31% *Macrorhabdus ornithogaster*, 17% Serositis/Peritonitis, 11/11% PDD, 9%	Underlying renal disease Concurrent systemic inflammation (liver, kidney, spleen, lungs)
Cockatoos	PDD, 56% Peritonitis, 11% Ventriculitis, 11%	 Concurrent systemic inflammation Concurrent systemic inflammation
Conures	PDD, 53% PV gland mineralization, 12% Ventriculitis and ulcerative V, 11%	 Underlying renal disease Concurrent fungal pneumonia, systemic disease, nephrosis
Eclectus	PDD, 29% Peritonitis, 20% Ventriculitis, 12%	
Lories & Lorikeets	Peritonitis, 36% PV gland mineralization, 29%	Concurrent systemic inflammation including mycobacteriosis Underlying renal disease
Lovebirds	*Macrorhabdus ornithogaster*, 36% PV *Cryptosporidia*, 14% Gastric carcinoma (PV), 12% PV gland mineralization, 10%	 Many also had concurrent AGY Older birds Underlying renal disease
Macaws	PDD, 53% Peritonitis, 11% PV mucosal mineralization, 7% Ventriculitis, 4%	
Parrotlets	*Macrorhabdus ornithogaster*, 60% Ventriculitis, 13%	
Canaries	*Macrorhabdus ornithogaster*, 39% Proventriculitis, 24% PV mucosal mineralization, 10% Gastric carcinoma, 9%	 Concurrent systemic inflammation
Finches	Yeast endoventriculosis, 25% *Macrorhabdus ornithogaster*, 19% PV *Cryptosporidia*, 16% Ventriculitis, 8% Gastric nematodes, 7%	 Concurrent systemic inflammation, hepatitis

Table 2. Medications Used for Treatment of Upper Gastrointestinal Disease in Birds.
(Additional antibiotics also affecting the upper GI tract are listed in Table 1 in companion article "Diseases Below Ventriculus." Drugs with effects on the lower GI tract are indicated with an asterisk (*).)

Drug/Herb	Dosage	Indication	Comments
Aminopentamide (Centrine)	0.05 mg/kg SQ, IM q12h x 3d	Regurgitation, prevents nausea	Central antiemetic
Ginger	150 mg/kg PO	Prevent nausea	Motion sickness, anesthesia-induced regurgitation
Metoclopramide (Reglan) *	0.5 mg/kg PO, SQ, IM, IV q8–12h	Regurgitation, upper GI hypomotility, (promotes peristalsis in duodenum and jejunim)	Ideally, administer 30 minutes before feeding Has local and central antiemetic properties Avoid if obstruction or bleeding is suspected Constipation possible with long-term use
Cimetidine (Tagamet)	5 mg/kg PO, IM q8–12h	Decrease gastric secretions in proventriculitis, gastric ulceration	
Bismuth subsalicylate (Pepto bismol)	1–5 mL/kg PO	Adsorbent, demulcent	
Charcoal, activated*	1 g/kg PO	Adsorb toxins (not corrosive, petroleum or heavy metals)	Can dilute 1 g charcoal with 5–10 mL water
Kaolin/pectin (Kaopectate)*	2 mL/kg PO q6–8h	Intestinal protectant	
Sucralfate (Carafate)*	25 mg/kg PO q8h	Esophageal, gastric, duodenal ulcers	If use with enrofloxacin, separate by 2–4 hours
Peanut oil	1 mLper 100 g PO q8h	Catharsis	Good adjunct for removing lead particles in ventriculus; Alternative is peanut butter and mineral oil 2:1
Psyllium (Metamucil)	0.5 tsp/60 mL handfeeding formula	Bulking agent, laxative (Impaction, passage of small objects)	Can add mineral oil; avoid concentrations >2% (risk of intestinal blockage)
Nystatin*	300,000 IU/kg PO q12h x7-14d	GI yeast (budding Candida)	Is not systemically absorbed
Fluconazole (Diflucan)*	5 mg/kg PO q12h x 7–14d	GI yeast (mycelial Candida)	Also, ketoconazole may be effective (more toxic), itraconazole (less effective against Candida)
Amphotericin B	100 mg/kg PO q12h x 30d	Avian Gastric Yeast	Is not systemically absorbed
Acetic acid (Apple cider vinegar)	1 tsp/pint drinking water x 10d	Gram-negative, yeast infections	
Amikacin	10 mg/kg PO	GI gram-negative bacteria	Useful for crop flush, dilute with saline; Is not systemically absorbed unless ulceration present
Celocoxib*	10 mg/kg q24h–25 mg/kg q12h x 3–6m	Primary treatment for PDD	Better COX-2 inhibition than meloxicam
Iohexol (Omnipaque)* 300 mg/mL	1 mL per 100 g PO	GI contrast agent	Use if suspect perforation or ulceration
Barium Sulfate 30%*	10–15 mL/kg PO	GI contrast agent	
CaEDTA	35 mg/kg SQ/IM q12h	Lead/Zinc chelator	Use until patient stable, then switch to oral
DMSA	35 mg/kg PO q12h	Lead chelator	3 rounds of 5 days on with 3 days of in between

DISEASES BELOW THE VENTRICULUS

Laura Wade, DVM, Diplomate ABVP (Avian)
Specialized Care for Avian & Exotic Pets
Broadway Veterinary Clinic, PC, Lancaster, NY

In this article, lower gastrointestinal tract organs below the ventriculus include the small intestine (duodenum, jejunum and ileum), large intestine (colon/rectum) and cloaca. Discussion focuses on more common intestinal and cloacal diseases seen in clinical companion avian practice. Cecal anatomy and physiology are briefly mentioned but specific diseases are not discussed in this article. Anatomy, physiology, and diseases of the pancreas are covered in a companion article in this proceedings by Dr. Echols.

CLINICAL EXAMINATION OF THE AVIAN PATIENT WITH LOWER GI DISEASE

History and Clinical Signs

Poor hand-feeding practices, inadequate quarantine procedures, poor sanitation, and inadequate diet are frequently implicated in gastrointestinal signs. Therefore, important components of evaluating a patient with lower gastrointestinal disease include dietary history (type of diet, changes, vitamin supplementation, water supply). Also, because infectious diseases and toxins are common causes, the presence and health status of other birds is especially useful. Diarrhea is the most consistent finding in birds with disorders of the intestinal tract. Weight loss, anorexia, maldigestion, melena, and voluminous droppings also occur.

Causes of diarrhea may be exudative (*Salmonella, Clostridia, Coccidia,* and *Histoplasmosis* sp), hypersecretory (enteropathic *E. coli*), malabsorptive (*Mycobacteria, Giardia,* and *Cryptosporida* sp), and osmotic (dairy products, abnormal disaccharide fermentation).

Diagnostics and Treatment

Because fecal samples are often readily available, basic diagnostic tests include: yeast/parasite analysis (fecal wet mounts and floats), and bacterial, fungal, protozoal cyst analysis (Gram's stain, Diff-Quik and acid-fast cytology). Depending on these preliminary findings and patient status, additional testing may include bacterial/fungal culture/sensitivity, complete blood count, plasma biochemistry profile and protein electrophoresis, toxicology (lead/zinc), microorganism polymerase chain reaction (PCR), coelomic radiography (including barium and iohexol contrast), coelomic endoscopy, and surgical biopsy/histopathology. Birds that die should have a complete necropsy evaluation, especially in flock situations. Because of the intimate association of the blood supply of the intestinal tract with the liver and kidney in birds, these organs may also be affected by intestinal disease. Depending on the clinical signs and results of diagnostic tests, appropriate medications may be administered (Table 1).

ANATOMY AND DISEASES OF THE SMALL INTESTINE

They pylorus joins the ventriculus to the duodenum, which is separated by a small pyloric fold that regulates passage of food into the small intestine where chemical digestion and absorption of food take place. The length of the small intestine is variable but shorter in birds than in mammals. In general, granivores, which eat a concentrated, high-energy diet have shorter small intestines than herbivores. The small intestinal mucosa contains smaller, thinner and more numerous villi in birds than in mammals. The intestinal nerve runs the length of the small and large intestine is unique to birds. It is thought to be analogous to the prevertebral ganglion and contains both sympathetic and parasympathetic autonomic fibers. Blood is supplied by the celiac artery (duodenum, ileum) cranial mesenteric artery (duodenum, jejunum), and caudal mesenteric artery (ileum). Often, intestinal divisions are not able to be seen grossly or histologically.

Duodenum

In the majority of species, the duodenum is a u-shaped loop on the right surface of the ventriculus with a proximal descending part and distal ascending part held together by a narrow fold of mesentery. The pancreas lies between the parts. Several bile and pancreatic ducts open near each other into the distal end of the ascending part in most species.

Jejunum and Ileum

In the majority of species, the jejunum and ileum are arranged in a number of narrow U-shaped loops (jejunal, ileal, axial, and supraduodenal) at the edge of the long dorsal mesentery in the right part of the abdominal cavity. The vitelline (Meckel's) diverticulum is the short, blind remnant of the yolk sac and yolk duct and can be used to divide the jejunum from the ileum. The axial loop has both jejunal and ileal components and the supraduodenal loop is the most distal loop of ileum and lies immediately dorsal to duodenum. The upper ileum is the most important site for absorption of digested fats, carbohydrates and proteins. Bile salts left over from digestion are absorbed in the lower ileum.

Small Intestinal Diseases

The majority of small intestinal diseases are due to infectious agents. The most common cause of diarrhea in pet birds is bacterial infection, especially gram-negative bacteria (Enterobacteriacae). *Campylobacter jejuni* can be found in psittacines, especially neonates. Primary and secondary gram-positive bacteria (*Enterococcus* and *Clostridia* sp) also should be considered. *Mycobacteria* sp primarily affect the gastrointestinal tract in birds and the intestine is the primary site of infection where the bacteria infiltrates the submucosa.

Primary fungal infections are rare; however, secondary invasion by *Candida* sp and others may occur. Budding yeast, and the presence of hyphae indicate active and invasive disease, respectively.

Viral infections include direct damage from adenovirus, herpesvirus, paramyxovirus, orthomyxovirus, circovirus, polyomavirus, parvovirus, picornavirus, reovirus, reticuloendotheliosis viruses (REV), rotavirus, lymphoid leukosis. Proventricular dilatation disease (PDD) causes segmental damage to intestinal smooth muscle, nerves, and ganglia and is thought to be due to a virus.

Intestinal parasites include cysts (*Coccidia* sp, *Cryptosporidia* sp, *Encephalitozoon hellum),* and flagellates (*Giardia, Hexamita,* and *Cochlosoma* sp. Nematodes are more common in Australian psittacines with ascarids and *Capillaria* sp found most frequently). Cestodes are common in insectivorous finches and parrots (cockatoos, African grey, and eclectus).

Ileus (intestinal hypomotility) may result from physical obstruction or extraintestinal compression and may cause fluid distension of the intestines. Causes of ileus include bacterial infection, septicemia, viral infection, including PDD, lead/zinc toxicosis, hypoxemia, peritonitis, anesthesia, foreign body, and neoplasia. Intussusceptions of the distal small intestine are less common in birds. Intussusceptions are more common in galliforms with enteritis and juvenile macaws and Amazons with hypomotility/infection.

Neoplasia of the small intestine include carcinoma, papilloma, leiomyoma/leiomyosarcoma, and lymphosarcoma.

ANATOMY AND DISEASES OF THE LARGE INTESTINE AND CLOACA

The ileum continues through a sphincter into the straight rectum (colon). Is relatively short compared with mammals and connects to the coprodeal compartment of the cloaca. Arising at the junction of the ileum and rectum are the ceca, which are small, rudimentary or absent in passerine, psittacine, and columbiform birds. The ceca assist granivorous and herbivorous birds in the breakdown of food and synthesis of vitamins by symbiotic bacteria. The celiac and cranial mesenteric arteries supply the ceca. The caudal mesenteric artery supplies the rectum and anastomoses with the cranial mesenteric artery at the ceca. The cloaca is innervated by the intestinal nerve and the cloacal ganglion/plexus, which arises from the pudendal nerve, and follows the ureter to the dorsolateral aspect of the cloaca.

Large Intestine

Unlike mammals, the avian rectum has numerous flat villi, very few crypts and very few goblet cells. The rectum exhibits antiperistalsis which allows urine from the urodeum to pass into the colon and ceca, where water and NaCl are reabsorbed.

Cloaca

The cloaca is the common pathway for the urinary, reproductive, and gastrointestinal tracts. The coprodeum is continuous with the rectum. The proctodeum opens externally through the vent. In the young bird, the bursa of Fabricius projects dorsally into the proctodeum and is involved in the developing immune system.

In male birds that have a phallus, the organ lies on the ventral lip of the vent in the proctodeum. The urodeum (middle compartment) empties the urinary and reproductive tracts.

Large Intestinal/Cloacal Diseases

Bacterial and fungal cloacitis is not common but may occur with cloacaliths, chronic cloacal prolapse and sporadically in females during reproductive activity. *Clostridia perfringens* can case necrotic enteritis characterized by foul-smelling feces in psittacines and is often found concurrently with *E. coli* infection. Slow gastrointestinal transit times and mucosal damage may be predisposing factors. Chronic *C. tertium* may cause megacolon. Cloacaliths occur when feces or urates solidify and collect in the cloaca and may impair defecation.

Cloacal prolapse may include oviduct prolapse in egg laying females and idiopathic coprodeal prolapse in male cockatoos. Over-bonding to humans and weaning concerns are likely predisposing problems. Intestinal prolapse is also possible with severe enteritis. Phallic prolapse occurs in waterfowl and ostriches with excessive sexual stimulation.

Neoplasia includes papillomas in the proctodeum, especially in South American species, and carcinomas.

REFERENCES

1. Gelis S. Evaluating and treating the gastrointestinal system. In: Harrison GJ, Lightfoot TL (eds): Clinical Avian Medicine, vol. 1. Palm Beach, FL: Spix Publishing, 2006, pp 411-440.
2. Lumeij JT. Gastroenterology. In: Ritchie BW, Harrison GJ, Harrison LR (eds.): Avian Medicine: Principles and Application. Lake Worth, FL: Wingers Publishing, 1994, pp 482-521.
3. Hoefer HL, Orosz S, Dorrestein GM. The gastrointestinal tract. In: Altman RB, Clubb, SL, Dorrestein GM, Quesenberry K (eds.): Avian Medicine and Surgery. Philadelphia: WB Saunders, 1997, pp 412-453.
4. Klasing KC. Avian gastrointestinal anatomy and physiology. Semin Avian Exotic Pet Med. 1999;8(2):42-50.
5. Hadley TL. Disorders of the psittacine gastrointestinal tract. Vet Clin Exotic Anim. 2005; 8(2):329-349.
6. Morrisey JK. Gastrointestinal disease of psittacine birds. Semin Avian Exotic Pet Med. 1999;8(2):66-74.
7. Rupley AE. Diagnostic techniques for gastrointestinal diseases of psittacine birds. Semin Avian Exotic Pet Med. 1999;8(2):51-65.
8. Schmidt RE. Pathology of gastrointestinal disease of psittacine birds. Semin Avian Exotic Pet Med. 1999;8(2):75-81.
9. Taylor M. The psittacine cloaca: a clinical review. Proc Annu Conf Assoc Avian Vet. 2002;265-269.
10. Carpenter JW. Exotic Animal Formulary, 3rd ed. Philadelphia: WB Saunders, 2005.

Table 1. Medications used for treatment of lower gastrointestinal disease in birds. Drugs with effects on the upper GI tract are indicated with an asterisk (*).

Drug/Herb	Dosage	Indication	Comments
Cisapride (Propulsid)*	0.5–1.5 mg/kg PO q8h	Lower GI hypomotility, including cloacal voiding abnormalities, may also affect PV via myenteric plexus stimulation	Do not use concurrently with azole antifungals or mycin antibiotics (ventricular arrhythmia potential); compounded
Lactulose	0.2 ml/kg PO q12h	Increase gram-positive GI bacteria, inhibit pathogenic bacteria (Clostridium, E. coli)	May delay gastric emptying time, shortens intestinal transit, stimulates colonic peristalsis
Nystatin*	300,000 IU/kg PO q12h x7–14d	GI yeast (budding Candida)	Is not systemically absorbed
Fluconazole (Diflucan)*	5 mg/kg PO q12h x 7–14d	GI yeast (mycelial Candida)	Also, Ketoconazole may be effective (more toxic), itraconazole (less effective against Candida)
Trimethoprim-sulfa*	30 mg/kg PO q12h 25 mg/kg PO q24h	Bacterial infections Coccidial infections	Maintain hydration, avoid in renal disease
Enrofloxacin (Baytril)*	15 mg/kg PO, SQ q12h 10 mg/kg q24h	Psittacines, passerines, columbiformes Raptors, waterfowl	Avoid IM injections and use in young birds
Amoxicillin*	100 mg/kg PO q8h		
Amoxicillin/clavulanate (Clavamox)*	125 mg/kg PO q8h		
Cefadroxil*	100 mg/kg PO q12h		
Tetracycline*	200–250 mg/kg POq12–24h 100 mg/gal drinking water x 5–10d		
Metronidazole (Flagyl)*	50 mg/kg PO q12–24h x 5-14d 25–50 mg/kg PO q12-24h x 5–7d	Anaerobic and hemorrhagic enteritis Trichomonas, Hexamita (use lower dose if BID)	
Ronidazole (Ridzol)*	Psittacines, columbiformes:100–200 mg/L drinking water x 7 d Passerines: 40 mg/L	Resistant flagellate infections	
Carnidazole*	20 mg/kg PO once (pigeons),q24h x 5d (raptors)	Trichomonas	
Sulfadimethoxine (Albon)	25 mg/kg PO q12h x5d	Coccidiosis	
Fenbendazole (Panacur)*	25 mg/kg PO, repeat in 14d 20–50 mg/kg PO q24h x 5d	Ascarids Capillaria (use lower dose for raptors, columbiformes)	Avoid in birds with developing primary feathers
Pyrantel pamoate*	7 mg/kg PO, repeat in 14d	Nematodes	
Ivermectin*	0.2 mg/kg PO, SQ, IM	Most nematodes (excellent Capillaria & Tetrameres; less effective against Ascaridia sp.)	Do not give by injection in passerines or psittacines; caution in toucans (sensitive to propylene glycol)
Praziquantel*	10–20 mg/kg PO, SQ, IM repeat 10–14d	Cestodes, trematodes	

MEDICAL SURPRISES IN THE COELOM

Laura Wade, DVM, Diplomate ABVP (Avian)
Specialized Care for Avian & Exotic Pets
Broadway Veterinary Clinic, PC, Lancaster, NY

The information in this article provides important background for the clinical cases described in this and subsequent articles in this proceedings.

THE AVIAN COELOM

The coelom is defined as "the body cavity" and in avian species consists of both the thoracic and abdominal cavities. Because birds lack a diaphragm, there is no separation of the thoracic and abdominal cavities as in mammals. The term *coelom* is preferred over *thorax* or *abdomen* to refer to the avian body cavity and abnormalities thereof (ie, coelomic fluid). However, the terms *thoracic* and *abdominal* may be used comparatively for parts of organs to distinguish between different anatomic locations (ie, thoracic esophagus, abdominal air sac). For the location of major organs within the coelomic cavity, see Figures 1, 2, and 3.

There are in fact, sixteen distinct and separate cavities enclosed within the avian body wall; eight are air sac cavities and eight are distinct coelomic cavities. As in mammals, birds have one pericardial and two pleural cavities. However, unlike mammals, birds have five peritoneal cavities (Table 1). Understanding the basics of the anatomy of these partitioned cavities is essential when interpreting coelomic tissue and fluid abnormalities in birds.

Pericardial and Pleural Cavities and Coelomic Air Sacs

The heart is contained within the pericardial cavity and the lungs are contained in the left and right pleural cavities. The avian pericardial cavity is essentially similar to that of mammals except that in birds, the lungs are so dorsal that they do not enclose the heart. Also, because there is no diaphragm, the avian liver extends on either side of the heart.

Because the avian lung is fixed and does not expand, there is limited pleural space compared to mammals. During embryonic development, dilations of developing bronchi extend from the lung and penetrate the pulmonary fold, forming coelomic air sacs.

The coelomic air sacs consist of three paired sacs: cranial thoracic (CrT), caudal thoracic (CdT), and abdominal (Abd); and two single sacs: clavicular (Clv) and cervical (Crv). Anatomically and physiologically, the sacs may be divided into two groups: cranial (Crv, Clv, CrT) and caudal (CdT, Abd) sacs. The Clv and crT air sacs arise from the medioventral secondary bronchi and receive air that has already passed through the lung during expiration. The caudal sacs arise from the lateroventral secondary bronchi (CdT) or the primary bronchus (Abd) and receive fresh air from the trachea during inspiration.

See Figures 2 and 4 for location of the CrT, CdT and Abd air sacs superimposed over the coelomic viscera. For location of the Crv and Clv air sacs, see also diagram (Figure 1) in companion article, "Tricks of the Non-coelom," in this proceedings.

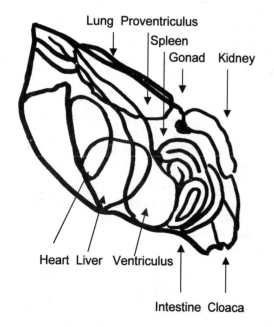

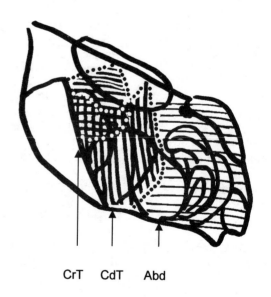

Figures 1 and 2. Lateral view of major organs of the coelomic cavity (Figure 1. left). Lateral view of air sacs superimposed over coelomic organs (Figure 2, right).

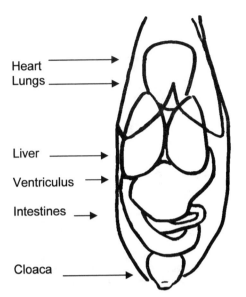
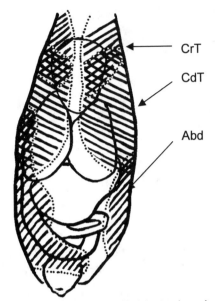

Heart
Lungs

Liver

Ventriculus

Intestines

Cloaca

CrT
CdT

Abd

Figures 3 and 4. Ventrodorsal view of major organs of the coelomic cavity (Figure 3, left). Ventrodorsal view of air sacs superimposed over coelomic organs (Figure 4, right).

Peritoneal Cavities

The detailed anatomy of the five peritoneal cavities is quite complex and is beyond the scope of this article. However, for clinical purposes, the peritoneal cavities are formed by five sheets of peritoneum (discussed below). The peritoneal cavities include: a midline intestinal peritoneal (IP) and lateral hepatic peritoneal (HP) cavities; the left and right HP cavities have dorsal and ventral portions. The IP cavity extends from the liver cranially and reaches the body wall caudally at the vent. The IP cavity can only be directly entered via an abdominal wall incision just cranial to the vent. The HP cavities extend from the liver to the caudal body wall and contain the liver lobes. The dorsal HP cavities are smaller and more cranial than the ventral HP cavities. Each individual peritoneal cavity is blind (separate) with one exception: the left dorsal portion of the HP cavity connects directly with the IP cavity.

One of the peritoneal sheets (combined dorsal and ventral mesentery) suspends the liver and intestines. Another sheet, the post-hepatic septum (PSH), separates the IP from the HP cavities. The clinical significance of this PHS partition is that it restricts the spread of disease between the cavities. Therefore, fluid accumulation from abnormal female ovulation (ie, egg-yolk) is found in the IP cavity and fluid accumulation from liver disease (ascites) is found in the HP cavity. Secondary tumors which spread across the coelom from the ovary or oviduct are often confined within the IP cavity and left dorsal HP cavity. The PSH also allows peritonitis caused by a foreign body to often be restricted to one peritoneal compartment. However, systemic disease which causes peritonitis may involve inflammation in all of the peritoneal cavities. Additionally, peritoneal fat deposits are stored in the PHS. When the bird is opened ventrally, very little of the stomach is seen because the abdominal organs are concealed by fat-laden post hepatic septum (and liver), especially in obese birds.

At the level of the liver and proventriculus a lateral abdominal wall incision enters dorsal HP cavities through the CrT air sac. The ventral HP cavities may be entered via a ventral abdominal wall incision. At the level of the ventriculus, a lateral abdominal wall incision enters the ventral HP cavities directly. Here the abdominal air sacs are within the IP cavity, which is medial to the ventral HP cavities.

Table 1. Major Cavities, Borders and Associated Structures within the Avian Coelom

Cavity	Pericardial (1)	Pleural (2)	Peritoneal (5)	
			Intestinal (1)	Hepatic (4)
Organs/structures contained within	Heart	Lungs	Intestines Gonads Abd AS	Liver Proventriculus (L, R dorsal) Vena cava (R dors)
Bordering organs/structures	Liver Cr/Cd TAS	Cr/Cd TAS	Kidneys Right wall of ventriculus	Cr/Cd TAS Left wall of ventriculus

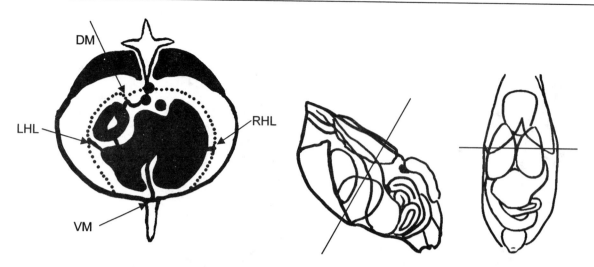

Figure 5. Transverse section through 5th thoracic vertebra just caudal to the heart, caudal view. Major organs (black) from dorsal to ventral are: lungs, proventriculus (left of midline) and liver (left and right of midline). Spaces separated by dotted lines include the left and right cranial thoracic air sacs (ventral to lungs and laterally), left abdominal air sac (just ventral of the 5th thoracic vertebra to the left of midline), and left and right dorsal and ventral hepatic cavities (medially, surrounding proventriculus and liver). Blood vessels (black dots) from dorsal to ventral include: aorta, celiac artery (midline) and vena cava (right of midline). Significant peritoneal sheets (solid black lines) include: dorsal and ventral mesenteries (DM, VM) and right and left hepatic ligaments (HL). Modified from King & McClelland.

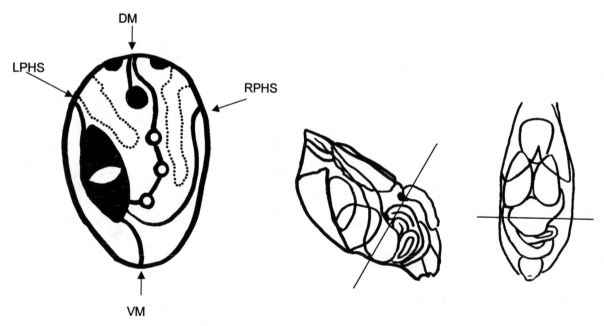

Figure 6. Transverse section several vertebrae caudal to section depicted in Figure 5, caudal view. Major organs (black) are from dorsal to ventral: kidneys, ovary (midline), intestines (midline), and ventriculus (left of midline). Spaces separated by dotted lines include the left and right abdominal air sacs. Significant peritoneal sheets (solid black lines) include: dorsal and ventral mesenteries (DM, VM) and right and left post-hepatic septum (PHS). Modified from King & McClelland.

REFERENCES

1. King AS, McLelland J. Birds: Their Structure and Function. East Sussex, England: Bailliere Tindall. 1984, pp 79-83.
2. Schmidt RE, Reavill DR. Thyroid hyperplasia in birds. J Avian Med Surg. 2002;16(2):111-114.
3. Helmer PJ, Carpenter JW, Hoskinson JJ. What's your diagnosis? J Avian Med Surg. 2000;14(3):200-203.
4. Powers LV. The avian spleen: anatomy, physiology and diagnostics. Compend Contin Edu Pract Vet. 2000; 22(9):838-843.
5. Powers LV. Diseases of the avian spleen. Compend Contin Edu Pract Vet. 2000; 22(10):925-933.
6. Latimer KS, Greenacre CB. Adrenal carcinoma in a budgerigar (Melopsittacus undulatus). J Avian Med Surg.1995;9(2):141-143.
7. Cornelissen H, Verhofstad A. Adrenal neoplasia in a scarlet macaw with clinical signs of hyperadrenocorticism. J Avian Med Surg. 1999; 13(2):92-97.
8. Ford SL. Wentz S, Garner M. Intracoelomic teratoma in a juvenile bald eagle (Haliaeetus leucocephalus). J Avian Med Surg. 2006;20(3):175-179.
9. Dennis PM. Bennett RA. Ureterotomy for removal of two ureteroliths in a parrot. J Am Vet Med Assoc. 2000; 217(6):865-868.
10. Wyre NR. Quesenberry KE. Bursal lymphosarcoma in a 4-year old Congo African grey parrot (Psittacus erithacus). Proc Annu Conf Assoc Avian Vet. 2007; 323.

TRAUMA TO THE COELOM

Laura Wade, DVM, Diplomate ABVP (Avian)
Specialized Care for Avian & Exotic Pets
Broadway Veterinary Clinic, PC, Lancaster, NY

When dealing with a severely traumatized bird, the most important first task is to assess the level of cardiorespiratory system compromise. Identifying possible causes and location of coelomic trauma is paramount to determining prognosis and guiding therapy. In most cases, the bird must be stabilized first via administration of pain medications, fluid support for shock/hypovolemia, and a low-stress, oxygen-rich environment prior to more extensive examination and diagnostics.

Trauma to the coelom may occur from blunt, compressive and penetrating injuries. Companion and wild birds frequently are injured by flying into objects, being stepped on, or attacked by predators. Air sac rupture, internal hemorrhage, pneumocoelom, and subcutaneous emphysema are possible complications. Radiographic abnormalities often include subcutanous and intracoelomic gas. These may manifest as increased visualization of the cardiac apex on the ventrodorsal view, increased prominence of the thoracoabdominal structures and gas lines between skeletal muscle and skin. Acutely, fluid accumulation (edema) in the lungs and air sacs may be detected by loss of normal pulmonary honeycomb appearance and generalized air sac opacification. Parabronchial ring shadows suggest subsequent inflammation of the lung.

BLUNT TRAUMA

Coelomic Air Sac Rupture: External Manifestation of Severe Coelomic Trauma

Coelomic air sac rupture appears clinically as a balloon-like deformity of the skin over the lateral flanks and lateral to the thoracic inlet. This is to be distinguished from cervicocephalic air sac "rupture" which involves the head and dorsal cervical region and has no communication with the coelomic air sac system. Common in Amazon parrots and cockatiels, cervicocephalic air sac distention is usually an external manifestation of infraorbital sinusitis. In contrast, coelomic air sac rupture is caused by blunt or compressive coelomic trauma or extension of air sac infection of the clavicular air sac from the lung. See the companion article "Tricks of the Non-coelom" in this proceedings for additional anatomic information on the anatomy of the extrathoracic diverticulae of this air sac.

On physical exam, a soft, air-filled swelling is palpable, which may be small and localized or more diffuse/generalized and may be unilateral or bilateral. Usually the external swelling is not clinically problematic when rupture occurs along the axillary fascial plane. External rupture occurring along the thoracic inlet fascial plane may cause compression on the crop or impede neck movement and may be more disruptive. Localization of the site of occlusion of normal airflow in traumatic cases may not be identifiable.

Treatment involves making a percutaneous fistula to allow for drainage of air. This relieves pressure to allow for healing. Using a hand-held pen-lite cautery or a 22-gauge needle placed in a lighter flame for several seconds, a small hole is created in the skin and the swelling immediately deflates. Use caution over important structures like the crop to not penetrate deeper than the surface layer. Surgical correction (Teflon stent) may be needed in chronic, recurrent cases. For wildlife and companion birds with a predator in the house that present with air sac rupture, administration of prophylactic antibiotics (Clavamox) is recommended, even with no visible puncture or scratch wounds. Use caution with administration of subcutaneous fluids with birds with air sac rupture; avoid the side with the rupture or use an alternate site.

Rule out trauma to a pneumatized bone (humerus or femur) and subcutaneous emphysema from other causes such as gas-producing bacteria or from a surgical incision.

PENETRATING FOREIGN BODIES

Gastrointestinal Foreign Bodies (Coelomic Trauma from the "Inside-Out")

Intra-coelomic (gastrointestinal-origin) items include fishhooks, nails, wires, and metal fragments. Ingested sharp foreign bodies may puncture the lower esophagus, proventriculus, or ventriculus, leading to hemorrhage, peritonitis, abscess formation, and adhesions to the liver and intestines. Endoscopy of the thoracic esophagus may be performed via flexible endoscopy through the oral cavity or rigid endoscopy through an ingluviotomy incision. If the foreign object has not completely passed through the esophagus, it may be able to be retrieved via the lumen. If the foreign body has passed into the cranial portion of the coelomic cavity, rigid endoscopy via the thoracic inlet may need to be performed. In most cases, once the proventriculus or ventriculus has been perforated, the prognosis is poor.

Penetrating Foreign Bodies (Coelomic Trauma from the "Outside-In")

Typical coelomic foreign bodies include extra-coelomic origin projectiles (gunshot, arrows, etc.). Infection is a possibility as the entry wound may allow pathogens to gain access to areas of devitalized tissue and contaminated feathers and skin can be drawn into the wound along with the object. Two-view, whole-body radiographs are obtained to attempt to localize the foreign bodies inside the coelomic cavity. Use of a rigid endoscope carefully placed through an entry wound can allow internal visualization of coelomic structures that may be damaged. Use of a rigid endoscope to aid in foreign body removal from a difficult to reach location in the respiratory tract was recently performed in a falcon.

Iatrogenic Foreign Bodies (Veterinarian-Induced Coelomic Trauma from the "Outside-In" and "Inside-Out")

Coelomic endoscopic examination and placement of an air sac tube are temporary foreign bodies deliberately inserted into the coelomic cavity. Attempts to minimize trauma and infection are crucial. Air sac tubes must be used for less than 5 days and ideally, less than 48 to 72 hours. Prophylactic antibiotics and possibly antifungals are warranted.

Care should also be taken when performing fine-needle aspirates and coelomic centesis, as there is potential for spreading fluid, infectious agents and neoplastic cells into new locations. Ideally, an ultrasound probe should be used to guide needle placement.

When performing rigid luminal endoscopy of the thoracic esophagus, proventriculus and ventriculus, extreme care must be made when approaching the ventriculus to avoid inadvertently perforating the proventriculus, especially in cases of wall thinning, such as suspected proventricular dilatation disease (PDD).

Any surgical exploration of the coelom, including liver biopsy and salpingohysterectomy, may disrupt coelomic cavities.

TRAUMA TO COELOMIC SUPPORT
Coracoid Abnormalities

The coracoid is the largest bone of the avian shoulder joint. It articulates firmly with the sternum on each side and keeps the thoracic cage from collapsing during flapping flight. During gliding flight, the coracoids also suspend the sternum, which supports the weight of the viscera. Luxations of the shoulder most often involve the coracoid. Front-on trauma to the shoulder may result in a fracture or luxation of the coracoid. Typically, the base of the coracoid becomes dislodged from the cranial end of the sternum. Depending on the severity, the displaced coracoid or fracture fragments may traumatize the nearby esophagus, heart and associated vessels and nerves.

Birds with a fracture of the coracoid can fly for short distances and have a strong flap but are unable to fly upward. They are unable to lift the injured wing (or wings) above the horizontal plane. Because of the collapse of the shoulder, the affected wing will be elevated above normal position, causing the unaffected wing to look drooped. Minimally displaced coracoid fractures should be maintained conservatively with a figure-of-8 wrap to immobilize the wing and with a wrap to the body wall to keep the wing in its normal anatomical position for 10 days. Ideally, twice-weekly passive physical therapy under anesthesia will help keep the pectoral muscle from developing fibrosis. After splinting, birds should have 2 weeks of cage rest, but complete healing often takes several months. Possible complications include compression of the trachea or esophagus by a large bony callus.

For severe subluxation, internal fixation (pinning) may be needed. This is a very difficult and potentially dangerous surgery but a recent report showed greater release rate of wild birds with coracoid fractures with surgical vs. conservative repair.

Trauma to Coelomic-Associated Pneumatic Longbones

Because the clavicular air sac has extrathoracic diverticula which extends into the pneumatized humerus, infection can quickly spread from the medullary cavity of the humerus to the lung and other coelomic air sacs. Open humeral fractures are frequently involved but closed fractures may be contaminated during surgery if improper technique is used.

Humeral fractures typically cause only a slight wing droop in most cases and may be diagnosed by palpation but their extent is determined by radiographs. Generally, humeral fractures tend to be open, spiral and unstable, with great displacement of the fragments. The longer it takes to stabilize a humeral fracture, the greater the likelihood of complications and reduction of flight capabilities. Regardless of size, minimally displaced, proximal humeral fractures often heal with a figure-of-8 + body wrap. The goal is to keep the humerus against the body but not overly flexed. Displaced fractures require internal fixation for the bird to regain the ability to fly. Mid-shaft humeral fractures are often too displaced for adequate fixation by a figure-of-8 bandage and surgical repair (type 2 external skeletal fixator with an intramedullary tie-in) is required. This is because the strong pull of the pectoral muscles rotate the proximal fragment dorsally and the triceps and biceps distract the distal fragment ventrally. Birds with recent open fractures should be placed on antibiotics, such as enrofloxacin or clavulinated amoxicillin. If open fractures are infected, ideally, cultures should be obtained and clindamycin should be used. Prophylactic antifungal medication with itraconazole should be considered to avoid development of *Aspergillus* sp air sacculitis.

There is also a pneumatic diverticula of the abdominal air sac into the femur. Open fractures and surgical manipulation of this bone may spread infection into the coelomic cavity.

REFERENCES

1. Harrison GJ, Lightfoot TL, Flinchm GB. Emergency and critical care. In: Harrison GJ, Lightfoot TL (eds): Clinical Avian Medicine, vol. 1. Palm Beach, FL: Spix Publishing, 2006, pp 214-232.
2. Bowles H, Lichtenberger M, Lennox A. Emergency and critical care of pet birds. Vet Clin Exotic Anim. 2007;10(2):345-394.
3. Chavez W, Echols MS. Bandaging, endoscopy and surgery in the emergency avian patient. Vet Clin Exotic Anim. 2007;10(2):419-436.
4. Gibbons PM, Horton S. What's Your Diagnosis? J Avian Med Surg. 2000;14(1):60-64.
5. Jekl V, et al. Endoscopic removal of a bullet from the cranial thoracic air sac of a peregrine falcon (*Falco peregrinus*). J Avian Med Surg. 2007;20(4):242-246
6. Lierz M. Diagnostic value of endoscopy and biopsy. In: Harrison GJ, Lightfoot TL (eds): Clinical Avian Medicine, vol. 1. Palm Beach, FL: Spix Publishing. 2006, pp 632-652.
7. Taylor M. Endoscopic examination and biopsy techniques. In: Ritchie BW, et al (eds.): Avian

Medicine Principles and Application. Lake Worth, FL: Wingers Publishing, 1994, pp 327-354.

8. Mitchell J, Bennet RA, Spalding M. Air sacculitis associated with placement of an air breathing tube. Proc Assoc Annu Conf Avian Vet. 1999;145-146.

9. Holtz PH. Coracoid fractures in wild birds: repair and outcomes. Aust Vet J. 2003;81:469-471.

10. Redig P. Anatomical and surgical considerations of the avian thoracic limb. Proc Annu Conf Assoc Avian Vet. 2000;429-438.

TRICKS OF THE NON-COELOM

Laura Wade, DVM, Diplomate ABVP (Avian)
Specialized Care for Avian & Exotic Pets
Broadway Veterinary Clinic, PC, Lancaster, NY

The cardiorespiratory organs reside in the pericardial and pleural cavities. Diseases that occur in these smaller, almost nonexistent coelomic cavities are often challenging to diagnose. Analysis of coelomic effusions may be useful in determining the nature and chronicity of coelomic diseases. With the more common use of computed tomography and magnetic resonance imaging, we will be able to better characterize these remote areas of the avian coelom.

PERICARDIAL AND PLEURAL CAVITIES AND COELOMIC AIR SACS

Disease of the Pericardial Mid-coelomic Cavity: Heart and Great Vessels

In birds, the right atrioventricular (AV) valve is actually a muscular flap and right heart disease is the predominant form of cardiac disease seen in birds. Hepatomegaly and ascites are common sequelae of right heart enlargement due to hepatic congestion. Ultimately, left heart failure and respiratory signs occur with severe, chronic heart disease. Radiographic enlargement of the cardiac silhouette may result from cardiomegaly (dilatation or hypertrophy), pericardial effusion (PCE), or superimposed mass. Echocardiography is needed to differentiate between these causes. Muffled heart sounds heard on auscultation may occur from hepatic congestion, coelomic fluid and PCE. Murmurs may occur from valvular dysfunction, including valvular endocarditis, stenosis (atherosclerosis) and severe anemia. Chronic inflammation or metabolic diseases may lead to stenosis of the semilunar valves.

Age and nutritional deficiencies over many years, combined with lack of exercise appear to play a role in the development of atherosclerosis in captive birds. Endothelial inflammation from toxins, immune complexes, hyperlipidemia and infections may be contributing factors. Atherosclerosis is more common in African grey parrots, macaws and Amazon parrots over 15 years of age. Lesions occur commonly in the aorta and brachiocephalic trunk, but may affect the coronary and axillary arteries. Sclerotization can cause plaque-like or diffuse hardening of the larger arteries (aorta and brachiocephalic trunk), which may lead to aneurisms. Radiographically, increased radiodensity/enlargement/ mineralization of the aorta may be seen as well as nodular densities (end-on arteries) cranial to heart. Birds with atherosclerosis often exhibit neurologic signs including lameness, lethargy, dyspnea, vomiting, ascites, and acute deaths (especially during stress/exertion).

The descending aorta contains aggregates of smooth muscle and is a common site of atherosclerosis. The avian arterial blood pressure is also high (140–250 mmHg), despite a slightly decreased total peripheral resistance compared mammals. This high blood pressure may cause aortic and auricular ruptures during stress or certain nutritional diseases (vitamin A deficiency). Birds with aneurysms seem to experience pain, and may exhibit voice change, coughing, dyspnea, regurgitation, weakness/collapse, and sudden death.

Diseases of the Pleural Mid-Coelomic Cavity: Lungs and Air Sacs

Understanding the anatomy of the avian lung and coelomic air sac is important to interpreting disease patterns (Figures 1 and 2). Pulmonary masses may originate from lung infection/inflammation due to viruses (polyoma, herpes, pox), bacteria (including *Mycobacteria* sp), fungi (*Aspergillus, Mucor* sp), protozoa (*Sarcocystis falcatula*), mites (*Steronstoma tracheacolum),* nematodes (*Cyathostoma* sp in raptors), toxins, inhalation of foreign material, and pulmonary neoplasia (fibrosarcoma, carcinoma). Pulmonary metastasis may also occur from adenocarcinoma, carcinoma, fibrosarcoma, hemangiosarcoma, liposarcoma, lymphosarcoma, melanoma, mesothelioma and osteosarcoma.

Air sacculitis may also be from bacteria seen in pneumonia (also Chlamydia), fungal, filarid nematodes (*Serratospiculum auraculata*) in falcons, and *Cyathostoma* in raptors. Neoplasia is rare. Air sac carcinoma typically involves fluid-filled cystic axillary masses or bony lesions of the right humerus and may invade the pulmonary parenchyma. There seems to be a higher incidence in large, white (*Cacatua* sp) cockatoos. There are 3 paired air sacs: cranial thoracic (CrT), caudal thoracic (CdT) and abdominal (Abd). Compared to non-psittacine species, the cockatoo has more extensive cranial and caudal thoracic air sacs and the abdominal air sac is smaller. The lines on the CrT air sac depict rib impressions.

There are 2 single (fused) air sacs: clavicular (Clv) and cervical (Crv). The clavicular and cervical air sacs have multiple diverticula. The clavicular air sac (Clv) originates from the cranial dorsal portion of the lung (medio-ventral secondary bronchi). The Clv is divided into two bilateral air sacs dorsal to the ventral thoracic inlet and fused together ventral to the thoracic inlet. The Clv connects to the cervical air sac (Crv) and has multiple intracoelomic and extracoelomic diverticulae (Figure 2). The Clv intrathoracic diverticulae surround the heart/great vessels, esophagus, and syrinx. Intrathoracic diverticula also extend into the sternum and sternal ribs (figure 2). The Clv extrathoracic diverticula invade fascial planes between skeletal muscle and skin in the thoracic inlet and axillary regions. The extrathoracic diverticula also invade the bones of thoracic girdle and shoulder joint (coracoid, furcula, scapula, humerus).

The cervical air sac (depicted by dashed line, figure 1) is the only air sac that does not connect directly to the lung; it is continuous with the clavicular air sac and extends along the vertebral column.

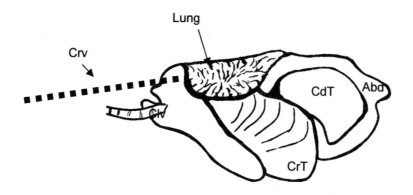

.**Figure 1.** Coelomic air sacs. This line drawing depicts the left lateral view of a latex cast of a sulphur-crested cockatoo *(Cacatua galerita)*. Adapted from Jaench, et al.[9]

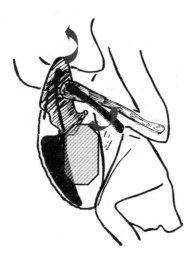

Figure 2. Anatomy of the clavicular air sac and intrathoracic and extrathoracic diverticula

COELOMIC EFFUSIONS

Some causes of coelomic effusions include: right heart failure, liver failure, mycobacteriosis, polyomavirus, viral serositis, reproductive tract disorders (egg-related peritonitis, cystic ovary), and coelomic neoplasia. Characteristics of the coelomic effusion may help determine possible etiology (Table 1). The presence of mononuclear white blood cells indicated mild irritation of the coelomic cavity, usually from a non-septic condition. The presence of heterophillic white blood cells typically is seen in exudates, often with acute inflammation. Degenerative heterophils with intracellular bacteria point to a septic condition. As the effusion becomes more chronic, increased numbers of macrophages, lymphocytes and plasma cells accumulate. Chronic/resolving hemorrhagic effusions show varying degrees of erythrophagocytosis (Table 2). Malignant effusions, typically show modified transudates, hemorrhagic effusions or exudates (with or without neoplastic cells) and result from blocked blood or lymphatic vessels. High protein transudates often result from hepatic neoplasia compressing outflow of the sinusoids.

Table 1. Coelomic effusions. Characteristics of Transudates, Modified Transudates, and Exudates.

	Transudate	Modified Transudate	Exudate
Total protein (g/dL)	<3	≤ 3	>3
Specific gravity	< 1.020	≤ 1.020	>1.020
Cells/µL	<1,000	1,000–5,000	>5,000
Disease processes	Cardiac insufficiency Hepatic cirrhosis Hypoproteinemia Overhydration	Cardiac insufficiency Cardiomyopathy Compressive tumor Organ torsion/inflammation Sterile irritants	Inflammatory Hemorrhage Neoplasia
Cells found	Macrophages Occasional mesothelial cells Lymphocytes Nondegenerate heterophils	Macrophages Reactive mesothelial cells	Macrophages Reactive mesothelial cells Red blood cells Lymphocytes Heterophils Neoplastic cells Organisms in phagocytes

Table 2. Coelomic Effusion Timeline. Presence of Thrombocytes and Nature of Erythrophagocytosis in First 72 Hours.

Thrombocytes		No Thrombocytes			
Erythrophagocytosis (RBC)			Erythrophagocytosis (iron pigment)		
0	24		48	72	96

REFERENCES

1. Mans C, Brown CJ. Radiographic evidence of atherosclerosis of the descending aorta in a grey-cheeked parakeet (Botogeris pyrrhopterus). J Avian Med Surg. 2007;21(1):56-62.
2. Brown CJ. Dilemmas of diagnosis in a psittacine bird: a miniature macaw with aortic aneurism. Proc Mid-Atlantic Assoc Avian Vet. 2007:159-175.
3. Vink-Nooteboom M, et al. Clinical diagnosis of aneurysm of the right coronary artery in a white cockatoo (Cacatua alba). J Sm Anim Pract. 1998;39(11):553-557.
4. Olgesbee BL. Aneurysm in right ventricle of a cockatiel. J Am Vet Med Assoc. 1998;212(11):1737-1742.
5. Sato Y, Aoyagi T, Miyano N. An occurrence of cardiac rupture in a capercaille (Tetrao urogallus) probably induced by myocardial infarction. Avian Dis. 2000;44:231-233.
6. Powers LV, Merrill CL, Degernes LA, Miller M, Latimer KS, Barnes HJ. Axillary cystadenocarcinoma in a moluccan cockatoo (Cacatua moluccensis). Avian Dis. 1998;42:408-412.
7. Garner MM. Air sac adenocarcinomas in birds: 7 cases. Proc Annu Conf Assoc Avian Vet. 2003;55-57.
8. Marshall K, Daniel G, Patton C, Greenacre C. Humeral air sac mucinous adenocarcinoma in a Salmon-crested cockatoo (Cacatua moluccensis). J Av Med Surg. 2004;18(3):167-174.
9. Jaensch SM, Cullen L, Raidal SR. Air sac functional anatomy of the Sulphur-crested cockatoo during isoflurane anesthesia. J Av Med Surg. 2002;16(1):2-9.
10. Cambell TW, Ellis CK. Avian and Exotic Animal Hematology and Cytology, 3rd ed. Ames. IA: Blackwell Pub. 2007:162-169.

WOUND MANAGEMENT IN EXOTICS AND WILDLIFE

Mark Bohling, DVM
College of Veterinary Medicine
University of Tennessee
Knoxville, TN

Veterinarians who treat non-domestic animals are often presented with patients that have a wide variety of wounds; management of these wounds often presents special challenges not seen with domestic species. Many different products and techniques are available for the management of wounds; a sound understanding of wound healing physiology is useful to guide the decision-making process as to the ideal way to manage each wound. This article begins with a review of wound healing physiology including a discussion of species differences and how those differences may affect wound management. A number of wound healing products, old and new, are then described along with their indications. Surgical management of wounds (primary and delayed closure) is often the most expedient method of wound management. Practical surgical techniques for wound management are described and illustrated with cases.

WOUND HEALING PHYSIOLOGY AS IT RELATES TO EXOTIC SPECIES

The basic principles of wound healing are already well known to most veterinarians and will be reviewed in only the briefest of ways. Wound healing has been traditionally divided into phases of inflammation, proliferation, and remodeling. More recently, it has been realized that while one of these processes may predominate during a particular time in healing, that in reality there is considerable overlap and a more accurate description of healing is of a group of processes rather than discrete phases. This knowledge is of particular importance to the fields of comparative wound healing and exotic animal practice, because it appears that most of the differences in wound healing that are seen across species lines are due to differences in the time of onset, duration, or intensity of the various healing processes. In other words, wound healing in various animal species looks different not because certain species possess unique healing mechanisms, but because they use the same mechanisms in different ways. The field of comparative wound healing is still in its infancy in veterinary medicine – very little is known about the specific details of healing in many species and most of what we apply in clinical practice is based on general knowledge of wound healing. This knowledge, gained from studies on other species, may be reasonably accurate in most instances, but in other instances, it could be quite wrong and even lead to less than optimal treatment planning. Acknowledging that our information is very incomplete at best, the following is a brief summary of some of the current knowledge in comparative wound healing:

Reptiles

It is generally agreed that wound healing in reptiles proceeds more slowly than in mammalian species; however, the rate of healing is heavily influenced by metabolic rate and thus ambient temperature. An ambient temperature increase from 21°C (70°F) to 30°C (86°F) resulted in an over 7 times increase in the rate of epithelialization of open wounds in garter snakes at 5 days post-wounding. Most veterinarians tend to leave sutures in place for rather prolonged periods in all reptile closures; although the limited experimental data suggests that this is not necessary, it is probably not particularly harmful, either. Bone healing is also an area of concern, particularly in chelonians since plastrotomy is often the only available coelomic approach. Current recommendations to leave patches in place for 1-2 years appear to be based on anecdotal reports of very slow bone healing; there is no experimental evidence to substantiate these recommendations.

Birds

In contrast to reptiles, clinical experience has shown that birds generally heal quite rapidly, in fact more so than some mammals. Again, there is little experimental data to substantiate this claim. With regard to exudation, wounds in birds are quite a bit more "dry" than in mammals, due to their primarily heterophilic acute wound response. The less fluid character of avian wound exudation can make wound drying and eschar formation more problematic with bird wounds, and makes moisture-retentive dressings particularly attractive for these species.

Variations Between Mammalian Species

Most small rodent and pocket pet species tend to heal rapidly as long as the wound is clean and uncomplicated, and not being traumatized by the patient. In contrast, at least one experimental report that compared several species indicated that healing in guinea pigs was slower than dogs, cats, rabbits or rats. In this report, the gain in breaking strength of sutured wounds was notably slower in guinea pigs than in the other species. As the authors observed no difference in the rate of fibroplasia between species, this difference may relate to the time of onset or rate of progression of the remodeling phase of healing.

OPEN WOUND MANAGEMENT IN EXOTICS

Open wound management for second intention healing has certain advantages: low cost, relative non-invasiveness, and in general, a high success rate. Disadvantages include slow progress, high labor requirement, and inferior cosmetic outcome in most cases. In addition, open wound management in exotics faces significant additional challenges involving the relative difficulty of handling and bandaging the patient, making the whole concept of "wound management" somewhat of a relative term. Perhaps "wound observation" would be a more accurate description in many cases! Nevertheless, certain interventions can be undertaken, even with uncooperative patients, and for the relatively few cooperative ones, open wound management can be performed much the same as for domestic species. The following "tricks of the trade" may be useful:

1. Use a wound-healing stimulant, even if you think it will not remain on the wound for long. Healing stimulants will help resolve the open wound faster, and that is an important goal. Besides, who knows, the patient may leave it alone, and even if not, the tiny amount in contact with the proliferating cells is what really matters, not having a big glob of stuff on the wound. Gels and other thick or sticky products (including very fine powders that may adhere to the wound due to wound fluid) may work well. Good choices include: tripeptide-copper complex (Iamin®), acemannan (Carravet®), in gel or lyophilized form, honey and other sugars such as maltodextrin powder (very fine and sticky), or table sugar with a wound disinfectant such as "sugardine" (sugar + betadine ointment) or "sugardene" (sugar + silver sulfadiazine ointment)

2. Less is often more; a bulky bandage may invite efforts by the patient to remove it. Consider instead a thin, light, moisture retentive covering such as Ioban® with Vi-Drape® applied to the periwound area beforehand to enhance tack and therefore retention of the dressing.

3. Remember, whatever you put "on" may end up "in" your patient and plan accordingly. All bandage materials should be nontoxic and able to pass the GI tract, and daily evaluation of the bandage should include a check of the housing area to see if removed bandaging has been consumed.

4. For patients that cannot be bandaged, look for other creative ways to clean and debride the wound and keep it moist (major goals of bandaging). Such methods can include: hydrotherapy/lavage debridement, medicated soaks/baths, and spray-on applications to deliver wound healing stimulants and antibiotics to the open wound. These techniques may be repeated as often as needed, up to several times per day.

5. Do not eschew the eschar. While "moist wound healing" techniques may be all the rage, (and largely with good reason as it does speed healing), we must not forget that healing still progresses under a scab, albeit a bit more slowly. Once granulation tissue has developed in the wound, it should be possible in many if not most cases to allow the scab to form and let nature finish the job.

SURGICAL MANAGEMENT OF WOUNDS IN EXOTICS

It has been said that "the best bandage for any wound is the other side of the wound," and this truism may be nowhere as true as it is for exotic animals. Management of open wounds for second intention healing is time consuming and involves increased risks of repetitive episodes of restraint, sedation, or anesthesia. In addition, the uncooperative nature of most exotic species and less-than-ideal environments (from a wound-healing standpoint) contribute to increased risks of failure to heal. In comparison, wound closure is rapid and takes care of the wound in a single episode. The difficulties encountered with open wound care on any veterinary patient are magnified with exotics, making surgical closure seem all the more attractive as an option. Balanced against this are the risks of anesthesia and the knowledge that the postoperative environment will most likely not be ideal for wound healing. Sound judgment must prevail as the risks and benefits of surgery vs open wound management are weighed. Certain surgical principles can be applied to closure of wounds in exotics to help maximize the odds of success. General surgical principles as applied to exotics:

1. Follow Halstead's principles to stack the odds in favor of rapid uncomplicated healing.
2. Over-engineer the repair to handle more than the expected level of stress
3. Minimize wound tension, particularly at the suture line—use methods to distribute the tension as widely as possible.
4. Use the simplest method when several options are available
5. Be realistic in your goals and expectations
6. Try to manipulate the postop environment to favor healing as much as possible; even if a perfect environment cannot be maintained, do what you can.
7. Make use of stimulants to wound healing in order to speed the process. Several products are compatible with surgical closures.

SPECIFIC COMMENTS REGARDING SURGICAL CLOSURES IN EXOTICS
Reptiles
1. Scaled skin edges naturally invert, thus reptiles require an everting closure. Good patterns include horizontal and vertical mattress patterns, either interrupted or continuous.
2. Monofilament sutures with low drag facilitate suture removal especially after shedding. Polypropylene and nylon are preferred.
3. In lizards and snakes, moderate to good skin stretch is available in the dorsoventral direction but skin recruitment in the craniocaudal direction is usually poor. If skin must be recruited from the craniocaudal plane, consider a 90° transposition flap that can be closed with dorsoventral traction.

Birds
1. The skin of most birds is very thin and delicate. Avoid putting it under tension in closure.
2. Buried absorbable closures are preferred where possible to avoid the stress of another vet visit for suture removal. Monofilament absorbable sutures such as polydioxannone or polyglecaprolate in sizes 4-0 to 8-0 are usually appropriate.
3. Skin grafting can be a very useful option in avian wounds when local tissues are inadequate for

closure. Donor skin may be harvested from wing or leg fold. The graft is prepared to be applied as a full-thickness meshed graft, in the same manner as for mammalian species. Time to graft "take" can be expected to be fairly rapid, owing to the thinness of avian skin with commensurately shorter distance for nutrient diffusion during the plasmatic imbibition phase of engraftment.

Small Mammals

1. Most surgeons tend to use suture that is larger than needed; skin and subcutis in small mammals can usually be closed very adequately with sutures no larger than 4-0 to 5-0. As with birds, an entirely buried closure is usually preferred.

2. Self-trauma of closures is a common problem; use of Elizabethan collars, body bandages, or similar restraints is generally recommended. Along similar lines, patients should be housed individually after surgery to prevent wound licking or other trauma by conspecifics.

3. Abcesses in rodents (particularly rabbits) tend to have a thick caseous exudate that is poorly responsive to standard open drainage techniques. Complete *en bloc* resection of these lesions with a conservative margin is more likely to yield good results in these cases. After excision, the lesion can be primarily closed or left to heal by second intention if not too large.

LEGAL ASPECTS OF ZOONOTIC DISEASES IN EXOTICS

Margaret E Cooper, LLB, FLS
c/o School of Veterinary Medicine
The University of the West Indies
St Augustine, Trinidad and Tobago, West Indies

It's not the best day for you, the senior veterinarian at an otherwise thriving exotic animal veterinary clinic. A client will shortly be bringing in a bird of prey that is "wheezing." A young child has arrived with a terrapin in his hand; his mother has sent a note because she herself is ill with vomiting and diarrhea. A physician has just telephoned saying that he has a patient with red marks on his arms—could it be related to the pet hedgehogs that he keeps? A family has arrived from overseas with their beloved juvenile monkey and they want you to be its vet, but you know that you often get cold sores in winter. They say that it was very sweet as a baby but it is getting a bit aggressive and has nipped one of the children. A client who says he is immunocompromised wants to know why you did not warn him of the additional health risks involved before he invested a lot of money in a parrot-breeding facility; now chlamydophilosis (*Chlamydophila psittaci* infection) has been diagnosed. Your clinic advises a local reptile breeder, the hygiene of the facility has been consistently poor over a long time and a routine veterinary visit is due. One of your staff has developed asthma and claims that it is work-related and a veterinary nurse/technician was bitten by a reptilian patient yesterday. On top of all this, your bright, newly qualified veterinarian has suggested that the practice is vulnerable to MRSA (meticillin-resistant *Staphylococcus aureus*). Finally, you read the report in Seminars in Avian and Exotic Pet Medicine that three out of four recipients of organs from one (deceased) donor died within a month of receiving their transplants, the cause of death in all cases being from lymphocytic choriomeningitis virus and the source was shown to be a pet hamster that belonged to the donor. A depressing day altogether, and maybe it is time to contact your lawyer.

ZOONOSES

The veterinarian is trained to treat disease and injuries in animals, not humans. However, in present times there is acute awareness that a significant number of animal diseases may infect humans. First named "zoonoses" by Virchow in 1885, these are currently defined by the World Health Organization as: "A zoonosis is any disease or infection that is naturally transmissible from vertebrate animals to humans.... Zoonoses may be bacterial, viral, or parasitic, or may involve unconventional agents." (http://www.who.int/topics/ zoonoses/en/). In this article the term *zoonoses* will be used in a slightly broader way to include:

- Other hazards that exotic pets present to humans, such as bites, stings and allergies (some of which can be associated with the spread of pathogens)
- Diseases and infections that may be contracted from captive invertebrates
- Diseases that pass from humans to animals

because the required physical precautions and the legal implications are usually comparable

For the most part, the veterinarian is concerned about maintaining the health of his or her patients. However, good clinics also consider the well-being of the client and provide advice on the potential effects of zoonoses—either information specific to the condition of a particular patient (eg, shown to be carrying salmonellae) or general guidance in care sheets or newsletters related to a particular species or health risk.

A number of zoonoses are recognized in veterinary practice in respect of conventional species but exotics are associated with additional diseases and potential physical injuries (http://www.oie.int/eng/publicat/ ouvrages/a_zoonoses2005%203vols.htm). Emerging zoonoses (either new diseases or a known agents appearing for the first time in a different species or place) have been overviewed. Although some may be of remote concern in day-to-day practice, a veterinarian is usually expected by clients to be well informed if public alarm is raised regarding diseases such as Ebola, a new strain of avian influenza, or monkeypox. The location (eg, urban or rural) of a clinic and its clientele (local or foreign) will dictate which zoonoses are most likely to be relevant but an exotic animal may have arrived from another environment (eg, imported) carrying more unusual agents.

LEGAL ISSUES

This article will consider the legal implications of zoonoses for the veterinarian in exotic animal practice. Despite the fact that each country has its own legal system and jurisdiction, there are a lot of common legal issues that will be familiar to veterinarians in any country. These matters fall broadly into two categories:

- Regulatory compliance and litigation
- Disciplinary supervision of the profession

In some countries, these issues are taken to high levels of implementation, while in others litigation (and even insurance) may be rare and disciplinary control minimal.

In applying law to any specific real-life situation appropriate legal, veterinary and other professional advice should be obtained.

REGULATORY COMPLIANCE
Animal Health

Some zoonoses are designated by animal health legislation as "notifiable" or "reportable" diseases, such as rabies or West Nile virus, and if their existence is diagnosed or suspected they must, by law, be reported to the relevant government authority. See:
http://www.defra.gov.uk/animalh/diseases/notifiable/in dex.htm;

http://www.oie.int/eng/maladies/en_classification2007
.htm?e1d7;
http://www.aphis.usda.gov/vs/nahss/disease_status.h
tm

Health and Safety

Health and safety welfare in the workplace or, as it is known in some countries, occupational health and safety (OSH), has a strong priority in most high-income nations. It impinges strongly on veterinary practice and the premises used. On the other hand, there are a lot of countries where such provisions are vestigial or not enforced.

Compliance with health and safety law is normally based on risk assessment together with guidelines, codes of practice and standard operating procedures (SOPs), protective equipment, training and supervision as appropriate. It includes providing staff with protection from the risk of zoonoses associated with exotic species by way of (for example) vaccinations, checking rabies titre, monitoring for *Herpes simplex* and *Staphyloccus aureus* or providing information—for example, the risk that *Pseudomonas* (not strictly a zoonosis) can be acquired either from amphibians or fish themselves or from the environment (eg, exposure during the cleaning of tanks).

Some zoonoses may require special awareness. There is particular concern at present regarding MRSA, for example. See Lloyd et al and http://www.defra.gov.uk/animalh/diseases/zoonoses/mrsa.htm; and http://www.bsava.com/resources/mrsa/mrsaguidelines/mrsaguidelines.htm), its transmission to and by animals, the need for prevention or eradication in the practice, and the special risks and concerns for vulnerable and immunocompromised people (eg, with cystic fibrosis) who keep pets (http://www.cdc.gov/healthypets /extra_risk.htm).

LITIGATION

In some countries there is a strong culture of litigation and professionals are (or feel) particularly vulnerable. Judicial decisions in respect of zoonoses are not likely to be common but it may be possible to extrapolate from other situations such as injuries. A wide range of veterinary law and litigation is discussed by Wilson and Dennis at http://www.vet.ksu.edu/studentorgs/VBMA/ppt/VeterinaryMalpractice.pdf.

Litigation by clients is based mainly in the civil law in which a claim for compensation may be made. These are most commonly based on the "torts" of negligence, strict liability for animals or malpractice (professional negligence).

Negligence

Where negligence is claimed, it is necessary to show three elements: that the veterinarian has a duty to the client or patient, that there was a failure in that duty and that the client suffered loss as a result. For example, failure to maintain proper barriers to the spread of an established zoonosis between patients hospitalized or attending a surgery

Strict Liability

It may be possible to construct situations in which strict liability (without the need to show negligence) for damage caused by exotics might be proved as a result of transmission of zoonoses by an animal already known to be infectious.

Malpractice (Professional Negligence)

This a special form of negligence in which a professional who offers a certain level of skill can be sued for compensation for injury, damage or loss suffered as a consequence if s/he fails to maintain the standard of competence normally expected of such persons. This might involve inadequate knowledge of relevant zoonoses leading to incorrect diagnosis and treatment.

DISCIPLINARY ACTION

Where the veterinarian has fallen short of the standards imposed by his or her veterinary professional body, disciplinary action may ensue. This may arise from a failure to meet practice standards, from an animal welfare issue, or improper conduct that is so serious as to bring the profession into disrepute.

EXPERT EVIDENCE

A veterinarian who is experienced in the treatment of exotic species may be asked to give evidence in court. This may be as a witness of fact relating to immediate observations of a patient; on the other hand, an expert opinion may be required to support or disarm evidence relating to, for example, the likelihood of the spread or transmission of a zoonosis.

It is a sad fact of a litigious society that clients and their lawyers are very eager to make a claim for compensation or to make a complaint to a veterinary disciplinary body. While there are situations where action is justified, clients, in their distress, may not always understand the fact that, when an animal dies in the hands of a veterinarian, there may be no fault involved. However, the veterinarian often has to bear the costs of defending his or her position and reputation. In either case, the veterinarian needs to be insured against the costs involved in investigation, advice, defense, and compensation.

CONCLUSION

The keeping and treatment of exotic animals involves risks of zoonoses and this may sometimes give rise to legal issues that concern the veterinarian. The key rules for dealing with such scenarios, which may help to reduce the risk of legal issues taking root, include the following:

- Maintain awareness of the zoonoses that different species, especially those that regularly come into the clinic, may harbor. This means reading the relevant literature, searching Web sites, and attending courses.
- Develop a relationship with exotic animal-owning clients; that means that you are consulted before a

new species is obtained or extra animals are added to a collection or significant changes to management are put in place.

- Provide general, accurate information on zoonoses for clients in the form of leaflets, newsletters, or other communications
- Where clients are likely to be at risk from zoonoses, formulate specific risk assessments for each situation (eg, listeriosis in sugar gliders). As far as possible, ensure that it is understood and followed by the client
- Establish a good relationship with others who may be able to assist in the prevention, detection, or amelioration of effects of a zoonotic outbreak. These include a laboratory with the required skills and interest and members of the medical profession.
- Ensure that your clinic/practice is OSH-compliant and zoonoses-aware by providing literature and information risk assessments and SOPs as well as training and continuing professional development for staff.
- Ensure that the practice is protected as far as possible by a package that provides adequate legal advice and insurance.

ACKNOWLEDGMENTS

The author thanks Professor J E Cooper for advice on this manuscript and the veterinary aspects of zoonoses and also the Medical Library of the University of the West Indies for use of its research facilities.

REFERENCES

1. Tseng, F, Lymphocytic choriomeningitis virus in organ transplant recipients – Massachusetts, Rhode Island. ProMed Mail, May 26, 2005. In Seminars in Avian and Exotic Pet Medicine, 2005; 14 (4) (October): 226.
2. Brown C, Emerging zoonoses and pathogens of public health significance – an overview. Rev sci tech Off int Epiz 2004; 23 (2): 435-442.
3. Desachy F, Les Zoonoses - transmission des Maladies des Animaux à l'homme. 2005; De Vecchi, Paris, France.
4. Schwabe, CW, Veterinary medicine and human health. 1964; Williams and Wilkins, Baltimore, USA.
5. Chitty J, Hendricks A, Zoonotic skin disease in small animals. In Practice 2007; 29: 92-97.
6. Cooper JE, Cooper ME, Introduction to veterinary and comparative forensic medicine. 2007; Blackwell Publishing, Oxford, UK.
7. NASPHV, Compendium of veterinary standard precautions: zoonotic disease prevention in veterinary personnel. 2006; National Association of State Public Health Veterinarians Veterinary Infection Control Committee.
8. Lloyd DH et al, Dealing with MRSA in companion animal practice. European Journal of Companion Animal Practice 2007; 17(1); 85-93.
9. Moore, JE Millar C, Reid, A, Elborn JS, MRSA in companion animals. Veterinary Record October 2006; 159: 605.
10. Wilson JF, Law and ethics of the veterinary profession. 1988, Priority Press, Yardley, PA.

CLINICAL PROCEDURES AND DIAGNOSTICS IN LIZARDS

Rob L. Coke, DVM
San Antonio Zoo
San Antonio, TX

Reptile medicine is a rapidly growing field with new developments in research and knowledge expanding the veterinarian's capabilities. The small animal practitioner may find reptile medicine daunting at first, but the basic understanding of small animal physiology and pathology creates a base on which to build the comparative differences of reptiles. In addition, the veterinarian needs to understand the background, natural history, and husbandry of reptiles, which play a most important role in disease and therapy.

HISTORY

As with other animals, obtaining a good history is the first step of the examination. Obtaining a full and detailed history is even more important in reptiles due to the impact that even the most basic environmental factors can have on the animal's health status. The history process begins at the front desk with recording the patient's basic data such as the identification of species, age, sex (if known), captive born/wild-caught, and where and when the individual was purchased.

The veterinary technician (or veterinarian) should then weigh the patient and inquire about the reason for the visit and any changes in behavior, water/food intake, time of occurrence/first symptoms, description of symptoms, and importantly what treatment(s) has the owner initiated. Background details about the environment of the patient should be noted including: temperature, humidity, light source and cycle, size of enclosure, single kept/group, an so on.

OBSERVATION

The first part of the exam is observation of the patient, either while the animal is still in a cage or on the exam table or floor. Different lizard species respond differently to stress such as hiding, "puffing up," hissing, or biting. Observation before the physical exam allows the veterinarian to assess problems or conditions that the owner is not aware or unbiased in their interpretation. A healthy lizard should be alert, interested in its environment, and actively moving about the enclosure or room. Movements should be even and smooth (even if fast) and they should be able to lift their heads and body off the ground during movement. They should be symmetrical in their confirmation and movement. A body condition assessment is also made.

PHYSICAL EXAMINATION

Proper restraint is essential for the safety of the patient and the examiner. Some lizard species are very small and delicate while others are large enough to require several handlers. Small lizards may be restrained with a single hand over the thorax and neck. The restrainer's fingers can hold and restrain the legs in-between fingers. Mid-sized lizards, such as iguanas (*Iguana iguana*), need to be restrained with one hand over the thorax and neck restraining the front legs and the head while the other hand holds the hind quarter over the pelvis, restraining hind legs and tail base. The hind legs are best controlled when stretched backward (watch the strong tail!). Very fast or aggressive lizards are examined in an enclosure or wrapped in a towel. Venomous species, such as the Gila monster (*Heloderma suspectum*), are dangerous and should only be restrained (and examined) by experienced individuals.

A complete physical exam is performed, not unlike that in small animals, where a systematic approach is used. For examination of head or oral cavity, restrain head behind jaw while holding onto the neck. The mouth may be opened with wooden or plastic instruments to avoid injuries of teeth, gingival, and tongue. The oral cavity should be assessed for bite abnormalities, dental disease, saliva character, tongue tone, or any other pathology. The nares should be examined for discharge and patency. The eyes should be examined externally for disease as well as internally with an ophthalmoscope. Ear canals should be evaluated for the presence of discharge, mites, or swelling. Auscultation of the heart and lungs may be performed if the patient is large enough for the proper size of stethoscope bell. A small, moistened cotton gauze over the skin will aid in reducing extraneous noise. Palpation of the trunk of the patient may aid in determining fullness of the gastrointestinal tract, urinary bladder, presence of masses, and gravidity. The cloaca should be examined for fecal staining or swelling. If large enough, digital palpation of the cloaca may determine kidney size, prolapse of organs (oviduct, hemipenis), fecal obstruction, or pelvic disease. Cloacal contents should be evaluated separately for feces, urates, and urine for abnormalities. A scan of the integument should reveal any presence of parasites, infection, or abnormal shedding. All the limbs should be evaluated for proper mobility and confirmation.

CLINICAL AND DIAGNOSTIC PROCEDURES

Ideally a minimum database of a complete blood cell count (CBC), a plasma biochemistry panel, and a urinalysis should be performed in all ill species. Also, a fecal specimen should be submitted and analyzed for internal parasites. In reptile medicine, the small size of patients (and client pocketbooks) may dictate a deviation from the desired norm.

Blood Collection

The clinician should have previously identified a laboratory that accepts and analyzes reptilian blood cell counts as well as biochemistries. In many cases, once the clinician has a blood sample, they need to prioritize which lab test should be run until the sample is exhausted. The amount of blood safely collected (ie, 0.5% to 0.8% body weight) from reptiles is less than what is acceptable for other species due to the relative lower amount of circulating blood volume. The location of venipuncture varies between species and clinician comfort and experience.

The ventral tail vein is the most common venous access point in those lizard species that have a large enough tail and lack tail autonomy. The patient is restrained on its back and the tail presented. Next palpate the muscles on the ventral tail on midline. Insert the needle in between the scales at a 70° to 90° angle. Advance slowly using light aspiration until the needle strikes bone, slowly retract and repeat at a slightly different angle in the vertical and/or horizontal plane. Alternatively, the vein can be accessed with the patient in dorsal recumbency on the exam table. The needle is inserted laterally at the muscular ridge along the side of the tail. Advance slowly using light aspiration until the needle strikes bone, slowly retract and repeat at a slightly different angle ventrally to hit the vein under the caudal vertebrae.

The medial abdominal vein lays in the region in-between the pelvis and the mid-point of the thorax and is formed from the confluence of blood flow from the abdominal fat bodies and ends in the liver. The animal is positioned on its back and the vessel may be seen readily in species with thin skin. A superficial blind venipuncture must be made in larger lizards with opaque skin.

Cardiac venipuncture is a delicate and potentially life-threatening venipuncture choice and should be reserved for "last resort." Under sedation, the heart's location can be determined by palpation or visual exam of the heart beats along the trunk. The needle is inserted between the ribs and the blood is aspirated slowly with each heart beat.

The jugular vein may be accessible in medium to larger lizards by a blind puncture in the region between the thoracic inlet and the angle of the mandible. Other locations such as the auricular vein in veiled chameleons (*Chamaeleo calyptratus*) and the cephalic veins of larger monitors (*Varanus* spp.) may also be used.

Fecal Examination

Reptiles have been kept in captivity and many species are being captive-bred each year. There are, however, hundreds of thousands of individuals that are imported into the Unites States. These wild-caught reptiles may play host to various external and internal parasites. Some of these parasites may be carriers for reportable foreign animal diseases (ie, Heartwater, *Cowdria ruminatum*, was found in ticks imported on Leopard tortoises (*Geochelone pardalis*)). Captive-bred specimens are not immune to internal parasites as evidenced by the prevalence of the host-specific *Isospora amphiboluri* in bearded dragons (*Pogona vitticeps*) and cross species infection of *Heximetra* from wild-caught panther chameleons (*Furcifer pardalis*) to captive-bred veiled chameleons (*Chamaeleo calyptratus*).

Methods of fecal examination for internal parasites include flotation, centrifugation, sedimentation, direct examination, aerobic culture and sensitivity, and cytology. The presence of external parasites is evaluated via visual exam plus magnification. The exact identification of a particular parasite to genus and species is not necessarily practical in clinical practice. Typically, identification of any parasites down to family group will aid in proper therapy. Many university parasitologists have interests in novel or unusual species of parasites and can be a resource to the private practitioner. Species identification will aid in life-cycle determination to facilitate specific therapy.

Identification of some parasites is important due to potential zoonosis from pentastomid parasites. These parasites seem to look like a cross between a helminth and an insect and belong to their own phylum. This group of parasites has proven to be very difficult to treat, often with egg shedding returning sometime after treatment. If accessible, surgical extraction of the individual parasites appears to be the current therapy.

Urinalysis

The analysis of urine of reptiles is complex with potential contamination with the co-production of uric acid, mixing of contents in the urinary bladder, and the mixing of fecal material in the cloaca. Some lizards may void their urine during stress of transport or when handled. To collect urine a sample may be pipetted from voided droppings, a glass or plastic tube inserted into the cloaca, or cystocentesis.

Radiography

Radiographs of lizards are a valuable and necessary part of the diagnostic puzzle. Internal organs are somewhat obscured due to the decreased amounts off coelomic fat. Standard two-view studies are appropriate to determine any marked roentgen signs. Horizontal lateral views are beneficial to isolate the lung fields in some species to determine pathology. Many lizard species are very active and restraint can be tricky to obtain diagnostic radiographs. Sedation may be required to allow for the proper positioning. Limbs may be adhered to the radiograph cassette with radiolucent tape.

Ultrasound

Ultrasonography has been used in lizards for many years as an obstetrical tool to determine follicular development or as a means to determine sex in juveniles of monomorphic species. Ultrasonography scans are a valuable tool to evaluate the heart, liver, kidneys, and other internal organs. Smaller lizard species may require machines with better detail and higher probe frequencies (> 7.5 MHz). Acoustic coupling gel must be used liberally to obtain better images due to rough scales. Water immersion of the patient and scanning through the water may be beneficial, but restraint of the patient may cause difficulties.

Endoscopy

Advances in instrumentation and decreased startup costs have made flexible and rigid endoscopy more practical to the veterinarian. Laparoscopic examination of the avian patient has been performed for decades with that knowledge and instrumentation being passed to the reptile practitioner. Larger lizard species are amenable to flexible endoscopy of the upper and lower gastrointestinal tract. Small diameter (2.7 mm) rigid endoscopes are capable of general laparoscopic examination of the coelomic cavity. The clinician is capable with the proper instruments to obtain biopsies from the various internal organs. Newer multi-port techniques have been described to perform more complex surgeries such as castration or ovariosalpingectomy.

Computed Tomography (CT) and Magnetic Resonance (MR) Imaging

Advanced imaging, once outside the realm of clinical practice, is becoming more accessible to the private practitioner though universities and regional specialty hospitals. CT scans allow detailed images of internal structures and new machines even perform calculations for digital 3-D anatomic models. CT scans can now be obtained faster with great images of the respiratory and skeletal systems. MR imaging provides excellent soft tissue detail but is limited by availability, cost, and long scanning times. Internal organs such as the liver, kidney, and brain are best examined with MR.

Electrocardiography (ECG)

Electrocardiography is still in the immature stages of diagnostic cardiology but is commonly used in cardiac monitoring while under anesthesia. Studies are emerging on standards and normals for a few reptilian species (ie, *Iguana iguana*). Dramatic changes may be determined for pathology but less subtle signs are difficult to interpret. Other factors such as temperature, anesthetics, and technique may alter normal cardiac physiology and any interpretation should be cautiously documented.

Coelomic Transillumination

Transillumination of the coelomic cavity can provide an inexpensive yet invaluable diagnostic tool. A pen light, finoff ocular transilluminator, or endoscopic light source is used to pass light through the coelomic cavity to visualize internal organs. Some species such as leopard geckos (*Eublepharis macularius*) are prime examples for diagnosis of such diseases as hepatomegaly, intestinal obstruction, follicular development, gravidity, dystocia, plus others. Care should be taken to prevent the light from burning the skin.

REFERENCES

1. Barten SL. Lizards. In Mader DR (ed): Reptile Medicine and Surgery. Philadelphia: WB Saunders, 2006, pp 683-695.
2. Burridge MJ, Simmons LA, Allan SA. Introduction of potential heartwater vectors and other exotic ticks into Florida on imported reptiles. J Parasitol. 2000; 86(4):700-704.
3. Coke RL. *Hexametra* transmission between wild-caught panther chameleons (*Chamaeleo pardalis*) and captive-born veiled chameleons (*Chamaeleo calyptratus*). Proc ARAV. 1997; 2-4.
4. Greiner EC, Mader DR. Parasitology. In Mader DR (ed): Reptile Medicine and Surgery. Philadelphia: WB Saunders, 2006, pp 343-364.
5. Hernandez-Divers SJ. Diagnostic techniques. In Mader DR (ed): Reptile Medicine and Surgery. WB Saunders, Philadelphia, PA. 2006; 490-532.
6. Klingenburg R. Understanding Reptile Parasites, 2nd ed. Mission Viejo, CA: Advanced Vivarium Systems, 2007, 200pp.
7. Koch TF. Evaluation of ECG parameters in green iguanas (*Iguana iguana*). Proc ARAV. 2007; 44.
8. Silverman S. Diagnostic imaging. In Mader DR (ed): Reptile Medicine and Surgery. Philadelphia: WB Saunders, 2006; pp 471-489.
9. Strik NI, Alleman AR, Harr KE. Circulating inflammatory cells. In Jacobson ER (ed): Infectious Diseases and Pathology in Reptiles. Boca Raton, FL: CRC Press, 2007, pp 167-218.

GECKOS: NOT JUST A COMMERCIAL ANYMORE

Rob L. Coke, DVM
San Antonio Zoo
San Antonio, TX

Leopard geckos (*Eublepharis macularius*) are popular reptiles in the pet trade due to their relatively small size of 8 to 10 inches total length (20–25 cm), relatively long life (up to 30 years for males but ~10–15 years for females), and excellent demeanor. They have been bred for the past 30 years and now come in a multitude of colors, patterns, and sizes. These "designer" geckos have provided a resurgence of breeding efforts of the past decade to create the next "it" colors and patterns.

NATURAL HISTORY

Leopard geckos belong to the gecko (Gekkonidae) family that encompasses species that inhabit all the continents with the exception of Antarctica. They belong to the subfamily of Eublepharidae that consists of terrestrial geckos that have movable eyelids. This group also lacks the adhesive sub-digital lamellae on their digits prohibiting them to be able to climb smooth vertical surfaces. They do possess small claws on each digit which assists in climbing around rocks and digging.

The leopard geckos inhabit the arid to semi-arid areas of Afghanistan, Pakistan, and India. They are often found in rocky habitats with hardened clay with sandy coverings to allow for burrows to be created in the rock crevices. Being a nocturnal species they sleep during the day in humid burrows and come out to hunt insect prey at night.

HUSBANDRY

Leopard geckos are easy to house in general with simple accommodations. Juvenile geckos and single adults may be housed in 10 gallon (38 L) or 20 inch (51 cm) long aquaria. When keeping a breeding pairs, a 20 gallon (75 L) or 30 inch (76 cm) long aquarium works well with larger sizes of enclosures directly proportional to larger breeding group sizes. The decorations may be very spartan for breeding setups with paper towels and plastic bowls. For display centerpieces in homes, the enclosure may be designed with rock formations, sand/soil, and small plants.

Leopard geckos are nocturnal and do not require the intense ultraviolet radiation as other heliotropic species. A full spectrum bulb of moderate wattage should be used to provide natural daylight cycles and to "show off" naturalistic enclosures. This bulb may provide some heat in conjunction with an under-tank heating pad to provide a daytime temperature of 75°F to 85°F (24°C to 29°C) with a focal heat region of 85°F to 90°F (29°C to 32° C). Night time temperatures may lower slightly by 5°F to 10°F (< 5°C). Humidity is generally low but geckos do require some periodic humidity to assist in shedding. Humidity can be provided though small plastic tubs with a hole access and filled with moist substrate, moss, coir, and so forth.

These terrestrial geckos are pure insectivores consuming any of the commercial prey insects of proper size in the pet market such as crickets, mealworms, etc. These insect food items need to be "dusted" with minerals/vitamins or fed with supplements (ie, Gut-Loaded) to fortify the nutritional contents of the insect's gastrointestinal tract. Breeders will often to leave out a small dish of a calcium powder with vitamin D3 supplement to allow the geckos (especially cycling females) to naturally consume their desired dietary intake. A small shallow dish of water should be provided and changes fresh daily. A small shelter should be provided to provide a visual barrier (ie, "hide box").

Leopard geckos become sexually mature at 3 to 5 months for males and 9 to 10 months for females depending on juvenile grown rates and time of year hatched. They do not fully mature in size and reproductive capacity until about 18 months. Male geckos can be differentiated from females by more prominent preanal pores, longer length, increased weight, and a more slender build. Breeders have found that they can combine one male gecko to 4 to 5 female geckos for optimal egg production. Female geckos may lay one to two eggs several times during the breeding season from January to September.

OTHER GECKOS

Crested geckos (*Rhacodactylus ciliatus*) are very popular in the current pet trade market and naturally inhabit New Caledonia and surrounding islands in Indonesia. They are semi-arboreal are can reach total lengths up to 8 inches (~20 cm). They require about 20 to 29 gallon (75 to 110 L) or up to 30 inch (76 cm) long/high enclosures. They are omnivores and nocturnal. They primarily eat a baby food mixture (2 parts fruit such as peaches or apricots to one part meat such as turkey or chicken) with added calcium and D3 supplement. They are offered supplemented insect prey several times per week.

African fat tail geckos (*Hemitheconyx caudicinctus*) have been kept for decades and are commonly seen in pet stores for sale. They originate from West Africa and may reach total lengths of 8 to 10 inches (20 to 25 cm). They are terrestrial and can be kept similar to leopard geckos described above. They are insectivores and nocturnal. They eat a diet that mostly consists of supplemented crickets, mealworms, and waxworms. Need a semi-dry habitat with a moist hiding area.

Day geckos (*Phelsuma* spp.) are a group of small brightly colored lizards from the island of Madagascar. They range from the smaller (~4 inches (~10 cm)) species such as the gold-dust day gecko (*P. laticauda*) to the larger (~11 inches (~28 cm)) grand day gecko (*P. madagascariensis grandis*). They require about 10 to 29 gallon (38 to 110 L) or up to 30 inch (76 cm) long/high enclosures depending on species. They are diurnal omnivores. They primarily eat a baby food mixture (two parts fruit such as peaches or apricots to one part meat such as turkey or chicken) with added calcium and

D3 supplement. They are offered supplemented insect prey several times per week.

Tokay Geckos (*Gekko gekko*) are a sporadically common species that is imported in large numbers. They are a nocturnal and arboreal gecko of Southeast Asia and Indonesia than can reach lengths of 10 to 14 inches (25 to 36 cm). They have been introduced into parts of Florida, Hawaii, and the Caribbean and have become an invasive species. They have a rather pugnacious personality and a vocalization that often sounds like a "bark." They eat a diet that mostly consists of supplemented crickets, mealworms, and waxworms. Need a topical habitat with a moist hiding areas and branches to climb.

CURRENT TOPICS OF MEDICAL CONDITIONS
Cryptosporidiosis

Over the past decade a serious disease has been noted in leopard geckos causing high morbidity and mortality. Originally this disease was called "skinny or pencil tail" or "wasting disease" due to the marked weight loss noted in these geckos. The affected geckos would also present with anorexia, regurgitation, and most importantly diarrhea. Cryptosporidium oocysts in the feces as well as histopathologic lesions of disease were determined as the etiology of the wasting condition.

Cryptosporidiosis in leopard geckos differs in the clinical disease and pathology seen in snakes with cryptosporidiosis. Much research has been done in the disease in snakes in determining that the causative agent is *Cryptosporidium serpentis* instead of *C. parvum* (seen in mammals). The pathology in snakes is primarily a proliferative gastritis with only occasional extension into the small intestine. In lizards, this disease has been unusually seen in the eustachian tube of an iguana, the salivary gland epithelium of an iguana, and the renal epithelium of an iguana and chameleon. In leopard geckos, the lesions present as a hyperplasia of the mucosa with mononuclear inflammation and are primarily seen in the small intestine with infrequent extension into the stomach or large intestine. *Cryptosporidium* spp. sporocysts were noted in association with the lesions typically in the apical cytoplasm of the lateral and apical enterocytes.

The oocysts are transmitted by direct fecal-oral routes in group situations. Fomite transmission is also common due to improper disinfection of the enclosures, water bowls, etc. Also, insect vectors may play a role as a direct mechanical transport from contact with contaminated fecal material to a naïve enclosure or as a paratenic carrier of oocysts if consumed. Oocysts can survive for months in the environment and most of the commercial disinfectants are ineffective at recommended concentrations. Studies have shown that only 5% ammonia and 10% formalin have some efficacy in disinfection of the oocysts.

Diagnosis of cryptosporidiosis in geckos may vary from easy, simple diagnosis to clinical frustration. Histopathology is the gold standard diagnostic method, but due to the patient size and poor condition is not practical as an ante-mortem test. Fecal flotation methods using a Sheather sugar solution may be employed but requires a sufficient number of oocysts in the sample and diligence in observation during scanning the slide to find the small oocysts. Acid-fast staining of fecal smears is the best practical diagnostic method. Unfortunately, this testing method is not as sensitive and requires timing of actual oocysts shedding and shedding of sufficient numbers to detect. Fortunately, geckos with the classical signs of weight loss and diarrhea often will shed thousands of oocysts and can be reliably determined through multiple fecal cytology acid-fast stains. Other methods such as immunofluorescent antibody stain (IFA) for *C. parvum* and enzyme-linked immunosorbent assay (ELISA) for *C. parvum* (or a special reptile specific test using anti-*C. serpentis* antibodies) may be used but does not seem to cross react with the *Cryptosporidium* spp. seen in Leopard geckos.

The species of Cryptosporidium that infects these geckos has not been definitively determined. There have been several species of Cryptosporidium described in a wide variety of lizard species. From morphometric and DNA analysis, the specific species that infects these geckos is not completely clear but is not *C. serpentis* and suspected to be *C. saurophilum*.

Therapeutics for Cryptosporidium-infected leopard geckos has traditionally been frustrating. Historically, there have been a multitude of drugs used in treating cryptosporidiosis in humans as well as reptiles including halofuginone, spiramycin, trimethoprim-sulfa, paromomycin, and many others. Azithromycin has been used successfully to clear clinical disease but not been 100% successful in recrudescence of oocyst shedding after cessation of drug administration. A novel therapy of hyperimmune bovine colostrum (HBC) was studied in leopard geckos which did decrease the number of oocysts but not a cure. Coccidiocidal drugs such as toltrazuril and ponazuril may be a better therapy for a possible cure but they have been sporadically used in reptiles with some success but no pharmacokinetic or pharmacodynamic studies have been published. One text (de Vosjoli and Tremper, 2005) mentions some success with nitazoxanide if given early in the disease progression,[3] but again no pharmacokinetic or pharmacodynamic studies have been published. Hopefully in the future, more investigators will try and fully evaluate more pharmaceuticals in reptiles to determine appropriate dosing and therapy. So far, the drugs used against Cryptosporidium are more prophylactic than therapeutic.

Shedding Problems

Although leopard geckos come from a mostly arid environment, they do require some moisture to allow for proper shedding. Their natural burrows in the rock crevasses are often relatively humid to their surroundings. In captivity, a small plastic enclosure with a moistened substrate such as moss, coir, etc should be provided to allow for natural selection of the enclosure during times of normal shedding (ecdysis).

Often leopard geckos will shed 95% of their surface area. The areas that do not seem to fully shed routinely are the digits. Retained skin layers on the distal digits over time will constrict down and accumulate over time. This will eventually cause necrosis and sloughing of the distal claw and digit. Bacterial infection of the remaining digit or foot is possible. High detail dental or digital radiographs may determine if any significant lesions or osteomyelitis is present. Treatment generally involves soaking the digits in isothermal water to moisten and loosen the skin. The gecko is then manually restrained or sedated (in severe cases) to "un-wrap" the skin or remove the digits if the damage is too severe.

"Metabolic Bone Disease"

Leopard geckos are nocturnal as a normal behavior; therefore, they do not need to bask in sunlight for the majority of a daylight cycle to metabolize vitamin D but must instead consume adequate amounts of it as well as calcium in their diets. They have been known to bask sporadically in the wild or in naturalistic enclosures. They will often consume their substrate to obtain enough calcium in their deficient diet which can lead to impactions described below. Insect diets are deficient in calcium and have an inverse calcium:phosphorus ratio (ie, less than 1:1). Insects must be "gut loaded" or dusted with an appropriate calcium and vitamin mix. Alternatively or additionally, a small shallow dish of calcium and vitamin mix may be added to the gecko's enclosure to allow for self feeding of supplement. Many breeders utilize this approach very successfully to maintain colonies in the hundreds of animals.

A leopard gecko with "metabolic bone disease" (MBD) from a total or relative calcium deficiency is the result of nutritional secondary hyperparathyroidism (NSHP). The most common clinical presentation is softened or "rubbery" bones where calcium has been removed in attempt to maintain blood concentrations. The dense bones are replaced with a fibrocartilage matrix in attempt to provide some stability. Unfortunately, the bone becomes distorted and decreases in functionality, especially the mandible which begins to restrict food intact through mechanical malfunction and pain from bending during mastication.

Therapy of NSHP revolves around basic nursing care of caloric supplementation and water intake. Many of these patients are anorexic and require syringe or tube feeding to maintain caloric intake. Artificial diets may be made from insect puree ("cricket and mealworm shake"), chicken baby food mixed 1:1 with liquid replacement diet (Ensure®, Abbott Laboratories, Abbott Park, IL), powdered replacement diet (Carnivore Care, Oxbow Enterprises, Murdock, NE), or a blended commercial insectivore diet (Mazuri® Insectivore Diet, PMI Nutrition International, St Louis, MO). Calcium supplementation is provided through calcium gluconate injections initially to oral calcium supplementation with calcium glubionate.

Sand Impaction

Leopard geckos may be housed on several substrates successfully, but keepers of these geckos should be very diligent in observation and food presentation for those kept on sand or sand alternative. Food items should be offered is shallow dishes to prevent accidental ingestion of sand during food consumption. Some geckos have been known to inappropriately ingest sand as a food substrate (pica). Keepers should monitor the fecal pellets for increased sand by mixing the pellets in water in test tube (or similar) which is parallel to methods used horses for the detection of sand ingestion. Careful observation of the food intake to prevent sand ingestion or early signs of anorexia or abdominal distention may prevent a full impaction.

Impacted leopard geckos may present with anorexia, decrease fecal output, and/or abdominal distention. Radiographs will often reveal radiodense material in the intestines. Abdominal trans-illumination may also reveal dense material in the intestinal tract. If instituted early in the disease process, oral fluid therapy in combination with gastrointestinal prokinetics (ie, metoclopramide, cisapride, fiber) may stimulate sand passage. If the sand has formed a full foreign body impaction, then surgical management of laparotomy with enterotomy to remove the contents is considered.

REFERENCES

1. Bradley T. Coelomitis secondary to intestinal impaction of Calcisand in a leopard gecko, *Eublepharis macularius*. Proc ARAV. 2000; 27.

2. Cranfield MR, Graczyk TK. Cryptosporidiosis. In Mader DR (ed): Reptile Medicine and Surgery. Philadelphia: WB Saunders, 2006, pp 756-762.

3. De Vosjoli P, Tremper R, Klingenburg R. The Herpetoculture of Leopard Geckos: Twenty-seven Generations of Living Art. Mission Viejo, CA: Advanced Visions, 2005; 259pp.

4. Frye FL, Garman RH, et al. Atypical non-alimentary cryptosporidiosis in three lizards. Proc ARAV. 1999; 43-48.

5. Graczyk TK, Cranfield MR, Bostwick EF. Hyperimmune bovine colostrum treatment of moribund leopard geckos (*Eublepharis macularius*) infected with *Cryptosporidium* sp. Vet Res. 1999;30(4):377-82.

6. Taylor MA, Geach MR, Cooley WA. Clinical and pathological observations on natural infections of cryptosporidiosis and flagellate protozoa in leopard geckos (*Eublepharis macularius*). Vet Rec. 1999; 145(24):695-9.

7. Terrell SP, Uhl EW, Funk RS. Proliferative enteritis in leopard geckos (*Eublepharis macularius*) associated with *Cryptosporidium* sp. infection. J Zoo Wildl Med. 2003; 34(1):69-75.

8. Upton SJ, McAllister CT, et al. *Cryptosporidium* spp. in wild and captive reptiles. J of Wildlife Dis. 1989; 25(1):20-30.

9. Xiao L, Ryan UM, et al. Genetic Diversity of *Cryptosporidium* spp. in Captive Reptiles. Appl Environ Microbiol. 2004; 70:891-899.

DRAGONS: FROM MEDIEVAL MYTH TO MODERN MEDICAL MARVEL

Rob L. Coke, DVM
San Antonio Zoo
San Antonio, TX

Inland bearded dragons (*Pogona vitticeps*) or "Beardies" have rapidly been gaining in popularity over the past decade due to their excellent demeanor and moderate size. They started to emerge on the pet scene in the early 1990s in the United States. They have broad requirements in diet and housing that make them attractive to novice and expert keepers alike. Their gentle dispositions, manageable size (up to 24 inches [~61 cm]), variety of colors and patterns (red to orange to yellow; blotched to stripped), hardy constitution, and long life span (>10 years) make them attractive to many a potential reptile owner.

NATURAL HISTORY

Bearded dragons belong to the agamid (Agamidae) family that encompasses many lizard species from Africa around Asia through Australia. The most common species seen in the United States is the inland or central bearded dragon (*P. vitticeps*). There are other species of Pogona that also appear in the pet trade on occasion such as the common or Eastern bearded dragon (*P. barbata*), the Rankin's or Lawson's dragon (*P. henrylawsoni*), and hybrids called "Vittikin" dragons.

The bearded dragon gets its name from the darkened area (more prominent in males) beneath the throat that works in conjunction with bone from the hyoid apparatus to "flare" forward as a means to ward off conspecifics or scare off predators. They will often continue this display with open mouth gaping and hissing. In captivity, the full behavior is often not observed unless during introductions of new individuals to a group or during extreme stress.

Bearded dragons (*Pogona* spp.) inhabit the hot, arid deserts to semi-arid scrub lands of southeastern Australia. They are adept climbers and movers spending their time navigating for basking sites on elevated rocks, or lower tree branches. One could easily find them basking on a fence post in the morning to warm up their core body temperature, and at dusk absorbing heat to maintain their core temperature during the cool nights. During the day, they often will estivate under rocks or in underground burrows. They are diurnal hunters that will search for prey such as opportunistic invertebrates and small vertebrates. As adults, they often forage on local plant leaves, fruits, and flowers.

HUSBANDRY

Juvenile bearded dragons found in most pet shops are approximately 6 inches (15 cm) long. Initially they can be housed in 20-gallon (75 L) or 30-inch (76 cm) long aquaria. However, this will only suffice as housing for a few months (or less if keeping more than one). Eventually the dragon(s) will need to be housed in much larger aquaria such as a 40-gallon (150 L) breeder tank or larger or custom built enclosure. Dragons may be housed in open top enclosures such as plastic tubs or cattle troughs. Large breeding facilities for dragons often house them outdoors in sectioned areas.

Provisions for lighting with ultraviolet light (UV-A and UV-B) need to be provided (12 to 14 hours per day) with special full spectrum fluorescent bulbs or recently developed mercury vapor bulbs designed for reptiles. Temperature gradients should be provided by heat lamps to achieve 85°F to 95°F (29°C to 35°C) with a basking site up to 105° F (< 41°C). Humidity is generally low, but dragons do require some periodic humidity which can be provided though small plastic tubs with a hole access and filled with moist sand, moss, or coir.

They are omnivores with juveniles receiving ~25% of their diet in veggies and adults receiving ~75%. The veggie part of the diet generally consists of ~75% dark green leafy veggies, ~20% color veggies, and ~5% fruits/treats. The rest of the diet is made up of insect prey such as crickets, mealworms, superworms, and waxworms. These insect food items need to be "dusted" with minerals/vitamins or fed with supplements (eg, Gut-Loaded) to fortify the nutritional contents of the insect's gastrointestinal tract. A small dish of water should be provided and changed daily.

Beaded Dragons become sexually mature at one to two years of age depending on juvenile grown rates and time of year hatched. Male dragons can be differentiated from females by more prominent femoral pores, wider head, and darker throat patch. Female dragons may lay a few eggs up to several dozen eggs per clutch several times during the breeding season.

OTHER DRAGONS

There are other famous dragons from the mythological (Chinese and medieval Europe lineages) to the mystical Puff the Magic Dragon. Closer to reality we have many "dragon" species that can be kept in captivity.

The Chinese water dragon (*Physignathus cocincinus*) has been around the pet trade for decades and is still popularly found in pet stores. They may live to around 15 years of age and may obtain a length up to ~36 inches (~91 cm). They are diurnal omnivores. Their diet consists mainly of insect prey with weekly offerings of a veggie mix.

Frilled dragons (*Chlamydosaurus kingii*) are unique in that they possess a larger (up to 12 inches (~30 cm)) cervical skinfold that encircles the neck that can be erected like a fan and vibrated to ward off enemies. They can reach total lengths up to ~30 inches (~75 cm) and require large enclosures with ample room for climbing. They are diurnal and insectivorous.

Recently the Mountain Horned dragon (*Acanthosaura capra*) has been imported in large numbers into the United States. They may obtain lengths up to around ~12 inches (~30 cm). They are diurnal insectivores. They need moderate humidity and climbing space. Most of the individuals seen in pet stores are wild caught and may contain numerous internal/external parasites.

Komodo dragons (*Varanus komodoensis*) are monitor species and generally only kept in zoological institutions or found in their natural habitat on the island of Komodo (and surrounding islands) in Indonesia. They are one of the most recognizable lizards in the world due to their large size of 6 to 10 feet (2 to 3 meters) and ~150 lbs (~70 kg), voracious appetite, and severe bacterial infections from their saliva in bite wounds.

CURRENT TOPICS OF MEDICAL CONDITIONS

There are many diseases noted in bearded dragons with each year bringing a better understanding of the etiology and the impact of co-factors such as husbandry and nutrition. This increase in knowledge will continue to grow and develop better diagnostics and therapeutics. Here are examples of just a few of the most significant and currently investigated diseases in bearded dragons:

Adenovirus

Although adenovirus (Agamid adenovirus 1 [AAdV1]) in bearded dragons has been noted for many years, the full significance and prevalence is recently becoming more evident. Adenoviruses are one of the larger, unenveloped DNA viruses. They are fairly resistant in the environment and require strict hygiene and extreme disinfection methods to control the spread of the virus.

Adenovirus infection has been noted in several Pogona species, such as the inland, common, and Rankin's dragons. It is unknown at this time if there are multiple strains of the virus present in the captive population or if the virus can be passed on to the offspring through the egg during egg deposition. Viral infections have been also noted co-infections with a dependovirus and coccidiosis. The disease state is also affected by other factors such as stressors from abnormal husbandry or nutrition. Most of the clinical cases have been noted in juveniles less than 12 weeks of age presenting with acute weakness and lethargy. The clinical course may progress to head tilting, circling posture, and eventually death. Histopathologic lesions of basophilic, intranuclear inclusions include hepatitis, enteritis, splenitis, esophagitis, and encephalitis.

Polymerase chain reaction (PCR) of cloacal swabs appears to be the most sensitive and currently the best diagnostic test modality. Blood is a poor sample choice due to low rate of viremia. Electron microscopy of the feces to look for viral particles is possible but is not very sensitive test when compared with PCR. Presence of virus in cloacal swabs is indicative of active viral shedding that subsequently contaminates the environment. Also, the presence of viral DNA does not necessarily indicate active clinical disease but may indicate a subclinical infection/carrier state.

Coccidiosis

Coccidiosis (*Isospora amphiboluri*) in bearded dragons is one if not the most common clinical diagnosis in bearded dragons. It is also one of the most frustrating diseases to manage for the veterinarian and the owner. The sporulated oocysts are about round to ovoid and 25 microns in diameter. The oocysts can be observed through direct microscopic examination of the feces and through classic concentration methods through floatation and/or centrifugation.

Classic coccidiostatic drugs (ie, sulfadimethoxine, amprolium, trimethoprim-sulfa) are effective in cessation of shedding but after the drugs are removed the shedding returns. Shedding adults will often be asymptomatic to periodic bouts of loose stools to anorexia. Neonates and juveniles may present with more severe changes and clinical disease may progress to death. Since traditional methods of therapy have not been effective, alternative natural methods such as oregano in the diet have been tried but found ineffective.

Coccidiocidal drugs are being investigated but no pharmacokinetic data have been published for any of these compounds. A recent abstract was presented using 15% ponazuril paste (Marquis®, Bayer Health Care, LLC, Shawnee Mission, KS) at 30 mg/kg PO every 48 hours for two treatments in bearded dragons. This drug has been on the market for several years for treatment of equine protozoal myeloencephalitis (EPM). No full investigation on side effects or toxic effects has been done for this drug in reptiles but the author reports clinical resolution of clinical signs and fecal shedding for up to a year.

Dermatitis

A skin condition bearded dragons known as "yellow fungus disease" (YFD) has been noted for the past few years by breeders and herpetoculturalists. Recent work in investigating this disease has determined that this pathology is related to *Chrysosporium* anamorph of *Nannizziopsis vriesii* (CANV), which is a ketatinophilic fungal disease that has been found to be pathologic to several reptile species. The clinical disease presents as a yellow discoloration to scaling of the dorsal skin (and ventrum). The lesions may become darker and necrotic then progress to a deeper dermal mycosis (granulomatous dermatomycosis). The disease has been noted to progress even further as a systemic mycosis with lesions in the internal organs such as the liver.

Therapy for fungal disease can be difficult due to the underlying causes or stressors that need to be corrected in conjunction with antifungal administration. Once the husbandry factors have been addressed and the patient has been stabilized with basic nursing care, then initiation of various antifungal medications either topical or systemic may begin. Itraconazole is currently the drug of choice for combating filamentous fungi such as CANV. Terbinafine has been used in avian medicine routinely for Aspergillosis, but no pharmacokinetic trials have been published in reptiles. Topical medications such as miconazole or clotrimazole may be used on superficial lesions. Deeper more extensive lesions may require surgical debridement and postoperative wound management.

REFERENCES

1. Bogoslavsky BA. The use of ponazuril to treat coccidiosis in eight inland bearded dragons (*Pogona vitticeps*). Proc ARAV. 2007; 8-9.

2. Bowman MR, Paré JA, et al. Deep fungal dermatitis in three inland bearded dragons (*Pogona vitticeps*) caused by the *Chrysosporium* anamorph of *Nannizziopsis vriesii*. Med Mycol. 2007; 45(4):371-6.

3. De Vosjoli P, Mailloux R, *et al.* The Bearded Dragon Manual. Mission Viejo, CA: Advanced Vivarium Systems, 2001, 174pp.

4. Johnson DH. An emerging dermatomycosis and systemic mycosis syndrome in bearded dragons. Exotic DVM. 2004; 6(3):75.

5. Kim DY, Mitchell MA, et al. An outbreak of adenoviral infection in inland bearded dragons (*Pogona vitticeps*) coinfected with dependovirus and coccidial protozoa *(Isospora* sp.). J Vet Diagn Invest. 2002; 14:332-334.

6. McAllister CT, Upton SJ, et al. A description of *Isospora amphiboluri* (Apicomplexa: Eimeriidae) from the inland bearded dragon, *Pogona vitticeps* (Sauria: Agamidae). J Parasitol. 1995; 81(2):281-4.

7. Mitchell MA. Evaluating oregano as a coccidiocide in the inland bearded dragon (*Pogona vitticeps*). Proc ARAV. 2003; 53.

8. Paré JA, Sigler L, et al. Microbiology: Fungal and bacterial diseases of reptiles. In Mader DR (ed): Reptile Medicine and Surgery. Philadelphia: WB Saunders, 2006, pp 217-238.

9. Wagner R, Dahlhausen R, Klein E. The detection of adenovirus infections in bearded dragons (*Pogona vitticeps*) with real time PCR. Proc ARAV. 2007; 19-22.

10. Wellehan JFX, Johnson AJ, et al. Detection and analysis of six lizard adenoviruses by consensus primer PCR provides further evidence of a reptilian origin for the Atadenoviruses. J Virol. 2004; 78:13366-13369.

CHAMELEONS: TECHNICOLOR BIOLOGY IN ACTION

Rob L. Coke, DVM
San Antonio Zoo
San Antonio, TX

NATURAL HISTORY

Old World Chameleons have long fascinated humankind with their independently rotating eyes, lightning fast tongues, and psychedelic color changes. Over the past few decades, chameleons have been kept as a temporary pet—living from a month to a couple of years. Within the last decade, increased information regarding proper nutrition, environmental conditions, and breeding has led to longer life spans with individual chameleons reaching 10 years old. Accompanying the increase in information, a multitude of captive-bred animals has entered the pet trade. Below are summaries of the three most commonly seen chameleons in the pet trade:

Panther Chameleon (*Furcifer pardalis*)

The Panther, or jungle, chameleon originates from the northern part of Madagascar. They are one of the most colorful chameleons sporting an array of colors from green to blue to red. They thrive in warm, humid climates with a moderate seasonal fluctuation in temperature. In the wild, they live in scrub forests (trees and shrubs up to three meters tall) and on the edge of larger forests. These chameleons are one of the species that are repopulating the areas where the rain forest has been destroyed. They are fiercely territorial, especially during breeding season. Their vibrant colors and hardiness are contributing to the increase in sales and captive ownership.

Veiled Chameleon (*Chamaeleo calyptratus*)

The veiled chameleon is indigenous to the Yemen coast of Saudi Arabia. This environment is a mixture of extremes ranging from the arid desert to the temperate mountains. These chameleons are generally a hardy species because they can tolerate either extreme; however, they do best somewhere in between these ranges. Among themselves, veiled chameleons are one of the most aggressive species; but towards humans, they are one of the calmer species. These are the hardiest of these chameleon species and make terrific pets.

Jackson's Chameleon (*Chamaeleo jacksonii xantholophus*)

The male Jackson's chameleon has three ominous looking horns protruding from his forehead. This variety of chameleon originates in Kenya. The Jackson's chameleon was recently introduced to Hawaii in the 1970s. The Hawaiian Islands support a thriving population of these chameleons even today. They are a true montane species coming from mountainous areas that have temperate days and cool nights. Therefore, they must not get too hot or too dry for prolonged periods.

MEDICAL HISTORY

A detailed and thorough history is invaluable in determining any potential disease in chameleons. Each client should complete a detailed history form containing questions on the caging, diet, prior medical history, etc. A client should be able to recall with some specificity the temperature ranges, cage dimensions, brand of lighting, and cage decorations.

A chameleon's diet plays a major role in its health. The veterinarian should not only elicit the types of food items (eg, crickets, superworms, waxworms) but also the percentages of each item eaten by the chameleon. The veterinarian should determine if the prey items have been "gut loaded," that is, fed calcium and vitamin-rich food sources. Are the prey items dusted with any supplements? If so, what products or brands?

EXAMINATION

As with any animal species, a thorough, systematic approach to the examination will provide clues to an appropriate diagnosis. Chameleons have sharp claws and the larger species have a noticeable bite. The patient should be examined for general demeanor as it climbs on a perch, and it should be restrained for the rest of the exam by grasping the head by the thumb and forefinger behind the eyes. This approach will enable control of the head. The palm of the hand should rest along the back allowing the fingers to catch the chameleon's feet.

DISEASES AND THERAPEUTICS
Eyes

Enophthalmia is a very common indicator of disease in chameleons. It is usually combined with other signs such as anorexia, dehydration, or emaciation. The "sunken eyes" are generally a poor prognostic indicator. Exophthalmia is another common sign of disease in chameleons. The swelling can come from the globe itself, the surrounding conjunctiva, or the retrobulbar space. The globe can increase in size due to uveitis or panophthalmitis and is best treated with systemic antibiotics to provide better antibiotic levels in the intraocular tissues.

Corneal damage can come from trauma secondary to shipping or aggression. Superficial lesions are responsive to topical treatments with common ophthalmic antibiotic preparations. Deep corneal lesions or lacerations may require enucleation if medical or surgical options fail. Due to the visual impairment even with mild disease, the chameleon is often anorexic, and supportive care (including syringe-feeding or hand-feeding) may need to be initiated.

If the globe of the eye looks normal, then the surrounding structures need to be addressed. Parasites that have migrating larval stages will sometimes stop within the conjunctival tissues, retrobulbar tissues, intraocular space, or the conjunctival sac. Surgical removal of the parasites may provide relief and return to normal visual function. Typical parasiticides may not completely remove these parasites and may cause toxic reactions from the decaying parasites. Conjunctival or retrobulbar abscesses may cause intense swelling around the eye. The infection may come from the conjunctiva itself or as an ascending stomatitis infection from the nasolacrimal duct. The abscess should be drained and cleaned with dilute chlorhexidine. The chameleon should be placed on broad-spectrum antibiotics preferably based on culture and sensitivity reports.

Oral Cavity

Chameleons naturally have pigmented gingiva. Many species of wild-caught chameleons have very xanthic (yellow) oral gingiva. Most captive-bred chameleons do not have the same degree of pigmentation and may be gray to pink in color. The variability in their normal coloration may be misinterpreted as a disease condition such as icterus or shock. The lateral commissures of the mouth have glands that produce a very musky, waxy residue that aids in fly/prey attraction. These areas need to be checked and periodically cleaned due to propensity to become infected.

Chameleons have a very primitive acrodont dentition, which is also found in frilled lizards (*Chlamydosaurus kingii*), bearded dragons (*Pogona* spp.), and water dragons (*Physignathus lesueurii*). The teeth are not within sockets but attached to the dorsal surface of the mandible and maxilla. This type of dentition seems to be predisposed to periodontal disease. Once the teeth are damaged, they are not replaced, unless the damage occurs while the chameleon is a very young juvenile. Care must be exercised with oral speculums not to damage the dental arcade.

Mild cases of periodontal disease may present as erythema to the gingiva or recession of the gum line. More severe cases can develop into stomatitis or even osteomyelitis. Stomatitis may also develop from infections by opportunistic pathogens from other causes such as stress, inappropriately decreased environmental temperatures, poor nutrition, or trauma. These underlying conditions need to be corrected before appropriate treatment can begin to work. Severe abscesses and deep lesions need to be cleaned and/or surgically debrided. In some cases, the area of the mandible will need to be debrided or even the rostral aspect removed. The cytology of the lesions should be examined to aid in determining an etiology. Organisms such as some anaerobes and *Mycobacteria* are more difficult to isolate in the laboratory, and cytology may be the only certain means for diagnosis. Organisms such as *Aeromonas*, *Pseudomonas*, and *Klebsiella* are commonly cultured from stomatitis lesions. The most important part of the culture is determining the sensitivities. The sensitivity helps determine antibiotic treatment. The appropriate antibiotic will need to be used for an extended period from 12 to 16 weeks. Follow-up cultures and sensitivities may need to be performed if the lesions do not heal in an appropriate amount of time.

The chameleon has a modified hyoid bone (entoglossal process) that acts as a firing pin for the projectile tongue. The tongue is accordion folded along the conical shaped bone. When firing, the accelerator muscle will contract down along the bone projecting the tongue towards its prey at over 5 meters per second. The tongue can extend roughly the length of the chameleon's body. The tip of the tongue contains a muscular tongue pad that contains microscopic ridges similar to the toe pads of arboreal geckos. The tongue pad contains glands that secrete mucin to aid in sticking to the prey. The lingual surfaces of the mandibular mucosa also contain glands that produce saliva that coats the outer surface of the tongue pad. The tongue pad also contains muscles (longitudinal adductor muscles) that contract to "grip" the prey. Once the tongue attaches to the prey item, the lateral surfaces of the tongue contain retractor muscles (hyoglossal muscles) that retract the tongue back over the entoglossal process.

This complex lingual system is prone to injury and can cause considerable morbidity. Most injuries come from infection or trauma. Injuries may come from trauma from the rough prey surface or prey bites. These injures under normal conditions should heal on their own. Under abnormal conditions, such as suboptimal temperatures or systemic disease, opportunistic bacteria may form lingual abscesses. These abscesses need to be opened and the chameleon placed on appropriate broad-spectrum antibiotics determined through culture and sensitivity results.

Trauma to the tongue can be due to muscle strain from hyperextension. A chameleon may miss the prey and attach to a fixed object (eg, cage wire or branch). The chameleon will attempt to contract the tongue but it is still attached to the fixed object. This causes micro tears in the delicate muscles. Most chameleons will then make subsequent attempts to snare prey and will either not be able to extend the tongue or weakly shoot part of the way. These chameleons need to rest from all attempts at remote capture of prey. These chameleons need 2 to 6 weeks of direct hand feeding. Direct hand feeding is presenting the prey item within 2 to 5 cm of the head. Sometimes presenting the prey inside the cage through the wire mesh is beneficial and may not stress the chameleon. Once the chameleon seems able to obtain prey easily in this manner then the distance can be slowly increased until normal distances are reached.

Musculoskeletal

Noninfectious diseases of the musculoskeletal system are common in chameleons. Metabolic bone disease (MBD) is one of the most common forms seen in practice. Clinical signs include lethargy, deformed/curled limbs, "rubber-jaw," stunted growth, or even death. MBD most commonly is the result of a nutritional secondary hyperparathyroidism (NSHP) resulting from a multi-factorial disease affecting calcium metabolism. The major contributing factors of MBD include insufficient dietary calcium supplementation, lack of available UV light source, insufficient vitamin D3, and excess of dietary phosphorus. Treatment of this form of MBD follows the same guidelines established for other lizard species. The goal of treatment is to establish a positive calcium balance by proper supplementation of calcium/vitamin D3 and exposure to UV light.

Other causes of noninfectious musculoskeletal disease include neuropathies and fractures. Neurologic diseases in chameleons are rare. Chameleons may allow one limb to dangle while resting on a branch. Some chameleons do this with no signs of physical disease. Others do this as early signs of gout or joint disease. Some wild-caught chameleons may have fractures or related soft tissue injuries. In the wild, the native collectors usually grasp the chameleon and force it from its branch. When the chameleon is out of reach, the collectors will use long bamboo shafts to beat and knock them off branches. Many of these injuries are associated with the carpal and tarsal joints. These injuries may be healed thru restrictive activity and possible splinting. Long bone fractures (non-pathologic) in chameleons are not very common due to their structural design, lightweight, and agility. Most fractures arise from traumatic falls or intraspecies aggression. These fractures may be healed by lightweight external fixation.

Osteomyelitis is a very devastating disease in chameleons. One of the most common locations is the mandible (described above). Untreated fractures, bite wounds, thermal burns, or joint injuries may lead to localized infections that spread into the bone or joints. Diagnosis can be derived from cytology or biopsy of the lesions. Use of different stains such as Wright's stain, gram stain, or acid-fast may rule in or out different causes such as bacterial, fungal, neoplastic, parasitic, or mycobacterial. Aggressive therapy is needed for these cases. Initial treatment lies with aggressive surgical debridement and deep antiseptic wound cleansing. In bacterial infections, a culture and sensitivity is extremely valuable in antibiotic selection. Treatment with appropriate antibiotics generally lasts for a minimum of 8 to 12 weeks and may last for 6 months. Even with appropriate treatment, amputation of the bone/limb may be required.

Genitourinary

The current market today in chameleons mainly revolves around breeding. This widespread breeding effort has led to an increased number of reproductive problems. One of the more common reproductive problems is dystocia or egg binding. Several improper husbandry factors have been identified as contributing factors. Some of the most common factors are an improper nesting site, lack of a nesting site, or inadequate nutrition (ie, calcium deficiency, decreased vitamin A). Other physical factors attributable to dystocia include uterine diseases, such as infection, stricture, rupture, torsion, or doubled egg.

The diagnosis of dystocia may be made through physical examination and radiographs. Differentiation of pre- or post-ovulatory stasis must be determined prior to medical treatment. Pre-ovulatory stasis may be treated with supportive care or surgical intervention; and if initiated early in the disease process, medical therapy may avert surgical intervention. Samples should be collected for evaluation, including complete blood cell count (CBC) and plasma biochemistries. Radiographs may be used to determine the cause of dystocia as well as assist in determining if the female is in pre- or post-ovulatory stasis. Any problems found in the diagnostics, such as dehydration or hypocalcemia, should be corrected prior to medical or surgical intervention.

REFERENCES

1. Barrie MT. Chameleon medicine. In Fowler ME, and Miller RE (eds): Zoo & Wild Animal Medicine: Current Therapy 4. Philadelphia: WB Saunders, 1999; pp 200-205.

2. Barten SL. Lizards. In Mader DR (ed): Reptile Medicine and Surgery. Philadelphia: WB Saunders, 2006; 683-95.

3. Coke RL. Old World Chameleons: Captive care and breeding. Bull Assoc Rept Amphib Vet. 1998;8(2):4-10.

PHARYNGOSTOMY TUBE PLACEMENT IN LIZARDS

Rob L. Coke, DVM
San Antonio Zoo
San Antonio, TX

INDICATIONS

Anorexia is a common disorder of reptiles. There are many facets of this condition that should be addressed by clinician and reptile owner. The background etiology includes a large list of problems and diseases beyond the full scope of this clinical topic.

Some species of lizards are anatomically designed in such a way that makes force feeding difficult or dangerous to the patient or caregiver. The strong jaw muscles of spiny tail lizards (*Uromastyx* spp.) and blue-tongue skinks (*Tiliqua* spp.) can make it nearly impossible to force their mouths open for syringe feeding. Many gecko species also have relatively strong jaw muscles, but the thin bones of their skull predispose them to fractures if their mouths are forcibly opened. Many of the larger monitor species (*Varanus* spp.) and iguana species (*Cyclura* spp.) have sharp teeth that can inflict severe damage to the person trying to force feed. The two venomous species of lizards, the Gila monster (*Heloderma suspectum*) and the Mexican beaded lizard (*Heloderma horridum*), are kept as pets/breeders throughout various parts of the United States. They pose an even greater challenge due to their strong jaw muscles and venomous bite.

Other conditions may require the use of a pharyngostomy tube in the nutritional management of a patient. A fracture of the maxilla or mandible may require fixation that may cause discomfort too great to masticate or a full-mouth fixation that prohibits opening of the oral cavity. Myositis, neuritis, or abscesses that involve the muscles of mastication may also require the use of a pharyngostomy tube to allow for caloric intake.

PROCEDURE

Typically, the patent is sedated or anesthetized for the procedure. In extreme cases, a local anesthetic protocol could be used in a severely debilitated patent but should be limited to such emergency cases. The patient can be masked for sedation with isoflurane or sevoflurane. Alternatively, propofol may be used intravenously for a period of short sedation for tube placement, radiographs, or phlebotomy. Monitoring equipment (eg, pulse oximetry, electrocardiography) should be used to evaluate the patient under sedation. Analgesics such as opioids or nonsteroidal anti-inflammatory drugs (NSAIDs) should be used appropriately depending on the status of the patient.

- The patient is placed in sternal or left lateral recumbency depending on the clinician's preference.
- The distance from the proposed pharyngostomy incision to the stomach is measured externally and marked on the tube.
- An appropriately sized curved mosquito hemostat is placed in the oral cavity.
- The tip of the hemostat is placed in the ventro-lateral aspect of the pharynx/neck. A scalpel blade is used to make a small skin incision, followed by soft issue dissection to exteriorize the hemostat. **NOTE:** Be careful not to cut the jugular vein which lies near the area.
- The end of the red rubber catheter is grasped with the hemostats and pulled through the oral cavity until the predefined length is reached.
- The tube is then reflected back into the mouth, down the esophagus, and into the stomach.
- A small section of white medical tape is attached to the red rubber catheter in a butterfly fashion to allow attachment of the tube to the patient. Preferably, the tape/tube is secured to the back of the lizard with nonabsorbable sutures. Alternatively suture material attached to the skin can then be attached to the feeding tube in a finger trap serried of knots.
- An intravenous (IV) injection cap is placed over the end of the red rubber catheter to seal the end.
- The patient should recover quickly and be able to move about shortly after the procedure.

AFTERCARE

Advantages of the pharyngostomy tube are the exact control over caloric intake/monitoring and the patient can eat around the feeding tube when it is ready to eat on its own. Unfortunately, the patient may not tolerate the tube by pulling it out, develop a local infection around the stoma, or food may clog the tube requiring multiple replacements. The natural diet of the patient should be considered to help select diet substitution items that can be passed through a small diameter tube:

- Carnivores are fed blended prey items (eg, rodent slurry) or tube fed a powdered replacement diet (Carnivore Care, Oxbow Enterprises, Murdock, NE).
- Herbivores may be fed a mixed veggie baby food mixed 1:1 with liquid replacement diet (Ensure®, Abbott Laboratories, Abbott Park, IL) or better a powdered replacement diet (Herbivore Care, Oxbow Enterprises, Murdock, NE).
- Omnivores may be fed a mixture of the herbivore diet above and the insectivore diet below.
- Insectivores may require actual insect prey items ("cricket and mealworm shake"), chicken baby food mixed 1:1 with liquid replacement diet (Ensure), powdered replacement diet (Carnivore Care), or a blended commercial insectivore diet (Mazuri® Insectivore Diet, PMI Nutrition International, St Louis, MO).

For further discussion on caloric requirements and/or other feeding recipes, please refer to the Nutrition chapter in Mader's *Reptile Medicine and Surgery*.

REFERENCES

1. Donoghue S. Nutrition. In Mader DR (ed): Reptile Medicine and Surgery. Philadelphia: WB Saunders, 2006, pp 251-298.

2. Coke RL. Pharyngostomy tube placement in a veiled chameleon. Exotic DVM. 2002;4(4):9-10.

OCULONASAL FLUSH IN CHAMELEONS

Rob L. Coke, DVM
San Antonio Zoo
San Antonio, TX

BIOLOGY

Old World chameleons (*Chamaeleo* spp.) have long fascinated humans due to their unique biology. Science has been fascinated with chameleons for the past century for their unique biology that is not seen in any other terrestrial vertebrate. The eyes of the chameleon act independently searching for prey. They rotate like turrets moving about 180° in the horizontal plane and 80° in the vertical plane. They are capable of spotting prey by scanning in short, rapid bursts called *saccadic movements*. The chameleon is unable to see well at night due to all cone retinas. This in combination with a deep fovea allows the chameleon to have excellent diurnal vision. The chameleon's lens is negatively powered which acts similar to a telephoto lens of a camera. The chameleon uses this optical power of each eye independently to triangulate the distance to the prey by the amount of accommodation. As the tracking progresses, the chameleon rotates both eyes towards its prey. The combination of accommodation and focus ability makes the chameleon one of the most accurate of all vertebrates. Clinical conditions involving the eye of the chameleon are one of the most frustrating conditions to pet owners and veterinarians alike. This condition is more of a syndrome of multiple etiologies than direct clinical sign with pathognomonic diagnosis.

ETIOLOGY

There have been a wide variety of etiologies proposed but none have been definitively proven. Chronic deficiency in vitamin A in the diet has been identified as one of the major factors of eye problems in chameleons. Historically, a non-peer reviewed article in a lay publication identified an edema condition with a commercial supplement that had "high" levels of vitamin A added to the diet in a small group of chameleons. This created fervor in the fledgling reptile supplement market to avoid preformed vitamin A and use its metabolic precursor beta-carotene instead. Without nutrition studies to evaluate the proper levels of vitamin A for all reptilian species, this issue remains unclear. Various veterinarians in the years following this "change" have started seeing an increase of ocular conditions. Although there have been some histopathologic reports to support a common diagnosis of squamous metaplasia secondary to hypovitaminosis A, not all reports do so. During the clinical examination, the clinician should take a very detailed nutritional history including prey items consumed and the brand and frequency of supplementation.

Exposure to various irritants also has been implicated in ocular problems. The manner of "watering" down enclosures may cause physical damage by pressure of the "jet' stream or temperature of the water from the spray hose (ie, too hot or too cold). Many chameleon husbandry texts recommend the use of live plants in the enclosure such as *Ficus* or *Pothos*. These plants produce a topical residue of insoluble oxalates. When misted, the water will pick up the oxalate compound which may be consumed or topically exposed to the eyes causing microscopic irritation. Increased frequency or times of "misting" the enclosures will help remove much of this material through dilution. Cleaning disinfectants (ie, bleach) should be thoroughly flushed after cage disinfection to avoid contact with the chameleon. Foreign debris such as sand or dust may also cause mechanical irritation once inside the conjunctival sac.

Other husbandry factors that may be negatively involved include improper temperature/humidity, decreased enclosure ventilation (ie, glass aquaria), and lack of exposure to sunlight. Watering systems must be periodically flushed and disinfected to remove organic buildup of mold and bacteria. Proper enclosures should be spacious with good ventilation with a means for proper temperature, humidity, and ultraviolet light (ie, natural sunlight, full-spectrum bulbs, or both).

EXAMINATION

A thorough ophthalmic examination by the clinician is required to determine the extent of disease or damage to the eyes. A complete physical examination, complete blood cell count (CBC), and biochemistry panel is also essential to determine concurrent diseases or signs that may have a significant impact on the presented ocular condition. The small eyelid opening relative to the eye globe makes the examination of the full extent of the sclera difficult. The cornea can be evaluated directly but may need microscopic evaluation via surgical head loops or ophthalmic instruments for a more complete assessment. Corneal staining under magnification is also beneficial to determine the level of damage present. Samples for cytology and aerobic cultures are collected at this time prior to flushing or therapeutics. Greatly distended tissues may require anesthesia (with analgesics) to obtain deep surgical samples. Radiographs of the head may reveal additional involvement of the soft tissue and areas of bone lysis due to invading osteomyelitis. Use of a digital radiograph system designed for dentistry is capable of ultra-detail images that can be manipulated to evaluate various densities of tissues as well as easily obtaining multiple image captures of various angles to determine if there is any evidence of bone involvement.

The initial stages of eye problems are often overlooked by owner and clinician. The chameleon may casually start rubbing its eyes on branches and leaves due to slight irritation of the conjunctiva. This will progress to a slight per-ocular edema with 0- to 2-mm ring around the orbital rim. As the condition progresses, crusting from serous to mucoid discharge will be noted around the tiny eyelids. The swelling will continue to progress until the one eye (or both) has fully filled with edema or purulent material from bacterial invasion. Due to the edema from the pressure or abscessation, the eyelids may rupture and drain. The eye globe during this time has sclera and conjunctival inflammation. The cornea may or may not have ulcerations due to mechanical trauma from rubbing. An alternative scenario seen by the author is a "dry" form where the conjunctival space is inflamed with debris but mostly desiccated with minimal eyelid swelling.

THERAPEUTICS

After the examination and clinical samples are collected, any abnormal findings should be addressed. The conjunctival space should be rinsed with an ophthalmic irrigating solution to remove any foreign, squamous, or inflammatory debris. The clinician should note if any of the solution is draining through the nasolacrimal duct. The nasolacrimal opening is located near the conjunctival fornix along the orbital rim at around the 8 (left side) or 4 (right side) o'clock margins. The nasolacrimal duct runs from the internal opening, through the inside of maxilla, and out to an opening inside the inner choanal space. If no or too little solution is noted, then consider the procedure below.

An oculonasal or nasolacrimal flush may be of benefit in cases of conjunctivitis to remove any excessive cellular debris or foreign material in the conjunctival space out the eyelid opening or nasolacrimal duct. Use of ophthalmic irrigation solution may be applied directly to the eyelid opening under digital pressure or through the assistance of a blunt tip nasolacrimal cannula, an olive tip tom cat urethral cannula, a very small metal ball tip feeding tube, or a small diameter soft tip rubber catheter. This cannula or catheter is attached to a syringe filled with irrigating solution and placed inside the eyelid opening, directed away from the cornea to avoid any damage. The fluid is injected in the space allowing the fluid and any debris to flow out the eyelid space. To flush the nasolacrimal duct, light digital pressure is applied to the eyelids to close them around the injection tube. Pressure is applied to the syringe plunger to force excess fluid into the conjunctival space hoping to dislodge any remaining material as well as force any debris stuck in the nasolacrimal duct to pass through allowing for proper drainage. The chameleon's head is placed in a downward position to avoid aspiration or drowning. Fluid from the internal choanal slit may be collected for cytologic or microbiologic analysis, if not already done so. In cases of suspected bacterial involvement, commercial liquid ophthalmic antibiotics (such as ciprofloxacin, gentamicin, or tobramycin) may be flushed in a similar manner.

Management of ocular conditions in Old World chameleons is difficult but plausible with aggressive case management. When used early in the disease process, it may prevent ocular or orbital damage and allows a non-surgical means of removing foreign debris from the conjunctival space and clearing the nasolacrimal duct. In severe cases, surgical exploration of the conjunctiva, abscess removal, and biopsies may be required in addition to medication. Nutritional support is often also required as many of these patients are visually impaired bilaterally.

REFERENCES

1. Barrie MT. Chameleon medicine. In Fowler ME, Miller RE (eds): Zoo & Wild Animal Medicine: Current Therapy 4. Philadelphia: WB Saunders, 1999, pp 200-205.
2. Coke RL. Old World Chameleons: Captive care and breeding. Bull Assoc Rept Amphib Vet. 1998;8(2):4-10.
3. Coke RL, Carpenter JW. Use of ocular/nasolacrimal flushes for treating periocular swelling in Old World chameleons. Exotic DVM. 2001;3(5):14-15.
4. Coke RL, Couillard NK. Ocular biology and diseases of Old World chameleons (Chamaeleonidae). Vet Clin North Am: Exotic Anim Pract. 2002;5(2):275-285.
5. Ott M, Schaeffel F. A negatively powered lens in the chameleon. Nature. 1995;373:692-694.

BASIC HUSBANDRY AND NUTRITION OF SNAKES

Orlando Diaz-Figueroa, DVM, MS
Diplomate ABVP (Avian Practice)
Lake Howell Animal Clinic, Maitland, FL

The snake has long been a contradictory species: you either love them or hate them. In the United States, these reptiles are popular pets. There is also a significant amount of energy placed into developing captive breeding programs to produce different color morphs for many species. In some cases, such as the ball pythons (*Python regius*), these color morphs can sell for $20,000 to $30,000 dollars each. In comparison to domestic mammals, snakes are long-lived. It is not uncommon for corn snakes (*Elaphe guttata guttata*) to live for 15 to 25 years and for ball pythons to live 35 to 45 years. Because of the longevity and value of these animals, more snakes are being presented to the veterinarian to manage medical and surgical problems, as well as for routine medical care. Veterinary personnel working with snakes should familiarize themselves with the specific husbandry and medical requirements of these animals so that they can make informed decisions regarding their management.

HOUSING REQUIREMENTS

Snakes are ectotherms and depend on the environmental temperature to regulate their **preferred body temperature (PBT)**. The PBT varies with species, age, season, and even time of day and is the temperature at which metabolism is optimal. The **preferred optimum temperature zone** (POTZ) is the temperature range that permits the reptile to achieve the PBT and should therefore be provided, if the snake is hospitalized, by the thermal gradient in the hospital vivarium. It is imperative that from the beginning, veterinarians are aware that behavior, physiology, pathology, and therapies are greatly influenced by temperature. Ophidia should be provided a secure enclosure that is large enough to establish an environmental temperature range that is appropriate for that species. The use of external heat sources (incandescent bulbs, infrared ceramics, heating pads or mats, warming cables, tubular heaters, convectors heaters, and natural sunlight radiation) which mimic radiant heat from the sun, are the preferred method for establishing the environmental temperature. In general, temperate and tropical species tolerate daytime ranges between 78°F and 86°F, whereas desert species generally tolerate a temperature range from 85 °F to 92°F. Evening environmental temperatures should be reduced by 10 °F to 15°F. Humidity is also an important environmental condition to monitor. Snakes maintained in low humidity environments may be predisposed to dehydration. Excessive humidity is frequently associated with dermatitis. Humidity levels should be based on the animal's natural history. In general, desert species tolerate humidity levels between 30% and 50%, subtropical species from 60% to 80%, and tropical species from 80% to 90%.

The shape and size of the enclosure should be selected based on the snake's biology. For example, a fossorial species should be housed in an enclosure that is long and wide. The height of the enclosure would not be as important for a fossorial species. In contrast, an arboreal species should be housed in a tall enclosure to ensure ample foliage can be placed into the enclosure. Because obesity is a common problem in large captive snakes, snakes should be provided ample area with an enclosure for physical activity.

Venomous snakes should be housed in enclosures that have restricted access to non-essential individuals. The enclosures should have two locking mechanisms, in case one locking mechanism fails. The enclosure should be designed so that the snake can be visualized from the outside of the enclosure. There should always be at least two people involved with the handling of a venomous snake. Appropriate tongs, hooks and collection tubes should be available for handling venomous snakes. Large, easy-to-read VENOMOUS SNAKE signs should be placed on the external walls of the enclosure. An emergency phone should be placed in the vicinity of the venomous snake enclosures with essential contact numbers. An anti-venom protocol should be developed with a local hospital.

All snakes should be quarantined for a minimum of 3 months prior to being introduced into a reptile collection. However, even a 3-month quarantine may be insufficient time to detect certain viral or bacterial diseases in which a snake is a latent carrier/subclinical. A thorough physical examination and appropriate diagnostic screening assays (eg, complete blood count, paramyxovirus titers) should be performed before the snake is placed into quarantine and prior to removing the animal from quarantine.

Vivarium

Glass aquaria are commonly used. Glass is a poor insulator and greater heat loss may lead to drastic temperature fluctuations. Plastic-coated wooden enclosures are popular, because they are more versatile by permitting the incorporation of additional ventilation panels, front access by sliding glass doors, and greater security. More recently, plastic and fiberglass enclosures are increasingly in demand. Their main advantage is that they can be thoroughly cleaned and disinfected without the risk of moisture damage associated with wooden enclosures.

Lighting

Most snakes do not have any significant requirement for broad or full-spectrum lighting.

Humidity

Humidity tends to be a function of temperature, water surface area, and ventilation. The major problem in most cases is the view that ventilation must be decreased to increase humidity. Consequently, such action result in stagnant air and an increase in bacterial and fungal infections, especially the integument, and the respiratory system. It is better to maintain ventilation and regulate humidity by providing a greater water surface area (shallow water containers and regular spraying) or an increase in water temperature by placing a heat mat under a shallow water container.

Water

For all snakes, fresh water should be provided at all times. Water bowls should be cleaned and disinfected periodically. A water container that is large enough for soaking should be provided. Vitamin-mineral supplements should not be added to the water. Palatability may be reduced and bacteria in the water may feed on the supplements resulting on bacterial bloom.

NUTRITION

Nutritional disorders are often caused by errors in husbandry; thus, history taking should include specific questions about management. Pertinent information includes the patient's origin (private breeder, importer, pet shop), whether the patient was born in captivity or caught in the wild, length of ownership, whether there are other reptiles in the home, and the disease history for the patient and the entire reptile collection. A dietary history allows the veterinarian to assess the animal's intake of energy and nutrients, and may provide information about the animal's clinical condition and behavior. It also may help in the early detection of nutritional problems before they become serious clinical disorders.

Attention should be given to the quality and wholesomeness of the food, cleanliness of feeding utensils and the skills and reliability of those responsible for feeding. The veterinarian should also determine whether the reptile has appropriate access to water.

When obtaining a dietary history, include the following:

- **Diet** – What is fed, how often and how much, how the food is prepared, where the food is placed in the habitat, when the food is removed and which food the reptile actually consumes
- **Supplementation** – Are supplements used, what type, how are they offered, how often, does the animal eat the food when the supplement is offered
- **Water** – How is water offered, frequency of water changes, and has the owner observed the animal drinking

Because the gastrointestinal tract of the snake is relatively short, it is important that these animals are provided a high quality diet in captivity. The diet should be based on the snake's normal feeding strategy. Most snakes seen by veterinarians feed on mammals. Boids (pythons and boas), rat and corn snakes (*Elaphe* spp), and gopher, bull, and pine snakes (*Pituophis* spp) are some of the more common snakes presented to veterinarians. Their diet consists of rats, mice, gerbils, rabbits, and young chicks. These prey items should be fed a high quality, complete ration to provide adequate nutrition. Trauma associated with feeding live prey is common. Therefore, training snakes to eat stunned, dead, or thawed frozen prey is preferred.

Caution should be used when feeding chicks or other birds to snakes because of potential exposure to salmonella. Boiling chicks before feeding may reduce the risk. Frozen rodents should be thawed rapidly in very hot water to minimize intestinal bacterial bloom.

Some snakes feeds on ectotherms, including crayfish, amphibians, fish, and other reptiles. Snakes that eat these prey items include indigo snakes (*Drymarchon* spp), ring-necked snakes (*Diadophis* spp), garter snakes (*Thamnophis* spp), hog-nosed snakes (*Heterodon* spp), water snakes (*Nerodia* spp), and king snakes (*Lampropeltis* spp). Freezing the prey item may eliminate nematode parasites; however, it will not usually eliminate bacteria and protozoa. Regular fecal examinations and deworming may be necessary to control protozoal parasites.

Ectotherm snakes should be trained to eat rodents. Initially, rodents can be scented with a more typical prey item. Supplementation is usually unnecessary if a portion of the diet is made up of rodents. Snakes that eat other snakes in the wild should be housed alone to prevent cage-mate predation.

Insect-eating snakes typically seen by veterinarians include worm snakes (*Carphophis* spp), ring-necked snakes (*Diadophus* spp), brown snake (*Storeria* spp), green snake (Opheodrys spp), and primarily fossorial snakes.

A variety of worms and insects should be offered, including crickets, mealworms, earthworms, nightcrawlers and wax-moth larvae. Insects should be fed a complete diet before they are fed to snakes. Insects should be dusted with a calcium and vitamin supplement weekly. Some of the larger snakes in this group may be weaned onto pinkie mice for added nutrition. Pinkies can be supplemented by dipping them into a liquid calcium supplement.

SUMMARY

Diversity among snakes challenges the veterinarian's ability to know the feeding management, estimate the nutritional requirements, and recommend appropriate diets for every species presented in practice. With the exception of field studies on free-living reptiles, nutritional research is limited. Thus, recommendations are based on knowledge of natural diets, feeding histories, clinical experience, and principles of comparative nutrition.

REFERENCES
1. Frye FL. Biomedical and Surgical Aspects of Captive Reptile Husbandry. Malabar, FL: Krieger, 1991, pp 52-53.
2. Obst FjJ Richter K, Jacob U. Atlas of Reptiles and Amphibians for the Terrarium. Neptune City, NJ: TFH Publications, 1988.
3. Jacobson ER: Snakes. Vet Clin North Am. 1993; 23: 1179-1212.

4. Donoghue S. Nutrition. In: Mader DR (ed): Reptile Medicine and Surgery, 2nd ed. Philadelphia: WB Saunders, 2006, pp 251-298.

5. Divers S. Basic reptile husbandry, history taking and clinical examination. In Practice 1996; 18:51-65.

LET YOUR FINGERS DO THE WALKING: HOW TO RESTRAIN AND EXAMINE SNAKES

Orlando Diaz-Figueroa, DVM, MS
Diplomate ABVP (Avian Practice)
Lake Howell Animal Clinic, Maitland, FL

The popularity of reptiles as pets is continuing to grow. Consequently, more reptiles are being presented to the veterinarian, and owners' expectations regarding their veterinary care are also increasing. More recent and continued strides have been made possible by the efforts of many clinicians and the establishment of the Association of Reptilian and Amphibian Veterinarians.

Snakes are members of the Class Reptilia and Order Squamata. Squamata includes the Suborders Serpentes (snakes) and Sauria (lizards). There are over 2,900 species of snakes in the world.

SNAKE ANATOMY

The anatomy of the snake, for the most part, is consistent across species. Therefore, developing a general understanding of organ location in one species will be beneficial when working with others. When evaluating the anatomy of the snake it may be best to separate the snake into four quadrants. The proximal quadrant of the snake generally contains the trachea, esophagus, parathyroid glands, thymus, thyroid, and the heart. The second quadrant contains the lung(s), liver, and continuation of the esophagus. The third quadrant generally contains the stomach, spleen, gallbladder, pancreas, proximal small bowel, adrenals, airsac, and gonads. Finally, the fourth quadrant contains the caudal small intestine, kidneys, cecum, colon, and cloaca. The quadrant system may be useful when attempting to identify an area to make a surgical approach for a specific organ system.

The integument of the snake is covered with two primary scale types, both originating from the epidermis. Small scales cover the dorsum and lateral surfaces of the snake, while larger scales cover the ventrum. Differences in scale shape, size, and texture are used to characterize different species. Reptile skin is relatively aglandular, although some reptiles have developed regionalized glands that are useful in attracting mates or used in defense against predators.

Ecdysis is a naturally occurring process in the snake that is regulated by the thyroid glands. Snakes should shed their entire skin, including their spectacles, in one piece, although large snakes (> 3 m) may shed their skin in pieces. Ecdysis generally takes approximately 14 days. A snake will become anorectic and avoid contact during the period of time leading up to an impending shed. Handling snakes during this period can be hazardous for the animal if the underlying epidermis is damaged.

Snakes do not have eyelids. To compensate, snakes produce spectacles or brilles. Spectacles are a modification of the epidermis and provide protection for the exposed anterior surface of the globe. Because they originate from the epidermis, the spectacles are routinely shed during ecdysis. Retention of the spectacles has been associated with the development of corneal disease and panophthalmitis.

The skeletal system of snakes is unique among the reptiles. The skull of the snake is kinetic and does not have a mandibular symphysis, which allows it to ingest prey items larger than would be possible by a reptile with a fixed skull. The vertebral column is comprised of several hundred vertebrate that show minimal regionalization. Snakes do not have a sternum. The ventral aspect of each rib is attached by muscle to the ventral scales.

Snakes do not have an external ear, tympanic membrane, or middle ear. The stapes (inner ear cavity) is in direct contact with the quadrate bone and transmits vibrations, which enables the snake to hear low frequency sounds (<600 Hz).

The glottis of the snake is located on the floor of the buccal cavity. The trachea of the snake has incomplete tracheal rings. Primitive snakes generally have two lungs, while more advanced snakes possess only one lung. The right lung is the primary lung in those species with two lungs. In general, the left lung is reduced or vestigial. Gas exchange occurs in the cranial compartment of the lung, while the caudal segment (airsac) serves to store air.

The digestive tract of the snake is a linear system that is modified to digest dense meals. The tongue is an important chemosensory structure. The tongue is inserted into the Jacobson's organ, located in the roof of the buccal cavity, to differentiate odors. Because snakes hunt by olfaction, they can be trained to readily accept pre-killed prey items. Venom glands are modified salivary glands that produce potent enzymatic compounds to assist with prey acquisition and digestion. The esophagus, stomach, small intestine, and colon are linear, losing much of the coiling frequently observed in omnivores and herbivores. The cloaca is comprised of the coprodeum, urodeum, and proctodeum. The coprodeum is located in the dorsal region of the cloaca and receives fecal material from the colon. The urodeum is located ventrally and serves as the site for collection of the urine from the ureters. The oviducts also open into the urodeum. The proctodeum is the collecting chamber for the urodeum and coprodeum.

The liver is a linear organ (single lobed) in the snake. The liver generally begins just distal to the heart and ends at the cranial segment of the stomach. In most species, the gallbladder is not directly associated with the liver. In most snakes, the pancreas, spleen and gallbladder form a triad and are caudal to the stomach, while some species have a combined hepatopancreas.

Snakes have metanephric kidneys that are linear and lobulated. The right kidney is cranial to the left kidney. Male snakes develop sexual segments to the kidneys during their reproductive cycle. Snakes do not have a urinary bladder.

RESTRAINT AND HANDLING

Nonvenomous snakes can be restrained by grasping the head of the snake at the level of the quadrate/mandible and supporting the snake's body. An additional handler should be used for every 3 to 4 feet of snake to support the spine. Snakes should never be draped over the neck of an individual.

Only trained professionals should handle venomous snakes. Hooks and tongs should be used to remove venomous snakes from their enclosure. Once collected from an enclosure, the snake should be directed into an appropriately sized clear plastic tube. The snake should be allowed to crawl to the midpoint of the tube and then prevented from advancing. This technique allows for safe management of the snake and allows veterinarians to grossly examine the snake and collect blood from the ventral coccygeal vein. Intravenous propofol (5 mg/kg) can be administered slowly via the ventral coccygeal vein to anesthetize the snake or isoflurane can be directed into the tube to anesthetize the snake.

PHYSICAL EXAMINATION

Physical examinations should be performed in a thorough and consistent manner. Unfortunately, there are times in a busy schedule when we may "cut corners" on our examinations to conserve time. Because many of the cases being presented are the result of multiple etiologies, time savings on the examination may result in the misclassification of a disease. There can be no substitute for a thorough physical examination.

Snakes as a group are relatively easy to evaluate with the standard examination techniques in practice for domestic pets. The aim of the physical examination is to localize any lesions or symptoms and to formulate a list of differential diagnoses. A systemic examination from rostrum to tail tip is always indicated whether the snake is being presented for postpurchase examination, yearly health examination, presurgical assessment, or because it is truly sick.

Always observe the snake from a distance prior to restraining it for a physical examination. Special attention should be given to mentation, respiration, and locomotion. The physical examination should be performed in a thorough and consistent manner. The spectacles should be clear with no apparent indications of a retained spectacle or subspectacular disease. A normal fluid layer under the spectacle drains through a duct to the cranial roof of the maxilla. When this nasolacrimal duct is blocked, the build up of fluids can cause a subspectacular swelling that often becomes infected, resulting in a subspectacular abscess. A baseline ophthalmic exam should be performed to evaluate the conjunctiva, cornea, and anterior chamber. Damage to the underlying cornea can result in panophthalmitis and ocular swelling, whereas retrobulbar abscessation results in protrusion of a normal sized globe. Other ocular pathologies can include uveitis, corneal lipidosis, and spectacular foreign bodies, including wood chip particles or other vivarium materials. The nares should be clear and free of discharge and retained shed. The infraorbital pits (where present) should be free from discharges or retained skin. The oral cavity should be opened using a soft, pliable speculum to permit an assessment of mucous membrane color and buccal examination for evidence of mucosal edema, ptyalism, hemorrhage, necrosis, and the presence of caseous exudates. White deposits may indicate uric acid deposition caused by visceral gout. The tongue should be identified and evaluated for function. The glottis should be free of discharge. The teeth should be closely inspected for fractures. The integument should be closely inspected for ectoparasites (especially the common snake mite, *Ophionyssus natricis*, and ticks), dysecdysis, traumatic injuries and inflammatory responses (dermatitis). Skin tenting and ridges may indicate cachexia or dehydration. The spine and ribs should be palpated. The epaxial muscle should be well developed. The spine will be prominent in snakes with muscle wasting. Palpation should be performed to assess the coelomic cavity for abnormalities. A thumb or finger can be used to gently palpate the viscera from the heart to the vent. Recently fed snakes have a midbody swelling associated with the prey in the stomach, and handling such individuals may lead to regurgitation. Eggs and preovulatory follicles may also be palpated. Any abnormal masses should be further evaluated using appropriate diagnostic tests. Examination of the tail length or probing of the hemipenes should confirm the gender. In males, the probe passes into the hemipenal sulcus to a depth of 7 to 15 subcaudal scales; in females, the probe enters the cloacal sac to a depth of 3 to 5 subcaudal scales. An audible ultrasonic crystal Doppler may be used to determine heart rate and evaluate the snake for cardiac irregularities.

DIAGNOSTIC TESTING

Snakes are stoic animals and can mask their illness. Hematologic samples can be collected to evaluate the physiologic status of a snake. Blood samples can be collected from the heart, jugular, or ventral coccygeal vein. Cardiocentesis is the most frequently used venipuncture technique in snakes greater than 200 grams. The heart is located approximately one quarter to one third the distance from the snout. Placing the snake in dorsal recumbency will facilitate direct visualization of the beating heart. Venipuncture requires a minimum of two individuals, one individual to restrain the snake and a second to collect the sample. The heart should be isolated using the index finger and thumb. A 1.0- to 1.5-inch 22- to 25-gauge needle fastened to a 3-mL syringe can be used to collect the sample. The needle should be inserted at approximately a 45° angle into the ventricle. The blood will flow into the syringe with each heartbeat.

The jugular veins are located cranial to the heart where the lateral and ventral scales meet. The snake should be placed in dorsal recumbency for the procedure. A 1.0- to 1.5-inch 22- to 25-gauge needle fastened to a 3-mL syringe should be inserted approximately nine ventral scales cranial to the heart on the medial aspect of the ribs.

The ventral coccygeal vein is located ventral to the caudal vertebral bodies. A 1.0- to 1.5-inch 22- to 25-gauge needle fastened to a 3-mL syringe can be used to collect the sample. The needle should be inserted along the ventral midline at a 45° angle between two ventral scales approximately one third to one half the distance from the vent. Special care should be taken when collecting samples from male snakes to avoid compromising the hemipenes. This is the preferred site for blood collection in venomous snakes.

Gastric lavage can be performed to collect samples from snakes that are regurgitating or with apparent gastric pathology. A red rubber feeding tube or stainless steel gavage tube can be used to collect the sample. The tube should be pre-measured to ensure placement into the stomach. Physiologic saline (5–10 mL/kg) can be used to perform the gastric lavage. A direct smear should be made from the sample and the remainder of the sample centrifuged to concentrate any pathogenic organisms.

An enema can be performed to collect samples from the colon and cloaca. A red-rubber feeding tube can be used to collect the sample. The tube should be coated with a sterile lubricant to facilitate passage. The tube should be inserted into the vent, through the proctodeum and coprodeum and into the colon. Physiologic saline (5–10 mL/kg) can be used to collect the sample. The sample should be centrifuged to concentrate microorganisms and cells into the pellet.

SUMMARY

Physical examination provides the veterinarian with a list of possible differential diagnoses and indicates which further investigations may be necessary to make a definitive diagnosis. Survey radiographs, ultrasonography, endoscopy, hematology, blood biochemistry, and microbiological and parasitologic investigations are all proven techniques that are used extensively in reptile medicine.

REFERENCES

1. Jacobson ER: Snakes. Vet Clin North Am. 1993;23: 179-1212.

REPTILE ZOONOSES: "DON'T KISS YOUR TURTLE"

Orlando Diaz-Figueroa, DVM, MS
Diplomate ABVP (Avian Practice)
Lake Howell Animal Clinic, Maitland, FL

With the growing popularity of exotic pets in the United States, the incidence of zoonotic diseases attributed to these pets should be expected to rise. Veterinarians play an important role in educating the public and should have an understanding of the epidemiology of these potentially devastating diseases. The purpose of this article is to introduce veterinarians to the most common zoonotic diseases encountered in reptile species.

BACTERIAL ZOONOSES

Salmonellosis

Salmonella spp. are gram-negative facultative anaerobes that are ubiquitous in the environment. These bacteria have been isolated from all of the different classes of animals. There are more than 2,400 different *Salmonella* serotypes, and they should all be considered pathogenic. Most animals appear to be asymptomatic reservoirs for this microbe. *Salmonella* spp. is primarily transmitted via the fecal-oral route or from contaminated fomites. Humans that contract salmonellosis from nontraditional species may experience headaches, nausea, vomiting, abdominal pain, enteritis, or septicemia. The incubation of *Salmonella* in humans is approximately 6 to 48 hours. Because of the inherent zoonotic risks associated with nontraditional species (eg, reptiles), ownership should be limited to cases that have adult supervision. Strict hygiene, including hand washing with soap, should be practiced to reduce the risk of exposure.

Individuals who are susceptible to *Salmonella* infections include the elderly, the very young, and those who are immunocompromised because of AIDS or immunosuppressive therapy. People with cirrhosis, diabetes, and sickle cell anemia are also particularly susceptible to severe *Salmonella* infection.

Salmonellosis in people usually manifests itself as diarrhea accompanied by abdominal cramps and fever. Salmonella can enter the bloodstream of people, become septicemic and cause meningitis, arthritis and other extraintestinal problems. Antibiotic treatment is usually limited to extraintestinal infection. Antibiotic given to people who have disease limited to the intestinal tract may prolong symptoms and can result in development of antibiotic resistant organisms.

Campylobacteriosis

Campylobacteriosis is a serious zoonosis. Although contaminated food (eg, poultry) is the primary source of *Campylobacter* spp., reptiles, such as chelonians, may harbor *Campylobacter jejuni* or *C. fetus*. The incubation of *Campylobacter* spp. is approximately 2 to 5 days. In general, the disease is self-limiting (10 to 14 days); however, it may persist in the immunocompetent host. Humans with compromised immune systems should limit contact with reptiles or other species of animals that have been identified as *Campylobacter*-positive.

Mycobacteriosis

Mycobacterium spp. has a cosmopolitan distribution. *Mycobacterium* spp. has been isolated from all of the major classes of animals. Many of the *Mycobacterium* spp. that can infect animals can also infect humans. *Mycobacterium* spp. can be transmitted to humans and herpetofauna through aerosolization of contaminated respiratory secretions or direct skin contact, soil, or water. Pet owners should always practice strict disinfection protocols when handling their pets and limit contact when they have an open wound on their hands. Reptiles and amphibians can harbor *Mycobacterium* species that can also be found as opportunistic pathogens in humans, especially those who are immunocompromised. Examples include *M. marinum*, *M. chelonei*, and *M. abscessus*.

Dermatophilosis

Dermatophilus congolensis is a gram-positive filamentous bacterium with a life cycle that involves the release of spores from the filaments and the development of these spores to form germ tubes and new filaments. In humans and animals it causes exudative dermatitis and, crusty scabs. It has been found in cattle, sheep, horses, and some 18 other animals including seals, lizards, and even in polar bears. Handling of infected animals by humans can result in human disease. It has been isolated from pet Savannah monitor (*Varanus exanthematicus*). In immunocompromised humans it can attack the brain, lungs, and kidneys.

Lyme Disease and Ehrlichiosis

Lizards are also bitten by *Ixodes* ticks that harbor bacterial infections such as *Borrelia*, which causes Lyme disease, and *Ehrlichia*, which causes ehrlichiosis in humans and other animals. While these diseases may not be zoonotic in the sense a human could not casually become infected from contact with the lizard, the ectoparasite of the lizard could, conceivably, vector the disease to humans. A great deal of care must be taken when treating or removing ticks from such animals.

Miscellaneous Bacterial Infection

Reptiles can harbor many other bacteria that potentially are human pathogens, including *Aeromonas* spp., *Citrobacter* spp., *Klebsiella* spp., *Proteus* spp., and *Serratia* spp. Prevention of all such enteric infections depends on meticulous hygiene and sanitation. Reptile cages should be cleaned frequently and waste disposed of in a sanitary fashion. Perhaps the most important means of prevention is hand washing after handling the reptile, its cage, or contents. This is most important for small children and others who are uniquely susceptible to infection.

PARASITIC ZOONOSES
Cryptosporidiosis

Cryptosporidiosis is a common zoonotic pathogen. *Cryptosporidium parvum* is a coccidian protozoan in the family Cryptosporidiidae, suborder Eimeriina. Affected animals may be asymptomatic or present with chronic diarrhea. Individuals with compromised immune systems should limit their contact with *Cryptosporidium*-positive nontraditional species. It has been isolated in many different hosts including mammals, birds, and reptiles. There has been no documented evidence that reptilian cryptosporidiosis is zoonotic.

Trichinella

In 1995, a new species of Trichinella (*Trichinella zimbabwensis*) was discovered in farmed Nile crocodiles (*Crocodylus niloticus*) in Zimbabwe, where the mode of transmission was the consumption of the meat of slaughtered crocodiles, used as feed. To determine whether *T. zimbabwensis* affects poikilotherm vertebrates in the wild, monitor lizards (*Varanus niloticus*) and Nile crocodiles were collected in Zimbabwe and Mozambique. In 5 (17.6%) of the 28 monitor lizards from Zimbabwe, *T. zimbabwensis* larvae were identified. For the wild Nile crocodiles from Mozambique, species-level identification was not possible, yet immunohistochemical analysis revealed that 8 (20%) of the 40 animals harbored non-encapsulated *Trichinella* sp. larvae, which probably belonged to *T. zimbabwensis*. This is the first report of *T. zimbabwensis* in wild reptiles, and the findings are consistent with reports that vertebrates with scavenger and cannibalistic behavior are the most important hosts of *Trichinella* spp. The wide distribution of monitor lizards and crocodiles in Africa and the development of national crocodile breeding programs in many African countries should be taken into consideration when evaluating the risk of transmission of this parasite to mammals, including humans.

Pentastomiasis

Pentastomida is a phylum of parasites intermediate between arthropods and annelids. A majority of pentastomes mature in the respiratory tract of reptiles, particularly snakes and varanids lizard. Pentastomes typically have an indirect life cycle. Humans, an aberrant host contract the infection by consuming water or foods contaminated with eggs eliminated in the saliva or feces of snakes, by consuming raw or undercooked snake meat, or by handling infected reptiles and then placing contaminated hands in the mouth. Other intermediate hosts are infected through ingestion of contaminated water, plants, or the snakes themselves. *Amillifer armillatus* is the most common genera identified from pythonids and viperids, *Kiricephalus* spp from culebrids, and *Porecephalus* spp. from boids and crotalids. The former is best known as a human pathogen. Larval and nymphal stages are found in various human organs, most often the mesentery. The infection is often diagnosed coincidentally on x ray because the organism can show up as radio-opaque c-shaped object. At present, no successful therapy exists against the larval forms in the incidental hosts. In snakes, pentastomes are difficult to treat with anthelminthic drugs because of the extraintestinal location of adult parasites. It may be possible to remove adult worms from the lungs of snakes endoscopically. The fact that humans can serve as incidental hosts for reptilian pentastomes should alert veterinarians to recognize the zoonotic potential of these parasites.

VIRAL ZOONOSES

West Nile virus (WNV) is a mosquito-borne flavivirus (Family *Flaviviridae*) that is transmitted by various species of adult *Culex* mosquitoes to a variety of mammals and birds. It emerged in North America in 1999 when it infected and caused the deaths of people, horses, and birds in New York. By the year 2001, WNV had spread into the southeastern US, including Florida. The continued expansion of WNV in North America presents an emerging threat to human and animal health in the Western Hemisphere.

Reptiles are known to be infected with several mosquito-borne viruses. Western equine encephalomyelitis virus (Family *Togaviridae*) was isolated from blood and found to overwinter in garter snakes (*Thamnophis* spp.) and the Texas tortoise (*Gopherus berlandieri*). Japanese encephalitis virus (Family *Flaviviridae*) was isolated from Chinese rat snakes (*Elaphe rufodorsata*) in Korea. In a survey in Venezuela, tegu lizards (*Tupinambis nigropunctatus*) were found to have antibody against eastern equine encephalomyelitis (EEE; Family *Togaviridae*) and Venezuelan encephalitis viruses (Family *Togaviridae*). In crocodilians, seropositive wild American alligators (*Alligator mississippiensis*) for EEE virus and farmed Nile crocodiles (*Crocodylus niloticus*) in Israel for WNV have been reported. Florida, Georgia, Louisiana, and Idaho have all experienced cases of WNV in alligators. Viremia data implicate the American alligator as a potential amplifying host for WNV in southeastern North America. In 2003, the first human case of WNV infection from a reptile occurred in Idaho. The mode of transmission did not come from the bite of an infected mosquito, but more likely from contact with the blood of infected, imported alligators.

Veterinarians may need to contact reptile owners about the possible role of the reptile in the disease and to encourage owners to house reptiles indoors during epizootic outbreaks. The potential role of reptiles and amphibians in the life cycle and epidemiology of WNV is not known.

Precautionary measures include mosquito abatement through habitat reduction, predation, and appropriate pesticide use; personal protection and use of mosquito repellents during outdoor activities.

TRAUMA (WOUND AND BITES)

All animal bites represent a potential for infection and sepsis. Any wound infection or necrotizing process in a reptile may contain potentially pathogenic organisms. A good example of this is stomatitis in snakes and lizards which may contain *Staphylococcus* spp., *Shigella* spp., or *Pseudomonas* spp., all which are potentially pathogenic to humans. Envenomation from poisonous reptiles can result in death or permanent disability. No one should keep poisonous snakes as pets, and veterinarians are justified in refusing to treat extremely dangerous animals in their private practice. In many states is illegal to possess such animals without special license.

Most cases of traumatic injury can be prevented by sound husbandry techniques, including appropriate caging and restraint procedures.

MISCELLANEOUS INFECTIONS

Mycotic agents commonly isolated from the diseased reptiles can also cause infection in humans. Zoonotic transmission of fungal agents, although possible, has not been documented.

PREVENTION

Proper cleansing and hygiene is essential for preventing zoonotic infections. Individuals who are immunocompromised for any reason should avoid contact with amphibians, reptiles, and any other animals known to transmit zoonotic infection.

Zoonotic infections from reptiles and amphibians are entirely preventable. In general zoonoses from these animals are rare and they represent a small fraction of all the infectious diseases which occur. Nevertheless, when they do occur, they often engender very negative publicity for reptiles so all hobbyists should be involved in disseminating information to prevent such infection from occurring.

REFERENCES

1. Johnson-Delaney, CA. Reptile zoonoses and threats to public health. In: Mader DR (ed.): Reptile Medicine and Surgery, 2nd ed. Philadelphia: WB Saunders, 2006, pp 1017-1030.

SNAKE CLINICAL PROCEDURES AND DIAGNOSTICS

Stephen J. Hernandez-Divers, BVetMed, DZooMed, MRCVS, Diplomate ACZM
College of Veterinary Medicine, University of Georgia, Athens, GA

There are very few pathognomonic signs in reptile medicine, and it is generally very difficult to make a diagnosis in the examination room. Definitive diagnosis is important to maximize therapeutic success, while reducing the negative impacts of providing veterinary care. In general, diagnosis relies upon the demonstration of a host pathological response (eg, cytology, histopathology, and serology) and the causative agent (eg, microbiology, toxicology). Diagnosis is often straightforward if appropriate samples can be collected, processed and interpreted. This article focuses on the most common techniques and procedures and is far from complete. Further details can be found in published texts.

CHEMICAL RESTRAINT

While some procedures can be performed in the conscious snake, sedation or anesthesia can facilitate procedures, and reduce trauma to the animal. A review of snake anesthesia appears elsewhere in these proceedings, and detailed reviews are available elsewhere.

HANDLING & EXAMINATION

A detailed review of husbandry and past medical history is required prior to physical exam. The head of an aggressive snake or a snake of unknown disposition should be identified and restrained before opening the transportation bag and removing the animal. Venomous snakes should be anesthetized prior to physical contact. In general, the head of the snake is held behind the occiput using the thumb and middle finger to support the lateral aspects of the cranium. The index finger is placed on top of the head. The other hand is used to support the serpentine body. Larger pythons and anacondas are powerful and potentially dangerous. When dealing with large, even docile boids, a second, third, or even fourth handler will be required to help control the body during the examination. It is usually safer and more convenient to sedate a large pugnacious snake than to struggle on and risk injury to the snake, client, or staff. A complete physical examination should be performed, starting if possible, with a hands-off approach to assess mentation and resting respiratory rate. The physical examination should start with a resting heart rate and be followed by an evaluation of neurologic function, muscle tone and strength, integument, infra-orbital pits (where present), nostrils, eyes, oral cavity, and cloaca. The entire head, body and tail should be palpated, and any internal abnormalities recorded as a percentage or fraction of snout-to-vent length. The gender should be determined from tail length/confirmation, or probing the inverted hemipenes.

DIAGNOSTIC IMAGING

Snakes can be difficult to position and restrain for radiographic examinations unless anesthetized. If the purpose of the examination is simply to rule out radiodense foreign bodies, the snake may be allowed to coil in its natural position while the radiograph is taken. If detailed examination of the skeletal, respiratory, and digestive system is desired, the snake must be extended. A plastic restraint tube can be utilized for this purpose; however, this may produce some radiographic artifact. In larger snakes, several films will be needed to radiograph the entire length of the body. It is important to properly label each exposure in order to keep track of all the different views. Lateral views are best taken using horizontal beams to avoid displacement artifact of the viscera. However, standard laterals with the snake taped in lateral recumbency can be useful especially where horizontal beams are not possible or safe to undertake. The interpretation of dorsoventral views is hindered by the spine and ribs, but can still be useful when dealing with obvious lesions including eggs and mineralized masses.

Traumatic fractures, spondylitis/spondylosis, osteomyelitis, and congenital abnormalities are common indications for examining the skeletal system of snakes. Fractured ribs with periosteal bone formation are a common finding in snakes. Another common finding is exuberant vertebral periosteal bone formation. On radiographs, this appears as several "fused" vertebrae. Common indications for radiographically evaluating the digestive system include hypertrophic gastritis, foreign body ingestion/impaction, constipation, hepatomegaly and other masses. Contrast studies are useful in diagnosing intestinal obstruction and constipation. In addition, contrast material in the gastrointestinal tract can often outline and help determine the origin of a non-specific intracoelomic masses; intraluminal or extraluminal. Cardiomyopathy has been reported in snakes, which can be indicated by cardiomegaly on radiographs. Metastatic mineralization of large blood vessels is often apparent around the heart due to the negative contrast afforded by the adjacent lung(s). The superimposition of other organs such as liver and stomach over the lung fields can make the radiographic interpretation of respiratory disease challenging. Common indications for evaluating the respiratory system are rhinitis, suspected neoplastic and infectious disorders of the trachea and lung, as well as abscesses or granulomas. The kidneys are not always radiographically evident, unless enlarged or mineralized. Disease processes that can cause renomegaly include renal gout and neoplasia. Eggs of oviparous species are leathery and poorly calcified, but can often be appreciated on plain radiographs. In viviparous species fetal skeletons become visible as they mineralize late in gestation. The hemipenes of some species may appear mineralized and can be detected radiographically.

Common indications for evaluating the reproductive system include dystocia, apparent infertility and reduced fecundity. The presence of any swelling is an indication for radiography. Abscesses, which can either be extracoelomic or intracoelomic and associated with a specific organ or the coelomic wall are common findings in snakes.

Ultrasonography is particularly useful for evaluation of soft tissues, especially the reproductive system, liver, and kidneys. Copious gel (or a water bath) is required to reduce artifact caused by air trapped under the scales. CT and MRI are used rarely, on a case by case basis.

BLOOD

The ability to collect quality blood samples is essential in any animal class. Complete or selective hematologic and biochemical evaluations are possible but the accuracy of results is often adversely affected by poor venipuncture, handling or laboratory skills. The production of poor quality blood data can be useless or even worse, misleading to the clinician. Likewise, the ability to administer intravenous medications, especially anesthetics, or place intravenous catheters also relies on proficient veniclysis technique. Venipuncture is generally a blind technique in snakes. Despite a continuous trickle of published blood ranges, there is still a relative dearth of hematologic or biochemical data for reptiles compared to domesticated animals. In addition, blood values can vary dramatically with species, environment, nutrition, age, breeding status, hibernation and disease status. Given this variability published ranges may be of limited value. More reliance should be placed upon establishing an individual's observed range and using serial sampling to monitor the progress of hematologic and biochemical changes rather than relying on a single result. The two common sites for venipuncture in snakes are the caudal (ventral tail) vein and the heart (Figure 1).

The caudal (tail) vein is accessed caudal to the cloaca, between 25 and 50% down the tail. It is wise to avoid the paired hemipenes of males (that may extend up to 14 to 16 subcaudal scales caudal from the vent), and the paired cloacal musk glands of both sexes (that may extend up to 5 subcaudal scales). The needle is angled at 45 to 60 degrees and positioned in the ventral mid line. The needle is advanced in a craniodorsal direction, while maintaining slight negative pressure. If the needle touches a vertebral body it is withdrawn slightly and redirected more cranially or caudally. This vessel is most easily entered in larger snakes and lymphatic contamination is possible but generally uncommon.

With the snake restrained in dorsal recumbency, the heart is located approximately 22% to 33% from snout to vent. The heart is palpated and immobilized. The needle is advanced at 45 degrees in a craniodorsal direction into the apex of the beating ventricle. Blood often enters the syringe with each heartbeat. It is wise to maintain digital pressure for 30 to 60 seconds following this technique. This technique has been employed in snakes of all sizes from 10 g neonates to 100+kg constrictors. Nevertheless, good chemical/physical restraint is essential if significant cardiac trauma is to be avoided.

INTEGUMENT

Dermatologic disease is a frequent presentation and there are various levels at which the clinician can intervene and collect biological samples. Shed skin, skin scrapes, impression smears, scale and skin biopsies can all be collected. The skin and associated structures are perhaps the easiest to sample for laboratory analysis due to their accessibility. However, they can also be the most demanding to interpret as contamination and secondary changes often mask the underlying primary complaint. Various ectoparasites may be clearly seen on

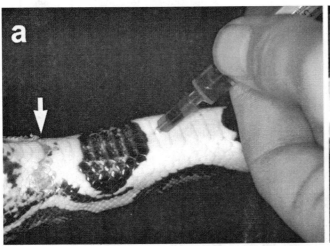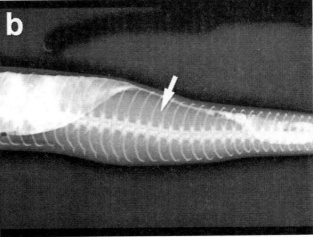

Figure 1. (a) Blood collection from the caudal (ventral tail) vein of a Boa constrictor – note the venipuncture site is in the ventral midline and caudal to the cloaca (*arrow*). (b) Dorsoventral radiograph of a corn snake following a barium enema – note the outline of a caudal mass, external to the intestinal tract. This well demarked and encapsulated mass was surgically excised, and proved to be a granulosa cell tumor

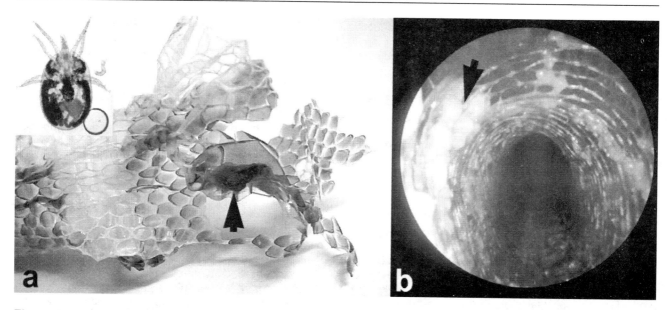

Figure 2. (a) Shed skin from a snake that was suffering from severe mite infestation and self-inflicted wounds from the intense pruritus. One of these lesions can be appreciated from the abnormal slough (arrow). Insert, the common snake mite, *Ophionyssus natricis*, was recovered from the shed skin. (b) Endoscopic view of a Ball python (*Python regius*) with granulomatous pneumonia (*arrow*). The diagnosis of pulmonary mycobacteriosis was made following biopsy as lung lavage proved unrewarding.

the surface of the skin, around nostrils, eyes, and skin folds (Figure 2). Mites, ticks, lice, maggots, flies can often be physically removed and submitted in specimen containers for taxonomic identification. The shed skin of reptiles is also a valuable asset and should be inspected for evidence of parasitism. Suspected mites can be collected direct from the snake using a wet cotton-tipped applicator, and transferred to a microscope slide for closer inspection and identification. Skin lesions are best cleaned and partially debrided using aseptic techniques prior to the collection of clinical samples. Microbiologic swabs should be taken from the periphery of the lesion but deep to any exposed areas. Impression smears can be taken after the lesion has been cleaned with sterile saline and gently dabbed dry with sterile gauze. Skin scrapes may be useful especially when dealing with drier more proliferative lesions. Where the clinician requires a skin biopsy the removal of a single scale may be all that is required as scales contain both epidermal and dermal elements. A small volume (0.02–0.1 mL) of local anesthetic (eg, 2% lidocaine) is injected subcutaneously in the area(s) of interest. Using aseptic techniques a single scale is then elevated and cut close to its insertion into the skin using a scalpel blade. If a larger sample is required then a combination of local, regional or general anesthesia and sharp excision or a skin punch biopsy instrument is effective. A single suture closes the deficit.

RESPIRATORY SYSTEM

The ability to diagnose pathologic changes within the respiratory system of snakes is often straightforward following lung lavage for the collection of cytologic and microbiologic samples. The collection of tissue biopsies

requires anesthesia and surgical or endoscopic techniques. The upper respiratory tract including the nares, buccal cavity, glottis and cranial trachea can be visualized and often sampled directly without anesthesia. Small diameter swabs permit the collection of samples, although the greatest concern comes from bacterial contamination by oral commensals. Swabs can be submitted for microbiology or rolled onto glass slides for staining and cytologic evaluation. The simplest method of obtaining a representative sample from the lower respiratory tract is by lavage. Although a lung wash or lavage can be carried out in the conscious reptile, the discomfort of such a procedure probably warrants some degree of sedation or light anesthesia. A sterile catheter of appropriate size is placed through the glottis (or better still through a sterile endotracheal tube pre-placed into the trachea) taking great care not to touch the oral membranes. The catheter is advanced caudal to the heart (>30% snout-vent) but in large specimens it may not be possible to reach the lung(s) and a tracheal lavage is performed. Once in place, 0.5 to 1.0 mL of sterile saline per 100 g bodyweight can be infused. Sample recovery is often aided by rotating the snake, and lifting the head and tail to accumulate fluid at the dependent area, near the catheter tip.

Lavage samples do not permit an appreciation of lung architecture. For this, and many other histopathologic exams, tissue biopsies are preferred. Surgical access to the lung can be achieved using a standard coeliotomy or transcutaneous pulmonoscopy. In snakes, the respiratory active anterior part of the lung is typically located between 12% and 45% snout-vent. However there is great species variation with regards to lung anatomy including the presence of a tracheal lung in some elapids and viperids, both left and right lungs in boids, and only a right lung in most other snakes.

GASTROINTESTINAL SYSTEM

In cases of severe diarrhea or regurgitation, material for laboratory submission will be forthcoming and may be collected and presented along with the animal by well educated owners or keepers. In addition, many reptiles will spontaneously defecate and urinate when handled during the examination process. It is important to appreciate that, like birds, the stools of reptiles are composed of fecal, urate and urine components and that the cloaca is a common chamber for the gastro-intestinal, urinary and reproductive systems. For example, watery stools due to polyuria must be differentiated from true diarrhea, and cloacal bleeding may be intestinal, reproductive or urinary in origin. Fecal material can be submitted for a variety of parasitologic, cytologic and microbiologic tests. The submission of only fecal material in appropriate sterile containers will prevent further mixing and contamination by urates and urine during transportation and processing. Microbiologic results from deposited feces should be interpreted with caution as contamination from other organ systems can occur in the cloacal proctodeum prior to elimination, while environmental contamination invariably occurs after elimination. The fresher the material, the more meaningful the laboratory results, although some parasitologic investigations (eg, helminth egg examination) can be performed on refrigerated material up to 4 weeks or more after elimination.

Unfortunately, the slow intestinal transit times of most reptiles often necessitate a more direct approach to obtain material. A cloacocolonic lavage can be performed on most conscious reptiles and provides the clinician with a diagnostic sample. A sterile lubricated round-tipped catheter is inserted into the cloaca and cranially towards the colon. A relatively large catheter should be used as this helps prevent kinking of the tube and perforation of the thin intestinal wall. On no account should the catheter be forced. Once in place, 0.5 to 1.0 mL sterile saline per 100 g bodyweight should be gently infused through the catheter and repeatedly aspirated until a sample is obtained. It is possible to infuse an additional 1.0 mL/100 g if no sample is forthcoming. The direct collection of fecal material from the distal colon using a lubricated gloved hand offers another practical option in large boids.

A similar technique can be used to collect samples from the stomach. A relatively large, round-tipped catheter can be inserted into the stomach of most conscious reptiles. The catheter should pass to the mid-body region before instilling 0.5 to 1.0 mL sterile saline per 100 g bodyweight. Such samples can be examined as a fresh wet preparation for parasites or stained to demonstrate micro-organisms. Microbiologic cultures are often worthy but care is required in their interpretation as contamination from the respiratory system and oral cavity is possible.

For the collection of gastric or intestinal biopsies, standard coeliotomy and excisional biopsies can be undertaken but endoscopy is much less invasive. In snakes the small intestine can be readily entered via the gastric pylorus. It is unwise to endoscopically biopsy the large bowel as the intestinal wall is often thin and easily perforated. Even excisional biopsies of the large intestine can be challenging to ensure adequate closure and the prevention of leakage.

URINALYSIS

The clinician may assess the osmoregulatory system of reptiles by sampling urine and biopsies from the kidney. Urinalysis is less helpful in reptiles than mammals. The reptilian kidney cannot concentrate urine and so urine specific gravity is of limited use in the assessment of renal function. Furthermore, renal urine passes through the urodeum of the cloaca before entering the posterior colon. Urine is therefore not necessarily sterile. The clinical picture is further complicated by the fact that electrolyte and water changes can occur across the cloacocolonic mucosa. Despite these biochemical drawbacks, urine samples are useful for cytological assessments of inflammation, infection, and for the identification of renal casts.

REPRODUCTIVE SYSTEM

The advent of minimally invasive endoscopic techniques has brought about an increase in urogenital evaluation and sampling. The rigid endoscope can be used to examine the cloaca and, if patent, the oviducts of female snake enabling the collection of exudates and retained egg material in some cases.

COELOMIC VISCERA

Visceral biopsy remains a powerful tool for conclusively reaching a diagnosis, indicating specific therapies and providing a more accurate prognosis. Fine needle aspirates are generally poorly diagnostic compared to tissue samples. Biopsies may be collected for histopathology and microbiology. Samples may be collected percutaneously (generally with ultrasound guidance from large organs like the liver), surgically (all organs), or endoscopically (all organs). Correlation between biochemical tests and histopathology are generally lacking but serial blood sampling and biopsy currently offers the best diagnostic and monitoring approach to hepatic disease.

Liver Biopsy

Blood biochemistry, radiography, ultrasonography and endoscopy may indicate the existence of a hepatopathy but they seldom provide the definitive diagnosis. The elongated liver of snakes is seldom totally visible from a single coeliotomy approach. Biopsies are best collected using ligation or wedge techniques to avoid post-biopsy hemorrhage. Endoscopic techniques are typically less invasive, permit closer examination of more of the organ and enable the collection of multiple biopsies

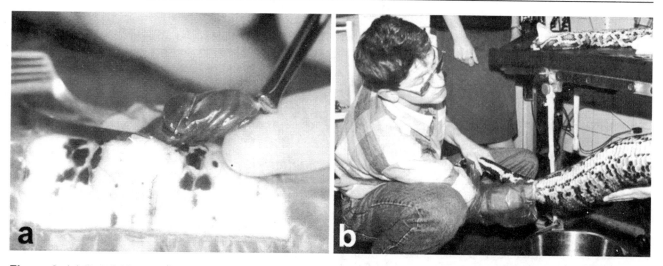

Figure 3. (a) Renal biopsy of a Boa constrictor following standard coeliotomy. In this case, vascular Hemoclips have been used to isolate a small kidney lobule prior to sharp excision. (b) Cloacocolonic internal examination in a large python using a lubricated gloved arm.

Renal Biopsy

A variety of infectious, degenerative and neoplastic renal diseases have been reported in snakes. The poor regenerative capabilities of the kidney make early diagnosis essential. The relatively poor diagnostic value of urinalysis and the late detection of renal disease by blood biochemistry further exemplify the importance of functional renal assessments and renal biopsy early in the diagnostic process (Figure 3). A standard coeliotomy between 85% and 95% snout-vent-length will generally access the kidneys, although ultrasonographic localization of the kidneys preoperatively is recommended to ensure surgical access where the left and right kidneys overlap. Excisional biopsies are easily collected by using suture or vascular clips to isolate a renal lobule. Snake endoscopy is more difficult that in chelonians or lizards due to the multiple fascial planes that have to be negotiated to reach the kidneys. However, evaluation of size, color and shape of the kidneys via smaller surgical entry is possible, and permits the collection of multiple small biopsies.

REFERENCES

1. Mader DR. Reptile Medicine and Surgery. Philadelphia, WB Saunders, 2006.
2. Raiti P, Girling S. Manual of Reptiles, British Small Animal Veterinary Association, Cheltenham, England, 2004.

TRIAGE OF SICK BOIDS (BOAS AND PYTHONS)

Dr Stephen J. Hernandez-Divers, BVetMed, DZooMed, MRCVS, Diplomate. ACZM
College of Veterinary Medicine,
University of Georgia, Athens, GA

Boas and pythons, members of the family Boidae (about 65 species in 16 genera), are commonly kept as pets and are frequently some of the most valuable reptiles presented in private practice. For example, the 'fire' and 'pie-bald' ball pythons (*Python regius*) currently sell for $4,000 to $10,000, while the so-called 'super jungle coral albino boa' (*Boa constrictor*) has a price tag of $20,000. Even if you don't particularly fancy the color mutants, the normal phenotypes that sell for under $100 are long-lived and many dedicated owners become attached to them, seeking veterinary care when their animal is sick.

Prevention is the key and owners of boids should be encouraged to seek professional preventative veterinary care, including quarantine protocols, routine blood work, fecal evaluations, etc. It is always easier dealing with an emergency for a snake that you already have baseline clinicopathologic data on.

More complete reviews of reptile critical care, emergency presentations and therapy is available from the references.

IT WAS FINE YESTERDAY...HONEST!

There are few true reptile emergencies. Many crises are really the terminal or near-terminal presentation of an unappreciated chronic process. Although the 'sudden' appearance of a mass, acute anorexia or vomiting and diarrhea can probably wait until the next scheduled appointment, acute/severe traumas (eg, injuries and burns) and severe changes in attitude or activity (eg, moribund) should be evaluated as emergencies. Having a reptile-friendly receptionist or technician can be helpful to filter calls from clients. During the initial phone call it is important that the owner is instructed how to properly transport a potentially large snake (eg, a large ice chest), while preventing sudden temperature changes. Husbandry and medical records (especially if a referral from another veterinarian), along with any vomitus, diarrhea, or unknown objects that may have appeared in the vivarium (eg, unfertilized ova, parasites) should also be brought with the animal to the clinic. An estimation of size and accurate identification of species is also essential, so that species-specific information can be perused and preparations made for the snake's arrival. Boids can exceed 600 cm (20 feet) and 150 kg, and therefore some advance preparation for hospitalization may be required.

INITIAL TRIAGE & PHYSICAL EXAMINATION

Upon arrival, the animal should be briefly examined to determine cardiovascular and respiratory stability, mentation, and evidence of trauma or hemorrhage. If cardiopulmonary-cerebral resuscitation, hemostasis or oxygen therapy are unnecessary, the snake can remain in the transportation carrier or moved to a hospital enclosure while a detailed review of husbandry, nutrition, and past medical history (including quarantine, preventative measures, home remedies, and treatments given by other veterinarians) is undertaken.

A detailed physical examination should follow established guidelines, with particular care given to resting respiratory and heart rates; neurologic evaluation; physical examination and palpation; oral examination including glottis; cloacal examination including temperature; and accurate weight. The tendency to rush through anamnesis and the physical, and move on to immediate diagnostic testing or therapy should be resisted. Differential diagnoses will often present themselves to the diligent clinician who is thorough in both historical review and physical examination.

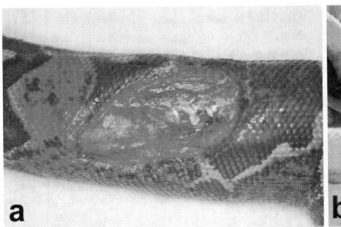 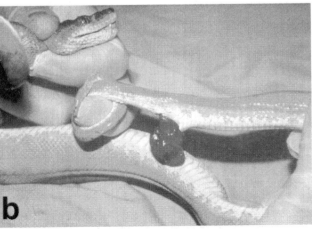

Figure 1. (a) One of several severe traumas caused by a live rat being left in the vivarium with this boa constrictor – note damage extends to and involves the spine. (b) Cloacocolonic prolapse in a green tree python.

CARDIOPULMONARY-CEREBRAL RESUSCITATION

The reptile should be examined for breathing and when no respiratory excursions are noted, cardiopulmonary-cerebral resuscitation (CPCR) should be initiated. The clinician should follow basic life support with the ABC (airway, breathing, circulation) approach of CPCR. Secure a patent airway by endotracheal intubation, and 100% oxygen should be initiated using an Ambubag (Ridge Medical) or ventilator (Small Animal Ventilator, Vetronics) connected to an oxygen outlet. Positive pressure ventilation is commenced at a rate of 4 to 6 breaths per minute, while peak positive pressure ventilation should not exceed 8 cm water. The heart is not easily auscultated using a standard stethoscope; however electronic stethoscopes and ultrasonic Dopplers are more rewarding. Electrocardiography (ECG) can be utilized to identify electrical activity. Dead reptiles may continue to exhibit cardiac electrical activity for many hours after CNS collapse. If no heart beat is detected, epinephrine can be administered endotracheally or intravenously; however, the author is unaware of any cases of recovery following true cardiac arrest in reptiles.

Pulmonary gas exchange and blood gases are difficult to interpret because of heterogeneous gas distribution within the lungs, arrhythmic breathing pattern, extrapulmonary gas exchange, cardiac and pulmonary vascular shunts. End tidal capnography during intermittent pressure ventilation may underestimate the true situation; however, the author has found pediatric mainstream capnography to be extremely valuable in monitoring ventilation. Pulse oximetry measures the hemoglobin absorbance and uses the ratio of oxyhemoglobin to deoxyhemoglobin to determine hemoglobin the saturation. Unfortunately, it is often difficult to obtain a reliable pulse wave, and the information provided for the hemoglobin saturation (SO_2) is based on the mammalian oxyhemoglobin dissociation curve. It remains unclear at this time whether pulse oximetry are accurate monitoring devices for use in snakes.

Doxapram can be given in cases of severe respiratory depression or arrest, and profound and immediate effects have been noted following IV administration. Boids typically have slow heart rates (30–70/min); however in cases of true bradycardia atropine is likely to be effective. If hypovolemia is suspected due to hemorrhage or severe dehydration, intravenous access (catheter or butterfly) should be placed (see catheter placement below) and fluids administered (see fluid therapy). The effectiveness of resuscitation can be assessed with the use of a Doppler probe placed at the base of the heart or peripherally (head or tail) to detect blood flow. The Doppler probe can sometimes be placed over a tail artery to assess pulse quality or determine systolic blood pressure (see shock resuscitation section). Trends in blood lactate and pH may be useful to assess improvement in circulatory status.

SHOCK, BLOOD PRESSURE, AND FLUID RESUSCITATION

Blood volume in healthy boids varies from 4% to 6%, and approximately 75% of body weight is water. Reptiles have an equal distribution of intracellular and extracellular fluid compartments (compared with mammals and birds; intracellular space contains 60% of fluid and the extracellular contains 40% of the total fluid volume). Approximately 30% of the extracellular fluid exists in the intravascular space and 70% within the interstitial space. The principles of water movement and fluid therapy are similar to that in other species.

The osmolarity of reptile plasma is typically lower than that of mammals, and consequently solutions osmotically balanced for mammals (eg, 0.9% normal saline) are likely to be mildly hypertonic for reptiles and may therefore further deplete the intracellular compartment. In addition, many arid species of snakes physiologically cope with dehydration by permitting major elevations of plasma osmolarity.

Blood pressure in reptiles is controlled by mechanisms similar to those described in mammals. Being ectotherms, normal blood pressure in snakes may be more profoundly affected by environmental parameters. The reptile's ability to mount an appropriate sympathetic response to hypovolemia requires a warm environment.

Monitoring blood pressure in reptiles during fluid resuscitation may be valuable. Indirect systolic Doppler blood pressure techniques have been tried but with no correlation to direct measurements. In snakes, the cuff is placed just distal to the cloaca and the probe detects blood flow from the caudal tail artery. Indirect systolic blood pressures have been reported between 40 and 90 mmHg. Some snakes withstand 4% graded hemorrhage until the cumulative deficit is 32% of total blood volume, and are able to maintain their initial blood volume throughout hemorrhage. Typically, 50% to 60% of the hemorrhaged deficit is transferred from the interstitium to the circulation throughout hemorrhage. Thus, fluid shifts between the intravascular and interstitial compartments significantly compensate for acute hypovolemia, but in some species do not result in a well regulated arterial blood pressure. Therefore, intravenous fluid therapy using crystalloids and colloids may be important for the treatment of hypovolemia.

Perfusion deficits are assessed using mucus membrane color, capillary refill time, blood pressure and heart rate. Bolus doses of warmed crystalloids (5–10 mL/kg) with colloids (3–5 mL/kg) can be given intravenously until improvements are detected. Some colloids such as oxyglobin (hemoglobin-based oxygen carrier) have also the added advantage of carrying oxygen to the tissue. The use of blood transfusions in reptiles has been anecdotally reported.

INITIAL DIAGNOSTICS

Having resolved any immediate cardiorespiratory emergency, initial diagnostic tests should be prioritized to those that can be undertaken in the conscious animal and that will have an immediate impact on directing initial therapy.

Blood

Blood should be collected as a priority for both a complete blood count and full biochemistry profile. Unless dealing with a small individual or a severe hemorrhagic episode, blood volume is usually not a limiting factor when dealing with these larger snakes. Blood is most often collected from the caudal (ventral tail) vein or the heart. The caudal vein is accessed caudal to the cloaca, between 25% and 50% down the tail. It is wise to avoid the paired hemipenes of males and the paired cloacal musk glands. The needle is angled at 45 to 60 degrees and positioned in the ventral mid line. The needle is advanced in a craniodorsal direction, while maintaining slight negative pressure. If the needle touches a vertebral body it is withdrawn slightly and redirected more cranially or caudally. This vessel is most easily entered in larger snakes and lymphatic contamination is possible but generally uncommon. If circulation is poor, it may be necessary to sample directly from the heart. With the snake restrained in dorsal recumbency, the heart is located approximately 25% to 33% from snout to vent. The heart is palpated and immobilized. The needle is advanced at 45 degrees in a craniodorsal direction into the apex of the beating ventricle. Blood often enters the syringe with each heartbeat. It is wise to maintain digital pressure for 30 to 60 seconds following this technique. Good physical restraint is essential to avoid significant cardiac trauma.

Full laboratory analysis, especially hematology, can take hours or even days if using an external laboratory and therefore quick assessment tests are often necessary:

- Packed cell volume (PCV), total protein (TP), and glucose can be quickly determined from 2 heparinized hematocrit tubes of blood using a microhematocrit centrifuge and glucometer. Serial evaluations are cheap and inexpensive.
- Blood smears can be stained with a Diff-Quik stain (Dade Behring), and an estimated total and differential leukocyte count can be performed within minutes. The total leukocyte count is determined by multiplying the mean number of leukocytes of ten fields (x40 objective) by 2000. Be aware that inaccuracy of up to 25% is not uncommon.
- Point-of-care analyzers (eg, I-stat, Abbot) can provide valuable data on blood pH, gases, electrolytes, lactate, and glucose, etc. However, these machines are calibrated for mammals, and not validated for reptiles.
- VetScan (Abaxis) can produce a reptile biochemistry panel (total protein, albumin, globulin, AST, bile acids, total calcium, phosphorus, uric acid, glucose, CPK, K^+, Cl^-, and Na^+) from 0.2 mL of whole blood in less than 15 min.

In-house laboratory results are used to direct therapy, and other supportive measures.

Diagnostic Imaging

Initial imaging should be obtained before giving bolus fluids because subcutaneous or intracoelomic fluids will make interpretation more difficult. In addition, studies should only focus on techniques that can be accomplished without the need for sedatives or anesthesia, and that will help stabilize the animal and direct emergency treatment. Dorsoventral and lateral (horizontal beam) radiographs and ultrasonograms can often be obtained to help assess gross abnormalities, eg, open versus closed fractures of the skull and spine, pulmonary versus gastrointestinal rupture, cardiomyopathy versus cardiac tamponade, tracheal chrondromas versus pulmonary consolidation, renal mineralization, etc. Emergency radiographs are often imperfect regarding positioning and subtle lesions may not be appreciated. It may therefore be advisable to repeat radiographs at a later date, when anesthesia can be safely undertaken.

Sample Collection

Sample collection should focus on those items that will be corrupted or altered by emergency therapy. Therefore, just as blood should be collected prior to fluid therapy, so exudates, fluids, and aspirates are collected prior to antimicrobial and anti-inflammatory use. Sample collection should again be restricted to procedures that can be performed with physical restraint alone, although, gastrointestinal, cloacocolonic, and lung lavage can usually be performed in sick lethargic snakes with minimal resistance. In the case of lung lavage, aspiration should precede saline infusion, because copious volumes of exudates may be aspirated directly from the lungs.

Samples for microbiologic and cytologic evaluation should be divided into those to be sent to a main laboratory and those for immediate in-house assessment. Gram stains can help direct initial antimicrobial choice, while cytology can confirm inflammatory and infectious host responses.

INITIAL TREATMENT
Temperature & Humidity

Moribund snakes cannot move or thermoregulate, and unless presented in a severely hypo- or hyperthermic state, should be immediately housed at the upper end of the species-specific preferred optimum temperature zone, commonly 29-30 °C (88-90°F). Unless species-specifc requirements dictate otherwise, 80% humidity should be provided.

Fluid Therapy

The parameters used for assessing hydration include mucous membrane moisture, skin elasticity, position of the ocular globe, PCV and TP. Many arid snakes have a high tolerance for dehydration and increases in plasma sodium and osmolarity. They are able to restore plasma

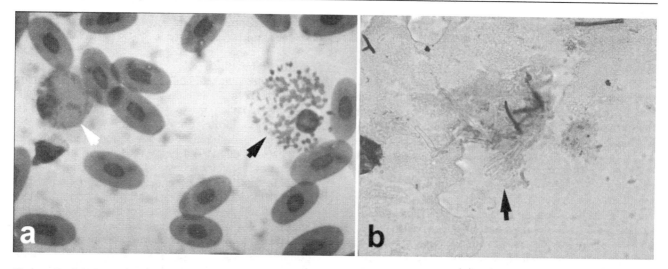

Figure 2. (a) Stained blood smear from a ball python demonstrating a reactive monocyte (*white arrow*) and toxic degranulating heterophil (*white arrow*), suggestive of severe inflammatory or infectious response. (b) Impression smear from an ulcerated wound indicating fungal elements (*arrow*) and the primary need for topical antifungal rather than antibiotic medication.

sodium through increased thirst and excretion of sodium from salt glands. Dehydration deficits should be restored using a crystalloid with an osmolarity comparable with normal reptile plasma (varies between 250 and 290 mOsm/L). The normal plasma sodium concentration varies with different species, but is generally between 142 and 165 mmol/L. Use of common mammalian isotonic crystalloids (Normal saline, 308 mOsm/L; Plasmalyte-A [Baxter], 294 mOsm/L; Normosol-R [Abbott], 294 mOsm/L) cannot be recommended because undiluted these fluids are relatively hypertonic for reptiles. Jarchow's modification (two parts of 2.5% dextrose in 0.45% saline and one part LRS, 278 mOsm/L) has been specifically recommended for reptiles in the past. The additional dextrose appears to be beneficial and once metabolized provides a net water gain which is particularly useful given that most reptiles present with water deficiencies. However, there may be little or no benefit of this self-made fluid when commercially available 2.5% dextrose in half-strength LRS (264 mOsm/L) is used as a replacement fluid. For meeting maintenance requirements, 2.5% dextrose in 0.45% saline (280 mOsm/L) also appears acceptable. Additional dextrose is given intravenously if the blood glucose is especially low. Reptiles produce lactate and use anaerobic metabolism during anoxia. Blood lactate levels also increase during shock with inadequate tissue perfusion. Lactate is rapidly metabolized to bicarbonate in the liver when tissue oxygen delivery is restored. Concerns over the use of lactate-containing fluids aggravating acidosis are largely unfounded in any snake with appropriate liver function. Fluid deficits can be replaced over 12 to 36 hours when lost acutely or more commonly over 48 to 96 hours for the chronically dehydrated snake. Maintenance fluid requirements are 5 to 15 mL/kg/day. Maintenance fluids are given orally when the reptile is able to assimilate oral nutrition and by

soaking the in warm fluids. Water absorption may take place through the cloaca during freshwater soaks. Intravascular catheter placement is difficult in snakes and largely restricted to the heart (critical and temporary only) or jugular veins (cut-down procedure but can be maintained for days to weeks).

Wounds

Acute and severe wounds can be caused by burns, exposed nails or screws, and rodent bites. Burns result in proteinaceous fluid loss and can quickly become severely infected and cause septicemia. While rodents can cause extensive trauma, down to the level of the spine. Emergency measures involve copious wound flushing and wet-dry dressings, fluid therapy, and antibiotic cover. Debridement and reconstruction occur later under anesthesia when the snake is stable.

Cloacal Prolapse

Unlike mammals and birds, dystocia is seldom an emergency presentation; however, straining can lead to cloacal prolapse. Prolapse can also be associated with environmental problems, parasites and intestinal disease, or extramural pressure associated with masses. Identification of tissue origin and viability are important. If the cloaca is viable, then copious flushing should be followed by lubrication and replacement. If impossible, the tissue can be lubricated with an antibiotic ointment and covered with plastic wrap (Cling Wrap®) until the snake can be stabilized for surgical cloacopexy or resection and anastamosis.

Neurologic Dysfunction

Most cases of severe neurologic disease are due to inclusion body disease, septicemia, or CNS trauma. If the cause is obviously traumatic, then intravenous methyl-prednisolone at 1 mg/kg IV may be tried; however, steroids are best avoided in reptiles.

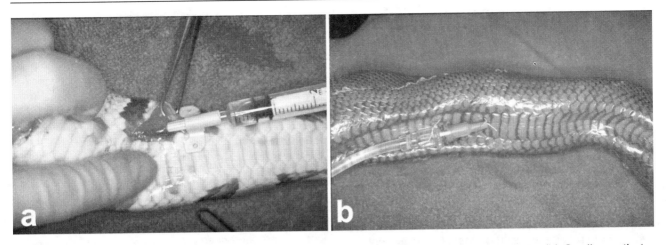

Figure 3. (a) Jugular catheter being placed into a moribund ball python under local anesthesia. (b) Cardiac catheter placed into the ventricle and sutured in place – the entire area is bandaged but the catheter is removed within 24 hours.

Drug Therapy

A complete listing of drugs is available elsewhere. However, the author's initial drug choices may include ceftazidime (gram-negative bacteria), penicillin (gram-positive bacteria and anaerobes), fluconazole or amphoteracin B (fungal), and meloxicam (NSAID) and/or morphine for analgesia.

FURTHER DIAGNOSTICS AND TREATMENT

Following initial stabilization over the initial 1 to 7 days, further case investigation and a definitive diagnosis should be pursued along established lines.[2, 3] Anesthesia, diagnostic imaging, endoscopy and surgery can be undertaken in an attempt to effect a cure.

REFERENCES

1. Martinez-Jimenez D, Hernandez-Divers SJ. Emergency care of reptiles. Vet Clin North Am Exot Anim Pract. 2007;10:557-585.
2. Mader DR. Reptile Medicine and Surgery. Philadelphia: WB Saunders, 2006.
3. Raiti P, Girling S. Manual of Reptiles. British Small Animal Veterinary Association, Cheltenham, England, 2004.
4. Diethelm G. Reptiles. In Carpenter JW (eds): Exotic Animal Formulary. St. Louis, MO: Elsevier Health Sciences, 2005, pp 55-131.

COLUBRIDS: COMMON CONDITIONS OF COMMON SNAKES

Dr Stephen J. Hernandez-Divers, BVetMed, DZooMed,
MRCVS, Diplomate ACZM
College of Veterinary Medicine,
University of Georgia, Athens, GA

Colubrid snakes belong to the family Colubridae, a truly huge and eclectic group composed of over 1700 species in 325 genera. Consequently, there are few characteristics shared by all members; some are oviparous, others viviparous; some are venomous, while others are constrictors. There is great variation in morphology, behavior, natural history, and therefore captive care requirements. The most commonly kept pet species include the rat (or corn) snakes, kingsnakes, milksnakes, racers, watersnakes, gartersnakes, bullsnakes, pinesnakes, and gophersnakes. Color mutants are common and have been developed through intensive (in)breeding, and may command high prices (eg, albino Arizona mountain x queretaro kingsnakes currently offered at $1000), while others may be sold for less than $10 (water snakes).

MEDICAL HISTORY

In addition to any immediate problem, a detailed anamnesis should include information on source and origin, captive husbandry, nutrition, quarantine and preventative medicine (Table 1). Space does not permit a detailed review of the diverse topic of captive colubrid management, and therefore readers are advised to consult the references.

Table 1. History Form

Reptile name or ID:		
Species, subspecies:		
Date of birth, age:		
Sex:		
Duration in owner's care/captivity:		
Origin (captive bred, wild import):		
Source (breeder, store):		
Enclosure/vivarium specifications:	Type (arboreal, terrestrial, aquatic)	
	Size	
	Construction (materials, fittings)	
	Décor and furnishings	
	Ventilation (mesh, grills)	
	Cleaning routine (agents used)	
Environment:	Heating equip	
	Heating control	
	Day-time temperature gradient	
	Night-time temperature gradient	
	Water temperature	
	Lighting equip (type, position, age)	
	Photoperiod	
	Humidity	
Diet:	Type and quantities	
	Frequency of feeding	
	When food offered	
	Changes of appetite	
Water:	Method of provision (spray, bowl)	
	Frequency of water changes, water quality	
	Changes in drinking behaviour	
Water and food supplements:	Type and frequency of use	
Breeding details:		
Other specimens in same vivarium:		
Other specimens in same room or air space:		
Disease history of presented animal:		
Details of any diseased in-contact animals:		
Quarantine protocol:		
Other details of relevance:		

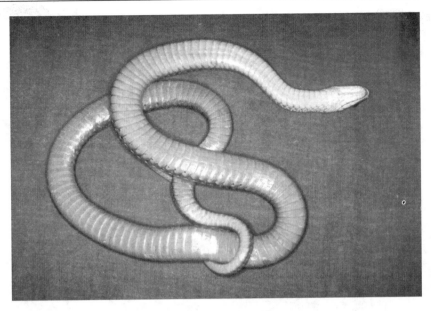

Figure 1. Hypovitaminosis B in a garter snake that was fed fish high in thiaminase, without additional thiamin supplementation.

PHYSICAL EXAMINATION

The head of an aggressive snake or a snake of unknown disposition should be identified and restrained before opening the transportation bag and removing the animal. In general, the head of the snake is held behind the occiput using the thumb and middle finger to support the lateral aspects of the cranium. The index finger is placed on top of the head. The other hand is used to support the serpentine body. An assessment of demeanor will quickly become obvious. Nervous or aggressive (nonvenomous) snakes can be restrained using plexiglass tubes or sedated prior to examination. A tame snake should be permitted to roam over the hands and arms thereby enabling the clinician to gauge muscle tone, propioception, and mobility. Propioception can be assessed by placing the snake in dorsal recumbency and monitoring the effort and ability of the snake to right itself. Systemically ill serpents will often be limp, lack strength, and be less mobile. Head carriage, body posture, cloacal tone, propioception, skin pinch, withdrawal, ocular and righting reflexes can be used to assess neurologic function.

The entire integument, particularly the head and ventral scales, should be thoroughly examined for evidence of dysecdysis (poor shedding), trauma, parasitism (especially the common snake mite, *Ophionyssus natricis*) and microbiological infection. If available, the recently shed skin should also be examined for evidence of retained spectacles. Skin tenting and ridges may indicate cachexia ('poverty lines') or dehydration while mites may congregate in skin folds, nostrils and ocular rims. The eyes should be clear, unless ecdysis is imminent. The spectacles covering the eyes should be smooth as any wrinkles usually indicate the presence of a retained spectacle. The subspectacular fluid drains through a duct to the cranial roof of the maxilla. When blocked, the build up of fluid cause a subspectacular swelling that often becomes infected resulting in a subspectacular abscess. Damage to the underlying cornea can result in panophthalmitis and ocular swelling, while retrobulbar abscessation will result in protrusion of a normal sized globe. Other ocular pathologies can include uveitis, corneal lipidosis, and spectacular foreign bodies including splinters of wood chip or other vivarium materials.

Examination of the oral cavity is often left until the end of the examination as many snakes object to such manipulation. However, even before the mouth is opened the tongue should be seen flicking in and out of the philtrum with regularity. The mouth can be gently opened using a tongue depressor or blunt sexing probe to assess the mucous membranes, teeth, and glottis. The pharynx and glottis should be examined for hemorrhage, foreign bodies, parasites and discharges. It is important to observe the glottis during respiration in an attempt to differentiate between discharges originating from the respiratory and gastrointestinal tracts. Unfortunately due to the stresses of examination, respiratory rates are often elevated in normal reptiles and therefore tachypnea may not be considered a definitive indicator of respiratory disease unless observed in the undisturbed snake. However, open mouth breathing is a reliable indicator of severe respiratory compromise. During the oral examination the patency of the internal nares and the state of the polyphyodontic teeth should be noted.

Working from cranial to caudal, the head and body are palpated for abnormal swellings, wounds and other abnormalities. The position of any internal anomalies, noted as a distance from the snout and interpreted as a percentage of snout-vent length (SVL), will enable an assessment of possible organ involvement. Depending

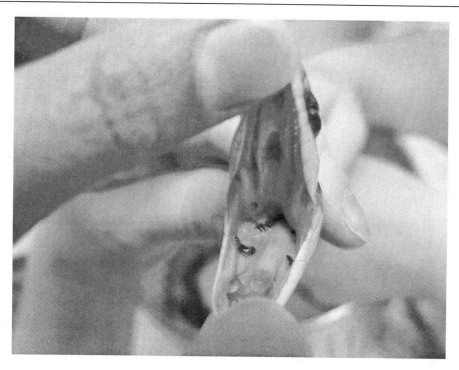

Figure 2. Digenic trematodes (Renifers) in the oral cavity of a wild-caught black racer.

upon the musculature, feeding habits and fat reserves of the snake, it may be possible to palpate the normal heart, stomach, liver, active ovaries, eggs, kidneys and fecal material. Recently fed snakes will have a mid-body swelling associated with the prey within the stomach, but handling such individuals may well lead to regurgitation. Eggs and pre-ovulatory follicles may also be palpated. The clinical examination should differentiate between coelomic (internal) and extracoelomic (subcutaneous) masses. The majority of subcutaneous masses are usually abscesses but parasitic cysts, blisters and neoplasia are occasionally seen. Internal masses may represent abscesses, neoplasia, granulomas, obstipation, organ hypertrophy, retained eggs or ova. The cloaca should have muscle tone and not be gaping open, be free from fecal staining with no discharges. Nervous snakes, especially colubrids will often expel the contents of their cloacal glands and cloacae in a defensive reaction to a perceived threat. This foul smelling material does not represent infection, but merely an annoyance as the smell is difficult to eradicate from clothing. Examination of the cloaca can be carried out using a dedicated otoscope or rigid endoscope. Digital palpation is often overlooked but is a useful technique. In small to medium snakes a latex-gloved, lubricated finger can be passed into the cloaca and may allow palpation of eggs, cloacoliths, fecoliths, or abscesses. Examination of the tail length or probing of the hemipenes (in males) should confirm the gender. The tail length (and the number of subcaudal scales) is always smaller in females than males but this method requires access to published information on tail length and scale counts unless both sexes are available for simultaneous examination. The hemipenes are entered by placing a blunt probe, lubricated with a water-soluble material, either side of midline, just inside the caudal cloacal rim. In males the probe passes to a depth of 6 to 14 subcaudal scales whereas in females the probe enters a cloacal gland to a depth of only 2 to 6 subcaudal scales.

COMMON PROBLEMS

Detailed descriptions of disease processes can be found in the references.

Table 2. Approximate Body Organ Position in Colubrids

Organ	Approximate % position from snout to vent
Heart	20-23
Right lung (excluding air sac)	22-32
Liver	30-48
Stomach	48-58
Left ovary	64-74
Right ovary	70-80
Left testis	69-74
Right testis	78-82
Left kidney	86-94
Right kidney	90-96

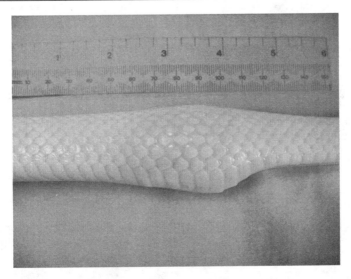

Figure 3. Intracoelomic mass (90% snout-vent) causing constipation in an albino Californian kingsnake. The mass proved to be a granulosa cell tumor and was successfully removed.

REFERENCES

1. Applegate R. General care & maintenance of milk snakes, Advanced Vivarium Systems Inc, BowTie Press, Irvine, CA, 1992.
2. Love K, Love B. Corn snakes: The comprehensive owners guide. Advanced Vivarium Systems Inc, BowTie Press, Irvine, CA, 2005.
3. Perlowin D. Garter snakes and water snakes, Advanced Vivarium Systems Inc, BowTie Press, Irvine, CA, 2005.
4. Perlowin D. Common kingsnakes, Advanced Vivarium Systems Inc, BowTie Press, Irvine, CA, 2007.
5. Gibbons JW, Dorcas ME. North American Watersnakes: A Natural History. University of Oklahoma Press, Norman, OK, 2004.
6. Richardson A. North American racer snakes, Capstone High-Interest Books, Mankato, MN, 2003.
7. McCracken HE. Organ location in snakes for diagnostic and surgical evaluation. In Fowler ME and Miller RE (eds): Zoo & Wildlife Medicine Current Therapy 4. Philadelphia: WB Saunders, 1999, pp 243-248.
8. Mader DR. Reptile Medicine and Surgery. Philadelphia: WB Saunders, 2006.
9. Raiti P, Girling S. Manual of Reptiles, British Small Animal Veterinary Association, Cheltenham, England, 2004.

Table 3. Differential Diagnoses by Clinical Signs (most common problems in **bold type**)

Clinical sign	Differential Diagnoses
Anorexia	Parasites: protozoa (***Cryptosporidia***, *Coccidia*, *Entamoeba*), helminths Gastrointestinal foreign body or impaction **Ecdysis and dysecdysis** **Stomatitis**, esophagitis, gastritis, enteritis **Pneumonia**, hepatitis, **nephritis (gout and neoplasia)** Systemic disease (eg, **septicemia**, toxemia, metabolic disease) Normal gravidity and **dystocia** **Seasonal (winter) anorexia** Intraspecific and interspecific aggression/suppression **Poor management, especially temperature**, photoperiod, inappropriate food offered Maladaption (especially recent wild imports, change of ownership)
Head and mouth signs	Tongue trauma or infection **Stomatitis (digenic trematodes)** **Respiratory disease** Pharyngitis Petechiae (septicaemia, poisoning) Pale deposits (urate tophi, abscessation) Submandibular cellulites

Table 3. Continued.

Regurgitation	**Stomatitis**, esophagitis, **gastroenteritis** Protozoal and helminth parasites especially *Cryptosporidia* Septicemia, intoxication, gastrointestinal foreign body, **abscess, neoplasia** **Poor management (inappropriate temperature, handling after feeding, rotten food item, insecurity)**
Coelomic mass or swelling	**Granuloma, abscess, neoplasia** Gastric hypertrophy (*Cryptosporidium serpentes*) Obstruction/constipation (parasites, too large a prey item, too frequent feeding, feeding dehydrated defrosted prey items, concurrent dystocia, foreign body)
Diarrhoea	Parasites (especially *Entamoeba*) Iatrogenic (medication, force-feeding, excessive oral fluid therapy) Gastroenteritis **Inappropriate temperature, rotten food item, inappropriate food item or change of diet**
Integumental signs	**Dysecdysis (mites** and rarely ticks, **low humidity and inappropriate temperature**, starvation) **Blister disease (too high humidity, unhygienic conditions)** Rodent trauma **Thermal burns**, chemical irritation Petechiae (septicemia, bacterial or viral dermatitis, transcutaneous hookworm (*Kalicephalus*) infection Bacterial and mycotic infections, including **abscesses** Myiasis Rostral abrasions due to repeated escape attempts
Ataxia, paresis, convulsions	Starvation, debilitation Hypoglycemia, **hypovitaminosis B1 (excess thiaminase in fish eating species)**, hypocalcaemia **Trauma** Meningitis (parasitic, bacterial, viral especially Paramyxovirus and boid inclusion body disease) Hepatic encephalopathy **Renal disease**, hyperphosphataemia Intoxication including medicines, eg, organophosphorus, ivermectin Septicemia, toxemia
Ocular signs	Intraocular – panophthalmitis, **subspectacular abscess** Extraocular – retrobulbar abscess (bacterial, fungal), ascending infection secondary to stomatitis or respiratory infection. Diffuse opacity – normal ecdysis Focal opacity – corneal scarring, corneal lipidosis, corneal foreign body **Wrinkled eye surface – retained spectacle (low humidity)**
Reproductive signs	**Infertile mating, laying unfertilised ova** – infertile male and/or female, unsuccessful copulation, inappropriate pre-breeding conditioning or poor seasonal stimulation, diseased reproductive tract Stillbirths – poor management of gravid female especially lack of suitable basking site or poor egg incubation, reproductive tract infection, trauma especially rough handling, lack of appropriate nest site **Dystocia** – obesity, incorrect temperature, lack of nest site, disturbance and other stresses, infertility, reproductive tract disease, egg/foetal abnormality, systemic or metabolic disease
Circulatory signs	True anaemia - hemorrhage, neoplasia, chronic disease, excessive blood collection Iatrogenic (false) anemia – lymphatic contamination during venipuncture, excessive rate of intravenous fluid therapy Petechiae – septicemia, toxemia Blood parasites – usually nonpathogenic Circulatory RBC Mitosis – normal **Cardiomegaly** – true cardiomyopathy, illusion due to starvation and emaciation, non-cardiac mass
Respiratory signs	Nasal discharge – rhinitis, pneumonia, stomatitis **Dyspnea – pneumonia**, airway obstruction, eg, stomatitis, normal wheeze upon disturbance or during ecdysis Glottal discharge – pneumonia (aspiration, bacterial, viral, parasitic)
Skeletal signs	**Spinal deformities** – trauma, osteomyelitis, **kyphosis, scoliosis**, metabolic bone diseases, **hypertrophic osteopathy**, congenital anomalies

SNAKE ANESTHESIA AND SURGERY

Dr Stephen J. Hernandez-Divers, BVetMed, DZooMed,
MRCVS, Diplomate ACZM
College of Veterinary Medicine,
University of Georgia, Athens

In general, performing anesthesia and surgery on a snake should be approached with the same principles as those used for domestic animals. However, there are obvious anatomic considerations, as well as unique aspects of patient preparation, positioning, and equipment with which the reptile clinician should be familiar.

ANESTHESIA

The secrets to successful snake anesthesia are an appreciation of anatomy, physiology, and detailed preparation. In particular, understanding the cardiorespiratory system, and the need to maintain appropriate species-specific temperatures throughout the entire hospital period, are essential. There are many ways to anesthetize a snake, and readers are directed to detailed reviews for complete coverage[4,5]; however, only the preferred options used by the author will be described here. Although nonvenomous snakes form the mainstay of the article, venomous-specific methods will be indicated; however, practitioners are advised to seek specialty training before working with these animals.

Pre-anesthetic Assessment

All snakes should be monitored from a distance (without handling) to record resting respiratory rate. A complete physical examination, including accurate weight and heart rate should also be conducted. The extent of pre-op blood testing will depend upon the situation, and can include hematology (ideally a complete blood count, but minimally hematocrit and estimated counts from a blood smear) and a biochemistry profile (including total protein, albumen, globulin, aspartate transaminase, bile acids, uric acid, and electrolytes). Consideration should be given not only to the amount of blood that can be safely collected from a healthy snake but also the potential blood loss from that snake during surgery. Total blood loss should not exceed 0.5 mL/kg. The VetScan VS2 analyzer (Abaxis) provides a full reptile profile with only 0.2 mL whole blood. Pre-anesthetic assessment of venomous species is typically restricted to visual appraisal.

Premedication

Given the preliminary findings reported by Sladsky, it seems dubious whether opiates are effective. Nevertheless, until confirmed, morphine at 1.5 mg/kg IM can be considered. In addition, meloxicam at 0.2 mg/kg IM is also useful, but should probably be given post-operatively if there are any doubts regarding hydration status and/or renal function. If infection has been confirmed (and culture has already been collected) then pre- and intraoperative antibiotics should be considered.

Premedication is generally ill-advised when dealing with venomous species.

Induction and Intubation

For small snakes (<500 g), it is frequently easier to place them into a ziplock bag, flush and fill the bag with 5% isoflurane or 8% sevoflurane, seal, and leave for 15 to 30 minutes in an incubator or vivarium (27-30°C, 80–88°F) for gaseous induction. This creates sufficient restraint for intubation (or easier intravenous access if deeper induction is necessary). For larger snakes, intravenous propofol (5–10 mg/kg) via the caudal vein or intracardiac injection facilitates intubation. For small snakes, uncuffed tubes are preferred for intubation using intravenous catheters or endotracheal tubes up to 2.5 mm in diameter. Tubes are typically taped (not tied) in place. For larger snakes, appropriately sized cuffed endotracheal tubes can be used but should be inflated with care, just enough to avoid gas leakage during ventilation. Maintain the snake in sternal and on a high level of anesthetic gas (eg, 4–5% isoflurane, 6–7% sevoflurane) until a surgical plane of anesthesia is achieved.

All venomous snakes should be transported to the practice in secure, double containers, that are locked and clearly marked. The inner container should be transparent and have a small hole drilled into one end to permit the insertion of an anesthetic gas line. This will permit induction without having to handle a dangerous species. When all righting reflexes have been lost, the snake can be removed using snake hooks, tongs and/or plastic tubes, taking all necessary precautions, and assuming that the snake is still conscious and capable of striking. Syringe cases are placed over the maxilla and mandible to cover the fangs, and the snake is carefully intubated using a long endotracheal tube. Evenomation is still possible from an anesthetized snake, and so a large syringe case (with the end cut-off) is placed over the endotracheal tube and snake's head to provide protection during the entire procedure.

Maintenance

The snake is positioned on a heated surface, with the forced warm air blankets appearing most effective at maintaining temperature (Bair Hugger, Arizant). A temperature probe is inserted into the esophagus or cloaca, and an ultrasonic doppler probe is taped over the heart or major peripheral artery. A pediatric, mainstream, end-tidal capnography unit is connected to the endotracheal tube, which is then connected to a ventilator and anesthetic machine. The Small Animal Ventilator (Vetronics) connects to an existing anesthetic machine, is simple to use, and effective. Starting from a maximum inspiration pressure of 2 cm water and expiration length of 2 sec, the maximum inspiration pressure is increased until normal coelomic breathing excursions are achieved. The rate at which inspiration occurs is controlled by the oxygen flow rate. The expiration length is then adjusted to initially equal the pre-anesthetic resting respiratory rate.

Vascular access can be achieved by placing an intravenous catheter into the caudal vein or, in an emergency, into the ventricle. For most noncritical cases, intracoelomic or subcutaneous fluids can be administered prior to surgery to ensure hydration, and repeated intraoperatively at a site distant to the surgical area. Accurate pulse oximetry readings can be difficult to maintain, but a reflectance probe inserted into the cloaca or esophagus, or a tongue clip probe across the mandible or maxilla is often successful. No values for MAC, isoflurane or sevoflurane, have been determined for any species of snakes; however, data from other reptiles suggests MAC values for isoflurane and sevoflurane of around 2 and 3, respectively.

Monitoring

Anesthetic monitoring should include an assessment of reflexes (eg, tongue, tail, vent, ventrum), ETCO$_2$, SpO$_2$, pulse or heart rate, ventilation depth and frequency, oxygen flow, and vaporizer setting, with a dedicated anesthetist to record and make adjustments to suit individual patient requirements. While it is impossible to give strict guidelines, the following are offered as mere guidelines;

- Heart rate: > 30, and not less than 60% of conscious values.
- SpO$_2$: readings often highly variable but monitoring the trend is more informative.
- ETCO$_2$: Maintain between 10 and 20 mmHg. Hyperventilation and values <10 mmHg are associated with respiratory alkalosis and prolonged apnea during recovery.
- Ventilation: Adjust depth and frequency to maintain appropriate ETCO$_2$, typically 1 to 4 breaths/min.

- Core temperature: 27–30°C, 80–88°F. Hypothermia leads to prolonged recovery.

Recovery

Before the end of surgery, anesthetic gas should be discontinued, and several minutes later, ventilation decreased to 0.25 to 1 breath/min in order to increase ETCO$_2$, decrease SpO$_2$, and induce spontaneous respiration. At the end of surgery, oxygen should be discontinued and replaced by air (ambulance bag), again at 0.25 to 1 breath/min. Once spontaneous breathing has returned, the snake should be moved to an incubator and continuously monitored. Venomous snakes should be extubated at this stage and placed in their original locked container and observed. Nonvenomous snakes can be extubated once righting reflexes or body movement has returned. However, they should still be monitored every 5 to 10 minutes as some individuals may regress and become apneic. Full anesthetic recovery has occurred once the snake is moving freely around the vivarium, and may take several hours.

SURGERY
Equipment

Proper surgical lighting and, for small snakes or microsurgery, magnification (operating loupes, Surgitel) are required. Radiosurgery (eg, Surgitron, Ellman) utilizes high frequency radiowaves to create hemostasis, is versatile and cost effective, and creates less collateral damage than CO$_2$ laser. Hemoclips (Weck closure systems) and LoneStar retractors are also invaluable (Table 1). Surgical instruments are listed in Table 2 and shown in Figure 1.

Table 1. Useful Equipment Suppliers

Lone Star retractor, 11211 Cash Road, Stafford, TX 77477
Surgitel loupes, General Scientific Corporation, 77 Enterprise Drive, Ann Arbor, Michigan 48103
Weck Closure Systems, 2917 Weck Drive, P.O. Box 12600, Research Triangle Park, NC 27709
4.0 MHz dual radiofrequency Surgitron, Ellman International, 1135 Railroad Ave, Hewlett, NY 11557
Adhesive surgical drape, Veterinary Specialty Products, P.O. Box 812005, Boca Raton, FL 33481

Table 2. Useful instruments for reptile surgery

Standard exotic animal surgery pack	Standard exotic animal microsurgery pack
Plain ophthalmic fine thumb forceps	Mini gelpi retractor
Adson ½ forceps, very fine	k-wire pin driver vice
Small scissors (top sharp tip, bottom blunt tip)	Doolen avian bone holding device
Castroviejo retractor	Stevens tenotomy scissors
Small suture scissors	Two balanced micro scissors
Derf needle holder	Doolen avian spay hook
Strabismus scissors	Extra delicate mosquito forceps, straight
Four curved ophthalmic mosquito forceps	Extra delicate mosquito forceps, curved
Twenty 3x3 gauze sponges	Sontec curved tying forceps
Twenty cotton tipped applicators	Ring-tipped thumb forceps with holes
Clear plastic adhesive drape	Two spring bulldog clamps
Vetrap 2"	Lonestar retractor

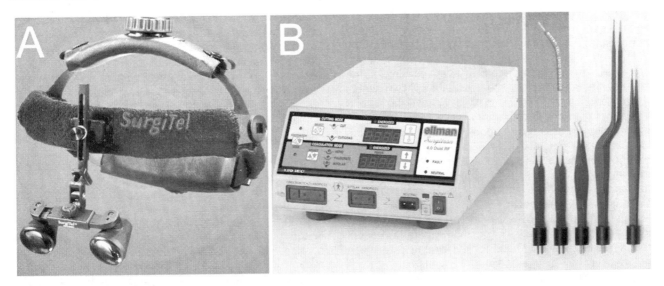

Figure 1. (A) Surgitel loupes mounted onto a headband provides a practical, comfortable and economical way to achieve focal magnification. (B) The 4.0 Mhz Surgitron unit is half the cost of a CO_2 laser and yet provides comparable fine cutting and a greater variety of instruments and hence applications in practice.

Preparation and Positioning

Consideration should also be given to appropriate surgeon and patient positioning to reduce surgeon fatigue, prevent patient compromise, and maximize surgical site access. Aseptic surgery should be carried out in an appropriately clean and sterile room by surgeons wearing surgical masks, hats, sterile gloves and gowns. The surgical site should be aseptically cleaned using chlorhexidine or povidone-iodine concentrate—a toothbrush is particularly useful for cleaning scaled skin. Transparent, adhesive drapes (Surgical drape, Veterinary Specialty Products) are preferred over cloth drapes.

SURGICAL PROCEDURES

Snake integument is composed of keratinized scales and thinner interscaler skin. Incisions should be made between the scales, thus making most surgical wounds scalloped. When reptile skin is incised, it has a tendency to invert. Therefore, everting suture patterns (eg, horizontal or vertical mattress) using polydioxione or nylon are recommended to ensure opposition of tissue without future dysecdysis. Fine polydioxione causes less reaction than polyglactin and is preferred for internal sutures. Skin sutures are typically removed after 6 to 8 weeks. Some of the most common surgical procedures performed on snakes are outlined below.

Wound Treatment

Wounds, usually grossly infected, are a frequent presentation, and given the caseous nature of the reptilian inflammatory response, surgical debridement is often always necessary. Sharp dissection is employed to remove all adherent necrotic and infected tissue that should then be submitted for histopathology and microbiology. The maintenance of topical medications, dressings and bandages can be challenging in some cases, and although slow, the ability of reptiles to recover from serious trauma is remarkable. Allogeneic and xerogeneic grafts have been documented in reptiles. Successful xerogeneic skin grafts using porcine small intestinal submucosa (Biosist, Cook Veterinary Products) have been reported in reptiles.

Cutaneous Abscess/Mass Removal

Subcutaneous abscesses are most common, neoplasia less so. Abscesses typically present as firm discrete swellings. If the skin is unaffected, a craniocaudal incision is made over the length of the abscess, and the skin reflected to facilitate complete removal of the abscess (including any fibrous). A piece of the abscess capsule should be submitted for bacterial and fungal culture. The underlying tissue is thoroughly irrigated with antiseptic solution. If the entire abscess including pyogenic capsule was removed, the skin can be closed in a routine manner. If there is any doubt the skin edges should be trimmed to leave an open wound that should be cleaned daily.

Subspectacular Abscess

Blockage of the lacrimal duct results in fluid accumulation between the spectacle and the cornea. Often this fluid becomes infected. A 30 degree wedge is removed from the ventral aspect of the spectacle. The caseous material is removed for cytology and microbiology, and the subspectacular space thoroughly flushed. The patency of the lacrimal duct must be assured. It is generally easier to catheterize the buccal opening of the duct as it emerges close to the cranial margin of the palatine teeth, and flush retrograde. The spectacle wedge incision is left open and frequent topical ophthalmic medication is recommended until the spectacle heals at the next shed.

Prolapsed Hemipenes

Snakes possess paired copulatory organs (hemipenes) that may by become prolapsed through the vent. If the tissue appears viable, it can be cleaned, moistened and gently replaced by inversion through the vent opening and caudally into the tail base. Two simple interrupted sutures can be placed across the lateral margins of the vent to prevent immediate recurrence for 2 to 5 days. A purse suture should not be utilized. If the tissue appears necrotic, hemipenal amputation is the treatment of choice. As the hemipenes do not contain a urethra, mattress sutures or circumferential ligatures can be placed at the base and the organ safely resected. Obviously, this procedure will compromise future breeding although snakes with a single remaining hemipenis can still breed. All affected animals will benefit from systemic antibiotics and topical wound care given the proximity of the surgical site to the cloaca.

Prolapsed Cloaca and./or Colon

Prolapse of the cloaca and distal colon are not uncommon. However, they are often treated inappropriately by replacement and purse-string sutures without due regard for the underlying cause. Minor prolapse can be replaced and two simple interrupted sutures can be placed near the edges of the vent to prevent recurrence. More severe prolapse is treated by transcutaneous cloaco- or colopexy, which is aided by using a rigid endoscope to visualize needle entry into the cloaca/colon. Uncommonly, this procedure will fail and a coeliotomy is required to anchor the colon to caudal ribs using nylon. In cases of severe cloacal and colonic necrosis, resection and end to end anastomosis is essential, and a combination of cloacal and coeliotomy approaches may be required. Great care is needed to identify and preserve the openings of the ureters and oviducts within the urodeum.

Coeliotomy

The elongated nature of snakes makes it impossible to make a single coeliotomy incision to access all major organs. Therefore, it is vital that the precise surgical site is accurately determined ahead of time using anatomy references, palpation, clinical pathology, and diagnostic imaging. A permanent marker is used to mark the surgical site, both on the snake and on white tape placed on the table (Figure 2). In general, the incision is made between the first and second rows of lateral scales, taking care to incise between the scales whenever possible. This ensures that the incision is positioned laterally and off the floor when the recovered snake is ambulatory. Radiosurgery, laser or blunt dissection is continued through the muscle layer, just ventral to the ribs. Entry into the coelom is made between the ribs and ventral musculature. It is often necessary to navigate through multiple fascial layers to gain access to the coelom, and extensive fat bodies can hinder visualization. A two-layer closure is routine with the

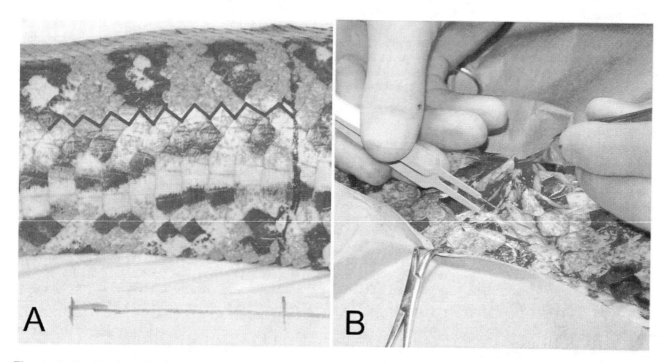

Figure 2. Positioning of a large snake in preparation for coeliotomy. The zigzag line indicates the preferred skin incision between the second and third rows of lateral scales. Note the tape marker on the table to remind the surgeon of the precise area of interest. (B) Using bipolar radiosurgery to incise through the coelomic musculature.

muscle layer closed using absorbable suture in a simple interrupted or continuous pattern. Skin closure is routine.

A variety of intracoelomic procedures can be attempted following successful entry into the coelom. These include, among others, salpingotomy (egg/ova/fetus removal), gastrotomy, enterotomy, pneumotomy, transmitter implantation, mass/tumor removal, and surgical biopsy.

POSTOPERATIVE CARE

All things being well, snakes are typically discharged the day after surgery, and rechecked a week later. Sutures are typically removed 6 to 8 weeks after surgey.

REFERENCES

1. Slatter D. Textbook of Small Animal Surgery. Philadelphia: WB Saunders, 1993.
2. Hernandez-Divers SJ. Surgery: principles and techniques. In Raiti P, Girling S (eds): Manual of Reptiles. British Small Animal Veterinary Association, Cheltenham, England, 2004, pp 147-167.
3. Bennett RA, Mader DR. Soft tissue surgery. In: Mader DR (eds): Reptile Medicine and Surgery. Philadelphia: WB Saunders, 1996, pp 287-298.
4. Mader DR. Reptile Medicine and Surgery. Philadelphia: WB Saunders, 2006.
5. Raiti P, Girling S. Manual of Reptiles. British Small Animal Veterinary Association, Cheltenham, England, 2004.

SNAKE RADIOLOGY: THE ESSENTIALS!

Stephen J. Hernandez-Divers, BVetMed, DZooMed,
MRCVS, Diplomate ACZM
College of Veterinary Medicine,
University of Georgia, Athens, GA

RESTRAINT AND POSITIONING

Snakes are relatively easy to position and restrain for radiographic examinations. Ultimately, anesthesia will provide the best positioning. If the purpose of the examination is to rule out radiodense foreign bodies, the snake may be allowed to coil in its natural position while the radiograph is taken. If detailed examination of the skeletal, respiratory and digestive system is desired, the snake must be extended. A plastic restraint tube can be utilized for this purpose; however, this may produce some radiographic artefact. The snake is introduced into a tube with a diameter that will not allow the snake to turn around and exit the tube. The radiograph is taken before the snake has an opportunity to back out. Snakes can also be restrained with heavy sand bags or tape but great care is required to avoid bruising. In larger snakes, several films will be needed to radiograph the entire length of the body. It is important to properly mark the snake and label each exposure in order to keep track of all the views. Lateral views are best taken using horizontal beams to avoid displacement artefact of the viscera. However, standard laterals with the snake taped in lateral recumbency can be useful especially where horizontal beams are not possible or safe to undertake. The interpretation of dorsoventral views is hindered by the spine and ribs, but can still be useful when dealing with obvious lesions including eggs and mineralised masses.

Table 1. Approximate Body Organ Position in Snakes

Organ	Approximate % Position from Snout
Heart	22–35
Lung(s)	25–50
Air Sac	45-85
Liver	35–60
Stomach	45-65
Spleen, pancreas, gall bladder	60–70
Small intestine	65–80
Kidneys	65–90
Colon	80-100

INTERPRETATION
Musculoskeletal System

Traumatic fractures, metabolic bone diseases, spondylitis/spondylosis, osteomyelitis, and congenital abnormalities are common indications for examining the skeletal system of snakes (Figure 1). Again, it is imperative to properly label each radiograph to document a lesion as it is difficult to discern by looking at the radiograph exactly where the lesion is located in the actual animal. Fractured ribs with periosteal bone formation are a common finding in snakes. Another common finding is exuberant vertebral periosteal bone formation. On radiographs, this appears as several "fused" vertebrae. Clinically, the animal is less flexible in the area that is affected and may display an angular deformity. The aetiology of this condition has not been conclusively documented, however, traumatic and/or infectious causes have been suggested.

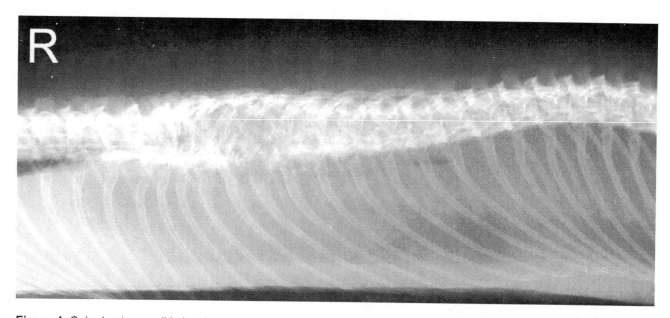

Figure 1. Spinal osteomyelitis in a boa constrictor.

Digestive System

The esophagus is not normally visualised unless gas or contrast material is present. The stomach is located in the middle third of the body. Often, the radiodense skeletal remains of recently ingested prey can be visualized. The liver is ventral to the lungs and caudal to the stomach. Ingesta of varying opacities can be observed in the small and large intestines in the caudal third of the body. The cloaca lies at the level of the last pair of ribs. The pancreas, gallbladder and spleen are not normally visualised. Common indications for radiographically evaluating the digestive system include hypertrophic gastritis, foreign body ingestion/impaction, constipation, hepatomegaly and hepatic masses. Contrast studies are useful in diagnosing intestinal obstruction and constipation. In addition, contrast material in the gastrointestinal tract can often outline and help determine the origin of a nonspecific intracoelomic masses; intraluminal or extraluminal.

Cardiopulmonary System

The heart generally lies at the end of the cranial third of the body. Cardiomyopathy has been reported in snakes, which can be indicated by cardiomegaly on radiographs. Metastatic mineralization of large blood vessels is often apparent around the heart due to the negative contrast afforded by the adjacent lungs.

The trachea can be visualized as a radiolucent line in the cranial third of the body extending from the head to the cardiac silhouette. The lungs are visualised caudal to the cardiac shadow in the middle third of the body, except in viperids and elapids where they can also be found cranial to the heart. Except in boas and pythons, the left lung is vestigial or absent and thus, not usually appreciated. In most species, the lung continues as a thin walled air sac into the caudal third of the body, extending in some almost to the level of the cloaca. The overlap of other organs such as liver and stomach over the lung fields can make the radiographic interpretation of respiratory disease challenging. Common indications for evaluating the respiratory system are rhinitis, suspected neoplastic and infectious disorders of the trachea and lung, as well as abscesses or granulomas (Figure 2).

Urogenital System

The kidneys of snakes are located dorsal to the intestinal tract in close association with intracoelomic fat bodies. They are not always radiographically evident, unless enlarged or mineralised. Disease processes that can cause renomegaly include renal gout and neoplasia.

The oviducts lie in the middle and caudal third of a coelom. Eggs of oviparous species are leathery and poorly calcified, but can often be appreciated on plain radiographs. Viviparous species (boas and viperids) do not produce eggs. In these species, fetal skeletons become visible as they mineralize late in gestation. The hemipenes of some species may appear mineralised and can be detected radiographically. A discrete soft tissue swelling at the level of the cloaca may indicate cloacitis, abscessation or fat deposition. Common indications for evaluating the reproductive system include dystocia, apparent infertility and reduced fecundity. It is important to note that dystocia is difficult to diagnose by radiology alone and a careful history, in combination with clinical signs and other diagnostic techniques such as ultrasound, is often necessary to make the final diagnosis (Figure 3).

Miscellaneous

The presence of any swelling is an indication for radiography. Abscesses, which can either be extracoelomic or intracoelomic and associated with a specific organ or the coelomic wall are common findings in snakes.

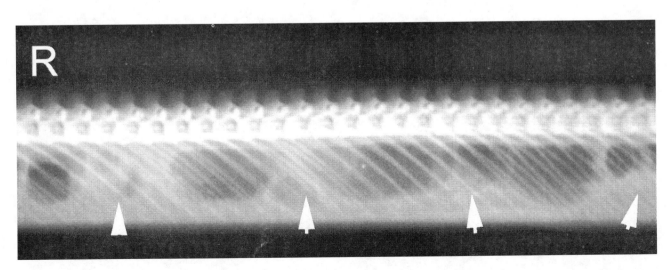

Figure 2. Multiple soft tissue opacities (*arrows*) within the lung fields of a ball python, later confirmed as pulmonary mycobacteriosis.

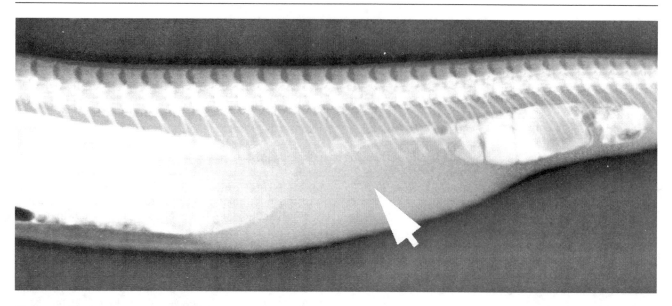

Figure 3. Barium contrast enema demonstrating compression of the lower intestinal tract due to a mass effect, which was later confirmed as an ovarian granulosa cell tumor.

REFERENCES

1. Hernandez-Divers SM, Hernandez-Divers SJ. Diagnostic imaging of reptiles. In Practice. 2001;23:370-391.

2. Mader DR. Reptile Medicine and Surgery. Philadelphia: WB Saunders, 2006.

3. Raiti P, Girling S. Manual of Reptiles, British Small Animal Veterinary Association, Cheltenham, England, 2004.

DYSTOCIA IN A GREEN ANACONDA
(*Eunectes murinus*)

Dr Stephen J. Hernandez-Divers, BVetMed, DZooMed,
MRCVS, Diplomate ACZM
College of Veterinary Medicine,
University of Georgia, Athens, GA

While egg retention is well documented in oviparous snakes, dystocia in viviparous snakes appears to be less common. In addition, dealing with giant species (which are still legal pets in most states) presents additional technical difficulties regarding handling, diagnostics, anesthesia and surgery. A case report involving a large anaconda is presented as an example. Reviews of snake reproduction and dystocia can be found in published texts.

CASE REPORT

An adult female green anaconda (*Eunectes murinus*) was quarantined following acquisition from another institution. Despite routine preventative medical procedures and assisted feeding, the snake failed to thrive in captivity. At the time of referral, the anaconda weighed 44.2 kg, and was estimated at 5.5 m (18 feet) in total length. The snake was alert but considered to be in poor body condition. Hematology and plasma biochemistry were unremarkable. The snake was premedicated with 40.5 mg butorphanol (Torbugesic, 10 mg/mL, Fort Dodge Animal Health) intramuscularly and anesthesia was induced with 280 mg intravenous propofol (Propofol, 10 mg/mL, Abbott Laboratories) into the caudal (ventral coccygeal tail) vein. Endotracheal intubation using a 4.5-mm cuffed tube facilitated maintenance of anesthesia using 2% to 5% sevoflurane (Sevoflo, Abbott Laboratories) in oxygen delivered by intermittent positive pressure ventilation. Anesthetic monitoring included pulse oximetry, Doppler, and esophageal temperature. Perioperative fluid support (160 mL/hr) was administered via a catheter inserted into the caudal vein. Survey (lateral, horizontal beam) radiographs indicated two retained fetuses 110 to 200 cm cranial to the vent. A standard surgical coeliotomy was undertaken. The first incision, started 72 cm cranial to the vent, and extended for 53 cm. Upon entry into the coelom the two oviducts were identified and exteriorized and a well-formed fetus was located lying between the two oviducts in an ectopic position. The second fetus was desiccated, had broken up into several sections, and was also located external to each oviduct. To remove all parts of this second fetus, a second incision (10 cm) was started 11 cm cranial to the first, and a third incision 9 cm was required 6 cm cranial to the second. The three surgical sites were irrigated with sterile saline. Coeliotomy closure was routine. The snake made an uneventful recovery and was discharged with ceftazidime (1 g Fortaz, GlaxoSmithkline), 20 mg/kg IM q 72 hrs for 5 treatments. The snake consumed a rabbit with minimal assistance 3 weeks after surgery. The snake voluntarily fed for the first time in over a year, 6 weeks after surgery. Sutures were removed 8 weeks after surgery. The anaconda has continued to improve and is now feeding regularly without assistance.

REFERENCES

1. Mader DR. Reptile Medicine and Surgery. Philadelphia: WB Saunders, 2006.
2. Raiti P, Girling S. Manual of Reptiles. British Small Animal Veterinary Association, Cheltenham, England, 2004.

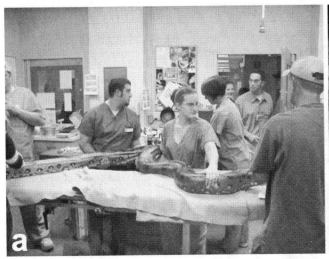
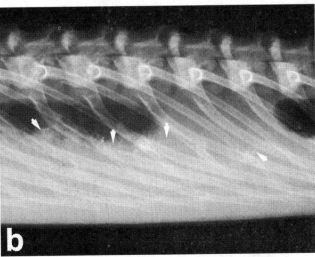

Figure 1. (a) Handling a large constrictor requires several experienced handlers, especially for accurate restraint for blood collection and anesthetic induction. (b) Lateral (horizontal beam) radiograph demonstrating the spinal column of a retained fetus (*arrows*).

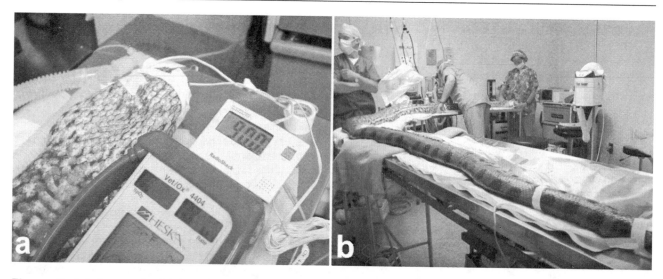

Figure 2. (a) Anaconda intubated and being maintained on sevoflurane on a rebreathing ventilator circuit – temperature and pulse oximetry readings are visible. (b) Surgical positioning of large snakes can be challenging, and in this case required the use of three surgical tables.

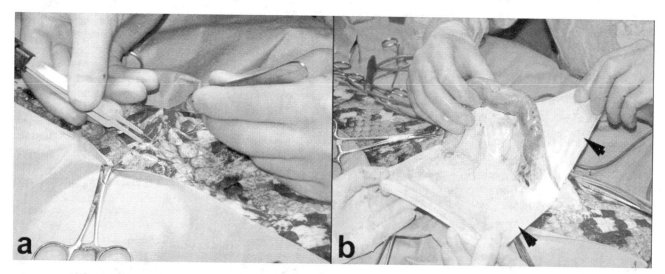

Figure 3. (a) A standard snake coeliotomy technique is used for giant snakes – bipolar radiosurgery is being used to ensure hemostasis. (b) Removal of a retained and mummified ectopic fetus lying between the two oviducts (*arrows*).

BASIC HUSBANDRY AND NUTRITION OF CHELONIANS

Charles Innis, VMD
New England Aquarium
Boston, MA

Proper husbandry is critical to the successful maintenance of reptiles in captivity. A number of thorough reviews of chelonian husbandry have recently been published. Strict attention must be paid to environmental temperatures, humidity, light quality, water quality, habitat complexity, and nutrition. Among the hundreds of turtle species, husbandry requirements vary extensively. Prospective turtle owners must familiarize themselves with the requirements of the specific species with which they wish to work prior to purchasing the animal.

Several issues must be addressed in selecting a potential species as a pet. First, the keeper must be sure that the species can legally be kept according to local, state, federal, and international law. Laws pertaining to the sale and ownership of pet reptiles vary tremendously among different states and cities. Several states have revised their legislation such that it is no longer determined which species *cannot* be kept as pets, but which species *can* be kept as pets. The list of species is revised on a yearly basis to reflect the current global status of the species. Information on the legal status of species at the state level may be obtained from state fish and wildlife departments. Local laws should also be investigated as some cities restrict ownership of certain large species.

Many reptile species have become threatened due to habitat loss and collection for the international food, skin, and pet trade. As such, the pet owner ethically should avoid keeping animals that have been collected from the wild. In addition to ethical concerns, wild-caught animals should be avoided as they are less likely to adapt to a captive life style and more likely to be harboring parasites than captive-bred animals. The pet owner should avoid the temptation to keep notoriously difficult or rare species, as well as the temptation to "rescue" ill animals from pet stores. Keeping such individuals is often very discouraging, and can introduce disease into an otherwise healthy collection.

In selecting a species as a pet, one should investigate those that are being bred in captivity in significant numbers and that have demonstrated longevity in captivity similar to that in their natural environment. Consideration should be given to the adult size of the species, and whether very large specimens can be humanely housed in a given geographic zone. For example, although the African Spur-Thigh Tortoise (*Geochelone sulcata*) is a friendly, hardy, inexpensive, captive-bred species, it is the third largest tortoise species in the world and cannot be humanely housed as an adult in the home of the average pet owner. It may make a fine pet in an outdoor corral in Arizona, but is impractical indoors in New England.

The following list of species includes those that are generally captive bred, and have proven in the author's experience to make good pets. This list is not meant to be all-inclusive, but rather a starting-point for the novice keeper. The keeper should be careful to choose captive-bred animals, as many of these species are available as both wild-caught and captive-bred specimens. Among land tortoises, redfoot tortoises (*Geochelone carbonaria*), Greek tortoises (*Testudo graeca*), and Russian tortoises (*Testudo horsfieldi*) make good pets. Among water turtles, painted turtles (*Chrysemys picta*), Reeve's turtles (*Chinemys reevesi*), and the New Guinea red-bellied turtles (*Emydura subglobosa*) are personable and relatively easy to care for.

Numerous sources for captive-bred reptiles have become available in the past ten years. Locally, reptile specialty pet stores often carry a wide range of healthy captive-bred specimens. In addition, the keeper should investigate classified advertisements in reptile pet magazines. Often, local breeders may be found through these advertisements and may allow the purchaser to handpick their animal. Direct contact with a breeder provides invaluable information on husbandry of the species. Other sources for captive-bred reptiles include numerous regional reptile shows, reptile Internet web sites, and large-scale national reptile breeders. Information on these sources can generally be found in reptile pet-magazines or on the Internet.

As ectothermic animals, reptiles must be able to move among various temperature zones to maintain their preferred body temperature. Inadequate temperatures promote poor immune response and poor digestive efficiency, and are a common cause of illness in captive reptiles. As such, heat sources appropriate to the species must be provided. One of the best heat sources for reptiles is simple incandescent lighting. Regular light bulbs in reflector-type fixtures focus heat into certain areas of the environment, simulating the heat derived in the wild from the sun. For most species, this is the most effective and natural way of heating in indoor environments. Temperatures below these lamps must vary with the ecology of the species. For example savanna tortoises may seek basking temperatures of 32–35°C, while some leaf-litter forest species may prefer to be at 20–25°C. In addition, some species must be kept very warm even at night, while others prefer a night temperature drop. Nighttime low temperatures should be maintained at 23–27°C for tropical species and 21–23°C for temperate species. In cases where night temperatures must be high, ceramic radiant heat emitters or heat panels may be installed to provide heat without providing light. Using light-emitting heat sources at night may adversely affect the animal's sleep cycle, immune response, and reproductive cycle.

Water heaters, such as those used in tropical fish tanks, may be useful to maintain stable background temperatures in aquatic environments. In general temperatures from 25–28°C are adequate depending on the species. Since these heaters are often made of ceramic or glass, one must ensure that they are located so that they cannot be broken by the turtles.

Most aquatic turtles need to be able to dry themselves completely while basking. Nonabrasive basking sites such as cork-bark or driftwood should be available. Aquatic plants such as *Anacharis* provide excellent hiding and resting areas.

Like the choice of heat source, the choice of enclosure will vary by species. Many small species can be maintained in traditional glass terrarium setups. The enclosure must be escape-proof for the kept species. Larger specimens may need to have custom-built enclosures or large commercially available enclosures. Large aquatic species need large pools such as those used in the aquaculture industry, and generally need some type of powerful filter system to maintain adequate water quality. A very effective filter system can be constructed using a pond pump, foam or mesh filter material, and a material such as lava rock to create surface area for biological filtration. In its simplest form, the pump is used to move water from the enclosure, through the foam, over the lava rock, and back to the enclosure. In this author's experience, tap water seems to be safe for aquatic turtles, although more conservative keepers may prefer to use aged tap water, bottled water, or reverse osmosis purified water.

Chelonians can be maintained indoors or outdoors, with each having its benefits. Indoor enclosures offer more safety and better climate control, while outdoor enclosures offer improved ventilation and exposure to natural sunlight. Both indoor and outdoor enclosures must be made predator-proof. Outdoor enclosures for small chelonians must include a secure wire bottom and top. The bottom may be covered with several inches of dirt and planted with grass creating an escape-proof enclosure. Where fire ants are a problem, appropriate control measures should be taken. Consider mammalian pets, especially canines and ferrets, to be a threat to small chelonians that are maintained indoors.

Enclosure substrate should be easy to clean and not harmful if ingested. Many types of bedding, including gravel, sand, crushed walnut shells, corn cob, and some bark mulch, are indigestible and often cause intestinal obstructions when they are ingested. Newspaper is a safe and effective substrate for most species. Other safe alternatives include non-frayed artificial turf or carpeting, paper towels, soil, hay, or large size bark mulch. In dry environments, alfalfa pellets such as rabbit food can be used as bedding. Substrates should be spot cleaned daily and replaced when heavily soiled.

Water must be made available as appropriate for the species. Many terrestrial turtles and tortoises will drink water from a shallow bowl. The animal must be able to easily access the bowl without spilling the water Spraying may also be required to maintain adequate humidity levels for tropical forest species. Areas of high humidity should be available, as even arid zone species will seek out such areas. Small plastic food storage containers can easily be modified to provide high humidity retreats. Recent evidence indicates that the commonly seen condition of "pyramiding," where the scutes of tortoises develop a conical appearance, may be caused by low environmental humidity.[5]

In addition to basking lights, full-spectrum lighting with ultraviolet B wavelengths is thought to be important for many species. Recent research has shown that UV exposure resulted in higher vitamin D levels in young red-eared sliders (Trachemys scripta elegans). The best source of UVB light is unfiltered natural sunlight. It is ideal to have an outdoor enclosure that can be used during mild weather. In the absence of natural sunlight, fluorescent or mercury vapor UVB-emitting bulbs should be provided. The lights should be located at a distance as specified by the manufacturer. UVB light is filtered out by glass or plastic, and UV intensity of most bulbs is reduced after 6 to 12 months of use.

Chelonians may be carnivorous, omnivorous, or herbivorous. Carnivores may accept earthworms, fish, killed rodents, insects, and commercial foods such as trout pellets. Herbivores require a high-fiber, high-calcium diet and should be fed greens such as kale, collards, endive, escarole, dandelion, clover, chicory, beet greens, and Swiss chard. These items are chosen to maximize the animal's calcium intake. High-fiber sources such as alfalfa pellets, chopped hay, and grass are also desirable. The concern about excessive levels of oxalates and thiocyanates in some greens has likely been overstated, and these greens are appropriate for chelonians as part of a balanced diet. Omnivores may be offered a mix of the carnivore and herbivore diet. In general, fruits are not tremendously nutritious and should be used as "dessert" in small amounts.

Unless whole rodents or fortified pellets are being consumed, vitamin and mineral supplementation may be needed. In particular, insects and plant matter are often deficient in mineral content. Reptiles that are not supplemented often suffer from calcium deficiency. Supplementation may be done by mixing a powdered calcium supplement with the food items, or by feeding insects a high calcium diet for several days before they are fed to the reptile ("gut loading"). Supplements should be used in moderation as oversupplementation can also occur. Multivitamin supplements in particular are often excessively high in Vitamin A and D and should generally be used only once weekly.

Proper husbandry and nutrition are the most important aspects of reptile preventive care. However, a number of other practices are recommended. Quarantine of new animals is extremely important. In general, a 2- to 3-month quarantine is recommended. Overzealous collecting and overstocking of environments should be avoided. During quarantine, fecal analysis should be performed several times to test for internal parasites. These parasites should be treated and eliminated if possible before release from quarantine. In some situations, further testing such as bloodwork may be recommended.

Finally, annual physical examination by a veterinarian is recommended for all pet reptiles. At the physical exam, the animal's growth and weight are measured, maintenance such as nail trimming and beak trimming is done, stool samples are checked, signs of illness may be detected, and a discussion of modifications of husbandry can occur.

Maintaining chelonians in captivity can be a rewarding and fun experience. By properly selecting a species, a specimen, and researching the species needs, the keeper may experience years of enjoyment.

REFERENCES

1. Gurley R. Keeping and Breeding Freshwater Turtles. Ada, OK: Living Art Publishing, 2003.
2. Highfield A. Practical Encyclopedia of Keeping and Breeding Tortoises and Freshwater Turtles. London: Carapace Press, 1986.
3. Mader DR (ed.). Reptile Medicine and Surgery. 2nd ed. St. Louis, MO: Elsevier, 2006.
4. McArthur S, Wilkinson R, Meyer J (eds.). Medicine and Surgery of Turtles and Tortoises. Cambridge, MA: Blackwell Science Ltd, 2004.
5. Wiesner CS, Iben C. Influence of environmental humidity and dietary protein on pyramidal growth of carapaces in African spurred tortoises (*Geochelone sulcata*). J Anim Physiol Anim Nutr. 2003; 87:66-74.

RESTRAINT AND PHYSICAL EXAMINATION OF CHELONIANS

Charles Innis, VMD
New England Aquarium
Boston, MA

Physical examination of chelonia should be conducted systematically, ensuring that each major organ system is assessed. Excellent accounts of chelonian medical evaluation have recently been published.

Small turtles should be weighed with an accurate gram scale. Larger turtles may be weighed using kilogram scales. Turtles should feel dense when picked up, similar to a rock of equal size. They should be reactive. They should protect themselves by withdrawal into the shell, or demonstrate a bright, alert, active posture. Underweight turtles may feel "empty" when picked up.

The head and limbs may be difficult to extract for examination. Experience, patience, and/or sedation may be required to perform a thorough examination. The limbs are palpated for muscle mass, strength, joint swelling, and bone structure. The nails are examined for overgrowth, hyperkeratosis, and so forth. The skin is examined routinely, specifically assessing the neck, axilla, and prefemoral regions for ticks, leeches, and fly larvae. The skin may show signs of hyperkeratosis, or flaking in long-term captive turtles kept on suboptimal diets. The cloaca is examined for evidence of inflammation or diarrhea. Some species can emit a foul odor when disturbed. In some cases the odor is produced by glands along the bridge of the shell. Turtles and tortoises will often defecate and urinate during examination. Use appropriate care, and save these diagnostic specimens for analysis.

Sexual dimorphism is usually apparent in sexually mature chelonians. Males generally have a longer tail with a more distal cloacal opening than females. The cloacal opening in males is often at or beyond the caudal carapace margin when the tail is pulled caudally and viewed ventrally. Males of many species also have a plastral concavity to facilitate mounting the carapace of the female for copulation. These rules do not hold true for all species, especially for plastral concavity, and other species-specific traits may be noted. For example, sexual dimorphism may be seen in the eye or skin color, adult size, or toenail length of some species. Common examples include the red iris of male eastern box turtles (*Terrapene carolina carolina*), elongated toenails on the forelimbs of male slider turtles (*Pseudemys* spp., *Trachemys scripta*), painted turtles (*Chrysemys picta*), and map turtles (*Graptemys* spp.), dramatically larger female versus male body size in map turtles and diamondback terrapins (*Malaclemys terrapin*), and more prominent mental glands, gular scutes, and body size, in male desert tortoises (*Gopherus agassizii*). In general males are more brightly colored than females. While sexual dimorphism is generally apparent in adult chelonians, it is much less apparent prior to puberty, and it can be difficult to ascertain the sex of juveniles. If desired, gender determination of juvenile turtles may be accomplished by coelioscopic examination of the gonad.

Respiratory exam includes assessment of respiratory rate, effort, and quality. Respiratory movements in most turtles are generated by slight to moderate rotational movement of the forelimbs and, or extension of the hind limbs. Pharyngeal pumping in most species has olfactory rather than respiratory function. Respiration should be silent or slightly audible and the mouth should be closed. Gasping or loud whistling is abnormal and may be a sign of rhinosinusitis or pneumonia. While some practitioners report that respiratory auscultation is useful in chelonia, the author has found this to be generally unrewarding.

The shell is examined for shape, symmetry, color, and density. The shell of mature specimens of most species should have strong bone density. Several species, including soft-shell turtles (several genera) and pancake tortoises (*Malacochersus tornieri*) have flexible shells. Several genera have normal plastron or carapace hinges that allow shell mobility. It is useful to palpate each scute, or keratin plate, of the shell, assessing for loose scutes, sensitivity, fluid, and so on. Ecchymoses or petechiae of the shell may be indicative of osteomyelitis, sepsis, or spirorchid trematode infection. Soft areas of the shell may be due to infection or secondary hyperparathyroidism. Long-term captive box turtles on suboptimal diets seem to develop a rounded, ball-shaped shell, rather the normal flat plastron and domed carapace. In these turtles, the limbs and head often seem disproportionately large in comparison the shell. This results in the soft tissues of the limbs, pelvis, and neck being exposed more than in a normal specimen.

Neurologic examination is conducted using standard principles. Observe the turtle walking around the exam room if cooperative. If possible, aquatic turtles should be observed while swimming. Abnormal buoyancy is common, and often indicates pulmonary, gastrointestinal, coelomic, neurologic, or metabolic abnormalities. Proprioception, withdrawal reflexes, and cranial nerve examination should be performed. Cardiac auscultation is difficult, but the heart rate, rhythm, and quality may be assessed with a Doppler monitor placed over the carotid artery or heart base. Use of Doppler monitor in the examination room is impressive to the client, and demonstrates a thorough examination. Coelomic palpation may detect eggs, bladder stones, masses, and organ enlargement. Palpation is accomplished via the prefemoral space. Depending on the size of the turtle, a single finger, multiple fingers, or the entire hand may be able to fir into the prefemoral space. The hind limb will need to be positioned in extension. Use caution in strong chelonians that may be able to crush one's fingers by withdrawing the hind limbs. In most cases, palpation will reveal only soft tissue.

The author prefers to examine the structures of the head as the last part of the examination, as the turtle is often significantly upset after head restraint, and may not allow further examination. Examination of the head is very important since many pathologic conditions affect the ears, eyes, nasal cavity, tongue, and oral mucosa. Restraining the head and opening the mouth requires some practice. Restraint of the head should not be done without sedation in dangerous species such as snapping turtles. In some cases, many of the structures of the head can be partially examined prior to restraint of the head (eg, eyes, nares). Ideally, the examiner patiently waits for the turtle to extend its neck, and then the examiner's thumb and index finger are swiftly moved to grasp the turtle's neck behind the jaw. The examiner's hand should come from behind the head to prevent the turtle from noticing the imminent restraint. It may take significant strength to maintain control of the head, and it may be helpful to brace the remaining fingers of the restraining hand against the anterior margin of the carapace. An alternate method of initial head restraint is to grasp the head with thumb and index finger on top of the head and between the rami of the mandible. This grip does not allow examination of the mouth, but can be used as a transitional hold prior to restraining the turtle behind the head. If head restraint is not possible because the turtle refuses to extend its neck, several options are available. In some cases, "tickling" the hind feet or tail of the turtle may cause it to extend the neck. Alternatively, placing the turtle on a flat surface for several minutes, or placing the turtle in shallow water may be helpful. Rocking the turtle side to side or front to back, while held in ventral recumbency may also help. If none of these techniques work, a curved-tip dental hand-scaler may be placed under the tip of the upper beak and carefully used to slowly and smoothly extract the head. In sea turtles, the head cannot be withdrawn and is easily accessible. After failing all of these methods, sedation may be considered.

Once the head is restrained, the eyes should be assessed for signs of inflammation, discharge, and corneal ulcers. Vitamin A deficiency, viral infection, and bacterial infection are common causes of inflammation of the eyes. Saline eye-wash solution may be useful to flush debris. Enophthalmia may be indicative of dehydration or cachexia. There is no external ear canal in turtles. The tympanum is just deep to the skin, and should be located by palpating for a soft spot on the side of the head. Asymmetry of the tympanum may be noted with otitis media. The nares should be examined for asymmetry and discharge because rhinosinusitis is common in chelonia. The conformation of the beak should be assessed. The keratin of the beak can become overgrown, and conditions such as prognathism may be seen. Turtles do not have teeth. Oral examination is performed in most cases with the head restrained. However, oral examination can sometimes be performed without head restraint. Some turtles will open their mouth as a defensive display (particularly if carefully coaxed). If the mouth must be manually opened, several techniques are useful. This, too, takes practice. In small sea turtles, some smaller species, or weak individuals, the mouth can often be opened by putting gentle ventral traction on the mandible, or by gently pulling the pharyngeal skin ventrally. If this is not successful, a tool is inserted along the edge of the mouth. As the turtle begins to open the mouth, the tool is quickly and smoothly repositioned transversely across the mouth. A number of tools will work well for this technique, but the author prefers a flat, stainless-steel dental spatula. Pen caps, blunted needles, or dental scalers may also be used. In the author's opinion, tongue depressors do not work well for opening turtle mouths.

Once open, the oral cavity is examined for mucous membrane color, mucosal plaques, glossitis, and stomatitis. Oral plaques have been reported in association with herpes virus and iridovirus infection of chelonia, and warrant biopsy for histopathology and molecular diagnostics. The glottis is located at the base of the tongue and should be examined for discharge. The paired choanae are located along the palate and should be evaluated for symmetry and discharge. Occasionally, discharge from the eustachian tubes may be visible in the caudal pharynx in cases of otitis media.

In some cases, chemical immobilization may be required for thorough physical examination of chelonia. Dissociative agents are useful for many procedures. Ketamine (20–100 mg/kg IM) and tiletamine/zolazepam (3–10 mg/kg IM) have both been used safely and effectively for many years. Chelonians often require treatment with the high end of the above doses. If sedation is inadequate, incremental doses up to the maximum dose may be given. Prolonged recovery may be seen with high doses of these drugs, but generally recovery occurs within two to twelve hours. Although spontaneous respiration often persists under the effect of these drugs, the patient should be monitored closely and ventilated if apneic.

Propofol (5–15 mg/kg IV or IO) has become a popular reptile anesthetic. Benefits of propofol include its rapid onset of action, relatively short residual effect, and cardiovascular-sparing effect. Drawbacks to the use of propofol include the necessity of IV or IO injection, relatively high cost, short shelf-life, and respiratory depressant effects. Medetomidine may be useful as an adjunct to other injectable anesthetics. Several studies in tortoises have found that medetomidine (25–100 µg/kg IM or IV) is a useful adjunct to ketamine (5–10 mg/kg IM or IV). By using medetomidine, a low dose of ketamine may be used, thus allowing for a more rapid recovery after reversal with atipamezole. The author has also used medetomidine (50 µg/kg IM) as an adjunct to tiletamine/zolazepam in several chelonian species, when standard doses of tiletamine/zolazepam provided inadequate restraint.

Neuromuscular blocking agents have been used for restraint of reptiles for nonpainful procedures. While these agents have not gained widespread acceptance, succinylcholine and gallamine have been used for procedures such as transport of crocodilians and intubation of chelonians. Rocuronium (0.4 mg/kg IM), has been studied in North American box turtles (Terrapene carolina ssp.). Initial clinical trials of this drug by the author indicate the drug to be useful in Mediterranean tortoises (Testudo sp.), but less effective at the proposed dose for tortoises of the genus

Geochelone. The effect of rocuronium is reversed by neostygmine and glycopyrrolate.

REFERENCES

1. Mader DR (ed.). Reptile Medicine and Surgery. 2nd ed. St. Louis, MO: Elsevier, 2006.
2. McArthur S, Wilkinson R, Meyer J (eds.). Medicine and Surgery of Turtles and Tortoises. Cambridge, MA: Blackwell Science Ltd, 2004.

CLINICAL PARASITOLOGY OF THE CHELONIA

Charles Innis, VMD
New England Aquarium
Boston, MA

Internal and external parasites, including ticks, insect larvae, protozoa, and metazoan worms are common in chelonia. The clinician must use judgement to assess the clinical implications of specific parasites. While wild turtles survive with a variety of parasites, turtles in captivity may be prone to superinfection under conditions of immunosuppression, crowding, and poor hygiene.

Ticks may cause localized inflammation, and may be vectors of disease. Ticks removed from imported chelonians should be submitted to the USDA laboratory in Ames, Iowa for identification. In the past, exotic ticks carrying the bacterial agent that causes heartwater disease have been found on tortoises imported into the United States from Africa. Introduction of such disease into the United States could be devastating for livestock. Ticks are most commonly found on the axillary and pre-femoral skin. Ticks may be removed using forceps. A commercially available permethrin spray (Provent-a-mite, Pro Products, Mahopac, NY) has been approved by the FDA for use in reptiles, and safety and efficacy studies against ticks have been conducted in tortoises. Sporadic reports of mite infestation of chelonia suggest that mites are much less of a problem for chelonia than for snakes and lizards.

Fly larvae are often found within the subcutaneous tissues of North American box turtles (*Terrapene* sp.). Large numbers of larvae can be found in some cases. The larvae are detected by examining the soft tissues of the neck and pre-femoral skin. Characteristic 1- to 2-cm soft tissue masses with a central orifice are present. Larvae must be manually removed. Leeches are commonly found on freshwater chelonia, and may be vectors of hemoparasites. They are removed manually.

Hemoparasites of chelonia do not always cause clinical signs. Intraerythrocytic parasites such as *Hemogregarina*, as well as extracellular hemoparasites such as *Plasmodium*, may be encountered during examination of blood smears. Anecdotal reports of anemia that resolved with treatment of hemoparasites suggest that these organisms may be problematic in some cases. Primaquine and chloroquine, at doses extrapolated from the treatment of malaria in birds, have been used in chelonians. Chloroquine is available for both intramuscular injection and oral administration. Previous reports of chloroquine's use in reptiles to treat *Plasmodium* infections have used a dose of 125 mg/kg PO every 48 hours for three doses. In humans a dose of 50 mg/kg per week is generally used to prevent malaria, while a dose of 50 mg/kg/day may be used in treatment of malaria. The author has used chloroquine in three chelonian patients at a dose of 50 mg/kg IM once weekly for three doses. One patient developed moderate ataxia in the limb used for injection after the second dose;

however, normal function was regained over several weeks, and it was unclear whether the drug was the cause of the problem. Other adverse effects, such as vision abnormalities seen in humans, were not detected but would be difficult to document in chelonians.

A systemic intranuclear coccidian parasite has been reported in chelonia over the past 15 years. Species affected have included the radiated tortoise (*Geochelone radiata*), impressed tortoise (*Manouria impressa*), leopard tortoise (*Geochelone pardalis*), Bowsprit tortoise (*Chersina angulata*), and Sulawesi tortoise. Organisms have been most commonly found in intestine, pancreas, liver, and kidney, with less frequent involvement of the eustachian tube, splenic macrophages, middle ear, lung, and stomach. Most cases were diagnosed post mortem. Intranuclear coccidia and *Mycoplasma* spp. were identified ante mortem from the nasal cavity of five Sulawesi tortoises (*Indotestudo forsteni*) affected by chronic rhinosinusitis and oronasal fistulae. Recent investigation identified this coccidian as a novel species, likely of a novel genus. Successful treatment of infected tortoises has not been described; however, toltrazuril has been used clinically in several unconfirmed cases. Ponazuril has recently shown promise for the treatment of coccidiosis in bearded dragons, and may have use in chelonia. However, the author is not aware of its use in chelonia at this time.

Entamoeba invadens may cause significant pathology in chelonians, particularly under conditions of immunosuppression. There appears to be a high prevalence of amoebiasis in recently imported Southeast Asian and African chelonians. After a lengthy collection and importation process, these animals are often emaciated, dehydrated, heavily parasitized, and suffering from various bacterial and fungal infections. Clinical experience in rehabilitating these animals has shown that eliminating *Entamoeba* infections appears to greatly increase survivorship. In addition, clearing *Entamoeba* infection from chelonians may be desirable if the chelonians are to be housed with more susceptible lizards or snakes.

The characteristic multinucleated cysts of *Entamoeba* are passed in feces and are directly infectious to a new host. Upon ingestion of the cysts, excystation occurs and motile trophozoites penetrate the wall of the gastrointestinal tract. While some infections remain within the GI tract, *Entamoeba* may spread to the kidneys or liver resulting in abscess formation. Symptoms of infection generally include watery, bloody, or mucoid diarrhea, anorexia, dehydration, and lethargy. Diagnosis of amoebiasis is generally made by detection of cysts or trophozoites on direct fecal wet mount or fecal floatation, although newer diagnostic modalities such as polymerase chain reaction (PCR) will likely be applied in the future.

The choice of medication for treating amoebiasis in humans often depends on the suspected location of the infection and the severity of the infection. Drugs are generally classified by their site of action and their ability to kill trophozoites and/or cysts. If a patient is an asymptomatic cyst shedder, a drug that is active within the intestine and effective against cysts is chosen. If the patient suffers from extraintestinal infection, combination therapy is generally used to kill migrating trophozoites as well as intestinal cysts.

The most commonly reported therapy for reptilian amoebiasis has been metronidazole given orally at relatively high doses and relatively infrequent intervals. However, recent pharmacokinetic studies in reptiles indicate that more frequent, lower doses may be more appropriate. Three reports of the pharmacokinetics of orally administered metronidazole in reptiles have been published; however, no pharmacokinetic study of oral metronidazole has been published for chelonian species. The pharmacokinetics of subcutaneously administered metronidazole have been recently described for the red-eared slider. The drug was absorbed well, but several turtles became ill during and after the study. Unfortunately the study design did not allow the authors to determine whether the illness was due to metronidazole, or was unrelated to the drug.

Treatment for *Entamoeba* should continue for at least 2 weeks, although much longer courses may be required. Unfortunately, although metronidazole in considered effective against amoebic trophozoites and is an effective extraintestinal amoebicide, it may be only partly effective or ineffective against amoebic cysts. As a result, combination drug therapy may be needed to completely clear an infection.

Iodoquinol or diiodohyroxyquin has been used to treat amoebiasis in humans, and has been used in many chelonian species. Many reptile practitioners may have unknowingly used this drug, as it is a component of Flagenase, a metronidazole suspension from Mexico that has often found its way into the hands of US veterinarians. Iodoquinol may be difficult to obtain. Compounding pharmacies may be able to obtain iodoquinol powder and formulate a palatable suspension. A dose of approximately 50 mg/kg orally once daily for 21 days has resulted in cessation of cyst shedding (not necessarily proving complete eradication) in the majority of cases. Adverse effects documented in humans, including neurologic signs, have not been observed, and necropsy of several treated animals has not shown lesions indicative of drug toxicity. Iodoquinol is thought to act mainly as an intestinal amoebicide, and is effective against both the trophozoite and cyst form.

Chloroquine is also labeled for treatment of extraintestinal amoebiasis and is effective against trophozoites. It is likely that chloroquine may need to be used in conjunction with a drug effective against cysts. Nevertheless, chloroquine is deserving of further investigation, particularly because of its potential convenience in chelonians as it is the only amoebicide that is available for IM injection.

Paromomycin is often used as part of combination drug therapy for treating human amoebiasis. Paromomycin is an aminoglycoside antibiotic that is theoretically not absorbed from the gastrointestinal tract. It is generally used as a lumenal amoebicide to eradicate amoebic cysts. Paromomycin has been used in reptiles for treatment of amoebiasis and cryptosporidiosis. Pare

reported elimination of cryptosporidium shedding in two Gila monsters treated with 300 to 360 mg/kg paromomycin every other day for 14 days. No adverse affects were noted. In addition, Lane and Mader report that Schweinfurth used paromomycin in snakes at a dose of 25 to 100 mg daily for 4 weeks to eliminate amoebiasis. The human pediatric dose of paromomycin is generally 30 mg/kg TID for 7 days. There are reports of renal failure in cats treated with paromomycin.

Use of diloxanide for treatment of amoebiasis has not been widely reported in reptiles, but the drug is often recommended in human cases. In humans, diloxanide may have fewer side effects in children than other amoebicidal drugs. Like paromomycin, diloxanide is a lumenal amoebicide, effective against the cyst stage. It may be used alone for treatment of asymptomatic cyst passers, or in combination with metronidazole for invasive amoebiasis. The human pediatric dose of diloxanide is generally 20 mg/kg SID for 10 days. Unfortunately, diloxanide is not readily available at this time in the US.

In addition to treatment with amoebicidal drugs, infected patients may also need nutritional support, antibiotics, and antifungal medications. A thorough assessment of the patient must be made, and amoebae treated with consideration of other concurrent disorders. Repeated evaluation of fecal samples over a several month quarantine period is required to ensure eradication.

Fatal *Cryptosporidium* infection of the small intestine has been described in several chelonian species. Paromomycin, as described above can be considered for these cases. In addition, there is a recent anecdotal report of the use of ponazuril to treat cryptosporidium infection in snakes. Hyperimmunized bovine colostrum has also been used in the management of *Cryptosporidium* infection in reptiles.

Some flagellated protozoa may be pathogenic to chelonia. In the author's experience, small numbers of flagellates found on fecal examination may not be problematic, particularly for herbivorous tortoises. However, flagellated protozoa such as *Hexamita* and *Myxidium* have been found to cause significant renal infection in some chelonia. Antiprotozoal therapy may be warranted if flagellated protozoa are found in chelonian urine.

Nematodes, such as the ascarid *Angusticaecum*, can cause disease in chelonia. In general, the author will seek to eliminate ascarids and strongyle-type nematodes from chelonia. There are rare reports of illness in chelonia caused by oxyurid (pinworm) nematodes. However, oxyurids are extremely common in herbivorous tortoises, and seem to cause no pathology in most cases. These can be difficult and frustrating to eliminate, and the author does not try to eliminate them if no clinical illness is present. Some authors postulate that pinworms may help to break down plant material in the large intestine of tortoises.

Acanthocephalans are commonly found in North American aquatic turtles, such as the red-eared slider. Their pathogenicity is unclear. Successful treatment of these parasites in turtles has not been reported, but they have been treated in some primates using albendazole.

Trematodes may be problematic for sea turtles and freshwater turtles. While in many cases these parasites seem to be found only incidentally at necropsy, there are numerous case reports of more severe disease. The most significant trematode infections in chelonia are caused by the cardiovascular trematodes, such as *Spirochis* sp. Much of the pathology associated with these worms is due to embolism caused by the trematode ova. Unfortunately, turtles that are clinically affected are often at an advanced state of disease, and carry a poor prognosis. One may attempt to treat them using principles for the treatment of heartworm disease of dogs, for example. Praziquantel, anti-inflammatories, and supportive care may be useful.

Diagnosis of gastrointestinal parasites may require fecal direct and floatation examination, fecal acid-fast cytology or ELISA testing (eg, *Cryptosporidium*), endoscopic gastrointestinal biopsy, etc. Once a diagnosis of parasitism is made, specific antiparasitic therapy may be selected. There is relatively little pharmacokinetic data available for anthelmintic use in chelonia; and there is even less safety and efficacy data. Oral praziquantel pharmacokinetics have recently been reported for loggerhead sea turtles (*Caretta caretta*). Fenbendazole has been used clinically in chelonia for many years; however, one recent report suggests that fenbendazole may have caused myelosuppression in Herman's tortoises (*Testudo hermanni*). However, an untreated control group was not utilized in this study. The author has had anecdotal success in treating oxyurid infection in several tortoises using fenbendazole administered per rectum. The dose and frequency of fenbendazole use is left to the discretion of the clinician. Some clinicians use it weekly, while others use it daily for 3 to 5 days. The author has used pyrantel (5 mg/kg PO q7d x 3–4 weeks) with apparent safety in efficacy several chelonian species. Ivermectin appears to be toxic to most chelonian species and should not be used.

The ciliated protozoan, *Nyctotherus*, is often seen in fecal examination of herbivorous tortoises. It does not appear to cause disease. The motile, ciliated stage of this organism is easily identified. The cyst stage of the organism is also seen commonly, and is a fairly large, slightly D-shaped, ovoid cyst, often with a single operculum at the tip of the long axis. Due to its resemblance to trematode ova of mammals, clinicians may be misled into treating with praziquantel. Trematodes are exceedingly rare in most tortoises. *Monocystis* is a parasite of earthworms that may be seen in fecal examination of chelonia that have been fed earthworms. It does not cause disease in chelonia. The ova of this organism resemble miniature *Trichuris* or *Capillaria* ova, and are often found in small packets of multiple ova.

Clinicians should thoroughly pursue the identification and characterization of chelonian parasites. Many of the parasitic diseases of chelonia that have been identified and characterized over the past two decades have been discovered due to the diligent effort of motivated clinicians.

References are available from the author upon request.

MEDICAL MANAGEMENT OF CHELONIAN GASTROINTESTINAL DISORDERS

Charles Innis, VMD
New England Aquarium
Boston, MA

The gastrointestinal tract of the chelonia is similar to that of other vertebrates, and suffers from similar disease states. The esophagus generally courses along the ventral medial or ventral right side of the neck, before coursing left toward the stomach. In sea turtles, the esophagus is lined with numerous, conical papillae. The stomach is similar to that of the dog or cat, beginning on the left, and exiting at the pylorus on the right. The duodenum and associated pancreas are also similar to dogs and cats. The distinction between duodenum, jejunum, and ileum may not be apparent. The large intestine has the typical ascending (right), transverse, and descending (left or midline) components. The large intestine of herbivorous chelonians, like that of horses, provides a site for microbial digestion of plant material. Disruption of intestinal motility or its microbial population may be detrimental.

Excellent reviews of the management of chelonian medical disorders have recently been published.[1,2] Common signs of gastrointestinal disease in chelonia include anorexia or hypophagia, diarrhea, vomiting or regurgitation, and reduced activity, As several of these signs are nonspecific indicators of chelonian illness, diagnostic testing may be needed to localize the problem to the gastrointestinal tract. It may be difficult to make the distinction between vomiting and regurgitation in chelonia, where it is difficult to assess the amount of abdominal effort put forth. Common causes of gastrointestinal signs in chelonia include inappropriate diet, foreign bodies, reduced motility, parasites, bacterial infection, and intestinal dysbiosis. Less commonly, intussusception, intestinal prolapse, viral infection, fungal infection, or neoplastic disease may be seen.

Assessment of chelonian gastrointestinal cases should follow standard medical principles. Tests such as fecal examination, radiographs, and endoscopy may be of use. While not often specific or sensitive for gastrointestinal disease, a complete blood count and plasma chemistry profile should be used to assess the general health of the patient.

Inappropriate or inadequate diets may cause gastrointestinal signs. This is particularly true for herbivorous chelonia. Much like herbivorous mammals, herbivorous turtles generally require a diet high in fiber and low in fat. Unfortunately, some herbivorous turtles seem to enjoy eating dog food and cat food. This often leads the owner to feed such diets to the exclusion of more appropriate diets. Most commonly, feeding high fat, low fiber diets to herbivorous turtles results in diarrhea; and could lead to more serious problems such as hepatic lipidosis. Veterinarians should counsel owners of herbivorous reptiles to feed appropriate items such as dark green, leafy vegetables; commercially made herbivore diets; grasses; and hay. Fruits, in general, may be considered as a "treat," but should not form the majority of the herbivore diet.

Pica is common in chelonia. Turtles often ingest stones, shells, pieces of metal, and so forth. In the wild, turtles have been observed ingesting bone fragments. It is possible that this behavior provides valuable mineral supplementation in the wild. In captivity, however, this most commonly leads to gastrointestinal impaction or obstruction. Substrates for chelonia should be carefully selected. Gravel, corn cob, and walnut shells often cause problems. Better choices include newspaper, soil, hay, or bark mulch. Areas where chelonia are allowed to wander should be free of dangerous ingestible items. One of the author's tortoise patients that was presented due to intermittent penile prolapse and straining later defecated the family cat's toy mouse. The penile prolapse immediately resolved.

Most, if not all, ill chelonia should have full body radiographs to look for gastrointestinal abnormalities, including foreign bodies. Protocols for gastrointestinal contrast studies of chelonia have been published, but such studies may be hindered by very long normal transit times for some species (days to weeks in some species). Management of gastrointestinal foreign bodies of chelonia follows standard medical principles, and will be affected by the location of the objects. In some cases, fluid therapy (parenteral and enteral), enemas, and warm water baths may be productive. Turtles will often drink copiously during bathing. This simple form of enteral fluid therapy should not be underestimated. If the turtle will not drink voluntarily, enteral fluid therapy may be provided in the form of water, fruit or vegetable juices, or sports drinks given by gastric intubation. Passage of a large number of foreign objects may take several weeks. If the patient is large enough, endoscopy may be of use. Alternatively, exploratory surgery via plastron osteotomy, pre-femoral coeliotomy, or supra-plastral coeliotomy may be required. Removal of fish hooks from the stomach or esophagus may be attempted using endoscopy with an over-tube. In some cases, the fish hook may be most easily removed by percutaneous palpation of the end of the hook, followed by a small incision to expose the barb of the hook. If the barb can be removed, the remainder of the hook may be removed per os or per cutaneously.

Reduced gastrointestinal motility is commonly seen in chelonia. This is often a nonspecific indicator of disease, and may be secondary to reduced food intake, physiological derangements (eg, dehydration), intestinal dysbiosis, and so on. Clinical signs include reduced fecal production, regurgitation, and anorexia. Radiographs are often helpful in detecting ileus or fecal impactions. Management of such cases should focus on identifying and medically managing the primary cause of the problem. Symptomatic treatment may include enteral and parenteral fluid therapy, enteral feeding, warm water baths, and enemas. Enteral feeding may be accomplished via per os gastric intubation, or by esophagostomy tube. Esophagostomy tubes may be placed relatively easily in chelonia. The patient is sedated if needed, and local anesthesia is used at the site of tube placement. Curved hemostats are placed into the mouth of the patient, with the tip directed to the site of tube placement. A 2- to 3-mm scalpel incision is made in the skin overlying the hemostat tip, and the hemostat tip is passed through the incision. A red-rubber feeding tube or similar item is grasped in the tip of the hemostats, and the hemostats are withdrawn into the mouth, passing the catheter caudally into the distal esophagus. The tube is secured at the incision using a small piece of surgical tape and suture. Esophagostomy tubes may be left in place for weeks to months in chelonia. Once feeling well, chelonians will often begin feeding voluntarily with the tube still in place. The tube is then removed by cutting the sutures and withdrawing the tube. In general, the esophagostomy site does not need primary closure, and heals rapidly by second intention. However, the clinician should use judgement in this regard.

The author has successfully utilized in-dwelling per cloaca colonic catheters in several large tortoises. A standard urinary catheter of appropriate size is placed into the colon via cloacal endoscopy, and held in place by suturing to the tail. The catheter can be used to deliver fluid therapy and/or medications directly to the colon. In the author's experience, the tortoise will defecate the tube after normal motility is achieved, and it can then be removed. Pharmacologic enhancement of motility may be considered; however, data on the efficacy of drugs such as metoclopramide, cisapride, and erythromycin in chelonia are lacking. In one preliminary study, these drugs had no effect on the transit time of gastrointestinal markers in one tortoise species. If one chooses to use such drugs, extrapolation of mammalian doses or metabolic scaling may be used.

A discussion of clinical parasitology of chelonia is provided elsewhere in this volume. Protozoan and metazoan parasites are common in chelonia. The clinician must use judgement to assess the clinical implications of specific parasites. For example, oxyurid nematodes, ciliated protozoa (eg, *Nyctotherus*), and flagellated protozoa are commonly detected in tortoise fecal examination, but very rarely cause disease. Several significant gastrointestinal parasites of chelonia include ascarids, Cryptosporidium, and Entamoeba. Diagnosis of gastrointestinal parasites may require fecal direct and floatation examination, fecal acid-fast cytology or ELISA testing (eg, Cryptosporidium), or endoscopic gastrointestinal biopsy. Once a diagnosis of parasitism is made, specific antiparasitic therapy may be selected. There is relatively little pharmacokinetic data available for anthelmintic use in chelonia; and there is even less safety and efficacy data. Oral praziquantel pharmacokinetics have recently been reported for loggerhead sea turtles (*Caretta caretta*). Subcutaneous metronidazole pharmacokinetics have recently been reported for red-eared sliders (*Trachemys scripta elegans*). Fenbendazole has been used clinically in chelonia for many years; however, one recent report suggests that fenbendazole may have caused myelosuppression in Herman's tortoises (*Testudo hermanni*). However, an untreated control group was not utilized in this study. The author has used pyrantel

(5 mg/kg PO q7d x 3–4 weeks) with apparent safety in efficacy several chelonian species. Ivermectin appears to be toxic to most chelonian species and should not be used.

Bacterial and fungal infection, as well as intestinal dysbiosis, may arise through similar pathophysiologic events. To date, there appear to be few known primary bacterial or fungal pathogens of the chelonian gastrointestinal tract. In most cases, bacterial and fungal gastrointestinal infections of chelonia are caused by overgrowth of normal gastrointestinal flora under conditions of a deranged intestinal milieu, parasitism, or immunosuppression. Fecal or gastric cytology may be useful to identify yeast or fungal infection, and inflammatory cells. Some clinicians feel that fecal cytology and cloacal culture are helpful for diagnosis of bacterial enteritis. In the author's experience, such tests often demonstrate a variety of gram negative organisms that may be considered normal flora (eg, *Salmonella, E. coli*). A better approach, perhaps, would be to obtain gastric or colon biopsies for histopathology and culture. This allows correlation of culture results with histopathology findings. A variety of antibacterial and antifungal therapies and routes of administration are used in chelonia. In general, antibacterials that have efficacy against gram negative bacteria are selected. Nystatin may be used to manage gastrointestinal yeast overgrowth. Pharmacokinetic studies of oral ketoconazole has been investigated in Gopher tortoises (*Gopherus polyphemus*), and subcutaneously administered Fluconazole has been studies in loggerhead sea turtles. Oral itraconazole pharmacokinetics have been evaluated in Kemp's ridley sea turtles (*Lepidochelys kempii*). The reader is referred to the previously published chelonian therapeutics literature for details. Re-establishment of "normal" gastrointestinal flora may be attempted. The efficacy of commercial probiotic agents is questionable, but they appear to be safe for chelonia. Some clinicians prefer to orally inoculate the patient with feces from healthy conspecifics. This is not without risk of transmitting undetected pathogens.

Intussusception and/or intestinal prolapse are occasionally seen in chelonia. Prolapse of any tissue from the cloaca should be thoroughly investigated to determine the tissue of origin, and the etiology of the problem. In the author's opinion, prolapse of a tubular organ from the cloaca will likely require definitive intracoelomic surgical management. While one may attempt to replace the organ per cloaca, this often does not address the primary problem and may simply hide necrotic tissue within the cloaca. Coelioscopy may be useful to identify the origin of the prolapsed tissue. With practice, the colon, urinary bladder, and oviducts can be identified via coelioscopy. If greater visualization and exposure is required, the procedure is converted to pre-femoral coeliotomy or plastron coeliotomy. In the author's experience, some portions of the chelonian gastrointestinal system are mobile enough to be partially exteriorized via pre-femoral coeliotomy. By using a rigid endoscope, the areas of interest are identified and grasped with endoscopic forceps. The tissue is then gently retracted to the body wall to allow for surgical manipulation. If successful, this approach avoids the more invasive technique of plastron coeliotomy.

Viral and neoplastic diseases of the chelonian gastrointestinal tract have been described. An adenovirus has recently been identified in Sulawesi tortoises (*Indotestudo forsteni*). The virus affects a number of tissues, and causes intestinal necrosis in some cases. The San Diego Zoo has reported several cases of lymphoma in Galapagos tortoises (*Geochelone elephantopus*).

The clinician may consider the use of other gastrointestinal medications such as sucralfate or H-2 blockers. The author has used these drugs clinically in chelonians, but safety, efficacy, and pharmacokinetic data are lacking.

REFERENCES

1. Mader DR (ed). Reptile Medicine and Surgery, 2nd ed. St. Louis: Elsevier, 2006.
2. McArthur S, Wilkinson R, Meyer J (eds). Medicine and Surgery of Turtles and Tortoises. Cambridge, MA: Blackwell Science Ltd, 2004.

CHELONIAN NECROPSY: ANATOMY AND COMMON FINDINGS

Charles Innis, VMD
New England Aquarium
Boston, MA

Excellent clinical reviews of chelonian anatomy, necropsy, and common pathologic conditions have been recently published. Necropsy is a critical diagnostic tool for the chelonian practitioner. The chelonian necropsy begins with a thorough external examination, including the shell, limbs, cloaca, skin, and structures of the head. The shell of the turtle is made of bone covered by keratin plates, or scutes. The number of scutes varies somewhat among species, and there are anatomic names for each scute. These names should be used to specify the location and extent of any shell pathology. The weight of the patient is recorded, and a variety of measurements (eg, straight carapace length, curved carapace length) are recorded if desired. Due to the high incidence of gross pathology of the oral mucosa, tongue, and nasal cavity, these areas should be specifically evaluated. Samples such as choanal cultures, nasal flushes, and so forth should be obtained before proceeding with the internal examination. In some cases, other diagnostics, such as radiography and computed tomography, may be desired. These techniques can help to direct the internal examination, and help to correlate clinical findings with necropsy results.

Exposure of the coelomic viscera is generally accomplished by removing the plastron, or ventral shell, of the turtle. In most cases, this is most easily accomplished using a bone saw or cast cutter to produce two longitudinal full-thickness incisions along each side, or bridge, of the shell. Take care to avoid lacerating the deeper viscera. In addition, a scalpel or scissors are used to incise the skin attachments to the plastron. Dissection then continues deep to the plastron, to separate the pectoral and pelvic girdles and associated musculature from the inner surface of the plastron. When the plastron is removed, the coelomic membrane should be visible. The large pectoral muscles will be evident, attached to the flat, triangular coracoid, and the elongated acromion process of the scapula.

Prior to entering the coelom, consider the general layout of the viscera to determine an appropriate point of entry. If obvious coelomic fluid is visible, collect this by centesis prior to entering the coelom. There are two bilateral paramedian veins that run longitudinally within the caudal coelomic membrane. These vessels can be avoided or ligated if desired, but this is not essential. When incising the coelomic membrane it is best to elevate it away from the underlying viscera. Since the urinary bladder of chelonia may be very large, it is easy to unintentionally lacerate the bladder during coelomic entry. This will immediately fill the coelom with non-sterile fluid. The coelomic membrane incision is extended anteriorly to the pectoral girdle. The pericardium is generally attached to the coelomic membrane just anterior to the liver, just deep to the the

coracoid. Consider pericardiocentesis if desired. A moderate amount of clear, colorless pericardial fluid may be normal in turtles (eg, 1–2 mL for a 1-kg turtle). Incision of the pericardium will expose the two atria and single ventricle of the heart. The incision is continued cranially along the skin of the ventral neck to expose the trachea and esophagus. In larger turtles, careful dissection will allow exposure of the thyroid at the base of the heart, and thymus along the ventral neck. If possible, the heart and great vessels should be dissected to evaluate the endocardium, valves, and any intravascular parasites.

Initially, the most obvious ventral coelomic viscera will be the liver, urinary bladder, and heart. The bladder is bilobed in most cases, and may be extremely large. It can be reflected caudally or removed at the discretion of the clinician. The sequence of visceral examination, and timing of organ removal is a matter of preference, but should generally follow methods used for other vertebrates. The gallbladder will be found on the right caudal dorsal surface of the liver. The liver may be removed to permit better visualization of the gastrointestinal tract. The esophagus generally courses along the ventral medial or ventral right side of the neck, before coursing left toward the stomach. In sea turtles, the esophagus is lined with numerous, conical papillae. The stomach is similar to that of the dog or cat, beginning on the left, and exiting at the pylorus on the right. The duodenum and associated pancreas are also similar to dogs and cats. The spleen is a red to purple globoid structure found on the right side, deep to the duodenum, suspended within the mesentery. The large intestine has the typical ascending (right), transverse, and descending (left or midline) components, and is often gas filled.

After removal of the digestive tract, liver, and bladder, the major remaining organs will be the gonads, kidneys, and lungs. The paired, dorsal, caudal gonads are identified easily in sexually mature turtles. Ovaries will generally contain numerous yellow follicles, while testes are elongated to ovoid and have a smooth tan to yellow surface. The gray to black epididymis is found attached to the posterior pole of the testicle. The kidneys are located in the most caudal, dorsal aspect of the coelom, and are actually retrocoelomic in most species. They can often be palpated just lateral to the colon, caudal to the gonads. Incision of the coelomic membrane will expose the roughly triangular kidney. The lungs are tightly adhered to the carapace and extend virtually the entire length of the carapace. They are relatively thin, membranous structures with relatively little parenchyma. The cut surface of the lung has a pink, honeycomb-like appearance. In large turtles, the adrenal glands may be identified along the cranial aspect of the kidney.

If clinical signs or diagnostic imaging results demonstrate other locations of interest, those sites should also be dissected (eg, osteolytic lesions of joints, caudal paralysis) Specific bones, shell, joints, muscle, spinal cord, etc. may warrant investigation. Bone marrow may be evaluated by submitting long bones, the bridge of the shell, or the jaw. The head of the turtle must be thoroughly examined. In small turtles, the entire head may be submitted intact for histopathology. In larger turtles, a variety of tissues, including the brain, eyes, ears, nasal cavity, tongue, and oral mucosa should be harvested.

Common gross pathology findings in chelonia include hepatic lipidosis, cachexia, granulomata, abscesses, oral or lingual plaques, cystic calculi, retained eggs, egg-yolk coelomitis, gout, gastroenteritis, and parasites. However, in many cases, no gross lesions are seen. Histopathology, microbiology, virology, parasitology, and molecular techniques should be used to obtain a thorough diagnosis. Complete investigation often results in documentation of previously undescribed disease entities. To allow for such investigations, clinicians should develop a good relationship with colleagues that provide such services. Consultation with these individuals prior to the necropsy will ensure proper tissue collection, fixation, and storage. At a minimum, representative tissue samples should be fixed in formalin and also frozen. Frozen tissues can be used for microbiology, virology, or molecular diagnostic techniques if histopathology indicates that this is warranted.

REFERENCES

1. Mader DR (ed). Reptile Medicine and Surgery, 2nd ed. St. Louis: Elsevier, 2006.
2. McArthur S, Wilkinson R, Meyer J (eds). Medicine and Surgery of Turtles and Tortoises. Cambridge, MA: Blackwell Science Ltd, 2004.

CHELONIAN EGG INCUBATION

Charles Innis, VMD
New England Aquarium
Boston, MA

Chelonian egg shells vary from flexible and leathery, to hard and brittle. The thinnest parchment shelled eggs are the most susceptible to changes in the hydric environment. Clutch size, egg size, and nesting frequency vary among species. Pancake tortoises (*Malacochersus tornieri*), bowsprit tortoises (*Chersina angulata*), Spider tortoises (*Pyxis arachnoides*), black-breasted leaf turtles (*Geoemyda spengleri*), Sulawesi forest turtles (*Leucocephalon yuwonoi*), and Central American wood turtles (*Rhinoclemmys* spp.) generally produce only one (rarely two) very large egg(s) per clutch, but may nest several times per year. At the other extreme, the large sea turtles, snapping turtles (*Chelydra serpentina* and *Macroclemys temmincki*), and softshell turtles (*Trionyx, Apalone,* and others) may lay dozens of eggs per clutch, with some sea turtles nesting several times per year.

Nesting is similar among most species, with the female excavating a terrestrial, flask-shaped nest with her hind feet, depositing her eggs, covering the nest, and departing without further maternal care. An exception to this general rule is the Burmese mountain tortoise (*Manouria emys* ssp.) that constructs a nest by gathering sticks, dirt, and leaf litter into a pile, and then guards the nest for several days to weeks after oviposition. Female western swamp turtles, *Pseudemydura umbrina,* dig their nest with their forelimbs. The northern long-necked turtle, *Chelodina rugosa,* may nest under water at sites that surface as the dry season progresses. Chelonian eggs typically do not survive submersion for extended periods, but, it is thought the *rugosa* eggs lie dormant until the water evaporates then development begins.

In most turtle species, the gender of the embryo is determined by the incubation temperature of the egg (temperature-dependent sex determination, TSD). In some species, higher temperatures produce males, while the reverse is true for other species. Most natural nests experience a range of temperatures, resulting in both male and female hatchlings. Some species show genetic sex determination rather than TSD.

After oviposition, eggs may be removed from the nest for artificial incubation. Several recent texts provide species-specific environmental requirements for incubation of chelonian eggs. In addition, these texts provide critical temperatures for TSD for each species, if known. It is difficult to generalize about egg incubation of the nearly 300 species of turtles, but several rules of thumb are provided herein.

For most species, incubation temperatures in the range of 82–86°F are appropriate. Some tortoise species may require higher temperatures, while some forest leaf-litter species may require lower temperatures. Temperature is maintained by locating the eggs in a thermostatically controlled room or incubator. Incubators are commercially available, or may be built with readily available materials. The specific design of the incubator generally depends on the desired humidity range for incubation.

As a rule of thumb, eggs that have flexible shells require higher humidity than eggs that have rigid shells. However, the microclimate of the species should also be considered. For example, tortoises from humid forest environments generally produce rigid shelled eggs, but still require high humidity. In general, flexible shelled eggs should be incubated in a high humidity environment (80–100%). Rigid shelled eggs, depending on the species may require high, low, or moderate humidity. The reader is advised to consult the species specific literature for details.

A simple high humidity incubator can be made using two plastic containers (one larger than the other), a submersible aquarium heater, water, a brick, and a thermometer. The brick is placed in the larger container, and water is added to the height of the brick. The smaller container is placed on top of the brick, and is filled with incubation substrate and eggs. The thermometer measures the temperature of the egg box. The heater thermostat is set at the desired temperature and fully submerged in the water. The egg box and outer container are both covered with lids with several ventilation holes. The heated water will create a humid, warm environment.

For incubation under dry conditions, commercial incubators may be used, or thermostatically controlled heat pads may be used to construct an incubator.

A variety of incubation substrates have been used successfully, including vermiculite, peat moss, gravel, soil, sand, etc. Some substrates do not retain moisture well and should only be used for low humidity incubation. Vermiculite is most widely used. Water is added to the vermiculite depending on the desired level of substrate water content. In general, a ratio of 1:1 water: vermiculite by weight is successful. If the substrate dries significantly during incubation, additional water may be added. Some keepers periodically spray the substrate with water. If desired, the entire egg box can be precisely weighed and water added as needed to maintain a constant weight. The eggs are generally partially buried in the substrate to allow visual monitoring of the eggs during incubation. Reptile eggs should not be rotated after the first few days of incubation, as the embryonic orientation may be disrupted.

Many chelonian eggs have a slightly yellow to orange hue when first oviposited. In many cases, fertile eggs will "chalk," or develop a flat white color over the first few days of incubation. This change is due to the initial development of extraembryonic membranes. In some species, this is first noted as a small circular white spot on the dorsal surface of the egg, which expands over several days to encompass the majority of the egg. In other species, this spot develops into a distinct white transverse band across the short axis of the egg.

Within several weeks, most eggs will show blood vessel development. Candling can be accomplished in a variety of ways, but an ophthalmoscope with transilluminator works well. One European institution has reported successful chelonian egg monitoring using an avian egg cardiac monitor.

Incubation length is highly variable among species. Most species require 2 to 4 months. In some species, it appears that the embryo may enter a diapause period that must be broken via environmental manipulation. For example, the spider tortoise (*Pyxis arachnoides*) from Madagascar seems to require an initial 3-month incubation, followed by a cooling period for 1 month, followed by 3 more months of higher temperature incubation. Failure to cool the egg seems to result in an indefinite delay in embryonic development.

Upon initial hatching, or pipping, the egg should be monitored closely. Turtles may take 1 to 2 days to emerge from the egg. During this time, the yolk sac remnant is generally resorbed. Disturbing the hatchling at this time may traumatize the yolk sac. Once emerged from the egg, the hatchling should be moved to a nursery enclosure appropriate for the species. Damp paper towels provide an excellent substrate for the first few days of life. Aquatic species are generally able to swim as soon as emerged from the egg.

REFERENCES

1. Gurley R. Keeping and Breeding Freshwater Turtles. Ada, OK: Living Art Publishing, 2003.
2. Highfield A. Practical Encyclopedia of Keeping and Breeding Tortoises and Freshwater Turtles. London: Carapace Press, 1995.

BASIC HUSBANDRY AND NUTRITION OF LIZARDS

Kevin Wright, DVM
Arizona Exotic Animal Hospital, LLC
Mesa, AZ

LIZARD DIVERSITY

Lizards are the most speciose group of reptiles in the world with over 3,000 species described by the end of the 20th century. They range in size from a Caribbean gecko that is about as long as a dime and lays an egg about the size of a BB pellet to the world famous Komodo dragon, about 10 feet long and exceeding 250 pounds in weight. Lizards may be food specialists, such as the Texas horned lizards and Australian moloch, which feed almost exclusively on ants, the Philippine monitors that feed on fruit, or the marine iguanas that feed on algae. There are lizards that burrow underground, live in trees, forage underwater in the ocean, or live underneath the flotsam along the high water mark of a tropical beach. Active body temperatures range from 22°C to 40°C within this group of reptiles, and some montane lizards have even been seen active on snow banks! Given this incredible diversity of natural histories, it is clearly impractical to do justice to the husbandry needs of this vertebrate group in a single lecture or paper. Instead, I will focus on a few of the key concepts of lizard husbandry

IDENTIFICATION

In order to give advice to a client, you have to be able to identify the lizard in front of you. Table 1 lists the lizard taxa that make up 90% of my lizard patients. Peruse some of the online classified ads, such as www.kingsnake.com, to find out what species are gaining popularity and help you to identify species that may be unfamiliar. Other sources include hobbyist magazines, field guides, and taxon-specific books about the natural history and husbandry of lizards.

Table 1. Lizards Often Seen in Private Practice

Family of Lizard	Common Names
Agamidae	bearded dragon, uromastyx, Asian water dragon
Chameleonidae	panther chameleon, veiled chameleon
Gekkonidae	leopard gecko, crested gecko
Iguanidae	green iguana, rock iguanas
Polychridae	green anole, brown anole
Scincidae	blue-tongued skinks
Teiidae	black and white tegu, red tegu
Varanidae	savannah monitor, Nile monitor, water monitor, "ackies" (Australian spiny-tailed monitors)

STRESS

If the captive environment and care routines do not support the natural behaviors of a lizard, it will become stressed. Although certain events such as cage cleaning and handling of a lizard often bring on an acute stress reaction, this is not necessarily detrimental to the overall health of the lizard. It is constantly living in a situation that is inappropriate in fundamental ways that bring on chronic stress, a debilitating condition that alters the endocrine system, suppresses the immune system, and overall increases the need for certain nutrients. A lizard that is in a state of chronic stress is more likely to develop abnormal behaviors, contract infectious diseases, and have trouble maintaining a normal weight, either becoming thin or obese. The vanguard of lizard preventive medicine is proper husbandry and nutrition.

IMPORTANT CONCEPTS IN LIZARD HUSBANDRY

There are certain ranges of environmental variables that optimally support a lizard's innate physiology to promote and sustain normal behaviors and health.

Preferred Operating Temperature Zone (POTZ)

As mentioned above, the Preferred Operating Temperature Zone (POTZ) is the range of temperatures that best support a lizard's physiology throughout its diurnal, season, and annual cycles. The core body temperature of a lizard varies based on its physiological needs. For example, a lizard that has just eaten a large meal often seeks out warmer temperatures than a lizard that has eaten recently because the enzymes that facilitate digestion work better at higher temperatures. Most lizards are cooler at night than during the day and that change in body temperature may facilitate some of the repair enzymes that are associated with sleep. A gravid female will often bask for longer periods of time than a nongravid female, and there are many other examples where a lizard seeks out a different core body temperature depending on a variety of factors. Since it is impossible to know what temperature is best for a lizard at any given time, the captive environment needs to provide a range of temperatures that allow the lizard to shuttle back and forth based on its innate physiological needs. Typically this is achieved by having a basking spot at one end of the cage to provide a warm area while the other end of the cage is allowed to be cooler. Unfortunately, the size of most cages tends to create fairly linear environment (hot end, cold end) which is somewhat different from the mosaic of temperatures a lizard would find in the wild. A much larger cage, one that has patches of warm and cool spots, some of which are in moist areas, some in dry areas, some in brightly lit areas, and some in darker areas, more closely replicates the natural environment, will promote a wider range of naturalistic behaviors and may be key to succeeding with species that have not historically done well in captivity.

Preferred Operating Illumination Zone (POIZ)

Illumination refers to the range of visible and near-visible electromagnetic radiation a lizard is exposed to in the course of its lifetime. Although we frequently only think of this in terms of light provided by the sun, night has a variable cycle of light provided by the moon. Illumination is a combination of the color rendering index of light provided, as measured in thousands of degrees Kelvin (°K), the wavelength of light provided, as measured in nanometers (nm), and the intensity of light. Intensity of light may be assessed in two ways. Radiant flux is the total power of light emitted at all frequencies and is measured in watts (w). Luminous flux is a weighted measure based on the optics of the human eye and what wavelengths are visible; it is measured in lumens. Lizards perceive light in the ultraviolet wavelengths that are invisible to human eyes. Thus a light source that appears white to the human eye may actually have a lot of ultraviolet in it that would alter the color perception of a lizard exposed to that light. These subtle differences in illumination may have profound impacts on why certain species of lizards do not thrive in captivity.

Illumination must take into account many factors to provide a light that allows the lizards to see things that are important to it: The colors of a mate or potential rival, the wax trails that reflect ultraviolet light and indicate a lizard has marked its territory, and the colors and movements of food items. It must provide physiologically relevant light, such as ultraviolet B, to support the metabolism of vitamin D and calcium. It may provide a source of heat. Typically, combinations of fluorescent and incandescent bulbs are needed in order to accommodate all these diverse needs.

Diurnal and annual cycles, important to establishing reproductive cycles, are established by the regularity of the photoperiod and the waxing and waning of day lengths as seasonally appropriate. Timers are needed for the lights to turn on and off regularly and establish the photoperiod—depending on human memory to do so will ensure that the photoperiod varies on a daily basis and may disrupt reproductive cycles.

Preferred Operating Humidity Zone (POHZ)

The POHZ is the range of environmental and atmospheric moisture needed to promote optimal health. This too varies depending on innate physiological needs. For example, a lizard that is shedding typically needs a more humid environment in order to successfully shed the skin over certain parts of its body, such as its toes and tail tips. Inappropriately low humidity often results in large sheets of shed skin remaining attached to its body. If exposed to a constantly high humidity, a lizard may develop skin infections and even slough some of the skin on the pads of its feet. There are some counterintuitive differences in humidity needs. Many desert lizards, such as gila monsters, have very permeable skin and quickly lose water when active above ground. The majority of their time is spent in burrows underground with very high relative humidity so this permeable skin allows them to actively uptake moisture from this environment. The cost is that they lose water rapidly above ground during the drier parts of the year. Conversely, many tropical rainforest lizards

have very water-resistant skin which helps protect them from aqueous desquamatization. Typically, the humidity will vary between day and night and between seasons. It is essential to know the natural history and climate patterns that a lizard would experience in the wild to offer the POHZ.

Preferred Operating Auditory Zone (POAZ)

The POAZ is the range of vibrations including audible noises that a lizard would experience in the wild. This is often overlooked as a source of stress in captive lizards. The common pet lizards come from wild habitats that are quiet other than bird vocalizations or insect noises. The bearded dragon living in a cage on top of stereo speakers is enduring vibrations that are completely outside the range of vibrations it would experience in the wild. More subtle vibrations may contribute to problems, such as a television playing late into the night, an aquarium pump that vibrates against the cage, or the buzzing of a fluorescent light ballast.

Preferred Operating Dimensions (POD)

Not all space is created equal. An enclosure that is perfect for a tree-dwelling day gecko is likely to be miserable for a ground-dwelling barking gecko.

For arboreal lizards, the cage needs to be vertically oriented with lots of climbable spaces that are vertical or angled. Horizontal perches should be placed a various heights. Hollow cork tubes, bamboo tubes, and PVC pipes may be used to create hiding spots throughout the upper reaches of the enclosure. Perches and climbable space needs to bring the lizard into all the various environmental zones described below (eg, basking spots, UVB illumination, etc.). Most arboreal lizards will do poorly if they perceive they are too close to the ground.

Terrestrial lizards need a horizontally oriented cage with a modest amount of height, perhaps only as tall as 1.5 times the lizard's total length although more height may be beneficial for some taxa. The more horizontal space, the wider range of microhabitats you can create by manipulating the environmental zones. Most terrestrial lizards need a little bit of variety in the enclosure, such as rocks, logs, or low-lying branches, and plenty of opportunities to hide in cork hollows or other furniture placed on the ground. Substrates that can be burrowed into are appreciated. Depending on the lizard, cypress mulch, washed clean play sand, or a "forest mix" of varying amounts of peat moss, orchid bark, and sand work well.

Fossorial lizards need a horizontally oriented cage with minimal height above the soil surface. The substrate needs to be appropriate. For many lizards, a forest mix that retains moisture and can sustain the shape of a burrow is important. For others, such as sand skinks, a looser sand mix is appropriate for them to "swim" around the enclosure.

Semi-aquatic lizards such as the caiman lizard (Teiidae) typically need a bathing area that is sufficient for them to fully submerge and swim a few body lengths. A bowl of water is usually not sufficient to keep these lizards healthy. Substrates need to be free of pests such as mites.

Preferred Social Environment (PSE)

The social needs of lizards are poorly understood. Many live in complex hierarchies and have territories they defend against intruders. Monogamy and parental behavior have been noted in some species. Some, such as bearded dragons and monitor lizards, appear to develop a true bond with their caregivers and even with cage mates of other species.

Common mistakes are to have too many lizards in a cage, to maintain incompatible species in the same room (eg, predator–prey), or to house incompatible age-classes together. If a lizard can sense a threat and cannot get away, it may be stressed.

Nutrition

The common pet lizards are typically insectivorous (eg, leopard geckoes), carnivorous (eg, monitors), omnivorous (eg, bearded dragons), or herbivorous (eg, uromastyx). High quality food items should be used.

Nutritional secondary hyperparathyroidism (NSHP), a type of metabolic bone disease, is still common among insectivorous and herbivorous lizards because their common food items have inappropriate amounts or ratios of calcium, phosphorus, or vitamin D3, or because they do not have access to ultraviolet B light. Young growing lizards need to feed more frequently and generally have a higher need for calcium, protein, and fat soluble vitamins. Gravid females typically share the needs of growing lizards. They are most at risk of developing NSHP.

A neonate that fails to thrive is often being underfed or is chronically dehydrated.

Freshly wild-caught lizards that are acclimating have different needs than well-adjusted, long-term captive wild-caught lizards or well-adjusted captive-bred lizards. More attention needs to be paid to providing adequate amounts of water-soluble vitamins and microminerals.

Some commonly available reptile supplements are lacking in key nutrients such as vitamin A. Given the lack of quality control of the reptile supplement industry, I often default to using iron-free human multivitamins instead.

FINAL THOUGHT

I believe that a veterinarian who invests the time to keep a few of the common species of pet lizards will be much more capable advisor for the client bringing in a sick lizard. So, if you've never had a bearded dragon of your own, go out and get one!

FROM TINY AND DELICATE TO LARGE AND CANTANKEROUS: THE JOY OF EXAMINING LIZARDS

Kevin Wright, DVM
Arizona Exotic Animal Hospital, LLC
Mesa, AZ

BEFORE THE EXAM

Your front desk staff needs to prepare the client so that you get the most out of your exam room time. When scheduling appointments, they need to extract the species name of the lizard from the client so you are able to read up on unfamiliar species. They also should tell the client that the lizard needs to be in a container when it comes to your clinic, for the safety of the lizard and the comfort of other clients. They should ask the client to bring in a few pictures of their set-ups for lizards. This may often tell you more about what sort of husbandry is actually being delivered to your patient than 30 minutes of questioning. A good idea is to have a standard husbandry questionnaire online and have your front desk staff ask the client to download this document and complete it to turn in at the appointment. A review of the completed husbandry history will help guide your exam of the lizard and conversation with the client.

Your exam room and hospital wards should be escape-proofed to contain small fast arboreal lizards. The ventilation grill and sink drain are two of the more common places that are overlooked when escape-proofing a room.

THE EXAM

If the lizard is in a clear-sided container, watch it closely before taking it out. A healthy lizard should watch you closely and lifts up it head and front legs. When walking, the belly should not drag on the surface. Normal breathing may be rapid in an excited small lizard or very slow and shallow in a calm large monitor lizard. Abdominal heaving and open-mouth gaping suggest extreme respiratory compromise. Tongue-flicking is a common way for healthy lizards to assess new situations. Look for any obvious asymmetries and gait abnormalities when the lizard moves. A monitor, tegu, or iguana often will turn and watch you, forming a semi-circle with its body and tail so it can whip you as a defensive move. It is not unusual for a lizard to urinate or defecate when it is handled. Males may evert their hemipenes when upset; some female lizards, particularly monitor lizards, may evert scent glands that are superficially similar to hemipenes.

Body Condition Scoring (BCS)

Assigning a BCS is often overlooked in the assessment of reptiles. I use a simple BCS scale, ranging from 1 to 5:

1. **Emaciated.** The dorsal processes of the spine, the ribs, and the pelvic bones are very prominent. The pectoral girdle may be obvious in some species, but this is often a more subtle abnormality than the pelvic girdle. The lateral processes of the tail are very prominent and the tail feels very loose and flexible. There is a depression on either side of the skull above and behind the eyes where the temporal muscles are wasted away. The eyes are sunken even in a well-hydrated lizard. The paralumbar fossa is deeply sunken in between the ribs and the hind legs suggesting depletion of the coelomic fat bodies. When the lizard is touched over any bones, there is little detectable soft tissue beneath the skin. It is often easy to feel points on the ventral aspect of the lumbar spine during ventrodorsal palpation of the coelom (abdomen). Overall, the lizard has lost over 15% of its bodyweight.

2. **Thin** is a weight of a lizard that is not eating a good diet regularly, although it may be a post-ovulation weight in an otherwise healthy female lizard. All of the major bone landmarks noted above are less prominent. The eyes may or may not be sunken. A small amount of soft tissue is palpable over the major bones. The paralumbar fossa may be even with the ribs or slightly depressed. The points of the ventral aspect of the lumbar spine are not readily detectable on ventrodorsal palpation. Coelomic fat bodies are difficult to detect via palpation but may be visible with transillumination of small lizards or via an ultrasonographic exam. Overall, this BCS is between 5% and 15% lighter than a normal lizard.

3. **Within Normal Limits**. This is the weight a lizard should be. There is good muscling over all the boney landmarks, the eyes are not sunken, and the coelom feels soft but full when palpated. The tail is firm and resists flexion or extension due to the lizard's strength. The paralumbar fossa is even with the ribs or slightly distended. The coelomic fat pads are readily palpated but do not occupy the majority of the coelomic volume. Healthy lizards often fluctuate 5% around their healthy weight as a normal physiological change. For "gorge eaters" like monitor lizards, the weight may fluctuate even more based on meal size or defecation.

4. **Heavy** is the weight of a lizard that has started to accumulate more than normal amount of fat. There is good muscling over all the boney landmarks and the eyes are not sunken. The coelom feels slightly distended when palpated. The tail bulges at its base and resists flexion or extension due to the lizard's strength. The paralumbar fossa is obviously distended. The coelomic fat pads are readily palpated and may occupy the majority of the coelomic volume. Overall, this BCS is between 5% and 15% heavier than a normal lizard.

5. **Obese** is a clearly overweight lizard. Laterally flattened lizards like monitors are unable to lifts their bellies off a surface when walking. The neck is the same diameter as the head or may be large with jowls starting to form. Legs are plump and there is an obvious bulging at the base of the tail. The tail may have fat folds when coiled. The coelomic fat pads are large and obscure palpation of other organs. Subcutaneous fat may be palpable. Some

lizards may have an indent on the ventral midline of the tail. These are lizards that are more than 15% above a normal body weight.

Getting Weights

It is a simple manner to get weights on medium-sized calm lizards, like leopard geckoes and bearded dragons. The lizard can be placed into a basket and weighed on a gram scale.

For small flighty lizards, like day geckoes (*Phelsuma*) a pre-weighed clear plastic bag is essential. The lizard's container should be placed inside the clear bag and the lizard allowed to climb into the bag. You can trap the lizard in a section of the bag and remove its traveling container, secure the mouth of the bag and then weigh the bag and lizard together. If the transport container was light enough, like a deli cup, you should weight the container and lizard first, get the lizard in the bag, and weigh the container by itself to get the lizard's weight. This second method doesn't work if the transport container is several orders of magnitude larger than the lizard. If a lizard weighs less than 10 grams, it is very difficult to get an exact weight due to the accuracy limitations of most durable gram scales.

Large lizards may be weighed on the typical cat scale found in a small animal clinic. Most will stand on the scale if their eyes are pressed close and held down firmly for a few seconds. Others may need to be placed into a pre-weighed pillowcase or other large container for weighing. Exceptionally large lizards, like adult water monitors (*Varanus salvator*) or blackthroat monitors (*Varanus albigularis*), may need to be weighed on larger scales, ones that read over 25 kg. Bathroom scales may be used but often accurate only to within 500 grams.

Restraint

Small lizards should be left inside the clear plastic bag for initial visual assessment. I prefer to catch the lizard through the plastic, then reach inside with my other hand to delicately lift it out. Most tiny lizards have tail autotomy, so you have to be careful not to grip it in a way that it will drop its tail. Some lizards, such as day geckoes, also slough their skin easily and cannot be restrained without damage. I always warn a client that this may happen before handling any lizard that is capable of dropping its tail or tearing its skin. Small lizards often may be transilluminated with a cool light source, such as the alternate fiberoptic head for an ophthalmoscope/otoscope. This will reveal much detail on the internal organs.

Medium-sized inoffensive lizards may simply be picked up in one hand and gently restrained with thumb and forefinger behind the neck or lightly gripping the thorax.

Large lizards and some medium-sized lizards can be dangerous. An angry adult bearded dragon can give a pretty severe bite to an unwary handler. Monitors, tegus, and iguanas can whip you with their tails, claw you with their sharp nails, bite exceptionally hard and tear out chunks of flesh, and slather you with their cloacal contents! They are best restrained by quickly immobilizing the head and tail. One technique is the "double peace sign" maneuver where you place the fork of your index and middle finger of one hand just behind the head and the same technique just in front of the back legs, quickly cupping the rest of your hand over the hind legs. If a lizard is too large for this technique, you use your whole hand to encircle the neck and the other hand in front of the hind legs and wrap the tail under the same arm immobilizing the hind end. Lightly pressing on the eyes may calm the lizard down. If the lizard resumes struggling, two cotton balls can be placed over the eyes and a quick throw of a wrap used to hold them in place. A welder's sleeve can give protection to the forearm and shoulder while leaving the fingers exposed and more dexterous.

Do not let the client handle a potentially dangerous lizard since you will be liable for any wounds they incur!

Nose to Toes (and Tail) Exam

A basic clinical skill is to completely survey a patient during your examination. I start with the nose and work backward to the tail, looking for asymmetries, ectoparasites such as mites and ticks, wounds and scars, lumps and bumps, hemorrhage or other discoloration, crepitation of joints, strength of muscles (eg, resistance to manipulation of feet or tail), and overall flexibility of the tail. Once I do this initial exam, I follow with a closer exam of the oropharynx, a nasal and ophthalmic exam, coelomic palpation, and, where large enough, a digital cloacal exam (which can identify enlarged kidneys in many species). If a lizard expels cloacal contents, that is saved. If feces are present, a wet mount and float are set-up for fecal parasite examinations.

A magnifying head set may be helpful. In large lizards, this may reveal otherwise overlooked details like early capillary blush within the scales, suggestive of septicemia or other systemic illness. It is helpful to appreciate features in tiny lizards, such as confirming the presence or absence of preanal pores. I have found that taking pictures with a digital camera capable of macrofocus and high resolution is extremely useful. Images can be readily enlarged over the magnification limits of the headset loupes. Recently, some handheld digital microscopes have come on the market that are useful.

Sex determination may or may not be possible as part of the examination. Some species have obvious sexual dimorphism, such as femoral or preanal pores, enlarged dorsal crests, or post-cloacal hemipenal bulges. A quick ultrasound with a 7.5 MHz probe may reveal ovarian follicles in mature female lizards. If you can identify the sex, it may help narrow your differential diagnoses.

COMMON PROBLEMS
Face
- Rostral abrasion
- Nasal discharge
- Sunken eyes

- Cloudy cornea or lens
- Periorbital swelling
- Mites and ticks (especially around eyes, ears, and submandibular skin folds)
- Deformed jaws
- Ulcerated gingiva, with or without tooth loss, with or without caseous exudate
- Abnormal tongue flick
- Pale mucus membranes with or without white shimmering deposits

Torso

- Unidentified coelomic mass
- Abnormal or absent coelomic fat bodies
- Ovarian follicles or ova
- Enlarged kidneys
- Deformities of the spine
- Hydrocoelom

- Skin lesions/discolorations
- Cloacal prolapse

Extremities

- Missing or deformed toes
- Missing nails
- Swollen bones
- Fractures
- Deformed long bones
- Swollen joints
- Masses

Tail

- Necrosis
- Lordosis/kyphosis
- Hemipenal plugs, infections
- Abscessed cloacal glands

CONSTIPATION IN BEARDED DRAGONS

Kevin Wright, DVM
Arizona Exotic Animal Hospital, LLC
Mesa, AZ

A common complaint for bearded dragons is failure to defecate (constipation) and a reduction or loss of appetite. Contributing factors that may be uncovered in the history are inappropriate substrate, poor diet with insufficient calcium, lack of sufficient green leafy produce (roughage) in the diet, inadequate water intake, poor hygiene, recent acquisition, onset of reproductive abilities, old age, prior trauma, stress caused by a recent move, new cagemates, or unusual activity near the cage. The patient may appear bright, alert, and well-fleshed, or weak, poorly responsive, and underweight, depending on the underlying condition and chronicity of the problem. A reasonable differential list for a bearded dragon with these signs includes constipation/impaction/GI foreign body, dehydration, gastrointestinal parasitism (eg, flagellated protozoa, amoebas, coccidia), nutritional secondary hyperparathyroidism (NSHP), renomegaly/renal failure, follicular stasis/dystocia, abscess/granuloma, anatomic malformations (eg, pathological fractures, fractures, pelvic deformities), intussusception, neoplasia, and idiopathic.

If there are obvious skeletal abnormalities, such as a curved spine, pelvis or long bone deformities, mandibular deformities, or inability to achieve an erect body posture, NSHP and fractures should be suspected. Radiographs may help assess if this is a recent or chronic phenomenon. Prognosis is poor with severe deformities of the spine or pelvis that narrow the pelvic canal significantly.

Palpation of the coelomic cavity is a key skill to master to help refine your differential list. In a healthy adult male bearded dragon, it is easy to palate the fat bodies on either side of the caudal coelom, the soft cylindrical colon curving around the caudal coelom, and a full stomach. A healthy female dragon offers the same palpable structures but you may also be able to feel ovulating ovarian follicles in the mid to cranial coelom or oviductal eggs throughout the coelom, depending on her reproductive status. Common abnormalities include an enlarged and firm cylindrical structure consistent with an impacted colon, a mass that cannot be ascribed to any of the other structures that is consistent with a gastrointestinal foreign body, an abscess/granuloma, a tumor, or, in the case of adult female dragons, an ovarian/oviductal abnormality.

Another key skill is the ability to successfully pass either your fingers or a tube through the cloaca and into the proctodeum (reptilian equivalent of the rectum). If you have very slender fingers, it is possible to perform a proctodeal exam on an adult bearded dragon. If the kidneys are enlarged, they often protrude so far into the pelvic canal that it is difficult to pass anything larger than a No. 8 French catheter into the cloaca and on into the proctodeum. However, for most other causes of constipation, by pressing just in front of the pelvic canal as you gently insert a lubricated red rubber catheter, you can guide it into the proctodeum and proceed to gently flush in warm water for either an enema or to obtain diagnostic samples. In cases of constipation with associated flagellated protozoa enteritis, amoebiasis, or sand impaction, the bearded dragon may often defecate large amounts after the enema. I recommend an immediate direct fecal exam on this fresh feces; you can also put some stool into a rubber glove filled with water for the "finger test" to determine if sand is present in any quantities.

If available, a quick ultrasonographic exam with a 7.5 to 10.0 MHz curvilinear probe can help identify if the mass is ovarian follicles or oviductal eggs. Follicular stasis typically appears as grape-like clusters in the mid to cranial coelom, often with many of the structures about 5 to 8 mm in diameter; typically both ovaries are readily imaged. There may or may not be free coelomic fluid readily detected. Unshelled oviductal eggs are larger and appear to be arranged in curving lines or occasional clumps throughout the coelom. Shelled oviductal eggs may show some mineral dense echoes, but are often too soft for this feature to be visualized. "Spaying" is recommended for prefollicular stasis; I typically perform a "spay" on dystocias too given the likelihood of recurrence. Enlarged kidneys suggestive of renal failure or renal gout may be imaged if you direct the probe caudally into the pelvic canal. Renomegaly carries a poor prognosis, especially if accompanied by hyperphosphatemia and hyperkalemia that do not respond to diuresis.

A reasonable supportive care plan for a constipated bearded dragon includes intracoelomic nonlactated fluids (1 part Normosol, 1 part of 0.45% NaCl, and 2.5% Dextrose) at a rate of 20 mL/kg every 24 to 72 hours, depending on state of dehydration. Intraosseous fluids may be needed to rapidly rehydrate extremely compromised bearded dragons but this is rarely necessary. Soaking in warm water (90°F) for 30 minutes daily will help with hydration and may stimulate defecation. Cisapride (1–4 mg/kg PO SID until defecating) may be helpful. Assist-feeding with canned pumpkin, peach baby food with 1/8 tsp of methylcellulose (eg, Citrucel™) per jar of baby food, or Critical Care for Herbivores™ (Oxbow Hay Company), or other high-fiber product may help stimulate normal defecation. Any diagnosed underlying conditions should be treated. A dose of metronidazole (50 mg/kg PO, repeated in 10 to 14 days) is often helpful in restoring the gastrointestinal flora. This dose is effective with most flagellated protozoa enteritis. For confirmed cases of amoebiasis, I use metronidazole 50 mg/kg PO SID for 5 to 10 days.

An enterotomy to remove impacted material may be performed but those patients carry a poor prognosis unless a GI foreign body is identified as a root cause.

In the event that there is no obvious underlying cause, or if the colon remains distended once the cause has been identified and treated, a bearded dragon may need long-term management with a high fiber, pulsed doses of cisapride and periodic enemas.

EUTHANIZING A SNAKE WITH THE OWNER PRESENT

Kevin Wright, DVM
Arizona Exotic Animal Hospital, LLC
Mesa, AZ

Although many veterinarians simply refuse to euthanize reptiles with the owner present, I have found that this is as important to some clients as it is for the dog or cat owner who has to make that same decision. By explaining fully what will happen and giving them a choice about whether to stay or go, I believe I give these clients peace of mind about their pets' final moments.

My conversation with the client strongly encourages them to say goodbye to the snake in the exam room after which I will take it back to "put it to sleep." If they ask for more information, I advise them that euthanasia of a reptile is not the same as being present when a mammal or bird is euthanized. To compare the two processes, I explain that when I euthanize a bird or a mammal, it will die fairly quickly once the barbiturate-based euthanasia solution is injected into its veins. The mammal or bird rapidly loses consciousness when the euthanasia solution has had a few heartbeats to circulate. The body may have a fluttering heart beat for a minute or so and there may be some agonal muscle movements and vocalizations at this time. A euthanized mammal may urinate or defecate as bowel and bladder control disappear when the body completely relaxes in death. I assure the client that the mammal is beyond any awareness or feeling at this point. I suggest that these last brief moments may be disturbing for an owner to witness even when they know their pet is no longer capable of feeling what is happening.

A snake, in contrast, lacks readily accessible veins to receive the viscous euthanasia solution injection. If I inject the solution into the heart, it causes a rapid death but sometimes it can be difficult to perform this procedure on a wide awake snake. The restraint necessary for a cardiocentesis may appear to be excessive to the owner; even though it is a procedure that is done routinely as part of diagnosing a condition, an owner may not wish their last contact with a snake to be present as this happens. A tail vein may sometimes be used in larger snakes, but I have found that euthanasia solution often extravasates during injection and I must end up using another route. A slower alternative is injection into the coelom; it is easier to perform but takes much longer to take effect. With either procedure, a snake or other reptile may have muscle movements long after its central nervous system is "dead"; muscle twitching may continue as long as several hours after the euthanasia solution has permeated its body. The muscle movement does not mean the snake is aware of what is happening; it is just the body finally letting go. After this explanation, I again strongly advise the client to say goodbye and leave the snake behind. I offer the option of them waiting in the room and having the body brought back to them but despite my efforts, on rare occasions a client will insist on being present in order to reach closure with the loss of their snake.

If the client still wishes to remain, I advise them that I will give the injection intracoelomically, a process that takes 20 to 45 minutes for full effect. I typically use 0.1 mL of euthanasia solution per g bodyweight. The client may hold the snake after the initial injection and a staff member will check in every 5 minutes to see the snake's status. Once the snake is limp, I will come in and evaluate whether additional solution is needed.

There are some cases where I feel that a cardiac injection is the best solution. I will give tiletamine-zolazepam (Telazol®; 25–40 mg/kg IM) first and explain that this is done so that the snake is easier to manage; it takes 20 to 30 minutes for effect. The client is allowed to hold the snake after the Telazol injection and a staff member checks back every 5 minutes or so until the snake is fully relaxed. I advise them that I will look for the heart once the snake is fully asleep. Thick-bodied snakes such as large pythons or boas can be difficult to find the heart without a Doppler and some are even difficult to find with a Doppler. With slender-bodied snakes like most of the common colubrids it is a little easier to find the heart either by palpation or a Doppler. I have a three strikes rule: if I am not able to aspirate blood from the heart and sustain an injection within three attempts, I go to the intracoelomic route. If I am able to administer an intracardiac injection, I administer at a moderate speed and periodically aspirate to make sure I am still getting blood. Within a minute or so, the snake will start to become even more limp. I tend to overdose with the euthanasia solution, usually giving 0.05 mL per 100 g bodyweight.

Euthanasia is never easy. Euthanizing a snake with the owner present is one of the bigger challenges we face for it is difficult for it to be done quickly and smoothly.

DIAGNOSTIC SAMPLING AND OTHER PROCEDURES WITH TURTLES AND TORTOISES

Kevin Wright, DVM
Arizona Exotic Animal Hospital, LLC
Mesa, AZ

GETTING STARTED

It is important to recognize that you can perform many of the same diagnostic procedures with a tortoise that you can with a dog or cat—just because the patient has scales and a hard shell doesn't mean you forget basic clinical techniques for working up a medical problem. What diagnostic samples are important varies based on the case you are working up and may include: 1) blood, serum, and plasma; 2) bacterial, fungal, and viral cultures; 3) feces; 4) urine; 5) cytology (fine needle aspirates, tracheal wash, touch preps, etc.); 6) biopsy samples; 7) external parasites; and 8) photographs of lesions.

Although some tortoises submit readily to common diagnostic procedures such as venipuncture and cloacal washes, a recalcitrant chelonian that retracts fully into its shell is all but impossible to sample without sedation or anesthesia. With these chelonian patients you are faced with a Catch 22 situation—you would like to have some physiological data such as blood work before proceeding with sedation anesthesia, yet in order to get the blood sample you need to chemically immobilize the tortoise. Before you proceed, you must explain to the client why you need the samples and what the risks are of sedating a chelonian to obtain these samples. It is an Arizona state law that such a written estimate have a signed consent before performing any services on an animal but your state may have different requirements. I insist that the client sign a written treatment plan (that includes an estimate of costs) as well as a separate sedation/anesthesia approval form before going ahead with any chemical immobilization.

SEDATION AND ANESTHESIA

It is important to have a tortoise at the correct core body temperature (typically at least 84 to 86°F) for immobilization to be predictable. If the core body temperature is much cooler, drug uptake and distribution may be slowed and yield inconsistent results such as delayed induction, insufficient analgesia and muscle relaxation, and prolonged recovery. Warm water bottles and safe surgical-quality heating pads can be used to provide warmth to a tortoise undergoing an immobilization.

At Arizona Exotic Animal Hospital, most of our chelonian patients are African spurred tortoises (better known as sulcatas), leopard tortoises, and Sonoran desert tortoises. Table 1 details some of the common anesthetic protocols we use.

Table 1. Sedation and Anesthesia Protocols for Chelonians

Ketamine 10 mg/kg IM Butorphanol 0.5 mg/kg IM	May give additional 5 mg/kg ketamine and 0.5 mg/kg butorphanol if sedation insufficient after 20–30 minutes	Light to deep anesthesia achieved and useful for many procedures such as placing esophagostomy tube. Intubate and use sevoflurane for longer procedures. Our most commonly used protocol
Butorphanol 0.5–1.0 mg/kg IM Metacam 0.2 mg/kg IM		Good moderate sedation for tortoises under 2 kg. Useful for venipuncture, tracheal washes, placing intraosseous catheters, cloacal flushes, and other diagnostic procedures.
Propofol 5–10 mg/kg IV	Delivered by subcarapacial vein	It is extremely difficult to hit a vein on a retracted sulcata. However, it is very easy to give this via jugular vein in desert tortoises.
Medetomidine 0.1–0.5 mg/kg IM	May be given with 5–10 mg/kg ketamine IM.	Has worked exceptionally well on some sulcatas over 20 kg. Use equal volume of atipamizole for reversal. One leopard tortoise induced with medetomidine died even with one dose of reversal. Intubation and respiratory support often needed.
Sevoflurane 4–5% in induction chamber	Leave tortoise in chamber for 3–5 minutes after full relaxation is apparent.	Works extremely well for small tortoises (under 200 g) for minor procedures. Provides 5–20 minutes of light anesthesia; longer and deeper anesthesia if tortoise is left in chamber longer. Isoflurane does not work well—tortoises hold their breath when they smell isoflurane but do not seem to do so with sevoflurane.

DIAGNOSTIC SAMPLING
Blood

Blood samples may be extremely useful to assess a tortoise's health through leukocyte differentials, complete blood counts, plasma or serum chemistries, and serology. Chelonian blood may coagulate, if collection is slow, particularly if the tortoise has an inflammatory disease. For this reason, I like to heparinize the syringe (and butterfly catheter if one is used) before collection but this does impact the staining characteristics of blood cells and renders the sample unusable for blood culture. It may also impact other diagnostic tests. Each diagnostic lab has different requirements for sample processing so check with your lab to determine their requirements before obtaining the sample.

The jugular vein is the preferred site of collection due to the large quantity of blood that can be collected rapidly, obviating the need for an anticoagulant in the syringe. The jugular vein often rolls if a needle larger than 25-gauge is used for venipuncture. Most Sonoran desert tortoises and redfoot tortoises can be handled for jugular venipuncture without sedation. I have an assistant hold the tortoise in right lateral recumbency with the forelegs pulled back while I hold the head in my left hand and gently extend the neck until it is straight. If the tortoise is tilted so that the head is below the body, it may help fill the jugular and make it easier to see. I may be able to hold off the jugular with my left index finger or I may have the assistant do that with a free finger. I like to insert the needle with the bevel facing up and I may or may not bend the needle slightly depending on how much space there is to work. After collection, I have the assistant hold off the vein for 1 to 3 minutes. Despite this, subcutaneous hemorrhage may cause some bruising and swelling at the venipuncture site.

For a complete blood count and plasma chemistries, I immediately make blood films followed by filling two hematocrit tubes. My next step is to place an adequate volume of blood into an appropriate anticoagulant tube, usually containing lithium heparin or sodium heparin. If serum is desired, such as for Mycoplasma serology, my next step is the serum separator tube.

My next favorite site is the subcarapacial vein, located beneath the nuchal scute or between the two midline cranial marginal scutes in tortoises that lack a nuchal scute. This works well in tortoises that are retracted in their shell if you have a long enough needle.

Lymph Contamination

There is an accessible vein on the lower aspect of the front limb where a large tendon dives into the back of the "wrist." This brachial vein is readily apparent in a large Galapagos and Aldabra tortoises that are stroked so they stand with legs extended. A smaller tortoise may sometimes be held in ventral recumbency with a front leg pulled forward and downward to access this vein. Although not as easy to find when a tortoise is in dorsal recumbency, this is an alternative method. Contamination with lymph is likely if the needle is moved around outside of the vein.

There are blood vessels on the dorsal and ventral aspect of the tail but I rarely use this due to likelihood of lymph contamination.

Cultures

Abscesses are common lesions noted on tortoises. If culture is desired, the skin should be aseptically prepared and a stab incision made. If the caseated abscess can be removed from the site, swab the outer layer of the abscess or the lining of the abscess capsule. Aerobic and anaerobic cultures are recommended.

Nasal flushes and tracheal flushes may yield appropriate material for culture. In my experience, culturing for Mycoplasma is often unproductive and does little to change my approach to a tortoise with minor nasal discharge. Tortoises with more severe respiratory diseases should have a tracheal wash submitted for culture. Sometimes it is necessary to drill a hole in the dorsal shell and use an endoscope to collect samples of lung tissue or exudate for culture.

Oral plaques and lesions are often the result of viral lesions but should still be evaluated for unusual bacterial or fungal specimens.

Cloacal cultures are often nondiagnostic except to confirm the presence of *Salmonella*.

Mycobacteria and fungi should always be suspected for granulomatous lesions that are widespread or are seemingly resistant to debridement and antibiotic therapy.

Feces

Fresh feces should be evaluated for parasites. I find direct fecal exams, with the feces diluted either with water or 0.9% saline, most productive. Although low levels of flagellated protozoa are normal for healthy tortoises, high numbers are of concern. *Hexamita* are always of concern given their propensity for invading the bladder and renal tissues and are readily distinguished from other flagellates by their rapid straight line travel across the field of view. Amoebas, particularly when coupled with abnormal amounts of RBCs and WBCs, are of concern. Pinworm ova are common in healthy tortoises, but other helminth parasites are of concern.

Feces that has been cooled or stored causes some protozoa to encyst and makes identification of significant parasites difficult. Some commensal ciliates encyst into structures that are commonly mistaken for trematode ova and I have seen many tortoises for second opinion that were being treated for "resistant flukes" that turned out to be ciliates.

Urine

If a tortoise urinates, I check the pH. Acidic pH suggests catabolic state from anorexia while an alkaline pH tends to suggest that the tortoise is still eating sufficiently.

Urine can also be assessed for casts, WBCs, and RBCs, as well as the presence of *Hexamita* and coccidia. Coccidia may be suggestive of a problematic disease, intranuclear coccidiosis.

Cytology

Fine-needle aspirates (FNAs) are often unrewarding because many masses are abscesses. Tumors may be productive but it is often difficult to make an interpretation other than an inflammatory mass or a suspected neoplasia unless there are extremely characteristic cells present. FNAs should be assess with acid fast stain to rule out Mycobacteia as well as a more conventional Gram stain and cellular stains.

Lesions in the oropharynx should be lightly debrided and the underlying tissue sampled to have a chance of detecting herpesvirus or other inclusions. Touch preps should be made on any ulcerative lesions, including organs prolapsed from the cloaca. In addition to standard stains, cloacal touch preps should be assessed by wet mount since nematodes may often be discovered this way.

Tracheal washes should be evaluated with acid-fast stain, gram-negative, and cellular stains.

Biopsy

Biopsies are more likely to be diagnostic than cytological specimens simply because histopathology is better documented.

Histopathology requires standard preservation of tissues in 10% buffered formalin. For shell lesions it is important to include underlying bone as well as adjacent apparently healthy tissue. Often the biopsy specimens must be collected via surgical endoscopy of the lungs, coelomic cavity, upper gastrointestinal tract, and cloaca, bladder, or proctodeum. Additional specimens should always be collected for culture and potentially samples for electron microscopy may be important. Any lesions noted during endoscopy should be photographed or videotaped in the event that a consultation with a referral veterinarian is desired.

External Parasites

Ticks, leeches, bot fly larva, and other ectoparasites are occasionally seen on chelonian patients. They may be preserved for identification. Restrictions on importation and interstate transport of some tortoises were enacted as the result of identifying ticks that were reservoirs for important foreign animal diseases.

Photographs

This is one of the most overlooked diagnostic tools in clinical practice. I highly recommend that a clinic have available a nice quality digital camera with high resolution and the capability for macrofocus. A ring flash is helpful for better illumination of some lesions. Digital photos can be readily enlarged allowing you to detect subtle lesions, such as petechia or septic blush that may not be readily visible with the naked eye. Photographing a patient on presentation and at recheck examinations will allow you to more objectively assess progress as well as giving a more comprehensive case to review if you consult another veterinarian.

CLINICAL MANAGEMENT OF BLADDER STONES IN TORTOISES

Kevin Wright, DVM
Arizona Exotic Animal Hospital, LLC
Mesa, AZ

Cystotomy to remove a bladder stone is the most common surgery of chelonians in our practice in the Phoenix metropolitan area. Although no pattern is evident as yet, our impression is that there are years where we see several stones in a month and other years where they are far less common. Nevertheless, we typically perform several chelonian cystotomies a year.

COMPOSITION OF BLADDER STONES

Tortoise bladder stones are largely composed of urates, compounds composed of uric acid and metals such as sodium, potassium, or calcium. The Sonoran desert tortoise (*Gopherus agassizii*) is the best studied tortoise with regard to physiology and is known to form nitrogenous wastes into urea or uric acid depending on their state of hydration. Urea is the main nitrogenous waste when a tortoise is well hydrated and has access to plenty of drinking water or moist food plants. Urea requires less energy to form than uric acid but it is more toxic than uric acid and therefore requires more water to keep it dilute enough to avoid damage tissue. Uric acid requires an additional investment of energy but is relatively insoluble in water and much less toxic than urea. Uric acid will crystallize out of solution at low concentrations and can be voided from the body in a paste that allows the tortoise to retain much more water per unit of nitrogen excreted than for urea. Thus, there is an advantage for a tortoise to excrete urea when water is abundant because more energy is conserved and used for other purposes and the nitrogenous wastes are eliminated from the body without reaching harmful levels. When water is not abundant, the energetic cost of searching for sufficient water to dilute the urea would outweigh any energy conserved by not converting the urea to uric acid. Xeric-adapted tortoises such as the Sonoran desert tortoise tend to produce uric acid preferentially as a nitrogenous waste product compared to rainforest tortoises such as redfoot tortoises (*Geochelone carbonaria*).

FORMATION OF BLADDER STONES

The exact pathophysiology of tortoise bladder stones is unknown. The bladder acts as a water storage organ during times of water stress and water can be extracted from the urine if needed. There are cilia lining the chelonian bladder that likely keep solid material in the bladder, such as microcrystals of urates, in suspension. Even when the urate levels are high, the suspension remains fluid and easier to void through the urethra than larger crystals—kind of like what a Slushee™ machine does with ice.

It seems likely that tortoises that do not drink enough water and do not urinate often may be more at risk. Dissolved solutes, such as, can become very concentrated in the urine of a tortoise that is not drinking and consequently not completely emptying its bladder on a regular basis. Theoretically, mineral crystallization results from urine retention leading to urine supersaturation with mineral constituents until an ionic balance appropriate for crystal aggregation occurs. An additional complication with tortoises and reptiles in general, is that urine is not sterile since the bladder communicates with the proctodeum (the opening of the gastrointestinal tract into the cloaca). Some organisms, such as the flagellated protozoa *Hexamita*, are often found in the urine of tortoises with bladder stones. (Since *Hexamita* is a well known pathogen of the urinary tract, treatment with metronidazole is needed when it is diagnosed.) It is possible that the bladder cilia are not functioning normally in tortoises that develop bladder stones. Tortoise urine is influenced by diet and water consumption and likely has many complicated interactions between nitrogenous wastes, electrolytes, proteins, other waste products, and bladder microbial populations. Extrapolating from mammals, certain proteins and ions within urine act as promoters or inhibitors to crystal formation; in tortoises, there may be substances that inhibit ciliary movements. Whatever the factors that promote uroliths in tortoises, once a nidus is formed that is too large to pass through the urethra, a bladder stone results.

COMMON PRESENTATIONS

In my experience, the Sonoran desert tortoise (*Gopherus agassizii*) and African spurred tortoise (*Geochelone sulcata*) account for the majority of bladder stone cases (uroliths). Since these are the most common species kept as pets in Arizona, it is not too surprising they account for the majority of our patients. Any species of tortoise may develop bladder stones. Nevertheless, when all of the commonly seen species of tortoises at our practice are included (eg, leopard tortoise *Geochelone pardalis*, European tortoises *Testudo* spp., redfoot tortoises *Geochelone carbonaria*, Indian star tortoises *Geochelone elegans*, and Aldabra tortoises *Geochelone gigantea*), the vast majority of bladder stone cases are desert tortoises and African spurred tortoises with leopard tortoises a distant third. Bladder stones have been found in juvenile tortoises fewer than 2 inches (5 cm) in length and adult tortoises weighing over 70 pounds (35 kg). Bladder stones may be hard and firm or hard and friable.

There is no single sign that indicates a tortoise has a bladder stone. Some tortoises may lose their appetites; others may simply be less active. More serious signs are straining or failure to defecate. Gravid females may repeatedly dig nests and strain to lay eggs without success. Some tortoises appear paralyzed or paretic in their hind limbs or may walk with an exaggerated limp on one or both sides, a sign sometimes described as a wheelbarrow gait. It is common that a tortoise is presented with another problem, such as an upper respiratory infection, and the bladder stone is detected in the course of the examination and diagnostics. Because this condition is so prevalent in my clinical practice, it is always on the differential diagnosis for any sick tortoises and is a compelling reason I recommend regular radiographic screening as part of the diagnostic work-up as well as part of the annual preventive medicine program for tortoises.

Although a bladder stone is an often painful condition in people, especially when small fragments break off and are voided through the urethra, a tortoise typically shows no signs of discomfort until the bladder stone has grown large enough to irritate and inflame the bladder, or compress its intestine, oviducts, or nerves enervating the hind legs.

DIAGNOSIS

Some bladder stones are so large that the tortoise's owner may be able to feel them but they may be mistaken for shelled eggs in a known female tortoise. Some bladder stones are just large enough for an experienced veterinarian to detect by palpating just in front of the hind legs. I have found that smaller bladder stones are easier to palpate if the tortoise is held with the head elevated so the body is between a 45° and 90° incline and I gently rock the tortoise from side to side. Stones that are too small to feel otherwise may lightly bounce off your fingertips. Some clinicians claim that detection of small bladder stones is enhanced by holding the tortoise with its hind end submerged in water but I don't see the logic in that.

Occasionally, if the stone has become lodged in the pelvic canal AND the tortoise is cooperative enough to allow a digital cloacal exam, it may be palpated by inserting a finger in the cloaca. However, radiographs (x-rays) are needed to determine the size and shape of the bladder stone (or stones) and if there are any other complications. As mentioned previously, since bladder stones are sometimes found as the underlying cause of a seemingly unrelated illness, I offer a screening radiograph as an option in the work-up of any sick Sonoran desert tortoise, African spurred tortoise, or leopard tortoise.

I typically recommend blood work, particularly looking at hematocrit, albumin, uric acid, calcium, and phosphorus, to assess a tortoise before surgery. A well-hydrated patient with elevated phosphorus and normal to low calcium may signal underlying renal disease, particularly when coupled with significant elevations of uric acid. Low hematocrit and low albumin often indicate poor surgical risk and signal poor post-operative healing. A dorsoventral (DV) radiograph and horizontal lateral are useful to identify the size of the stone as well as surgical landmarks so you do not accidentally cut into the pelvic or pectoral girdle during plastronotomy. A urinalysis can help clarify if the tortoise has been eating or not; a healthy tortoise has urine with an alkaline pH, a tortoise in a catabolic state typically has neutral to acidic urine. A wet mount of the urine may pick up *Hexamita* and other abnormalities.

In some cases, other illnesses may have to be managed before a tortoise can undergo surgery. Rehydration may be needed and diuresis to assess if phosphorus is reversibly elevated. Assist feeding with

Critical Care for Herbivores (Oxbow Hay Company) may be helpful to promote an anabolic state. Antibiotics and anti-inflammatories may be needed to manage existing infections. However, in some cases the patient has to go to surgery with a less than ideal physiological state simply because the stone is large enough to preclude much improvement otherwise.

Since tortoise bladder stones cannot be dissolved medically, surgery is required for a cure. In rare cases, the bladder stone may be removed by manipulation through the cloaca. Some bladder stones may be removed by placing the tortoise in a lateral position and making an incision in the inguinal skin just in front of a hind leg with the bladder wall exteriorized and stay sutures placed. Most cases require that a portion of the plastron shell is removed temporarily so that the bladder may be accessed ventrally. In these cases, an epoxy patch is used to hold the cut shell in place during post-operative healing. The patch will need to be changed several times before the shell is healed. It may take over a year for some tortoises to fully heal. During surgery, I examine the different internal organs and biopsy any that look abnormal. If these tissues are submitted to a pathologist, the knowledge gained may help with long-term management of the tortoise.

Postoperatively, tube-feeding EXPAND and injectable fluids EXPAND may be needed for nutritional support and pain relievers may be prescribed to help the tortoise feel better. I usually surgically implant an esophagostomy tube in debilitated tortoises so that they can more easily receive oral medication and nutritional support for a long time postoperatively. Some tortoises may need to be hospitalized for several days until they are passing urine and stool regularly. In some cases cisapride (1 mg/kg PO SID) may be needed to promote defecation. Most tortoises will be put on enrofloxacin (10 mg/kg IM SID x 14 days) and ampicillin (20 mg/kg IM SID x 7–14 days) but large sulcatas have bad reactions to injectable enrofloxacin and are usually managed with amikacin (2.5 to 5 mg/kg IM q 48–72 hours) and ampicillin. The tortoise is scheduled for recheck appointments 7 to 10 days postoperatively and thereafter every 2 to 4 weeks so that the incision can be monitored and, in the case of a plastron surgery, the shell patch can be changed as needed. Occasionally, the bone underlying the patch may die and need to be removed. A bandage is then used until a firm fibrous substitute for the shell has formed. In time, this will become bone and covered with keratin. At these recheck exams, I often do bloodwork, urinalysis, and fecals to assess how the tortoise is recovering.

A tortoise recovering from bladder surgery should be isolated so it may be carefully monitored. It is essential to keep the cage warm. A basking light, typically a 60- to 100-watt spotlight, should be set-up on one end of the tank. The temperature underneath the spotlight should reach 95–100°F. The other end of the cage should be about 15–20°F cooler. I recommend that the owner uses an infrared (laser) thermometer to directly measure the temperature of the tortoise. If it spends all its time under the light, the cage may be too cool. If it spends all its time at the cool end of the cage, the basking spot may be too hot. Some source of floor heat, such as a heat tape, is useful for night-time heat. Ultraviolet B light may stimulate healing. ZooMed's *Reptisun 5.0 UV Bulb* or *10.0 UV Bulb* and T-Rex *Active UV Heat* appear to be excellent sources of ultraviolet-B light. They should be set up to illuminate the area around the basking light. The *Active UV Heat* can serve as the basking light. These bulbs need to be replaced every 6 to 12 months, even if they are still shining, because their ultraviolet output decreases over time. The tortoise should have a shallow water bowl for drinking but it should not be soaked until the incision has healed or the patch has been on long enough that there is good granulation tissue beneath. The appetite needs to be closely monitored. When the tortoise begins feeding on its own, its feeding tube may need to be removed. It is also important to monitor urine and fecal output throughout recovery.

HOW I TREAT HERPESVIRUS IN TORTOISES

Kevin Wright, DVM
Arizona Exotic Animal Hospital, LLC
Mesa, AZ

Herpesvirus causes lesions in the mouth and choana of tortoises and may also cause a more generalized illness. The herpetic tortoise is often reluctant to eat or drink, has a runny or crusty nose, has drool or a crusty mouth, has an audible whistle or gurgling nose while breathing, and may open-mouth breathe or gape. You may see white or yellow material lining the inside of the mouth and tongue. Other signs are closed or swollen eyes, lethargy, and hiding a lot. In rare cases, a tortoise may circle or have uncoordinated movement. Some tortoises die without obvious signs.

All species of tortoises are susceptible to herpesvirus infection. However, it is more commonly a problem with Russian tortoises (*Testudo horsfieldii*) and Greek tortoises (*Testudo graeca* spp.) that are still imported from the wild in large numbers. Since herpesviruses can live quietly in a tortoise and erupt when the tortoise is under any stress, it can even cause illness in long-term captives. Even captive-bred tortoises have herpesviruses and may be asymptomatic carriers. There is no such thing as a *Testudo* that is guaranteed to be free of herpesvirus

I typically recommend bloodwork, fecal parasite exam, urinalysis, and radiographs to assess an ill tortoise's overall health and rule out other causes for the illness. Although it is difficult to definitively identify herpesvirus, the clinical signs are classic in most tortoises. I will clean and debride the plaques lining the mouth and often flush the choana with an antibiotic and anti-inflammatory solution (2.27 mL enrofloxacin, 0.4 mg dexamethasone sodium phosphate, and 0.8 mL saline). This may be needed every 48 to 72 hours. I start antiviral therapy with a drug called acyclovir (80 mg/kg PO SID) using a compounding pharmacy so that the drug is delivered to the client's house by mail. (In Arizona, there are many compounding pharmacies so a client may drive to pick up the acyclovir.)

Enrofloxacin (10 mg/kg IM SID) may be needed to manage bacterial infections that develop in areas damaged by the virus such as the mouth and upper airways. Oral lysine has been proven to help manage mammalian herpesvirus so I have started offering Viralyse (1.25 mL/kg PO SID) as part of the treatment. Tube-feeding or an esophagostomy tube may be needed for administration of oral medications, liquid diet, and anti-inflammatories such as Metacam (0.1–0.2 mg/kg PO SID). Some tortoises may need to be hospitalized so I may do more aggressive treatments such as daily debriding of the mouth, regular fluid therapy, nebulization, and different antibiotics.

A tortoise's chances depend on how long it was sick before treatment was started and whether or not it has any other ongoing disease such as parasites or malnutrition. Advanced cases in which the tortoise has been sick long enough to lose weight carry a poor outlook. With early detection and aggressive care, over 90% of tortoises recover with proper care at home. If there are other tortoises in the home, it is likely that they have already been exposed to the herpesvirus, or were themselves the carrier that infected the sick tortoise, and should be closely watched for signs of illness.

Isolate the sick tortoise and all tortoises that have had close contact with it. Chlorine bleach diluted 1 part to 30 parts water is very effective disinfectant for tools, water bowls, and cages. Outdoor enclosures with dirt and plants are likely contaminated for a year or more and should not be used to house clinically healthy tortoises. A client should wear disposable gloves or wash hands with warm water and soap after handling an infected tortoise and should not wear the same shoes when servicing an infected enclosure as when they service pens of healthy tortoises.

A client handout with treatment instructions for herpesvirus in tortoises is shown in Figure 1.

Figure 1. Client handout on herpesviruses in tortoises.

TREATMENT OF INSTRUCTIONS FOR HERPESVIRUSES IN TORTOISES

Herpesvirus spreads by direct contact between infected tortoises. All *Testudo* carry herpesvirus which can be deadly to different species of tortoises. Aggressive medical management is necessary for treatment. Despite this, some tortoises do not survive.

My tortoise's drug treatment plan is as follows:

ANTIVIRAL DRUG:

Acyclovir (_____ mg/mL) — Give ____ mL by mouth once daily for ___ days.

ANTIBACTERIAL DRUG:

Enrofloxacin (____ mg/mL) — Give ___ mL by injection into the muscle once daily for ____ days. Alternate injection sites each time.

OR

_____ — Give _____mL by injection into the muscle every ____ hours for ____ days. Alternate injection sites each time.

OR

_____ — Give _____ mL by mouth every ____ hours for ____ days.

INTRACOELOMIC FLUID THERAPY:

Give _____ mL of reptile fluids into the body cavity every ____ hours for ____ days.

OTHER MEDICATIONS:

OTHER TREATMENTS:

DENTAL DISEASE IN FERRETS: MORE SERIOUS THAN WE THOUGHT

Cathy A. Johnson-Delaney, DVM, Dipl. ABVP (Avian)
Eastside Avian & Exotic Animal Medical Center
Washington Ferret Rescue & Shelter
Kirkland, WA

While most practitioners are familiar with dental disease and oral health issues in dogs and cats, many do not provide the same thorough dental examinations and care for ferrets. Ferrets, as carnivores, develop many if not all of the common dental disorders as do dogs and cats. An oral examination should be included in all physical examinations, and at least annual prophylaxis provided. Owners can be taught how to care for their ferret's teeth at home to provide continued care.

DENTITION AND ORAL ANATOMY

The ferret is a strict carnivore and has teeth and jaw structure to accommodate such a diet. The jaws are short with the articular condyle of the mandible fitting into a transverse articular fossa. This has a postarticular process preventing dislocation upon wide opening for a strong bite. The tooth-bearing arcades of the jaws are approximately equal in length, but the lower arcade is narrower and fits medially to the upper arcade. This allows for the shearing motion during chewing. The six upper incisors are slightly longer than the six lower incisors. The second incisors of the mandible are set back from the others. The mandibular canines close in front of the maxillary canines. While usually there are four premolars in Carnivora, only three are present in the ferret. The first premolar has been lost in development. The last maxillary carnassial tooth (third cheek tooth) is the fourth premolar. It has three roots. There is a single molar in the maxillary arcade that has three roots. It is wider in the buccolingual breadth compared with the mesiodistal length making it appear to be rooted at right angles to the rest of the teeth. It has a narrow depressed waist that separates its lingual side from the buccal side of the crown. There are two small cusps on the buccal part and a single cusp on the lingual part. This tooth may be overlooked in an awake ferret examination due to its location. The large mandibular carnassial tooth (fourth cheek tooth) is the first molar. All living mustelids only have the first molar in the maxilla and both the first and second molars in the mandible. The crown of the first mandibular molar has a crown with three distinct cusps. Two form the blades of the carnassial and the smaller, lower cusp in conjunction with the second molar, interlocks with the cusps of the maxillary molar. The first mandibular molar has two roots, although sometimes there is an accessory slender central root present. The second mandibular molar is a small tooth with a single root and a simple crown with a minor ridge and cusplets.[2] It does not occlude with any maxillary teeth, but helps with the crushing function for the caudal cusp of the first mandibular molar. Congenitally this tooth may be missing in many pet ferrets. There is speculation that it is in the evolutionary process of becoming lost or vestigial as has happened in other carnivores. Mustelids crush their food using the post-carnassial molars. The domestic ferret has 28 to 30 deciduous teeth (di3–4/3: dc1/1: dm3/3). The permanent dental formula is I3/3: C1/1: PM3/3: M1/2 = 34.

Ferrets have relatively large oral cavity. The labial commissures extend farther caudally than the carnaissal teeth.[1] The orbicularis oris muscle is moderately well-developed. The lower lip is closely attached to the mandibular gum, with little flexibility. The opening of the parotid duct is at the level of the maxillary carnassial tooth. The mandibular gland opens on a sublingual papilla and joins with several small ducts from the sublingual gland. The molar or buccal gland's duct opens into the oral cavity just opposite the mandibular molars. The zygomatic gland has several ducts opening opposite the upper cheek teeth. Duct openings should be examined routinely during any oral examination or procedure.

Periodontal and gingival tissues and structures are similar to that of other carnivores. Oral flora, pH, and enzymes have not been characterized as they have in other species such as dogs. Using dog and cat dentistry as guidelines for veterinary and home care appears to be relevant.

DENTAL DISEASE CONDITIONS

As mentioned previously, there may be congenital lack of mandibular second molars. There may also be supernumerary teeth, most commonly found between the first and second maxillary incisors. Dental disease includes dental calculus, osteomyelitis/periodontal disease association with tooth infection and/or gingival infection or inflammation, fractured teeth, necrotic teeth, tooth damage from chewing on cage bars, dental abscesses, wear from diets or toys, and teeth lost due to a variety of disease processes including malnutrition, renal disease, and neoplasia.

CALCULUS

Calculus is defined as the mineralized buildup of plaque on tooth surfaces. It is often referred to as "tartar." The plaque itself is a buildup of saliva, bacteria, cellular and food debris, epithelial cells, and bacterial by-products. The pH of the saliva as well as enzyme content, and enzyme release from the bacteria, as well as content of the diet and consistency of the diet influence the degree of plaque buildup. However, plaque appears in pet ferrets whether fed kibble, canned diet or "dook" soup. The domestic ferret fed a processed diet appears to lack some of the dietary components that inhibit plaque buildup in wild mustelids. The conformation of the mouth itself may influence the buildup as the bite may allow pocketing of material. The author has not found studies done on the natural flora, pH (particularly in periodontal and gingival sulci), and enzyme characterization and levels. These, in combination with diet content, would aid in development of effective prophylaxis treatments.

Calculus and plaque left on tooth surfaces extended into the gingival pockets, and accumulates, causing gingivitis. Gingivitis left unchecked along with calculus and time contribute to periodontal disease where the tissue destruction extends into the periodontal ligaments and the bone itself. As this process continues, infection and inflammation can involve the tooth root and abscess, with permanent damage occurring to the tooth. There is also considerable pain with this process. Many ferrets presented for anorexia have severe dental disease that makes eating not only painful, but likely distasteful as well.

ABSCESSES

As mentioned above, abscess of a tooth may come from diseased gums, periodontal tissues, and underlying bone. Infection may also enter the tooth from the pulp cavity if it becomes exposed due to fracture or caries. In many cases by the time the abscess is discovered, the tooth is not longer viable, and there is enough periodontal disease and bone loss to make root canal and tooth retention not an option. Root canal in the ferret is difficult due to the extremely small size of the pulp cavity and in the canines, the added curvature. Radiographs are helpful to exam the roots and underlying structures. Abscesses should be drained, necrotic teeth and tissue removed, and in many cases packed with antimicrobial saturated hemostatic gel (Gel Foam, Pfizer, New York, NY) The gums may be sutured loosely over the opening not only to hold the gel in place, but to prevent impaction with food materials. Parenteral antibiotics, pain medications, and oral rinses will generally be successful.

FRACTURED AND LOST TEETH

One of the most common presentations is fracture of the tips of the canine teeth, particularly the maxillary canines. Pet ferrets frequently bite and pull at their cage bars when they want out. They also fracture teeth during falls and during play when they hit walls and other obstacles. If presented immediately after the fracture and the pulp cavity is exposed, and the tooth is still viable, a superficial pulpectomy can be done in the canine tooth. This involves using a high speed burr into the pulp a few millimeters below the exposed surface, drying and sterilized on the pulp chamber, and filling with a composite as is done in other species. The danger is in overheating the pulp cavity and thence destroying the pulp in the process, which will lead to eventual necrosis. The author prefers to try and preserve canine teeth if possible particularly in young ferrets, but despite "drilling and filling" many proceed to fracture them again or progress to necrosis. Parenteral antibiotics should be instigated as well as oral rinses when doing endodontic procedures. Unfortunately, many fractures are unnoticed by owners, or owners are unaware of the pulp cavity exposure when the tip becomes fractured, and the tooth is non-viable or in the process of dying (painful upon cold probing usually) when the ferret is presented. Ferrets also lose teeth from dental disease, periodontal lesions, severe trauma to the tooth or from metabolic disease that causes bone loss. These may have not been noticed by the owner. It is important to determine if there are retained roots and eliminate the possibility of deep abscess. Radiographs are very useful to determine if remnants of teeth exist.

DIAGNOSIS, ASSESSMENT, AND TREATMENT

The author has developed a grading system to assist in determining a dental program for each ferret.[3] Stage 1 is gingivitis, with inflammation of the gingival due plaque. Some of the plaque may be mineralized (calculus), although buildup is usually fairly minimal. The gingiva will be erythematous, and may be slightly swollen along the edge abutting the teeth. These usually do not bleed when the pockets are probed.

Stage 2 is early periodontitis. The gingivitis has progressed to actual infection of the gums, periodontal tissues and even the bone, although the teeth are still firmly attached, and on radiographs roots are still viable. There may be gumline abscesses at this point and there may be some gingival recession or periodontal pocket formation. Up to 25% of the dental attachments may have been lost. For oral examination and probing in the awake ferret at this stage, the author first applies an oral lidocaine 2% gel (lidocaine gel, Henry Schein, Melville, NY) to the gingival areas.

Stage 3 is moderate periodontitis. Bleeding usually occurs during dental probing and affected teeth may have up to 50% loss of attachments. There may be root exposure. Some teeth may be slightly loosened. Abscesses are frequently found around the roots and accumulations of food and debris encountered in the periodontal/gingival pockets. Most ferrets require light sedation, parenteral analgesia, and topical dental anesthetics for a full oral exam at this stage.

Stage 4 is advanced periodontitis. There is greater than 50% loss of attachments, tooth roots are usually exposed due to gum and bone recession. on radiographs, tooth roots will show the lack of attachment and often degree of abscessation or destruction (lysis), and loss of viability. There is often blood and pus surrounding the tooth. The tooth may also be loose. This condition is painful and further examination requires heavy sedation, analgesia, or anesthesia. Teeth may be lost at this stage even if periodontal treatment is initiated using protocols used in dogs (including resection of gums, packing with an antibiotic gel, parenteral/oral antibiotics, brushing of the teeth).

Cleaning of ferret teeth should be done at least annually under anesthesia. Deep planing of the teeth and removal of calculi can be done utilizing a McColl's scaler which will fit under normal ferret gingiva. After gingival recess planing has been done, further removal of plaque can be done utilizing an ultrasonic dental cleaning system or by further hand scaling. Polishing of the teeth can be done utilizing a prophy cup on a low speed handpiece with a mild abrasive polish (Zircon-F, Henry Schein, Melville, NY). After rinsing and removal of debris, the teeth can be dried thoroughly and either a fluoride paste, varnish (several brands as used in dogs, Henry Schein, Melville, NY) can be applied or a sealant (Oravet, Merial, Duluth, GA) can be used.

If extractions of teeth are necessary, the author advocates first locally blocking the area with lidocaine 2% (volume dependent on size of the dental area and weight of the ferret; for most teeth 0.05–0.1 mL is adequate), then gingivectomy. Incise the periodontal tissues. In some cases, it may be necessary to remove some alveolar bone. Once the ligamentous tissues have been severed, the tooth can be easily elevated using a fine-tipped elevator or 18-gauge needle (for the smaller teeth), and extracted often with just hemostats. If there is an open alveolus (as with the canine teeth), the cavity may be packed with a hydrostatic gel or synthetic bone matrix material (Consil Bioglass, Nutramax, Baltimore, MD). The gums can be sutured with 4-0 or 5-0 absorbable suture on a fine swaged-on taper point needle. Suturing the gums encourages healing and decreases debris being introduced. Analgesics, nonsteroidal anti-inflammatory drugs (NSAIDs), and often antibiotics will be used post extraction. Owners are usually instructed on how to apply a mild chlorhexidine rinse to the sutured area twice daily for up to a week as well.

Home dental care should include the continued application of Oravet (if that was used) on a weekly basis. If teeth are not sealed, then owners should be instructed on how to brush their ferret's teeth. The author uses cotton swabs and an enzymatic toothpaste (CET, Virbac, Fort Worth, TX) in either malt or poultry flavor. Most pet ferrets do not mind tooth brushing as they like the taste of the toothpaste. Follow-up examinations should be done on a regular basis.

CONCLUSION

Dental disease is extremely common in pet ferrets and should be included as part of a regular wellness program as it is in other animals. Diagnosis, treatment and prevention are similar to other carnivores.

REFERENCES

1. Evans HE, An NQ: Anatomy of the ferret. In Fox JG (ed): Biology and Diseases of the Ferret 2nd ed. Baltimore: Williams & Wilkins, 1998; pp 19-69
2. Church B. Ferret dentition and pathology. In Lewington JH (ed): Ferret Husbandry, Medicine and Surgery 2nd ed. Edinburgh, UK: Saunders Elsevier, 2007; pp 467-485.
3. Johnson-Delaney CA. Ferret dental disorders: pictorial of common clinical presentations. Exotic DVM. 2007:9:40-43.

NEW FERRET TRICKS: EMERGING DISEASE PRESENTATIONS

Cathy A. Johnson-Delaney, DVM, Dipl. ABVP (Avian)
Eastside Avian & Exotic Animal Medical Center
Washington Ferret Rescue & Shelter
Kirkland, WA

The domestic ferret, *Mustela (putorius) furo*, is a highly inbred animal that is extremely popular as a pet. In the past 10 years, there has been a large increase in the number of pet ferrets available in pet stores in the United States. Predominantly they are from one commercial breeder, but there are other commercial breeders and small, individual breeders as well. Most of the diseases discussed are being seen in ferrets from different sources, although in the pet trade different shipments may be mixed. There has also been a move by all suppliers to neuter/spay and descent the ferrets at 3 to 4 weeks of age. The implications of surgery at that age on the immune system and disease exposure has not been studied (or at least appeared in the published literature). The alterations to the growth and development of the ferret may also be affected (as is being studied with adrenal disease). Regardless, this practice will continue. Ferrets are shipped usually at 6 to 8 weeks of age, and usually they have received only one vaccination, canine distemper. They are due for the rest of the series, and most do not get it, as pet stores repeatedly (erroneously) tell people "they've had their shots." Completion of distemper vaccination and rabies is frequently done after the ferret is 6 months to a year old, or has developed other medical problems. Most pet ferrets during their lifespan will develop dental disease, neoplasia, cardiomyopathy, and some form of gastrointestinal disorder. The pet ferret has one of the highest tumor rates of any mammal. These serious illnesses are in addition to the usual ferret follies: ear mites and trauma of multiple types. We do advise ferret owners to establish a savings account for their ferret's medical needs.

Many of the disease problems we are currently seeing need to be characterized and studied. Practitioners with cases are encouraged to tabulate their data and coordinate this with the pathologists or clinicians trying to discern the etiology, treatment, and prevention. Networking through online veterinary exotics discussion groups is extremely helpful as it establishes a pattern from which we can look at epidemiology.

FERRET INFECTIOUS PERITONITIS (CORONAVIRUS–FIP)

Ferrets are susceptible to coronavirus infections: experimentally to SARS (severe acute respiratory syndrome) and FECV (ferret enteric coronavirus). FECV is the cause of epizootic catarrhal enteritis (ECE) in ferrets. Lesions are only in the gastrointestinal tract, with virus found in the saliva, feces, and enterocytes. Feline coronavirus (FCOV) is responsible for a feline enteric self-limiting disease and the mutated form is responsible for feline infectious peritonitis (FIP). The agent responsible for the "FIP-like" disease in ferrets appears to be a variant of the FECV virus, and is being called ferret systemic coronavirus (FSCV). Gross, histologic, and immunohistochemical features of FSCV are identical to FIP.[1,2]

Clinical signs include weight loss (in some severe), anorexia, palpable intra-abdominal mass or masses, lethargy, vomiting, splenomegaly, dehydration, bruxism, renomegaly, sneezing/nasal discharge, systolic heart murmur, urine discoloration, dyspnea, peripheral lymphadenomegaly, rectal mucosa erythema, rectal prolapse. Central nervous system signs are seen in some ferrets and include acute or progressive hind limb paresis or paraparesis, ataxia, seizures, abnormal posture, opistothonus, abnormal gait, and proprioceptive deficits. Some ferrets have fevers ranging from 103°F to 105.4°F.

PATHOLOGY

On biopsy or necropsy, the primary gross lesions are circumscribed to coalescing white, tan or slightly pink irregular nodules or foci of white discoloration ranging from 5 to 30 mm in greatest dimension on the surface and within the parenchyma of spleen, liver, kidneys, lung, mesentery, and lymph nodes.[1] Splenomegaly, renomegaly, hepatomegaly, and ascites have also been noted.

Histologic lesions have been detected in the mesentery/peritoneum, lymph nodes, spleen, kidneys, liver, lung, intestine, pancreas, stomach, brain, and adrenal glands. Other notable lesions include nonsuppurative meningoencephalitis and suppurative or nonsuppurative tubulointerstitial nephritis.[1] Coronavirus antigen was detected in all tissues with lesions, however the staining reaction was most prominent in lymph nodes, splenic lymphoid follicles, and all foci of pyogranulomatous inflammation.[1]

CURRENT ASSESSMENT AND VIROLOGY

FSCV has similar gross and histologic lesions to those in cats with FIP. It resembles the "dry form" of FIP with widespread nodular foci on serosal surfaces and within the parenchyma of thoracic and abdominal viscera. There is also nodular enlargement of mesenteric lymph nodes. Clinically, some practitioners have reported effusions in the body cavities resembling the "wet form," but this has not been the predominantly reported or documented finding. Designating "wet" or "dry" forms is somewhat arbitrary as many cats exhibit lesions consistent with both forms during the course of the disease. This is likely the case in ferrets. As more cases are collected, more effusive cases may be documented.

On sequencing, there is slight cross-reactivity in some samples with the FECV-specific primers that may indicate sequence conservation between nucleocapsid genes of FSCV and FECV. Further genomic sequencing of the virus is required. In conclusion, the relatively recent recognition of this disease in pet ferrets suggests a recent mutation or shift in the FECV resulting in the systemic disease. This is similar to the mutations that occurred in FCOV preceding the development of FIP-1

DISSEMINATED IMMUNOPATHIC MYOSITIS

Disseminated immunopathic myositis (DIM) was not described prior to 2003. It is characterized by a fatal, inflammatory condition of the muscles. Ferrets have typically been between 3 and 24 months of age, with the average age being 10 months. There is no sex predilection and ferrets have been from a variety of breeders.

The clinical presentation is one of rapid onset, characterized by high fever (105–108°F), anorexia, and reluctance to move. There may be variable lymphadenopathy and splenomegaly. Hematology usually shows a neutrophilic leukocytosis. Serum chemistries may show an elevated AST, hyperglycemia, and hypoalbuminemia. Most ferrets have some degree of dehydration and are losing weight and condition. Some ferrets with DIM also show diarrhea, mild serous nasal discharge, and have increased heart and respiratory rates. Radiology and ultrasonography usually show no abnormalities. Biopsies of skeletal muscle from the hind leg or lumbar region, lymph nodes and/or any masses may be useful for antemortem diagnosis and prognosis. If necropsy tissues are submitted, esophagus, heart, skeletal muscle (several sites), diaphragm, lymph nodes, spleen, bone marrow are most definitive, although full tissue submission is preferred.

Many therapies have been attempted in efforts to reduce the fever and inflammation associated with this disease, but rarely has there been recovery. Antibiotic therapy including penicillins, cephalosporins, fluoroquinolones, doxycycline, clarithromycin, azithromycin, trimethoprim-sulfa, aminoglycosides, metronidazole, and chloramphenicol has been unsuccessful. Treatment with steroidal and nonsteroidal anti-inflammatory drugs (NSAIDs) also has had little effect. Other drugs including antifungal and antiviral agents have been ineffective in controlling signs of DIM. Interferon-alpha at a dose of 600 IU/day has been shown to reduce the fever in a few cases temporarily. Cyclophosphamide has also been without much success. As most ferrets require fluid therapy, nutritional supplementation and analgesia as the disease progresses, many owners elect euthanasia following the biopsy diagnosis. To date, the author has not successfully treated this: all patients succumbed.

PATHOLOGY

Gross lesions include atrophy of skeletal muscle throughout the body including the esophagus (described as red and white mottling, dilatation). Histologically there is moderate to severe suppurative to pyogranulomatous inflammation of skeletal muscle and fascia of the esophagus, heart, limbs, body wall, head and lumbar regions. There is myeloid hyperplasia of the spleen and/or bone marrow. On electron microscopy lesions include mitochondrial swelling, intracellular edema, disruption of myofibrils and Z bands.[3]

At this time, the etiology of DIM is unknown. No pathogen has been isolated in any of the confirmed cases by bacterial or viral cultures, EM, immunohistochemistry, or polymerase chain reaction testing for a wide variety of known pathogens. One vaccine from one manufacturer is the only known commonality. This vaccine is no longer available, and so it is unknown if we will continue to see this syndrome. We have not had any cases presented in the past year. In an experimental trial using the canine castration vaccine, this myofasciitis syndrome was reproduced in the entire group, suggesting that it is an immunological response to an initial inflammatory stimulation.

APLASTIC ANEMIA/BONE MARROW

This condition has been seen repeatedly in ferrets across the country. Cases are being tabulated, but so far, the only discernible pattern is that the ferrets are under 18 months of age. They are presented due to lethargy and anorexia, but upon physical examination are found to have pale to white mucus membranes. Some have moderate splenomegaly, but other physical parameters appear normal. Packed cell volumes are less than 10%. Bone marrow aspirations have shown erthyrocytic aplasia. These ferrets tend to have normal white blood cell counts, and serum chemistries are often normal. Although transfusions are done, erythropoietin therapy is usually ineffective. High doses of corticosteroid have been tried to try an rule out an immune-mediated disease: this has also seemed ineffective. Etiology is unknown, but collection of case information and full necropsy work needs to be done.

ACUTE HEMORRHAGING SYNDROME

This syndrome has manifested within the past year and seems to occur mainly in recently shipped ferrets or ones recently placed in pet stores. One of the major pet store chains alerted veterinarians to it in their August newsletter (Edling T, PetCo Newsletter) These young kits have acute hemorrhage, often first as epistaxis, and from oral ulceration. Hemorrhages can also be seen from the rectum, and petechiation may appear on the skin. Hemorrhage within the abdominal cavity has also been seen. Immediate therapy with parenteral vitamin K and supportive care appears to have stopped the hemorrhaging if caught early, but many literally bleed out no matter what treatment is attempted. If possible, blood can be drawn for a coagulation profile antemortem: it is speculated that this may be a hemophilia disease. Normal coagulation parameters on ferrets need to be collected and then compared. If you encounter this, please collect blood for a coagulation profile, attempt therapy, and contact Dr. Drury Reavill, who is coordinating the pathology work.

AMINO ACID METABOLISM ABNORMALITIES

Two conditions are being found in ferrets that appear to be genetic metabolism pathway abnormalities. One is cysteine metabolism, which results in cysteine urolithiasis. Ferrets that have shown this condition have all been on novel protein diets. L-carnitine metabolism abnormality is being linked to skeletal muscle weakness in older ferrets, particularly in the hind legs. Supplementation with L-carnitine has ameliorated the most severe symptoms, but further characterization of this needs to be done. Dr. Michelle Hawkins is working on various genetic disease issues in ferrets. If you encounter urolithiasis in ferrets, stone analysis can be performed at the University of California, Davis. Contact Dr. Hawkins concerning the case.

CONCLUSION

A number of emerging diseases in ferrets need to be researched prior to effective treatments or preventive measures can be accomplished. Practitioners need to share case information particularly with pathologists and investigators if we are to solve these clinical dilemmas.

REFERENCES

1. Garner MM, Ramsell K, Morera N, et al. Clinico-pathologic features of a systemic coronavirus-associated disease resembling feline infectious peritonitis in the domestic ferret (*Musteal putorius*). Vet Pathol, in press.
2. Martinez J, Ramis AJ, Reinacher M, Perpiñan D. Detection of feline infectious peritonitis virus-like antigen in ferrets. Vet Rec. 2006:158:523
3. Garner MM, Ramsell K, Schoemaker NJ, et al. Myofaciitis in the domestic ferret. Vet Pathol. 2007:44:25-38.

UPDATE ON THE FERRET GENOME PROJECT

Cathy A. Johnson-Delaney, DVM, Dipl. ABVP (Avian)
Eastside Avian & Exotic Animal Medical Center
Washington Ferret Rescue & Shelter
Kirkland, WA

Because adrenal disease is so widespread in pet ferrets, a genetic basis for the large numbers of affected ferrets is being investigated, primarily by Dr. Michelle Hawkins and her team at the University of California, Davis, and Dr. Robert Wagner at the University of Pittsburgh.

The hypothesis is that if an aberrant/mutated tumor suppressor gene or genes is/are present, hyperplastic tissue with stimulation progresses to adenoma, then eventually adenocarcinoma, following models in other animals and humans. The genes may be defective, or the regulation of the genes may be defective. The hypothesis also includes the possibility of multiple tumor suppressor genes "oncogenes" being involved. A completed study looked at tumor markers in ferrets, based on the work in gonadectomized DBA/2J mice that develop adrenocortical tumors expressing transcription factor GATA-4. 86% of the ferret adrenocortical carcinomas, particularly in areas of myxoid differentiation expressed GATA-4. Normal adrenocortical cells lacked GATA-4 expression. Two other markers of adrenocortical tumors in gonadectomized mice that are co-expressed with GATA-4 are inhibin-alpha and LH receptor. These were co-expressed in some of the ferret tumors. No GATA-4 expression was observed in three cases of nodular hyperplasia; however patches of anaplastic cells expressed GATA-4 in 50% of the tumors classified as adenomas. The conclusion was that GATA-4 does function as a marker of anaplasia in ferret adrenocortical tumors. The relevance of this shows that there may be a way of tracking and marking the tumors (prognostication for the practitioner when advising the client), and pathways of cancer development in the ferrets is similar to that of other species. This also is suggestive of a genetic root to the development of the disease, as GATA-4 is a protein marker.

GENETIC RESEARCH

In humans, the appearance of benign or malignant proliferations within two or more endocrine glands is nearly always genetically determined and is termed multiple endocrine neoplasia (MEN) syndrome. There are three currently accepted human familial syndromes in which there is a progression from hyperplasia to neoplasia in endocrine tissues: MEN types 1 (MEN1), 2a (MEN2a), and 2b (MEN2b). MEN1 syndrome usually is characterized by parathyroid hyperplasia, pancreatic islet cell and/or pituitary tumors. Up to 40% of MEN1 patients also develop adrenal, thyroid or thymic tissue tumors. MEN2a and MEN2b syndromes are characterized primarily as medullary thyroid cancer (MTC) with or without pheochromocytomas and parathyroid adenomas. MEN1 and MEN2 are inherited as autosomal-dominant genetic traits. The MEN1 gene is ubiquitously expressed and is not limited to organs affected by the syndrome. A number of different mutations have been described for the MEN1 gene in humans. As there seems to be a similarity between the endocrine neoplasm patterns in the ferret and the human MEN1 syndrome, research being conducted by Dr. Hawkins is first looking for a homologous gene in the ferret to the human MEN1 gene.

DNA has been collected from buccal swabs and flash frozen tumor tissue. Polymerase chain reaction (PCR) primers from human, dog, and cow were used. Tissue culture of cancer (adrenal, thyroid and/or pancreas) cells has not been as good at yielding chromosomes for karytyping due to the clumping during tumor growth. Ferret whole blood also provided enough material for analysis. G-band karyotyping is being done using standard cytogenetic methods.

Affected ferret's chromosomal material was sequenced and both an MEN-1 and a Ret oncogene have been sequenced. The MEN-1 has a 99.40% homology with the dog MEN-1; 97.70% homology with the human gene, and 98.10% homology with bovine. The Ret has a 100% homology with dog, 97.60% with cat, 94.00% with human, but only a 75.90% with mouse. So far, no mutations have been identified. There is 100% conservation of nucleotide base pairs for both genes in all individuals, with 0% variability. This is extremely unusual as genetic material usually even among purebreds and genetically designed mice, for example, has some degree of variation.

Dr. Wagner's research has been concentrated on the p53 tumor suppressor gene and the CHEK-2 oncogene in tumor tissues. At this writing, identification of some aberrant p53s has been found.

For all of the genetic work, population genetics and an evaluation of kinship is ongoing. This looks at a panel of 30 microsatellite DNA cancer genes such as found in material from sea otters and mink, other members of the Mustelidae. A partial cancer pedigree needs to be constructed within worldwide ferret populations. Genetic material from ferrets around the world, and if possible from breeders where there are several generations of non-affected ferrets is needed. To date, material looked at from affected ferrets worldwide has virtually no genetic variation. It may be necessary to look at the genetics of the European polecat, *Mustela putorius*, that is the direct ancestor of the domestic ferret.

If genetic variation is so limited, identification of non-aberrant genes and/or regulators becomes problematic. Ferrets will need to be found without the abnormalities. Tissue typing for histocompatibility proteins should also be done to continue work on the genetic pedigree. Therefore, at present, clinicians need to continue to identify medical and surgical management of neoplasia for the individual ferret.

REFERENCES

1. Schoemaker NJ, Hawkins MG. Hyperadrenocorticism in ferrets: clinical updates. Proc Assoc Avian Vet: Assoc Exotic Mammals, Providence, RI, 2007: 79-84.

POSTSURGICAL DISASTERS: MANAGING COMPLICATIONS OF ELECTIVE SURGERIES

Cathy A. Johnson-Delaney, DVM, Dipl. ABVP (Avian)
Eastside Avian & Exotic Animal Medical Center
Washington Ferret Rescue & Shelter
Kirkland, WA

Everyone who has done elective surgeries on small mammals has had postsurgical complications. These include death 1 to 2 hours or within 24 hours of apparent successful surgery and anesthetic recovery; wound dehiscence, hemorrhage, sepsis at the incision site or in the body cavity following gastrointestinal tract manipulation, pregnancy resulting from incomplete or re-grown vasectomies, and postsurgical hypoglycemic ferrets. Analysis of what went wrong, along with new methods for monitoring and taking pre-emptive steps, should help to decrease complications. This presentation is a culmination of 27 years of exotic pet practice experience.

UNEXPECTED DEATH: SUCCESSFUL SURGERY AND RECOVERY?

There are a number of factors that must be considered other than the surgery itself that contribute to a successful outcome. These include ventilation, oxygenation, maintenance of blood pressure, circulation including renal perfusion, and body temperature maintenance. In many of our small patients, we may not be providing for these as we might in a larger animal such as a dog or cat. Yet these parameters may be even more important given the higher metabolic rate, greater surface area, and frequent lack of good ventilation/oxygenation (not intubated). Many of our small herbivores have relatively small thoracic cavities in relation to their abdomens. In dorsal recumbency, the heavy intestinal tract may exert pressure on the diaphragm (particularly if the body is slanted with the head downward), as well alter abdominal blood circulation. Rabbits, guinea pigs, chinchillas, and even hamsters then may be less than optimally able to expand their lungs and provide oxygenation. It is difficult to intubate guinea pigs due to the ostium, but with practice it is possible. It is also possible to intubate rabbits, chinchillas, rats, prairie dogs, and most rodents with practice. The laboratory animal industry has developed not only methodology but the equipment needed to do so. Ventilators are also available for these small animals as they have been developed for research. Unfortunately, most of the ones designed for rats and mice may be out of the price range of most practitioners. Small animal ventilators (BAS Vetronics, Bioanalytical Systems, West Lafayette, IN; and Hallowell Ventilator, Hallowell Engineering & Manufacturing Corp, Pittsfield, MA) are available that work well with rabbits, ferrets, and other small exotics. Capnography is an excellent way to monitor CO_2 levels and hence ventilation. Capnography is preferable to pulse oximetry. Pulse oximetry probes may be difficult to place in many of our small patients, and they also frequently compress the tissue and become nonfunctional. These may require frequent readjustment. Monitoring the patient with electrocardiography in my opinion is mandatory. Not only does ECG act as a direct heart rate monitor, usually with audible beeping, but frequently have respiratory monitors as well. The ECG also is the first indicator of abnormalities in conduction occurring either due to anoxia or electrolyte imbalances (T-wave elongation or alteration), arrhythmias, and if the vagal reflex (going into cardiac arrest) has been triggered. With ECG monitoring you can act quickly with repositioning the animal, ventilating, intravenous intervention with appropriate agents (such as lidocaine or atropine), decrease level of anesthesia, increasing local analgesia or correction of electrolyte imbalances, although usually in our small patients intra-surgery blood gases and electrolyte analysis are not done.

Maintenance of blood pressure and core body temperature appear to be key elements of the "post-surgery/anesthesia" deaths. During anesthesia, core body temperature begins to drop, and may drop precipitously if a body cavity is opened. The smaller the animal, the more rapid and dramatic the temperature drop. A warm water circulating blanket or under-patient heating apparatus does not maintain body temperature well in most. Many patients have lost body temperature during the preparation process: particularly if large areas are shaved and alcohol applied. Under-the-patient heating systems are not very effective at bringing the body temperature back up to preanesthetic normals. The forced-warm air systems (Bair Hugger, Avizant Healthcare, Eden Prairie, MN) are superior in warming the hypothermic patient back to normothermia and maintaining core body temperature for even prolonged surgeries. Small pads can be made using towels that can then be laundered and re-used. The towel is sewn to create a ridged effect when air is blown in, Velcro is used to fasten it around the hose from the warming unit. Holes are punched on the side of the towel that the patient lays on. Blood pressure can be monitored using Doppler monitors (Parks Medical Electronics, Aloha, OR or Nadeco Minidop, Jorgenson Labs, Burlington, WI), placed on tails (ferrets, rats, wallabies, monkeys) or forelimb in other small animals. The pulse can usually be found in the carpus area. Mean arterial pressure (systolic) should be established pre-anesthetic, and monitored periodically throughout the procedure. Full anesthetic recovery includes return of the blood pressure to pre-anesthetic levels. It is interesting to note that painful stimuli may cause blood pressure to increase even during surgical anesthesia, and administration of some medications, such as meloxicam (Metacam, Merial, Duluth, GA) during recovery may decrease blood pressure. It is always advantageous to have intravenous or intraosseous access during surgery for continuous fluid infusion. Fluid rate can be increased if blood pressure drops, or if colloids, transfusions, and/or additional medications need to be administered to maintain cardiac output during the surgery. Intravenous catheters may be difficult to place in short-limbed small animals such as guinea pigs, although it is possible using the saphenous or jugular vein. The jugular vein access usually requires a cut-down procedure. Intraosseous catheterization is feasible in the tibia or femur of many small animals. Fluid administration should be calculated prior to the surgery. If it is not possible to have direct venous access, particularly for short procedures such as castration, subcutaneous fluids should be administered. Fluids should be warmed; fluid bags and lines can be heated and insulated. Choice of fluids is based on the animal's condition and type of surgery to be done. For non-herbivore small animals including Callitrichids, the author adds dextrose particularly if fluids are to be given subcutaneously rather than intravenously. The amount is empirical: 1 mL of 50% dextrose to 19 to 29 mL of an isotonic crystalloid fluid. Utilizing this type of fluid has prevented postoperative hypoglycemia in small omnivores and carnivores that prior to this often had severe hypoglycemic episodes during recovery. Hypoglycemia coupled with lowered blood pressure, hypothermia, decreased ventilation during anesthesia that has led to decreased oxygenation and perfusion (lactic acid build-up) are all factors that can be implicated in the death after successful anesthesia recovery.

Bottom line: we need to practice the level of anesthesia monitoring and pre-, intra- and postoperative procedures and monitoring as we do in other animals in specialty surgical practices. It is also critical to minimize stress prior to anesthesia; elevations of heart rate, blood pressure, cortisol, epinephrine, even histamine due to anxiety, fear, pain or illness sets up instability in the cardiovascular system prior to any anesthesia or surgical procedure. Utilizing antianxiety medications such as midazolam or diazepam as part of the preanesthetic regimen eases induction and stabilizes cardiovascular parameters. Pre-emptive pain control as well as intraoperative pain management (use of local, epidurals, incisional blocks) can be done as easily in any of these animals as it is done in dogs, cats or humans. Postoperative pain and anxiety management increases the likelihood of a full recovery. Despite years of doing so, "just masking an animal down with isoflurane" is detrimental to the events the cardiovascular, nervous, and system directly affected by the surgery will experience. There is rarely if never any reason not to administer an analgesic and/or an antianxiety/relaxant medication. If attention is paid to the above parameters, unexpected deaths can greatly be decreased.

DEHISCENCE

With rodents and rabbits, opening of the surgical incision is often due to the animal chewing out sutures. Generally if an incision is painful, the animal will groom it and work on it to try and eliminate the irritant. Good, balanced pain control before and after surgery is essential. In addition, there are several techniques that can lessen the chances of the animal reopening the site, or the site dehiscing on its own.[1] Do multiple layer closures. With small animals sometimes it seems enough to just close the body wall then the skin, but instead, the body wall (plus pleura or peritoneum if body cavity is opened) should be closed; then use the fascia/muscle sheaths to created an overlapping layer for the second, then a subcuticular suture pattern for skin closure, with tissue glue to close gaps. For rats and mice, skin staples work well, and rats tolerate staples better than skin sutures. I recommend using a combination of horizontal mattress suture for the center of the incision, interrupted sutures at each end, then short sections of continuous sutures, with different patterns overlying each other. If the animal manages to get past the subcuticular layer, they will encounter more difficulty getting further, and if observed regularly, probably won't totally get into the site. But with adequate pain control, most do not bother the site. The addition of topical anesthetic cream frequently to the incision along with blocking the incision itself, adds to the systemic analgesia. The dorsal approach for ovariohysterectomy in rats, guinea pigs, and other rodents also decreases the likelihood of dehiscence as the heavy abdominal organs are not pressing on the incision site. Collars should be used sparingly on rabbits and rodents that practice cecotrophy as they prevent the nightly ingestion of the cecotrophs. Without cecotrophy within a few days the gastrointestinal tracts and metabolism of rabbits and these rodents may start into dysbiosis and nutrient depletion. Topical bitter taste deterrents can be made using any ophthalmic base ointment or antiseptic cream with a small amount of crushed metronidazole. This can be applied as needed to the incision site. Ferrets rarely bother incision sites or pull out sutures. Dehiscence may occur due to too much activity before the incision has healed. Three-layer closure plus skin sutures using 3-0 suture material generally are enough. However, if there is neoplastic infiltration in any of the closure layers, or excessive amounts of fat included in the suture lines, the closure may break down.

HEMORRHAGE

Hemorrhage of the body wall, body cavity, or from tissues thought ligated or hemostatically clipped adequately can occur upon recovery and increase in blood pressure and as the body returns to normothermia. This is a major reason that blood pressure and body temperature need to be closely monitored and maintained throughout surgery. If liver disease is present, addition of vitamin K parenterally perioperatively may also help to decrease hemorrhage. If presurgery liver disease is known, a coagulation panel should be run to determine if there is a risk of hemorrhage.

SEPSIS

With rabbits and rodents that are hindgut fermenters, the cecum can be a source of leakage of bacteria and toxins, particularly if there has been dysbiosis or stasis prior to the surgery. Manipulation of the large hindgut not only directly inflicts trauma on the serosal surface, often with serosal hemorrhages and bruising, but can result in areas of ischemia and decreased vascular perfusion. With the likelihood of clostridial organisms and other potential coliforms that produce enterotoxins, this vascular and wall trauma may allow bacteria and/or toxin production and dissemination. There is also the possibility of torsions and vascular occlusions with gastrointestinal manipulations. Powder from gloves can contribute to areas of irritation and adhesions. Rabbits are prone to forming adhesions, which can provide an environment for bacterial colonizations. Close attention to keeping the tissues moist with sterile saline, rinsing of gloves, minimal manipulation and touching of the gastrointestinal tract, sterile instrumentation, drapes and surgical skin preparation should be standards of surgery. Depending only on postoperative antibiotics as a substitute for good technique is not acceptable. For herbivore surgeries where the hindgut was manipulated, consideration to providing anticlostridial therapy should be considered. Fluid therapy and getting the animal eating as soon as possible will also decrease sequellae from gut trauma.

VASECTOMIES

Vasectomy surgeries are often done in ferrets and nonhuman primates. It is important to not disturb the vascular supply to the testicles or cause torsion during the elevation of the vas. Ligation of the vas proximally and distally, with at least 0.25 to 0.5 cm of vas removed in between the ligatures will decrease the likelihood of reconnecting. I also like to tack each end to the serosal tissue adjacent to the ligated ends. Adequate time must also be allowed before the male is back with females, as there can be some residual sperm in the urethra. Usually 30 to 45 days is enough, but a urine sample cytology can be used to check for the presence of sperm.

OCCULT ISLET CELL DISEASE/HYPOGLYCEMIA

In ferrets, a blood glucose level is usually checked prior to major surgery. There may be no history of any signs of "insulinoma" or hypoglycemic episodes. During any abdominal surgery, checking visually and by palpation the pancreas often detects some nodules or small masses. Even in surgeries where the pancreas grossly appears normal, there can in fact be hyperinsulin-secreting areas. If regular electrolyte fluid therapy is done, coupled with fasting of at least 2 hours prior to surgery, by the time the ferret is recovering from anesthesia, it may be severely hypoglycemic. One way to prevent this is to include dextrose in the pre-, peri- and postoperative fluid therapy, plus get the ferret to eat at least a small amount of "soup" or Nutrical (Evsco, Buena, NJ) as soon as it can lick it off a spoon or tongue depressor. Taking a blood glucose during recovery is also suggested for ferrets over 4 to 5 years of age.

CONCLUSION

Applying thorough pre-, peri-, and postoperative techniques utilized in small animal surgeries for dogs and cats are appropriate for our small exotic mammals. Consideration of anatomical and metabolic differences as well as balanced anesthesia and analgesia will greatly diminish the number of postoperative complications. Using vascular, microsurgical and other small, atraumatic instruments, sutures (non-chromic gut, always swaged-on) and magnification will also contribute to successful outcomes rather than disaster.

DIAGNOSTIC DEAD ENDS?
SO WHAT'S THE NEXT STEP?

Cathy A. Johnson-Delaney, DVM, Dipl. ABVP (Avian)
Eastside Avian & Exotic Animal Medical Center
Washington Ferret Rescue & Shelter
Kirkland, WA

FERRETS

Islet cell neoplasia has been reported in ferrets between the ages of 3 and 8 years, with the most common onset being 4 to 5 years of age. Both sexes are affected. The history varies from acute onset to a chronic course of weeks to many months, with episodes that may last from several minutes to several hours. The episodes usually end with spontaneous recovery, or after administration of an oral sugar solution, fruit juice, or syrup by the owner. Owners will report the glazing over of the eyes, collapse, increased salivation, gagging, tearing at the mouth (nausea), weakness of the hind legs, and ataxia. There may be a gradual weight loss. Between episodes, the ferrets act normally. Physical examination may reveal no abnormalities, although many have varying degrees of splenomegaly. Other neoplasias occurring simultaneously are common: adrenal neoplasia, lymphoma, and various skin tumors. Additional disease such as cardiomyopathy may be present. Fasting time should be fairly short (no more than 4 to 6 hours, or less if signs of hypoglycemia ensue) and done under close observation for signs of hypoglycemia. More than one test is usually done with concurrent insulin levels.

A full diagnostic work-up of the ferret should be done, including a complete blood count (CBC) and chemistries. There may be increases in alanine aminotransferase (ALT) or aspartate aminotransferase (AST) reflecting hepatic lipidosis secondary to chronically low blood glucose concentration or liver metastasis. Radiographs may show other problems. Abdominal ultrasound may highlight large tumors. Medical management includes using prednisone and/or diazoxide orally in conjunction with dietary management. Ferrets with mild to moderate clinical signs may be controlled by prednisone therapy alone, in peroral (PO) dosages ranging from 0.5 to 2 mg/kg every 12 hours. Start with the lower dosage, and increase if necessary. Diazoxide (Proglycem, Baker Norton Pharmaceuticals, Miami, FL) is a benzothiadiazine derivative which acts by inhibiting insulin release from the pancreatic beta cells, by promoting glyconeogenolysis and gluconeogenesis by the liver, and by decreasing the cellular uptake of glucose. Usually diazoxide at 5 to 10 mg/kg every 12 hours PO is added to the protocol when prednisone alone is not adequately controlling the hypoglycemia. The dosage may need to be increased gradually with the maximum of 60 mg/kg per 24 hours divided every 8 to 12 hours. Recently doxorubricin has been tried and shows some promise. Famotidine at 2.5 mg/ferret one to two times a day may be helpful with the stomach upset and nausea which accompanies the islet cell disease.

Ferrets naturally infected with *Helicobacter mustelae* have a predominantly mononuclear gastritis. Infected ferrets produce elevated immunoglobulin G (IgG) titers to *H. mustelae*. Ferrets also generate autoantibodies to gastric parietal cells. Infection is life-long and the severity of the gastritis increases with age. It may play a role in the development of inflammatory bowel disease and gastric carcinoma.

Samples may be obtained by gastric endoscopic biopsy for microbiology and histology. The Warthin-Starry and H&E stains are used for assessment of colonization and mucosal histopathologic morphology respectively. Serum antibody titers can be done although serum antibody to *H. mustelae* is not protective because ferrets with high titers are already colonized by the organism and have associated gastritis. ELISA titers also rise with age and chronicity of infection. *H. mustelae* can be cultured from feces. Real-time polymerase chain reaction (PCR) (Research Associates Laboratory [RAL], Dallas, TX, 972-960-2221, www.vetdna.com) is available. This test confirms the presence of *H. mustelae* DNA and provides the practitioner data on the quantity of organisms. Immunohistochemical staining to demonstrate the presence of *Helicobacter* organisms in biopsy samples, gastric and fecal swabs is also available from RAL. This test can also be used to monitor treatment. Collection of the gastric swab for either immunohistochemical staining or PCR can be done with a standard culture swab extended with sterile tubing passed in an intubated, anesthetized ferret. The stomach is gently manipulated externally to allow contact between the swab and gastric mucosa.

Ingestion of foreign materials is common. Symptoms vary depending on volume ingested and presence of complete or partial blockage and if pre-existing ulcers or other pathology is present. The most common symptoms are anorexia, vomiting, nausea, and lethargy, which are sometimes accompanied by stress-related diarrhea and weight loss. In some ferrets, however, small amounts of material ingested over several days eventually leads to obstruction, ulceration, or penetration. Gastric distention, gastrointestinal pain, or presence of the foreign material may be palpated. Plain radiography may reveal GI gas patterns typical of obstruction. Definitive diagnosis is made at exploratory surgery.

RABBITS

Respiratory diseases are a major cause of morbidity and mortality in rabbits. Pasteurellosis is the primary respiratory disease, but many other pathogens can play a role in the disease complex. The term "snuffles" can refer to any upper respiratory disease (URD). Comprehensive studies have shown that rabbits can resist infection even if housed with infected rabbits, spontaneously eliminate *Pasteurella multocida*, become chronic carriers, develop acute disease, develop bacteremia and pneumonia, or develop chronic disease. The pathogenesis depends on host resistance and virulence of the strain. Many rabbits carry *Bordetella bronchiseptica* and *Moraxella catarrhalis* in the nares. The prevalence of *P. multocida* infection varies between rabbitries. It increases with the age of rabbits in facilities where the disease is endemic. There is an inverse relationship between *P. multocida* and *B. bronchiseptica* infections in rabbits. Weanlings have higher infection rates with *B. bronchiseptica*. *P. multocida* predominates in adults.

Clinical signs include URD (rhinitis, sinusitis, conjunctivitis, dacryocystitis), otitis, pleuropneumonia, bacteremia, and abscesses (subcutaneous tissues, organs, bones, joints, genitalia). The nasolacrimal duct can be occluded. In many rabbits, the signs of rhinitis subside or disappear as the infection continues in the paranasal sinuses or middle ears. Mucosal erosion and nasoturbinate atrophy occurs with chronic infection. Otitis media can be asymptomatic or if the inner ear is affected, torticollis, nystagmus, and ataxia can develop. The tympanic membrane may rupture. Radiographs: increased soft tissue density within the bulla with bone thickening. Chronic infection in the thoracic cavity may be caused by *P. multocida* or *Staphylococcus* spp. Pleuropneumonia, pericarditis, and abscessation around/in the lungs and heart may occur.

B. bronchiseptica is a common inhabitant of the respiratory tract of rabbits. The nares and bronchi become colonized. Usually respiratory disease is not associated with infection, but predominant recovery of this organism in a rabbit with URD points to it as the causative agent. Some strains are cytotoxic and enhance colonization by toxigenic *P. multocida*. *B. bronchiseptica* can be considered a co-pathogen or a predisposing factor in *P. multocida* infections.

GUINEA PIGS

Vitamin C deficiency may be an underlying etiology or contribute to any infectious illness in the guinea pig. Additional vitamin C should be included as part of any medical therapy. *Streptococcus* spp, *Staphylococcus aureus,* and *Chlamydia psittaci* are also common pathogens involved in conjunctivitis.

Guinea pigs should not be housed with animal species which carry *Bordetella bronchiseptica*. (rabbits, cats, dogs, pigs). It is a common etiology of conjunctivitis combined with vitamin C deficiency. Bordetellosis will cause signs of respiratory distress, weight loss, and even sudden death. Radiographs are useful to see the extent of pneumonia.

RAT AND MOUSE

Many infectious agents affect both rats and mice. Few colonies that provide animals for the pet trade are respiratory pathogen free. *M. pulmonis* infections may present with dyspnea, respiratory distress, nasal discharge, and torticollis (otitis interna). Diagnosis: culture, serology, and histopathology of the lung and/or ear. Treatment is with doxycycline at 2.5 mg/kg PO every 12 hours or 250 mg/liter drinking water. While the tetracyclines may control and manage the disease, they probably do not eliminate it. Tylocin has been used in the past, but it is no longer as effective. Sendai virus infections may be present. Diagnosis is through serology and histopathology of lung. Treatment: supportive care.

Usually it resolves within about a week in adults. It may exacerbate *M. pulmonis* infection. The cilia-associated respiratory (CAR) bacillus is another respiratory pathogen. Its pathogenicity without *M. pulmonis* co-infection is unclear. Diagnosis should include serology and special histopathology stains. Treatment is supportive, with doxycycline or tetracycline to treat the concurrent *M. pulmonis* infection. CAR is persistent and does not clear. *Corynebacterium kutscheri* infection in rats may just be respiratory, while it is systemic in mice. Diagnosis should include culture and histopathology. Treatment consists of doxycycline, tetracycline, or chloramphenicol to control symptoms. This is also a persistent infection unlikely to be cleared with treatment, just managed. Owners with pet rats and mice that have respiratory problems need to know that periodically they will need to manage the clinical symptoms. They must recognize when symptoms occur so that treatment can minimize the chances of progression to pneumonia. If they add a new rodent to the household, it is likely to trigger flare-ups in the resident rodents, plus the new animal may break with it, too. Most rat owners learn how to work with this. Eventually, there is enough lung pathology that many succumb in older age to pneumonia/fibrosis (unless neoplasia or urolithiasis is the cause of death).

ANOREXIA IN RABBITS AND RODENTS

Rabbits that are presented with or without malocclusion but with painful abdomens, anorexia, diarrhea, or lack of stool need treatment prior to correction of the oral problems. Immediate administration of analgesics and fluids often results in the rabbit beginning to eat and the gastrointestinal tract beginning to move. A detailed history and physical examination including auscultation of the abdomen allows the practitioner to evaluate degree of gastrointestinal distress. Radiographs are useful to determine ileus. Contrast series may be utilized to determine an impaction. Most trichobezoars will move once hydration is corrected and sufficient roughage is available. Use of motility enhancers may be tried if no impaction is present. Once pain is alleviated and hydration corrected, walking and some food intake will encourage gastrointestinal motility. While not proven, probiotics are often administered per os or intrarectally. These are primarily *Lactobacillus* spp. which are not the primary microflora of the rabbit. Vitamin B complex may be given to stimulate appetite. As hepatic lipidosis may be present, it is advantageous to get food into the anorexic rabbit as soon as possible. If the rabbit does not immediately start eating hay, a gavage of diluted Critical Care (Oxbow Pet Products, Murdock, NE) is given.

Rarely is surgery necessary to relieve an impaction, but if a necrotic or ischemic section of the gut is suspected, surgery may be necessary to resect the bowel. Prognosis is guarded primarily because of endotoxins produced by *Clostridium* sp. present in most herbivore gastrointestinal tracts.

Cavies are cecotrophic, strict herbivores. Dental disease is leading cause of anorexia. Two conditions involving the gastrointestinal system are seen frequently, and both may be linked. The first is anorexia. The clinician needs to determine if the anorexia is primary (refusal to eat a new brand of pellets), with subsequent malocclusions, and hindgut dysbiosis (change in microflora) and motility, or if the anorexia is secondary to a hindgut disorder or dental disease. Second is diarrhea. It needs to be determined if it subsequent to other disease or if it is a primary gastrointestinal (GI) disease. Changes in diet, stress, illness, anesthesia, or reproduction may alter gut motility and/or gut microflora causing diarrhea. Clostridial infections secondary to antibiotic therapy is frequently the cause. Broad-spectrum antibiotics administered subcutaneously or intramuscularly are less likely to cause problems to the GI tract. Fecal/rectal cultures, gram stains, and parasite evaluation (coccidia) along with history and complete physical examination including the teeth should be done. Diarrhea associated with an overgrowth of *Candida albicans* has been seen in cavies on prolonged antibiotic treatment.

REFERENCES

1. Harcourt-Brown F. Textbook of Rabbit Medicine. Oxford, UK: Butterworth Heinemann; 2002.
2. O'Malley B. Clinical Anatomy and Physiology of Exotic Species: Structure and Function of Mammals, Birds, Reptiles, and Amphibians. London, UK: Elsevier Saunders; 2005.
3. Johnson-Delaney CA. Exotic Companion Medicine Handbook for Veterinarians. Lake Worth, FL: Zoological Education Network: 1996, 1997.

E. CUNICULI: WHAT'S NEW? CLINICAL UPDATE

Cathy A. Johnson-Delaney, DVM, Dipl. ABVP (Avian)
Eastside Avian & Exotic Animal Medical Center
Washington Ferret Rescue & Shelter
Kirkland, WA

Encephalitozoon cuniculi, a microsporidian, obligate, intracellular protozoan parasite, is widespread in pet rabbits. It is considered an opportunistic infection as it does not always cause identifiable clinical signs. When it does, rabbits may exhibit neurologic signs including head tilt, ataxia, nystagmus, and hind limb paresis or paralysis and urinary incontinence. Rabbits may also have some degree of renal disease: a nonsuppurative, granulomatous nephritis that progresses to interstitial fibrosis.

DIAGNOSTIC TESTING

Serodiagnosis is problematic since many seropositive rabbits are totally asymptomatic. Studies published for various rabbit populations show that immunoglobulin G (IgG) titers may be higher in symptomatic rabbits, but the difference is not useful for clinicians to use the titer level as confirmation of infection. An IgG seropositive status may represent chronic infection, clearance with seroconversion, incidental exposure to the organism, or a possible cross-reaction with another antigenically similar protozoan.

Immunoglobulin M (IgM) titers were thought to reflect acute infection (experimentally infected rabbits showed IgM titers between day 17 through 38), and it was hoped that this could be used for diagnosis. Polymerase chain reaction (PCR) to detect *E. cuniculi* spores in the urine of infected animals was thought to be a method to improve sensitivity and specificity of testing. Dr. Carolyn Cray of the University of Miami Miller School of Medicine, Miami, FL, was also working on correlation of titers, PCR, and protein electrophoresis to aid in the diagnosis of active infection. Study results showed that IgM titers were more likely to be positive in *E. cuniculi* suspect rabbits, but some low titers were found in normal rabbits. IgG titers were consistently higher in infected versus non-infected rabbits, but alone a titer level is not conclusive.

Protein electrophoresis (EPH) appears to be useful as one of the diagnostic tools to diagnose *E. cuniculi* infection. Changes in the globulin fractions were consistently found in *E. cuniculi* suspect rabbits. There was a significant increase in gamma globulins in rabbits studied in the UK. In the US, both beta and gamma globulins had significant increases.

Work is still ongoing concerning PCR identification of spores in the urine. At present, a definitive antemortem diagnosis of *E. cuniculi* is still inconclusive: combined usage of serology, PCR, and EPH may be indicated.

Ultrasonography of the kidneys and guided biopsies with histopathology may also confirm the presence of *E. cuniculi*. It is also useful to assess how much damage has occurred. But many asymptomatic rabbits will have "lumpy bumpy" kidneys and live their full lifespan without renal failure.

TREATMENT

In rabbits presented with neurologic signs, the goal is to stop the progression of signs, and support the rabbit while antiprotozoal medication decreases the activity of the parasite. The goal is a good quality of life for the rabbit. Several different drugs and regimens have been used to varying levels of success, some of which is based on efficacy in humans. As diagnosis is presumptive, it is prudent to treat with an antibiotic initially that has central nervous system activity. Chloramphenicol at 50 mg/kg subcutaneously (SC) every 12 hours for 7 days is suggested. If the rabbit is having seizures, diazepam may be used at 0.1 to 1.0 mg/kg intramuscularly (IM) or SC depending on the severity of the seizures or muscle spasms. Meloxicam can be used at 0.2 to 0.5 mg/kg PO or SC every 24 hours for headache, pain associated with head tilt and in particular pain of muscle cramping. Meclizine has been used in rabbits that are anorexic to decrease the nausea associated with the neurologic vestibular signs at 12.5 to 25 mg/kg PO every 12 to 24 hours. In severe head tilt, some rabbits traumatize the "down" eye: eye lubricating ointment and owner diligence may be needed to prevent corneal abrasion and foreign body introduction into the conjunctiva. Assist-feeding may be needed using softened pellets, hay or other greens, and Critical Care (Oxbow Pet Products, Murdock, NE). Adjunctive nutraceuticals may include omega 3-6-9 fatty acids, vitamins B6 and B12, and vitamin E, which have been linked to circulation, muscle and neurologic function. Fluid therapy may also be necessary if the rabbit is having problems drinking due to the head tilt or paresis. Owners may also need to clean the rabbit's perineal area frequently due to urinary incontinence or accumulation of fecal material as some ill rabbits have a difficult time grooming. It may be necessary to clip the hair in long-haired breeds to prevent accumulations and dermatitis.

To try and eliminate or decrease the organism, benzimidazole anthelmintics have had the best success. Several have been used and reported in the literature. The author uses oxibendazole at 30 mg/kg PO every 24 hours for the first 1 to 2 weeks, then 10 mg/kg orally (PO) every 24 hours indefinitely as signs stabilize. Albendazole has been used at 30 mg/kg PO every 24 hours for 30 days then reducing it to 15 mg/kg PO every 24 hours for an additional 30 days; or at 10 to 15 mg/kg PO every 24 hours for up to 3 months. Fenbendazole has been used at 20 mg/kg PO every 24 hours for at least 30 days, and longer if signs persist. Cessation of benzimidazole treatment often is empirical as the veterinarian needs to work with the owner to assess the degree of improvement and when the signs have stopped improving. There is no definitive way to check the efficacy of the drugs other than clinical appearance. The author likes to recheck rabbits at least at 2-week intervals to assess condition and owners are encouraged to weigh the rabbits daily as food and water intake may be altered.

In summary, a definitive antemortem test for *E. cuniculi* is still not available. Serodiagnosis along with protein electrophoresis and response to benzimidazole anthelmintic treatment may be all the practitioner can offer the client. Ruling out other causes of the clinical signs should also be done. Supportive care for the rabbit as well as some remission of signs is part of the disease management program.

REFERENCES

1. Cray C, Arcia G, Schneider R, et al. Application of serodiagnostics and PCR for the diagnosis of *Encephalitozoon cuniculi.* In Proceedings of the Association of Avian Veterinarians, Association of Exotic Mammal Veterinarians Scientific Program, Providence, RI, 2007, pp 85-87.

2. Deeb BJ, Carpenter JW. Neurologic and musculoskeletal diseases. In Quesenberry KE, Carpenter JW (eds): Ferrets, Rabbits and Rodents Clinical Medicine and Surgery, 2nd ed. St Louis, MO: Saunders, 2004, pp 203-210.

3. Carpenter JW. Rabbits. In Exotic Animal Formulary, 3rd ed. St. Louis, MO: Elsevier Saunders, 2005, pp 409-444.

THERE'S MORE THAN ONE WAY TO DO IT: SURGICAL CASTRATION TECHNIQUES

Angela M. Lennox, DVM, Diplomate ABVP (Avian)
Avian and Exotic Animal Clinic of Indianapolis
Indianapolis IN

Castration techniques for exotic mammals include scrotal, prescrotal, and abdominal approaches. These can be further classified as open or closed. Technique depends on the anatomy of the patient, and in many cases, is largely surgeon preference. Familiarity with alternatives will allow the surgeon flexibility to select the most appropriate technique when faced with an unfamiliar species or an anatomical peculiarity.

FERRETS

Few veterinarians in the US castrate male ferrets, as the majority arrive in the pet store already neutered. The urogenital anatomy of the male ferret is similar to that of other canids, with the penis situated cranial to the scrotal sac. Both scrotal and prescrotal techniques are described, with the use of suture, hemostatic clips, or even "self-tying" the vas deferens to the vessels. In the scrotal approach, the incisions are left to heal without suture; while the pre-scrotal skin and subcutaneous incision is sutured with 4-0 or 5-0 absorbable suture.

In the ferret, indications for castration include prevention of pregnancy, and reduction of very strong odor and aggression. It should be noted that neutering of both male and female ferrets is linked to adrenocortical neoplasia.

RABBIT

The urogenital anatomy of male rabbits presents a peculiarity unique among placental mammal species but common in marsupial species. The penis is located caudal to the testicles, which lie cranial to the penis in two separate hemiscrotal sacs. Another very important anatomical peculiarity, similar to rodent species, is that he inguinal canal remains open throughout life, and the testicles are free to move from the hemiscrotal sacs to the abdominal cavity, making rabbits (and rodents) "functional cryptorchids." Position of the testicles depends on many factors including body position, body temperature, breeding activity, gastrointestinal tract filling, and the amount of abdominal fat. The testicles are elongated and not round. The epididymis is clearly visible at the caudal pole of the testicle, but not as developed as in rodent species. There is fat surrounding the testicles, but much less than in rodent species. The glans of the penis is not well developed, is point shaped, and covered by a prepuce.

The two main anatomical peculiarities of male rabbits have important implications in regard to surgical techniques. The open inguinal canal is breached during surgery, and must be closed in order to prevent open communication between the hemiscrotal sac and the abdominal cavity, and potential herniation of abdominal viscera (intestine, bladder) into the hemiscrotal sac. The position of the penis caudal to testicles allows the surgeon to choose a prescrotal approach and a single incision on the midline as an alternative to a scrotal approach

Castration in the rabbit is indicated for prevention of pregnancy, and reduction of urine spraying, social aggression, and unwanted sexual behavior. It should be kept in mind that many owners maintain single intact male rabbits who do not exhibit undesirable behaviors. Therapeutic castration is indicated in cases of testicular disease including infection and neoplasia, and for correction of hemiscrotal herniation and true cryptorchidism.

Prescrotal Approach

The rabbit is placed under general anesthesia in dorsal recumbency, and the prescrotal area shaved. For this technique, it is not necessary to attempt to shave and prepare the thin, delicate skin of the hemiscrotal sac. The surgical site is prepared for surgery. A 1.5- to 2-cm skin incision is made on the midline, just cranial to the base of the hemiscrotal sacs. Blunt dissection of the subcutaneous tissue, fat, and inguinal fascia reveals the vaginal processes caudal to where they enter the abdomen through the inguinal canal. In mature rabbits with abundant subcutaneous fat, identifying the vaginal processes may be slightly difficult. The surgeon can easily identify these by gently massaging the testicles back and forth from the hemiscrotal sac to the abdomen and visually identifying them as they pass through the transparent vaginal processes. The vaginal process is bluntly dissected from surrounding soft tissues and isolated.

At this point the procedure is continued by opening the vaginal process, or leaving it closed, thus proceeding as an "open" or "closed" technique. In the open technique, the vaginal process is exteriorized and 3-0 to 4-0 absorbable suture material passed around it and tied loosely or secured with a hemostat. The vaginal process is incised with blunt scissors to prevent iatrogenic damage to the vessels of the spermatic cord. The testicle is exteriorized through the incision, and the spermatic cord and vessels sutured. The remaining suture used to pass around the vaginal process is tied securely proximal to the incision in order to close the vaginal process. The procedure is repeated on the contralateral vaginal process, and skin incision closed routinely.

For the closed technique, the isolated vaginal process is bluntly dissected caudally while pulling gently, which inverts the scrotal sac. The vaginal process containing the testicle, deferens and vessels are ligated. A hemostat or blunt probe is used to replace the inverted scrotal sac, and the incision closed as above.

Both techniques produce some degree of inversion of the scrotum, which should be manually restored to normal position with gentle traction at the conclusion of the procedure.

Scrotal Approach

Both open and closed scrotal approaches to castration of the rabbit have been well described. The major disadvantage of the scrotal approach is challenging surgical preparation, as it is difficult to completely remove hair and adequately prepare the site for sterile surgery. However, most surgeons are familiar with this approach, and for experienced surgeons, complication rate is low.

Opening the vaginal process (open technique) allows direct visualization and ligation of the spermatic cord and vessels, but necessitates closure of the vaginal process at the end of the procedure. In the closed technique, the vaginal tunic is closed and spermatic cord and vessels simultaneously ligated.

Abdominal Approach

The rabbit under general anesthesia is placed in dorsal recumbency. The caudal area of the abdominal surface is surgically prepared routinely. Celiotomy is performed on the caudal midline 4 to 5 cm cranially to the hemiscrotal sacs. The urinary bladder is exposed, exteriorized and reflected caudally. The deferens are gently retracted, and testicles are exteriorized. Dissection of the tail of the epididymis from the caudal pole of the everted hemiscrotal sac and ligation of the spermatic cord are performed as shown before, through the celiotomy access. Suturing of the abdominal wall and the overlying soft tissues is performed routinely.

GUINEA PIGS

In general, techniques for the rabbit are similar to those for the guinea pig, with a few important differences. The penis of the guinea pig is positioned cranial to the testicles; therefore the prescrotal technique cannot be performed with a single midline prescrotal incision. Instead, two parallel incisions are made slightly lateral to the midline in order to access both vaginal processes.

OTHER RODENTS
Prairie Dog

The male prairie dog does not have a scrotal sac. During breeding season, the testicles are often palpable beneath the perineal skin and subcutaneous tissues; however, access is challenging. The author prefers a "scrotal" approach in mature animals during the breeding season. The testicles are located and isolated beneath the subcutaneous tissues, and ligated routinely.

The other most commonly described technique is an abdominal approach. The patient is prepared for caudal abdominal surgery under general anesthesia. Celiotomy is performed on the caudal midline 4 to 5 cm cranial to the perineum. The urinary bladder is exposed, exteriorized, and reflected caudally. The deferens are gently retracted, and testicles exteriorized. The tail of the epididymis is dissected from the caudal pole of the everted hemiscrotal sac and spermatic cord and vessels ligated. Closure of the surgical site is routine.

MARSUPIALS
Sugar Glider

Orchiectomy is performed in the sugar glider for prevention of unwanted pregnancy, to reduce territorial aggression and for reduction of strong, objectionable musky odor. The anatomy of the male marsupial is unique, with testicles contained in a pendulous scrotal sac. Techniques described include a single scrotal incision and ligation with small hemostatic clips or fine absorbable suture (4-0 to 5-0); and scrotal ablation with the incision made along the pendulous stalk.

It should be noted that some breeders and distributors of gliders are castrating very young animals simply by clamping and cutting the scrotal stalk, or by applying various types of bands, all without benefit of anesthesia or analgesia.

Virginia Opossum

Orchiectomy is seldom performed in this species, and anatomy and technique are similar to that described above for the sugar glider, with the exception that the scrotal sac and testicles are much larger than in the sugar glider.

REFERENCES

1. Capello V. Comparison of common surgical procedures in small mammals: surgical techniques for orchiectomy of the pet rabbit. Proc Int Conf Exotics 2005, on-site supplement, 9-18.
2. Donnelly TM. Basic anatomy, physiology and husbandry. In Quesenberry KE, Carpenter JW (eds.): Ferrets, Rabbits and Rodents: Clinical Medicine and Surgery, 2nd ed. Philadelphia: Saunders, 2004, pp 136-146.
3. Duncan AE, Ramsay EC. A technique for rabbit castration. JSEAM 1993;3(2):116-118.
4. Harcourt-Brown FM. General surgical principles and neutering. In Harcourt-Brown FM (ed.): Textbook of Rabbit Medicine. New York: Butterworth-Heinemann, 2002, pp 352-360.
5. Hoyt RF Jr. Abdominal surgery of pet rabbits. In Bojrab MJ (ed.): Current Techniques in Small Animal Surgery, 4th ed. Philadelphia: Williams & Wilkins, 1998, pp 777-790.
6. Jenkins JR. Soft tissue surgery. In Quesenberry KE, Carpenter JW (ed.):: Ferrets, Rabbits and Rodents: Clinical Medicine and Surgery, 2nd ed. Philadelphia: Saunders, 2004, pp221-230.
7. Mandel M. Indications and procedure for castration of the domestic rabbit. Vet Med Small Anim Clin. 1976;71(3):365.
8. Millis DL, Walshaw R. Elective castrations and ovariohysterectomies in pet rabbits. J Am Anim Hosp Assoc 1992;28(6):491-498.
9. Okerman L. Anatomical peculiarities. In Okerman L (ed.): Diseases of Domestic Rabbits, 2nd ed. Oxford: Blackwell Scientific Publications, 1994, pp 10-13.
10. Okerman L. Trauma and surgical intervention. In Okerman L (ed.): Diseases of Domestic Rabbits, 2nd ed. pp. 128-130. Blackwell Scientific publications, Oxford, 1994, pp 128-130.
11. Popesko P, Rjtovà V, Horàk J. A Colour Atlas of Anatomy of Small Laboratory Animals. Vol. I: Rabbit,

Guinea Pig. London: Wolfe Publishing Ltd, 1992, pp 122-123.

12. Ludwig L, Aiken S. Soft tissue surgery. In: Quesenberry KE, Carpenter JW (eds): Ferrets, Rabbits and Rodents: Clinical Medicine and Surgery, 2nd ed. Philadelphia: WB Sauders, 1994, pp 121-134.

Table 1. Techniques for Castration of Small Exotic Mammals

Class	Species	Approach	Comments
Carnivore	Ferret Skunk Fox	Scrotal Prescrotal	Techniques similar to that performed in dogs and cats
Herbivore	Rabbit	Scrotal Open Closed	True aseptic surgical preparation is difficult
		Prescrotal Open Closed	Can be performed with single incision Improved aseptic surgical preparation; avoids incision into delicate hemiscrotal sac. Procedure is generally longer than scrotal approach
		Abdominal	Indicated for true cryptorchids
Herbivore	Guinea Pig	Scrotal Open Closed	True aseptic surgical preparation difficult
		Prescrotal Open Closed Abdominal	Improved aseptic surgical preparation: avoids incision into delicate hemiscrotal sac. Procedure generally takes longer than scrotal approach
Herbivore	Prairie dog	Scrotal	No true scrotum or hemiscrotal sac; easier during breeding season
		Abdominal	Preferred approach is animal is immature, many prefer this technique routinely
Herbivore	Most rodents	Scrotal Open Closed Prescrotal	See comments above for guinea pig
Marsupial	Sugar glider Virginia opossum	Scrotal	Scrotum is pendulous; some prefer scrotal ablation

CRITICAL RODENTS AND OTHER SMALL EXOTIC MAMMAL EMERGENCIES

Angela M. Lennox, DVM, Diplomate ABVP (Avian)
Avian and Exotic Animal Clinic of Indianapolis
Indianapolis, IN

A common scenario for all exotic pets is chronic disease presenting as an acute onset of illness. Many rodents and smaller exotic pets fall into the category of prey species, with inherent instincts to hide illness until unable to do so. Therefore, any animal presented in acute crisis must be carefully evaluated for long-term chronic underlying illness.

Common underlying factors in diseases affecting these species are malnutrition and improper husbandry, especially in those with difficult husbandry requirements, for example, sugar gliders. All efforts at diagnosis and treatment must include careful investigation into husbandry and explicit recommendations for correction based on the most recent understanding of the needs of these species.

The principles of emergency care and stabilization are the same as those established in human and more traditional pet medicine: airway and cardiac support, control of hemorrhage, correction of underlying fluid and electrolyte abnormalities, and restoration of normothermia.

Some patients require sedation, or even general anesthesia to reduce pain and stress associated with critical care procedures. Sedatives and anesthetic agents must be chosen carefully to reduce the risk of exacerbating the condition or causing death.

AIRWAY SUPPORT

Intubation of these species for direct establishment of an airway is possible in theory with use of the endoscope and/or specialized laboratory animal rodent intubation instruments. However, this is often not a realistic option for the practitioner, especially in the critical patient. Emergency tracheal intubation via tracheotomy may be an option in very small animals using a standard tracheotomy approach and small endotracheal tubes, IV catheters, or red rubber catheters. The author has no experience with a small rodent patient post recovery of placement of a tracheostomy tube, but assumes the risk of tracheal damage and/or stricture to be high.

In less severe cases oxygen can be delivered via facemask or while the animal is resting quietly in an oxygen chamber.

CONTROL OF HEMORRHAGE

Blood volume of mammals is estimated at 7% to 10% of body weight, and it is estimated normal healthy individuals can tolerate an acute loss of approximately 10% of blood volume. Direct pressure is often the most effective means to control hemorrhage. Silver nitrate and coagulative powder products may be used for nail hemorrhage. More severe bleeding may require ligation of the compromised vessel.

Treatment for blood loss includes blood transfusion or the use of colloids with oxygen-carrying ability such as Oxyglobin.

Rough guidelines for the indication for blood transfusion are similar to those used in other species and include acute blood loss resulting in packed cell volume (PCV) below 20%, or chronic blood loss with PCV below 12% to 15%. Overall patient condition (bright and alert versus pale and depressed) is also important when considering transfusion.

With the exception of the ferret, small exotic companion mammals are known to have distinct blood types. However, the likelihood of transfusion reaction after a single transfusion is unlikely. The risk of reaction must be weighed against the risk of withholding transfusion.

Sources of blood donors include the ill pet's housemates, or pet stores. The author keeps a list of owners willing to provide blood donors in exchange for clinic credit. Blood is collected from healthy donors under sedation with 1 mL acid citrate dextrose (ACD) per 10 mL blood, maximum 10% of blood volume based on calculated body weight. Blood is administered via intravenous (IV) or intraosseous (IO) catheter.

An example of blood transfusion following hemorrhage in a rodent or other small exotic mammal is outlined below:

- Control external hemorrhage with direct pressure, or consider a bandaging technique.
- Administer a sedative if needed to facilitate handling (midazolam .25 mg/kg IM). Administer general anesthesia if necessary, weighing the risk of a potentially hypotensive anesthetic procedure against the risk of stress and manual restraint.
- Place a 25- to 22-gauge IO catheter into the tibia or humerus of the recipient after installation of lidocaine as a local block.
- Place a catheter cap or injection port, and secure the catheter with tape
- Administer midazolam .25 mg/kg to a healthy same species donor and then mask induce with an inhalant anesthetic agent.
- Collect blood from the donor (7–10% of body weight) via the vena cava into one or several 1- to 3-mL syringes prepared with sodium citrate 1 cc/ 10 mL blood.
- Administer whole blood via the IO catheter manually over 3 to 5 minutes, or with a small precision infusion pump.

Optimal fluid therapy is critical for treatment of hypovolemic shock and correction of dehydration. While little information exists on specific guidelines for treatment of hypovolemic shock in these species, information can be extrapolated from work with other species, including the guinea pig, rabbit, and ferret. For these species, Lichtenberger recommends rapid intravenous infusion of warmed isotonic crystalloids at 10–15 mL/kg, followed by colloids (Hetastarch, 6%, Braun Medical, Irvine, CA) at 5 mL/kg over 5 to 10 minutes. After achieving systolic Doppler blood pressure of above 40 mmHg, aggressive external heat support is initiated until rectal body temperature reads at least 98°F. Boluses of isotonic crystalloids (10–15 mg/kg) and colloids (5 mL/kg) are continued until systolic Doppler blood pressure reads above 90 mmHg. At this point dehydration deficits are calculated and corrected using isotonic crystalloids over a 6-hour period in cases of acute disease, and 12 to 24 hours in more chronic diseases cases.

Vascular Access

Intravenous catheterization is difficult for species smaller than guinea pigs. However, vascular access is feasible with intraosseous access, via the tibia or humerus. The author prefers the use of standard IV needles (27–22 gauge), which are placed, secured with tape and fitted with a standard catheter infusion cap. Confirmation of correct placement can be assumed by stability of the catheter and failure to accumulate fluids in soft tissues, but absolute confirmation requires radiographs of the catheter in situ in two views.

Fluid infusion is accomplished via intermittent administration via a small volume syringe, as larger syringes produce excessive pressure. It is often difficult to use an infusion pump in conjunction with a small IO catheter.

Small needles used as catheters occasionally occlude with bone or blood clots, which can be removed using very fine sterilized cerclage wire as a stylette.

Measurement of Blood Pressure

Measurement of systolic Doppler blood pressure has been reported in these species, and has been found to be similar to that in other small mammals. Practitioners may find this more challenging in smaller individuals, in particular hedgehogs and sugar gliders, but like every challenging technique improves with practice. For some very small or active patients it may be more feasible to monitor blood pressure trends with the aid of anesthesia or sedation. Measurement of indirect systolic blood pressure is accomplished with pediatric blood pressure cuffs and a Doppler vascular monitor. In most exotic mammals, the cuff is placed at the humerus, and the Doppler placed in a shaved area just above the ventral forelimb footpad. Several manufacturers offer blood pressure cuffs for human digits, which can be easily adapted to limbs of small exotic mammal patients.

When blood pressure measurement is unsuccessful, practitioners may be forced to make judgment calls regarding perfusion status based on patient response and parameters such as capillary refill time, turgor of visible surface vessels, temperature, and heart rate.

RESTORATION OF NORMOTHERMIA

Normal rectal body temperature of small companion mammal species vary widely. Measurement of body temperature is not difficult in debilitated animals. The author recommends a constant readout flexible temperature probe that can be inserted rectally, and taped into position. Depending on size, probes may not be practical in smaller species. Methods for external rewarming include heating pads, warm water bags or bottles, forces air warming devices, radiant heat sources, and commercial small mammal incubators. Internal rewarming can be accomplished via infusion of warmed IV fluids, which has been shown to be extremely important for the prevention of an afterdrop effect, or return of cool fluids to the body core and worsening of condition when external warming is used alone.

SEDATION AND GENERAL ANESTHESIA FOR CRITICAL PATIENTS

The introduction of a number of sedatives and anesthetics with wider margins of safety has greatly increased success in exotic companion mammals. It should be kept in mind that any anesthetic procedure in a critical patient should be planned carefully, with evaluation of the risk of anesthesia vs. risk of attempting a potentially stressful or painful procedure without anesthesia. Anesthetic agents are discussed fully in Dr. Marla Lichtenberger's articles in these proceedings.

The author prefers the use of midazolam as a sedative agent in critical patients. This drug has a relatively wide margin of safety, and often greatly facilitates diagnostic and therapeutic procedures such as venipuncture, collection of radiographs and administration of medications. This drug combined with local infusion of lidocaine and an analgesic (butorphanol, buprenorphine) often facilitates placement of an intraosseous catheter. Additional anesthesia can be provided with an inhalant agent such as isoflurane or sevoflurane.

Most exotic animal practitioners are familiar with the use of isoflurane and sevoflurane in practice. It should be kept in mind, however, that both have dose-dependent vasodilation properties, which lead to hypotension. Therefore, the risk of adverse anesthetic outcome is greater when these drugs are used at higher flow rates, which is often necessary when they are used alone. Isoflurane and sevoflurane also require higher flow rates to avoid a pain response, and provide no residual analgesia when discontinued. The use of preanesthetic agents and analgesics provides a more balanced anesthetic approach, and reduces the risk associated with higher dosages of any one drug.

Drugs such as ketamine and medetomidine should be avoided in critical patients, especially those with cardiovascular compromise. The author and several others (Lichtenberg) have been using intravenous etomidate in critical patients with success. More information on these drugs, plus recommended dosages is presented in Dr. Lichtenberger's articles in this proceedings.

REFERENCES

1. Lennox AM. Emergency and critical care in sugar gliders (*Petaurus beviceps*), African hedgehogs (*Atelerix albiventris*) and prairie dogs (*Cynomys spp.*). Vet Clin North Am Exotic Pet Pract 2007;10(20).
2. Lichtenberger M. (ed). Emergency and critical care. Vet Clin North Am Exotic Pet Pract 2007;10(20).

IN-HOUSE DIAGNOSTICS: WHAT THE EMERGENCY CLINICIAN NEEDS TO KNOW

Angela M. Lennox, DVM, Diplomate ABVP (Avian)
Avian and Exotic Animal Clinic of Indianapolis
Indianapolis, IN

Collection of blood for diagnostic testing can be challenging in exotic pet mammals, especially in smaller species. Modern technologies allow acquisition of useful information from very small samples, but samples still must be of high quality and meet minimum volume requirements. The challenge of blood collection is compounded in critically ill, hypovolemic, and/or hypothermic patients. In many cases, initial therapy must precede sample collection.

Volume of sample is limited by patient size. A common guideline is to collect no more than 10% of blood volume. Total blood volumes vary from species to species but can generally be assumed to be 6% to 8% of body weight. Clinical judgment may necessitate adjustments to recommended volume limits.

Samples can be run with in-house equipment or sent to reference laboratories familiar with diagnostic testing in these species. The most compelling advantage of in-house diagnostic testing is rapid results. Abaxis (Abaxis, Union City, CA) in-house blood chemistry analyzer can run a chemistry panel in 13 minutes on whole blood samples, and practical minimum volume is 0.15 cc of high quality whole blood. Reference laboratories will often analyze smaller samples, but may use dilution techniques. Individual laboratories should be contacted for instructions on submission of low-volume samples for analysis.

When sample volume does not allow clinical chemistry or complete blood count, a manual complete blood count (CBC) can be obtained on a single drop of blood collected into a heparinized hematocrit tube. Information that can be obtained from a manual in-house CBC includes hematocrit, differential white blood count, and analysis of both red and white blood cell morphology and characteristics, complete blood count utilizing a hemocytometer, and measurement of total serum solids.

Sample collection in small exotic mammals requires practice. Collection site depends on species, patient condition and practitioner preference. The following guidelines are offered based on the author's personal preference and experience, and others may advocate other sites or techniques. The "correct" technique is that which results in consistently good results with optimal patient safety.

RISKS OF BLOOD SAMPLE COLLECTION

Venipuncture inherently involves some degree of risk, including risk of injury or death caused by restraint and handling. Risks from blood collection itself include vessel laceration and hemorrhage, infection, inadvertent damage to adjacent soft tissue structures, and sudden hypotension due to decreased blood volume. Careful patient evaluation, restraint and technique help minimize risk. In the author's opinion, it is best to delay blood sample collection in patients that are hypothermic, hypovolemic, and/or severely depressed. Many patients benefit from gentle warmth and fluid administration for 4 to 6 hours, with frequent re-evaluation.

RESTRAINT

While restraint is relatively easy in larger species such as ferrets and rabbits, it is increasingly challenging in smaller species. The method often depends upon the preferred collection site. In some cases, sedation or anesthesia is appropriate and necessary, especially when considering collection from the vena cava in species other than the ferret. Guidelines for safe sedation and anesthesia are discussed below.

In the author's experience, most ferrets can be safely restrained manually for blood collection by scruffing and stretching, or by rolling the patient in a towel with the head, neck, and forelimbs exposed. It should be noted some ferrets will not tolerate this form of restraint and may require sedation or anesthesia as discussed below. Rabbits are prone to self-injury during restraint and handling, especially luxation and subluxation of the vertebrae caused by kicking with powerful rear legs. Restraint, therefore, must minimize this risk. The author prefers using a burrito-style towel wrap with either the head or caudal portion of the rabbit exposed, depending on desired collection site. Again, sedation can greatly reduce stress of handling.

Guinea pigs and larger rodents can often be restrained by simply grasping them securely around the shoulders and thorax or with a towel wrap. It becomes exceedingly difficult to safely manually restrain species smaller than the guinea pig for blood collection, and safe sedation and/or anesthesia become even more important.

SEDATION AND ANESTHESIA FOR VENIPUNCTURE

For individuals where manual restraint for sample collection is difficult and risky, or patient struggling is excessive, sedation and/or anesthesia should be considered. The risk of sedation and anesthesia must be balanced against the risk of foregoing diagnostic blood testing. A number of sedation and protocols can be considered, and method should be chosen depending on a number of factors, including overall patient condition. Methods include simple sedation and anesthesia with injectable and/or inhalant agents. The author has found administration of intravenous (IV) or intramuscular (IM) midazolam at 0.25 mg/kg combined with butorphanol at 0.4 mg/kg IV or IM extremely useful to reduce stress for simple procedures such as sample collection and catheterization in exotic companion mammals. It should be noted that collection from the vena cava in smaller patients requires anesthesia to prevent patient injury.

BLOOD SAMPLE COLLECTION SITES

Sample site is based on clinical experience and practitioner preference. Author preferences are listed in Table 1. The greatest limiting factors with regard to site selection are patient size and ability to safely restrain.

Table 1. Suggested Blood Collection Sites for Selected Exotic Mammal Species, in Order of Author Preference

Species	Method	Comments
Ferret	Cranial vena cava Jugular Tail vein	Vena cava approach especially easy and safe due to particular anatomy of the ferret, even with manual restraint
Rabbit	Auricular or Central ear artery Lateral saphenous Medial femoral Cranial vena cava Cephalic	Reported risk of vessel damage with auricular method, rare in author's experience Restraint relatively easy Restraint relatively easy Manual restraint for vena cava approach extremely stressful and not recommended Reduced size makes adequate sample collection difficult
Guinea Pig	Lateral saphenous Cranial vena cava Cephalic	Restraint relatively easy, is located more proximally than expected. Shaving enhances visualization. Manual restraint for vena cava approach is extremely stressful, and potentially dangerous, and therefore not recommended Reduced size makes adequate sample collection difficult
Rodents	Cranial vena cava Lateral saphenous Tarsal vein Lateral tail vein	Manual restraint for vena cava approach is extremely stressful and potentially dangerous, and therefore not recommended Note: Manual restraint for collection from any site increasingly difficult
Hedgehogs, gliders	Cranial vena cava	Manueal restraint for vena cava approach is extremely stressful and potentially dangerous, and therefore not recommended Manual restraint impossible in all but extremely debilitated patients

Notes on Sample Collection from the Vena Cava

Exotic practitioners have utilized the vena cava as a safe and effective method of sample collection for many years. Careful understanding of the anatomical relationship of the vessel, the heart, and external landmarks greatly reduces risk. In the ferret, the vena cava is exceptionally long due to relative caudal placement of the heart in the thoracic cavity. The cava is surrounded and protected by fat, and is accessible just below the notch of the sternal manubrium. Correct needle placement is very shallow, and poses no risk to inadvertent penetration of the heart.

The cava is shorter in other species, and the distance between accessible vessel and the heart is progressively smaller as patient size decreases. Use of small, short needles (1/2- and 5/8-inch, 25- to 27-gauge) reduces risk. In all but very small guinea pigs, these needles will prevent inadvertent puncture of the heart. In other smaller species, however, risk of cardiac penetration is greater, and the practitioner must avoid advancing the needle into the thoracic cavity. While not ideal and absolutely to be avoided, it should be noted that in most cases, inadvertent cardiac puncture is not associated with severe complications or death in the still, anesthetized patient. It should be stressed that sedation and often general anesthesia are absolutely required for collection from the vena cava. A possible exception is venipuncture of calm, well-restrained ferrets.

The general procedure for vena cava puncture is as follows:

- Isolate the center of the cranial sternum and manubrium
- Insert a 25- to 27-gauge needle to the right or left of the manubrium at a slight angle aiming for the opposing hip
- Advance the needle while applying negative pressure, redirecting slightly until a flash of blood is detected. The vessel is very close to the surface under the cranial sternum, and it is not necessary to advance the needle very far
- Blood should flow readily after detecting the flash. Failure to flow often means the needle was advanced into and through the vessel, or the bevel is obstructed by the vessel wall. Pull out, rotate and/or redirect slightly until blood flow improves

SAMPLE HANDLING

Analysis of blood samples is markedly impacted by sample quality. Poor sample quality will result in no results (sample failure) or inaccurate results. When working with small exotic companion mammals, the author prefers collection using smaller sized needles and heparinized syringes (1 cc syringe with 27- to 25-gauge needles), or in case of particularly small vessels, venipuncture with a needle only, and collection from the hub into heparinized hematocrit tubes. While the use of heparin may interfere with some analytes, collection without heparin resulted in unacceptably high rate of coagulated samples, and samples containing large fibrin clots. Samples for in-house analysis are processed immediately (preparation of blood film, determination of packed cell volume [PCV] and total serum solids, and in the author's practice chemistry panel run on whole blood using an in-house analyzer [see above]).

Samples intended for outside laboratory analysis should be processed and delivered per reference laboratory instructions and recommendations for the handling of smaller samples.

SAMPLE ANALYSIS

While a full complete blood count and chemistry panel are ideal, the minimum database for the critical care patient is PCV/total serum solids (TSS), examination of the blood film (differential), blood glucose, and blood urea nitrogen (BUN).

In the critical care setting, in-house testing represents a significant advantage over submission of samples to reference laboratories in terms of speed of test results. In-house testing allows analysis and decision making prior to initiation of specific therapy. Critical patients can seldom wait hours to days for test results. As mentioned above, several in-house chemistry analyzers can perform speedy analysis of small test samples. The author prefers the Abaxis in-house chemistry analyzer, which can accept samples as small as 0.15 mL high quality whole blood. In-house hematology analyzers have for the most part not been validated in exotic pet species, but can be useful as well.

Comments on specific analytes are listed below:

PCV and Total Serum Solids

Determination of PCV with total serum solids can reveal anemia, or conversely suggest dehydration, and are important when planning treatment. In general a low PCV and TSS suggests anemia due to blood loss whereas a low PCV and elevated TSS suggests anemia due to other causes. Normal PCV with elevated TSS suggests dehydration.

Blood Smear (Differential)

The blood smear is evaluated for rough cell numbers and cell quality. Abnormalities such as left shift, white cell toxicity and absence of polychromasia in the face of anemia are important in the evaluation of the critical patient.

Glucose

Exotic companion mammals are prone to stress hyperglycemia. If the glucose is higher than 300, measurement of blood glucose should be repeated and/or evaluated with urine glucose. As in small mammals, diabetes is documented with repeatable high blood glucose with a glucosuria.

Hypoglycemia is seen occasionally, especially in any sick anorectic animal. Pancreatic islet cell tumors of ferrets (insulinoma) are of special concern, and commonly produce mild to profound hypoglycemia. Diagnosis is based on measurement of hospital-monitored fasting blood glucose of 65 mg/dL or lower. Most experts recommend fasting for 6 hours; however blood glucose should be measured at the first indication of symptoms suggesting hypoglycemia, including weakness, lethargy, nausea, drooling, and hind limb weakness.

Measurement of glucose is straightforward. Practitioners have investigated the use of human hand-held glucometers, especially in patients requiring serial or repeated monitoring. It should be kept in mind that many human units are not calibrated to be accurate at levels typical of hypoglycemia exotic mammals. Any hand-held device should be checked against standard measurement of glucose to determine accuracy at lower glucose levels.

Blood Urea nitrogen (BUN)

BUN is reduced in patients with liver disease and elevated in patients with pre-renal, renal, or post-renal azotemia. A quick estimate of the BUN can be obtained by placing a drop of blood on a commercially available Azostick (Bayer, Pittsburgh, PA) and evaluating the color change. Because this test is subject to operator error and the subjective ability to assess color changes, actual measurement of BUN is preferred. Assessment of BUN can be very helpful in evaluating animals with vomiting and anorexia, as the underlying cause of illness may be renal disease rather than primary gastrointestinal disease. Whenever possible, a urine sample should be obtained prior to administering fluids. Concentrated urine with an elevated BUN is consistent with dehydration, whereas isosthenuria with azotemia generally indicates primary renal disease.

OTHER DIAGNOSTIC TESTS

Additional tests are performed based on history, physical exam, and results of other diagnostic testing. Routine hematology and chemistry analysis includes a CBC and at a minimum liver enzymes, glucose, BUN, creatinine, calcium, phosphorus, albumin, and electrolytes. Hematology and biochemistry tests are important in the diagnosis of infectious, metabolic, inflammatory, and some toxic diseases.

ANESTHESIA AND ANALGESIA FOR THE CRITICAL PATIENT

Marla Lichtenberger, DVM, Diplomate ACVECC
Thousand Oaks Pet Emergency Clinic
Thousand Oaks, CA

Pain is present with many diseases as well as in association with surgical and traumatic conditions. The demonstration of pain is not always obvious; therefore, an animal should be assumed to be experiencing pain in any condition expected to produce pain in humans. The assessment and control of pain is an art as well as a science. Clinicians should keep in mind that the art of pain management is a continual learning experience requiring assessment and therapeutic adjustment for individual animals even when they are undergoing similar surgical procedures. Therefore, standard or rule-of-thumb analgesic and anesthetic protocols are not always appropriate.

If we accept that animals can experience pain, then how do we determine if a ferret or rabbit is or is not painful? It is likely that the tolerance of pain by ferrets and rabbits varies greatly between individuals, as it does in other species. This coupled with ferrets' innate ability to mask significant disease, and probably pain, make it difficult to assess pain. Compared with dogs and cats, very few investigations have been carried out on the assessment and alleviation of pain in ferrets and rabbits. Most likely, as in cats, the mainstay of pain assessment in ferrets, rabbits, and birds appears to be behavioral.

There are certain behaviors that are commonly seen in ferrets and rabbits suffering acute trauma or postoperative pain. Such ferrets and rabbits are often depressed, immobile, silent, and appear and distanced from their environment. They do not respond normally to petting or attention; ferrets and rabbits tend to hide when experiencing pain. They may also hyperventilate. In the my clinic, I have found that ferrets and rabbits have a very similar response to pain as is seen in cats.

MULTIMODAL APPROACH

The process of nociception and pain involves many steps and pathways, so one analgesic agent is unlikely to alleviate pain completely. An effective management plan includes drugs of different classes, each acting at a different part of the pathway; this is termed *multimodal analgesia*. For example, a ferret can be premedicated with an opioid, which will modulate pain; ketamine can be used as a part of the induction protocol to reduce wind-up; a local anesthetic block could be incorporated to inhibit transmission; and a nonsteroidal anti-inflammatory drug (NSAID) can be added pre- or postoperatively to alter transduction. This approach also allows smaller doses of each drug to be used as the effects are additive and may reduce any undesirable side effects from larger doses of individual drugs.

Constant rate infusions (CRIs) are delivered intravenously at a constant rate, frequently over a long period of time. Constant rate infusions have several advantages. They allow the drug to be titrated to effect resulting in a reduction in the total amount of drug used, frequently resulting in fewer side effects, less "rollercoaster" analgesia, fewer hemodynamic effects, and more cost effectiveness. Disadvantages include a slow rise in plasma concentrations to therapeutic levels, which is why a loading dose of the drug is frequently given prior to starting the CRI.

The easiest way to administer a CRI is via an automated mechanical pump system. In veterinary medicine, syringe pump systems are the most common delivery system and are mandatory for the small volumes used for rabbits and ferrets. These are small pumps that can utilize a 1 cc to 60 cc syringe for delivery of the drug through an intravenous extension line. The syringe pump is advantageous because it allows very small volumes of drug to be delivered at a constant rate infusion.

PAIN MANAGEMENT OPTIONS IN THE RABBIT AND FERRET

There is no doubt that pain management for rabbits and ferrets in clinical practice is presently inadequate. The ferret and rabbit have an undeserved reputation for adverse respiratory depression after opiate treatment. In the author's opinion, the ferret and rabbit become very comfortable and sleep normally after administration of opioids postoperatively. Birds have mainly kappa pain receptors and therefore respond to kappa agonist drugs for pain relief. Rabbits are very sensitive to the side effects of most drugs. Ferrets are deficient in the glucuronidation pathway as are cats, and inappropriate dosing of NSAIDs can lead to toxicity. Fear of these adverse effects has resulted in many ferrets and rabbits not receiving analgesics after surgery or trauma. Drugs used in rabbits and ferrets are discussed in the next section.

ANESTHETIC/ANALGESIC DRUGS USED IN FERRETS AND RABBITS

The five major classes of analgesics employed for acute pain management are considered in this section. Drugs and dosages used by the author in ferrets and rabbits are discussed.

Opioids

Ferrets and rabbits continue to have an undeserved reputation of having "repiratory depression" after administration of opioid drugs. Resting very quietly without pain is being interpreted as respiratory depression. When used appropriately, opioids can be administered to ferrets and rabbits and are safe and effective for alleviating pain. Opioids in general have a very wide margin of safety and excellent analgesic properties. In veterinary medicine, the most commonly used opioid CRIs are fentanyl, hydromorphone, morphine, and butorphanol. Some animals may respond better to one opioid over another depending on individual variability, breed, species, and source of pain.

Butorphanol continues to be the most commonly used opioid in ferrets despite recent questioning of its analgesic properties. Described as an agonist-antagonist agent, its agonist activity is exerted at the kappa receptors and its antagonist actions are demonstrated at the mu receptors. Opioid drugs in this class exert a ceiling effect, after which increasing doses do not produce any further analgesia. Butorphanol appears to be an effective visceral, but a poor somatic, analgesic. Butorphanol is a poor analgesic choice for surgery patients where there will be somatic and visceral pain, however. Its ceiling effects limits its use to minor procedures, and the frequent dosing required is inconvenient and expensive. When used in the author's clinic for treatment of pain in the ferret and rabbit we prefer to use it as a CRI, instead of repeated dosing. Higher doses repeated throughout the day are used in avian medicine for pain relief.

Hydromorphone and fentanyl are mu receptor agonists. They are excellent analgesics for visceral and somatic pain. Intuitively, CRIs are necessary when using rapidly metabolized opioids, such as fentanyl, for operative and postoperative analgesia.

Tramadol (opioid-type drug) is another possible drug to be used orally for postoperative pain control. No studies have been done on use of this drug in the ferret. Tramadol binds to opiate receptors and also inhibits reuptake of norepinephrine and serotonin. The agent thus stimulates two endogenous, antinociceptive mechanisms in the spinal cord and the brain stem.

Nonsteroidal Anti-inflammatory Drugs (NSAIDs)

NSAIDs are excellent agents for alleviation of acute postoperative and traumatic pain. As in other species there are concerns about preoperative use of NSAIDs in ferrets. The main concern relate to inhibition of prostaglandin synthesis, which may lead to gastrointestinal erosion, impaired renal function, and bleeding. The limited ability for glucuronide conjugation in ferrets can prolong the duration of action of the NSAIDs, but with appropriate changes in dose and dosing intervals they can be used safely. The advantages of this category of drugs are their long duration of action and that no Drug Enforcement Administration (DEA) paperwork is required. In young ferrets with no evidence of renal disease, this group of drugs is a good choice.

Injectible carprofen has become available in the United States, but it is unlikely to be labeled for use in ferrets. Carprofen is not a potent inhibitor of prostaglandin synthetase and has proved to be a safe agent in ferrets. Ketoprofen (Ketofen®, Fort Dodge Animal Health) is available as an injectible agent, but because of its COX-1 inhibition, should be reserved for postoperative administration. Meloxicam (Metacam®, Boehringer Ingelheim Vetmedica) is recently available as an injectible and oral form, and is the most commonly used NSAID in the ferret. It has primary COX-2 inhibition. NSAIDs should not be used in animals with preexisting renal disease, hypovolemia, or bleeding disorders or if severe surgical hemorrhage is anticipated. Flunixin meglumine is an NSAID and is a very potent inhibitor of cyclo-oxygenase. Recommendations for its use in rabbits and ferrets with gastric stasis and septic

shock are common in literature. This is most likely due to its use in horses in colic. The author warns against its use with preexisting renal disease, hypovolemia, or bleeding disorders as with only NSAIDs. Newer NSAIDs that are specifically COX-2 inhibitors may be safer to use in ferret and rabbits than use of flunixin.

Local Anesthetics

Local anesthetic agents can be employed successfully in ferrets. The two most commonly used agents are lidocaine (Lidocaine HCl oral topical solution, USP 2%, Hi-Tech Pharmacal Co.) and bupivacaine. An advantage of this group of drugs is their low cost and uncontrolled status. A complete sensory block prevents nerve transmission, making use of these agents one of the most potentially practical pre-emptive techniques. Local anesthetics can be infiltrated into the surgical skin site, or discrete nerve blocks can be preformed.

Alpha-2 Agonists

Alpha-2 agonists as medetomidine (Domitor®, Pifizer Animal Health) possess analgesic, sedation, and muscle-relaxant properties. These drugs are usually reserved for healthy animals because of the cardiopulmonary depression that accompanies their use. Microdose medetomidine preserves the blood pressure effects in healthy animals with good cardiac output, and provides good analgesic, sedation and muscle relaxation when used with a tranquilizer and opioid. These drugs have not been used by the author in ferrets.

NMDA Antagonists (Ketamine)

The NMDA receptor plays an important role in the central sensitization, and there is much interest in developing drugs that can inhibit this receptor. In veterinary medicine a commonly used NMDA antagonist is ketamine (Vetaket®, Lloyd Laboratories), which may be effective at preventing, or at least lessening, wind-up at subanesthetic doses. When used with gas anesthesia and opioids there is a reported opioid-sparing and gas anesthetic-sparing effect seen. The interesting thing about ketamine is that minute amounts of it need to be used via a CRI to have analgesic effects. Therefore, the cardiovascular effects that commonly occur with the anesthetic doses of ketamine do not occur at the analgesic dose. Ketamine is an excellent adjunct to opioid therapy and frequently allows reduction in the opioid dose being administered.

The author uses micro-dose ketamine continuous rate infusions (CRIs) with opioid CRIs during surgery in the ferret. When the CRIs are combined there is a overall gas anesthetic-sparing affect. The common side effects of gas anesthesia are hypotension and are avoided when combined with ketamine/opioid CRIs.

ANESTHESIA INDUCTION AGENTS IN RABBITS AND FERRETS
Etomidate/Propofol

Etomidate (Amidate®, BenVenue Laboratories) is an imidazole derivative that undergoes rapid redistribution and hepatic metabolism, resulting in rapid recovery following a single bolus. Etomidate induces minimal cardiovascular and respiratory depression and has a wide margin of safety. Etomidate is frequently used in the author's clinic in patients that have poor cardiovascular function. We routinely combine diazepam with etomidate induction in compromised patients. The recommended dose of etomidate after a benzodiazepam premed (ie, diazepam 0.5 mg/kg intravenously) is 1.0 mg/kg.

Propfol (Rapinovet®, Abbott Laboratories) is chemically unrelated to other anesthetic drugs. It has a fast onset and short duration of action. Apnea following administration of propofol is common and is more pronounce with rapid injection of the drug. The author uses propofol as an induction agent in the stable ferret patients at a dose of 4 to 6 mg/kg intravenously.

EPIDURAL ANESTHESIA/ANALGESIA IN RABBITS AND FERRETS

Epidural drugs achieve pain relief with less to no systemic effects as compared with drugs administered intramuscularly or intravenously. This factor is important in small mammals when the administered drug has negative side effects, such as cardiac and respiratory depression. Epidural drugs may decrease recovery time, which is always an advantage when working with ferrets and rabbits. The improvement in recovery time occurs because of the decreased percentage of gas anesthesia needed when used in conjunction with an epidural anesthetic.

In most small mammals, after epidural injection of lidocaine, analgesia develops within 10 to 15 minutes and lasts 60 to 90 minutes. Bupivacaine can provide up to 6 to 8 hours of surgical analgesia. Ferrets have been treated with lidocaine 1.5% at 0.4 mL/kg. Bupivacaine can provide up to 5 to 6 hours of surgical analgesia. Morphine at 0.22 mg/kg that is administered into the epidural space provides prolonged postoperative analgesia for up to 24 hours.

INTUBATION TECHNIQUES FOR INHALATION ANESTHESIA

- **Ferrets**
  - Endotracheal intubation in the ferret is done in the same way as is described in cats and dogs.

- **Rabbits**
  - Use of a semi-flexible fiberoptic endoscope (Focusscope) inserted into the endotracheal tube (2.0–2.5 mmID) from its adapter end, and the tip of the scope is positioned to within 1 to 2 mm of the beveled end of the tube, The semi-flexible endoscope has a portable handheld light source. The endoscope and ET tube is advanced over the base of the tongue until the tip of the epiglottis is visible through the soft palate. The tip of the scope is advanced in a dorso-caudal direction, lifting the soft palate and thus allowing the epiglottis to fall forward. The tube is advanced into the laryngeal opening and the ET (endotracheal tube) tube is advanced over the scope into the trachea. The endoscope is removed.
  - **Nasotracheal Intubation.** The rabbit is held in extreme extension. An 8 French (small rabbits <1 kg) or 2-mm ET tube is passed medially and ventrally into the nose. The ventral meatus is entered while the ET tube is passed into the larynx and trachea.

- **Small Mammals**
  - Small mammals may be intubated using the same technique described above for rabbits. When a flexible endoscope is not available, most small mammals are anesthetized and maintained with inhalant anesthesia using a mask.

- **Dental Nerve Blocks**
  - This is a local block procedure that is used along with opioids and NSAIDs for dental procedures. Anesthesia used is lidocaine 2% is mixed with bupivicaine 0.5% in a ½ cc syringe with a 25-auge needle. For each kilogram body weight mix 0.05 mL of lidocaine with 0.18 mL of bupivicaine and 0.27 mL of sterile water (can increase amount of sterile water to increase the total volume to be given). The total volume will be divided into the number of sites to block. The 5 dental blocks will be described in the lecture and consist of the infraorbital, palatine, mandibular, maxillary, and mental nerve blocks.

References are available from the author upon request.

THE CRITICAL RABBIT:
HOW TO KEEP THEM ALIVE

Marla Lichtenberger, DVM, Diplomate ACVECC
Thousand Oaks Pet Emergency Clinic
Thousand Oaks, CA

Although the principles for emergency and critical care are universal in all species, the small size and predisposition to stress creates a unique set of challenges when dealing with rabbits, ferrets, and other small mammals. This article provides basic nutrition, restraint, physical exam, blood collection, diagnostic and therapeutic procedures for the rabbit. Guidelines for monitoring and treatment of hypovolemic shock in small mammals will be discussed.

PHYSICAL EXAM AND HISTORY

Timothy Hay should be fed ad libitum. The rabbit can be fed fresh greens, such as dandelion greens, parsley, mustard greens and collard greens at ½ cup per day of packed greens. The maximum amount of pellets (fiber content greater than 19%) should be 1/8 cup per 5 kg body weight per day and fed at night.

Physical Examination

Critically ill rabbits may not tolerate excessive handling and should be observed in the carrier before physical exam. General attitude, respiratory pattern, and fecal and urine output can be assessed. The veterinarian can determine respiratory rate by observing nasal movements. The rabbit is a prey species and conceals any signs of illness to escape predation.

Examine rabbits on a skid-free surface and place a towel under the body or wrap a panicky rabbit in a towel. Keep a hand under the rabbit at all times, even if recumbent. Normal body temperature is 101–104°F (38.3–39.8°C). Avoid heat lamps in rabbits since they have thin skin. Hypothermic rabbits should be maintained in an incubator. The normal heart rate is 180 to 325 beats per minute. Smaller rabbits have higher heart rates. Normal systolic blood pressure is between 90 and 120 mmHg. The perfusion status of a critically ill rabbit can be assessed by determining capillary refill time (CRT), color of mucous membranes, heart rate, blood pressure, and temperature. The hydration status is determined by moistness of the mucous membranes, skin tenting and turgor of the eyelid.

The heart and lungs should be auscultated for any abnormalities as assessed in dogs and cats. The abdomen is palpated for any distention, pain, or masses.

The teeth are always examined using a otoscope or human nasal speculum.

CLINICAL TECHNIQUES IN RABBITS
Venipuncture

Although several sites are available for venipuncture (ie, ear vein, jugular vein, cephalic vein, and lateral saphenous), the author prefers the lateral saphenous. Vessels in the ears are easily visualized but collapse and have an increased risk of thrombosis and sloughing in small rabbits. Jugular venipuncture may be difficult in obese rabbits and those with large dewlaps. The cephalic vein is maintained for catheter placement. The saphenous vein is most commonly used for collection of blood. The rabbit can be restrained in lateral recumbency and the rear leg is held off above the hock. A 25-gauge needle and 1-cc syringe are used to withdraw the blood sample.

Intravenous catheters of either 24- or 26-gauge can be placed in most small rabbits, and 22-gauge catheters can be easily placed in rabbits over 3 kg. The cephalic or saphenous veins are well suited for indwelling catheters. When intravenous catheterization has failed or the veins are too small or fragile to place an intravenous catheter, then an intraosseous catheter is extremely beneficial. The proximal femur or the proximal tibia are recommended sites to place a 20-gauge, 1.5-inch spinal needle. The greater trochanter of the femur or proximal tibia is preferred.

GASTROINTESTINAL PROBLEMS IN THE RABBIT

- Nearly all the disease problems in rabbits are directly or indirectly related to diet. The two most common rabbit emergency problems that result in anorexia are gastric stasis and malocclusion involving the incisors, cheek teeth, or both.
- Gastric stasis is one of the most common syndromes in rabbits and is characterized by anorexia, decreased or no stool production, and a large stomach filled with dough-like stomach contents and hair. Nearly all of the important disease problems that rabbits experience are directly or indirectly related to diet. Rabbits that are fed a high-carbohydrate, low-fiber diet cause a disruption of gastrointestinal motility and frequently leads to gastric stasis. There is a loss of liquid from the material in the stomach and the resultant dehydrated mass of gastric ingesta may not be passed by the rabbit. The material in the stomach usually consists of ingested food with or without hair.
- Malocclusion of either the incisors, the cheek teeth, or both is common in rabbits. Incisor malocclusion is usually apparent to the owner, while malocclusion of the cheek teeth is rarely obvious to the owner. Rabbits usually present with a history of anorexia and weight loss.

Pathophysiology

- Rabbits are herbivores, and hindgut fermenters. Their digestive system is driven by the presence of fiber in the diet, which allows efficient digestion of the nonfiber portion of food. High-fiber diets stimulate cecocolic motility, and have a low level of carbohydrate and thus decrease the risk of enterotoxemia caused by carbohydrate overload of the hindgut. Frequently, a reduction in the amount of fiber in the diet, an increase in carbohydrate consumption, and disruption of gastroenteric motility lead to alterations in the cecal pH and disruption of the complex bacterial flora of the hindgut. The spore-forming anaerobes, consisting mostly of

Clostridium sp, and coliform species as *E. coli* increases the population of normal organisms decrease. This will lead to enterotoxemia, sepsis and death.

- Hepatic lipidosis develops rapidly when a rabbit stops eating, and reversing this process can be difficult. The author uses the same principles as used in the cat for anorexia and gastric stasis. The etiology for gastric stasis in the rabbit is often a low fiber diet but is also commonly seen with stress (as occurs in the cat).

- The pelleted diets fed exclusively are high in calories (high in digestible carbohydrates), high in protein, and highly digestible, and designed to increase weight in growing rabbits raised for meat. These diets, when fed exclusively or in large quantities, cause gastrointestinal complications such as gastric stasis, obesity and malocclusion (decreased grinding action that keeps the occlusal surface evenly worn).

- Malocclusion of the incisors is frequently a genetic trait. Malocclusion of the premolars and molars is common in middle-aged to older animals and may result from many factors. It leads to overgrowth and sharpening of the lateral (upper arcade) and the medial (lower arcade) edges. Common causes of malocclusion are:
  - Genetic factors leading to a mandible that is too narrow or too short, resulting in misalignment of the teeth.
  - Decreased chewing action of rabbits fed an all pellet diet.
  - Trauma and infections can increase the risk of malocclusion problems.

Clinical Findings

- Anorexia for more than 2 days' duration.
- Malocclusion identified on oral exam.
- Weight loss may be noted in some rabbits.
- Ptyalism and ocular discharge (upper cheek teeth are very close to the nasolacrimal duct) should make the clinician think of dental disease.
- When gastric stasis is present, a firm, dough like mass is often palpated in the cranial region of the abdomen. Gas may be palpable in the stomach or intestines. The number of fecal pellets is significantly reduced or absent. The stools passed are much smaller than normal or may contain hair.

Differential Diagnosis

- Gastric or intestinal obstruction can be caused by a large mat of fur or rarely by some ingested foreign material like carpeting or bedding. Rabbits present with an acute abdomen that is painful, bloated and with a tympanic stomach. The rabbit is usually in shock. Decompression of the stomach is required by passage of a nasogastric (NG) tube. Radiographs may show a dilated, fluid-filled stomach or cecum. Animals must be treated for shock and then taken to surgery. The prognosis for surgery is poor.

- Enterotoxemia from other causes as reproductive disorders, bacterial enteritis, or pneumonia
- Parasites

Diagnostic Tests

- Radiology may or may not be helpful in diagnosis of gastric stasis because the mass of food and hair appears similar to normal ingesta. However, visualization of a large, ingesta-filled stomach on a radiograph of a rabbit that has been anorexic suggests the presence of gastric stasis.

- CBC and serum chemistries are performed to evaluate the rabbit for other causes of gastric stasis as infections, hepatic, or renal disease. A minimum data base (ie, blood glucose, PCV/TP and azotick) should be performed immediately. This will alert the veterinarian for possible hypoglycemia secondary to anorexia, dehydration, azotemia, and anemia.

- Evaluation of the teeth:
  - Incisors are relatively easy to evaluate. The lower incisors should oppose the peg teeth and the four main incisors should have a beveled cutting edge as described above.
  - Cheek teeth are more difficult to evaluate without general anesthesia. Initially an otoscope is used to evaluate the cheek teeth for the presence of points. Palpate the ventral line of the mandible. It should be smooth along the ventral aspect of the mandible. If any bumps are palpated they likely indicate cheek tooth root disease. Skull radiographs under general anesthesia is required when dental disease is suspected. Four vies are taken: dorsoventral, lateral, right lateral oblique, and left lateral oblique. Mask anesthesia with isoflurane and subsequent intubation is recommended. The author commonly uses propofol intravenously through a butterfly catheter (6 mg/kg IV) with or without gas anesthesia. Teeth specula and cheek dilators developed by Dr David Crosley (Jorgenson Labs, Loveland, CO). These are helpful in getting a good look at rabbit cheek teeth crowns. In most cases the upper cheek teeth develop spurs on the lateral aspect while the lower teeth develop spurs medially. These can cut into the cheek gingival or the tongue causing anorexia and a lot of pain.

Treatment

- Stop all inappropriate antibiotics as ampicillin, amoxicillin, or clindamycin.
- Fluid therapy. Perfusion and dehydration are corrected initially.
- Treat hypoglycemia when <70 mg/dL by adding 50% dextrose to the fluids to produce a 2.5% dextrose solution. When the animal is symptomatic with seizures and hypoglycemia, treat with a 1:1 solution of 50% dextrose with saline at 1 cc/kg BW IV. The author has also seen hyperglycemia in a stressed rabbit (up to 385 mg/dL) and hypoglycemia

in rabbits that were anorexic for greater than 2 to 3 days).

Placement of a Nasogastric Tube

- Placement of a nasogastric tube for nutrition and rehydration of the stomach contents. The tube can be used for a primary gastric stasis, anorexia or after performing dental procedures.
  - o The use of a 5-8 French Argyle® tube (The Kendall Co., Mansfield, MA) is chosen. The length necessary to reach the stomach is determined by measuring from the tip of the nose to the last rib. Do not use a stylet since the esophagus of the rabbit can be perforated with any additional force. A local anesthetic (2% lidocaine gel or ophthlamic anesthetic) is placed into the rabbit's nostril. The rabbit must be properly restrained, protecting its back, and the head is ventrally flexed by an assistant. The tube is passed ventrally and medially into the ventral meatus. The end of the tube is advanced until it enters into the stomach.
  - o Verification of placement is determined with a radiograph.
  - o Feeding procedure. A 35-mL syringe is used for slow bolus delivery of a liquid diet. The liquid diet used for the rabbit is the enteral nutrition (Herbivore Enteral Nutrition, Walk About Farms, Pembroke, VA). The diet contains some fiber, though not enough to meet the needs of a rabbit requiring long term feeding (greater than 2–3 days). A 2-kg average adult rabbit requires approximately 175 kcal/d. The feeding schedule using the enteral herbivore diet consists of mixing 10 cc /kg of water with 7 cc/kg of fiber diet. The slurrey is given into the NG tube with a syringe every 6 hours. The tube should be flushed with 5–6 cc of tap water after each feeding. In the author's experience most rabbits will start to eat and produce stools after 1–2 days. The tube can remain in place until the rabbit eats on its own and stool production begins.

- o Gastrointestinal motility is induced with cisapride 0.5 mg/kg liquid suspension into the NG tube every 8 hours.
- o Pain or discomfort may require the use of analgesics as butorphanol at 0.2–0.3 mg/kg IV, IM or SQ.

Treatment with Force Feeding

- Syringe feeding the critical care herbivore diet (Oxbow) may be optimal for the mildly ill patient with adequate perfusion parameters and normal hydration. These animals may be sent home with instructions for care by the owner. The directions for quantities to feed are written on the can. The syringe tip fits into the diasterna, the large space between the incisors and premolars. The rabbit can be wrapped in a towel if it is uncooperative. This may be very stressful to a rabbit and therefore is not recommended in the moderately to severely ill patient.

Treatment of Dental Malocclusion

- A slow speed drill with a straight handpiece using a #8 HP bur is the instrument of choice to trim incisors and remove points form cheek teeth. Alternatively some authors recommend the use of a rongeurs (Jorgenson Labs, Inc., Loveland, CO). If there is radiographic evidence of mild root disease (increased lucency at the tips of the roots) but there is no evidence of infection, burring the crowns to the gum line may be all that is required. If there is evidence of osteomyelitis (lysis and proliferation of bone surrounding a tooth), the tooth should be removed. For more advanced dental procedures in the rabbit the reader is referred to other sources and should be carried out in a step-wise fashion
- Broad spectrum antibiotics are used after invasive dental procedures:
  - o Enrofloxacin 5–15 mg/kg PO q 12–24 hours.
  - o Trimethoprim sulfa 15–30 mg/kg PO q 12 hours.

References are available from the author upon request.

THE CRITICAL FERRET: HOW TO KEEP THEM ALIVE

Marla Lichtenberger, DVM, Diplomate ACVECC
Thousand Oaks Pet Emergency Clinic
Thousand Oaks, CA

RESTRAINT

When ferrets are critically ill, they will require minimal restraint. The active ferret should be scruffed by the back or the neck. This elicits relaxation and a yawning reflex. When the ferret must be totally immobilized, anesthesia is required.

PHYSICAL EXAMINATION

Ferrets with respiratory distress may tolerate only brief periods of handling and should be placed in an oxygen-rich incubator before a full physical exam is attempted. Common signs of nausea in the ferret are bruxism, ptyalism, and pawing at the mouth. Posterior paresis in a ferret can be a manifestation of weakness from any cause, hypoglycemia or neurological disease.

The normal body temperature is 100 to 103°F (37.7–39.4°C). Ferrets do not like to have their temperatures taken and often require grasping both the nape of the neck and around the hips to secure the hindlimbs. Cataracts are common in juvenile and adult animals. Testing of hydration status is evaluated by moistness of the mucous membranes and skin turgor of the eyelids, since tenting of the skin can be inaccurate. Normal perfusion is assessed by a capillary refill time of 1 to 2 seconds, pink mucous membranes, normal heart rate, and blood pressure. The heart rate is normally 180 to 250 beats/min. but varies with the ferret's normal marked respiratory sinus arrhythmia. The heart is located caudally in the thorax and auscultation for arrhythmias or murmurs warrants auscultation between the 7th and 10th intercostal space. The blood pressure can be easily performed by use of Doppler on the distal paw or ventrally on the base of the tail. Normal systolic blood pressure is 90–120 mmHg.

Palpation of the abdomen is important. Palpate for the presence of foreign bodies, abnormal kidneys, presence of adrenal masses or an enlarged bladder. Splenomegaly is a normal finding in the ferret but marked splenomegaly may warrant further evaluation with an ultrasound exam. Most ferrets are neutered at 6 weeks of age and are tattooed on the right ear pinna at the same time. A swollen vulva in a neutered female ferret may indicate adrenal disease, or the presence of an ovarian remnant. Male ferrets have an os penis, and the prepuce is located ventrally on the abdomen. Alopecia at the tip of the tail may be incidental or an early sign of adrenal disease. Symmetrical, bilateral alopecia or thinning of the hair coat starting at the base of the tail and progressing cranially is a common finding in ferrets with adrenal disease.

CLINICAL TECHNIQUES

Venipuncture

Blood is most easily collected from the jugular vein, or vena cava. In the author's practice, venipuncture via the vena cava is most commonly used. Ferrets are wrapped tightly in a blanket up to their front legs. Ferrets are held in dorsal recumbency with the forelimbs pulled caudally over the thorax and the head extended. Needle penetration is performed in the notch between the first rib and manubrium of the sternum. A 25-gauge needle attached to a syringe, is held at a 45-degree angle with relation to the skin, and directed toward the contralateral hip. The needle is inserted to the hub and the plunger is pulled back as the needle is slowly removed. A small amount of blood for blood glucose may be taken from the lateral saphenous using a tuberculin syringe. This small needle will prevent collapse of the vein.

Catheter Placement

Peripheral catheterization can be performed in a critically ill ferret, but very active ferrets may require anesthesia. Use a 22- or 24-gauge peripheral catheter for placement in the lateral saphrenous or cephalic vein. To facilitate IV catheter placement, first puncture the skin over the vein, being careful to avoid the vein. Secure catheter in place with tape or suturing a butterfly tape to the skin.

An intraosseous (IO) catheter can be placed in the humerus, femur, or tibia using a 20- or 22-gauge, 1.5-inch spinal needle. The soft tissue and periosteum can be blocked with local anesthesia. The technique for placement is the same as described for a dog or cat.

Uretheral Catheterization

Most cases of urethral catheterization involve the male ferret as the result of cystic calculi or hyperplastic or cystic prostatic tissue at the neck of the bladder. Catheterization of the male ferret is difficult due to the J-shaped os penis and small diameter of the penile urethra. The ferret should be placed in dorsal recumbency and the aseptically prepare the prepuce. In some of the larger ferrets a 3.5-Fr red rubber tube is placed. The smaller ferrets may require placement of a 22-gauge jugular catheter. Suture the catheter to the prepuce and the skin and connect to a closed suction system. If a catheter can not be placed then a percutaneous cystoscopy needs to be done as described in the dog and cat. This catheter can be left in place until surgical correction of the cystic calculi or adrenalectomy takes place.

MONITORING AND TREATMENT OF HYPOVOLEMIC SHOCK IN THE FERRET

Blood Pressure Monitoring

Although there are several indirect or noninvasive methods (ie, oscillometric and Doppler) available, it is sometimes impossible to obtain a reading on exotic patients. The Doppler method is more versatile than the oscillometric method, and is the method used by the author for all exotic patients. The ultrasonic Doppler flow detector (Parks Medical Electronics Inc., Aloha, OR) uses ultrasonic waves to detect and make audible blood flow in an artery distal to the blood pressure cuff. The ferret, rabbit, or small mammal is placed in lateral recumbency. A pneumatic cuff is placed above the carpus, tarsus or on the tail base in a ferret. Hair is shaved between the carpal/tarsal pad and pads of the feet. The transducer probe crystal is placed on the shaved area (digital branch of the radial artery) in a bed of ultrasonic gel and taped or held in place. The cuff bladder is inflated to a suprasystemic pressure with cut-off of the Doppler signal. The cuff is deflated with the first sound heard and marked as the systolic pressure.

Fluid Therapy

The blood volume in the ferret and rabbit is 50 to 60 mL/kg in contrast to 90 mL/kg in the dog. When intravascular volume deficits result in poor perfusion, it has been recommended in the past that crystalloids be administered fast in volumes equivalent to the animal's blood volume. However, resuscitation with crystalloids alone can result in significant pulmonary and pleural fluid accumulation. The resultant hypoxemia contributes to the shock pathophysiology.

Rabbits, ferrets and small mammals are difficult to resuscitate from hypotensive episodes. In the rabbit, when baroreceptors have detected inadequate arterial stretch, it has been found that vagal fibers are stimulated simultaneously with sympathetic fibers. As a result, the heart rate may be normal or slow, instead of the typical tachycardia demonstrated by the dog. This baroreceptor response may be similar in the ferret and other small mammals. In the author's experience, normal ferrets and rabbits have heart rates between 180 and 240 beats per minute (bpm), systolic blood pressure between 90 and 120 mmHg, and temperatures between 100 and 102°F (37.7—38.8°C). Most ferrets, rabbits and small mammals presented for hypovolemic shock demonstrate heart rates less than 200 bpm, hypotension (systolic blood pressure less than 90 mmHg), and hypothermia (temperature < 98° F [36.6°C]).

Because cardiac output is a function of contractility and rate, the compensatory response to shock normally seen in dogs and birds is most likely blunted in ferrets, rabbits and small mammals. The hyperdynamic signs of shock seen in the dog and birds are not typically seen in the cat, ferret, rabbit and small mammals. Shock in the cat, rabbit, ferret and small mammal is most commonly decompensatory, manifested by normal or slow heart rate, severe hypothermia (<98°F or 36.6°C), weak or nonpalpable pulses, and profound mental depression. The mucous membranes are gray or white and capillary refill is not evident. The bradycardia and low cardiac output contribute to hypothermia, and hypothermia accentuates the bradycardia.

The hypothermia most likely plays a significant role in the poor compensatory response and to the difficulty in providing adequate fluid resuscitation without causing pulmonary edema. The theory is that as the rectal temperature falls, the adrenergic receptors become refractory to catecholamines. This leads to the normal or slow heart rate and most likely impaired compensatory vasoconstriction, in spite of the presence of norepinephrine and epinephrine. Part of the resuscitation plan in the rabbit, ferret and small mammal must include rewarming. Once the rectal temperature approaches 100°F, it appears that the adrenergic receptors begin to respond to catecholamines. Temperatures during this rewarming phase must be checked frequently in all exotic species to prevent hyperthermia.

Resuscitation from hypovolemic shock can be safely accomplished with a combination of crystalloids and colloids and rewarming procedures. This animal must be handled as little as possible. Placement of an IV or IO catheter will facilitate fluid administration. Initial blood work is done to determine the packed cell volume (PCV), total protein (TP), glucose, and azostick. In the hypovolemic ferret, rabbit, and small mammal, a rapid infusion of isotonic crystalloids is administered at 10 to 15 mL/kg. Hetastarch is administered at 5 mL/kg over 5 to 10 minutes. The blood pressure is checked and once it is above 40 mmHg systolic, then only maintenance crystalloids are given while the patient is aggressively warmed. The warming procedures should be done within the next 30 minutes to 1 hour with warm water bottles and warming the IV fluids. Active re-warming is required for patients with moderate to severe hypothermia and core temperatures below 95°F. Active external rewarming can be accomplished by hot water bottles, heated blankets or a forced warm air blanket. Active external re-warming can be accomplished by hot water bottles, heated blankets, or a warmed incubator for small animals. Forced air enclosed around the patient has proved effective in core re-warming in humans. Temperatures increased from 92°F to 99°F in 1 hour at the Animal Emergency Center using the forced air system (Thermacare®, Gaymar Industries Inc., Oakland Park, NY), which is a system of disposable plastic and paper covers and a heat source that directs warm air across the skin. This system simultaneously provides convective heat transfer and shielding against radiant heat loss.

If cardiac function is normal, and glucose, acid-base and electrolytes abnormalities have been corrected, treatment for nonresponsive shock is continued. Oxyglobin® has not been approved for use in the cat, ferret, rabbit or small mammal, but has been used successfully at our hospital when given in small volume boluses. Cats, ferrets, rabbits, and small mammals do not tolerate rapid, large volume boluses as given in the dog and birds. Cats and ferrets appear to be more predisposed to rapid onset of pulmonary edema when large volume boluses are given (this is assumed to occur in the other small mammals). At the Animal Emergency Center, we titrate 2 mL/kg boluses given over 10 to 15 minutes until normal heart rate and blood pressure (systolic blood pressure greater than 90 mmHg) are obtained. This is followed by a continuous rate infusion of oxyglobin® at 0.2 to 0.4 mL/kg/h.

References are available from the author upon request.

THE CRITICAL MAMMAL DISASTER: PART 1

Marla Lichtenberger, DVM, Diplomate ACVECC
Thousand Oaks Pet Emergency Clinic
Thousand Oaks, CA

Angela M. Lennox, DVM, Diplomate ABVP (Avian)
Avian and Exotic Animal Clinic of Indianapolis
Indianapolis IN

ANESTHESIA AND ANALGESIA OF THE CRITICAL EXOTIC MAMMAL PATIENT

Introduction in all Species

Pain is present with many diseases as well as in association with surgical and traumatic conditions. The demonstration of pain is not always obvious; therefore, an animal should be assumed to be experiencing pain in any condition expected to produce pain in humans. The assessment and control of pain is an art as well as a science. Humans and animals express three types of opioid receptors, mu, kappa, and delta. The authors have used this information for clinical use of opioids in small mammals. Clinicians should keep in mind that the art of pain management is a continual learning experience requiring assessment and therapeutic adjustment for individual animals, even when they are undergoing similar surgical procedures. Therefore, standard or rule-of-thumb analgesic and anesthetic protocols are not always appropriate.

If animals can experience pain, then how do we assess pain in ferrets, rabbits, and other exotic companion mammals? It is likely that the tolerance of pain by these animals varies greatly from individual to individual. Furthermore, these animals innate ability to mask significant disease and pain, make it difficult for us to assess their degree of pain. Compared with dogs and cats, pain in ferrets, rabbits and other companion mammals is far more difficult to assess. As in cats, the mainstay of pain assessment in these animals appears to be behavioral observation.

Behaviors that are commonly seen in exotic companion mammals suffering acute trauma or postoperative pain include depression, and sitting immobile, silent, and distanced from their environment. They may stand with their eyes half-closed and do not groom. Rabbits and ferrets may exhibit bruxism. They often do not respond normally to petting or attention. Many of these species will hide when experiencing pain.

Multimodal Analgesia in All Species of Birds and Small Mammals

The process of nociception and pain involves multiple steps and pathways, so a single analgesic agent is unlikely to alleviate pain completely. An effective pain management plan should include drugs of different classes with each acting at a different step of the pathway; this is termed multimodal analgesia. For example, a ferret can be premedicated with an opioid, which will modulate pain; ketamine can be used as a part of the induction protocol to reduce wind-up; a local anesthetic block could be incorporated to inhibit pain transmission; and a nonsteroidal anti-inflammatory drug (NSAID) can be added pre- or postoperatively to alter pain transduction. This approach also allows smaller doses of each drug to be used as the effects are either additive or synergistic and reduce any undesirable side effects from larger doses of individual drugs.

Pain Management Options in the Rabbit and Ferret

There is no doubt that ferret and rabbit pain management in clinical practice is presently inadequate. Traditional thought is that these animals have adverse respiratory depression after opiate treatment, but in the authors' opinion, these species become very comfortable and sleep normally after administration of opioids postoperatively. Rabbits are more sensitive to the side effects of most opioids. Ferrets are deficient in the glucuronidation pathway as are cats, and inappropriate dosing of NSAIDs can lead to toxicity. Fear of these adverse effects has resulted in inadequate analgesia after surgery or trauma..

Local Anesthetics

Local anesthetics agents can be employed successfully in ferrets. The two most commonly used agents are lidocaine (Lidocaine HCl oral Topical Soln, USP 2%, Hi-Tech Pharmacal Co.) and bupivacaine (Bupivacaine HCl, 0.5%, Abbott Laboratories). Suitable dosages and anticipated duration of action are shown in Table 1.

Use of local anesthetics for incisional line blocks, wound infiltration, nerve ring blocks, topically or epidural anesthesia is recommended by the authors. For incisional line blocks before surgery the authors use a 25-gauge, ¼-inch needle to infiltrate the subcutaneous tissue and skin. The local anesthetics are used as part of the multimodal approach to analgesia. The calculated dose of the drugs should not exceed the doses listed in Table 1. Local analgesic protocols (eg, ring blocks, incisional blocks) are commonly combined with other drugs (ie, opioids, constant rate infusions (CRIs)) for multimodal analgesia.

An advantage of local anesthetics is low cost and non-controlled drug status. A complete sensory block prevents nerve transmission, making use of these agents attractive for practical pre-emptive techniques. Local anesthetics can be infiltrated into the surgical skin site, or discrete nerve blocks can be preformed. The addition of an opioid to the mixture of local anesthetics for local blocks mixture potentially lengthen the median duration of analgesia (addition of morphine to the lidocaine/bupivacaine mixture prolonged analgesia 10 hours longer with the morphine, and 9 hours longer with the buprenorphine). With the conclusion that adding an opioid to the local anesthetic mixture lengthens the duration of analgesia. In the authors' experience the analgesia is prolonged significantly when an opioid is added to the local block. In another study buprenorphine-local anesthetic axillary perivascular brachial plexus block provided postoperative analgesia lasting three times longer than local anesthetic block along and twice as long as buprenorphine given by intramuscular (IM) injection plus local anesthetic-only block. This supports the concept of peripherally mediated opioid analgesia by buprenorphine. This study was performed in humans with the dose of buprenorphine was 0.3 mg mixed with the lidocaine/bupivicaine as given above.

Dental Blocks

There are five important dental blocks for small mammals. All five blocks incorporate lidocaine and bupivacaine mixture as given above for the ring block. The total dose of the mixture is drawn up into a syringe and 1/5th of the total dose is given into each of five sites. Use a 25- to 27-gauge needle with a 1-cc syringe.

The following techniques can be used to provide regional anesthesia for rabbits and other small mammals (Dr Dale Kressin, personal communication,). Kressin recommends the following protocol for dental blocks.

Infraorbital Nerve Block. The infraorbital nerve arises from the maxillary branch of the trigeminal nerve. This nerve provides sensory fibers to the upper incisor teeth, the upper lip and to the adjacent soft tissues. The zygomatic nerve also arises from the maxillary nerve just proximal to the infraorbital nerve. This nerve also supplies sensory fibers to the lateral aspect of the face.

The infraorbital foramen is located approximately 5 to 12 mm dorsal to the crestal bone adjacent to the upper first premolar (cheek) tooth, at the lateral aspect of the skull. The foramen is not as easily palpated as in the dog. The facial tuber is a palpable bony prominence at the mesial (rostral) aspect of the zygomatic bone and is approximately 4 to 10 mm ventral to the infraorbital canal. The infraorbital nerve can be blocked by infusion of the local anesthetic at this foramen.

Mental Nerve Block. The mental nerve arises from the mandibular nerve, as it extends into the mental foramina to form the mental nerve. The mental nerve supplies sensory fibers to the ventral and lateral aspect of the mandible, the lip, the lower incisor and motor fibers to local muscles.

The mental nerve exits the mental foramen located at the dorsal lateral aspect of the body of the mandible. The foramen is rostral (2–4 mm) to the first mandibular premolar (cheek tooth) and located ventrally in the dorsal third of the body of the mandible. The mental nerve can be blocked by infusion of local anesthetic at this foramen.

Mandibular Nerve Block. The mandibular nerve arises from the trigeminal nerve and supplies sensory and motor fibers to the ventral mandible as well as the muscles of mastication. The mandibular nerve provides sensory fibers to the mandibular molar and premolar (cheek) teeth as well as adjacent tissues.

The mandibular nerve enters the mandibular foramen on the medial surface of the mandible. An intraoral approach to block this nerve is not practical in the rabbit as in other species, due to the limited access of the oral cavity. An extraoral approach should be made with great care to avoid neurovascular structures (facial vessels and nerves) at the ventral aspect of the mandible. The mandibular foramen is approximately midway between the distal aspect of the last molar (cheek) tooth and the ventral aspect of the mandible. In addition, the foramen is approximately 2 to 5 mm distal to the third molar tooth. After this location is determined, an appropriate length infusion needle can be "walked along" the medial aspect of the mandible to the mandibular foramen for infusion of the local anesthetic. This will effectively block the mandibular premolar and molar (cheek) teeth.

Maxillary Nerve Block. The maxillary nerve supplies sensory fibers to the upper premolar and molar (cheek) teeth and adjacent tissues. Intraoral approaches to the maxillary nerve have not been attempted by this author due to the limited access to the oral cavity. In large breed rabbits the maxillary nerve can be blocked using a "caudal infraorbital" strategy. A 27-gauge needle is advanced 1 to 2 cm into the infraorbital canal. The syringe is aspirated to ensure the needle is not in a vessel lumen. Firm digital pressure is placed over the rostral end of the infraorbital canal while slowly infusing the local anesthetic. This block will anesthetize all ipsilateral premolar and molar (cheek) teeth and the adjacent periodontal tissues. In small rabbits and other small mammals, it may not be possible to thread the needle into the infraorbital canal. It these cases, the author will place the needle at the rostral entrance to the canal, apply firm digital pressure, and infuse the local anesthetic. Application of "splash blocks" of the local anesthetics to the periodontal ligament and adjacent soft tissues may also augment regional anesthesia.

Palatine Nerve Block. The sphenopalatine nerve ends within the sphenopalatine ganglion. Three nerves extend from the ganglion to regional tissues. The nasal cavity is innervated by the nasal rami, the rostral or anterior hard palate by the nasopalatine nerve and the posterior hard palate via the anterior palatine nerve. The oral cavity of the rabbit limits easy visualization; however, the anterior palatine nerve can be blocked as it exits the larger palatine foramen. This foramen is located half way between the palatal aspect of the third upper premolar (cheek) tooth and the palatal midline. Infusion of a local anesthetic will block this nerve and the palate of the ipsilateral side.

Intratesticular Block

The authors recommend that castration in small mammals can be performed with a IM preoperative injection of buprenorphine (0.02 mg/kg) with midazolam (0.25 mg/kg) IM. Mix 0.1 mg/100 g body weight bupivacaine (0.5%) and 0.1 mg/100 g body weight of lidocaine (2%) with buprenorphine 0.0003 mg/100 g body weight. This can be diluted in saline to have a final volume of 1 mL. Use a 25-gauge 5/8-inch needle for guinea pigs or rabbits and a 27-gauge 5/8-inch needle for a mouse or gerbil. Place the needle through the testicle starting from the caudal pole aiming for the spermatic cord. It is desirable for the needle to exit the testicle proximally as it is the spermatic cord that will be ligated. Aspirate before injection. Inject, expressing firm backpressure, while withdrawing the needle, Expect to use about one third of the drug volume per testicle leaving the organ firmly turgid. Repeat for the other testicle and the remaining drug can be used to place a dermal incisional block. This will provide analgesia for 22 hours (Dr. Stein, personal communication, 2006).

Alpha-2 Agonists

Alpha-2 agonists such as medetomidine (Domitor, Pifizer Animal Health) possess analgesic, sedation, and muscle-relaxant properties. The higher dose (30 µg/kg) drugs are usually reserved for healthy animals because of the cardiopulmonary depression that accompanies their use. One study in healthy rabbits found that the combination of medetomidine and ketamine showed the best sedation, while medetomidine-fentanyl-midazolam had the least cardiovascular effects, and xylazine-ketamine had the greatest cardiovascular side effects.

Micro-dose medetomidine (1–3 µg/kg) minimally affects the blood pressure in animals with normal cardiac output, and provides good analgesic, sedation and muscle relaxation when used with a tranquilizer and opioid. Medetomidine requires only a slight alpha-2-adrenoceptor availability to decrease noradrenaline turnover and very low doses of medetomidine result in sympatholysis. Therefore, patients who require a high level of sympathetic tone to maintain blood pressure may not tolerate medetomidine (ie, animals in shock and in compensated hear failure). In conscious dogs intravenous medetomidine at 1.25 µg/kg increased blood pressure by 15% and decreased heart rate by 26% and cardiac output by 35%.

In postoperative patients sympathetic tone was not entirely abolished by medetomidine. Only the unwanted increases in heart rate and blood pressure were attenuated. Medetomidine has no effect on cortisol levels. Alpha-2 agonists are commonly used in human medicine to decrease the stress response. Their use in small mammals for the inhibition of the stress response may be warranted. The authors recommend micro-dose medetomidate for use in small mammals, with the caution not to use this drug in any animal with a compromised cardiovascular system.

NMDA Agonists

Ketamine is commonly used for induction of anesthesia in small mammals. Reports in human and veterinary medicine indicate variable patient response following ketamine administration which is related to the status of the cardiovascular system at the time of ketamine administration. Ketamine used for induction is well tolerated in the stable patient. Patients that exhibit significant preexisting stress or a patient with hypertrophic cardiomyopathy have an increased risk of cardiovascular destabilization following ketamine administration. Ketamine increases sympathetic tone causing an increase in heart rate, myocardial contractility, and total peripheral vascular resistance. The authors feel that high-dose ketamine used for induction of anesthesia in a stressed small mammal (especially the rabbit) may cause an increased risk of destabilization. The authors avoid using ketamine as an induction agent for the stressed critically ill rabbit. The

NMDA receptor plays an important role in the central sensitization, and there is much interest in developing drugs that can inhibit this receptor. In veterinary medicine a commonly used NMDA antagonist is ketamine (Vetaket®, Lloyd Laboratories), which may be effective at preventing, or at least lessening, wind-up at sub-anesthetic doses. When used with inhalant anesthesia and opioids there is a reported opioid-sparing and inhalant anesthetic-sparing effect seen. The interesting perspective about ketamine is that the minute amounts used via a CRI route induce analgesic effect. Micro-dose ketamine does not cause an increase in sympathetic tone and are frequently used for analgesia with a CRI (given below).

Constant Rate Infusions

CRIs have several advantages over bolus delivery when treating with an analgesic. When using a CRI the drugs can be titrated to effect, resulting in a reduction of the total amount of drug used, fewer side effects, less "rollercoaster" analgesia, fewer hemodynamic effects and improved cost-effectiveness. One disadvantage to CRI is a slow rise in drug plasma concentration to therapeutic levels, which is why a loading dose of the drug is frequently given prior to starting constant rate infusion. Another disadvantage of CRI is the need of a pump, which is the easiest way to administer a CRI. Syringe pumps, most of which use a 1-cc to 60-cc syringe for drug delivery through an IV extension set, allow constant-rate delivery of very small volumes of drug. When these CRIs are combined, there is an overall inhalant anesthetic sparing effect. A common side effect of inhalant anesthesia is hypotension, which is avoided when inhalant anesthesia is combined with ketamine/opioid CRIs. The dose of fentanyl used by the authors is much lower than previously reported for use in small mammals. The authors do see a much greater depressive effect in small mammals when using the high dose ranges of fentanyl. We have not seen fentanyl-induced ileus or other gastrointestinal side effects in small mammals when using the lower end of the dose given in Table 1, when combined with ketamine. The multimodal approach of using two or more drugs combined allows for lower doses with fewer side effects of both drugs than when either drug used alone. We commonly use the lower CRI doses for butorphanol-ketamine CRIs or fentanyl-ketamine CRIs in rabbits with gastric stasis pain (Table 1). Ketamine is an excellent adjunct to opioid therapy and frequently allows reduction in the opioid dose being administered.

Inhalants

Based on available research in dogs, cats and ferrets, there are advantages of both sevoflurane and isoflurane depending in the circumstances. Isoflurane has the advantage if cost is a issue. Sevoflurane may have an advantage if mask induction is necessary or if the anesthetist needs to adjust the depth of anesthesia. Mask induction and changing of the depth of anesthesia are very important in exotics. Sevoflurane has a much less pungent odor. No differences in the speed of recovery were noted in ferrets in a controlled study. In most animals and birds the MAC for isoflurane is between 1.28 and 1.63, and for sevoflurane the MAC is between 2.10 and 2.60. Isoflurane and sevoflurane both have dose-dependent vasodilation properties leading to hypotension. Neither drug has any analgesic properties following termination of the anesthesia.

Epidural Anesthesia/Analgesia

Epidural drugs achieve pain relief with less or no systemic effects as compared with drugs administered intramuscularly or intravenously. This factor is important in small mammals when the administered drug has negative side effects, such as cardiac and respiratory depression. Epidural drugs may decrease recovery time, which is always an advantage when working with ferrets, rabbits, and other small mammals. The short recovery time occurs because of the inhalant sparing effect induced with an epidural anesthetic.

The local anesthetics lidocaine and bupivacaine are the most commonly used for epidural analgesia. Using local anesthetics can result in sensory, motor and autonomic blocks. This may be prevented by administering the diluted dose and lower dose recommended by the author and given in Table 1. When placing epidural needle as described below, the clinician should lower the local anesthetic dose by ½ when cerebrospinal fluid (CSF) fluid is seen in the hub (CSF fluid may only fill the hub with use of a stylet – see placement below).

In most small mammals, after epidural injection of lidocaine, analgesia develops within 10 to 15 minutes and lasts 60 to 90 minutes Bupivicaine can provide between 4 and 8 hours of surgical analgesia. It may exert analgesic effects with minimal motor blockage when used in dilute concentration. This dilution may be obtained by mixing 1 part of 0.25% bupivicaine (0.125% bupivicaine at 0.1 mg/kg) with 1 to 3 parts of an opioid by volume and administered at the desired opioid dose. The principal advantages of local anesthetics are the potential for complete regional anesthesia, and marked potentiation of the analgesic effect of the epidural opioids. Morphine (Morphine Sulfate inj preservative free, USP, Baxter Healthcare) at 0.1 mg/kg that is administered into the epidural space provides prolonged postoperative analgesia for up to 24 hours. Morphine is the least soluble opioid and this characteristic delays the epidural and systemic absorption of the drug. The peak analgesic effects may be delayed for 90 minutes following injection, and some analgesia may be present for 6 to 24 hours. It is important to administer it immediately after induction of anesthesia because of the relatively long latency to peak analgesia. Bupivacaine or lidocaine can be administered with morphine epidurally so that analgesia onset is shortened to 15 to 30 minutes and duration for 8 to 24 hours. In humans, postoperative neural blockage has also been associated with attenuation of the stress response, improved respiratory function, and improved hemodynamic stability.[8]We notice marked improvement in postoperative recovery in small mammals after receiving epidural analgesia prior to abdominal surgery or surgery on the rear limbs. When included as part of a patient management strategy, these epidural analgesic techniques as part of the multimodal approach may reduce morbidity and mortality.

The lumbosacral space is the preferred site of injection because of the relatively large space between L7 and S1. In most ferrets the dural sac terminates just cranial to that location (L7-S1). The absence of a complete dural sac at the LS junction reduces the likelihood of subdural injections. The dural sac of many rabbits extends to the sacrum, and attempts at epidural injection of the LS space in this species may result in subdural injections. Most subdural injections will also be subarachnoid, and injected medications will enter the CSF. Possible complications of subarachnoid injection include leakage of CSF, mitigation of the drug to the brainstem, and complete spinal blockage when using local anesthetics. We recommend the use of a 25-gauge hypodermic needle for epidural injections in small mammals and finds the length of the needle rarely enters past the epidural space. A stylet can be cut from orthopedic wire, sire sutures and then sterilized. It is important to have a stylet because it prevents a skin plug from clogging the needle which can prevent visualization of the CSF fluid. If a skin plug were injected into the epidural space, it could serve as a nidus for infection and inflammation. The disadvantage of using a hypodermic needle versus a spinal needle is that the bevel is longer with cutting edges on the hypodermic needle and this will not allow you to sense the pop when the needle passes through the ligamentum flavum. Care should be taken to avoid cutting and traumatizing the spinal cord during the insertion. The authors recommend aspiration with a syringe after placement of the needle. If CSF is seen in the hub of the needle, half of the dose that was intended for epidural administration should be administered instead.

The procedure for epidural anesthesia is similar to that described for dogs and cats. A 25-gauge needle is advanced trancutaneously at a 90 degree angle to the skin in the center of the LS junction. If bone is encountered, the needle is walked cranially or caudally to find the LS space. In small mammals, using a sharp 25-gauge needle, the resistance or "pop" through the ligamentum flavum is minimal. Confirm epidural placement with the use of a syringe and negative suction. There will be no CSF in the hub of the needle.

CESAREAN SECTION ANALGESIA AND ANESTHESIA PROTOCOLS IN SMALL MAMMALS
Stable Patient

Preoperative Drugs. The patient is sedated with midazolam IM, an IV catheter is placed and the animal is started on crystalloids. In some of the smaller mammals (eg, guinea pig, hedgehog), intravenous catheterization is difficult. Inhalant mask anesthesia will decrease the stress of this procedure. The ferret and guinea pig will need a small cut down (use 22-gauge needle bevel to make a hole at catheter entrance) to avoid burring the catheter on entering the skin. Bloodwork, radiographs

Table 1. Analgesic Drugs Used in Small Mammals

The following drug doses are those that are used by the authors in small mammals. Very few pharmacological studies have been done with regard to the listed drugs in the ferret and rabbit.

Drug	Pre-op Dose for Rabbit/Ferret	Induction Dose for Ferret/Rabbit	CRI Dose/Post-op for Rabbit/Ferret
Tranquillizers			
Diazepam	0.5 mg/kg IV		
Midazolam	0.25–0.5 mg/kg IM/IV		
Opioids			
Butorphanol	0.2–0.8 mg/kg SQ, IM or IV		0.1–0.2 mg/kg loading dose, then 0.1–0.2 mg/kg/hr
Fentanyl	5–10 µg/kg IV		Intraop: 5–20 µg/kg/hr w/ ketamine CRI Postop: 2.5–5 µg/kg/hr w/ ketamine CRI
Hydromorphone	0.05–0.1 mg/kg IV		0.05 mg/kg IV loading dose, then 0.05–0.1 mg/kg/hr
Tramadol			Post-op-10 mg/kg PO q 24 hr
NMDA Antagonists			
Ketamine		4–10 mg/kg IV	Intraop: 0.1 mg/kg IV loading dose, then 0.3–0.4 mg/kg/hr w/ fentanyl CRI Postop: 0.3–0.4 mg/kg/hr w/fentanyl CRI
Propofol		4–6 mg/kg IV	
Etomidate		1–2 mg/kg IV w/ benzodiazepine	
Alpha-2 agonists			
Medetomidine	1–2 µg/kg IM, IV		1–2 µg/kg q 4-6 hr IV
NSAIDs			
Carprofen			4 mg/kg PO q 24 hr
Ketoprofen			Postop 1–2 mg/kg q 24 hr
Meloxicam			0.2 mg/kg (first dose) SQ, IV, PO and then 0.1 mg/kg q 24 hr (rabbit 0.3 mg/kg q 24 hr)
Local Anesthetics			
Lidocaine			Local infiltration Introp: 1 mg/kg at incision site or ring block
Bupivicaine			Local infiltration Intraop/postop: 1 mg/kg at incision site or ring block
Epidurals			
Morphine preservative -free		0.1 mg/kg epidural w/ or w/o bupivacaine preop	
Bupivicaine 0.125%		0.1 mg/kg epidural w/ or w/o morphine	

and other diagnostics can be done at the same time. When an IV catheter can not be placed, the use of an IO catheter should be attempted.

Induction. Propofol or etomidate IV or intra-osseously (IO) and an epidural injection of morphine and bupivicaine is given.

Maintenance. The animal is intubated or masked and maintain on oxygen. A lidocaine/bupivacaine incisional block is performed. After the fetuses are removed the patient is started on isoflurane or sevoflurane inhalant. The patient is given buprenorphine or hydromorphone IV.

Postoperatively. One dose of NSAIDs can be given postoperatively and the animal may be sent home on tramadol (Table 1).

Critically Ill Surgical Patient

Prior to surgery any preoperative perfusion deficits are corrected. The small mammal is rehydrated over 6 to 8 hours. The animal is treated with sedative-analgesics (ie, opioid and midazolam) as required for pain during resuscitation. In some of the exotic patients, such as the guinea pig, intravenous catheters are difficult to place while they are conscious. They have short legs and pull away when the catheter is inserted into the skin. The mammal can be anesthetized with an inhalant using a mask. This will decrease the stress on the mammal. Blood pressure can be taken at that time. The mammal is taken off of anesthesia after catheter placement and stabilized on fluid therapy. Many critical mammals are hypothermic and will need heat support. When blood pressure is stabilized the mammal is taken to surgery.

Preoperative Drugs. One half hour prior to surgery the dose of the small mammal is given a preoperative loading dose of fentanyl IV along with ketamine microdose (1 to 2 mg/kg IV). A CRI of fentanyl and ketamine is prepared.

Induction. The animal is induced with etomidate (1–2 mg/kg) IV and midazolam (0.25 mg/kg) IV and intubated if possible, otherwise maintained on mask with inhalant. An epidural injection of morphine +/- bupivacaine can be used in the painful animal (Table 1).

Maintenance Anesthesia. The CRI of fentanyl and ketamine is started at the lower CRI dose (Table 1). The fentanyl/ketamine CRI requires that a loading dose of the drugs be given prior to starting the CRI (Table 1). The dose can be mixed with saline in a syringe. The CRI can be piggy-backed with a Y connector to the crystalloids and/or colloids being administered during surgery.

The animal is maintained on sevoflurane at the lowest possible concentration. Using the CRI of fentanyl/ketamine lowers the inhalant concentration. The maintenance isoflurane or sevoflurane is at 1 and 2 %, respectively. A lidocaine and bupivacaine incisional block is used (Table 1). Isotonic crystalloids (LRS, Plasma-Lyte® R, Normosol®R) are used as a constant rate infusion at 10 mL/kg/hr with colloids at 0.8 mL/kg/hr during surgery.

Hypotension during Surgery. If hypotension occurs during the surgery, the inhalant anesthesia is reduced first, while the CRI is increased. The animal should also be treated for hypovolemia if there is blood loss or fluid deficits are suspected until the blood pressure is normal. Checking blood glucose, PCV/TP and blood gas analysis intraoperatively is recommended. Monitoring devices such as the pulse oximeter, end tidal CO_2, temperature, ECG rhythm and rate are checked for abnormalities.

Postoperatively. Continue the CRI of fentanyl for 12 to 36 hours postoperatively or until the patient is stable. NSAIDs can be given if perfusion, hydration, gastrointestinal and renal function are normal.

CASE EXAMPLE: URINARY OBSTRUCTION IN A FERRET

This case is aimed at treatment of a critically ill ferret with UO (urinary obstruction) by correcting perfusion, dehydration, azotemia, electrolyte, acid–base abnormalities and placement of a urinary catheter. The use of percutaneous cystostomy tubes for patients in which urethral catheterization fails will also be discussed. Electrocardiogram and blood pressure monitoring are used for treatment of the ferret presenting with UO. Definitive treatment for adrenal gland disease and prostatomegaly are listed.

Diagnostic and treatment protocol for urinary obstruction in the ferret: (Note dosages used are listed in Table 1.)

1. Place an IV (intravenous) catheter using the cephalic or saphenous vessel.
2. Anesthesia for placement of a urinary catheter is always required in the ferret. The ferret is first given analgesia using butorphanol intravenous [IV]) or fentanyl IV. In the unstable cardiovascular patient, the author prefers etomidate IV with either diazepam IV or midazolam IV because of the minimal cardiovascular effects of these drugs. Other choices include a combination of: ketamine (5 mg/kg IV) with diazepam or midazolam IV or propofol (4–6 mg/kg IV) with diazepam or midazolam IV. Most ferrets should be intubated and maintained on isoflurane or sevoflurane for extended anesthesia time.
3. Heat support using a forced air warmer, heating pad or warm water bottles is required during the procedure. Due to small size, ferrets commonly become hypothermic under general anesthesia.
4. Monitoring

Electrocardiogram (ECG)

If hyperkalemia is present without an arrhythmia and perfusion is normal (ie, normal BP and heart rate), forced diuresis and relief of the obstruction is generally effective at correcting the potassium excess. Treat for hyperkalemia (as given below) if an arrhythmia is present. In the author's experience hyperkalemia is the most life threatening consequence of UO.

Hyperkalemia may result in ECG changes. These changes include loss of the P wave, widening of the QRS complex, peaked T wave, and a short QT interval; as the QRS and T waves merge, a sine wave is recognized. In the authors experience the severity of the ECG of hyperkalemia does not correlate with the magnitude of change in the plasma potassium level, and therefore treatment of hyperkalemia should be guided by monitoring the ECG with return of normal rhythm.

Treatment for Hyperkalemia

Calcium gluconate is given at a dose of 50 to 100 mg/kg slowly IV with continuous ECG monitoring. This antagonizes the membrane effects of hyperkalemia by decreasing the threshold potential and re-establishing the potential difference between resting membrane potential and threshold potential. This protects the myocardial muscle but does not decrease the serum potassium concentration. The effects will last about 20 to 30 minutes.

Regular insulin administered at a dose of 0.2 to 0.2 U/kg IV stimulates cell membrane sodium-potassium-adenosine triphosphatase and causes potassium to move intracellularly. Insulin administration should be followed by a glucose bolus of 1 to 2 g/U of regular insulin given to prevent hypoglycemia. This treatment should begin to lower potassium concentration and return of normal rhythm in 2 to 5 minutes. The ferret should be continued on a 2.5% dextrose solution in the IV fluids. Monitor blood glucose during the treatment to prevent hypoglycemia, which is of particular concern in the insulinomic ferret.

Doppler Blood Pressure

Correction of hypotension using crystalloids (15 mL/kg) and colloids (Hetastarch at 5 mL/kg) boluses are used once the obstruction is relieved and given below under fluid therapy.

Unblock the Urethra

- Relieve the obstruction by catheterization (eg, Slippery Sam, 3 French or red rubber, 3.5 French) and retropulsion with hydraulic forces using a sterile physiological solution. An indwelling catheter should be placed and sutured to the prepuce as discussed elsewhere. The catheter is connected to a closed collection system. If a catheter cannot be placed use of a percutaneous cystostomy tube is recommended. Cystocentesis is not recommended because it can lead to rupture of the urinary bladder and uroabdomen.
- Percutaneous cystostomy tube placement (prepubic catheterization)
  - Temporary cystostomy is performed to provide cutaneous urinary diversion in ferrets with urinary obstruction until definite treatment allows decrease in size of the prostate.
    - Make a small midline incision adjacent to the prepuce in male ferrets
    - Locate the bladder and place stay sutures and a purse-string into it
    - Place the tip of the Foley catheter (silicone, 5 French catheter) into the abdominal cavity through a separate incision in the abdominal wall. A second

incision for the catheter uses the tunneling effect principle; a better seal of catheter into the abdominal wall.

- Make a small stab incision within the purse-string suture (while suctioning the urine out of the bladder) and place the Foley catheter into the bladder lumen
- Inflate the balloon with saline and secure the catheter by tieing the purse-string suture around catheter
- Tack the bladder to the body wall with several absorbable sutures
- Close the initial incision and tack the catheter to the skin by placing sutures through a piece of tape attached to the catheter
- The catheter is removed after treatment is performed for prostatomegaly and the ferret is urinating on his own (usually requires 1 to 3 days). Catheter removal is performed by simply removing sutures in the skin, and deflating the foley catheter. The wound will heal by second intention.

Fluid Therapy

- Perfusion abnormalities (ie,, hypotension) are corrected first with crystalloids and colloids.
- Rehydration requirements are calculated by % dehydration and multiply by body weight in kilogrammes (5 kg cat that is 8% dehydrated will require 5 x 8/100 liters = 0.4 liters to correct the deficit). This should be administered over 6 hours. Output is measured every 1 to 2 hours once the animal is rehydrated. Output must be at least 1 to 2 mL/kg/hr, otherwise fluid input is adjusted with outflow during the diuresis phase. The fluids are adjusted by determining the urine produced and add the insensible loss (1 mL/kg/hour). Medical management for adrenal gland disease is initiated at this time. Fluids can be gradually discontinued when hydration and urine production are restored (fluids in and urine out are matched), correction of urinary obstruction takes place (ie, ferret is urinating normally), blood urea nitrogen, creatinine, acid–base and electrolytes are normal and patient is eating and drinking.
- If the clinician chooses surgical management for adrenal gland disease (given below), then surgery is performed only after hydration and urine production is restored (fluids in and urine out are matched), blood urea nitrogen, creatinine, acid–base, and electrolytes are normal. In the authors experience this requires about 24 to 36 hours for stabilizing the ferret prior to surgery.

Diagnostics

- Chemistry panel
  - Azotemia (ie, increased blood urea nitrogen, creatinine) is present in most cases of UO in the ferret and will be corrected with fluid therapy after relieving the obstruction.

- Acid-base and electrolytes
  - The most common abnormalities are metabolic acidosis and hyperkalemia. The hyperkalemia should be corrected immediately when electrocardiogram changes are present (as given above). The author uses fluid therapy to correct the metabolic acidosis.
- Urinalysis with culture and sensitivity since urinary tract infection often accompanies UO.
- Ultrasound to evaluate kidneys, bladder and prostate

Pain Relief and Sedation in the ICU

The author commonly uses the following drugs for sedation, pain relief and restraint (most ferrets will try to remove the percutaneous cystostomy tube without proper sedation and analgesia) after placement of the catheter.

- Narcotics
  - Butorphanol continuous rate infusion (CRI) at 0.025–0.1 mg/kg/hr
  - Fentanyl CRI at 2.5–5 µg/kg/hr
- Ketamine CRI (mix together with one of the narcotics) at 0.4–0.8 mg/kg/hr
- Tranquilizer such as diazepam/midazolam (0.25–0.5 mg/kg) as needed

TREATMENT FOR ADRENAL GLAND DISEASE

Treatment options for adrenocortical tumors are surgical removal/debulking, or medical management. Surgery offers the only potential cure for adrenal disease; however, local invasion of neoplasia of the right adrenal gland into the vena cava and the presence of ectopic adrenal tissue makes complete cure unlikely. Surgery is delayed until correction of electrolyte, acid/base, fluid and perfusion abnormalities. Medical treatment has not been proven to slow growth of the tumor, but can be effective in relieving clinical signs.

- **Adrenalectomy.** Techniques for adrenalectomy in the ferret have been described. In cases of secondary prostatic enlargement, it is important to collect biopsies and culture and sensitivities of prostate tissue.
- **Medical Management.** A number of drugs have been proposed for control of the symptoms related to adrenal disease, including leuprolide acetate (Lupron, TAP Pharmaceuticals) and melatonin. Other drugs are currently under investigation, including desorelin implants. Research currently supports Lupron as the most effective currently available drug for medical management of adrenal disease. A recent study indicated that while melatonin was effective in reversal of alopecia, effects were temporary in most cases (nine months).

REFERENCES

1. Lichtenberger M (ed): Emergency and Critical Care. Vet Clin North Am Exotic Anim Pract. 2007;10(2).
2. Ramer J, Benson K, Morrisey J, Obrien R, Paul-Murphy J. Effects of melatonin adinistration on the clinical course of adrenocortical disease in domestic ferrets. J Am Vet Med Assoc. 2006;229(11):1743-1748.

THE CRITICAL MAMMAL DISASTER: PART 2

Marla Lichtenberger, DVM, Diplomate ACVECC
Thousand Oaks Pet Emergency Clinic
Thousand Oaks, CA

Angela M. Lennox, DVM, Diplomate ABVP (Avian)
Avian and Exotic Animal Clinic of Indianapolis
Indianapolis IN

OVERVIEW OF GASTROINTESTINAL EMERGENCIES IN THE RABBIT

Gastric stasis is a common syndrome in rabbits and is characterized by anorexia and decreased to no stool production. Palpation often reveals gastrointestinal gas, and/or and enlarged food and hair packed stomach. There are many underlying disease conditions that can result in gastric stasis, including primary gastrointestinal disease, stress, or any conditions resulting in decreased food intake or anorexia. Gastrointestinal motility disorders and stasis are often directly caused or exacerbated by inappropriate diet. A secondary complication of decreased food intake is hepatic lipidosis, which can be difficult to reverse once established.

Pathophysiology of Gastric Motility Disorders

Rabbits are herbivores, and hindgut fermenters. Their digestive system is driven by the presence of fiber in the diet, which allows efficient digestion of the non-fiber portion of food. High-fiber diets stimulate cecocolic motility. Reduction in fiber content and/or increased carbohydrate consumption can decrease gastroenteric motility, leading to alterations in the cecal pH and disruption of the complex bacterial flora of the hindgut. Spore-forming anaerobes (in particular *Clostridium* sp) and coliforms such as *E. coli* multiply as the population of normal organisms decrease. This can lead to enterotoxemia, sepsis, and death.

The natural diet of the rabbit is high-fiber hay. Many commercial pelleted diets are lower in fiber, and can contain excessive carbohydrates in the form of grains and dried fruit. Some diets are designed for rapid growth in rabbits intended for food or fur, and are inappropriate for long-term optimal health of pet rabbits.

Differential Diagnosis for Gastric Stasis in the Rabbit

- Gastric or intestinal obstruction. True foreign body obstruction is rare in rabbits, but can be caused by hair or ingested foreign material such as carpeting or bedding. Rabbits present with an acute abdomen, characterized by pain, and gas accumulation. The rabbit is usually in shock. Radiographs may show a dilated, fluid-filled stomach or cecum, depending on the location of the obstruction. These patients must be treated for shock and stabilized prior to attempting surgical resolution. Decompression of the stomach may be required, and is accomplished by passage of a nasogastric tube. Post-surgical prognosis is reported to be poor.
- Gastrointestinal stasis secondary to other underlying disease processes
- Gastrointestinal stasis secondary to stress-related anorexia

Diagnostic Tests

1. Radiology may or may not be helpful in diagnosis of gastric stasis because the mass of food and hair may appear similar to normal ingesta. However, visualization of a large, ingesta-filled stomach in a rabbit that has been anorexic suggests the presence of gastric stasis. Small amounts of gas distributed throughout the gastrointestinal tract are usually normal; large accumulations of gas in the stomach, intestines or cecum are abnormal.

2. CBC and serum chemistries. A minimum database includes blood glucose, PCV/TP and BUN/creatinine, and should be performed as soon as possible to detect hypoglycemia secondary to anorexia, dehydration, azotemia, and anemia.

3. Dental evaluation (see comments on dental disease below):
   - Incisors are relatively easy to evaluate. The lower incisors should oppose the secondary incisor teeth (peg teeth), and the four primary incisors should be of normal length and shape.
   - Cheek teeth are more difficult to evaluate without general anesthesia. Initially an otoscope is used to evaluate the cheek teeth for the presence of gross abnormalities such as marked alterations to the occlusal plane (wavemouth, stepmouth, lingual or buccal points). It should be kept in mind that it is possible to miss dental lesions using this technique, and when patient condition allows, rabbits with suspected dental disease must be evaluated with a full oral exam under anesthesia and radiographs. Palpation of the mandible may reveal masses consistent with abscesses, or deviations in the ventral margin, suggesting mandibular tooth root disease. Skull radiographs under general anesthesia are required when dental disease is suspected. The minimal database for evaluation of the rabbit skull is lateral, ventrodorsal, and both right and left oblique views. Premedication with midazolam, followed by mask anesthesia with isoflurane and subsequent intubation is recommended. Alternatively, the author commonly uses propofol intravenously via a butterfly catheter (6 mg/kg IV) with or without gas anesthesia. Equipment designed for evaluation of the rabbit and rodent oral cavity are ideal, and include a variety of speculums, and cheek dilators. (Jorgenson Labs; Universal Surgical, www.universalsurgical.com).

Treatment

1. Discontinue any inappropriate antibiotics as ampicillin, amoxicillin, or clindamycin.

2. Begin fluid therapy. Correction perfusion abnormalities and dehydration (see fluid therapy of rabbits). Treat hypoglycemia when blood glucose is less than 70 mg/ml by adding 50% dextrose to fluids to produce a 2.5% dextrose solution. For cases of hypoglycemic seizure, treat with a 1:1 soluion of 50% dextrose with saline at 1 mL/kg IV. The author has also seen hyperglycemia in rabbits experiencing stress (up to 385 mg/dL). Most cases of hypoglycemia appear in rabbits that have been anorexic for greater than 2 to 3 days.

3. Begin nutritional support.

Syringe feeding. This procedure is appropriate for the mildly to moderately ill patient with adequate perfusion parameters and normal hydration. Critical Care herbivore diet (Oxbow Hay Company) is ideal for this purpose. Patients may be sent home with instructions for care, and directions for mixing and use are written on the product packaging. The tip of an oral feeding syringe is gently introduced into the diastema (the large space between the incisors and premolars) and food introduced as the rabbit swallows. Some rabbits willingly accept syringe feeding. Those that do not should be wrapped securely in a towel and fed as above. Syringe feedings is not recommended in severely debilitated rabbits, or those that strongly resist and show evidence of stress.

Feeding via nasogastric tube. This procedure is recommended for moderately to severely debilitated patients, or those who strongly resist or become stressed by syringe feeding. The nasogastric tube provides nutrition, and allows rehydration of firm stomach contents.

The author recommends a 5-8 French Argyle® tube (The Kendall Co). The length necessary to reach the stomach is determined by measuring from the tip of the nose to the last rib. A stylet is not recommended due to risk of perforation of the esophagus. Apply a drop of local anesthetic (2% lidocaine gel or ophthlamic anesthetic) into the rabbit's nostril. Restrain the rabbit carefully, ensuring protection of the back. An assistant flexes the head ventrally while the tube is passed ventrally and medially into the ventral meatus. The end of the tube is advanced until it enters into the stomach.

Verification of placement is determined radiographically.

Feeding procedure: A 35-mL syringe is used for slow bolus delivery of liquid diet. In the authors' experience most rabbits begin to eat and pass stool within 1 to 2 days. The tube can remain into place until the rabbit is eating and passing adequate stool. Options for feeding solutions include:

- Enteral nutrition (Herbivore Enteral Nutrition, Walk About Farms). This diet contains some fiber, though not enough to meet the needs of a rabbit requiring long term feeding (greater than 2 to 3 days) A 2-kg average adult rabbit requires approximately 175 Kcal/d. These needs can be met by feeding a mixture of 10 mL/kg of water and 7 mL/kg of fiber diet every 6 hours. The tube should be flushed with 5 to 6 mL of tap water after each feeding.

- Critical Care (Oxbow Hay Company). This diet is nutritionally complete, but will not pass through smaller bore catheters without first thoroughly grinding the diet in a commercial coffee grinder. It is advisable to test the ground diet through a similar bore tube before attempting to feed a rabbit with the tube in place.

- Gastrointestinal motility is induced with cisapride 0.5 mg/kg liquid suspension into the nasogastric tube every 8 hours. Cisapride is difficult to find commercially, but can be ordered through a compounding pharmacy.

- Pain or discomfort often requires the use of analgesics as butorphanol at 0.2 to 0.3 mg/kg IV, IM or SQ.

Plan correction of underlying dental disease (see comments below). The ultimate goal of dental treatment is to return the teeth to normal length and shape, and to treat secondary complications such as infection. The return of teeth to normal length and shape is best accomplished with a straight higher speed dental handpiece with a silicon or metal bur. Clipping teeth with a rongeur or similar instrument is not recommended due to risk of iatrogenic damage such as fracture of the reserve crown. These instruments cannot return the tooth to normal shape, and in fact may leave sharp, irregular occlusal surfaces.

Teeth that are loose or infected should be extracted. Treatment of dental abscesses are described in detail elsewhere. Broad spectrum antibiotics may be indicated after an invasive dental procedures. Commonly used choices include enrofloxacin at 5–15 mg/kg PO q12–24h, and trimethoprim sulfa at 15–20 mg/kg PO q12h. It should be noted dental abscesses and osteomyelitis are often complicated by the presence of anaerobic organisms. In these cases, injectable penicillin may be a better choice.

Dental Disease as an Underlying Cause of Gastric Stasis in Rabbits

Dental disease is common in pet rabbits. Disease may affect the incisors, cheek teeth, or both. Severely maloccluded incisors are often recognized by owners; however, disease of cheek teeth may produce more subtle clinical signs. More common presenting clinical signs include weight loss, decreased appetite or anorexia, ptyalism, teeth grinding and epiphora.

Disorders of the incisors can be primary (fracture, congenital jaw malformation and malocclusion), or secondary to disease and overgrowth of the cheek teeth. Disorders of the cheek teeth can be primary (fracture, elongation and malocclusion due to inappropriate wear as a result of inappropriate diet), or secondary to congenital malocclusion of incisors. Inappropriate wear and elongation of cheek teeth can also result from any condition resulting in reduction of normal jaw motion, such as infection and trauma.

Typical Clinical Findings
1. Anorexia for more than 2 days' duration.
2. Malocclusion identified on oral exam.
3. Weight loss in some rabbits.
4. Ptyalism and epiphora in some rabbits (maxillary incisors and maxillary cheek teeth are very close to the nasolacrimal duct) should make the clinician think of dental disease.
5. Gastric stasis suggested by the presence of a firm, doughlike mass palpable in the cranial region of the abdomen. Alternatively, gas may be palpable in the stomach or intestines.
6. Reduced production of fecal pellets. The stools passed are much smaller than normal or may contain hair.

OVERVIEW OF URINARY TRACT EMERGENCIES IN THE RABBIT

Differential Diagnosis
1. **Excretion of porphyrin pigments.** Both normal and diseased rabbits can produce urinary pigments that appear brown to dark red, which is often difficult to distinguish from blood.
2. **Uterine adenocarcinoma.** This is the most common neoplasm in the rabbit. It most often affects intact female rabbits greater than 3 years of age. A fluctuant, lobulated mass may be palpable in the caudal abdomen. Radiographs and abdominal ultrasound can help detect an abnormal uterus. Treatment is ovariohysterectomy, which can be curative if performed early in the course of the disease. Pre-surgical radiographs of the thorax should be performed to screen for metastasis to the lungs.
3. **Cystitis.** Diagnosis is based on culture of urine collected via cystocentesis. Treatment is based on sensitivity results, but care must be taken to avoid drugs contraindicated in the rabbit, for example erythromycin and oral penicillins. Cystitis can accompany urolith disease.
4. **Urolithiasis.** This disease is common in rabbits, and the exact cause is uncertain. Rabbits normal excrete calcium via the urinary tract, and the presence of calcium "sand" in the urine can be a normal finding. This must be distinguished from distinct uroliths, which may be present in the urethra, bladder, ureters or kidneys. The accumulation of large amounts of calcium crystal in the urine (bladder sludge) can be a consequence of dehydration, poor diet and lack of exercise.

Diagnostic Tests
1. CBC and chemistry panel.
2. Complete urinalysis
3. Abdominal radiographs
4. Ultrasound

Treatment
Urolithiasis. Urinary tract disorders such as cystitis and urolithiasis can result in hematuria and should be diagnosed as in small animals. The exact cause is unknown, but may be partly due to diets high in calcium (eg, alfalfa). Some rabbits have a moderate amount of calciuria that should not be confused with discrete calculi on radiographs and ultrasound. Treatment is surgical and since underlying etiology is uncertain, it is unclear whether or not dietary modification is likely to aid in prevention. There is considerable debate over the role of dietary calcium in formation of uroliths in the rabbit.

Pyelonephritis. Commonly seen in middle to older aged guinea pigs. The symptoms include dysuria and hematuria that sometimes require long-term antibiotics. A culture and sensitivity of the urine should be done in order for selection of the appropriate antibiotic.

Bladder sludge in rabbits is secondary to poor diet, decreased exercise, and fat. Sludge causes bladder detrusor muscle atony.

- Treatment
  - Uropropulsion
  - IV fluid diuresis
  - Bladder manual expression

REFERENCES
1. Harcourt-Brown F. Textbook of Rabbit Medicine. Elsevier Science Limited. 2002.
2. Capello V, Gracis M, Lennox AM (ed): Rabbit and Rodent Dentistry Handbook. Zoological Education Network. Blackwell Publishing, 2005.
3. Lichtenberger M (ed): Exotic animal practice. Vet Clin North Am Exotic Pet Pract. 2007;10(2).

INTERPRETING THE CHEMISTRY PROFILE IN FERRETS

Joerg Mayer, Dr.vet.med., MSc
School of Veterinary Medicine
Tufts University, North Grafton, MA

While the ferret is not considered to be a particularly exotic pet and in general its clinical medicine is very similar to feline clinical medicine, the interpretation of the ferret chemistry profile deserves special attention as there can be several pitfalls if ferret profiles are interpreted by comparing with cat or dog normal values. This article focuses on some of the most important clinical pathology parameters and their interpretation.

As in other species, an exact diagnosis of a clinical problem should never be based on blood work alone, but should include an evaluation of other diagnostic tools such as biopsies. One abnormal parameter is rarely pathognomic for a problem, and often two or three clinical pathology parameters need to be assessed in order to better locate the potential origin of the clinical problem, especially if it is subclinical. If several different parameters are significantly altered, a preliminary diagnosis can be with a high degree of certainty and then pursued with further diagnostics. Further diagnostics approaches, eg, biopsies, should be recommended. The lecture presents clinical cases, which highlight the need to harvest biopsies early on in the diagnostic process in order to come to a definitive diagnosis and to establish an accurate treatment plan early on.

Recommended reading for a detailed discussion on GI and liver diseases of ferrets includes the chapter "Ferret gastrointestinal and hepatic diseases" in the new edition of *Ferret Husbandry, Medicine and Surgery*[2] or the 2006 American Ferret Association (AFA) proceedings.[1]

PARAMETERS TO EVALUATE DIFFERENT ORGAN FUNCTION

Pancreas
- **Glucose**
  - Normal values 90–200 mg/dL
  - An extremely important parameter, as insulinoma is the most common form of cancer affecting the ferret in the US
    - Extremely common in ferrets older then 4 years; blood glucose should be checked at least once a year
  - Care has to be taken when using a human glucosometer as these devices will artificially read out lower values then the true value, usually 15–20 mg/dL lower)
    - In addition, the (in)accuracy of these units is around 20 mg/dL
  - The fasting glucose (4- to 6-hr fast) should be between 90–120 mg/dL
  - If animal has been fasting for longer periods of time, the glucose will be low and is not considered diagnostic for insulinoma
  - If the animal has eaten within the last 4 hours and the glucose is below 90 mg/dL (< 60 mg/dL on the human glucometer) this is diagnostic for insulinoma
  - Blood glucose alone is diagnostic for insulinoma; no other parameters need to be taken into consideration
  - Repeated levels above 350 mg/dL might indicate diabetes mellitus (rare in my experience)
    - It can also develop after a partial pancreactomy was performed.

Liver
- **ALT (Alanine Aminotransferase)**
  - Liver specific in ferrets (not in rabbits!) is released when liver cells are damaged. Activity in liver is 3–10 times higher than in other tissues (in ferret)
    - Normal value 80–290 IU/L
    - High normal value than in other species
    - Steroids can increase ALT very fast.
    - Hepatic lipidosis, lymphocytic hepatitis, other forms of hepatitis often produce:
      - Up to 800 mg/dL
      - With alkaline phosphatase (ALP) up to 100 mg/dL
      - Increase in aspartate aminotransferase (AST) as well
      - Same occurs in gastritis
    - Careful when diagnosing primary liver disease on blood work alone
    - Check for increased billirubin, low total protein and icterus
    - Suggest biopsy in order to characterize liver lesion
      - Lymphocytic hepatitis
      - Suppurative hepatitis
      - Vacuolar hepathopathy
      - Hepatic lipidosis
      - Cirrhosis
      - Hepatic neoplasia
      - Billiary cystadenoma

- **Gamma Glutamyltransferase (GGT)**
  - The biliary system is the primary source of plasma GGT. In addition to biliary GGT, significant levels of renal epithelial GGT can be found in the urine
  - Normal around 5 IU/L
  - Over 10 IU/L high index of suspicion for liver problems
    - Need to differentiate nature of elevation
    - Recommend abdominal ultrasound +/- ultrasound-guided biopsy of liver to rule out primary liver pathology
    - Liver involvement is sometimes secondary to ascending inflammation from gut

- Suggest exploratory with multiple biopsies (GI tract, liver, lymph node)

Kidney
- **Blood Urea Nitrogen (BUN)**
  - BUN measures the amount of urea nitrogen, a waste product of protein metabolism, in the blood.
  - Normal range 10–40 mg/dL
  - I consider BUN a relatively insensitive test for evaluating renal disease in ferrets due to:
  - Pre-renal factors influencing the BUN in ferrets include
    - High-protein diet
    - Tendency to develop gastric ulcers very fast
  - Post-renal elevations include urinary tract problems such as
    - Urinary obstructions.
    - Infections (prostatitis, etc.)
    - Often due to adrenal disease!!
  - Might go up to 200–300 mg/dL with normal or mildly elevated creatinine
  - Drug interaction
    - Drugs such as steroids or NSAIDs may cause GI ulcers, therefore increasing the BUN value
    - Levels have been shown to decrease with the administration of diuretics, aminoglycosides, amphotericin B, and chloramphenicol (not a ferret-specific fact)

- **Creatinine**
  - Creatinine is a nitrogenous waste product produced by the breakdown of creatine, which is an important part of muscle. A serum creatinine test measures the amount of creatinine in the blood and is an indirect indicator of renal glomerular filtration rate and can estimate renal function.
  - It has been demonstrated that creatinine is an insensitive indicator of renal failure in ferrets perhaps related to their capacity for **extrarenal** elimination of creatinine. Ferrets also have a considerably lower and narrower range of creatinine in the blood than other mammals.
  - Narrow range at normal 0.2–0.6 mg/dL
  - Is considered relatively insensitive as an indicator of renal failure
  - The normal creatinine level averages approximately half the level of the dog and cat
  - If > than 0.8 mg/dL, then renal suspect
    - Elevations of BUN up to 300 mg/dL have been seen with a mild increase of creatinine. to 2–3 mg/dL
    - Three-fourths of renal function must be lost before abnormalities in creatinine concentration are seen
    - In contrast to BUN, creatinine is not influenced by diet or GI ulcers

- Lab artifacts
  - Elevated levels: False-high serum test values can result when using Jaffe's reaction, a chromogen color reaction when the sample contains non-creatinine chromagens, such as ketones, glucose, fructose, ascorbic acid, protein, urea, and ascorbic acid
  - Decreased levels: Creatinine deteriorates in plasma samples older than 24 hours leading to unreliable results. Bilirubin can also cause sampling errors.
- **Phosphorus, Calcium, Potassium**
  - These three parameters can be used to assess renal function in conjunction with BUN and creatinine
  - Suspect true renal failure if:
    - Phos > 10 mEq/L AND
    - Cal < 8 mg/dl AND
    - Potas > 6 mEq/L

Gastrointestinal Tract
- **Lipase**
  - Enzyme that breaks down triglycerides into monoglycerides and free fatty acids
  - Normal values 0–200 U/L
  - While in other species, lipase is primarily produced in the pancreas, with a small amount being produced by the gastric mucosa, it appears that the ferret produces more lipase in the stomach than in the pancreas
    - Therefore, elevations of lipase appear more diagnostic for GI problems than for pancreatic problems.
  - Elevated if > 500 IU/L from commercial labs or > 1000 IU/L from the IDEXX Vet-test)
  - Significant elevation most commonly seen cases of mild to severe GI disease like inflammatory bowel disease (IBD) and/or eosinophilic granulomatous disease
    - Check globulin for evaluation as well
    - Run CBC to check for peripheral eosinophilia
  - In my opinion, lipase is one of the most commonly underused clinical pathology parameters
  - Steroids will increase lipase levels in other species (dogs, etc)
    - Most likely in ferrets as well.
- **Globulin**
  - Globulins are proteins that are mostly involved the immune defense system. Any protein that is not albumin is classified as a globulin
  - Normal values 2–2.9 mg/dL
  - Often elevated with chronic inflammatory conditions such as IBD
    - Check lipase for elevation in cases of IBD

- Most confirmed cases of IBD have high levels (> 3–5 mg/dL)
- Consider Aleutian disease if elevation goes beyond 6 mg/dL
- Increases in dehydration
- Decreased globulins are generally the result of decreased production (ie, liver failure) or increased loss
- Lipase and globulin should always be interpreted with each other to check for signs of IBD
- I usually recommend GI biopsies to diagnose IBD in these cases
- It has been speculated that chronic unmanaged cases of IBD might develop into GI lymphoma
- Potential laboratory error: Globulin levels are often calculated by subtracting albumin from the total protein. Any error in the measurements of albumin or total protein will give you erroneous globulin levels

REFERENCES

1. Burgess M. Gastrointestinal and hepatic diseases. In: A Comprehensive Veterinary Symposium, Advanced Course. Management of the Ferret. AFA Meeting, Pittsburgh, Pennsylvania. 2006, pp 79-97 (order online at www.ferret.org).
2. Lewington J. Ferret Husbandry, Medicine and Surgery, 2nd ed. St. Louis, MO: Saunders/Elsevier, 2007.
3. Hamosh M, Henderson TR, Hamosh P. Gastric lipase and pepsin activities in the developing ferret: nonparallel development of the two gastric digestive enzymes. J Pediatr Gastroenterol Nutr. 1998;26(2): 162-166.

SURGICAL TECHNIQUES FOR SPAYING RABBITS AND RATS

Joerg Mayer, Dr.med.vet., MSc
School of Veterinary Medicine
Tufts University, North Grafton, MA

RABBITS
Indications
- Intact females have a high rate of uterine adenocarcinoma , as high as 80% by age 3 years and older
  - Very high incidence of systemic metastasis (mainly lung and liver)
- Intact females are impossible to keep together due to constant fighting
- High reproductive rate
  - Females can conceive within 24 hours post partum

Anatomy
- The vaginal body is very long and more flaccid than in other species.
- The vagina fills with urine during micturition.
- Two cervices (bicornute cervix or cervix duplex) are present as normal anatomy.
- The ovarian vessels are very well developed.
- The bladder receives a branch from the uterine artery.
- The uterine horns and the uterine blood vessels are often encased in large amounts of fat, especially in older females.
- The large intestine, especially the cecum, is in close proximity to the surgery site.

Preparation
- All forms of stress should be avoided prior to surgery
  - House rabbit in a quiet ward
  - Avoid barking dogs
  - Try not to house a ferret directly next to a rabbit
  - Avoid olfactory or direct visual contact between the rabbit patient and prey species
- In older intact rabbits, do perform radiographs and/or an ultrasound exam prior to surgery to check for subclinical uterine neoplasia or metastasis.
- Ideally a CBC and a chemistry panel should be run prior to anesthesia.
- Ensure that the doe is optimally hydrated:
  - Maintenance fluids are approximately 120 mL/kg/day

Procedure
- Generally very similar to a cat spay. Approach by ventral midline incision
- Make a 1- to 2-inch incision between umbilicus and pubis
  - Make incision closer to umbilicus as ovarian ligaments are not 'stretchable'
- Cervices will be visible immediately in the incision

- Do NOT use spay hooks of any kind
- Avoid manipulation of GI tract at all costs.
- Follow uterine horn cranially to ovary
- Ovary is extremely small in relation to uterine horn, and yellow
  - Left ovary is close to kidney
- Identify ovarian artery and ligate immediately
  - Hemoclips will speed procedure up
- Bluntly dissect along uterine horn
  - Radiocauthery can be used on smaller uterine vessels
- Repeat procedure on other side
- In young animals transection of uterine horn can be made cranial to cervix
  - Will leave cervix behind and may provide an additional barrier against bacterial contamination from vagina
- In older animals remove cervices completely
- Transection is performed in vagina (ovario-vagino-hysterectomy)
  - Reduces the chance of a subclinical uterine cancer in remnant tissue
- Close incision in a three-layer fashion
  - Use an intradermal suture pattern

Follow-up
- Make sure animal is eating, urinating and defecating

Possible Complications
- Intestinal adhesions
  - Fibrin clots
- Ligation of a ureter
- Leakage of urine from vaginal stump
  - If cervix is completely removed
- Uterine cancer in the residual tissue
  - If cervices are not removed

RATS
Indications
- Intact females have a high incidence of mammary cancer (adenoma/adenocarcinoma)
  - As high as 66% by about 2 years of age (21 months)
  - Spayed rats have a significantly lower rate of mammary cancer.
  - If mammary cancer develops it usually has a low incidence of systemic metastasis (eg, lung and liver)
- High reproductive rate
  - Note: Intact female hamsters normally have a vaginal discharge
    - Often mistaken for pyometra

Anatomy
- The ovaries are located caudal to the kidneys in a large fat pad
- The uterine horn wraps around the ovary
- The ovarian vessels are not well developed
- The ovarian ligament is very long and the ovary is easily exteriorized

Preparations
- Evaluate patient thoroughly for subclinical forms of respiratory disease or heart disease in older animals (over 2 years old)
- Ideally a minimal screen (hematocrit, total solids, blood glucose and blood urea nitrogen) should be run prior to anesthesia
- Make sure animal is optimally hydrated
  - Maintenance is approximately 100 mL/kg/day

Procedure
Ventral Approach
- Very similar to cat spay
- Approach by ventral midline incision
- Make a 1-inch incision between umbilicus and pubis
- The cervix will be immediately visible in the incision
- Follow uterine horn cranially to ovary
- Identify vessels in mesovarium and ligate
  - Hemoclips will speed procedure up, otherwise use 5-0 Maxon or PDS
- Bluntly dissect along uterine horn
  - Radiocauthery can be used on smaller uterine vessels
- Repeat procedure on other side
- In all animals transection of uterine horn can be made cranial to cervix
- Will leave cervix behind and may provide an additional barrier against bacterial contamination from vagina
- Close in a two- or three-layer fashion
  - Use an intradermal suture pattern
  - Apply lidocaine to suture site to decrease frequency of self-mutilation

Dorsal Approach
- Developed in lab animal medicine where ovariectomy is a common procedure
- Ovaries and part of the uterine structures can be accessed dorsally
- A dorsal approach offers a number of advantages to the ventral approach
  - Less invasive
  - Less painful
  - Smaller incision
  - Less likely to see postsurgical incision complications due to self-mutilation or contamination with soiled bedding material
- Make a half-inch skin incision on midline, directly over the spinal column, between the last rib and pelvis.
- The skin incision can then be moved to the left or right side about 1 cm lateral to the spinal processes to access the body wall.
- Move the skin incision laterally to one side and bluntly dissect through the body wall.
- A large fat deposit is usually seen when dissecting through the body wall and the ovary sits within this fatty tissue.
- Exteriorize the ovary and the uterine horn and place a hemoclip around the uterine horn prior to excising it.
- The body wall can be closed with a 5-0 Maxon or PDS or can be left open.
- Repeat the procedure on opposite side.
- Close skin with an intradermal suture pattern.

Follow-up
- Make sure animal is eating, urinating, and defecating.
- Recheck suture site frequently.
- Keep separate from other cage mates, as they sometimes 'groom' suture out.

Common Complications
- Suture removal by animal
- Inadequate pain management often responsible for self-mutilation

REFERENCES
1. Capello V. Surgical techniques for neutering the female pet rabbit. Exotic DVM. 2005;(7.5):15.
2. Johnson-Delaney C. Ovariohysterectomy in a rat. Exotic DVM. 2002;(4.4):17.

ADVANCED DIAGNOSTIC IMAGING IN EXOTIC MAMMALS

Joerg Mayer, Dr.med.vet., MSc
School of Veterinary Medicine
Tufts University, North Grafton, MA

While standard radiographic and ultrasound imaging techniques are common diagnostic tools in exotic animal medicine, the use of more advanced imaging techniques such as computed tomography (CT) and magnetic resonance imaging (MRI) currently appear to be underutilized for exotic patients. Although radiographs are often considered the first choice for the initial imaging modality in the exotic patient, very often a second imaging technique is needed, especially in cases where the clinical signs suggest a condition for which radiographs may not produce adequate imaging to rule out the suspected problem, eg, a gastrointestinal blockage due to a plastic foreign body. It is therefore often useful to combine different imaging modalities in order to improve the accuracy of the diagnosis and ensure that the limitations of one imaging modality are overcome by a second mode of imaging.

ULTRASOUND

Ultrasound is considered a standard diagnostic approach in traditional pet species, and should be more commonly used in exotic species. New publications are appearing every year highlighting the significant diagnostic benefits of this tool for soft tissue imaging. Ultrasound should be considered for every pathologic process that might have a soft tissue component. In addition, in dogs, cats, and large animals, US can also be used to assess for osteomyelitis, bone involvement of soft tissue tumors, assess fracture healing, or to guide biopsies. The noninvasive character, as well as the ability to obtain real-time images with magnification and to assess blood flow using color and spectral Doppler, make this tool truly indispensable. The most common uses of ultrasound as an imaging technique include documentation of pregnancy; monitoring of the reproductive cycle; evaluation of the internal organs for shape, size, architecture, and homogeneity; echocardiography; and as a guide for invasive techniques such as Tru-cut biopsies or fine needle aspirates. Ultrasound images allow visualization of small details that might not be seen in survey radiographs. For example, small (<3 mm), bladder stones that can cause significant urinary tract problems in the guinea pig, may not be visible on plain radiographs even though they are radiodense. For this reason it is advisable to routinely perform ultrasound examinations on small mammals showing signs of urinary tract disease that have negative findings on radiographic images.

The two major disadvantages of ultrasound are the inability to completely image bony structures, and the fact that the ultrasound waves will not travel through air, making it difficult to examine birds, because of their air sacs, or mammals with large amounts of gas in the GI tract, eg, herbivores. However, imaging of the surface of normal bony structures (or deeper bony structures in cases of disruption due to neoplasia or infection) is sometimes possible.

COMPUTED TOMOGRAPHY

While traditional radiographic images are easily obtained in almost every clinic, accessibility to CT scanners is less common, although they are becoming more available. While the actual CT image is produced by traditional x-rays, the process of acquiring it is dynamic. The x-rays are passed through the patient in a full 360-degree circle by rotating the x-ray producing tube, with the x-ray detectors positioned opposite, around the patient. As the x-rays pass through the patient, they experience differential attenuation based on the density of tissues they encounter along their path. Contrast in a CT image is based upon this differential attenuation. Radiolucent tissues, such as air-filled structures, attenuate fewer x-rays and appear darker, while more radiodense tissues, eg, bone or metal, attenuate more x-rays and appear whiter. The dynamically acquired images can then be visualized as variably sized slices or summed to provide reconstructions in various planes. One of the downfalls of CT is the significantly higher amount of radiation experienced by the patient compared with that of traditional radiography. In order to obtain information regarding dynamic processes in the body, intravenous iodinated contrast media, eg, iodine, can be used to improve the contrast between different body tissues. With the addition of specialized software, a 3D model of the animal or lesion can be created in order to demonstrate the spatial correlation of pathologic processes. This tool has significant benefit for accessing a mass or structure when planning radiation treatment or surgery.

The average time to obtain a scan in a modern CT unit is about 10 minutes, and the patient needs to be anesthetized to prevent blurring due to movement. When contrast is used, the scan is repeated, effectively doubling the time of anesthesia. From start to finish, a complete session usually requires the patient to be under general anesthesia for approximately 45 minutes.

The most significant advantage of CT images over traditional radiographs is the fact that each slice, which can be as thin as 1 mm, provides superior information about the tissue in question over traditional radiographs due to the fact that no superimposition of tissues hinders the interpretation. In addition, images obtained from the CT scan can always be modified later, and also maintain the original 3D character of the structures imaged. The most significant disadvantages of the CT scan over traditional radiographs are the increased costs associated with the imaging, less accessibly to the equipment, and the need for prolonged anesthesia during the scan.

One of the most useful applications of CT scans is in the diagnosis of dental problems in small mammals. The benefit here lies in the ability to completely assess the involvement of tooth, tooth root and surrounding structures such as the mandible or the maxilla in the problem. Very often important information about the relationship of the teeth and their environment gets lost in traditional radiographs due to superimposition of structures encountered in a two-dimensional image. In general, a CT scan provides excellent images of all bony structures. With 1-mm-thick slices of the skull, small fractures are easily appreciated. Subtle bony lysis of turbinates due to chronic upper respiratory tract infections, abnormalities of the tympanic bulla cavities due to chronic ear infections, and even skull tumors can easily be detected and assessed, all of which might not be easily appreciated with traditional radiographs.

Similar to ultrasonography as an adjunct to radiography, CT scans are an equally valuable modality for imaging small changes that cannot be seen with traditional radiographs. CT should be considered especially when lung metastases are suspected in cancer patients. Radiographs will often miss even large numbers of small nodules, which will become immediately apparent on a CT scan.

Evaluation of the brain parenchyma is also significantly better on CT scan than with radiographs, and so, a CT scan should be recommended for any pathologies involving the head, including trauma. The abdomen should also be scanned in cases where an abdominal ultrasound exam was inconclusive. The application of CT scans in neurology cases are of interest when imaging the spinal canal or in head trauma cases due to superior image contrast over radiography, and the fact that even critical patients can undergo this relatively short procedure in comparison to an MR scan. The use of iodine intravenous contrast material can enhance and differentiate between cystic or solid lesions as well as gain an idea of vascularity or aggressiveness of a lesion, eg, tumors, and to document physiological processes such as elimination via the kidneys.

MAGNETIC RESONANCE IMAGING (MRI)

MR images are obtained by placing the animal into a very strong magnetic field (up to 100,000 times stronger than the earth's magnetic field) and visualizing the movement of the hydrogen atoms in the body in reaction to the magnetic field changes. This is obviously an oversimplification of a very complicated process, but the imaging therefore does not require any radiation or other form of ionizing rays, and is non-invasive making obtaining the image relatively risk-free.

An MRI scan is the diagnostic imaging modality of choice for neurologic problems since MR images of the central nervous system (CNS) are of superior quality to CT images. The second largest practical use of MRI scans is in the imaging of certain soft tissues such as joints and muscles. As with CT scans, the use of contrast material (Gadolinium) can be used intravenously to make interpretation of the images more diagnostically valuable. Use of contrast material is considered a routine procedure for MRI scans in order to compare pre- and post-contrast images, while the use of contrast with CT scans is considered to be elective.

While the image quality of the MRI scan is superior to any other imaging modality, there are significant disadvantages associated with this procedure. While the images of the neurologic tissues are significantly better with MR, the prolonged scanning time compared with a CT scan, which produces less detailed images, prevents the MR scan from being the imaging modality of choice for critical neurological patients. Very often a CT scan is preferred for unstable patients due to the speed of the procedure, and therefore, less anesthetic time. In addition to the longer scan time, the costs associated with MR are also much higher than for a CT scan. In addition, the local availability of MR scanners is often less than with CT. However, because MR scanners are becoming physically smaller, and less expensive, they are now being installed in many referral centers.

When scanning very small exotic patients such as small rabbits or rats, care must be taken to check with the radiologist about the resolution of the image obtained with the available magnet to see if the procedure will result in a diagnostic image of the tissue of interest. A MR scanner equipped with a magnet of 1.3 Tesla field strength appears to be suitable to image the brain of smaller mammals such as small rabbits or ferrets. However, 'weaker' magnets with a field strength of only 0.2 to 0.4 Tesla will have significantly less resolution. Larger field strengths have a larger signal to noise ratio permitting not only higher resolution images, but faster scan times. Scan times have been significantly reduced with new sequences and higher field strengths so that length of scan time is becoming less problematic This is similar to a camera taking pictures with 1 mega-pixel or 6 mega-pixels resolution. These images may not have enough resolution to be diagnostically useful in the smaller patients.

OTHER "NEW" MODALITIES

While CT and MR imaging modalities are not new to human medicine or traditional pet medicine by any means, their use in exotic or nontraditional pets is vastly underutilized. In addition, other imaging modalities exist which may have value in exotic patients. CT and MR scanners combined with other specific equipment can be used to detect and trace radioactive material as it is injected into the patient, eg, **positron emission tomography (PET) scans**, and have been used in some cases to diagnose clinical problems in exotic patients. PET scans are also being used to assess pain in birds. Scintigraphy is an additional imaging modality and its use has recently been used by the author in the diagnosis of hyperthyroidism in a Guinea pig. In addition, the use of **thermography** in the early detection of rabies in a raccoon was recently published. At Tufts University we are currently experimenting with the clinical application of thermography as a clinical tool in exotic animal medicine.

Without a doubt, advanced imaging techniques in exotic pets are becoming more and more popular. It is in the best interest of the patient, the client, and the veterinarian to be aware of these different modalities, and to recognize their applications and limitations in order to integrate them successfully into the routine workup of challenging cases.

REFERENCES

1. Souza MJ, Greenacre CB, Jones MP, Hadley TL, Adams WH, Avenell JS, Wall JS, Daniel GB. Clinical use of microPET and CT imaging in birds. Proc Annu Conf Assoc of Avian Vet. 2006, pp 13-16.
2. Paul-Murphy J, Sladky KK, McCutcheon RA, et al. Using positron emission tomography imaging of the parrot brain to study response to clinical pain. Proc AAZV, AAWV, AZA/NAG Joint Conf. 2005, pp 140-141.
3. Dunbar M, Maccarthy KA. Use of infrared thermography to detect signs of rabies infection in raccoons (*Procyon lotor*). J Zoo Wildlife Med. 2006;37:518-523.

ANNOYING RESPIRATORY TRACT DISEASES IN RATS

Joerg Mayer, Dr.med.vet., MSc
School of Veterinary Medicine
Tufts University, North Grafton, MA

Chronic respiratory tract infection is a common clinical presentation in rats of all ages. Very often treatment fails to alleviate the clinical signs, or provides only temporary relief due to a variety of reasons. Very commonly the respiratory signs are caused by a mixture of pathogens including both bacteria and viruses. The sialodacryoadenitis virus (SDA) is a virus commonly involved in causing respiratory signs in young rats, whereas adult rats are often symptomless carriers. The SDA virus is a coronavirus that affects both lacrimal and salivary glands, as well as the upper respiratory epithelium, causing respiratory signs. In these cases the clinical signs usually only last for about 3 weeks, and the affected animals recover spontaneously. Clinical improvement is often erroneously attributed to the antibiotics given. Other viruses causing clinical signs in adult animals include Sendai virus, which is a parainfluenza virus; rat parvovirus; pneumonia virus of mice, which is a paramyxovirus; and hantavirus, which has been associated with human deaths. These viruses are just one of the many reasons why this clinical condition is often not controlled by antibiotics.

One of the most commonly discussed pathogens associated with chronic respiratory tract infections in rats is *Mycoplasma pulmonis*. Unfortunately, this pathogen is extremely difficult to treat, and in most cases, the animal cannot be cured because the organism cannot be completely eliminated from the body. *Mycoplasma* can cause a significant granulomatous response in the lower respiratory tract and cause respiratory distress due to mechanical problems in addition to the inflammatory response. Radiographs can often visualize these granulomas and help determine the prognosis.

Very often chronic respiratory tract problems are secondary to inappropriate husbandry set-ups. Use of enclosures without adequate air circulation, such as an aquarium, combined with infrequent cleaning of the droppings and the urine, will lead to an increase in the ammonia concentration at the bottom of the enclosure. Ammonia fumes are extremely caustic to the respiratory tract tissue, and therefore predispose the animal to chronic respiratory tract disease.

Treatment of chronic respiratory tract disease cases is often unrewarding since the disease is frequently caused by both a combination of viral and bacterial pathogens and environmental problems. Antibiotics most often used are enrofloxacin, alone, or in combination with tetracyclines. Enrofloxacin (Baytril) is effective in treating lower respiratory tract bacteria, and tetracycline has the added benefit of exhibiting an anti-inflammatory activity in addition to being an antibiotic. Obtaining an anti-inflammatory effect this way is preferable to exposing the animal to large doses of steroids over a prolonged time. While in some cases steroids might decrease the respiratory signs in an affected animal, the side effects of these drugs, eg, immune suppression, are often serious and so their use is not beneficial to the animal in the long term, and the use of steroids should be avoided whenever possible.

Unfortunately, in many cases, large masses filled with pus are already present in the lungs before presentation, making the antimicrobial treatment minimally effective. In order to reach a high enough concentration of the antibiotic in the lower respiratory tract to be effective, nebulization therapy can be used in addition to oral or injectable drug therapy. Care must be taken to select a nebulizer, which produces a small enough particle size (<3 microns) to reach the alveolar space. The use of bronchodilators, eg, aminophylline, can be used during the nebulization session or given orally since very often animals affected with chronic respiratory tract problems have breathing difficulties due to severe bronchospasm as a sequel to the chronic inflammatory processes. When using nebulization treatments it is also helpful to decrease the mucus producing biofilm that often covers the respiratory tract and prevents the drugs from contact with functional tissue. Hypertonic saline (9%) used in the nebulizer will break down the biofilm and its use will very often show significant benefits.

No matter what treatment options are used, it is important to communicate with the owner about the possible etiology, especially husbandry issues, and the chronic and often lifelong nature of the problem. An educated owner will be able to avoid future problems relating to husbandry and will better understand the often poor response to treatment.

EXTRACTION OF INCISORS IN RABBITS

Joerg Mayer, Dr.med.vet., MSc
School of Veterinary Medicine
Tufts University, North Grafton, MA

INDICATIONS

The most common indication for the extraction of incisors in rabbits is malocclusion. This is often due to trauma or due to congenital problems. However, other causes, such as malocclusion due to molar teeth pathology or abnormal chewing, are possible. Cutting an elongated tooth with a tool such as a nail cutter carries a large potential to damage the incisor teeth. The teeth might be permanently damaged and need to be extracted as well as the opposing teeth. The use of instruments to cut teeth in rabbits is therefore not recommended.

INSTRUMENTATION

Specialized instruments (ie, Crossley luxator) for the removal of incisor teeth (and molar teeth) exist and can be ordered through veterinary supply catalogues (eg, www.universalsurgical.com). Many people successfully use an 18-gauge needle as an elevator/luxator instead of or in combination with specialized equipments.

The author recommends using inhalation anesthesia and having the animal intubated in order to avoid aspiration and to be able to keep the animal anesthetized safely for the entire length of the procedure. Using a facemask to deliver the inhalation gas is not recommended due to the requirement to access the upper incisors without interference from the mask.

PROCEDURE

The author prefers to start with the extraction of the lower incisors as these teeth are easier removed in comparison with the upper ones. Initially, the surgery site is cleaned with a disinfectant such as Betadine solution on a cotton tip applicator; then a scalpel blade or a hypodermic needle is used to separate the periodontal ligaments from the tooth. This process requires the deep insertion of the needle or blade between the gingival and the tooth. The separation of the ligaments has to be done very thoroughly and needs to be performed 360 degrees around the tooth. It is important not to rush through this step as the successful completion of the following steps requires a complete separation of the ligaments from the tooth. After the ligaments have been loosened, the Crossley luxator is inserted between the two teeth and the gingiva to continue the separation and

to break the remaining fibers. The luxator is inserted and careful pressure is applied to move the teeth medially and laterally from different insertion points (medially and laterally). The tooth should be moved slowly but with a certain amount of force. Once the tooth is moved to the side, it is best to keep the tooth locked in the moved position with a medium amount of pressure in order to slowly break or weaken all the fibers and ligaments. The risk of this procedure is that the tooth will either break when too much force is applied in the lateral direction, or that the tooth is not completely freed of ligaments for the entire length of the root. Once this procedure has been repeated a few times (tooth deviated into different directions) and the tooth feels loose in the socket, extraction forceps can be used to gently remove the tooth from the socket. Very often in addition to the pulling movement a rotating motion needs to be applied while pulling the tooth gently out of its socket. If the tooth does not come out readily, more ligaments need to be broken down with the luxator. Never force a tooth out of the socket with the extractor. Very often the tooth will break when too much force is applied during the extraction, which will result in a regrowth of the tooth.

Once the tooth has been extracted it should be carefully inspected and hopefully the pulp is visible on the base of the tooth root. After the tooth has been removed, it is good practice to try to destroy any germinal cells possibly left behind in the alveolus. An electocautery with a ball-tip probe can be inserted into the socket and the remaining germinal tissue can be destroyed by thermal damage. Alternatively, mechanical destruction of the cells can be tried by repeatedly inserting the 18-gauge needle forcefully into the socket. The alveolus can be closed using absorbable suture in cases in which the extraction was complete and there is no suspicion of infection. The skin should be closed with a purse-string pattern. The surgery site should be monitored for swelling and discharge by the owner. The animal should start eating the same day.

The same procedure is repeated for the upper four (!) incisors. The procedure appears to be bloodier for the upper incisors and requires more time due to the need to remove the very small peg teeth, which can readily break during the procedure if not carefully handled.

It is important to pay attention to the nasal cavity and try to keep it clear from blood clots as the rabbit is an obligate nasal breather and respiratory distress could result from nasal passage obstruction, which is only evident after the extubation. It is good practice to plan to have the animal under anesthesia for about 2 to 3 hours depending on the ease of the removal and the skill of the surgeon.

REPRODUCTIVE SURGERY OF SMALL EXOTIC MAMMALS

James K Morrisey, DVM, Diplomate ABVP (Avian)
Cornell University
Ithaca, NY

Castration and ovariohysterectomy of small exotic mammals such as ferrets, rabbits, and rodents is a common practice and can easily be incorporated into the routine procedures offered to these clients. This article reviews these two procedures in the most common species, and offers advice for small mammal surgeries in general. Anesthesia is beyond the scope of this article but care should be taken in terms of maintaining body temperature using convective heating pads, warm water heating pads, or similar devices. Surgical time should be kept to a minimum to help prevent hypothermia and low blood pressure. Alcohol should be avoided when preparing the animal for surgery as it also decreases body temperature. Blood loss is usually minimal with these procedures but the surgeon should keep a strict eye on how much is lost to know if replacement methods are necessary.

For all species, the same instruments used in cats and dogs work well for neuters. Debakey forceps are useful for grasping the ovarian structures atraumatically within the deep abdomen of these species. Fine surgical instruments are helpful but not necessary, especially when dealing with the rodents. Small suture material such as 3-0 to 7-0 will be used so it may be helpful to have fine needle drivers. All suture mentioned is on a small taper needle and is a synthetic absorbable suture such as polydioxanone (PDS®) or polyglactin (Vicryl®) unless otherwise mentioned. Magnification can be beneficial by using either hobby loupes or head loupes.

FERRETS

Most ferrets are spayed or neutered and descented at 3 to 6 weeks of age; however, the number of private breeders is increasing so it is possible to see unaltered ferrets. These animals should be neutered by 6 to 8 months of age. Castration of ferrets is very similar to cats. The testicles are located ventral to the anus and caudal to the penis. The area is aseptically prepared for surgery and a short, linear incision is made in the center of each scrotal sac. The castration can be performed closed or open. The 'self-tie' technique used in cats doesn't work in ferrets because the testicle cannot be extracted very far from the scrotum. I prefer a closed technique so will clamp and double ligate the spermatic cord using 3-0 to 4-0 suture. Chromic gut sutures can be used for ferrets but not other small mammals. Closure of the incisions is not usually necessary.

Female ferrets should be spayed between 6 and 8 months of age before their first heat. Ferrets are induced ovulators and can develop severe anemia secondary to bone marrow suppression from hyperestrogenemia if not bred during their first heat or spayed before this time. The ferret uterus is bicornuate similar to that of the cat and the surgical procedure is likewise similar to the cat.

A ventral midline incision is made and the ovaries identified. There may be significant fat around the ovaries, making it difficult to view the vasculature; so care should be taken when exposing the vessels to avoid the ureters, which course medial to the ovaries. In young animals or animals in estrus, the vessels may be too friable to clamp with hemostats so ligatures can be placed without clamping. The ovarian vessels are double ligated using 4-0 suture. The suspensory ligament is usually slack and easily torn with blunt dissection. The uterine arteries and uterine body can be double ligated with 3-0 sutures. Closure of the abdomen is routine with 4-0 suture in the linea and then a subcuticular suture using 4-0 or 5-0 suture. Skin sutures are not necessary.

RABBITS

Routine castration of rabbits should be performed between 4 and 6 months of age to avoid urine spraying and other secondary sexual characteristics. The testicles are found in separate, hairless scrota on either side of the perineal mound at the level of the penis or slightly cranial to it. The testicles descend at about 12 weeks of age. Sexing rabbits before this time can be difficult, but look for a vertical genital opening in females and a round opening in males. Rabbits have open inguinal rings so the testicles may easily retreat into the abdomen, especially during surgery. If this occurs, place the flat of your hand on the ventral abdomen and gently roll it towards the tail to push the testicles back into the scrotal sacs. The area is aseptically prepared for surgery, taking care with the clippers not to lacerate the thin skin of the rabbit. A ventral incision is made over the testicle from about the center of the testicle to the palpable head of the epididymis. The castration can be performed open or closed, again I prefer closed. A small towel clamp can be used to grasp the ligament of the head of the epididymis so that tension can be placed on the testicle as it is dissected from the surrounding fascia. There is a large epididymal fat pad located in the inguinal tunic that can be removed if performing an open castration or left intact if doing a closed technique. A hemostat can be used to clamp the tunic and 3-0 or 4-0 suture can be used to ligate in the crushed band of tissue. This is repeated and the testicle then removed. If an open technique is used, the superficial inguinal ring should be closed using 4-0 suture. The scrota can be left open or tissue glue can be used to close the incision site.

The rabbit uterus is bicornuate but has two cervices, no uterine body, and a long vaginal vestibule. Spaying rabbits is recommended because of the very high incidence of uterine disease, including adenocarinoma, pyometra and endometritis, in unspayed females. Rabbits should be spayed between 3 and 6 months of age. The mesometrium is the primary site of fat storage in rabbits so it's beneficial to perform the surgery before significant amounts of fat accumulate. A ventral midline incision is made from 1cm cranial to the brim of the pelvis and 1cm caudal to the umbilicus. The aponeuroses of the abdominal muscles can appear to be linea, so make sure you are on the midline before incision the linea alba. Take care when cutting the linea as the cecum is large and is often pressed against the body wall. The reproductive tract is easily visualized in rabbits just cranial and dorsal to the bladder. The bladder should be emptied before surgery for better visualization. The reproductive tract can exteriorized easily but is more fragile than other species. The ovaries are surrounded by a long, dark red oviduct that is somewhat friable. The vessels can be difficult to visualize because of the fat surrounding them and should not be crushed with a hemostat before ligation as they easily tear. Instead, make a window through the fat on either side of the vessels and pass your ligature through these windows. There will be vessels that connect to the ovary from the dorsal body as well as a vessel within the ovarian ligament. Once the vessels are double ligated with 4-0 suture, a hemostat can be placed at the base of the oviduct to prevent hemorrhage from the tract when the ovarian vessels are transected. Once the ovarian vessels are ligated the tract can be flipped caudally and the large uterine vessels exposed. These vessels lie a few centimeters from the vagina and cervices and will need to be double ligated separately using a 4-0 suture. Then the cervices can be removed together by ligating across the distal vagina. There should be two ligatures placed here, one circumferential and one transfixing suture. The cervices can also be left intact and separate ligatures placed distal to each cervix and the uterus removed in two separate pieces. The linea is then closed with simple interrupted sutures because of the weight of the cecum on the incision. Subcuticular sutures are also placed to avoid the animal chewing out any skin sutures.

HYSTRICOMORPH RODENTS

Hystricomorph rodents such as guinea pigs and chinchillas are more easily neutered than spayed. The testicles lie on either side of the perineal area in pouches called post anal sacs. Both species have open inguinal rings so the same precautions should be taken in rabbits to either perform a closed castration or close the inguinal ring. A closed castration is easier and allows for a smaller incision. Guinea pigs reach sexual maturity as early as 3 months in males so castration should be done between 3 and 6 months of age. The boars are placed in dorsal recumbency and the area around each sac is prepared for surgery. Careful palpation is necessary so the penile body is not confused with a testicle. The incision should be made at the cranial aspect of the scrotal sac and the testicle pushed into view. As with rabbits, grasp the ligament of the head of the epididymis using towel clamps and free the testicle from the surrounding fascia with blunt dissection. Be gentle to the tissue to avoid post-operative swelling and inflammation. The spermatic cord is crushed using a hemostat distal to the epididymal fat body and the cord is double ligated using 3-0 or 4-0 suture. I have had problems with Monocryl® in guinea pigs, although other clinicians have used it routinely without problems. Once the testicles are removed the skin should be closed with a subcuticular pattern using 4-0 or 5-0 suture. It's more important to close these incisions since the testicles tend to lie or

drag on the ground more than other species. Both species are prone to sterile abscess after surgery and should be placed on anti-inflammatories for 7 to 14 days (meloxicam 0.3 mg/kg PO q24h).

Spaying guinea pigs and chinchillas is somewhat difficult because of the deep abdomen and short ovarian ligaments. Breaking these ligaments, as with a dog spay, is not possible as it is likely to rupture the vessels. Chinchillas have two cervices like the rabbit but a shorter uterine body so the cervices are usually left intact and the uteri removed separately. Both species accumulate fat in the mesometrium making it difficult to visualize vessels around the ovaries. Again, a ventral midline incision is made from the umbilicus to the pubis. Care should be taken in incising the linea to avoid the underlying cecum and bladder. Ovaries are located by following the uterus cranially. Ligatures should be placed around the ovarian vessels without crushing them by making two windows in the fat. The vessels are more easily visualized on the medial side of the mesovarium. Double ligate the vessels using 4-0 or 5-0 suture. The suspensory ligament is easily broken down to visualize the uterine vessels. The uterine vessels can be double ligated with the uterus, or separately like the rabbit using 3-0 or 4-0 suture. In guinea pigs the entire uterus and ovaries are removed together but in chinchillas each side can be removed separately. Closure is similar to the rabbit mentioned above.

MYOMORPH RODENTS

Spaying and neutering small rodents like rats, mice, hamsters and gerbils is a less common practice although recent evidence demonstrated that spaying rats greatly reduced the incidence of mammary tumors. The testicles of males are generally large and they have open inguinal rings. These species have a well-defined scrotal sac that is located caudal to the anus under the tail. There are three approaches to castration, a single midline incision at the base of the testicles, two incisions over each testicle or removing the caudal end of the scrotum. I prefer a closed castration that is performed by an incision in each scrotum. The incisions can be made on the caudal-dorsal portion of the scrotum to avoid damage to the incision from dragging it along the ground. The technique is the same as the guinea pig and chinchilla with the tunic and skin being closed with 4-0 or 5-0 suture. Tissue glue can be used to close the incision if it is less than 1 cm.

The rat is the only myomorphic rodent that is spayed with any regularity. The rat has a long bicornuate uterus with well-developed uterine horns and a short uterine body. The long suspensory ligaments make ligation of the ovarian vessels easier using 4-0 or 5-0 suture. There is less fat in the mesometrium as well so visualization is also easier. The small size of the structures makes the use of a head loupe or other magnification beneficial but not required. The uterine vessels can be ligated with the uterine body. The linea is closed with 4-0 to 5-0 suture and the subcutis with 5-0 to 7-0 suture. Tissue glue can be used to close any defects in the skin but skin sutures should not be used as they are often chewed out.

EVERYTHING YOU WANTED TO KNOW ABOUT ADRENAL DISEASE IN FERRETS

Nico J. Schoemaker, DVM, PhD,
Diplomate ECAMS and ABVP-Avian
Division of Avian and Exotic Animal Medicine
Faculty of Veterinary Medicine
Utrecht University, Utrecht, The Netherlands

Adrenal disease can refer to changes to the adrenal cortex and/or to the adrenal medulla. The most common form of adrenal medulla pathology is a pheochromocytoma. These rare tumors are usually much larger than tumors of the adrenal cortex and can remain unnoticed for a long time. Although cases have been reported where pheochromocytomas have been diagnosed based on histologic characteristics of the adrenal tumor, measurement of urinary metanefrine is necessary to confirm the diagnosis. To the author's knowledge this type of confirmation has not yet been performed in ferrets. The most common form of adrenal disease in ferrets is hyperadrenocorticism, also referred to as adrenocortical disease, in which the adrenal cortex is affected. The outermost layer of the adrenal cortex is the zona glomerulosa, which produces mineralo-corticoids (primarily aldosterone). The zona fasciculata consists of an outer and inner part, and produces glucocorticoids (cortisol and corticosterone) and androgens. The most interior zone is the zona reticularis, which is extremely variable in its prominence and cellular composition. This zone contains the smallest cells of the adrenal cortex and produces primarily androgens. Thus, in principle, three distinct syndromes may arise in adrenocortical hyperfunction: hyperaldosteronism, hypercortisolism, and hyperandrogenism.

Primary hyperaldosteronism or Conn's syndrome is the most common form of hyperadrenocorticism in cats, usually due to excessive secretion of mineralocorticoids by an adrenocortical neoplasia or bilateral adrenocortical hyperplasia. The exact pathogenesis of primary hyperaldosteronism remains to be elucidated.

Hypercortisolism or Cushing's syndrome is the most common form of hyperadrenocorticism in dogs, and also occurs frequently in humans. In these species, hypercortisolism most frequently results from excessive secretion of adrenocorticotropic hormone (ACTH) by a pituitary adenoma. ACTH-independent hypercortisolism may be due to excessive secretion of glucocorticoids by a benign or malignant adrenocortical tumor. However, ACTH-independent hypercortisolism may also occur as a result of expression of aberrant or overactive eutopic hormone receptors. In humans, various membrane-bound receptors, functionally coupled to steroidogenesis, have been reported, including gastric inhibitory polypeptide, catecholamine, vasopressin, serotonin, and luteinizing hormone (LH) receptors. LH-dependent hypercortisolism has been reported in several women. In addition to LH-dependent hypercortisolism, virilizing and feminizing LH-dependent adrenal tumors have been reported in humans.

HYPERADRENOCORTICISM

In neutered pet ferrets hyperandrogenism is the most common form of hyperadrenocorticism. In ferrets, plasma androstenedione, 17-hydroxyprogesterone and estradiol concentrations are increased. It has been reported that approximately 85% of ferrets with hyperadrenocorticism have enlargement of one adrenal gland without atrophy of the contralateral adrenal gland. In the other 15% of cases bilateral enlargement is present. After surgical removal of a unilateral adrenal tumor, the disease commonly recurs due to involvement of the contralateral adrenal gland. The adrenal glands have been histologically classified as (nodular) hyperplasia, adenoma and adenocarcinoma. The histologic diagnosis, however, does not provide information on functionality of the tumor, nor does it provide any prognostic information. No relationship has been found between pituitary and adrenal tumors in ferrets. At this stage, pituitary tumors should be regarded as incidental findings.

Different etiologies have been suggested for the high occurrence of hyperadrenocorticism in ferrets. These include (early) neutering of ferrets, housing ferrets indoors, and genetic background.

In recent years, evidence has been gathered that increased concentrations of gonadotropins, which occur after neutering (due to the loss of negative feedback), stimulate the adrenal cortex, eventually leading to an adrenocortical neoplasm.

- First, the initial signs of hyperadrenocorticism occur only during the breeding season, when plasma concentrations of gonadotropic hormones are high.
- Second, in the US, where the neutering of ferrets is common practice, hyperadrenocorticism is common, whereas hyperadrenocorticism is seldom diagnosed in the United Kingdom, where ferrets are usually not surgically castrated.
- Third, a significant correlation has been found between the age at neutering and age at onset of hyperadrenocorticism.
- Fourth, the depot gonadotropin-releasing hormone (GnRH)-agonists leuprolide acetate and deslorelin have been used successfully in the treatment of this disease.[6,7]
- Finally, luteinizing hormone (LH) receptors have been detected in the adrenal cortex of ferrets. These receptors are considered to be functional, because plasma concentrations of adrenal androgens increase after intravenous injection of a GnRH agonist.[4]

There remains debate, however, if the neutering has to take place at an early age for this disease to occur. In the US, ferrets are commonly neutered at an age of 6 weeks. In the Netherlands, however, most pet ferrets are neutered between 6 and 12 months of age. Since the prevalence of hyperadrenocorticism in Dutch ferrets is approximately 0.55% (95% confidence interval: 0.2–1.1%), it is likely that this disease is just as common in the Netherlands as it is in the US. The age at which ferrets are neutered is therefore not likely to have an influence in the development of these tumors.

The hypothesis that ferrets that are being kept indoors have a higher chance of developing hyperadrenocorticism compared with ferrets housed outdoors is in line with the above mentioned hypothesis. Ferrets that are kept indoors will be more under the influence of light—and thus gonadotropins—than ferrets that are housed outdoors. This applies to neutered as well as intact ferrets. The fact that adrenal gland disease is less common in the United Kingdom can therefore be explained by the fact that many ferrets are still being kept outdoors without being neutered.

A genetic background can play a role in the etiology of this disease as well. In the US, a specific breeding facility, which provides an estimated 80% of all American ferrets, has been blamed for the high occurrence of hyperadrenocorticism in American ferrets. If this claim would be accurate, than why is the prevalence of hyperadrenocorticism so high in the Netherlands, where ferrets do not have the same genetic background as ferrets from this facility? Although the breeding facility cannot be blamed for the high incidence of hyperadrenocorticism in ferrets, this does not mean that a genetic background for the disease is not possible. In humans three different hereditary syndromes have been recognized in which multiple endocrine neoplasms are seen (MEN1, MEN2a and MEN2b). Since insulinomas and adrenal gland tumors are frequently seen simultaneously in ferrets, a condition similar to MEN in humans may exist. Research at the University of California, Davis is in progress to determine if this is indeed the case.

Clinical signs of hyperadrenocorticism in ferrets include symmetrical alopecia, vulvar swelling in neutered female ferrets, recurrence of sexual behavior after neutering, urinary blockage in males (due to peri-prostatic or peri-urethral cysts), occasional mammary gland enlargement in female ferrets, and pruritus. The skin is usually not affected, although some excoriations may be seen. Alopecia usually begins in spring, which coincides with the start of the breeding season, and may disappear without treatment. The next year the alopecia usually returns after which it usually does not resolve spontaneously at the end of the breeding season. Polyuria and polydipsia are reported in ferrets with hyperadrenocorticism. It is not clear, however, whether adrenal hormone production is responsible for these signs, or if these (elderly) ferrets have concurrent kidney disease. A case of LH-dependent hypercortisolism (Cushing's disease) has been diagnosed by the author. The major complaint in this ferret was severe PU/PD. Only a minimal amount of alopecia was found in this ferret. The diagnosis in this case was confirmed by a plasma ACTH-concentration which was below the detection limit, an increased urinary corticoid creatinine ratio, and a rise of the plasma cortisol concentration after the administration of human chorionic gonadotropin (hCG). During ultrasonographic examination an enlarged right adrenal gland was detected while the left adrenal gland could not be located. Polyuria and polydipsia

resolved within 3 weeks after the administration of a deslorelin implant (see later). Plasma and urinary hormones had returned to normal 3 months after the initial diagnosis. It was striking to find that the right adrenal gland had diminished in size, while the left adrenal gland now had a normal appearance, suggesting that the left adrenal gland was initially atrophic. Two years after diagnosis the ferret is still doing fine without recurrence of symptoms.

When considering predisposing factors, age appears to be an important factor, which is in its turn linked to age at neutering (as mentioned earlier). In the US, diagnosis of hyperadrenocorticism in ferrets is already possible at an age of 2 years. In the Netherlands, however, most cases of hyperadrenocorticism are seen in ferrets older than 3 years of age. Although initial reports suggested that the majority of ferrets with adrenocortical disease were females, a Dutch study could not confirm this sex predilection. In the author's practice there is actually a tendency of seeing more male than female ferrets with hyperadrenocorticism.

The most important differential diagnoses for a ferret with signs of hyperadrenocorticism are a non-ovariectomized female or a ferret with active remnant ovaries. Severe alopecia and pruritus in a ferret, however, has also been seen due to a food allergy. Hormone analysis in blood and urine, as well as an abdominal ultrasound could not confirm the presence of a hyperfunctioning adrenal gland in this case. All signs in this ferret resolved after it had been converted to a different brand of ferret food.

Although many advanced techniques can be used in diagnosing hyperadrenocorticism in ferrets, the clinical signs remain the most important. Further confirmation can sometimes be obtained by palpating a (tiny) firm mass craniomedial to the cranial pole of the kidneys, representing the enlarged adrenal gland(s). The right adrenal gland is more difficult to palpate due to the overlying right caudate process of the caudate liver lobe. Hormones that are commonly elevated are androstenedione, estradiol, and 17-hydroxy-progesterone. Blood can be sent to the University of Tennessee for analysis of these hormones. Dehydroepiandrosterone sulfate used to be included in this panel, but is currently no longer incorporated. Elevation of one or more of these hormones is considered to be diagnostic for hyperadrenocorticism. However, plasma concentrations of androstenedione, estradiol, and 17-hydroxyprogesterone in intact female ferrets are identical to those in hyperadrenocorticoid ferrets. It is therefore likely that this hormone panel does not aid in differentiating between a ferret with hyperadrenocorticism and one with an active ovarian remnant. The author therefore does not routinely measure these hormones in the diagnosis of this disease. He does, however, measure plasma concentrations of androstenedione (the only androgen in the panel and precursor of estradiol) for the evaluation of hormonal treatment.

ACTH stimulation tests and dexamethasone suppression tests—as commonly used in dogs with

Cushing's syndrome—are not considered diagnostic in ferrets. In addition, plasma concentrations of ACTH and α-MSH in hyperadrenocorticoid ferrets were found to be identical to those from healthy neutered ferrets. It was concluded that these hormones, therefore, could not aid in diagnosing hyperadrenocorticism in ferrets.

Plasma cortisol concentrations have, just as in dogs, been found to be of no use for the diagnosis of hyperadrenocorticism in ferrets. In dogs, it has become standard to measure the urinary corticoid-creatinine ratio (UCCR), in combination with a high dose dexamethasone suppression test (HDDST). An increased UCCR has also been found in ferrets with adrenocortical disease. The HDDST demonstrated that the hyperadrenocorticism is of adrenal and not pituitary origin. This is in agreement with the fact that no functional pituitary tumors have been found in hyperadrenocorticoid ferrets. Although the UCCR is elevated in ferrets with adrenocortical tumors, the UCCR is considered to be of no diagnostic value because this ratio is also increased in intact ferrets during the breeding season, and in ferrets with an active ovarian remnant.

The most useful tool in diagnosing hyperadrenocorticism in ferrets is abdominal ultrasonography. One has to remember, however, that with this technique only the size of abdominal organs is visualized. This technique does not provide any information on hormone release. It is therefore possible that only one adrenal gland is enlarged, while both adrenal glands contribute to the androgen release. Ultrasound is especially of great value prior to surgery, if you want to determine which adrenal gland is affected, or if an ovarian remnant is present. In this way the owner can be informed about the potential surgical risks that may be encountered. Another advantage of this technique is that other abdominal organs can be evaluated during the same procedure.

It has been reported that adrenal glands may remain undetected during an ultrasonographic exam. It is especially difficult to distinguish an adrenal gland from an abdominal lymph node. By using specific landmarks, however, the adrenal glands can fairly easily be detected in nearly 100% of the cases. The left adrenal gland is located lateral to the aorta, at the level of the origin of the cranial mesenteric and celiac arteries. The right adrenal gland is more difficult to locate. Since this adrenal gland lies adjacent to the caudomedial aspect of the caudate process of the caudate liver lobe, the liver may be used as an acoustic window. The three major vessels (aorta, portal vein and caudal vena cava) in that area are located. The vena cava is the most lateral and dorsal of the three. In addition, the portal vein has a much wider diameter compared to the caudal vena cava. The right adrenal gland is attached to the dorsolateral surface of the caudal vena cava, at the level of and/or immediately cranial to the origin of the cranial mesenteric artery. The adrenal glands of ferrets with hyperadrenocorticism have a significantly increased thickness, have a rounded appearance, a heterogeneous structure, an increased echogenicity, and sometimes contain signs of mineralization.

When attempting to treat a ferret with hyperadrenocorticism, the most ideal treatment would probably be a combination of surgery and placement of an implant containing deslorelin (a depot GnRH analogue). Many different factors influence the eventual choice of treatment. An owner may decline surgery based on criteria such as the age of the ferret, presence of concurrent disease (cardiomyopathy), risk of surgery when the right or both adrenal glands are involved, and financial limitations. When an owner chooses for only surgery, gonadotropin release will persist, resulting in continued stimulation of the remaining adrenal gland. Disadvantage of hormonal therapy (use of a depot GnRH agonist such as leuprolide acetate) may be the price of this drug and the fact that it needs to be repeated on a regular basis. Once the deslorelin implants become registered for use in animals the latter disadvantage will be diminished. Autonomous production of steroids by the adrenal gland may result in loss of response to treatment with a depot GnRH agonist.

Surgical removal of the left adrenal gland is fairly easy. The adrenal gland is dissected out of the retroperitoneal fat and the *Vena phrenicoabdominalis* is ligated. The location of the right adrenal gland makes it much more difficult to remove. The close proximity to the liver and the dorsolateral attachment to the caudal *Vena cava* would make a dorsal approach more logical. This is in fact the surgical approach to the adrenal glands in humans. In ferrets, however, an abdominal approach is most commonly used. During resection of the right adrenal gland, either a part of the adrenal needs to be left attached to the *Vena cava*, or part of the wall of the vein has to be removed. Ligation of the caudal *Vena cava* is only possible if this vein is already occluded for a major portion of its diameter and collateral veins have opened up. If this is not the case there is a great risk of hypertension distal to ligation which may lead to acute kidney failure. Although the author is not in favor of removing bilateral adrenocortical tumors, different surgical protocols have been proposed. Many advise to leave part of an adrenal gland behind, while others advise to remove both adrenal glands. It would seem likely that hypoadrenocorticism would occur after removing both glands, but this seems to occur only in a minority of cases. Accurate diagnosis of an Addisonian crisis, including an ACTH stimulation test to confirm the diagnosis, has not been published. It appears, however, that short-term treatment with cortisone and fludrocortisone seems to be sufficient in most cases.

The most effective drugs at this moment are the depot GnRH-agonists of which leuprolide acetate (Lupron Depot, TAP Pharmaceutical Products) is the most well known. Deslorelin is another pharmaceutical GnRH-analogue. This drug is commercially available as implant for chemical castration of male dogs in Australia (Suprelorin®, Peptech Animal Health, Australia). Advantages of these implants over leuprolide acetate are that the drug does not need to be reconstituted, lasts much longer than the depot injections, will be registered for use in animals, and will probably be cheaper. These implants have already been used in ferrets with hyperadrenocorticism and seem to be very effective. Once this drug becomes commercially available in Europe and the US, it is likely that this will become the drug of choice. Approximately 10% of ferrets seem to develop adrenal carcinomas after 1.5 to 2 years of treatment. More research will be necessary to determine why these tumors are seen, and how high the frequency actually is.

Until the deslorelin implants are commercially available leuprolide acetate provides a suitable alternative. The Lupron 30-day Depot formulation is given in a dose of 100 µg IM for ferrets less than 1 kg and 200 µg IM for ferrets over 1 kg. This drug will suppress adrenocortical hormone release for at least 1 month in ferrets and may even last up to 3 months. Some veterinarians use a 3-month formulation (which is 3 times as expensive), but this drug does not seem to work 3 times longer than the 30-day formulation.

It may seem strange that a depot GnRH-agonist is used in ferrets with hyperadrenocorticism, when the increased release of GnRH and gonadotropins, which occur after neutering, are responsible for the disease in the first place. To understand the mechanism behind this treatment, it is important to know that pituitary and hypothalamic hormones are released in a pulsatile fashion. Gonadotropins are only released when GnRH is secreted in pulses. The depot GnRH-agonist overrides the pulsatile release, thereby blocking the release of gonadotropins. The administration of a depot GnRH agonist therefore results in an initial single release of gonadotropins followed by baseline concentrations.

Melatonin has also been proposed as therapeutic option for hyperadrenocorticoid ferrets. Mink which receive such an implant develop appealing thick furs. This has also been reported in ferrets. Melatonin supposedly suppresses the release of GnRH. Researchers showed in the early eighties of the last century that ferrets, which were kept under 8 h light : 16 h darkness (8L : 16D), would come into estrus only 7 weeks later than ferrets exposed to long photoperiods (14L : 10D). It is therefore debatable if melatonin is indeed capable of suppressing the release of gonadotropins. Clinical improvement, however, is seen in hyperadrenocorticoid ferrets either receiving 0.5 mg melatonin daily PO or an implant containing 5.4 mg melatonin. In the study in which melatonin was given orally, however, hormone concentrations, in general, rose and the tumors continued to grow. This treatment may therefore pose a risk to the ferrets as their condition deteriorates, which remains unnoticed by the owner. Another point to consider is that melatonin can be purchased in drugstores in the US. Home-medication with melatonin may therefore delay the initial presentation of ferrets with hyperadrenocorticism to veterinarians.

As described above, the most common medical treatment option for ferrets with hyperadrenocorticism is the use of a depot GnRH agonist. Ketoconazole and mitotane (o,p'-DDD) are well known drugs for treating hypercortisolism in dogs and humans. These drugs have also been tried in ferrets, but both were not considered very effective and should be considered obsolete.

In recent years Trilostane (Vetoryl®, Arnolds Veterinary Products/Dechra Veterinary Products), a 3β-hydroxysteroid dehydrogenase (3β-HSD) blocker, has become an important drug for treating pituitary-dependent hyperadrenocorticism in dogs. Since 3β-HSD is necessary for the synthesis of androstenedione and 17-hydroxyprogesterone it is tempting to speculate that this drug would be very effective in treating ferrets with hyperadrenocorticism. In a pilot study 5 mg trilostane was given orally once daily to a ferret with hyperadrenocorticism. Within a month the owner complained that the alopecia and vulvar swelling in the ferret increased. Plasma hormone analysis showed a decreased 17-hydroxyprogesterone concentration, but increased concentrations of androstenedione, estradiol, and dehydroepiandrosterone sulfate. These results can be explained by the fact that a decrease of 3β-HSD may lead to an activation of 17,20-lyase, and thus the androgen pathway. In another hyperadrenocorticoid ferret in which the depot GnRH agonist did not seem to work anymore, no improvement was seen after a month of treatment with trilostane. The hormone concentrations in this ferret did not decrease or increase in this ferret during the treatment with trilostane. More research is necessary before this drug can be safely used in ferrets.

REFERENCES

1. Kuijten AM, Schoemaker NJ, Voorhout G. Ultrasonographic visualization of the adrenal glands of healthy and hyperadrenocorticoid ferrets. J Am Anim Hosp Assoc. 2007;43:78–84.
2. Quesenberry KE, Rosenthal KL. Endocrine diseases. In: Quesenberry KE, Carpenter JW (eds.): Ferrets, Rabbits and Rodents; clinical medicine and surgery, 2nd ed. Philadelphia: WB Saunders. 2003, pp 79–90.
3. Schoemaker NJ, Schuurmans M, Moorman H, et al. Correlation between age at neutering and age at onset of hyperadrenocorticism in ferrets. J Am Vet Med Assoc. 2000;216:195–197.
4. Schoemaker NJ, Teerds KJ, Mol JA, et al. The role of luteinizing hormone in the pathogenesis of hyperadrenocorticism in neutered ferrets. Mol Cell Endocrinol 2002;197:117–125
5. Schoemaker NJ, Wolfswinkel J, Mol JA, et al. Urinary excretion of glucocorticoids in the diagnosis of hyperadrenocorticism in ferrets. Domest Anim Endocrinol. 2004;27:13–24.
6. Wagner RA, Bailey EM, Schneider JF, Oliver JW. Leuprolide acetate treatment of adrenocortical disease in ferrets. J Am Vet Med Assoc. 2001;218:1272-1274.
7. Wagner RA, Piché CA, Jöchle W, Oliver JW. Clinical and endocrine responses to treatment with deslorelin acetate implants in ferrets with adrenocortical disease. Am J Vet Res. 2005;66:910-914.

ADDITIONAL READING

1. Nico Schoemaker's PhD thesis on hyperadreno-corticism in ferrets can be found online at: http://igitur-archive.library.uu.nl/dissertations/2003-1128-094343/inhoud.htm.

HOW I WORK UP THE FERRET WITH HIND LIMB WEAKNESS

Nico J. Schoemaker, DVM, PhD,
Diplomate ECAMS and ABVP-Avian
Division of Avian and Exotic Animal Medicine
Faculty of Veterinary Medicine
Utrecht University, Utrecht, The Netherlands

Many terms, such as *ataxia* and *posterior paresis*, are used when a ferret has a decreased ability to use its hind legs. It is important to realize that these terms implicate different problems and thus also can originate from different lesions.

The official definition of *paresis* is "partial paralysis"—that is, a partial loss of voluntary movement, which is commonly accompanied with deficits in proprioception. The definition of *ataxia* is "loss of the ability to coordinate muscular movement," and it may be of vestibular, cerebellar, or proprioceptive (that is, spinal column and periphery) origin. In both cases the neuromuscular system is involved, thus it is clear that both deficits of neurologic and muscular origin can result in onset of a certain degree of paresis (paralysis) or ataxia.

Hind limb weakness can also have systemic causes, which is often the case in ferrets. The most frequent diagnosis in these cases is insulinoma, but many other differentials should be considered (Table 1). It should also be noted that lameness caused by orthopedic problems can mimic weakness in the hind legs, and distinction between the two is thus very important.

CLINICAL APPROACH

History – As with all of your patients, a thorough history of the case should be obtained. Within the history, it is important to focus on the progression and localization of the disease. Since insulinoma is the most important differential diagnosis, I often ask specific questions towards this diagnosis. It is therefore important to know if the weakness is gradually getting worse, is stable, and/or is it only seen at certain periods (that is, associated with prolonged periods of not eating,

Table 1. Differential Diagnosis of Hind Limb Weakness in Ferrets

Systemic causes	Hypoglycemia	Insulinoma Food deprivation / anorexia Vomiting Sepsis Neoplasia Severe hepatic disease
	Cardiac disease Hypoxia Anemia Thromboembolism Addison's disease (electrolyte imbalance) Toxin ingestion (ie, ibuprofen) Proliferative bowel disease Severe debilitating disease	Severe splenomegaly Inguinal/sublumbar lymphadenopathy Cystic/renal calculi Peritonitis Prostatic enlargement Urinary blockage
Neurologic causes	Central nervous location	Hernia nucleus pulposi Central neural trauma Plasma cell myeloma Spinal cord lymphoma Chordoma Tumor of the plexus choroideus Aleutian disease
	Peripheral nervous location	Polyneuropathy Myasthenia gravis
Orthopedic causes	Fracture Myositis (Poly)arthritis	

which resolves after a meal). The latter is indicative of an insulinoma. A constant, deteriorating weakness of the hind limbs, on the other hand, does not fit within the history of a ferret with insulinoma. It is also important to ask for signs of nausea (ie, salivation and pawing at the mouth), which may occur as a result of adrenalin release. In humans, adrenalin release is seen during the early stages of hypoglycemia. Another important question is whether the ferret is periodically seen with a glazed look in its eyes.

Taking the other potential diagnoses into consideration it is important to ask routine internal medicine questions inquiring about diet, appetite, water intake, urination, vomiting, stool consistency, and power of endurance. It is also important to know if other signs are present apart from the hind limb weakness, such as head tilt, leaning, or circling. This may help you to differentiate between a systemic and a neurologic disease.

Physical Examination – A complete physical examination is then performed on the ferret. It is important to observe the respiration while the animal is in a calm state. This should therefore be performed prior to handling of the ferret. During the examination special attention should be focused on the circulatory system. The heart frequency should not exceed 250 beats per minute, while a firm femoral pulse should be palpable. During auscultation no heart murmurs should be heard, and mucous membranes should be moist and pink. A thorough abdominal palpation is always included in the general physical exam of ferrets.

When the history and the initial physical exam point towards an insulinoma, a fasting blood glucose (see later) will be measured at this stage. When the blood glucose is within normal limits, or when the history and exam point towards a neurologic condition, a neurologic exam is performed. First, inspection of locomotion can provide valuable information. Is the back still arched? Is there paresis or paralysis? Are only the hind limbs involved, or is there paresis of the front legs as well? This is followed by the postural reactions. Just as in the other companion animals it is possible to test the knuckling-over reflex, to test tactile and optical placement of the legs, and hopping. The most commonly tested spinal reflexes are the patellar ligament reflex, and the flexor reflex. Finally, pain perception is evaluated.

Blood Examination – Since an insulinoma is high within the probability list, a glucose measurement should be included in any ferret with hind limb weakness. It is important to realize a couple of things when measuring blood glucose. First, blood glucose values can be normal after a meal. Food should therefore be withheld from the ferret for at least 4 hours. Second, it is important to realize that most in-house glucose meters—especially those intended for use in human diabetic patients—are calibrated to measure normal to high blood values. These meters have a tendency to underestimate the actual blood glucose in the low range. When you measure a value within the normal range, you can assume that this value is correct. When you measure a

borderline low value, however, you should consider that the value may still be within the reference range. In these cases you can either prolong the fasting of the ferret for another hour, or send the blood to an official lab. When you send the blood to an outside lab, the blood should either be collected in a NaF tube, or the plasma should be separated from the erythrocytes as soon as possible to prevent continued use of glucose by these cells. It is important to know that blood collected in a sodium fluoride (NaF)-coated tube cannot be used for the in-house assays.

Since hypoglycemia can also be the result of other conditions than an insulinoma, it is advised to perform a complete blood count (CBC) and full plasma chemistry panel (including urea, calcium, sodium, potassium, inorganic phosphorus, aspartate aminotransferase (AST), bile acids, total protein, and protein electrophoresis). The plasma chemistry panel will also assist you differentiating between systemic causes when glucose levels are within the reference range.

There is debate whether measuring insulin is of use. Insulin could either be elevated, but it may also be within the reference range. It is tempting to believe that a ferret cannot have an insulinoma, when the insulin is within normal limits. This is actually not true. When plasma glucose concentrations are low, insulin should be below the detection limit of the assay. If insulin is still within the reference range, it is actually too high! Although measuring insulin has its value, the author does not routinely measure insulin as this assay is not run on a regular basis in the Netherlands, and it would take too long for the results to arrive. Since the other causes of hypoglycemia can usually be ruled on the basis of the ferret's history, physical exam and plasma chemistry at tentative diagnosis of insulinoma can be made.

A hypergammaglobulinemia is suggestive of Aleutian disease. A positive antibody test (counterimmuno-electrophoresis [CIEP] or enzyme-linked immunosorbent assay [ELISA]) strengthens the diagnosis. The diagnosis can be confirmed by demonstrating infiltration of tissues (spleen, kidney, liver) by round nucleated inflammatory cells in cytologic samples of these organs.

Diagnostic imaging – Diagnostic imaging is of no use in diagnosing an insulinoma in ferrets. The texture of insulinomas resembles that of surround fat, and as the tumor is so small it cannot be distinguished during an ultrasonographic exam. This is in contrast to dogs in which metastases of insulinomas can be found in the liver during an ultrasonographic exam. When an insulinoma is not likely the cause of the hind leg weakness an ultrasonographic exam can be of great value to evaluate abdominal structures. Echocardiography is also of great use in diagnosing cardiac disease in ferrets.

Spinal radiographs may be of use to locate intervertebral disk disease by looking at the intervertebral space. The latter decreased space, however, is usually barely detectable due to the size of the animals. Myelography, computed tomography (CT), or magnetic resonance imaging (MRI) may assist in locating the herniated nucleus pulposi. Contrast enhancement may be necessary. Due to the size of the animal it is important to contact the radiologist prior to referral to ask whether the resolution of the equipment is sufficient for animals of this size. Spinal radiographs can be very useful in detecting osteolysis when neoplasias are responsible for the hind leg weakness.

Miscellaneous Tests – Cerebrospinal fluid (CSF) may be collected in the atlanto-occipital region and between L5 and L6. The CSF may be submitted for culture and cytology. Finally, an electromyogram can be performed to see whether there is denervation or other neuromuscular abnormalities.

TREATMENT

Insulinoma – Treatment of an insulinoma is possible by surgical resection of the tumor or by medical intervention. Within the pancreas multiple primordial insulinomas may be present, explaining why there is such a high recurrence rate after nodulectomy of an insulinoma. It has therefore been proposed to perform a partial pancreatectomy. Although it is impossible to locate any primordial tumors, a mean disease-free state after surgery of about 1 year, and a survival time of 22 months is reported after a partial pancreactectomy. Be aware, however, not to remove too large a portion of the pancreas, as this may induce diabetes mellitus. Another important aspect to consider is the location of the insulinoma: when it is found in the corpus of the pancreas, surgical removal is not possible due to proximity to the pancreatic duct.

Prednisone and diazoxide are the drugs that are described for the medical management of insulinomas. Although prednisolone is recommended in most textbooks as drug of first choice, the author believes that this should be diazoxide, as this drug inhibits insulin release. Expense is often given as reason why prednisone is chosen over diazoxide. Although the drug is certainly more expensive than prednisone, the low weight of ferrets minimizes the amount of drug needed. The total expense is therefore limited. Compounding the drug with methylcellulose makes it also easy to give to ferrets.

Prednisone, which induces gluconeogenesis, seems to be very effective in practice, and side effects are hardly ever seen. The author, however, has seen a case of iatrogenic Cushing's disease in a ferret with long-term treatment of prednisone.

Treatment is started at a dose of 5 mg/kg diazoxide (PO, q12h). The effect of treatment may be evaluated based on disappearance of clinical signs as well as plasma glucose concentrations. Blood should be collected 4 hours after giving the diazoxide. During this period food should be withheld from the ferret. Although it has been mentioned that the dose of diazoxide may be increased to 30 mg/kg q12h, there is no actual upper limit of the dose. Potential gastrointestinal side effects (ie, vomiting, diarrhea), can easily be treated by lowering the dose of diazoxide, and adding prednisone (0.2–1 mg/kg PO, q24h) to the treatment regimen. Medical management is usually sufficient for a period of 6 to 18 months.

Other Conditions – A discussion of all the treatment options for all differential diagnoses of hind leg weakness is beyond the scope of this article. In ferrets with cardiac disease, it is important to decrease the work load of the heart. Diuretics, such as furosemide, are very useful. In addition, digoxin, angiotensin-converting enzyme (ACE) inhibitors, and pimobendan may be of use in regulating heart rate and blood pressure. Choice of one of these drugs is dependent on the outcome of the ECG and ultrasound.

MISCELLANEOUS

Aleutian disease is uncommon in ferrets, but frequently mentioned within the differential diagnosis in ferrets with hind limb weakness. At least three different strains, with differing virulence, have been identified in ferrets since the late 1970s. Most ferrets in which antibodies are found by CIEP will not develop any signs of disease. Different outbreaks, however, have been reported in which serious disease was seen in many ferrets. Up to 2005, Aleutian disease was seldom diagnosed in ferrets in the Netherlands. In 2005 and 2006, however, a Dutch ferret veterinarian (Hanneke Moorman) saw that in her practice many young ferrets died with unclear signs. Based on results obtained from the University of Georgia, she was able to diagnose a ferret with Aleutian disease. A serologic survey among Dutch ferrets showed that 66 of 1436 (4.6%) had a positive CIEP titer. She collected follow-up information on 22 of the CIEP-positive ferrets. One and a half year after initial diagnosis, ten ferrets had died of the disease. The most prominent clinical signs in these ferrets were; chronic wasting, paresis and/or paralysis of the hind legs, urine and fecal incontinence. Some ferrets also showed signs of pneumonia, vomiting, diarrhea, uveitis, and fever. Since the ferrets were either imported from New Zealand, or had been in contact with ferrets from New Zealand, the import of these ferrets was discontinued. As of 2007, Aleutian disease did not seem to be a problem any longer in the Dutch ferret population.

HOW I WORK UP PU/PD IN A FERRET

Nico J. Schoemaker, DVM, PhD,
Diplomate ECAMS and ABVP-Avian
Division of Avian and Exotic Animal Medicine,
Faculty of Veterinary Medicine,
Utrecht University, Utrecht, The Netherlands

Polyuria and polydipsia (PU/PD) is not easy to notice in an individual ferret when it is housed in a group. This may be one of the reasons why some textbooks mention that kidney disease in uncommon in ferrets. Only in a case of severe polydipsia does the owner notice that the ferret is continuously found near the water bowl or bottle. To confirm that the ferret indeed has polydipsia, it is best to ask the owner to measure water consumption for a couple of days. Although no references for normal water consumption in ferrets are published, it is safe to assume that water consumption over 100 mL/kg/day is excessive.

Based on the differential diagnosis of PU/PD in dogs and cats,[5] a list can be compiled for the ferret (Table 1). It is useful to have this list as a guide when working up the case.

One of the more common differentials in dogs and cats, diabetes mellitus, is considered extremely rare in ferrets. In addition, no information could be found on diabetes insipidus and the possible use of a modified water deprivation test in ferrets. In dogs, hepatic failure is associated with hypercortisolism and a disturbance of vasopressin release. Up to now the author has not seen any association between PU/PD in a ferret and hepatic failure.

HISTORY

Within the history and signalment it is important to know the age and sex of the ferret, and whether it has been neutered. The latter is especially important to know in case pyometra is suspected. It is also important to inquire about the appetite of the animal, and if the ferret has lost weight. Further questions should be directed towards progression of the signs and if the ferret has received any medication, or could have consumed any of the toxins mentioned in the differential list. Since melena may be seen in severe cases of kidney disease, the owners should be asked about the color and odor of the feces.

PHYSICAL EXAMINATION

A general physical exam should be performed in all ferrets. Special attention should be directed towards the color of the mucous membranes and the skin turgor (to look for signs of anemia and dehydration) and oral lesions. Pyometra is seen in ferrets in estrus. Inspection of the vulva in intact ferrets is therefore also necessary. Further examinations (ie, blood and urine examination) will always be necessary to direct you to a more definitive diagnosis (see below).

BLOOD EXAMINATION

In case of chronic renal failure the packed cell volume (PCV) may be decreased due to a reduced secretion of erythropoietin by the renal medulla. Measurement of the PCV in combination with reticulocytes is therefore advised. In addition, glucose, urea, calcium (Ca), phosphorus (P), sodium (Na), potassium (K), alanine aminotransferase (ALT), total protein, albumin, and bile acids should be measured. Measurement of creatinine has been found to be ineffective in evaluating kidney disease in ferrets. The author has indeed seen ferrets with chronic interstitial nephritis that had creatinine values within the reference range.

It is very suggestive that renal disease is present when P (measured in mmol/L) is higher than Ca (measured in mmol/L), while the latter value is within the reference range. Divide the mg/dL P by 3 to estimate the mmol/L P, and divide the mg/dL Ca by 4 to estimate the mmol/L Ca.

No information on diabetes insipidus has been published in ferrets. Information on plasma and (urinary) osmolality is therefore also not available in ferrets.

URINALYSIS

Urinalysis should consist of at least the specific gravity (SG), pH, protein, glucose, hemoglobin and sediment. We have lately also started to measure creatinine in the urine. Although no reference values have been established, extreme high urinary protein/creatinine ratios have been found. In these cases, however, the urinary protein was also very high. The extra value of this measurement is therefore not clear at this stage. It is noteworthy to warn for associating glucosuria with diabetes mellitus. Glucose may also be lost through the kidneys when there is a disturbance in absorption in the proximal tubule. This condition is referred to as Fanconi's syndrome.

In most PU/PD cases the urinary corticoid/creatinine is not measured. The author has seen a case, however, in which a ferret had severe PU/PD, without any abnormalities in the blood and urine analysis. We were able to confirm that this ferret had a luteinizing hormone (LH)-dependent hypercortisolism based on an increased urinary corticoid/creatinine ratio, decreased plasma ACTH and an increase of plasma cortisol after intramuscular stimulation with human chorionic gonadotropin (hCG). Ultrasonographic examination further confirmed the presence of a unilateral adrenal tumor and atrophy of the contralateral adrenal gland.

Glomerular Filtration Rate

Under laboratory conditions, references for endogenous and exogenous creatinine clearance as well as inuline clearance have been established to determine the glomerular filtration rate (GFR) in ferrets.[1] For the endogenous creatinine clearance the ferrets were kept in metabolic cages, while for the other clearances the animals were kept under anesthesia for 24 to 48 hours. The latter may explain why the author has not found any reports on measurement of the GFR in clinical cases in ferrets.

SUGGESTED READING

1. Esteves MI, Marini RP, Ryden EB, Murphy JC, Fox JG. Estimation of glomerular filtration rate and evaluation of renal function in ferrets (*Mustela putorius furo*). Am J Vet Res. 1994;55:166-a72.
2. Fisher PG. Exotic mammal renal disease: causes and clinical presentation. Vet Clin Exotic Anim. 2006;9:33–67.
3. Fisher PG. Exotic mammal renal disease: diagnosis and treatment. Vet Clin Exotic Anim. 2006;9:69–96.
4. Pollock CG. Urogenital diseases. In: Quesenberry KE, Carpenter JW (eds.): Ferrets, Rabbits and Rodents: Clinical Medicine and Surgery, 2nd ed. Philadelphia: WB Saunders, 2003, pp 41-49.
5. Taylor SM. Polyuria and polydipsia. In: Ettinger SJ, Feldman EC (eds.):Textbook of Veterinary Internal Medicine, 5th ed. Philadelphia: WB Saunders, 2000, pp 85–89.

Table 1. Differential Diagnosis for PU/PD in the Ferret

Primary Polyuria
- Osmotic diuresis
  - Diabetes mellitus (rare in ferrets)
  - Primary renal glucosuria, Fanconi's syndrome
  - Postobstructive diuresis
- ADH deficiency – central diabetes insipidus (no reports found in literature)
  - Idiopathic
  - Trauma induced
  - Neoplastic
  - Congenital
- Renal insensitivity to ADH – nephrogenic diabetes insipidus
  - Primary nephrogenic diabetes insipidus (no reports found in literature)
  - Secondary nephrogenic diabetes insipidus

Renal insufficiency
Pyelonephritis
Pyometra
Hypercalcemia (e.g. due to lymphoma)
Hypokalemia
Hyperadrenocorticism (e.g. Cushing's disease)
Hyperthyroidism (no reports found in literature)
Hypoadrenocorticsm (no primary cases reported in the literature)
Hepatic insufficiency (uncertain whether this is also true for ferrets)

        Drugs (Cadmium, cholecalciferol, diquat herbicides, ethylene glycol, mercury, nephrotoxic antibactrials [bacitracin, polymyxin-B, gentamicin, neomycin], NSAID's, oxalic acid, phenolics, rhubarb, zinc)

Primary polydipsia
- Psychogenic (behavioral)
- Encephalopathy
- Neurologic
- Fever
- Pain

MANAGING THE FERRET WITH THE ENORMOUS SPLEEN

Nico J. Schoemaker, DVM, PhD,
Diplomate ECAMS and ABVP-Avian
Division of Avian and Exotic Animal Medicine
Faculty of Veterinary Medicine
Utrecht University, Utrecht, The Netherlands

The spleen in ferrets is usually large to huge in size. Based on the frequency of seeing large spleens in ferrets, one may actually speculate that a large spleen is normal for ferrets. The differential diagnosis includes extramedullary hematopoiesis, lymphoma, myeloid tumor, hemangioma, hemangiosarcoma, Aleutian disease, and idiopathic hypersplenism.

In the majority of cases an enlarged spleen is an incidental finding during a physical exam. The inexperienced veterinarian may consider the "abdominal mass" a point of concern. The more experienced veterinarian will take different points under consideration before being concerned about the mass. One of the first things to consider is: "Why is the animal presented to a veterinarian and can the "mass" be linked to this complaint?" In a ferret with symmetric alopecia, for instance, signs cannot be explained by the finding of an enlarged spleen. Anorexia and abdominal enlargement, on the other hand, may be associated with the spleen. Another point to consider is: "How large is the spleen and are any irregularities palpable?" In extreme cases, the spleen may fill up most of the abdominal cavity. In case of lymphoma or other neoplasia, the border of the spleen will loose its sharp edges and lumps may be identified during abdominal palpation.

HISTORY

Clinical signs that are often associated with an enlarged spleen are abdominal enlargement, difficulty ambulating, anorexia, pale mucous membranes (or pale eye color in albino ferrets), and lethargy. Since many of these signs are nonspecific, a complete history should be taken including all of the regular internal medicine questions.

PHYSICAL EXAMINATION

The most important part of the physical examination is the abdominal palpation. This is often most easily performed with the one-hand technique, whereby the thorax is supported in one hand, while the abdomen is carefully palpated with the other. Special attention should also be paid to the circulatory system (pulse frequency, heart murmurs, and mucous membranes), and lymph nodes.

SPECIFIC TESTS

On radiographs an enlarged spleen may be identified. However, no information will be obtained with this technique regarding texture and masses that may be present within the spleen. The most important method to evaluate the spleen is ultrasonography. This technique enables accurate visualization of size and texture of the spleen, as well as additional structures within the abdomen. A homogeneous texture and smooth edges of the spleen are more often associated with benign processes, such as extramedullary hematopoiesis. A mottled appearance or areas of poor echogenicity are suggestive of a neoplasm. Fine-needle aspiration biopsies can usually be performed without the guidance of ultrasound. The disadvantage of taking biopsies in this fashion is that a normal area of the spleen may be sampled, while pathology is present within other areas of the spleen. The author therefore only takes samples under ultrasound guidance, with the ferret under anesthesia with isoflurane. The needle is directed to the affected area, increasing the likelihood of obtaining a diagnostic sample. In case of lymphoma, a homogenous population of (atypical) lymphocytes will be found. A mixed population of lymphocytes and leukocytes points towards a reactive spleen, while a population of mature and immature erythrocytes is suggestive of extramedullary hematopoiesis. A lymphocytic-plasmacytic infiltrate may be an indication for Aleutian disease.

Since hypersplenism has been associated with anemia, leukopenia, and/or thrombocytopenia, it is advised to obtain a complete blood count in ferrets with a large spleen. It is also important to include a reticulocyte count to determine if there is sufficient erythropoiesis.

MANAGING THE LARGE SPLEEN

In the majority of cases no interference is necessary when a large spleen is found. The cause for the extramedullary hematopoiesis is unknown, but it usually does not pose any threat to the well-being of the ferret. When the spleen is so large, however, that it fills up the entire abdominal cavity, a splenectomy may benefit the ferret. The author was initially taught that the erythrocytes produced by extramedullary hematopoiesis in the spleen did not come into the circulation, but has discovered since that this is not the case. Removing a spleen may therefore have serious consequences to the turnover and production of erythrocytes. A bone marrow sample therefore should always be taken prior to removal of the spleen to ascertain adequate erythropoiesis.

In case of lymphoma or other neoplasms, the spleen should be surgically removed. It is important to know whether metastasis or other organs are involved, which can be evaluated by use of diagnostic imaging techniques such as survey radiographs and ultrasound. In those cases, additional chemotherapy may be necessary.

Hypersplenism

Hypersplenism has been described as a rare condition in ferrets in which excessive destruction of circulating blood cells takes place within the spleen. The presence of a cytopenia combined with normal, active bone marrow, in absence of an infection, neoplasm or other cause of a cytopenia, would be suggestive of hypersplenism.[1] The suggested treatment is splenectomy.

The author has seen a case resembling hypersplenism. The animal was a 5-year-old, male neutered ferret that was presented with lethargy, difficulty ambulating,, and a distended abdomen. Abdominal palpation revealed an enormous spleen. Complete blood count (CBC) revealed a packed cell volume (PCV) of 27%, a white blood count (WBC) of 2.0 x 10^3/µL, a thrombocyte count of 122 x 10^3/µL, and a reticulocyte count of 38.4%. One week later the PCV was 26%, the WBC 1.0 x 10^3/µL and the thrombocyte count 29 x 10^3/µL. The reticulocyte count was 35.3% at this time. It was then decided to evaluate the bone marrow by use of an aspirate biopsy, which was considered within normal limits. Based on these findings hypersplenism was the tentative diagnosis, and the spleen was surgically removed. One month after surgery, however, the ferret's hematologic values had not improved: the PCV was 21% and the WBC 2.1 x 10^3/µL. The thrombocyte count had increased to normal values: 709 x 10^3/µL. The reticulocyte count, however, had decreased dramatically to 1.9%. By removing the spleen we had thus converted a regenerative anemia into a nonregenerative anemia. Histology of the spleen only showed extramedullary hemotopoiesis. Despite many efforts, we were not able to find a specific cause for the anemia and the ferret died 5 months later.

SUGGESTED READING

1. Hillyer EV. Part II of cardiovascular diseases. In: Hillyer EV, Quesenberry KE (eds.): Ferrets, Rabbits and Rodents; Clinical Medicine and Surgery, 1st ed, Philadelphia: WB Saunders,1997, pp 71–76.
2. Morrisey JK. Part II of Cardiovascular diseases. In: Hillyer EV, Quesenberry KE (eds.): Ferrets, Rabbits and Rodents; Clinical Medicine and Surgery, 2nd ed, Philadelphia: WB Saunders, 2003, pp 66–71.

WORKING UP PRURITUS AND SKIN DISEASES

Nico J. Schoemaker, DVM, PhD
Diplomate ECAMS and ABVP-Avian
Division of Avian and Exotic Animal Medicine
Faculty of Veterinary Medicine
Utrecht University, Utrecht, The Netherlands

Skin diseases are common in exotic companion mammal medicine. Some of the diseases are infectious, with potential transmission towards the owners, while others have a metabolic etiology. A list of commonly found dermatologic conditions in exotic companion mammals can be found in Table 1. The approach to skin diseases in exotic companion mammals is similar to that of skin diseases in other companion animals.

SIGNALMENT Before being able to establish a diagnosis it is necessary to know some basic background information of your patient. It is foremost important to know what species you are dealing with. Certain diseases, such as syphilis, are very common in one species, while they are seldom diagnosed in other species. Sex predilection is also important for certain dermatologic conditions (eg, symmetric alopecia in female Guinea pigs with cystic ovaries). Another important factor is age. A study among Dutch ferrets has shown that symmetric alopecia and swelling of the vulva in female ferrets under the age of three is most likely due to a functional remnant ovary, while in ferrets over 3 years of age hyperadrenocorticism is more likely.

HISTORY

As with all patients, a thorough history provides you with very valuable information. Important questions that should be asked are:

- Where and when was the animal purchased? Certain dermatologic diseases are seen at an early age and most often directly after purchase (eg, dermatophytosis, the different types of mange and *Treponema paraluis cuniculi*).
- Does the animal have pruritus? With this question you can general differentiate between an infectious cause (bacterial, parasitic or fungal infection) and a metabolic cause (often hormonal). Infectious diseases are commonly associated with pruritus, while animals with a hormonal skin disease do not have pruritus. It is good to realize that hyperadrenocorticism in ferrets is an exception to this rule. Although pruritus is a common finding in this condition, it is not known what the triggering factor is for the pruritus.
- Do any of the other animals (if present) or any person in the household also have cutaneous symptoms? With this question you will also get an indication whether you are dealing with an infectious cause. If lesions are seen in persons in the household, it is likely you are dealing with dermatophytosis, although ectoparasites in humans may result in self-limiting erythematous papules as well. Children especially are sensitive in developing skin lesions due to dermatophytosis which may be located on the hands, arms, and in the neck. The latter is often seen when rabbits are carried against the body of the child.
- What is the progression of the disease? Are the clinical signs static, are they constantly getting worse, or are there periods of improvement? Dermatophytosis for instance may be self-limiting, with flare-ups during times of immune suppression.
- Has any medication been given to the patient? This may either be to treat or prevent the skin disease, but may also be unrelated to the cutaneous lesions.

Table 1. Skin Diseases Found in Exotic Companion Mammals

Species	Skin Disease	Pruritus?
Guinea pig	*Trixacarus caviae*	Yes
	Chirodiscoides caviae	Yes (mild)
	Trichophyton mentagrophytes	Yes
	Trichofolliculoma	No
Rat	*Notoedris muris*	Yes
	Myobia musculi	Yes
	Myocoptes musculinus	Yes
	Radfordia affinis	Yes
Rabbit	*Psoroptes cuniculi*	Yes
	Treponema paraluis cuniculi	No
	Cheyletiella parasitivorax	Yes (mild)
	Trichophyton mentagrophytes	Yes
	Pododermatitis	No
Ferret	*Otodectes cynotis*	Yes (sometimes)
	Hyperadrenocorticism	Yes (sometimes)
	Microsporum canis	Yes (mild)

PHYSICAL EXAMINATION

Cutaneous signs may be a reflection of systemic disease. It is therefore mandatory that in every patient which is presented with skin disease a physical examination is performed.

DERMATOLOGIC EXAMINATION

After an inspection of the animal from a distance, a closer inspection of the hairs, skin (including the pinnae), and mucous membranes is performed. Attention is paid to the quality of the hairs; is there (symmetric) alopecia, or are any broken hairs found? Are any lesions present? If so, how should they be characterized (papule, pustule, vesicle, wheal, nodule or tumor)? Are there any scales or crusts present? Are there signs of hypo- or hyperpigmentation? All lesions should be recorded in the file, which can then be used as a reference at return visits.

Specific Tests

Deep skin scrapings are performed in the majority of dermatological cases in search of a parasitic infestation. Scrapings should be performed in at least three different locations. Cytologic evaluation of the skin is possible by performing either direct impression smears, or tape preparations. The latter is commonly used to diagnose the yeast *Malassezia* spp. We have frequently attempted to find this yeast in association with hyperadrenocorticism in ferrets, but did not succeed.

To determine if the patient is infected with superficial ectoparasites (eg, lice and fur mites) the fur can be vacuumed while a tissue is held in front of the hose. The collected material can then be examined under a stereomicroscope or placed on a slide with KOH for evaluation under a regular microscope.

For direct visualization of ear mites in ferrets and rabbits it is most often sufficient to look into the ear with an otoscope or endoscope. In the author's experience, however, mites can be missed. In case no mites are seen, it is necessary to collect some cerumen and exam this under a microscope.

A Wood's lamp is seldom of use in exotic animal medicine. The great majority of fungal diseases in this group of animals are caused by *Trichophyton mentagrophytes* which is not detected by the Wood's lamp.

The most successful way to diagnose fungal infections is by using the McKenzie toothbrush method. For this technique the hair is brushed with a new toothbrush after it has been taken out of its sealed package. The brush may be sent directly to an official lab, or the hair and scales which were caught in the tooth brush are brought onto a culture medium. Sabouraud's agar to which a color indicator is added (Dermatophyte Test Medium [DTM]) is commercially available enabling in-house testing. In case of dermatophytosis the agar will change color during the growth of the fungus. This test method, however, does not enable you to differentiate between the different dermatophytes.

When all tests are unsuccessful in determining the cause of skin disease, a skin biopsy is the next step. Specific biopsy punches are available to obtain high quality skin biopsies with sharp borders. I prefer to bring all patients under general (isoflurane) anesthesia to obtain the biopsies, but in docile animals local anesthesia can also be used. Be careful with local anesthetics such as lidocaine, as most standard preparations have a high concentration of the active ingredient which may easily result in an overdosage (stay below 4 mg/kg BW). To obtain the best results, multiple biopsies (from different stages of the disease) should be taken within the border of the lesion. At the border most of the active process is ongoing which will provide the pathologist with extra information.

In case of skin tumors, such as trichofolliculomas in guinea pigs and sebaceous epitheliomas in ferrets, the entire tumor may be removed and sent in for histological examination.

The etiological agent for syphilis in rabbits is *Treponema paraluis cuniculi*. The typical lesions are found on the nose and in the anogenital region. Although the clinical signs are very suggestive of the disease, confirmation is not easy with any of the above described techniques. In these rabbits, serology is necessary to confirm your diagnosis. It has been described that the spirochete can be visualized with special silver stains in a biopsy. Serology, however, is the preferred method of diagnosis.

Allergies

In dogs and cats allergies are responsible for a great deal of the dermatologic cases seen in practice. In a ferret a food-related dermatological case has been reported, which responded to a commercial hypoallergenic diet for cats. The author has also seen a ferret with severe alopecia and pruritus. This ferret was initially suspected of hyperadrenocorticism, but all diagnostic tests could not confirm this diagnosis. After the owner changed the diet from a commercial cat food into a commercial ferret food, complete resolution of all signs occurred.

Alopecia, crust formation, and erythema can be seen in rabbits on all four feet, while no dermatophytes can be cultured. Thus far no cause for this clinical presentation has been reported. Although no hypoallergenic diets are available for rabbits, the author has seen improvement of clinical signs in these cases after placing the rabbit on a diet containing only hay and vegetables.

No intradermal skin tests have ever been described in exotic companion mammals.

NON-TYPICAL PRESENTATION OF DERMATOLOGICAL CASES

In our clinic we frequently have Guinea pigs presented with anorexia as their main complaint. As dental disease is high on the differential list for anorexia in this species an oral examination is required. Except for the expected cases of dental disease, we frequently see that the Guinea pig has hairs between the teeth and gingival. These Guinea pigs often do not have any signs of dental disease. The owner, in these cases, will often mention within the history that the animal licks its fur. The latter is a sign of mild pruritus, and prompts us to vacuum the fur in search for *Chirodiscoides caviae*. In case this fur mite is not found, a McKenzie toothbrush hair sample should be collected. Although *Trichophyton mentagrophytes* usually gives severe pruritus, cases with mild pruritus are also seen.

Example Case: "Speedy"

Speedy is a 4-year-old, male rabbit which was found in the wild at a very young age. His weight is 1.5 kg and is housed together with two other pet rabbits.

At first presentation he had a history of progressive alopecia, scaling, pruritus (in the form of licking the paws), thickening of the skin, and becoming less active. Since the rabbit did not want to be touched anymore, it was believed that the skin was very painful. This had been going on for at least 2 months. The two other rabbits, as well as the owner did not have any cutaneous complaints. The practitioner had performed multiple skin scrapings, but did not find any burrowing mites. Treatment with ivermectin also did not improve the condition. A fungal culture was inconclusive and it was decided to treat this rabbit with griseofulvin (25 mg/kg q24h). Improvement was seen and treatment was discontinued after 7 weeks when all signs seemed to have resolved. One month later, however, all clinical signs reappeared and treatment with griseofulvin was unsuccessful.

Clinical signs at presentation consisted of scattered alopecia of the entire body, spots of crusts and scales over the entire body with strong emphasis on the pinnae, and erythema on the abdomen (Figure 1). Again, skin scrapings as well as a vacuum sample did not reveal any mites and it was decided to take multiple skin biopsies. Pending the results the animal was treated with prednisolon (for possible autoimmune dermatosis), trimethoprim/sulfamethoxazole (for secondary bacterial infection), and fenbendazole (as precaution against *E. cuniculi* due to the prednisolone treatment). The initial histological result was: perivascular and interstitial dermatitis, with crusts suggestive of an allergic dermatitis. It was not considered to be typical of an auto-immune dermatitis. We then asked the pathologist to consult a pathologist with a specific interest in dermatology and ask if this would fit within the disease: sebaceous adenitis. The final diagnosis indeed was a chronic manifestation of sebaceous adenitis, as the biopsies did not contain any sebaceous glands.

CONCLUSION

Most dermatologic cases in exotic companion mammals can be diagnosed by taking skin scrapings, fungal culture, and vacuuming the fur. If these tests do not result in a diagnosis, it is advised to take skin biopsies and treat on the basis of these results.

SUGGESTED FURTHER READING

1. Paterson S (ed): Skin Diseases of Exotic Pets. Blackwell Publishing, 2006.
2. Schmidt RE (ed): Dermatology. Vet Clin North Am Exotic Anim Pract. 2001;4(2).

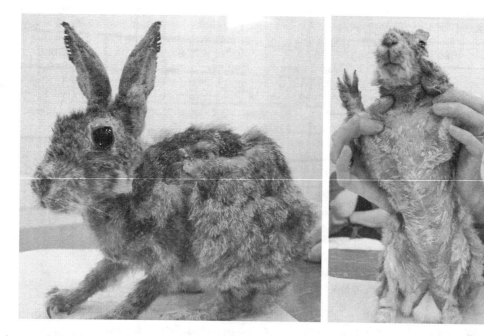

Figure 1. A 4-year-old rabbit with scattered alopecia, crust formation, thickening of the skin and erythema. Skin biopsies revealed that this rabbit had a chronic form of sebaceous adenitis.

EXOTIC COMPANION MAMMAL ZOONOSES: SMALL ANIMALS CAN HAVE BIG CONSEQUENCES

Nico J. Schoemaker, DVM, PhD,
Diplomate ECAMS and DABVP-Avian
Division of Avian and Exotic Animal Medicine
Faculty of Veterinary Medicine
Utrecht University, Utrecht, The Netherlands

Nearly two thirds of human diseases can be transmitted to animals. As veterinarians, however, we tend to use the term *zoonosis* when infections are transmitted from animals to humans.

An estimated 75% of emerging infectious diseases are zoonotic, mainly of viral origin, and likely to be vector-borne. Among the major causes of these emerging diseases are alterations in human behavior and modifications to natural habitats, consumption of bushmeat and other wild animals, development of ecotourism, access to petting zoos, and ownership of exotic pets. For exotic pet veterinarians, the latter two are the most important factors to consider.

Bacterial gastroenteritis and dermatophytosis are considered to be the most common zoonoses in exotic pets. Many other zoonotic diseases are diagnosed sporadically, but may have a detrimental outcome for the person who is infected. Besides knowledge of potential zoonotic diseases, it is important to know which measures should be taken to prevent infection. A selection of potential zoonotic agents, which have been found in exotic pet mammals, is given below.

BACTERIAL DISEASES
Salmonella spp

An estimated 3% to 5% of all cases of salmonellosis in humans are associated with exposure to exotic pets. A large portion of these cases are linked to exposure to reptiles, and, to a lesser extent, sugar gliders and hedgehogs. The most common symptoms in humans are headache, malaise, nausea, fever, vomiting, abdominal pain, and diarrhea. Symptoms usually occur within 12 to 24 hours after infection. Although most infections may be treated adequately, mortality in immunocompromised individuals has been described.

In the hedgehog *Salmonella tilene* and *S. typhimurium* are the most common pathogens associated with disease in humans. In East Anglia, however, the potential zoonotic *S. enteritidis* (PT11) has also been isolated from hedgehogs.[6] Human health officials are concerned about the prophylactic use of antibiotics in exotic pets by breeders and wholesalers, as this may lead to antibiotic-resistant *Salmonella* strains. The use of prophylactic antibiotic treatments should therefore be discouraged and limited to clinical cases, with a proper indication. Care should be taken that the dose, course duration and route of administration are correct to avoid suboptimal therapy.

Streptobacillus moniliformis (Rat Bite Fever)

Streptobacillus moniliformis, the causative agent for rat bite fever, can either be spread through rat bites or through water and/or (unpasteurized) milk contaminated by rats. Although up to 50% of rats have been reported to carry the bacterium in the nasopharynx or excrete it via the urine, infections occur only sporadically. The incubation period is 1 to 10 days in humans. Besides a fever, most human patients show an erythematous rash and arthritis of multiple joints. In severe cases endocarditis may occur. The bacterium seems sensitive to macrolides and tetracyclines.

Francisella tularensis (Tularemia)

The first reports of tularemia are were lemmings in Norway (lemming fever) and Californian ground squirrels in the Californian county Tulare. In the US, wildlife reported to be carriers of the bacterium consist of ground squirrels, cotton-tail rabbits, hares, and jack rabbits. In Europe, rabbits, water rats, and other rodents may carry the bacterium. Transmission occurs usually through tick bites (or other biting insects) [type 2], but may also be associated with hunting (contact) [type 1] or consumption of infected material [type 3]. Airborne infections [type 4] may occur through inhalation of contaminated dust of infected hay. The latter route seems to be the most likely when dealing with privately kept species.

The infection causes ulceroglandular, plaque-like lesions. The incubation period is 2 to 6 days. If left untreated lesions may persist for months. Treatment with aminoglycosides, eg. streptomycin, is recommended for a period up to 14 days. For endemic areas, vaccination may be considered.

Although the infection seems to be most commonly associated with wildlife, a 24-year-old man seroconverted during an outbreak of tularemia in prairie dogs (caused by *Francisella tularensis holartica* [type B], the less virulent strain); this man only showed atypical signs of the disease.

PARASITIC DISEASES
Baylisascaris procyonis

Baylisascarus procyonis is a roundworm that is commonly found in raccoons (up to 70% and 90% in adults and juveniles, respectively). These animals are increasingly kept as exotic pets in the Netherlands, but also live in close proximity to homes in the US. Raccoons can shed enormous amounts of eggs. When these eggs are consumed by an animal, other than a raccoon, the larvae will migrate through tissues and may eventually invade the eyes and brain (5% to 7% of cases). The latter may lead to severe disease and even death. Currently, there is no effective treatment available for the larval stage of *B. procyonis*.

Although only a few cases of larval migrans have been reported in humans, it should be discouraged to keep raccoons as pets. For the same reason, feeding raccoons in your back yard is not advised, as this will increase the risk of contaminating the yard with *B.*

procyonis eggs, which may survive in the environment for extended periods of time.

Encephalitozoon cuniculi

Encephalitozoon cuniculi is a microsporidial infection that is commonly associated with disease in rabbits. In humans, severe neurologic disease has been reported due to infection with *E. cuniculi*. Besides neurologic signs, AIDS patients were shown to display signs of hepatitis and nephritis. *E. cuniculi* could be isolated from the urine of some of these patients. The isolates were identified to be of rabbit origin. It should therefore be discouraged to AIDS patients to keep rabbits as pets.

Treatment of *E. cuniculi* is difficult because of its intracellular location. Albendazole is considered to be very efficacious against *E. cuniculi*, and may eliminate the infection completely.

VIRAL DISEASES
Rabies

Rabies is caused by a Lyssavirus. The virus replicates in all warm-blooded animals, and infection is fatal in nearly all cases. Transmission of the virus usually occurs when the infected animal is moribund. Each year, between 50,000 and 60,000 people die from rabies. Over 90% of these deaths occur in the tropics, resulting from canine bites. In Northern America, however, bat bites are responsible for more than 90% of human infections in the past 15 years. Of the confirmed rabies cases in animals in Northern America, over 60% consists of raccoons and skunks, and another 20% of different species of bats. In 2005, a rabbit was confirmed to have died from rabies as well.

Veterinarians who work with wildlife and exotic animals should be vaccinated in areas where rabies is endemic. Even when you have been vaccinated, treatment against rabies should commence directly after possible exposure to the virus. Exposure may either consist of a bite from a rabid animal, or contact with saliva of such an animal. It is therefore advised to never touch a bat, whether it is dead or alive. Rabies immune globulin and rabies vaccine are included in the treatment protocol.

Treatment should not only be given to people with known contact to the virus but also when a bat is found within the room of a sleeping person, an unattended child, and/or a mentally disabled or intoxicated person.

During a resent joint OIE/WHO/EU conference the Director General of the World Organization for Animal Health (OIE), Dr. Bernard Vallat said; "It is the prime responsibility of the veterinary profession to apply its knowledge and skills in animal disease control in order to create a buffer between the animal source of the disease and susceptible human beings."

As exotic animal veterinarians we should at least vaccinate all dogs, cats, ferrets, raccoons, skunks, fennic foxes, and other canids which come into our practice.

Lymphocytic Choriomeningitis (LCM)

Lymphocytic choriomeningitis (LCM) is caused by an Arenavirus. LCM is a common infection in laboratory mice, rats, and hamsters, but is rarely transmitted to humans. Approximately 5% of wild house mice are infected with LCM. Excreta of these mice are considered the most likely source of transmission of LCM infections in pet rodents and humans. Approximately 5% of humans have antibodies against LCM, indicating that they have once been infected with the virus. The great majority of LCM infections is benign and may give rise to symptoms such as fever, malaise, coryza, muscular pain, and bronchitis. Meningeal forms are also possible and may include headache, paralysis, and personality changes. In rare instances severe meningo-encephalomyelitis may lead to death of the patient.

LCM infections can be passed from a pregnant woman to her unborn child. Intrauterine infections may lead to hydrocephalus and retardation of the infant.

Monkey Pox

In 2003, a total of 71 persons were infected with monkey pox. These people had either been in direct contact with prairie dogs or had been on the premises where prairie dogs were kept. The incubation period ranged from 1 to 31 days.

These prairie dogs appear to have been infected by Gambian giant rats and dormice, which had been imported from Ghana. The presence of monkey pox was confirmed in prairie dogs, a Gambian giant rat, some dormice and rope squirrels. Because many of the imported rodents could not be traced, no human cases of monkey pox infection could be directly linked to these other rodents.

This case series illustrates the risk of importing animals and the need for a thorough tracing system of animals during the distribution process from the time of import until the sale to the end-user.

FUNGAL DISEASES
Dermatomycosis

Dermatophytosis is probably the most common zoonotic disease transmitted by pet exotic mammals. The most common dermatophyte in exotic pets is *Trichophyton mentagrophytes*. Infection may take place either through direct contact with an infected animal, which may be an asymptomatic carrier, or via an infected environment. The typical lesions in humans are centrifugally growing, roughly circular areas of variable erythema, scaling and desquamation. A central healing area may be present. While *Microsporum canis* generally causes a mild inflammation, *T. mentagrophytes* frequently produces more severe lesions.

Infections in humans are generally self-limiting, and respond well to topical imidazole treatment. Terbinafine is an allylamine antifungal that has proven to be effective local as well as systemic, often with a more rapid response time and/or higher response rate than the imidazoles.

PREVENTION OF ZOONOSIS

Of the list of potential zoonotic agents, many are not frequently associated with infections in humans. The humans which are at greatest risk are YOPI's (ie, young [below 5 years of age], old, pregnant, immuno-compromised). It should be advised that people who belong to this group do not keep exotic pets, especially those which are less frequently kept.

The infections which do occur frequently (eg, dermatophytosis, salmonellosis) can often easily be prevented by taking proper hygienic measures. It is surprising to see how little educational information was available in petting zoos before the year 2000. Minimal recommendations should include no eating and drinking while animals are being handled, and washing of the hands after handling animals (ie, facilities should be present). In addition, cages of exotic pets should not be cleaned in sinks where food may be prepared for human consumption.

As practitioners we should function as role models. Wash your hands after each animal examination, wear scrubs or a lab coat when working with animals, do not allow drinking and eating in the clinic (a separate area should be present). Before eating, drinking, or smoking, take of your scrubs and wash your hands. In the Netherlands some practices have developed a "no lab coat" policy. The idea behind this policy is to lower anxiety of the animals while being examined. From a hygienic standpoint, however, this policy should be discouraged as this highly potentiates the risks of transmitting zoonoses.

REFERENCES

1. Avashia SB, Petersen JM, Lindley CM, et al. First reported prairie dog–to–human tularemia transmission, Texas, 2002. Emerg Infect Dis. 2004;10:483-486.
2. Blanton JD, Krebs JW, Hanlon CA, Rupprecht CA. Rabies surveillance in the United States during 2005. J Am Vet Med Assoc. 2006;229:1897-1911.
3. CDC. Update: Multistate outbreak of monkeypox – Illinois, Indiana, Kansas, Missouri, Ohio, and Wisconsin, 2003. MMWR. 2003;52:642-646.
4. Chomel BB, Belotto A, Meslin F-X. Wildlife, Exotic Pets, and Emerging Zoonosis. Emerg Infect Dis. 2007; 13:6-11.
5. Palmer SR, Soulsby L, Simpson DIH (eds): Zoonosis; Biology, Clinical Practice, and Public Health Control. Oxford University Press, 1998.
6. Riley PY, Chomel BB. Hedgehog zoonoses. Emerg Infect Dis. 2005;11:1-5.
7. Sorvillo F, Ash LR, Berlin OGW, et al. *Baylisascaris procyonis*: An emerging helminthic zoonosis. Emerg Infect Dis. 2002;8:355-359.
8. Woodward DL, Khakhria R, Johnson WM, Human salmonellosis associated with exotic pets. J Clin Microbiol. 1997;35:2786-2790.

THE FLORIDA PANTHER: BIOMEDICAL INVESTIGATION AND GENETIC RESTORATION

Mark W. Cunningham, DVM
Florida Fish and Wildlife Conservation Commission
Gainesville, FL

The Florida panther is one of the most endangered mammals in the world and is a case study in the obstacles facing remnant populations. These obstacles are not only associated with small population size, such as reduced genetic variation and inbreeding depression, but also with the increasing impact of human activities experienced by virtually all wildlife populations. Anthropogenic factors such as habitat destruction and fragmentation reduce population size and restrict gene flow. Human activity may also reduce the quality of habitat or force wildlife to use less suitable habitat. Poaching, vehicular collisions, and other human activities can cause direct mortalities. Environmental contaminants, domestic animal diseases, exotic species, and introduction of foreign parasites and diseases are also having an increasing effect on today's wildlife populations. The Florida panther is impacted by virtually all of the above-mentioned anthropogenic effects; and management goals of panther restoration are directed towards ameliorating these impacts.

Historically the Florida panther occupied the entire southeastern United States and was contiguous with other cougar subspecies to the north and west. However, by the 1970s hunting and habitat destruction had reduced the panther to a remnant population occupying the Big Cypress and Everglades ecosystems of south Florida. Indeed the persistence of this population was uncertain until a survey documented at least two Florida panthers in the early 1970s.[1] This discovery led to an intensive long-term demographic and biomedical research project beginning in 1981. Veterinarians have played an important role in this project and recovery effort, assisting in panther capture and immobilization, emergency treatment and rehabilitation, research into genetic and disease threats, and management of disease outbreaks.

A significant proportion of the panther population is currently radio-instrumented, and captures are performed approximately every 2 years to replace radio-collars. The capture event is inherently a risk to the panther, and is achieved using trained hounds to tree the cat, followed by immobilization using a 3-mL dart and CO_2 powered rifle.[2] The panther usually trees between 15 and 50 feet high but occasionally bays on the ground. Before and/or after the panther is darted the area below the tree is cleared and a net and, depending on height, a crash bag are deployed.[3] Frequently the cat will come down or jump from the tree after being darted–either treeing again or baying on the ground.

There is the potential for injuries or complications at any stage of the capture. A panther may be anesthetized but remain in the tree—potentially resulting in hypoxia if ventilation is impaired. Pneumothorax, spinal injury, or other trauma may be associated with the fall following immobilization. Finally, running immediately after injection of immobilization drugs may result in hyperthermia, dog bites, drowning, and fractures. Drugs and equipment are present at all captures to reduce the likelihood and/or treat these injuries or complications. Additionally, contingency plans are in place for the removal of injured panthers to captive treatment facilities. At capture panthers undergo physical examination and are vaccinated against feline rhinotracheitis virus, feline calicivirus, feline panleukopenia virus, feline leukemia virus, and rabies. They also may be dewormed with praziquantel and ivermectin. Blood and other tissues are collected for CBC, serum chemistry, genetic analysis, environmental contaminants, and archiving.[4]

Early research findings painted a grim picture for the panther—environmental contaminants, anthropogenic mortality factors, inbreeding depression, lack of genetic diversity, and a host of other problems indicated the panther was in an extinction vortex and not likely to persist.[5] Environmental contaminants were and continue to be a threat to the Florida panther. In some areas of panther range mercury (Hg) concentration in panther hair has been as high as 150 ppm, and levels as high as 40 ppm have been detected in neonatal panther kittens. DDE and PCB levels have also been detected at levels as high as 100 ppm in fat. The source of these contaminants is believed to be bioaccumulation through the aquatic food chain.[6] Panthers feeding primarily on raccoons (and occasionally alligators) may have a greater risk for accumulation of these toxins compared to panthers feeding on ungulates.[9] Although a direct link has not been demonstrated,[7] Hg toxicosis is the suspected cause of death of one panther and may have contributed to the deaths of at least three others.[6] Further, sub-lethal Hg, DDE, and PCB concentrations may work with other stressors to reduce fitness and productivity.

Trauma is the most important mortality factor in the Florida panther—a large proportion of which are anthropogenic.[7] Intraspecific aggression—panthers killing panthers—was the most important mortality factor for radio-collared Florida panthers accounting for 40% of deaths in this cohort.[7] This primarily involves adult resident males killing dispersing juvenile males. However, with increasing frequency adult males have been killing adult females—many of whom have dependent kittens. The cause of this is unknown but may be related to increasing panther density. Vehicular collision was second in importance as a morality factor accounting for 19% of radio-collared panther mortalities.[7] Highway underpasses and fencing have greatly reduced panther and other wildlife vehicle-related mortality in areas where they exist. Indeed, since establishment of these underpasses no panthers have been killed on Interstate 75, historically the site of numerous road kills. However, as panther range expands mortalities are occurring at an increasing rate in areas without underpasses. Increasing traffic volume and a growing panther population are also contributing to the annual increase in panther highway mortality. The importance of illegal kills to the panther population is largely unknown; however, at least seven deaths due to poaching have been documented.[7] Complete necropsy of all panthers found dead helps to identify illegal kills and increased numbers of law enforcement personnel may help to reduce poaching. As with intraspecific aggression, the loss of females to vehicular collision and poaching may also result in the loss of dependent kittens.

Rehabilitation of orphaned kittens and injured panthers has helped reduce the impact of these mortality factors on the populations. Orphaned kittens and injured panthers, when possible are captured, raised in large wooded enclosures, trained to hunt, and released back into the wild as subadults. This effort has been quite successful with 11 of 13 panthers re-establishing themselves in the population. Panthers whose injuries are too severe or kittens that are too habituated to humans to release are kept in captivity as part of a captive population.

Protein electrophoresis and mitochondrial and minisatellite DNA analyses indicated the Florida panther is among the most genetically depauperate of any free-ranging felid population.[8] Small, isolated populations such as the panther face a number of demographic, environmental, and genetic threats. Random fluctuations in demographic variables, environmental fluctuations, and catastrophes can have severe impacts on small populations. Additionally, inbreeding and loss of genetic variation is inevitable in small isolated populations, and breeding between closely related panthers has been documented.[8] Inbreeding often results in inbreeding depression which may be manifested as congenital anomalies, reduced reproductive success, reduced neonatal survival, and immunoincompetence.

The Florida panther is believed to suffer from inbreeding depression, examples of which include atrial septal defects, cryptorchidism, poor semen quality, and immunosuppression.[8-11] These anomalies have impaired the health of individuals and consequently have had an impact on the population. Atrial septal defects are believed to have contributed to the deaths of three panthers,[9] and at least three panthers have been bilaterally cryptorchid and considered sterile.[10] Finally, reduced genetic variation may also increase the vulnerability of a population to infectious diseases. Together inbreeding depression and reduced genetic variation limit a population's ability to adapt to or compensate for demographic and environmental changes—resulting in an ever-increasing likelihood of extinction.

To reverse this downward spiral, a plan for genetic introgression was developed by the Florida Fish and Wildlife Conservation Commission and the U.S. Fish and Wildlife Service.[12] The plan called for a 20% introgression using cougars (*Puma concolor stanlyana*) from Texas—a subspecies that was historically contiguous with the Florida panther. This artificial restoration of historic gene flow was accomplished with the release of eight adult female cougars into South Florida in 1995. These pumas, for the most part, successfully established home ranges, bred, and reared kittens. This management action has greatly reduced the impact of inbreeding depression. The genetic restoration program and other management actions have been hugely successful and the panther population has rebounded from fewer than 30 to over 100. However, habitat loss has continued and the panther population likely has a greater density—increasing the risks of infectious diseases.

Infectious disease transmitted from domestic animals is an increasing threat to the panther population. As the panther expands its range and human encroachment into panther habitat increases there is increasing exposure of panthers to domestic animals. Feline leukemia virus (FeLV) has recently emerged as an important threat to the panther. Routine testing by ELISA for FeLV antigen in captured panthers had been negative since testing began in 1978. However, during the 2002–2003 capture season two panthers tested positive. This led to an investigation into the epizootiology of the disease and an evaluation of management methods.[13] Retrospective analysis of archived tissues indicated increasing exposure to the virus beginning in the late 1990s. The finding of FeLV antibodies without FeLV antigen also indicated that panthers could be exposed to the virus but not become persistently infected. However, at least 5 panthers were known to have become viremic, and at least 3 died due to FeLV-related diseases. All viremic panthers were clustered in the northern portion of panther range (Okaloacoochee Slough ecosystem [OKS]). Management of the epizootic began with vaccination, with efforts initially targeting panthers in a band between OKS and the remainder of the population. As of April 2007, approximately 40% of the population has received at least one FeLV inoculation.[13] Most importantly, no viremic panthers have been detected since July 2004.

Management efforts to reverse the decline of the Florida panther have largely been successful. The population may have reached a low of as few as 20 individuals, many of whom suffered from severe inbreeding depression. However, genetic introgression, construction of underpasses, management for greater prey densities, and other conservation efforts have resulted in a three- to fourfold increase in the panther population. Nevertheless, the panther must still contend with continued habitat loss and emerging threats such as FeLV. Further, without the establishment of additional populations, the panther population will inevitably be small due to limited available habitat. For these reasons continued intense management of the panther population is necessary to ensure their long-term survival.

REFERENCES

1. Nowak RM, McBride R. Status survey of the Florida panther. *In* World Wildlife Fund Yearbook 1973-1974. Danbury, CT: Danbury Press, 1974, pp 112-113.

2. McBride RT Jr, McBride RT. Safe and selective capture technique for jaguars in the Paraguayan Chaco. Southwestern Naturalist (in press, 2007).

3. McCown, JW, Maehr DS, Roboski J. A portable cushion as a wildlife capture aid. Wildlife Society Bulletin 1990;18: 34-36.

4. Roelke ME. Florida panther biomedical investigation, final performance report. Endangered species project E-1-11 7506. Florida Game and Fresh Water Fish Commission, Tallahassee, FL, 1990, 175 pp.

5. Seal US, Lacy RC, et al. Florida panther population viability analysis. Report to the US Fish and Wildlife Service. Captive Breeding Specialist Group, Species Survival Commission, IUCN, Apple Valley, MN, 1998.

6. Roelke ME, Schultz DP, Facemire CF, Sundlof SF, Royals HE. Mercury contamination in Florida panthers. A report of the Florida Panther Technical Subcommittee to the Florida Panther Interagency Committee, 1991, 25 pp.

7. Taylor SK, Buergelt CD, Roelke-Parker ME, Homer, BL, Rotstein DS. Causes of mortality of free-ranging Florida panthers. Journal of Wildlife Diseases 2002;38:107-114.

8. Roelke ME, Martenson JS, O'Brien SJ. The consequences of demographic reduction and genetic depletion in the endangered Florida panther. Current Biology 1993; 3: 340-350.

9. Cunningham MW, Dunbar MR, Buergelt CD, et al. Atrial septal defects in Florida panthers. J Wildlife Dis.1999; 35:519-530.

10. Mansfield KG, Land ED. Cryptorchidism in Florida panthers: Prevalence, features, and influence of genetic restoration. J Wildlife Dis. 2002; 38: 693-698.

11. Barone MA, Roelke ME, Howard J, et al. Reproductive characteristics of male Florida panthers: Comparative studies from Florida, Texas, Colorado, Latin America, and North American Zoos. J Mammalol. 1994; 75: 150-162.

12. Seal US. A plan for genetic restoration and management of the Florida panther (*Felis concolor coryi*). Report to the Florida Game and Fresh Water Fish Commission, Conservation Breeding Specialist Group, SSC/IUCN. White Oak Conservation Center, Yulee, Florida, 1994, 23 pp.

13. Cunningham MW, Brown M, Shindle D, et al. Epizootiology and management of feline leukemia virus in the Florida panther. J Wildlife Dis. Submitted for publication, 2007.

EMERGING DISEASES OF WILDLIFE WORLDWIDE

Kirsten Gilardi, DVM, Diplomate ACZM
Wildlife Health Center - School of Veterinary Medicine
University of California, Davis
Davis, CA

The role that free-ranging wildlife plays in the occurrence and emergence of disease in domestic animal and human populations is being increasingly recognized by governmental agencies charged with protecting the public's health and by the public itself. Diseases affecting North American wildlife such as chronic wasting disease, bovine tuberculosis, and West Nile virus figure prominently in our scientific journals and in the media. In contrast, the public remains less aware of many other emerging diseases of wildlife of similar importance in terms of their impacts. Several diseases of wildlife documented and described for the first time in the last decade or so are causing declines in populations (eg, facial tumor disease in Tasmanian devils), significant economic losses (eg, viral hemorrhagic septicemia of fish), or are threats to human health (eg, harmful algal blooms, or HABs). Other diseases are ones we have known something about for quite some time (eg, lead toxicity in birds), but that are now impacting new taxa, or occurring in new habitats or geographic locations. The following select diseases illustrate the variety of new disease impacting free-ranging wildlife populations, and demonstrate in some cases the ways in which human actions have directly or indirectly contributed to the emergence of these diseases.

FACIAL TUMOR DISEASE IN TASMANIAN DEVILS

Orofacial tumors (undifferentiated subepithelial sarcomas) were first reported in wild Tasmanian devils in 1996. In less than a decade, the disease spread across >50% of the devil's range, and over 50% of trapped animals in some areas are affected by the disease.[1] Only adults are affected, and the disease is invariably fatal, with mortality occurring presumably due to the impact of the tumors on the ability of the devil to see and feed, leading to starvation. Tumors are spread by direct transmission of whole tumor cells from an infected host to another devil via bite wounds, which is similar to the mode of transmission for canine transmissible venereal tumors (via allograft). The disease has caused significant declines in the Tasmanian devil population, with losses up to 80% in some areas. No reservoir species have been identified. The impact of this disease on Tasmanian devils has led the State Government of Tasmania to list the species as threatened.

LEAD TOXICITY IN TERRESTRIAL BIRDS

The banning of the use of lead shot to hunt waterfowl and aquatic birds in many parts of the world (including in the United States and Canada) has significantly reduced the incidence of lead toxicity in these species. However, lead ammunition is still used to hunt terrestrial species (eg, deer), and as a result, terrestrial birds continue to be affected by lead poisoning through ingestion of hunter-killed carcasses and gut piles.[2] This is especially true of raptors and scavengers, including the California condor: indeed, losses of California condors from lead poisoning was the primary reason for the decision to capture all remaining free-ranging California condors out of the wild. Lead toxicity has even been documented in upland game birds and columbiformes that ingest spent lead pellets as grit. The extent to which lead toxicity due to lead bullet fragment ingestion was impacting the Stellar's sea eagle and white-tailed eagle populations led Japan to ban the use of lead ammunition to hunt deer on the island of Hokkaido.

VIRAL HEMORRHAGIC SEPTICEMIA (VHS) OF FISH

This highly contagious rhabdoviral disease was first isolated from wild Atlantic cod in 1979, and has since been detected in over 40 species of wild and farmed marine fish.[3] In North America, VHS first appeared in 1988 in adult coho salmon in Washington State. The viral disease has decimated farmed salmon stocks and wild Pacific herring, Pacific hake, and walleye pollock populations. The virus then invaded freshwater systems: it was first detected in the Great Lakes in 2003, and by Spring 2007, had hopped overland to invade inland freshwater lakes in Wisconsin, New York, and Michigan. In these lakes, VHS has been implicated as the cause of precipitous declines in top predators like muskellunge, a prized sport fish in the region.

AVIAN VACUOLAR MYELINOPATHY

This neurologic disease of bald eagles, American coots and other species of waterfowl first emerged in 1994. It affects migrating and wintering birds using reservoirs in the southeastern United States. It is believed that initially coots and waterfowl are infected from an environmental source, and then bald eagles are affected after eating diseased coots or other waterfowl species. AVM-affected birds are ataxic, unable to perch, swim in circles, or collide with objects during flight. Histologically, affected birds exhibit vacuolation of the white matter of the central nervous system. The etiology of AVM is unknown: researchers suspect a natural neurotoxin, perhaps associated with underwater vegetation like *hydrilla*, an introduced aquatic plant.[4]

CHYTRIDIOMYCOSIS IN AMPHIBIANS

Batrachochytrium dendrobatidis is a chytrid fungus that was first detected as a major cause of mortality in frogs in Australia in the 1990s. The fungus produces motile spores that disperse in water and invade the oral cavities of larvae and the epidermis of mature frogs. Since first detected in Australia, the fungus has caused major die-offs of frogs in the US, Mexico, Europe, New Zealand, and South America, likely due to repeated introductions of the fungus to naive areas. The fungus has been detected in frog populations that are not exhibiting widespread mortality, however, suggesting that some populations or species are resistant to disease while others are extremely sensitive. On a global scale, chytridiomycosis is of significant concern in light of the fact that up to one third of all amphibian species are threatened with extinction due to habitat loss, harvest, invasive species, environmental contaminants, climate change, and disease. In fact, the Wyoming Toad (*Bufo baxteri*) has been driven to near-extinction by the disease. Some conjecture that global climate change may be creating local environmental conditions that may allow *B. dendrobaditis* to invade, persist, and spread.

MYCOPLASMA CONJUNCTIVITIS

Mycoplasma gallisepticum conjunctivitis was first recognized in wild house finches in 1994 in the eastern United States. The disease in wild birds was caused by a novel strain of *M. gallisepticum*. Within three years, the disease had spread over the entire eastern range of the house finch, causing a severe decline in the wild finch population. Mycoplasma conjunctivitis was first documented in the western United States (in Montana) in 2002, and reached the West Coast (in Oregon) in 2004.[5] The disease is now endemic in house finches, causing seasonal peaks in morbidity and mortality and thereby limiting house finch populations. It has also been documented to cause diseases in other passerines.[6]

HARMFUL ALGAL BLOOMS (HABS) IN MARINE WILDLIFE

Since the 1980s, there have been numerous reports of marine mammal and seabird mortality events caused by brevetoxin, saxitoxin and domoic acid. These neurotoxins are produced by marine diatoms (algae); wildlife are exposed when they ingest prey items (fish, shellfish) that have consumed or concentrated the toxin-laden algae. It is the general consensus that these HABs have increased in both frequency and distribution worldwide. For example, in Puget Sound, Washington, *Pseudonitzschia*, which produces domoic acid, has been documented in the water for decades, but a toxic bloom of the diatom required closure of shellfish harvest beds for the first time in 2003. Since 1998, hundreds of California sea lions have been affected by domoic acid, and in fact, domoic acid toxicity has been a significant cause of reproductive failure in California sea lions in some years.[7] In the winter and spring of 2007, hundreds of coastal marine birds stranded in Southern California with neurologic disease during a *Pseudonitzschia* bloom that caused some of the highest concentrations of domoic acid ever measured in seawater. Scientists link the increase in HABs with changes in coastal land use as well as climate change effects in the ocean.

NSAID TOXICITY IN ASIAN VULTURES

The first decade of the 21st century has seen the first ever occurrence of a man-made pharmaceutical compound threatening a free-ranging wildlife species with extinction. Populations of *Gyps* vulture species went into steep decline in the 1990s, with Oriental white-backed vultures reduced by more than 95%. The cause of mortality was renal failure and visceral gout, due to ingestion of Diclofenac™, a nonsteroidal anti-inflammatory drug (NSAID) administered in large quantities to cattle in Pakistan, India and Nepal.[8] Vultures, which in India and surrounding south Asian countries feed primarily on livestock carcasses, were dying of acute renal failure. Researchers, using liquid chromatography and mass spectroscopy, detected diclofenac residues in the kidneys of every vulture carcass examined.

These diseases are just a few examples of the many infectious and non-infectious agents affecting the health of free-ranging wildlife worldwide. While pathogens and disease are a normal aspect of the ecology of wild animals, the extent to which human-induced changes in land use, management, and climate are modulating these natural host-pathogen processes is of concern. The veterinary community is urged to work closely with biologists, food producers, policy-makers and the public to work towards better balancing the needs for habitat and food of both wildlife populations and human communities,

REFERENCES

1. Hawkins CE, Baars C, Hesterman H, et al. Emerging disease and population decline of an island endemic, the Tasmanian devil *Sarcophilus harrissii*. Biol Conservation. 2006; 131(2): 307-324.
2. Fisher IJ, Pain DJ, Thomas VG. A review of lead poisoning from ammunition sources in terrestrial birds. Biol Conservation. 2006: 131: 421-432.
3. Gagne N, MacKinnon AM, Boston L, et al. Isolation of viral haemorrhagic septicaemia virus from mummichog, stickleback, striped bass and brown trout in eastern Canada. J Fish Dis. 2007; 30(4): 213-223.
4. Fischer JR, Lewis-Weis LA, Tate CM, et al. Avian vacuolar myelinopathy outbreaks at a southeastern reservoir. J Wildlife Dis. 2006; 42(3): 501-510.
5. Ley DH, Sheaffer DS, Dhondt AA. Further western spread of Mycoplasma gallisepticum infection of house finches. J Wildlife Dis. 2006; 42(2) 429-431.
6. Farmer KL, Hill GE, Roberts SR. Susceptibility of wild songbirds to the house finch strain of *Mycoplasma gallisepticum*. J Wildlife Dis 2005; 41(2): 317-325.
7. Brodie EC, Gulland FMD, Greig DJ, et al. Domoic acid causes reproductive failure in California sea lions (*Zalophus californianus*). Marine Mammal Sci. 2006: 22(3): 70-707.
8. Oaks JL, Gilbert M, Virani MZ, et al. Diclofenac residues as the cause of vulture population decline in Pakistan. Nature 2004; 427: 630-633.

DERELICT FISHING GEAR AND MARINE WILDLIFE: IMPACTS & SOLUTIONS

Kirsten Gilardi, DVM, Diplomate ACZM
Wildlife Health Center - School of Veterinary Medicine
University of California, Davis
Davis, CA

Derelict fishing gear—nets, lines, pots, traps, and other gear that is lost in the ocean—impacts marine wildlife, underwater habitat, and people. Derelict gear sits on the seafloor, gets caught on rocky reefs, or floats in the water column, where it entangles or traps marine life, is swallowed, or endangers boats and people, especially divers. Since the 1950s, commercial and recreational fishing gear has been made of synthetic materials that do not decompose in seawater for years. Leaving fishing gear in the ocean is usually not intentional. However, unfortunately ropes attaching a piece of gear to a vessel or a float fail or get cut by another boat's propeller; and stormy weather can roll a pot, trap, or net far from where the fisherman first put it in the water, so that he/she can't find it upon returning to harvest the catch.

Rehabilitators and veterinarians treat hundreds of coastal birds and marine mammals every year for gear-related injuries. Most beach visitors have at some point observed a bird with a hook and line hanging from its bill or wrapped around its foot. Entanglement in man-made debris (primarily fishing gear) was the cause of injury in 107 live stranded pinnipeds admitted to the California Marine Mammal Center between 1986 and 1998,[1] and between 1988 and 1995, 3 of 11 Guadalupe fur seals stranding in California were entangled in debris.[2] In just one year, approximately 1% of the New Zealand fur seal and Australian sea lion populations living on an island off the coast of South Australia were affected by fishing gear entanglement, with the authors of the study estimating that fishing gear entanglement causes 1400+ mortalities in seals and sea lions in Australia every year.[3] And finally, in Hawaii, derelict fishing gear is the most serious human-related threat to the fragile coral reefs of the Northwestern Hawaiian Islands (NWHI), where derelict gear abrades, enshrouds, encrusts and breaks the corals. It also endangers wildlife like the endangered Hawaiian monk seal: between 1982 and 2000, biologists documented over 200 Hawaiian monk seal entanglements in derelict gear, 25 seals in 1999 alone.[4]

Impacts of derelict fishing gear on the Hawaiian monk seal and coral reefs prompted the federal government to start a major clean-up operation in the NWHI in 1998; since then, well over 500 tons of fishing gear and other debris have been removed from the island chain. Washington State started a derelict fishing gear removal program in 2002 in order to address the problem of thousands of abandoned crab pots and hundreds of lost nets in Puget Sound which were ghostfishing or drowning wildlife.

In order to reduce the impact of derelict fishing gear on marine wildlife in California, the UC Davis Wildlife Health Center's SeaDoc Society launched the California Lost Fishing Gear Recovery Project in (www.lostfishinggear.org). SCUBA divers survey the seafloor for lost gear; once gear is located, divers disengage it from the reef and raise it to the sea surface, where it is winched on board a boat and transported back to the mainland. To date we have retrieved over 11 tons of commercial fishing gear from critical wildlife habitat in Southern California. As well, we have removed thousands of feet of fishing line and hooks from the water around public fishing piers, and have set up fishing line recycling bins on several of these piers (this recycling effort is modeled on a very successful program developed here in Florida: www.brevardcounty.us/mrrp). We are currently conducting a retrospective review of data at wildlife rehabilitation centers to determine baseline rates of injury in California coastal wildlife due to fishing gear entanglement and ingestion, so that we may look at rates of injury after the pier clean-up and prevention program to determine overall efficacy of our project.

REFERENCES

1. Goldstein T, Johnson SP, Phillips AV, Hanni KD, Fauquier D, Gulland FMD. Human-related injuries observed in live stranded pinnipeds along the central California coast 1986–1998. Aquat Mammals. 1999; 25(1): 43-51.
2. Hanni KD, Long DJ, Jones RE, Pyle P, Morgan LE. Sightings and strandings of Guadalupe fur seals in Central and Northern California, 1988 - 1995. J Mammalogy. 1997; 78(2): 684-690.
3. Page B, McKenzie J, McIntosh R, et al. Entanglement of Australia sea lions and New Zealand fur seals in lost fishing gear and other marine debris before and after government and industry attempts to reduce the problem. Mar Poll Bull. 2004; 49(1-2): 33-42.
4. Boland RC, Donohue MJ. Marine debris accumulation in the nearshore marine habitat of the endangered Hawaiian monk seal, *Monachus schauinslandii,* 1999-2001. Mar Poll Bull. 2003; 46(11): 1385-1394.

WHAT YOU NEED TO KNOW ABOUT AVIAN INFLUENZA IN WILD BIRDS

Jonathan Sleeman, MA, VetMB, Dipl. ACZM, MRCVS
Virginia Department of Game and Inland Fisheries
Richmond, VA

INTRODUCTION TO AVIAN INFLUENZA

Avian influenza is usually an inapparent infection of wild birds that is caused by type A strains of influenza viruses. They consist of a collection of slightly different viruses rather than a single virus type. The virus subtypes are classified based on two types of surface antigens, hemagglutinin (H) and neuraminidase (N). There are currently 16 H and 9 N recognized subtypes, and all subtypes are known to infect wild birds, thus providing an extensive reservoir of influenza viruses circulating in bird populations. Avian influenza viruses are able to change their genetic components by antigenic drift (ie, accumulation of mutations in the genetic makeup of the virus) and antigenic shift (ie, the process by which two different strains of influenza combine to form a new subtype having a mixture of the surface antigens of the two original strains, or by re-assortment that mixes any of the other eight viral segments). Different combinations of the two antigens appear more frequently in some bird groups. For example, in waterfowl the H3, H4, and H6 are the predominant subtypes, whereas the H11 and H16 are the predominant subtypes in gulls. H9 and H13 were thought to be the predominant types in other shorebirds; however, recent research indicates that there may not be any subtype predominance, and the subtypes vary each year.

Avian influenza viruses are also classified as low pathogenic (LPAI) or highly pathogenic (HPAI) based on genetic comparisons with known isolates and the viruses' ability to cause high mortality in domestic poultry. HPAI viruses are associated with the H5 and H7 subtypes; however, not all H5 and H7 subtypes are highly pathogenic but most are thought to have the potential to become so. The avian influenza viruses in wild birds are almost exclusively low pathogenic subtypes that pose no threat to human or domestic animal health. In fact, prior to the HPAI H5N1 avian influenza outbreaks (see below) the only mortality event in wild birds caused by a HPAI was a die-off of common terns in South Africa during 1961 in which a H5N3 subtype was isolated.

Low pathogenic avian influenza viruses are most often found in migratory *Anseriformes* (ducks, geese and swans), especially mallards. Other wild birds yielding influenza viruses include various species of *Charadriiformes* (gulls, terns, and shorebirds) as well as quail, pheasants and ratites. LPAI viruses survive well in cold fresh water and the virus is maintained in wild birds by fecal (or contaminated water)–oral routes of transmission. Observable signs of illness due to LPAI have not been described for wild birds. These viruses are found worldwide, and can be found throughout the year in waterfowl. The highest prevalence in waterfowl occurs during late summer and early fall. In Charadriiformes, the prevalence is highest in spring during migration, and to date a high prevalence has only been reported in ruddy turnstones from the Delaware Bay area.

Wild birds represent the historic source of type A influenza viruses for domestic bird and mammalian species. After the movement of these viruses from wild to domestic animals or humans, the virus may evolve to become a new host-adapted virus. These new viruses would differ from the original wild bird strains and would no longer be associated with wild bird populations. Fortunately, this movement and adaptation from wild birds to new host species is a rare event.

HIGHLY PATHOGENIC H5N1 AVIAN INFLUENZA (HPAI H5N1)

HPAI H5N1 is a highly pathogenic H5N1 avian influenza virus that emerged in Asia and at least two clades have persisted since 1996–1997. It has now caused the largest and most severe avian influenza outbreak in poultry on record. Extensive outbreaks were detected in Southeast Asia in 2003, and have now spread throughout a large geographic area in Asia, Europe and Africa. To date, nine Asian countries have reported outbreaks, and the virus has become endemic in some domestic poultry (primarily populations of chickens and domestic ducks) in several of the initially affected countries. In July 2005, the virus spread geographically beyond its original focus to affect poultry and wild birds in the Russian Federation and Kazakhstan. Almost simultaneously, Mongolia reported detection in wild birds. In October 2005, the virus was detected in the Middle East and spread to Africa and various European countries.

In 1997, a human death resulting from HPAI H5N1 infection was reported in Hong Kong and as of July 2007, 318 cases with 198 deaths have been reported to the World Health Organization. Human cases have been reported in Asia, Africa, the Pacific, Europe and the Near East, and almost all have been linked to direct contact with infected poultry. Indonesia and Vietnam have reported the highest number of human cases.

During 2002–2003, wild bird mortality in Hong Kong was attributed to infection with HPAI H5N1. In May 2005, HPAI H5N1 was reported to be the cause of a large die-off of bar-headed geese in Qinghai, China in which 5% to 10% of the local population may have perished. Most of the wild birds confirmed as infected with HPAI H5N1 either were displaying clinical signs consistent with HPAI infection, or were moribund, or dead. Wild bird mortality associated with HPAI H5N1 has continued through 2007, and the virus has now been isolated in over 90 species of wild birds and mammals. This extent of mortality in wild birds is highly unusual and unprecedented. Experimentally, clinical signs in wood ducks and laughing gulls included cloudy eyes, ruffled feathers, weakness, incoordination, tremors, seizures and death. Torticollis was also seen in gulls. Other species did not develop clinical signs but did shed virus. In the same study, gross pathologic lesions in wood ducks were multiple petechial hemorrhages in the pancreas, whereas gulls had more extensive petechiation in the ventriculus (gizzard), heart, cerebrum, and pancreas.

Role of Migratory Birds

The role of migratory wild birds in the movement and transfer of this Eurasian strain of HPAI H5N1 is not clear. While the virus has been detected in an increasing number of wild birds, the pattern and timing of several outbreaks have not coincided with periods of major migratory movements or known migration routes. However, there are reports of wild bird mortality associated with outbreaks of HPAI H5N1 in poultry, and the expansion in distribution of HPAI N5N1 throughout Asia to Europe and Africa suggests that domestic flocks are being infected with this virus through contact with migratory birds. In addition, phylogenetic studies of the viruses from different outbreaks in birds have found that viruses from the most recently affected countries are almost identical to viruses recovered from dead migratory birds at Qinghai Lake, China.

There is concern that bird migration may be a possible route of introduction of HPAI H5N1 into North America. Some migratory bird species do move between North America, Asia, and Europe. North American birds that over-winter in Asia may come into contact with infected birds during the winter months, and in spring infected migratory birds returning from Asia can potentially interact with other North American wild birds as they co-mingle on the breeding grounds. However, genetic studies of avian influenza viruses from Europe, Asia and North America suggest that there is very limited exchange of strains of virus between continents. Thus, based on the known epidemiology of low pathogenic avian influenza viruses, the introduction of HPAI H5N1 into North America via migratory birds would be a low probability event. Illegal smuggling of birds and poultry products, travel by infected people or people traveling with virus-contaminated articles are more direct, and more likely, routes of introduction of this virus to the United States.

Another concern is the possibility of HPAI H5N1 being maintained in wild bird populations. There is limited information with which to assess this, but experimental studies have demonstrated bird-to-bird transmission of HPAI H5N1 in young mallards. Other experimental studies have consistently demonstrated higher respiratory, rather than cloacal, shedding of the virus. LPAI viruses are associated with cloacal shedding and fecal-oral transmission via contaminated water. Thus, it is uncertain if the extent of fecal shedding of HPAI H5N1 is consistent with the ability to be transmitted via the fecal-oral route in a natural setting, and subsequently be maintained in wild bird populations. In addition, these viruses do not appear to be as resistant in the environment as naturally occurring LPAI viruses. To date, the detection of HPAI H5N1 in wild birds has always been associated with morbidity and mortality of wild birds, and there has not been any detection of the virus as a result of surveillance of asymptomatic live birds that were not spatially associated with poultry outbreaks. Consequently, the potential for this virus to be maintained in wild bird populations has not been proven.

Close contact with infected poultry has been the primary way that people have contracted HPAI H5N1 virus. While there are no confirmed reports of people being infected with HPAI H5N1 from wild birds, it is probable that seven human cases in Azerbaijan were exposed to the virus as a result of de-feathering dead swans. In the United States there is currently no public health risk associated with HPAI H5N1 and wild bird contact, and there is no indication that wild birds in North America are infected with HPAI H5N1. However, basic hygiene is recommended when handling any wild animals or carcasses. People should avoid direct contact with any birds that are found dead. Dead birds that are encountered should not be picked up. The location should be accurately documented and the appropriate state or federal wildlife agency should be contacted to determine if testing is warranted. If the birds need to be disposed, then they should be handled with disposable gloves or a shovel should be used to maintain a barrier. The dead birds should be placed in a trash bag or double shopping bag, tied off, and placed in the garbage bin. Alternatively, the birds may be buried but not in a plastic bag or cover. Hands should be washed with warm water and soap, and the shovel cleaned with 10% bleach. Hunters should wear some basic protection such as gloves, and keep tools and work surfaces clean when preparing game animals. Hunters should also follow basic hygienic precautions such as hand washing, proper food preparation, and thorough cooking of game meat.

Surveillance for HPAI H5N1 in Wild Birds in the United States

Due to the concern that migratory birds may introduce HPAI H5N1 into North America, wild bird surveillance for avian influenza has been dramatically increased since 2005 and 2006. This surveillance is a coordinated effort between various state and federal government agencies and is based on *The US Interagency Strategic Plan: An Early Detection System for Asian H5N1 Highly Pathogenic Avian Influenza in Wild Migratory Birds* that was developed by the US Departments of Agriculture, and Interior, with input from the Department of Health and Human Services, Association of Fish and Wildlife Agencies, and others. The goal is to detect, as early as possible, the unlikely introduction of the Eurasian strain of HPAI H5N1 into North America by migratory wild birds. Species for sampling were selected based on their potential risk for being exposed to, or infected with, HPAI H5N1 because of their migratory patterns. It is thought that the most likely entry points are via Alaska or the Greenland/Northeastern Canada corridor. Thus, birds that migrate from these areas, birds that have the potential to be in contact with species that migrate from these areas, or are considered a sentinel species due to their susceptibility to HPAI H5N1 have been (and will continue to be) sampled for this virus. Sampling strategies include investigation of morbidity and mortality events, active surveillance of live birds and hunter-killed birds, surveillance of sentinel species, and environmental sampling. To date, more than 147,849 birds in every US state and Canadian province have been tested, and HPAI H5N1 has not been detected in North America. This surveillance will continue during 2007-2008 and as long as the risk remains.

PANDEMIC RISK

A pandemic can start when a new influenza subtype emerges, it infects humans causing serious illness, and there is efficient and sustained human-to-human transmission. HPAI H5N1 meets the first two conditions, but not the latter. The risk that this virus will acquire the ability to transmit efficiently from human-to-human as a result of genetic changes (mutations within the virus or recombination or re-assortment with a human influenza virus) will persist as long as the virus continues to circulate in birds. If this were to occur it would be considered a new virus and it would no longer require an avian source.

References are available from the author upon request.

CAN WE MANAGE CHRONIC WASTING DISEASE?

Terry J. Kreeger, MS, DVM, PhD
Wyoming Game and Fish Department
Wheatland, WY

Jonathan Sleeman, MA, VetMB, Dipl. ACZM, MRCVS
Virginia Department of Game and Inland Fisheries
Richmond, VA

Chronic wasting disease (CWD) is a fatal brain disease of white-tailed deer, mule deer, elk, and moose. Chronic wasting disease is classified as a transmissible spongiform encephalopathy (TSE). There are many TSEs that affect humans and other animal species. Examples of human TSEs are sporadic Creutzfeldt-Jakob disease, variant Creutzfeldt-Jakob disease, kuru, familial Creutzfeldt-Jakob disease, and fatal familial insomnia. The cattle TSE is bovine spongiform encephalopathy, or more commonly called "mad cow disease." Scrapie is the TSE of sheep and goats.

The agents of TSEs (prions) are thought to be abnormal isoforms of a normal extracellular glycoprotein, but agents such as viruses have not been disapproved. Prions are neither bacteria nor viruses. They are proteins devoid of nucleic acid. In conspecific strains, prions have identical amino acid sequences as normal cellular proteins, but in a different conformation. The functional role of the normal cellular protein is unknown, but it may be involved in copper homeostasis or intercellular communication. The abnormal prion causes a conformational change in the normal cellular protein whereby the normal alpha helical content of the protein diminishes and the amount of beta sheet increases. When the prion is injected directly into the brain of a test animal, spongiform encephalopathy occurs. If the test animal is devoid of normal protein, injection of the abnormal prion results in no pathology.

CLINICAL SIGNS OF CWD

In cervids, the general clinical signs of end-stage CWD include emaciation, poor body condition, rough hair coat, behavioral changes (hyperactive when constrained; reluctance to move; ears droop), excessive salivation, excessive urination, excessive drinking (or staying close to water sources), lethargy (but will react when approached closely), teeth grinding, and death. As with other TSEs, a relatively long incubation precedes the clinical phase of CWD; most infected animals that are harvested by hunters outwardly appear to be normal and in good physical condition.

EPIZOOTIOLOGY OF CWD

In North America, all native cervids (elk, mule deer, white-tailed deer, moose) with the exception of caribou have been diagnosed with CWD, which can occur both in wild populations and in captivity. Although fawns and calves may have evidence of CWD-associated prion accumulation, clinical disease usually does not occur for at least 12 months after experimental exposure, and perhaps longer after natural infection. Either sex can contract CWD, but there is a slight bias towards males. CWD is one of two contagious prion diseases (the other is scrapie). The route of natural exposure is unknown, but the oral route is known through experimentation. The source of infectivity is unknown, but it could be prion-infected saliva, urine, feces, or contaminated feed or soil, or insects or other vectors. Transmission is lateral; that is from one animal to another, or indirectly from an infected animal to the environment to an uninfected animal. Prevalence of CWD may be quite high (>50%) when animals are held in captivity.

HUMAN HEALTH

Bovine spongiform encephalopathy (BSE) was first recognized in 1986 in the United Kingdom. BSE was associated with cattle consuming feeds possibly containing scrapie-infected meat products. Human consumption of BSE-infected beef resulted in variant Creutzfeldt-Jacob disease in 1995. Whereas sporadic Creutzfeldt-Jakob disease occurs in about one in one million people (usually in advanced age, 55–70 years), variant Creutzfeldt-Jakob disease occurs in younger people (19–39 years). Because BSE and CWD are both TSEs, there is a concern that humans can contract CWD.

The case rate for Creutzfeldt-Jakob disease in Wyoming and Colorado is less than the national average, yet CWD has been in these states for more than 25 years. Thus, there is no epidemiologic evidence that CWD affects humans. In addition, some very compelling research using transgenic mouse models for both cervids and humans, indicated that there is a substantial species barrier for transmission of CWD to humans. Currently, the scientific community thinks that it is unlikely, but not impossible, for humans to contract CWD from eating infected deer or elk.

LIVESTOCK HEALTH

Unlike with humans, there is direct experimental evidence regarding CWD and domestic cattle. In parallel studies conducted in Wyoming and Colorado, 10 cattle given a single oral inoculum of CWD showed no signs of disease and 20 cattle living amongst CWD-infected deer and elk also showed no signs of disease. However, when the CWD prion is injected directly into the brain of cattle, some neurologic pathology has been noted. Nonetheless, these data strongly support that it is very unlikely that cattle can contract CWD from either deer or elk.

WILDLIFE HEALTH

A common mantra for management of CWD is: 1) prevent spread by containing the disease, 2) control CWD by reducing prevalence, and 3) eventually eradicate the disease. However, it has also been a common rule that once a disease has become established in wildlife, it is very difficult to eradicate. Thus, there is no substitute for prevention. Disease control in wildlife can be difficult, costly, long-term, and may inflame the public.

The "chronic wasting" syndrome was first recognized in Colorado in the late 1960s, but may well have been occurring there and elsewhere prior to that time. CWD is now found in Colorado, Wyoming, Nebraska, South Dakota, Kansas, Utah, New Mexico, Wisconsin, Illinois, West Virginia, New York, Saskatchewan, and Alberta.

Understandably, management of CWD has varied from state to state and province to province. Two factors have probably directed the management of CWD more than any others: 1) CWD could eventually result in the decimation or even extermination of a given cervid population and 2) like BSE, humans could contract CWD and develop some form of TSE. Mathematical models have indicated as CWD prevalence increases within a population there is a concomitant decrease in numbers, perhaps eventually leading to local extinction. Currently, there is no known confirmation of these predictions based on field data. However, there are indications that CWD can affect the age structure of the population by reducing the proportion of older animals. Eventually, these changes may have profound effects on a population.

WISCONSIN CWD MANAGEMENT

CWD was discovered in south central Wisconsin in 2002. The state launched an aggressive CWD management program with the goal of eradicating CWD. This program included increased hunting, unlimited bag limits, free licenses, rewards, and other actions to reduce deer numbers and prevalence. Initially, the target population density goal was five deer per square mile. Despite these efforts, deer numbers actually increased from 26/mi² in 2002 to 38/mi² in 2005 in the disease eradication zone. As of May 2007, the Wisconsin Department of Natural Resources estimated that deer populations have not been significantly lowered in the disease eradication zone. However, no new cases were detected outside of the CWD zone in 2006 and government sharpshooters killed 987 deer to remove 23 positive animals (2.3%). Still, CWD prevalence in the disease eradication zone has not decreased. Rather, it has increased slightly since 2002. Although initially high, hunter enthusiasm for killing large numbers of deer has declined since initiation of the CWD eradication management plan. As of 2006, Wisconsin has spent more than $27 million for CWD management. This equates to $31,579 per positive CWD deer removed.

COLORADO CWD MANAGEMENT

Colorado probably is the leader in researching and implementing various CWD management actions. The state attempted deer herd reductions in a few areas to reduce prevalence; although this approach received moderately good public support, it was discontinued because managers could not demonstrate that reducing local deer numbers consistently resulted in lowered disease prevalence. Preliminary results from a test-and-remove experiment indicated that this method might reduce prevalence as well as remove positive animals from the population, but the approach was expensive and time-consuming to implement, and application appeared most useful in urban settings.

Colorado's current CWD management approach is to 1) eliminate CWD suspects; 2) enforce longstanding cervid feeding prohibitions; and 3) prevent spread of CWD via human activity (ie, rehabilitation, captive wildlife movements, improper carcass disposal).

The Colorado Division of Wildlife's philosophy on CWD management is that eradication is infeasible because of persistence of the CWD prion in the environment. Control of the disease is also problematic because of difficulties as to where to start within the state and how to measure efficacy. The state also believes that the usual approach (ie, killing deer) is probably ineffective and that there are no clearly effective tools or technology, nor vaccines, preventative, or curative treatments.

PRINCIPLES OF CWD MANAGEMENT
Surveillance

Management actions that do appear to have merit include statewide surveillance, not only to track prevalence rates, but to identify new areas outside of the core endemic area. However, cost-effective surveillance approaches are needed to sustain long-term monitoring of areas where CWD has not been detected.

Hot Spots

When new areas ("hot spots") outside an endemic area are identified through surveillance, agencies can initiate increased animal harvest in the hopes of locating and eliminating all CWD positives or, at the least, obtain better data on true prevalence rates in the area. Prevalence rates often give an indication of how long the disease has existed in the area; if the disease appears to have been in existence for several years there is little, if anything, agencies can do to eliminate the disease. As currently practiced, this approach has yielded mixed success.

Game Ranch Programs

The Animal and Plant Health Inspection Service of the federal government has drafted a nationwide program to monitor CWD in cervid ranches. The goal of this program is to identify ranches with CWD and eliminate all positive animals, as well as to invoke controls on animal movement within and among the states. Because the animals are in captivity and can be observed and tested routinely, there is a high likelihood that this program will be successful in greatly reducing, if not eliminating, CWD from cervid ranches.

Check Hunter Kill

Although it probably will never be known whether humans can contract CWD, there will be a certain segment of the hunting population that will have lingering concerns and will have a desire to have their deer, elk, or moose tested for CWD. This is a service that most state wildlife management agencies do or could provide.

Ban Artificial Feeding

Artificial feeding of animals, primarily in the wintertime, concentrates animals in a very small area, which increases the likelihood of disease transmission, whether it is CWD or any other disease. Prohibiting the private feeding of game animals will decrease this artificial concentration and thus should decrease the probability of disease transmission.

Remove Obviously Affected Animals

Killing and removing any cervid showing obvious signs of CWD is a standard policy of virtually all states and provinces. This is because these animals may be actively shedding the CWD prion into the environment and transmitting the disease to other animals plus removal eliminates any role the carcass may have in disease transmission.

Carcass Transport Control

Research conducted in Colorado has demonstrated that a CWD-infected carcass left in the environment can transmit the disease to other animals. Thus, controls should be implemented to restrict movement of possibly infected carcasses from a CWD area to an uninfected area or require/encourage proper disposal of the carcass.

Research

In the past few years, much has been learned about CWD, but a tremendous amount is still unknown. Effective CWD management probably will never be implemented without knowing precisely how the disease is transmitted from one animal to another. Because of the interest in human TSEs, there has been increased research in vaccinations or treatments. From a wildlife management agency viewpoint, the one big question yet unresolved is what impact CWD has on free-ranging populations of deer, elk, or moose.

ROADBLOCKS TO CWD MANAGEMENT

There are major obstacles to successful control of CWD in free-ranging populations. The most intractable of these is probably the persistence of the CWD prion in soil. Exactly how long the CWD prion remains infective is unknown, but recent research regarding the scrapie prion indicated that it can persist in the soil for at least 16 years. Thus, agencies may be successful in reducing or eliminating a population from a given area, only to have the infection began anew when re-populated by animals outside of the eradication area.

The unimpeded movement of infected wild animals is also problematic. Elk have well documented migration behaviors. Recent research conducted in Wyoming on white-tailed deer documented a one-way, 150-mile movement of a CWD-infected doe. If CWD becomes established in a large area, it would be virtually impossible to stop or impede the movement of infected animals and the establishment of CWD in new areas.

The inability, thus far, to specifically identify how CWD is transmitted from one animal to another will continue to prevent meaningful management intervention. Research is currently being conducted in Wyoming and Colorado to identify the method of transmission, as well as to develop sensitive assays capable of detecting the prion in a variety of substrates.

THE FUTURE

It is probably safe to predict that CWD will continue to spread in the wild. However, there is hope that CWD will be significantly decreased or eradicated in game ranches. There probably will be increased barriers to movement of carcasses from states having CWD to uninfected states or provinces. There will be a continued demand by hunters to have their harvested animals checked for CWD. If no effective tools are developed for the control of CWD, checking hunter-killed animals and minimizing potential human exposure (or at least ensuring hunter participation in controlling infected cervid populations) may ultimately be all that can be done.

CONSERVATION MEDICINE APPROACH TO MANAGING WILDLIFE DISEASES

Jonathan Sleeman, MA, VetMB, Dipl. ACZM, MRCVS
Virginia Department of Game and Inland Fisheries
Richmond, VA

Emerging infectious diseases are commonly defined as infectious diseases whose incidence has recently increased or threatens to increase in the near future. There are various categories including new infectious agents that result from changes or evolution of existing organisms (eg, highly pathogenic H5N1 avian influenza and multi-drug resistant tuberculosis); known infections spreading to new geographic areas, species, or populations (eg, chronic wasting disease, and West Nile virus); previously unrecognized infections appearing in areas undergoing ecological transformation (eg, Ebola virus and severe acute respiratory syndrome, or SARS); and old infections re-emerging (eg, bovine tuberculosis). In recent history there has been an unprecedented number of new infectious diseases that have been identified, and many of the emerging diseases that are threats to human, animal, and ecosystem health are of wildlife origin. In fact, it has been estimated that approximately 75% of emerging diseases are zoonotic in origin.

Globalization can be defined as increasing global connectivity, integration, and interdependence in the economic, social, technological, cultural, political, and ecological spheres. While globalization can increase economic prosperity as well as opportunity, especially among developing nations, enhance civil liberties, and lead to a more efficient allocation of resources, it can also result in unsustainable harm to the biosphere. Globalization and the associated human activities create a global environmental situation that favors disease emergence. Examples of these human activities or "drivers" of emerging infectious diseases include ecological alterations (climate change, loss of habitat and biodiversity as well as invasive species); human demographic and behavior changes; international travel and trade; microbial adaptation and change; and lack of resources to prevent and control these diseases, as well as breakdown of public health measures due to war and natural disasters.

Disease prevention is the desired method to protect the health of wildlife populations as once a disease has been introduced into a population it can be very difficult, if not impossible, to control or eradicate. There are very few effective wildlife disease management tools available to wildlife veterinarians, managers, and conservationists. The few options available (eg, population reduction, use of vaccines or other biologics, and environmental modification) are expensive, lack any assurance of success, and can be unpalatable to the general public. Historically, disease control and prevention has focused on the immediate cause of ill-health, ie, controlling the infectious or toxic agent and mitigating the effects on the host. However, intervening at the level of the "driving forces" or "pressures" that promote the emergence of health threats will be the most effective point of control. For example, in developing countries it is often poverty, or lack of economic opportunity, that drives the depletion of natural resources that result in environmental degradation that is responsible for the emergence of an infectious agent and subsequent threat to the health of wildlife and human populations. Thus in this example, focusing on poverty reduction and sustainable development should eliminate the drivers of these diseases and prevent emerging disease outbreaks. Consequently, it is vital that relevant national and international policies such as agricultural, economic, energy, environmental, health, housing and development, trade and transportation policies, among others, appropriately balance the need for economic development with the need to protect human, wildlife, and ecosystem health. Ensuring this balance is met as well as focusing on long-term action directed at mitigating the effects of the drivers of emerging diseases will not only be the most cost-effective method to prevent the emergence of wildlife diseases, but will have multiple benefits for wildlife, humans, and the shared ecosystems.

Additional measures needed include the promulgation of laws and regulations that enforce this balanced approach, public education, and development of enhanced biosecurity measures. In addition, risk analysis, early-detection disease surveillance, and rapid response systems will be essential to allow robust and effective responses to wildlife disease outbreaks. Considerable research is also necessary to ensure that decisions at all levels are science-based as well as to develop new disease diagnostic, surveillance, and management tools. One of the biggest impediments to successful wildlife disease management is the lack of capacity to effectively address wildlife health issues, and the Association of Fish and Wildlife Agencies has developed a *National Fish and Wildlife Health Initiative for the United States* with the goals of developing and enhancing federal, state, and territorial fish and wildlife management agency capacity to effectively address health issues, and develop and implement a national strategy to address health issues involving free-ranging fish and wildlife through management, surveillance, and research (www.fishwildlife.org). International capacity building will also be vital.

Conservation medicine is a relatively new interdisciplinary scientific field that studies the relationship between human and animal health, and environmental conditions. Conservation medicine is at the nexus of the fields of human, animal, and ecosystem health, requires professionals from diverse disciplines to work together to address these new disease threats to human and animal health from anthropogenic ecological changes, and provides a theoretical framework with which to address the problems of emerging infectious diseases and wildlife disease management discussed above. Animal health and human health are inextricably connected through the ecological realities governing life on our planet, and we need to define the appropriate balance between the needs of people, wildlife, and domestic animals in the face of finite energy, land and resources. Nothing less than the integrity of the biosphere is at risk.

REFERENCES
1. Taylor LH, Latham SM, Woolhouse ME, Risk factors for human disease emergence. Philos Trans R Soc Lond B Biol Sci. 2001;356:983-989.
2. Wobeser GA. Essentials of Disease in Wild Animals. Blackwell Publishing, 2006.
3. Corvalan CF, Kjellstrom T, Smith KR. Health, environment and sustainable development. Identifying links and indicators to promote action. Epidemiology. 1999;10:656-660.
4. Aguirre AA, Ostfeld RS, Tabor GM, House C, Pearl MC (eds.): Conservation Medicine: Ecological Health in Practice. Oxford University Press, 2002.

WILDLIFE ZOONOSES WITH AN EMPHASIS ON BIOTERRORISM AGENTS

Jonathan Sleeman, MA, VetMB, Dipl. ACZM, MRCVS
Virginia Department of Game and Inland Fisheries
Richmond, VA

Zoonotic infections are diseases that occur primarily in wild and domestic animals that can be transmitted to humans. Infectious pathogens that originate in wildlife have become increasingly important in recent decades. The emergence and re-emergence of these wildlife zoonoses is associated with a range of causal factors, and most of them are a result of human activities such as increasing human populations, global human travel and trade of wildlife, changing land use patterns, and other environmental changes. In addition, there is the increasing threat of acts of bioterrorism, ie, the deliberate release of biological agents as weapons with the aim of causing illness and death in people, animals, or plants. Four of the six Category A, or high priority agents that pose the highest risk to the public and national security are also considered wildlife zoonoses, and include anthrax, plague, tularemia, and viral hemorrhagic fevers.

Veterinarians are often considered a source of information by the general public as well as clients on all topics relating to animal health and zoonotic diseases. While all persons who feel they have been exposed to a zoonotic pathogen should be immediately referred to his or her health care provider so that a diagnosis can be made and the correct treatment prescribed, it is important that veterinarians are able to give advice regarding the potential risks, what to do in the event of exposure, assist in early recognition of disease as well provide information to help prevent exposure. Consequently, this article emphasizes practical information and advice that veterinary practitioners can give to their clients and the general public regarding measures that can be taken to prevent or reduce exposure to zoonotic pathogens. In addition, some wildlife species are highly susceptible to the high-priority bioterrorism agents mentioned above and unusual morbidity and mortality of wildlife may provide an early warning of an act of bioterrorism, prior to recognition of illness in humans. In order to realize the role of wildlife as sentinels of bioterrorism events, it is important that veterinarians are aware of the clinical signs of infection with these agents in wildlife. The recognition of these early warnings will allow rapid reporting to the appropriate authorities and protection of the public's health.

RABIES

Rabies is an acute encephalomyelitis caused by viruses belonging to the genus *Lyssavirus* in the family *Rhabdovirus*. It is one of the oldest recognized infectious diseases and has a global distribution except for Antarctica. The *Lyssavirus* genus contains at least seven antigenically distinct viruses which are maintained in different reservoir hosts. Within each serotype or genotype there are also a number of variants that are maintained by different hosts. All mammals are considered susceptible; however, terrestrial carnivores and bats are the major reservoirs. The major terrestrial reservoir species in North America are the raccoon (*Procyon lotor*), skunks (*Mephitis mephitis* and other species), foxes, (*Vulpes vulpes, Urocyon cinereoargenteus*, and *Alopex lagopus*) and coyote (*Canis latrans*). These species are responsible for maintaining distinct rabies strains in various geographic regions of North America. In contrast, rabies in insectivorous bats, caused by several bat-adapted strains, occurs throughout the continental United States.

Rabies virus is shed in the saliva and is usually introduced by a bite wound. Rare forms of transmission include a contaminated scratch or wound, mucous membrane exposure, aerosol, laboratory accident or organ transplantation. Incubation is variable, but is usually less than 3 months. The clinical course of the disease is short and once clinical signs develop it is invariably fatal. Animals with rabies will typically have markedly abnormal behavior which is often classified into two forms. "Dumb" rabies is characterized by aimless wandering, lethargy, ataxia, hind leg weakness, paralysis, and loss of awareness. Other signs include pruritis, hyperexcitability, hyperesthesia, photophobia, hypersalivation, dysphagia, change in phonation, and mydriasis. Less frequently in some species "furious" rabies may occur with vicious attacks on any object and self-mutilation. Both forms ultimately result in seizures, coma, and death.

Rabies is only transmitted when the virus is introduced into bite wounds, open cuts, or onto mucous membranes from saliva or other potentially infectious material such as neural tissue. People are usually aware if they have been bitten; however, because bats have small teeth the bite marks may be small and easily missed. Consequently, if a person awakens to find a bat in the room, or if a bat is near a child or mentally impaired or intoxicated person then rabies exposure should be suspected. Persons who have been exposed should be advised to wash the wound thoroughly with soap and water and should be referred to his or her physician and state or local health authorities. The wild animal suspected of having rabies should be killed without damage to the brain and placed in double layered bags for submission to a diagnostic laboratory. Latex gloves should be worn when handling the carcass which should be refrigerated. It is vital that the veterinary practitioner obtain a detailed case history including names and contact information of persons exposed as well as the identity of any exposed domestic animals. Diagnosis of rabies in animals is done post mortem using fluorescent antibody testing on central nervous tissue.

People should be advised to not approach or handle unfamiliar wild or feral animals especially if they appear friendly. Wild animals should not be fed, or unintentionally attracted to human inhabited areas, for example, due to open garbage cans or litter. People should not bring wild animals into their homes or try to nurse sick animals. People should be advised to call animal control or the state wildlife agency regarding sick, injured or nuisance wildlife. "Bat proofing" houses and community buildings may also help prevent exposure. This can be achieved by caulking or filling any holes that are larger than a quarter-inch diameter. Window screens, chimney caps, and draft-guards beneath doors to attics should be used as well as ensuring that all doors to the outside close tightly. Attics can be bat-proofed by covering outside entry points by hanging bird netting or plastic sheeting. When the bats leave the holes can be permanently sealed. The best time to bat-proof a home is in the fall and winter as most bats will leave to hibernate.

Considerable resources are dedicated to controlling rabies in free-ranging wildlife populations. Currently, the United Stated Department of Agriculture Animal and Plant Health Inspection Service Wildlife Services program is distributing oral rabies vaccines in an effort to create rabies-free barriers in various regions of the US. The vaccine consists of a live vaccinia vector with a rabies virus glycoprotein spliced into the vaccinia virus. Although the vaccinia virus is highly attenuated it does present a remote risk to immunocompromised persons, particularly those who have skin disease or are pregnant. The plastic vaccine sachets are ice-cubed size and are coated with a sticky, scented substance. Some are placed inside fish meal polymer baits. The baits have a toll free number (1-877-722-6725) printed on them for people to call in the event of human or domestic animal contact. People should be advised not to touch the bait and wash their hands after handling one. There is no harm from touching an intact bait. Pet owners should be warned not to attempt to remove a bait from an animal's mouth as a bite wound from an animal that has broken the sachet may result in exposure to the vaccine. Contact with the liquid vaccine inside the sachet should be reported to the local health department. In addition, the exposed area should be washed thoroughly with soap and water. Vaccine consumption is not harmful to animals, and does not interfere with the regular rabies vaccination schedule; however, some diarrhea may develop if multiple baits are consumed.

ANTHRAX

Anthrax is caused by the bacterium *Bacillus anthracis*. Anthrax has been reported in a wide range of species, but herbivores especially cervids and bovids are most susceptible to fatal disease. Carnivores are more likely to develop chronic form of disease. Anthrax is an extremely rapid disease and animals will die within a few hours of illness. Fever, weakness, dyspnea, and hemorrhage from orifices are common observations. Often anthrax occurs in numerous animals simultaneously resulting in a sudden die-off. The natural reservoir of anthrax is the soil, particularly areas with neutral to alkaline soils with high organic content. Accidental ingestion of spores by grazing animals is the most common route of transmission, but once infection has started, bacteria can be spread from animal to animal by biting flies or mechanical means.

Transmission to humans typically occurs as a result of incidental contact with infected animals or contaminated animal products or as a consequence of fly bites. Symptoms in humans vary according to the type of anthrax. Cutaneous anthrax presents as a small sore that develops into a non-painful blister and ulcer with a black central area. The symptoms of gastrointestinal anthrax include, nausea, hemorrhagic diarrhea, and fever whereas signs of inhalation anthrax will include respiratory signs such as coughing, chest discomfort, shortness of breath, fatigue, and myalgia.

Anthrax can be used as a weapon, and this occurred in the US in 2001. Anthrax was deliberately spread through the postal system by sending letters with powder containing anthrax and resulted in 22 cases of human infection.

TULAREMIA

Tularemia is a serious life-threatening human disease caused by the bacterium *Francisella tularensis*. At least two subspecies are recognized: *Francisella tularensis* biovar *tularensis* (also known as type A) and *Francisella tularensis* biovar *palaeartica* (or type B). Type A is considered the more virulent subspecies. *Francisella tularensis* has one of the broadest host ranges of all bacteria, but is primarily a disease of lagomorphs and rodents. In North America, tularemia most commonly involves cottontail rabbits (*Sylvilagus* sp), black-tailed rabbits (*Lepus californicus*), snow shoe hares (*Lepus americanus*), beaver (*Castor canadensis*), and muskrat (*Ondatra zibethicus*). Clinical signs in wildlife species are often variable, but may include lethargy, ataxia, stupor, and infected animals are often more easily caught compared with healthy animals. Tularemia is highly infectious and can be transmitted by all known epidemiologic routes including arthropod vectors, direct contact with infected blood or tissues, through intact skin or wounds, through ocular mucous membranes, inhalation and ingestion. Symptoms in people will vary depending on the route of exposure but include ulceroglandular and glandular syndromes typified by fever and swollen lymph nodes or oropharyngeal form typified by pharyngitis and tonsillitis. Typhoidal tularemia presents with fever, chills, headaches, diarrhea, myalgia, arthralgia, progressive weakness and may be accompanied by bronchopneumonia. Pneumonia is usually a sequel to inhalation exposure. The practitioner should advise the general pubic to avoid touching and handling sick animals, especially lagomorphs and rodents, and wear latex gloves and wash hands thoroughly after handling animal carcasses. Game meat should be cooked well. Persons frequenting areas with arthropod vectors should take the appropriate precautions (see section on Tick-Borne Diseases). Finally, people should be advised to avoid areas where tularemia is known to be occurring in wildlife.

Francisella tularensis could be used as a bioterrorism agent as it is very infectious, and only a small number of organisms (10–50) can cause disease. If *F. tularensis* were used as a weapon, the bacteria would likely be made airborne for exposure by inhalation. People who inhale an infectious aerosol would experience severe respiratory illness, including life-threatening pneumonia and systemic infection, if left untreated. The bacteria that cause tularemia occur widely in nature and could be isolated and grown in quantity in a laboratory, although manufacturing an effective aerosol weapon would require considerable sophistication.

PLAGUE

Plague is a rare bacterial disease caused by *Yersinia pestis* and there is a long history of human outbreaks. Its importance is illustrated by the fact it is one of very few international quarantinable infectious diseases of people. It is flea transmitted and perpetuated by rodents. Infection in humans can result in severe disease with a high case fatality rate. In North America, plague is mostly confined to the southwestern areas with most cases reported from New Mexico, Arizona, Colorado, and California. Periodically there are outbreaks among more susceptible species of rodents such as prairie dogs (*Cynomys* spp) ground squirrels (*Spermophilus* sp), and fox squirrels (*Sciurus niger*) and these die-offs are often the first indication of plague activity in an area. Public education, particularly for hunters, trappers and other outdoor recreationists and restriction of activities in areas with active plague are important preventive strategies. People should also be advised to not touch dead animals, and make homes and human-inhabited buildings rodent-proof (see section on Hantavirus Pulmonary Syndrome). Persons frequently outdoors should take the appropriate precautions to prevent flea bites (see section on Tick-Borne Diseases). Cats are very sensitive to plague and can bring infected fleas into homes. Consequently, domestic pets should be treated for fleas and not allowed to roam freely.

Yersinia pestis could be used as a bioweapon in an aerosol attack that could cause cases of the pneumonic form of plague. Clinical signs would develop 1 to 6 days after becoming infected. Once disease develops, the bacteria could spread to other persons in close contact. Because of the delay between being exposed to the bacteria and becoming sick, people could travel over a large area before becoming contagious making control of the disease more difficult.

HANTAVIRUS PULMONARY SYNDROME (HPS)

This disease is caused by infection with a variety of hantaviruses, was first recognized in 1993 in the Southwestern United States, and this outbreak was later found to be caused by the Sin Nombre virus. Since then, several pathogenic hantaviruses have been identified in the US, and each virus has a single rodent host. All hantaviruses known to cause HPS are carried by New World rats and mice of the family *Muridae*, subfamily *Sigmodotinae*. The deer mouse (*Peromyscus maniculatus*) is the host for Sin Nombre virus. The deer mouse is common and widespread in rural areas throughout much of the US. Other hantaviruses associated with sigmodontine rodents and known to cause HPS include New York virus, which is hosted by the white-footed mouse (*Peromyscus leucopus*); Black Creek Canal virus, which is hosted by the cotton rat (*Sigmodon hispidus*); and Bayou virus, which is hosted by the rice rat (*Oryzomys palustris*). Nearly the entire continental US falls within the range of one or more of these host species. Early symptoms in humans include fever, headaches, myalgia, nausea, vomiting, diarrhea, dizziness and chills. Later symptoms include severe respiratory distress due to pulmonary edema and can be rapidly fatal. Humans are exposed through the inhalation of aerosolized rodent urine, feces and saliva as well as handling rodents. Prevention involves excluding rodents from homes and buildings including shelters and cabins, as well as watching for signs of rodent infestation and promptly removing any infestations. Homes should be kept clean and food covered in rodent-proof containers. Garbage should also be secured. All entry holes to buildings wider than ¼ inch should be sealed. Spring-loaded rodent traps and Environmental Protection Agency (EPA)-approved rodenticides can be used to reduce infestations. Predators such as non-venomous snakes and raptors are excellent natural methods to reduce local rodent populations. Infested areas can be cleaned using 10% bleach solution. Workers who regularly handle rodents are at increased risk for this disease, and should contact the Centers for Disease Control and Prevention (CDC) for more detailed safety precautions (www.cdc.gov).

ARTHROPOD-BORNE VIRAL ENCEPHALITIS

There are a number of arthropod-borne viruses in North America that cause encephalitis in humans including St. Louis encephalitis, Eastern (EEE) and Western equine encephalitis, LaCrosse encephalitis, Jamestown Canyon encephalitis (JCE) and most recently West Nile virus (WNV). Infection with these diseases is most often asymptomatic, or results in transient, mild clinical signs such as fever, headache, nausea, vomiting, and lymphadenopathy. Rarely, mostly older people will develop severe illness including high fever, neck stiffness, stupor, disorientation, coma, tremors, convulsions, vision loss and paralysis. The most severe encephalitis is caused by EEE which can have a case fatality rate of 50%. The arboviruses are maintained in complex cycles involving different wild vertebrate hosts (eg, birds, rodents and deer for JCE) and a variety of mosquito species, and humans will acquire infection through the bite of infected mosquitoes. The most effective way to avoid WNV and the other arboviruses is to prevent mosquito bites. People should be advised to use insect repellent containing an EPA-registered active ingredient. It is important that the directions on the package are followed. Many mosquitoes are most active at dusk and dawn and avoiding outdoor activities during these times is advisable; otherwise persons should wear long sleeves and trousers. Houses and other buildings should be mosquito proof including appropriate screens on doors and windows. Finally, it is advisable to remove potential mosquito breeding sites by eliminating standing water from flower pots, buckets, wading pools, blocked gutters and drains, and other containers including water bowls and bird baths. Holes should be drilled in any receptacle that could collect water, such as tire swings, to allow drainage.

There is currently no evidence that WNV can be transmitted directly through handling infected birds or handling and consuming infected meat; however, people should be advised not to handle live or dead wild birds directly with bare hands. The local health department or state wildlife agency should be contacted for advice on reporting and disposing of the carcasses. Hunters and trappers should wear gloves when handling and cleaning animals and meat should be cooked thoroughly.

TICK-BORNE DISEASES

There are an increasing number of tick-borne diseases that appear to be increasing in prevalence in certain regions of North America. These diseases occur most commonly from May to September when ticks are most active. Lyme disease is caused by the spirochete bacterium *Borrelia burgdorferi*, and is found most commonly in the northeast from Massachusetts to Maryland as well as the upper Midwest. Human ehrlichiosis is a recently recognized tick-borne disease caused by at least two types of bacteria that infect leukocytes. The distribution of human infections correlates with the distribution of the tick vectors and human cases have been reported in the southeast, northeast, upper Midwest and west coast. For *Ehrlichia chaffeensis*, the causative agent of human monocytotrophic ehrlichiosis, white-tailed deer (*Odocoileus virginianus*) are the primary reservoir and the geographic distribution of naturally infected animals was found to be a good sentinel system for predicting risk for human infection. Rocky Mountain Spotted Fever (RMSF) is caused by the bacterium *Rickettsia ricketsii*, and occurs most commonly in the southeastern and south-central states. In addition, babesiosis is caused by hemoprotozoan parasites of the genus *Babesia*. *Babesia microti* and *Babesia divergens* have been identified in most human cases and occurs most frequently in the northeast and Midwest. All these diseases have complex life cycles involving many species of wild mammals, birds and possibly reptiles as natural reservoirs for these organisms and different species of ticks as vectors. Furthermore, white-tailed deer are not important reservoirs for Lyme disease, but are important in the epidemiology of the disease as the primary host for adult *Ixodes scapularis*, which is the main tick vector in the northeastern, central, and southeastern states.

Despite the number of tick-borne diseases and their complex epidemiology, prevention and control is the same for these diseases and relies on methods to limit exposure to ticks. Ticks prefer wooded and bushy areas with high grass and leaf litter and people should be advised to avoid tick-infested areas, especially during May to September. Insect repellents with 20% to 30% DEET (*n, n*-diethyl-*m*-toluamide) applied to the skin can be used to prevent tick bites. Use DEET with caution on children. In addition, permethrins can be applied to clothing but should not be applied directly to skin. Persons at risk should be advised to wear long trousers, long sleeves and socks as well as light colored clothes to help detect ticks more easily. Eliminating gaps in clothing such as tucking pant legs into socks can also be helpful. After being outdoors, all parts of the body should be carefully checked especially haired areas. Outdoor clothes should be thoroughly washed and dried to kill any ticks. Ticks should be removed from the body immediately using fine-tipped tweezers. The tick should be grasped as close to the skin as possible and pulled upward with steady, even pressure. The tick should not be jerked or twisted to prevent the mouthparts remaining in the skin. Ticks should not be handled with bare hands and care should be taken not to puncture the body. After removing the tick, the areas should be disinfected and some people may wish to freeze the tick for later identification should illness occur within 2 to 3 weeks. Other community-based methods such as the application of acaricides and landscape manipulation can be applied if the risk warrants these more intensive and expensive measures. Deer movement and population control is another strategy and this is initiated at a local level in consultation with the state wildlife agency. Activities that can artificially increase deer populations such as feeding should be discontinued. There are some new tools available such as bait boxes that will treat wild rodents with an acaricide and they are available from licensed pest control companies, and research is continuing to investigate other tick control measures such as treatment of deer with acaricides as well as biological control measures.

POLYARTHRITIS IN ALASKAN ARCTIC FOXES (*ALOPEX LAGOPUS PRIBILOFENSIS*)

Terry R Spraker, DVM, PhD, Diplomate ACVP
College of Veterinary Medicine and Biomedical Sciences
Colorado State University, Fort Collins, CO

Paula White, BS, MS, PhD
Monterey, CA

As far back as the late 1700s, arctic foxes (*Alopex lagopus*) have been commercially farmed for their fur. Despite hundreds of years of captive husbandry and intensive management associated with fur-farming of *Alopex* throughout their range, there has been little investigation into naturally occurring disease in this species. To date, only a few diseases have been described in *Alopex*. These primarily include conditions that negatively impact reproduction because these conditions decreased commercial harvest of pelt. Other diseases and parasites that are potentially dangerous to humans or domestic animals (eg, rabies, canine distemper, parvovirus, *Echinococcosis*) have been documented in arctic foxes.

A previously unrecognized condition characterized by failure to shed the winter pelage and lameness has been observed in the Pribilof Island Arctic foxes (*Alopex lagopus pribilofensis*) from the Saint Paul Island, Alaska. The Pribilof fox (*Alopex lagopus pribilofensis*) is a subspecies of the arctic fox that occurs on the Pribilof Islands, Alaska. This condition is called Shaggy Lame Fox Syndrome, denoting the primary clinical signs. Sick foxes are usually observed in the summer. The first clinical sign usually observed is lameness in all four limbs. The foxes do seem to warm out of the disease. This can be observed in early spring. As the disease progresses there is a failure of the fox to shed its winter hair coat. Because of this the foxes appear extremely shaggy. These foxes appear to have a difficult time walking and finding food, ultimately resulting in death by starvation and associated complications in most, but not all cases. Also due to the polyarthritis the foxes seem to have a difficult time catching food. Approximately 30 of these affected foxes have been found and examined at necropsy. Prominent gross lesions included severe polyarthritis, small irregular and pitted kidneys, and overgrown nails of the forelimbs. The polyarthritis is characterized by swollen joints with mild to severe exostosis with a minimal increase in joint fluid. Histologic lesions (26 foxes) included a generalized vasculitis, severe polyarthritis with lymphoplasmacytic synovitis, tenosynovitis, bursitis, and periosteal proliferation, renal cortical infarctions, myocarditis with myocardial infarctions, and meningoencephalitis with cerebral infarction. The etiology and pathogenesis of Shaggy Lame Fox Syndrome is not known at the present time. The gross and histologic lesions combined with the microbiological results suggest that Shaggy Lame Fox Syndrome may be an immune-mediated bacterial disease. *Streptococcus bovis* was isolated from the swollen stifle joint from one fox that appeared to be an extremely early case.

ECOLOGICAL IMBALANCES AND THE DECLINE OF ALASKAN NORTHERN FUR SEALS

Terry R. Spraker, DVM, PhD, Diplomate ACVP
College of Veterinary Medicine and Biomedical Sciences
Colorado State University, Fort Collins, CO

The largest northern fur seal (*Callorhinus ursinus*) rookeries in the world are located on two of the five Pribilof Islands (St. Paul and St. George), Alaska (57°15'N/170°20'W). These two islands comprise roughly 72% of the world's breeding population.[5] Fur traders nearly annihilated the seals in the early 1800s and a second time in the early 1900s. When the harvest of fur seals for their pelts was discontinued for a time; the population rebounded both times.[9]

The fur seal population was estimated to be approximately 2 to 2.5 million animals in the 1950s and 1960s. A deliberate population reduction was conducted during 1956–1968 which included the killing of tens of thousands of adult females. This was followed by a decline in pup production starting in 1958 and continued through the early 1970s.[9] The population was relatively stable for the next 10 years, but seemed to start declining again. This decline in population starting in the early 1980s has been unexplained.[5,6]

A brief description of the life history of the northern fur seal may be helpful for interpretation of conditions found during this study. Northern fur seals are sexually dimorphic (adult males weighing 4 to 5 times as much as females) and have a highly polygamous breeding system.[1,8] Fur seals are pelagic during the late fall, winter and early spring of each year. Adult males leave the islands in the fall and stay in the North Pacific and Bering Sea until they return to the islands in mid to late May to set up defend territories. A breeding bull usually maintains his territory for 8 to 10 weeks.

Adult females usually leave the Pribilof Islands in late October to early December and travel south through the Aleutian Island passes into the North Pacific. They migrate as far south as California remaining in deep water off the continental shelf during winter.[6] Some females go as far west as Japan and Russia. Pregnant females return from their winter feeding areas, arriving on the islands in mid June and early July.[2,3] Females have high site fidelity and usually go to the rookery on which they were born. They give birth to a single pup 1 to 2 days after arrival on the rookery. The pup nurses and remains close to its mother during the first week of life. The female copulates on day 5 to 6 following parturition. Within a day or two after the female is bred, she will leave for her first post-parturient foraging trip. Depending on where she feeds and her success, she will be gone 4 to 8 days.[1,3,7] The female then returns to nurse her pup and alternates 1- to 2-day visits to shore with foraging trips to sea which last from 6 to 10 days.[3,7] Because females nurse only their own offspring, pups fast when their mothers are at sea. This pattern of behavior will continue throughout the summer and fall.

Pups are weaned in late October to early December when they are approximately 120 to 150 days old.[3]

When pups are 4 to 5 months of age they leave the rookeries and are pelagic for 6 to 30 months; then return to the rookeries of birth as 1, 2, or 3 year olds. "On land" juvenile males are found within regions on the periphery of rookeries called "haul-out areas." Young females usually stay within or just on the intersection of the rookeries and haul-out areas. The first breeding of the females is at 3 to 4 years of age and usually occurs within rookeries but sometimes takes place within haul-out areas. Following breeding they usually remain in the rookeries. For the first 8 to 9 years of life the males remain in haul-out areas while ashore during the summer and fall (June to October/November), but are pelagic over winter in the Bering Sea or North Pacific. During the summer and fall the activities of the subadult males alternates between sleeping and playing on haul-out areas and foraging trips at sea. Males can not hold a territory until they are 9 to 10 years of age and the typical age of territorial males is 10 years.[1,3,4,8]

The primary goal of this study was to identify causes of "on land" mortality of pups, subadult and adult northern fur seals in order to ascertain if disease was a significant factor contributing to this nearly 30-year of unexplained decline of the population.

Pre-weaned northern fur seal pups (*Callorhinus ursinus*; *n* = 2,822) were examined at necropsy from 1986 through 2007 on St. Paul Island (57°15'N/170°20'W), one of the islands of the Pribilof Archipelago, Bering Sea, Alaska. Five general categories of mortality were identified: emaciation (1,501 pups, 53%), trauma (514 pups, 18%), perinatal mortality (539 pups, 19%), infectious diseases (82 pups, 3%), and miscellaneous causes (186 pups, 7%). In the miscellaneous category a condition of unknown etiology characterized by multifocal necrotizing myopathy and cardiomyopathy (92 pups, 3%) was found. A multicentric ganglioneuroblastoma was found in one pup, an extremely rare congenital tumor. Evidence was not found to implicate mortality of pups prior to weaning as an important factor in the decline of northern fur seals that has been occurring since the early 1980s.

Ninety-eight subadult male northern fur seals (*Callorhinus ursinus*) were examined at necropsy from the Pribilof Islands, Alaska from 1986 to 2007. A variety of fatal and nonfatal conditions were found. Fatal conditions: hyperthermia, blunt trauma, entanglement, and bite wounds. Nonfatal conditions: seizures, orange discoloration of the blubber, neoplasia, and parasitism. Of the 85 animals that had fatal conditions 82 were directly or indirectly associated with activity of man. Adult seals (n=179) also were examined. The sex of these animals: 132 females and 47 males. Females were collected from the rookeries (n=110), isolated beaches (n=2) and the subsistence harvest (n=20). The causes of death of the females collected from rookeries: bite wounds/cellulitis (81/74%), dystocia (18/16%), blunt trauma (2/2%), neoplasia (2/2%), miscellaneous (7/6%). One of the females found on an isolated beach was killed by a gun shot to the abdomen; the other was clubbed on an isolated rookery by a person in the fall of 2005. The causes of death in bulls: bite wounds and secondary infections (38/81%), pulmonary edema (3/6%), retrobulbar abscesses (1/2%), massive fractures of the liver with hemoperitoneum (1/2%), gun shot (1/2%), fell from a cliff resulting in brain stem hemorrhage and pulmonary edema (1/2%) and accidentally clubbed in the subsistence harvest (2/4%). The overall degree of "on land" mortality of subadult and adult northern fur seals was extremely low and does not play a role in the present day decline in the population.

This investigation does confirm that infectious diseases are not a problem with "on land" mortality in Northern fur seals. Moreover, overall "on land" mortality is extremely low and does not play a role in this 30-year decline. The primary problem appears to be lack of recruitment of the 2- to 3-year-old seals (especially the females). Not enough of the pups return from their first 1.5 to 2.5 years at sea. The most likely problem is the nutritional status of these pups during their pelagic travels. They experience malnutrition and probably become emaciated and hypothermic and drown out at sea. One problem appears to be not enough food for the pups during their first 1.5 to 2.5 years of pelagic travels. These animals range through out the entire Bering Sea and North Pacific. Therefore, alteration of the fishing activity in these regions may be the only management strategy that may help to increase the population of northern fur seals.

SELECTED REFERENCES

1. Bartholomew GA, Hoel PG, Reproductive behavior of the Alaska fur seal, *Callorhinus ursinus*. J Mammalogy. 1953;34: 417-436.
2. Bigg MA, Migration of northern fur seals (*Callorhinus ursinus*) off Western North America. Canadian Technical Report Fish and Aquatic Science No. 1764, 1990.
3. Gentry RL, Holt JR. Attendance behavior of northern fur seals. In: Gentry RL, Kooyman GL (eds.): Fur Seals: Maternal Strategies on Land and at Sea. Princeton, NJ: Princeton University Press, 1986. pp 41-60.
4. Johnson AM, Annual mortality of territorial male fur seals and its management significance. J Wildlife Management. 1968; 32: 94-99.
5. Loughlin TR, Antonelis GA, Baker JD, York AE, Fowler CW, R.L. DeLong RL, Brum H. Status of the northern fur seal population in the United States during 1992. In: Sinclair EH (ed.): Fur Seal Investigations, 1992. NOAA Tech. Memo. NMFS-AFSC-45. 1994, pp 9-28.
6. Ream RR. Northern fur seal status and life history. 2005; available at: http://nmml.afsc.noaa.gov/AlaskaEcosystems/nfshome/presentations/PIC2005htm
7. Robson BW, Gobel ME, Baker JD, Ream RR, Loughlin TR, Francis RC, Antonelis GA, Costa DP. Separation of foraging habitat among breeding sites of a colonial marine predator, the northern fur seal (*Callorhinus ursinus*). Canadian J Zool/Rev Canadienne De Zoologie. 2004;82:20-29.
8. Scheffer VB. Relative growth in the northern fur seal. Growth. 1953;17:129-145.
9. York AE, Hartley JR, Pup production following harvest of female northern fur seals. Canadian J Fisheries Aquatic Sci. 1981;38:84-90.

OF A DIFFERENT FEATHER: MEDICAL TECHNIQUES FOR BIRDS OF PREY

John E. Cooper, DTVM, FRCPath, FIBiol, FRCVS
Diplomate ECVP
School of Veterinary Medicine,
The University of the West Indies
St. Augustine, Trinidad and Tobago

Birds of prey (raptors)—Orders Falconiformes and Strigiformes—have been kept in captivity for the purpose of falconry for hundreds, possibly thousands, of years. Some species have also long been valued as specimens for display in public and private zoological collections. In recent years increasing numbers of raptors have been maintained for aviculture, for scientific research and (as sick, injured, or "orphaned" birds) for treatment and rehabilitation back to the wild.[1]

Although many aspects of medical treatment apply to both Orders of raptors, there are some anatomic and physiologic features of owls that can make them different as patients.[1,2]

Medical attention for falconiform birds of prey has a long history. Falconry texts dating back five hundred to a thousand years, in Arabic and other languages as well as in English, provided detailed advice on how to recognize certain diseases[1] and, while many of the methods of treatment that were then advocated are much outdated, some of the authors' recommendations for prevention and for keeping hawks healthy are still sound.

The past 35 years have seen an unprecedented amount of research on both infectious and noninfectious diseases of birds of prey coupled with the appearance of several authoritative books and many theses and scientific publications.[1,3-5] As a result, raptor medicine is now a discipline in its own right, on a par with other areas of exotic animal veterinary work.

Medical attention for birds of prey can conveniently be divided into two types: (a) preventive, and (b) therapeutic.

Preventive medication for raptors remains limited in scope. Vaccines have been developed and used for certain infectious diseases, such as avian pox. Prophylactic anthelmintics, antibiotics, and certain other agents have a place, from time to time, in the event of an outbreak of disease or when birds are being translocated or quarantined. Nutritional supplements probably help to protect birds of prey against certain disorders and immunostimulants may be beneficial but little controlled scientific research on this and similar topics has been reported.

The value of therapeutic medication in raptors, on the other hand, is increasingly being substantiated as a result of properly performed studies. Nevertheless, despite such work, it must be borne in mind that most medicinal agents that are administered to birds of prey, whether in North America, Europe, or elsewhere, are not specifically licenced for them. Therefore, caution must always be exercised in their use and the client made aware of the possible dangers or side effects. Special care needs to be taken with agents that are new on the market that appear to have potential for the treatment of raptors but have not been properly evaluated and assessed by colleagues. In such circumstances in the United Kingdom, use of a consent form is advocated, whereby the bird's owner signs to confirm that s/he understands the situation and accepts possible risks.

For this and other reasons, it is important that at least a provisional, preferably a definitive, diagnosis is made before specific treatment is given. This implies full clinical examination, supporting investigations such as radiography, ultrasonography and endoscopy, and the performance of laboratory tests. Even standard procedures, such as the administration of antibiotics, should, whenever possible, follow the taking of a swab and carrying-out of a sensitivity test. At the very least, there should be examination of a stained smear to see what sort of organisms appear to be involved and whether or not inflammatory or other cells are present.

Nonspecific therapy, such as the administration of fluids and electrolytes, or the palliative treatment of wounds, on the other hand, can and often should be carried out at an early stage, especially if the bird's survival or welfare is compromised. For example, stabilization of an incoming sick raptor should be considered an essential prerequisite to specific medical or surgical treatment of the bird. This must encompass fluids and electrolytes and can include the administration of corticosteroids (dexamethasone), iron dextran, B-vitamin complex, high calorific enteral preparation, and enrofloxacin or other antibiotics.[6]

Another important, sometimes essential, part of non-specific therapy of birds of prey is pain relief. The past few years have seen the appearance, use and testing of a number of efficacious analgesic agents. The correct use of these will not only enhance the welfare of the bird but also encourage feeding, preening, and other important activities that may aid recovery.[1]

One of the key components of supportive therapy for birds, especially but not exclusively wild bird casualties, is nursing. This is a practical subject, as much an art as a science. It is often the bird's owner or the nurse/technician who has the particular skills that make for successful nursing of the sick raptor. Our understanding of its value has advanced greatly in recent years.

Nursing of a bird of prey can be divided into five main areas:

- Thermoregulation, usually implying the provision of warmth
- Minimizing physical, visual, and audible stressors
- Metabolic management
- Carefully formulated administration of analgesics (see earlier)
- Continuous or regular monitoring of the bird

Minimizing stressors is an adjunct to any treatment and is particularly important when dealing with casualties. A bird that is regularly disturbed by noise or bright lights will become stressed. It may also damage itself as a result of its attempts to move away from the stressor(s). If the raptor is of a diurnal species it is often best to keep the patient hooded, or in a closed, padded, cardboard box or dark cupboard, except when feeding or treatment has to be carried out. In all such cases a balance has to be struck between the wish to reduce stressors and the need for regular monitoring.

Medical treatment of a sick raptor usually entails handling and this serves as a stressor, to the detriment of the bird. Any handling or more prolonged restraint should be carried out proficiently and must always be limited in duration. Equipment that is likely to be required, such as syringes, needles, and specimen bottles, must be to hand before the procedure starts.

Medication of birds of prey can be carried out using a variety of routes and techniques: orally (in the food or by hand), by intramuscular, intravenous, subcutaneous, or intraosseous injection, intratracheally, or by nebulization. Each has its own advantages and drawbacks. As a general rule, any raptor that may need to be treated should be weighed and given a health check prior to medication.

Medicines for birds of prey can be broadly categorized as follows:

- Antibiotics
- Antifungals
- Antiprotozoals
- Anthelmintics
- Acaricides and insecticides
- Anesthetics, tranquilizers, etc.
- Analgesics
- Hormones and similar agents
- Nutritional/metabolic agents
- Antiseptic, disinfectants and wound-cleaning preparations
- Miscellaneous agents

When calculating dosages of medicinal agents, attention has to be paid not only to the weight (body mass) of the bird of prey but also to its metabolic rate (MR). As a general rule, the MR of a bird increases as its body weight declines. The result is that in a small raptor the agent is likely to be absorbed, metabolized, and excreted more rapidly than in a larger bird. It is therefore good practice not to base dosages on body weight alone.

Use of allometric scaling[7] permits more correct calculation of dose and helps to determine how frequently the medicine needs to be administered for optimal effect.

Some standard agents appear to be contraindicated or are known to be significantly toxic in raptors (and sometimes other avian species). For instance, particular care should be taken with the use of gentamicin, procaine penicillin, amphotericin B, ketoconazole, and mebendazole. Other drugs may have local rather than systemic effects on the bird; for instance, tetracyclines can cause significant muscle damage when given intra-muscularly.

Emergency medication is an important consideration when working with raptors. It will be needed, for example, if respiratory or cardiac arrest occurs during anesthesia. The veterinarian who deals regularly with birds should have to hand an emergency kit and formulate, for immediate use in the practice, resuscitation protocols for both respiratory and cardiac arrest.

Emergencies are not confined to cases that are undergoing anesthesia. The problems that are seen frequently in raptors and that warrant urgent attention[3] include low condition/anorexia, respiratory disease with dyspnea; nervous disorders, and life-threatening hemorrhage. Detailed clinical investigation of such cases is often unwise because of the risk of jeopardizing the patient's survival.

The critically sick raptor may be treated while conscious but sometimes light isoflurane anesthesia can be beneficial because it minimizes stress during evaluation and therapy. Under such circumstances anesthesia must be carried out with caution and with concurrent use of nitrous oxide if this is available.

The correct treatment of a sick raptor can be further complicated by other factors. For example, some falconers, bird-keepers, and rehabilitators use or ask their veterinarian for homeopathic or other non-conventional ("complementary and alternative") medicines.

The practitioner may or may not agree personally with the use of such therapy and with the current emphasis in veterinary medicine on employing "evidence-based" therapy, using such methods may present practical, ethical, and legal dilemmas.

For centuries before the advent of modern therapy, falconers treated their birds with traditional medicines: locally concocted compounds that included herbs and minerals. There is some anecdotal ('non-evidence-based'!) indication that a few of these were efficacious. Some falconers, especially but not exclusively in Arabia, still use such traditional medicines to treat their birds but in very few cases have any of these substances been scientifically assessed. Some in fact are known to be dangerous—ammonium chloride, for example.[8]

Despite great advances in recent years, the medical treatment of birds of prey continues to present the veterinarian with challenges and dilemmas. The practitioner who treats these valuable and important patients' needs to be familiar with the literature, must adopt a scientific but cautious approach to the choice and mode of administration of agents, and should combine all of this with a properly formulated cost–:benefit analysis.

REFERENCES

1. Cooper JE. Birds of Prey: Health & Disease. Oxford: Blackwell, 2002.
2. Hoomeijer J, Zwart P, Eulen. In Gabrisch K Zwart P (eds.): Krankheiten der Wildtiere. Hannover: Schutersche, 1987.

3. Redig PT, Ackermann J. Raptors. In Tully TN, Lawton M, Dorrestein GM (eds.): Avian Medicine. Oxford: Butterworth-Heinemann, 2000.

4. Samour JH. Avian Medicine. London: Mosby, 2000.

5. Lumeij JT, Remple JD, Redig PT, Lierz M, Cooper JE. Raptor Biomedicine III. Zoological Education Network, Lake Worth, FL, 2000.

6. Forbes N. Chronic weight loss, vomiting and dysphagia. In Beynon PH, Forbes NA, Harcourt-Brown NH (eds.): Manual of Raptors, Pigeons and Waterfowl. Cheltenham, UK: British Small Animal Veterinary Association, 1996.

7. Pokras M, Karas AM, Kirkwood JK, Sedgwick CJ. An introduction to allometric scaling and its uses in raptor medicine. In Redig PT, Cooper JE, Remple JD, Hunter DB (eds.): Raptor Biomedicine. University of Minnesota Press, 1993.

8. Samour JH, Bailey TA, Keymer IF. Use of ammonium chloride in falconry in the Middle East. Vet Rec. 1995;137:269-270.

CRAWLING INTO YOUR CLINIC SOON: MEDICAL HUSBANDRY OF TERRESTRIAL INVERTEBRATES

John E. Cooper, DTVM, FRCPath, FIBiol, FRCVS
Diplomate ECVP
School of Veterinary Medicine
The University of the West Indies
St. Augustine, Trinidad and Tobago

The invertebrates, the animals "without backbones," constitute nearly 90% of the animal kingdom and there are millions of different species, many of them still unknown to science.

To the veterinary profession invertebrates have traditionally been considered as pests, parasites, and intermediate hosts of parasites. The aim of most veterinarians has been to kill or to destroy them, with little attention usually paid to their biology or contribution to biodiversity.

In recent years thinking has changed and a more enlightened approach has evolved. While some taxa of invertebrates are still considered to be "pests" necessitating control, there has been increased interest in studying host–parasite relations and in applying this information to more rational treatment strategies.

Certain terrestrial species of invertebrates are important because they contribute to the well-being of humans. Examples include the honey-bee (*Apis mellifera*) and the silkworm (*Bombyx mori*), giant land snails (*Achatina* and *Archachatina* species) and various other edible species of insect (especially members of the Lepidoptera, Orthoptera and Isoptera). Veterinary attention for such species is sometimes needed.

Some invertebrates benefit humans indirectly because they are managed as part of a conservation or education program: for example, the farming of butterflies or the captive-breeding of endangered species of snails. These animals will come under the scrutiny of the veterinarian when they are in ill health or fail to thrive or if, as in the United Kingdom, such collections are open to the public and therefore required by zoo legislation to be inspected.[1]

INVERTEBRATES OF PARTICULAR VETERINARY IMPORTANCE

The categories of terrestrial invertebrates that are of particular relevance to veterinary practitioners comprise those species that are kept as "companion animals." Although there has long been interest in keeping and breeding certain insects, such as butterflies, recent years have seen an increase in the maintenance of more "exotic" species, such as scorpions, mygalomorph spiders, praying mantis, and giant cockroaches.

Veterinary attention for such companion animals is increasingly sought and the profession is expected to be able to provide advice. A number of textbooks and papers have been published on the care of these creatures and new ones are appearing regularly.[2–7] Another facet of the profession's responsibility towards invertebrates is attention to the large numbers that are kept for research. Here disease control is an essential part of good management and a prerequisite to good science.

THE APPROACH TO TREATING INVERTEBRATES

Any captive invertebrate is dependent upon its keeper and there is a clear need to ensure not only that it remains in good health but also that its welfare is not unduly compromised. A key part of working with such animals is for the veterinarian to be familiar with their biology and natural history and to make every effort to gain practical experience of handling them. This will also impress the client. The best way of achieving this is to keep some invertebrates oneself.

MANAGEMENT

Captive invertebrates vary greatly in requirements, depending on whether, for example, they are terrestrial or aquatic, breathe atmospheric air or use gills, or live in temperate or tropical areas.

Important considerations in the management of captive invertebrates are to provide the animals with:

- An **environment** that simulates that in the wild, especially in terms of temperature, relative humidity and substrate. For example, desert species such as certain scorpions may need sand and a dry environment while arboreal invertebrates such as stick insects will probably require foliage and possibly a higher relative humidity.

- A **diet** that is either "natural" or contains the appropriate nutrients for that species. Invertebrates vary greatly in their feeding habits. Some taxa, such as spiders, are obligate carnivores and require living prey. Others, such as the larvae of butterflies, feed only on certain plants. A few—for example, cockroaches—will eat a variety of different foods of both plant and animal origin. Some herbivorous species are very selective, with (for example) larvae of certain moths feeding on only one food plant. Other Lepidoptera may be more catholic in their tastes and will accept a variety. If there is doubt over the best vegetation or prey species to give invertebrates, a selection should be offered.

- **Adequate space** and opportunity for the animals to perform most normal functions. Invertebrates that can fly need to be able to do so. Spiders that build large webs should have an appropriately sized enclosure.

Record-keeping is a crucial part of good management of invertebrates.[1] It should be coupled with a comprehensive health program.

HANDLING AND RESTRAINT

Methods of handling and restraint depend upon the species. Some invertebrates have to be manipulated with care because they are toxic or can present other dangers. Gloves, nets, and plastic/cloth bags are useful aids to handling.

Restraint of invertebrates can be physical—an extension of handling—or chemical, using "anesthetic' agents such as isoflurane, carbon dioxide, or (for aquatic species or life stages of otherwise terrestrial invertebrates) benzocaine or tricaine methane sulfonate (see below). Physical restraint must be carried out with care as many invertebrate species are delicate. Some are readily damaged by a fall: rupture of the chitinous exoskeleton of spiders, for example, can lead to rapid, often fatal, loss of hemolymph.[2] Lepidoptera, in particular, will readily lose limbs or surface scales if they are roughly handled.

Chemical restraint often has much to commend it and can be used safely and effectively to facilitate the examination of dangerous species.

ANESTHESIA

Anesthesia of invertebrates follows basic principles.[8] The animal should be examined carefully before induction. Assessment of depth of anaesthesia is often not easy. Some species and individuals will take time (hours, not minutes) to recover.

Hypothermia can be used to facilitate the handling of invertebrates and to take samples but it can prove fatal in some sensitive species, such as solifuges, and should never be employed for procedures that may cause pain.

DISEASE CONTROL

Many diseases of invertebrates are recognized and these can be broadly divided into those that are infectious and noninfectious. Often there is overlap. For example, damage to an animal's calcareous or chitinous exoskeleton may permit the ingress of infectious agents. There are few specific therapies for infectious diseases (see later) and exclusion of pathogens should be the aim. Noninfectious conditions are often attributable to suboptimal environment and attention to management can halt morbidity and/or mortality.

Infectious agents that can cause disease in invertebrates include metazoan parasites (mites, hymenopterous and dipterous insects) as well as viruses, fungi, bacteria and other organisms. Spread of pathogens is enhanced when large numbers of invertebrates are kept together—in a laboratory or butterfly house, for example.[1]

Signs of ill health in terrestrial invertebrates include anorexia, lethargy, change of color, discharges, and dysecdysis (difficulty in shedding the skin). Behavioral changes may also be seen; for example, mealworms (Tenebrio molitor) will assemble on the surface of their container if the carbon dioxide concentration is high. However, some apparently aberrant behavior may be perfectly normal; for example, a mygalomorph spider that is shedding its skin may lie on its back and appear to be dead or dying.

A full investigation of any incident involving morbidity or mortality of captive invertebrates must be carried out promptly and details taken of the history and method of management. The animals should be handled and examined individually. Even small invertebrates can be seen in some detail using a hand lens. Clients who keep invertebrates should be encouraged to maintain detailed records and also to save shed skins and empty egg and pupal cases so that these can examined later by the veterinarian for parasites or lesions.

Exclusion of infectious diseases from collections of invertebrates hinges upon:

- Quarantining all incoming stock
- Isolating sick animals
- Practicing good hygiene

The veterinarian who deals with invertebrates, especially in large collections, should familiarize him/herself with the ways in which the various pathogens can spread and infect stock and take appropriate precautions. For example, the larvae of butterflies are susceptible to attack by parasitic wasps and flies and exclusion of the adults of these is essential. This is likely to require double layers of fine netting. Eggs of incoming insects may be contaminated with micro-organisms, necessitating their being washed, on arrival and when transferred elsewhere, in dilute hypochlorite.

TREATMENT

Treatment of individual invertebrates is certainly possible but is generally restricted to the larger species. Wounds can be cleaned and escape of hemolymph stemmed. Minor surgery is feasible and may include the amputation of limbs or the debridement of wounds and infected orifices. Anesthesia may be needed (see earlier).[8]

Little is known about the efficacy or safety of most agents that might be used to treat captive invertebrates although some proven data are available on the use of antibiotics and certain other drugs in honey bees and a few laboratory species. Increasingly, clinical reports are appearing of the safe and apparently successful use of a variety of medicinal compounds in a range of different invertebrates.[6] Whenever a new product is being tried, initial test therapy on a small number of animals in the group or, if there is only one patient, on some other healthy invertebrates, is advisable.

Changes in management will often arrest mortality in captive invertebrates. For this reason, if a number of animals are affected the veterinary surgeon should suggest that some are separated and kept under different conditions pending proper diagnosis. Altering the temperature, relative humidity, or terrain may in itself prove beneficial.

Hygienic precautions play an important part in disease control, especially among arthropods where many micro-organisms are recognized pathogens. In a few cases there may be a risk of transmission of infectious agents to the keeper. Regular cleaning of cages and the removal of sloughed skins and feces will go a long way towards minimising the risk of this or an epizootic in the animals. Care must be taken over some species, however; giant land snails (Achatina species), for example, appear to prefer "dirty" conditions and will often thrive in the presence of decaying vegetation. Similarly, over-ripe fruit is a favored food of adult

Lepidoptera and is regularly provided in many butterfly houses. One must, therefore, be selective when implementing apparently standard hygienic measures.

DIAGNOSTIC TESTS

Diagnostic samples can be taken from invertebrates.[9] Swabs and brushings, for example, can be cultured or examined directly. In some cases it may be possible to withdraw blood (hemolymph) or remove biopsies. Laboratory techniques developed for work on insect pests can often be used or modified for veterinary diagnostic purposes.[10]

NECROPSY

Post-mortem examination of invertebrates can prove useful and is recommended as a routine.[9] Even if the veterinarian is not familiar with the pathology of the species he or she should know something of the normal anatomy, be able to detect gross lesions, to demonstrate the presence of parasites, and to take appropriate samples for microbiology and histopathology.

EUTHANASIA

Individual invertebrates can be killed physically but these animals are then unsuitable for *post-mortem* examination. It is preferable to use gaseous agents, such as isoflurane or carbon dioxide. The United Kingdom's Federation of Zoos (now BIAZA) has produced guidelines on this and other subjects relating to the humane care of invertebrates.[1]

CONCLUSION

The veterinary profession has had a rightful and long-standing concern about invertebrates as parasites and pests. Now, however, veterinarians are beginning to recognize that many such insects, other arthropods, and molluscs are of intrinsic interest and may be of service to the human race. The provision of medical care to such a diverse group of animals is not easy but brings with it much interest and intellectual stimulation and the opportunity for the practitioner to contribute to new fields of animal health and welfare.

REFERENCES

1. Collins NM (ed.): The Management and Welfare of Invertebrates in Captivity. London: National Federation of Zoological Gardens, 1990.
2. Cooper JE. A veterinary approach to spiders. J Small Anim Pract. 1987;28:229-239.
3. Cooper JE. Wirbellose (Invertebraten). In Gabrisch K, Zwart P (eds.): Krankheiten der Wildtiere. Hannover: Schlütersche, 1987.
4. Cooper JE. Invertebrate care. Vet Clin North Am Exotic Anim Pract. 2004;7:473–486.
5. Frye FL. Captive Invertebrates: A Guide to Their Biology and Husbandry. Melbourne, FL: Krieger, 1992.
6. Lewbart GA (ed): Invertebrate Medicine. Ames, IA: Blackwell Publishing, 2006.
7. Williams DL. Invertebrates. In Meredith A, Redrobe S (eds): Manual of Exotic Pets. Gloucester, UK: British Small Animal Veterinary Association, 2002.
8. Cooper JE. Invertebrate anaesthesia. Vet Clin North Am Exotic Anim Pract. 2001:4:57–67.
9. Cooper JE, Cunningham AA. Pathological examination of captive invertebrates. Int Zoo Yb 1991;30:137–143.
10. Davidson EW (ed.): Pathogenesis of Invertebrate Microbial Diseases. Totowa, NJ: Allanheld & Osmun, 1981.

THE EXOTIC SIDE OF CSI: FORENSICS IN NON-DOMESTICATED ANIMALS

John E. Cooper, DTVM, FRCPath, FIBiol, FRCVS
Diplomate ECVP
Margaret E. Cooper, LLB, FLS
School of Veterinary Medicine,
The University of the West Indies
St. Augustine, Trinidad and Tobago, West Indies

"CSI" – CRIME SCENE INVESTIGATION!

The very words conjure up a picture of murder, mystery, police officers, and poison analysis. Few would normally associate such activities—and all else that is part of modern forensic science—with contemporary veterinary practice. Nothing, however, could be further from the truth.[1-3] Forensic veterinary medicine is here to stay!

So what is exactly is "forensic veterinary medicine"? It can be defined as the application of veterinary knowledge to the purpose of the law: it therefore can also concern such matters as civil actions, insurance claims, and allegations of professional misconduct.

Certain aspects of animal forensic work may be the responsibility of the specialist pathologist, toxicologist, or DNA technologist, but veterinary practitioners increasingly need to have some familiarity with the subject and to be able to deal adequately with a case when it is first presented.

SCOPE OF FORENSIC VETERINARY MEDICINE

There has been an unprecedented increase in litigation relating to animals over the past few years. Domesticated animals attract the majority of criminal cases at present and these usually concern such issues as ownership, provenance, aging and parentage, causes of ill-health or death, and health and welfare.

Exotic species, ranging from touracos to tarantulas, are increasingly the subject of litigation and here legal cases generally fall into the following categories.

Circumstances of Death

This category relates to the situation in which a dead animal is investigated with a view to determining the circumstances—cause, mechanism, and manner—of its death. Essentially one or more of the following questions is being asked about the dead animal:

How did it die? *Why* did it die? *When* did it die? *Where* did it die? *Who* might have been involved?

Animal Welfare

In animal welfare cases the forensic veterinarian usually investigates whether an exotic animal is being (or has been) subjected to unnecessary pain, stress, neglect, or starvation.

Abuse

This is a field in which forensic evidence from veterinarians is becoming very important. These cases concern the links between child abuse and domestic violence.[4] Although investigation of alleged assaults on domesticated animals is at present the main focus of such work, there is increasing evidence that attacks on exotic species may be associated with a propensity to be violent to human beings.

Conservation

Legal cases that fall in this category come under what is generally termed "wildlife crime" (see later)—that is, activities that threaten wild animals, plants, or their habitats and which constitute an offense under national, regional, or international law.[5] The financial value of many exotic species means that they may be taken illegally from the wild, moved from one country to another, or kept in captivity without the necessary authorization. .

Animals as Sentinels

Sometimes animals form part of a forensic investigation because they can provide important data that is relevant to other species. For example, pet birds may be found dead or dying in a house following a fire or explosion. Clinical examination, necropsy, or sampling of such birds can yield information as to why and when the accident occurred and possibly detect evidence of materials (chemicals or explosives) that might have been responsible.

APPLICATION TO EXOTICS

Exotic animals present particular challenges in forensic cases. Their wide anatomic, physiologic, and taxonomic diversity means that the veterinarian who is involved in such work must have some knowledge of comparative biology and of natural history. In an investigation identification of exotic species or their derivatives can depend as much upon such simple but skilled techniques as microscopical examination of hair, feathers or scales, as it may on the use of molecular techniques.

Important forensic needs such as aging of wounds and lesions are likely to be complicated in exotics by their disparate physiological features, such as whether the species is ectothermic or endothermic. Even the differentiation of *ante-mortem* lesions and *post-mortem* changes can present problems in some taxa and there appear to be few authoritative texts available to guide the veterinarian other than some work on certain selected species.[6]

In general, published information on forensic aspects of exotic animals is either sparse or nonexistent. This deficit is likely to be rectified as a result of the growth of interest in what is being termed "comparative forensic medicine." This emerging discipline has been defined as being concerned with forensic studies on different vertebrate and invertebrate species of animal, including humans, and the application of such work to the provision of scientific information to judicial and other processes.[1] Such a comparative approach is of particular relevance and potential value to those who are concerned with exotic species and free-living species but, because it also opens up possibilities for proper scientific study, is important to all who are involved in animal forensics. An urgent need, if the quality of evidence in animal forensic cases is to be improved, is good quality research, including the development and use of live, dead, and computer-generated models that can be used to test hypotheses and to develop improved investigative techniques. .

THE VETERINARIAN AS A WITNESS

There are two scenarios whereby a veterinarian may become involved in a forensic case. The first of these is where he or she is invited to examine an animal or a sample or to give an expert opinion on a report. In such instances, before agreeing to accept the case, the veterinarian should consider whether:

- He or she wants to act as an expert witness
- The undertaking is feasible and realistic in terms of time and outlay and what is required of him or her.

The second scenario is when the veterinarian has no option, no choice. He or she may be a witness of fact (for example, on account of seeing an incident or dealing with the animal when it was first presented) or be called under a subpoena to give evidence. In such circumstances the veterinarian is committed to appearing in court or providing an oral/written statement.

Regardless of whether the veterinarian has agreed willingly to appear in a case involving exotic species or wildlife, the following guidelines are likely to prove useful:

- Familiarize yourself with the species of animal involved, in particular its anatomy, physiology, normal behavior, and diseases.
- Where your knowledge or experience is limited, be prepared a) to seek advice from others, including non-veterinarians, b) to carry out a *full* literature search, if necessary in different languages, and c) to extrapolate, with care, from similar species or previous cases.
- Proceed with caution and record everything you do, preferably in the presence of a colleague who can testify to your findings.

FORENSIC TECHNIQUES

In most exotic animal forensic cases investigation involves a combination of the following:

- A visit to the scene of the alleged crime and an assessment of what is seen or found
- Interviewing people who are, or are believed to be, involved
- Clinical examination of live animals
- Postmortem examination of dead animals
- Collection and identification of specimens, including derivatives and samples for laboratory testing
- Correct storage and dispatch of specimens for laboratory testing
- Laboratory tests

- Production of report(s)

Crime scene investigation, part of the title of this presentation, is, indeed, often an important component of forensic work with exotic species. Sometimes the crime scene is very similar to that portrayed in the CSI series—an area where an animal's dead body has been found under suspicious circumstances, for example. The location needs to be cordoned and contained in the same way as it would if a human cadaver was under investigation. However, there are many variants. The advent of computer-generated criminal activity, which sometimes involves animals, brings to the crime scene a new and very different dimension! Scenes of crime that involve wildlife are often in isolated areas—for example, in forest or on mountains, where rare species have been killed, captured, or poached. Here the veterinarian needs ingenuity, adaptability, and a willingness to work in the field, often using portable equipment or a mobile laboratory.[1]

Routine clinical and *post-mortem* veterinary diagnostic techniques have a major part to play in forensic investigations in animals. However, they usually have to be supplemented with a range of more specific tests that include laboratory tests (see later), radiography, ultrasonography and other imaging methods, and DNA technology. Forensic entomology can prove important in animal forensic investigations.[7] Insects are the prime invertebrates of importance, as they are in human work,[8] but millipedes, spiders, ticks and mites can play a part. The veterinarian must either have access to a person with experience of invertebrates or have such knowledge him/herself.[1]

The collection, submission, processing, and storage of specimens ("evidence") are of the utmost importance in legal cases. The samples as well as the results may need to be produced in court. Essential requirements are the use of standard techniques following established protocols, meticulous investigation, a reliable chain of custody (evidence), proper selection, labeling and transfer of samples, and accurate record-keeping.

Although forensic medicine offers exciting challenges, it is not seen by most academic institutions as a bona fide discipline within the veterinary curriculum and is rarely given recognition as a specialist subject. This lack of status, coupled with the shortage of literature and data, hampers the ability of the veterinarian to contribute much needed skills and knowledge.

The next few years are likely to see an escalation in lawsuits concerning exotic animals. This is attributable to various factors, among them an increasing tendency for owners of animals to resort to litigation, the financial value of many species, the global trade (some of it illegal) in wildlife, and greater public concern over conservation and environmental issues.

There are also likely to be more contested insurance claims and a greater tendency for owners of exotic species to threaten or to bring disciplinary proceedings against veterinarians who are perceived to provide inadequate or unprofessional services. These developments all imply that the practitioner who is dealing with less familiar species must be better prepared. This means, in particular, ensuring that proper records are kept, that sound protocols and established chains of custody are followed, and that all in the practice are conscious of the potential of a legal action, when admitting, examining or treating suspect, unusual, or particularly valuable animals.

If the veterinary profession is to play its full part in forensic medicine, increased pressure needs to be put on professional bodies and regulatory authorities to recognize this new discipline and to provide adequate training and support for its advancement.

CONCLUSION

Forensic work can be fun and challenging. It introduces a new dimension to veterinary practice and to dealing with the myriad of species that constitute "exotics." However, this area of work is not for the faint-hearted. It will bring the practitioner into contact with the less savoury aspects of human nature and in court is likely to expose him or her to strong, sometimes aggressive, interrogation and penetrating enquiry during cross-examination.

Nevertheless, this is all constitutes part of the judicial process and veterinarians, as professional people, have an essential and growing role to play in ensuring that justice is done. "CSI" is, therefore, very relevant to exotic animal practice and seems set to become even more so.

REFERENCES

1. Cooper JE, Cooper ME. Introduction to Veterinary and Comparative Forensic Medicine. Oxoford: Blackwell, 2006.
2. Cooper JE, Cooper ME. Legal cases involving birds: the role of the veterinary surgeon. Vet Rec. 1991; 129:505-507
3. Cooper JE, Cooper ME (eds): Forensic veterinary medicine. Special issue. Seminars Avian Exotic Pet Med. 1998; 7 (4).
4. Munro HMC, Thrusfield MV. "Battered pets": Features that raise suspicion of non-accidental injury. J Small Anim Pract. 2001;42:218-226.
5. Wobeser G. Forensic (medico-legal) necropsy of wildlife. J Wildl Dis. 1996;32:240-249.
6. Frye FL. Establishing the time of death in reptiles and amphibians. Proc Assoc Rept Amph Vets. 1999; 23-25.
7. Stroud RK, Adrian WJ. Forensic investigational techniques for wildlife law enforcement investigations. In Fairbrother A, Locke LN, Hoff CL (eds.): Non-infectious Diseases of Wildlife. Ames, IA: Iowa State University Press, 1996.
8. Smith KV. A Manual of Forensic Entomology. London: British Museum of Natural History, 1986:

THERMOGRAPHY — NOT JUST AN EXPENSIVE TOY

Gregory J. Fleming, DVM
Veterinary Services, Disney's Animal Kingdom
Lake Buena Vista, FL

The use of thermal imaging technology has grown over the last 10 years in zoological settings and has been widely used in human medicine since the 1960s to diagnosis inflammation, nerve, fever, and musculoskeletal injuries. One of the main advantages of thermal imaging is that it can be done remotely (1–20 meters) and thus does not require handling or immobilizing the subject under review. The technology can also be adapted to evaluate reptile enclosures to develop thermal gradients used in behavioral thermoregulation.

HOW IT WORKS

Infrared thermal imaging is the graphic display of infrared radiation emitted from objects. Infrared radiation is emitted from living and nonliving objects as photons that pass harmlessly through the atmosphere. An infrared imaging radiometer, (thermal imaging camera) can detect these photons, whether they are emitted from an object or a reptile. When these photons hit the electrically charged detector plate, within the camera, electrons on its surface are displaced and the difference in the electrical current is measured and used to calculate the radiant energy.

This energy reading is then converted into thermal data by the thermal camera software. The camera used in this study was the Inframetrics PM280 (Inframetrics, N. Billerica, MA). The photon detector plate of this camera contains approximately 65,000 pixels (picture elements) with each pixel capable of recording a temperature. The information captured by the camera can be viewed as still images or as real-time high-resolution videotape (30 frames/sec). Images can also be viewed as black and white or color in a variety of palets. Stored images can be further analyzed using proprietary software (Thermogram Pro 95®, Inframetrics) to obtain spatial and temporal analyses

In environments with static ambient temperatures, the body surface will come to thermal equilibrium with skin temperature. In the absence of environmental influences or injured or diseased tissues, mammalian skin temperatures tend to be symmetrical between the left and right sides of an animal. Thus any deviation from a symmetrical pattern may require a closer look. In mammals, the surface heat is derived from local circulation and tissue metabolism. Heat moves from areas of higher temperature at the body's core to areas of lower temperature at the surface. Surface skin temperatures are altered by heat losses through conduction, convection, infrared radiation, and evaporation. The thermal imaging camera detects radiant energy loss at the surface of the skin only, not deeper structures.

Thermal changes visible using infrared thermal imaging in mammals are due to a variety of causes including disease processes, inflammatory response, muscle and nerve injury, and a variety of environment forces. For example, muscle atrophy is associated with less muscle activity and lower amounts of metabolic activity, resulting in a lower temperature. A compressive nerve injury resulting in damage to a motor nerve fiber may be accompanied by over-activity of the sympathetic nerve fibers and vasoconstriction resulting in a cooling of the skin. Inflammation derived from a septic joint or trauma may also be visualized; however, deep abscess, or internal inflammation may not be visualized. A recent study showed that raccoon infected with rabies, in a laboratory setting could be distinguished from none infected animals via thermography. This was accomplished by rises in body temperature and thus nose temperature of late stage infected raccoons.

Other disadvantages are that the unit may not be used in direct sunlight (outside) as the light photons will affect the image. As well, hair and feathers block heat loss and will block the emissivity of an object masking skin surface temperatures. Wet or damp skin may also disrupt the image, as the water will draw heat from the skin, masking the true temperature of the skin. The biggest disadvantage to using thermography is that the units may be expensive. ranging from $30,000 to $40,000. However, many universities, veterinary schools, and private equine veterinarians have access to this technology and are more than often happy to assist in helping make a diagnosis.

In summary, thermography has been used in zoos to successfully diagnose lameness in hoof stock and long-legged birds, abscesses in a variety of mammals, elephant foot and trunk problems, marine mammal dental issues, and evaluation of reptile environments. Used under the correct conditions, thermography is one more additional diagnostic tool that can be added to the battery of diagnostic imaging modalities available to veterinarians.

REFERENCES
1. Arena PC, Warwick C. Miscellaneous factors affecting health and welfare. In: Warwick C, Frye FL, Murphy JB (eds.): Health and Welfare of Captive Reptiles. London: Chapman and Hall, 1995, pp 263-283.
2. Avery RA. Field studies of body temperatures and thermoregulation. In: Gans C (ed.): Biology of the Reptilia, Vol 12. New York: Academic Press, 1982.
3. Bartholomew GA, Tucker VA. Control changes in body temperature, metabolism and circulation by the agamid lizard, Amphibolurus barbatus. Physiol Zool. 1963;36:199-218.
4. Barnes RB. Determination of body temperature by infared emission. J Appl Physiol, 1967;22:1143-1146.
5. Bennet RA. Anesthesia. In Mader DR (ed.): Reptile Medicine and Surgery. Philadelphia: WB Saunders, 1996, pp 241-247.
6. Coulson RA, et al. Biochemisry and physiology of

alligator metabolism in vivo. Am Zoo. 1989;29:921.

7. Coulson RA, Hernandez T. Alligator Metabolizm: Studies on Chemical Reactions in Vivo. London: Pergamon Press, 1983.

8. Coulson RA, Coulson TD. Effect of temperature on the rates of digestion, amino acid absorption and assimilation in the alligator. Comp Biochem Physiol. 1986;83A:585-588.

9. Diefenbach CO. Thermal preferences and thermoregulation in *Caiman crocodilius*. Copeia. 1975;530-540.

10. Dowling P, et al. Thermographic and electromyographic evaluation of a lumbosacral spinal injury in a cow. Prog Vet Neurol:. 1991;2:73-76.

11. Glassman AB, Bennet CE. Response of the alligator to infection and thermal stress. In: Throp JH, Gibbons JW (eds.): Energy and Environmental Stress in Aquatic Systems. Washington, DC: Technical Information Center, US Department of Energy, 1978.

12. Grenard S. Handbook of Alligators and Crocodiles. Malabar: Krieger Publishing, 1991.

13. Hamilton BL. An overview of proposed mechanisms underlying thermal dysfunction. In: Abernathy M, Uematsu S (eds.): Medical Thermography. American Academy of Thermology, Washington DC, 1986, pp 6-18.

14. Hertz PE, Heuy RB, Steenson RD. Evaluating temperature regulation by field-active actotherms: the fallacy of the inappropriate question. American Naturalist. 1993;142: 803

15. Heatwole H, Taylor J. Ecology of Reptiles. Surrey Beatty and Sones Ltd. Chipping Norton, New South Wales, Australia, 1987.

16. Lane TJ. Crocodilians: In: Mader DR (ed.): Reptile Medicine and Surgery. Philadelphia: WB Saunders, 1996, pp 78-94.

17. Loughmiller, JA, Spire MF, Dritz SS, Fenwick BW, Hosni MH, Hogge SB. Relationship between mean body surface temperature measured by use of infrared thermography and ambient temperature in clinically normal pigs and pigs inoculated with *Actinobacillus pleuropnemoniae*. Am J Vet Radiol. 2001;62;676-681.

18. Norris KS. Color adaptation in desert reptiles and its thermal relationships. In: Milstead WW (ed.): Lizard Ecology: A Symposium. University of Missouri Press, Columbia, 1967, pp 62-229.

19. Plough FH, et al. Temperature and water relations. In: Plough FH (ed): Herpetology. Upper Saddle River, NJ: Prentice-Hall, 1998.

20. Porter WP, Gates, DM. Thermodynamics equilibria of animals with environment. Ecol Monogr. 1969;39:227-244.

21. Purohit RC, McCoy MD. Thermography in the diagnosis of inflammatory processes in the horse. Am J Vet Res. 1980;41:1167-1174.

22. Purohit RC, et al. Value of clinical thermography in veterinary medicine. Auburn Vet. 1977;33:104-108.

23. Spire MF, et al. Use of infrared thermography to detect inflammation caused by contaminated growth promotant ear implants in cattle. J Am Vet Med Assoc, 1999;9:1320-1324.

24. Stnttgen G, Flesch U. Dermatological Thermography. Weinheim, Germany: VCH Verlagsgesellschaft mbH, D-6940; 1985, pp 13-31.

25. Stnttgen G, Turner TA. Thermography as an aid to the clinical lameness evaluation. Vet Clin North Am (Equine Practice). 1991;7:311-337.

26. Terpin KM, Spotila JR, Foley RE. Thermoregulatory adaptations and heat energy budget analysis of the American alligator, *Alligator mississippiensis*. Physiol Zool. 1979;52:296-312.

EXOTIC HOOF STOCK ANESTHESIA AND ANALGESIA: BEST PRACTICES

William R. Lance, DVM, MS, PhD, Diplomate ACZM
Wildlife Pharmaceuticals, Inc.
Fort Collins, CO

Veterinary care of non-domestic hoof stock has become more common practice through the integration of veterinary medicine in state and federal natural resource management programs, zoological collections, exotic animal ranching expansion, and hobby collections of exotics. Likewise, veterinarians are expected to have the knowledge and capability to safely anesthetize and handle these animals.

Anesthesia of exotic hoof stock requires the knowledge of not only the pharmacology of the drugs used but also the variation in dose response among families, genera, species, and, in some cases, even sub-species of this group of animals. The second challenge is matching the pharmaceutical tools available with the environment and conditions surrounding the animal and the procedures or events preceding, during, and following the anesthesia. An anesthesia protocol available and practical in a small fenced captive environment in many cases may not be applicable in a free-ranging or large pasture enclosure. It is the combination of all these factors that will dictate what is the "best practice."

BACKGROUND

The quality of anesthesia and analgesia achievable in non-domestic hoof stock today has only been possible through the availability of new, more receptor-specific, and highly potent, agonist reversible pharmaceuticals combined with our expanding knowledge of the receptors within the central nervous system. In the infancy of exotic animal handling, the first widely used drug was a potent neuromuscular blocking agent, succinylcholine chloride that produced muscular immobilization but no analgesia or loss of consciousness. This was used on numerous animals successfully and was thought to be the 'best practice' until the advent of the first potent opiate agonist M99 (etorphine hydrochloride) and its specific antagonist M50/50 (diprenorphine hydrochloride) in the early 1970s. M99 and M50/50 revolutionized anesthesia and handling of wildlife for the following 25 years as it allowed the safe, reversible anesthesia of species that previously could only be captured by physical means (elephant, giraffe, zebra, rhinoceros).

During the years between 1970 and 2000, the pharmaceutical industry serving veterinary medicine has provided a virtual tool chest of drugs with application to exotic hoof stock anesthesia that includes xylazine, ketamine, medetomidine, tiletamine, zolazepam, fentanyl, butorphanol, carfentanil, thiafentanyl, azaperone, and the specific antagonists yohimbine, tolazoline, atipamezole, and naltrexone. Although there are others used, these drugs are most commonly in current use in various combinations and dose forms and provide the basis for non-domestic hoof stock anesthesia and analgesia today.

With these pharmaceuticals, the standard of care in non-domestic anesthesia and analgesia must include rapid non-traumatic induction, adequate muscle relaxation for manipulation, acceptable levels of cardiovascular and respiratory function, adequate anxiolysis and analgesia, rapid and safe recovery, and proper levels of post procedure analgesia or sedation if required. The veterinarian and staff must have the knowledge, pharmaceuticals and support equipment to achieve a "best practice" outcome.

CERVIDS

The family Cervidae is represented as an indigenous group on all major continents except Africa and Australia. The cervids vary greatly in size, environmental adaptations, and response to anesthesia protocols.

The selection of the protocol to be used in a given species will be dictated by whether rapid induction is absolutely essential and, if rapid recovery is required, by the animal's situation.

If rapid induction is required, then the potent opiates are almost always used. When using opiates in cervids or any hoof stock, remember that more have been killed by under-dosing than overdosing. Under-dosing with opiates (etorphine, carfentanil, thiafentanyl) in all non-domestic hoof stock results in a prolonged induction hyperextension-type running which leads to malignant hyperthermia commonly triggering the capture myopathy complex. The rule with opiates in cervids and any hoof stock is always dose high and reverse as needed once the animal is down. It has been shown that small amounts of naloxone IV can be used to manage opiate respiratory depression in elk.[1]

The North American cervids, white-tailed deer (*Odocoileus virginianus*), mule deer (*Odocoileus hemionus*), elk (*Cervus elaphus*), caribou (*Rangifer tarandus*), and moose (*Alces alces*)) can be anesthetized with a variety of combinations of opiates, alpha-two agonists, dissociatives, and tranquilizers. Alpha-two agonists (xylazine and medetomidine) are to be avoided in moose since they tend to promote relaxation of the cardia of the rumen with regurgitation and inhalation of rumen contents as the animal becomes recumbent.[2] Although mule deer and white-tailed deer belong to the same genera, they have a different response to pharmaceuticals. The published literature should always be reviewed before going to the field.

The current area of active investigation for improved anesthesia of North American cervids is focused on a balanced protocol combining opiate agonist/antagonist with butyrophenones and potent alpha-2 agonists. A combination of butorphanol, azaperone, and medetomidine produces a safe and reversible anesthesia without hyperthermia and good analgesia in white-tailed deer, mule deer, elk, and moose. This combination can be delivered with a low volume dart.

Most of the European and Asian members of the Cervidae can be successfully anesthetized with combinations of carfentanil or thiafentanyl with an alpha-2 agonist or combinations of tiletamine/zolazepam with medetomidine. The species that are known to present difficulties are fallow deer (*Dama dama*), Pere David's deer (*Elaphurus davidianus*), and Eld's deer (*Cervus eldi*). There is not an anesthesia protocol for fallow deer that is dependable and predictable in all situations.[3] The potent opiates produce severe hyperthermia in this species and their response to most alpha-2/dissociative combinations varies with individuals and circumstances. Pere David's deer tend to use water containments for safety and many after darting run to the nearest body of water. Eld's deer have demonstrated uncontrollable seizures resulting in death following use of alpha-2 antagonists.

BOVIDS

The family Bovidae encompasses the vast majority of the species of large hoof stock that are encountered in the wild and confinement. Like the cervids, their response to anesthesia and the challenges to anesthetic management can be as varied as their size and the habitats they occupy. Many bovid species pose special problems or have special requirements.

Bighorn sheep (*Ovis canadensis*) and mountain goats (*Oreamnos americanus*) in the free-ranging state are a challenge in that most cases they are in a steep precipitous habitat that requires the induction time be minimized before the animal goes over a cliff or into more dangerous conditions. This dictates the use of the potent opiate group, carfentanil or thiafentanyl. To reduce induction time even more, the use of up to 7000 units of hyaluronidase in each dart is recommended. Bighorn sheep have exhibited acute pulmonary congestion resulting in death when anesthetized with medetomidine/ketamine combinations.

Bison (*Bison bison*) are difficult to immobilize or capture with predictability except with the potent opiates. Carfentanil and thiafentanyl are both highly effective in bison.[4] The response of bison to the common alpha-2 agonists and various combinations is variable. The **"never do this"** is to try to immobilize a bison with xylazine alone. It will always turn out bad. European wisent (*Bison bonasus*) respond to these drugs in a similar pattern as bison.

The African buffalo (*Syncerus caffer*) historically were anesthetized with etorphine but with the advent of thiafentanyl, it has become the drug of choice combined with azaperone and hyaluronidase as it produces shorter induction time. The large wild cattle of Southeast Asia, banteng and gaur can now be effectively handled with carfentanil combined with low doses of alpha-2 agonists.

The antelope group contains members such as the large common and giant eland, greater and lesser kudu, gemsbok, waterbuck, nyala, sable, roan, plus numerous smaller species of the mini-antelope such as the duikers (*Philantomba*, *Cephalophorus* and *Sylvicapra* spp), suni (*Neotragus moschatus*) and klipspringer (*Oreotragus oreotragus*). As a broad statement, thiafentanyl, usually combined with azaperone, is now the drug or combination of choice for this group with some significant exceptions.[6] These drugs have taken much of the fear and risk out of anesthesia of sable and roan. When dealing with giant eland, they are prone to violent regurgitation and inhalation of rumen contents with fatal consequences. When handling this species with any combination, endotrachial intubation immediately is the rule.[10] Lesser kudu respond differently to drugs than greater kudu. Gemsbok, if not under thiafentanyl combinations with medetomidine, may strike out at handlers with their horns upon approach.

ANTILOCAPRID

The American pronghorn (*Antilocapra americana*) occupies its own family and genera and as might be expected has its own unique response to anesthesia. Until the advent of the potent opiates, the pronghorn was difficult if not impossible to safely capture or anesthetize. Although carfentanil is effective, the current drug of choice for pronghorn is thiafentanyl.[8] Recent fieldwork indicates that a combination of butorphanol, azaperone, and medetomidine may have application to pronghorn anesthesia.

CHARISMATIC MEGAFAUNA

Elephant, rhinoceros, and giraffe, sometimes referred to as the "charismatic megafauna," occupy different families and genera but present similar challenges in anesthesia. All three groups are exquisitely sensitive to the potent opiates, present anesthesia management challenges, and physical manipulation obstacles.

The first potent opiate, etorphine, opened the doorway for anesthesia of these animals. As experience with etorphine grew, it became obvious that the quality of anesthesia and management of side effects, eg, rumen bolus eructation in giraffe, were necessary.

In elephants, etorphine combined with azaperone is still a drug of choice, but thiafentanyl combined with azaperone has proven to provide an improved induction time and quality of anesthesia.[11] With thiafentanyl, most elephants tend to go to the preferred lateral recumbency position on initial induction.

Rhinos are the most sensitive of this group to opiates with the white rhino being more sensitive than the black rhino and present the challenge of management of respiratory depression and depressed PO_2 during anesthesia. White rhino in captivity can be immobilized by as little as 1 mg of etorphine or less. Etorphine as well as thiafentanyl with azaperone is the most common combination used. In the field, the addition of hyaluronidase (2000 units) to the dart is recommended to shorten induction time. Recent fieldwork indicates that combining etorphine with the opiate agonist/antagonist butorphanol and midazolam improves respiratory function dramatically (Citino, personal communication, 2007). It is accepted procedure to always have supplemental oxygen available for intranasal delivery during anesthesia to improve blood oxygen levels.

Giraffe have been an anesthetic challenge from the advent of the first available drugs. Under etorphine in the field giraffe once sternal or lateral commonly regurgitate a rumen bolus that is promptly inhaled resulting in foreign body pneumonia. Hyperthermia is also a common problem in giraffe with etorphine. In the last 10 years protocols using medetomidine and ketamine have been safe and effective in giraffe, especially in captive environments. Recently, the use of thiafentanyl combined with azaperone has produced the most effective routine protocol for capture in the field (Raath, personal communication, 2007). Once the giraffe is sternal, the animal is blindfolded, the thiafentanyl rapidly reversed with naltrexone, and the giraffe loaded into the transport trailer.

EQUIDS

The wild non-domestic equids (zebra, wild ass, and Przewalski horse), containing seven species are the most challenging group regarding consistent, predictable, quality anesthesia. There is tremendous variation in opiate response within the zebras. Some species may respond to thiafentanyl (mountain zebra) while others are totally refractory to it (Burchell's and Grevy). As a rule for zebra, etorphine is the drug of choice combined with azaperone. In this group it is important to never under-dose as they are prone to prolonged induction and hyperthermia. Przewalski horse (*Equus caballus*) can be effectively immobilized with a medetomidine/ketamine combination under confined conditions.[9]

In almost all instances, once the equid is sternal or lateral, it will be necessary to supplement the protocol with intravenous propofol to achieve satisfactory muscle relaxation.

THE OTHER 'STUFF"

It is essential that every hoof stock anesthetic procedure have the capability to manage hyperthermia (water for cooling, chilled IV fluids, etc.) supplemental oxygen available and the equipment necessary for endotracheal intubation to maintain airways and manage rumen content regurgitation. Hyperthermia and hypoxia are the most common complications of exotic hoof stock anesthesia.

REFERENCES

1. Moresco A, Larsen RS, Sleeman JM, Wild MA, Gaynor JS. Use of naloxone to reverse carfentanil citrate-induced hypoxemia and cardiopulmonary depression in Rocky Mountain wapiti (*Cervus elaphus nelsoni*). J Zoo Wildl Med. 2001; 32:81-89.
2. Kreeger TJ. Xylazine-induced aspiration pneumonia in Shira's moose. Wildl Soc Bull. 2000; 28:751-753.
3. Kreeger TJ, Arnemo JM. Handbook of Wildlife Chemical Immobilization, 3rd ed. 2007, p 186.
4. Kock MD, Berger J. Chemical immobilization of free-ranging North American bison (*Bison bison)* in Badlands National Park, South Dakota. J Wildl Dis. 1987; 23:625-633.
5. Wilson SC, Armstrong, DL, Simmons LG, Morris DJ, Gross TJ. A clinical trial using three regimens for immobilizing gauer (*Bos gaurus*). J Zoo Wildl Med. 1993; 24:93-101.
6. Pye GW, Citino SB, Bush M, Klein L, Lance WR. Anesthesia of eastern giant eland (*Taurotragus derbianus gigas*) at White Oak Conservation Center. Proc AAZV, AAWV, NAZWV Joint Conf. 2001;226-231.
7. Kock MD, Meltzer D, Burroughs R (eds.): Chemical and Physical Restraint of Wild Animals. IWVS (Africa), Greyton, South Africa 2006, pp 161,165.
8. Kreeger TJ, Cook WE, Piche´ C, Smith T. Anesthesia of pronghorns with thiafentanil or thiafentanil plus xylazine. J Wildl Manage. 2001; 65:25-28.
9. Matthews NS, Petrini KR, Wolff PL. Anesthesia of Przewalski's horses (*Equus przewalskii przewalskii*) with medetomidine-ketamine and antagonism with atipamezole. J Zoo Wildl Med. 1995;26:231-236.
10. Geoffrey et al., 2001.
11. Raath, 2007.

Additional reference information available from the author upon request.

GET A HAND ON YOUR PATIENT: PRIMATE RESTRAINT AND ANALGESIA

Hayley Weston Murphy, DVM
Zoo New England, Boston, MA

It is essential that any personnel working with nonhuman primates (NHP) be well versed in primate behavior, husbandry and enrichment requirements, zoonoses, and noninfectious hazards. A rigorous program of veterinary care, as well as a well-established occupational health and personnel protective equipment training program needs to be in place before any NHP is handled.

NON-HUMAN PRIMATE RESTRAINT

Any time a NHP is handled, appropriate protective clothing, a HEPA mask (protective against TB), primate gloves, and eye shields should be worn. Any persons with open skin lesions should avoid contact with NHP or their body excretions. Whenever possible, chemical restraint should be used to minimize the risk of injury and zoonotic disease to the handlers, veterinarian and NHP. A large portion of the NHP medical examination may be done before ever having to restrain the animal. A complete medical history—including any pre-existing diseases, assessment of anesthetic risk, temperament, and previous history of anesthetic problems is needed before proceeding with a NHP examination—with or without sedation or anesthesia. In order to minimize anesthetic time and risk, much of the examination can be done by keen observational skills and a good history from the owner or animal caretaker. Once again, whenever possible, chemical restraint should be used for the actual physical examination. The type of restraint used for routine procedures will vary greatly depending on the size, health and temperament of the NHP, the owner/caretaker, and the clinical setting.

Non-human Primates Weighing <12 kg

A squeeze cage, where either the back or front is moveable and able to squeeze the primate against the bars for easy injection, is preferable. Not many veterinary clinics have these cages available, although if a large percentage of clients own NHP as pets, they are well worth the investment. At least one handler, plus the veterinarian, is needed for adequate restraint. The owner of the primate should not be one of the handlers. For a physical examination on a small primate, a restraint chair or pole may also be utilized. If the NHP must be held, a safe way to do this is to firmly grasp the animal from behind, just proximal to the elbows. The arms should be gently rotated so that the elbows are almost touching behind the animals back. Excessive force may result in fractures, especially in severely debilitated and undernourished animals. Once the arms have been properly restrained, the ankles should be grasped and the legs extended until the NHP is in a stretched position.

Non-human Primates Weighing 12–15 kg

At least two handlers are needed and anesthesia is highly recommended. It is very important to never underestimate the strength of these animals. Heavy leather gloves may be worn, although restraint may be difficult with these on and they may provide a false sense of security. Many NHP have penetrated such gloves with their teeth. The use of nets, pole syringes, grab poles and rabies poles may be sufficient to give the veterinarian time to quickly inject the NHP with a tranquilizer. Non-human primates are very intelligent and have been known to grab syringes and redirect them towards the handler or veterinarian! They also have a tremendous memory and what works once, may not work again.

NHP Over 15 kg

Unless severely debilitated, these animals should always be chemically restrained in order to prevent human injury.

CHEMICAL RESTRAINT AND ANESTHESIA

The species variability as well as the clinical presentation of the NHP will greatly influence the drug choice and dosages needed. Almost all drugs used will be off-label. The mental state of the animal needs to also factor into the drug and dose needed. An extremely agitated NHP that is anticipating a procedure may need a much larger dose than expected. On the other hand, a severely debilitated, depressed animal may require much less. The incredible size range variation in this group of animals also needs to be considered when dosing any drug. In general, smaller and younger primates require larger doses per kilogram body weight than do larger and older animals. Fasting may be problematic in small primates due to hypoglycemia and size considerations for tracheal tubes ranging from 300 gm marmosets to 40kg baboons or bigger also need to be accommodated.

Premedications

The use of premedications may make anesthetic induction smoother, both from a handling point of view as well as decreasing the amount of drug needed to induce anesthesia. Commonly used preanesthetics include acepromazine at 0.2–1.0 mg/kg PO, SC, or IM; diazepam at 0.1–1.0 mg/kg PO, IM, or IV; and midazolam hydrochloride at 0.05–0.5 mg/kg IM, IV. In a healthy animal, the owner may give these premedications at home approximately 30 minutes before presentation at the veterinary clinic. It must be stressed to the owner that they cannot be given in a large volume of food or liquid because of increasing the chances of regurgitation and vomiting during anesthetic induction. Atropine sulfate at 0.02–0.04 mg/kg IM or glycopyrrolate at 0.005–0.01 mg/kg IM can be given for prevention of bradycardia and hypersalivation.

Tranquilizers and Anesthetics

In very small NHPs, anesthetic chamber induction may be performed. It is important to remember that stress and hyperthermia may occur, at least initially. The chamber also must be secured and escape proof. Intramuscular dosing is the only practical route to use on most non-human primates. This limits the choices of drugs to those that can be given in small volumes and that are not muscle toxic. Unless the NHP has been trained to accept hand-injections, some type of mechanical restraint or remote injection device must be used. Mechanical restraint may include trained handlers, nets, squeeze cages, etc., or a pole syringe. Pole syringes can prove very dangerous due the NHP's ability to grasp objects quickly and redirect them to the injector! Remote drug delivery systems can also be used effectively. These include the use of blow darts and tranquilizer guns. Once again, NHP have been known to throw the tranquilizing darts back at the veterinarian, sometimes with very accurate aim! Remember that dosages may vary widely depending on animals' size, age and temperament. (See Table 1 for drug listing).

- **Ketamine hydrochloride** has traditionally been the drug of choice. It is generally safe, inexpensive, and allows for adequate restraint for minor procedures or to enable safe handling until animal can be placed on inhalant anesthesia. The dose range varies from 5 to 40 mg/kg IM depending on size and temperament with the larger animals (apes) getting closer to 5 mg/kg and smaller NHP (marmosets and tamarins) getting 20 mg/kg. If the volume to be administered is large, the dose can be split up into multiple sites or a fraction of the initial dose may be enough to facilitate physical restraint and subsequent dosing. Ketamine is also available in more concentrated solutions, greater than the standard 100 mg/mL, from compounding pharmacies. One disadvantage of ketamine is the lack of a reversal agent. It also has been known to cause seizures in lemurs.

- **Tiletamine and zolazepam** (Telazol®: Fort Dodge Animal Health) is licensed for use in non-human primates. Standard dosing of Telazol is 2–6 mg/kg IM. Recovery time from Telazol tends to be somewhat prolonged when compared with ketamine and animals may be ataxic so injuries may occur during this time. There is no reversal agent for tiletamine, but flumazanil, a benzodiazepine receptor antagonist (0.025–0.2 mg IV every 30–60 sec until desired effect; maximum dose 1 mg [human dose]) can be used to reverse the zolazepam. The short half-life of flumazanil (approx. 1 hr) makes repeated dosing sometimes necessary.

- **Medetomidine** (Dormitor®: Pfizer Animal Health) combinations have recently gained popularity in the literature for anesthesia in NHPs. Dosages range from 0.05 to 0.1 mg/kg PO, IM, or IV. Medetomidine alone has been proven effective as a sedative-analgesic in a number of other species, but has not worked well as a complete immobilizing agent in NHP. In addition to the profound sedation and analgesia seen with alpha 2-agonists such as medetomidine, significant effects on the cardiovascular system are also seen and need to be considered before this drug is chosen. Intense vasoconstriction with compensatory bradycardia may be seen. Reversal of medetomidine with atipamezole (Antisedan®: Pfizer Animal Health) at approximately four to five times the dose of medetomidine (0.15–0.3 mg IV, IM, SC) or a partial dose IV and the rest IM is an advantage of these combinations.[3]

- **Medetomidine–k**etamine combinations for induction followed by isoflurane anesthesia have been proven to be safe and effective in NHPs. Drug volumes and inhalation gas concentrations needed are both decreased with minimal cardiovascular side effects seen. Reversal of the medetomidine portion of this combination should be rapid, smooth, and complete.

- **Medetomidine–zolazepam and tiletamine** combination has been evaluated as an immobilizing agent in Southeast Asian primates. This combination produced smooth inductions and complete immobilizations with minimal cardiovascular side effects.[2]

- Once an animal has been anesthetized, endotrachael intubation and IV catheter placement should commence. It is important to remember blood-borne pathogen safety guidelines whenever NHP blood/body secretions are encountered. In larger NHPs, head and neck extension is needed to keep the endotrachael tube from kinking and occluding the airway and care must be taken not to place the tube past the bronchial bifurcation. NHPs tend to have very short tracheal lengths before bronchial bifurcation occurs. In small NHPs such as marmosets and callitrichids, hypothermia while under anesthesia can be life-threatening and should be prevented with supplemental heating devices.

Analgesics

Analgesics should be routinely used whenever pain is present or anticipated. Oral dosing once the animal goes home can be used; however, it can sometimes be very difficult to medicate NHPs orally. The discriminating primate may detect even the most carefully disguised drug. There are compounding pharmacies available that will make up medications in a variety of flavors and formulations. If a procedure is scheduled enough in advance, these compounded formulations are usually the easiest way to medicate the NHP. Cutaneous pain control methods such as fentanyl patches are generally not successful because they need to be applied prior to the procedure and it is hard to adequately restrain the NHP from peeling them off. Some oral analgesics that owners may use at home include acetaminophen (5–10 mg/kg PO q 6 h); acetylsalicylic acid (5–10 mg/kg q4-6h PO); Carprofen (Rimadyl®, Pfizer Animal Health) 2–4 mg/kg PO q 12—24 h); and ibuprofen (20 mg/kg q24h PO). For injectable analgesics, see Table 1.

Recovery

After an anesthetic protocol has been completed and the recovery time is started, it is important to remember to place the animal in an escape-proof and safe environment. Animals should be placed in right lateral recumbency with their right arm extended if at all possible (the recovery position) and extubation should occur only after a complete swallow reflex is obtained. If the animal is a colony animal and must go back in with its group, care must be used in re-introduction, especially if animal has been out for an extended period of time or is still not fully recovered.

REFERENCES

1. Carpenter JW, Mashima TY, Rupiper DJ. Exotic Animal Formulary. Greystone Publications. 1996, pp 272-274
2. Fahlman A, Bosi EJ, Nyman GN. Immobilization of Southeast Asian Primates with medetomidine, zolazepam and tiletamine, and reversal with atipamezole. Proc Am Assoc of Zoo Vet. 1999: 334.
3. Horne WA. Norton TM, Loomis MR. Cardiopulmonary effects of medetomidine-ketamine-isoflurane anesthesia in the gorilla (*Gorilla gorilla*) and chimpanzee (*Pan troglodytes*). Proc Am Assoc Zoo Vet. 1997:140-142.

Table 1. Some Commonly Used Anesthetics and Analgesics in NHP

AGENT	DOSAGE	COMMENTS
Acepromazine	0.5–1.0 mg/kg PO, SC, IM	Preanesthetic, tranquilizer
Bupivacaine 0.25%	1 mg/kg locally	Intercostal nerve block
Bupivicaine hydrochloride 0.5%	1.2 mg/kg	Epidural analgesia
Buprenorphine	0.005–0.03 mg/kg IM, IV q6–12h	Analgesia Opioid agonist-antagonist
Butorphenol	.01–0.2 mg/kg IM, SC, IV q12-48h	Analgesia. May cause profound resp. depression in NHP
Diazepam	0.5–1.0 mg/kg PO 0.25–0.5 mg/kg IM, IV 0.1–0.5 mg/kg IM	Sedation Seizures, muscle relaxation Lemurs-prevent ket. Induced seizures
Flunixin meglumine	0.3–2.0 mg/kg SC, IV q12-24h	Analgesia
Ketamine	5 mg/kg IM 10–15 mg/kg IM 20 mg/kg IM	Great ape/follow w/inhalant anes. Medium sized primates (10-30kg) Marmosets/tamarins
Ketamine (K)/ Acepromazine (A)	(K) 4mg/kg/ (A) 0.04mg/kg IM	Lemurs
Ketamine/ Diazepam	(K) 15 mg/kg/ (D) 1 mg/kg IM	Anesthesia
Ketamine (K)/Xylazine (X)	(K) 10 mg/kg/ (X) 0.5 mg/kg IM	Anesthesia
Medetomidine (M)/ Ketamine (K)	(M) 40 µg/kg/ (K) 2–6 mg/kg IM	Anesthesia
Medetomidine	0.04–0.1 mg/kg PO, IV, IM	Anesthesia induction
Medetomidine (M)/ Telazol (T)	(M) 0.02–0.06 mg/kg/ (T) 0.8–2.3 mg/kg IM	Anesthesia
Midazolam	0.05–0.5 mg/kg IM, IV	Pre-anesthetic / lemurs
Morphine sulfate	1–2 mg/kg SC, IM q4h	Analgesic
Naloxone	0.01–0.05 mg/kg IM, IV	Narcotic reversal
Oxymorphone	0.03–0.2 mg/kg SC, IM, IV q6-12h	Analgesic
Propofol	1–4 mg/kg IV 0.4–0.6 mg/kg/min IV infusion	Induction Maintenance
Tiletamine/zolazepam (Telazol)	1–20 mg/kg IM 2–6 mg/kg IM 4–10 mg/kg IM	Wide ranges for different species variation

MY PATIENT IS SEDATED, NOW WHAT: PRIMATE CLINICAL TECHNIQUES

Hayley Weston Murphy, DVM
Zoo New England, Boston, MA

The order Primata is large and has over 200 species of primates, including humans. Veterinarians who elect to see non-human primates (NHP) in their veterinary practice have a responsibility to become educated in the specialized behaviors and needs of the many different species of NHP. One of the most critical of these concerns is becoming familiar with zoonoses of NHP and how to handle the NHP in order to screen for these diseases and others without unduly endangering the animal, the owner, staff, and other patients and owners. It is important to remember that experience with one species of NHP does not necessarily mean that another species of NHP can be approached in the same fashion.

It is beyond the scope of this report to cover, in depth, all of the zoonotic diseases transmissible from NHP to humans. It would be negligent not to state that any keeping of NHP as pets should be strongly discouraged, both from an animal health and welfare point of view, as well as a human health concern. It should also be pointed out that seeing NHPs in a private veterinary clinical setting should be approached with caution. Only a well-equipped practice, with staff that have been properly trained in primate handling and have been informed about and screened for zoonotic disease, should take on this challenge. Even then, the occupational health and safety hazards, ethical and legal ramifications can be enormous.

CONSIDERATIONS FOR NON-HUMAN PRIMATE PHYSICAL EXAMINATION

Staff Training/Safety

Any employees that are asked to work with NHPs need to be properly trained in an occupational health and safety plan and safe work practices to minimize the risks of physical injury and disease transmissions. Some of the topics that need to be discussed include NHP behavior, personal hygiene, housekeeping, specialized restraint equipment, personal protective equipment, blood-borne pathogen training, personal health screening as well as response procedures if an injury/ exposure should occur. Human health recommendations for all NHP handlers, including veterinarians and staff, include the following: health screens including a health questionnaire that is reviewed by an occupational health expert, up to date immunizations (may vary depending on risk exposure), serum banking, and tuberculosis testing. Completion of all training programs must be documented before any contact with NHPs occurs and must be ongoing to address staff changes, as well as reviews and changes in protocols as needed. [2]

The most common routes of exposure to potential zoonoses in NHP handlers are scratches, needle sticks, cuts, bites, and mucous membrane exposure. Every clinic that sees NHPs must be prepared to deal with accidental exposures and have a readily accessible and well-stocked primate exposure/bite kit. The likelihood of transmission of disease depends on several factors, including kind and severity of injury/exposure, health status of individual injured as well as that of the NHP involved. Defining this risk involves close communication with an occupational health expert familiar with both the person and NHP. Every facility/clinic must have a primate exposure/bite kit that should include the following: a 10% buffered bleach solution, an antiseptic skin cleanser, a sterile ophthalmic cleansing solution, Iodophor surgical scrub, disposable latex gloves, sterile gauze and irrigation syringe, sterile bowl, safety glasses/face shield, phone numbers and directions to local emergency rooms, and step by step instructions. Wounds should be scrubbed vigorously with an antiseptic cleanser first. Then, using gloved hands saturate gauze sponges in bowl with the 10% buffered bleach solution and vigorously scrub and soak wound for a full 15 minutes. Irrigate deep wounds with this also via syringe. Loosely cover the wound and proceed to emergency room. For eye splashes, irrigate the eye with clear water or sterile ophthalmic solution for a full 15 minutes before proceeding to the emergency room. The animal involved should also be identified and appropriate testing done to determine any zoonotic risks. At a minimum, antimicrobial therapy should be initiated and the occupational health expert and employees supervisor should be notified immediately.

Equally important is education of NHP owners about the risks to themselves and their pets. Complete necropsies should always be done in the event of an animal death to rule out potential unknown health risks to caretakers and owners.

Primate Taxonomy

Understanding primate taxonomic categories will help in determining specific husbandry and veterinary needs. It is important to understand these categories when discussing zoonoses, specialized husbandry and dietary needs, and social complexities. While all NHP carry zoonotic diseases, the phylogenetic closeness of the Old World primates makes their zoonoses of particular concern. In general, the order primates share many behavioral and anatomical features that make them somewhat unique in the animal kingdom. Among these features are: well-developed manual dexterity, extreme strength for body size and agile reflexes, and a well-developed sense of sight and good hand-eye coordination. They have highly developed cerebral cortices, long infant dependency periods, and tend to have very complex social organizations. Physically, NHPs are set apart by their prehensile, opposable thumbs, tactile pads and nails on fingers and toes, a precise grip and extremely mobile, strong arms. They have large eyes with binocular vision. All of these physical and mental adaptations make the husbandry and veterinary care of NHP complex and demanding.

Clinical Adaptations

The examination room should be equipped with securely locking doors and escape proof, locked windows. The counters should be cleared and everything needed for the examination (capture nets, primate gloves, towels, squeeze cage, pole syringe, and sedative dose drawn up) should be placed in the room before the NHP enters the room. Re-capping of injection needles should be avoided and a secure biohazard sharps container should be present at all times. Once the NHP is in the room the doors should not be opened again until the primate is properly restrained. Many NHPs are excellent escape artists and this skill should not be taken lightly.

Pre-examination Considerations

A large portion of the NHP medical examination may be done before ever having to restrain the animal. A complete medical history including any pre-existing diseases, assessment of anesthetic risk, temperament, and previous history of anesthetic problems is needed before proceeding with a NHP examination, with or without sedation or anesthesia. In order to minimize anesthetic time and risk, much of the examination can be done by keen observational skills and a good history from the owner or animal caretaker. Whenever possible, chemical restraint should be used for the actual physical examination.

Which sedative or anesthetic used to enable a thorough physical examination will depend on several factors including previous medical and anesthetic history, current health status, and temperament and drug delivery options. Any time a NHP is handled, examined or its cage cleaned, appropriate protective clothing, respiratory and mucus membranes protection, and primate bite gloves should be worn. Whenever possible, chemical restraint should be used to minimize the risk of injury and zoonotic disease to the handlers, veterinarian and non-human primate. All work should be done in a well-ventilated area that has UV exposure and air exchanges >6/min.

Physical Examination

Once the animal is safely restrained/anesthetized, a complete physical examination should be done, including a thorough dental and ocular exam, cardiac and gastrointestinal (GI) evaluation. GI examinations should include direct and indirect fecal screens (floatation as well as centrifugation techniques) and fecal cultures. Blood work should include a complete blood count (CBC), serum chemistry, as well as species

appropriate viral screening and possibly serum mineral analysis. Whole body radiographs should also be taken to look for any suspicious thoracic lesions, diaphragmatic hernias, nutritional bone diseases, or other radiographic abnormalities.

Every NHP should have a tuberculosis screening, with frequency determined based on exposure risks. Current methods of TB screening include using 0.1 mL of a 1:10 dilution of mammalian tuberculin (Tuberculin mammalian, Human Isolates Intradermic sold by Synbiotics Corp.) equivalent to 1500 or more units of old tuberculin . A 25- to 27-gauge, ½-inch needle is used to inject the tuberculin intradermally, usually in the upper eyelid. The nipple can be used as a secondary confirmatory site. The test should then be read at 24, 48, and 72 hours. This test can give false-positive and false-negative results but any reaction should be considered positive until further diagnostics can be run and the animal should be immediately quarantined. A valuable ancillary test is the use of a rapid whole blood interferon-γ (WB-IFN-γ test – Primagam). This test measures cell-mediated immune responses in NHPs. The test kit also contains tuberculosis antigens (Bovine PPD, Avian PPD and Nil antigen control). Primagam® is available from Prionics AG Wagistrassa 27A. 8952 Schlieren-ZU Rich. Switzerland Phone +41 44 200 20 00; Fax +41 44 200 20 10 or www.info@prionics.com. Other diagnostic tests may include radiographs, sputum, fecal and blood cultures, gastric lavage for cytology and culture, and comparative TB tests.

Some NHPs may also be predisposed to certain diseases that may require additional diagnostic tools. Examples of these are the prevalence of cardiac disease in the apes, GI blockages due to parasitism in smaller primates and GI ulcerations in stressed animals.

REFERENCES

1. Murphy, H.W., Miller, M., Ramer, J., Travis, D., Barbiers, R., Wolfe, N.D., Switzer, W.M.
2. Implications of simian retroviruses for captive primate population management and the occupational safety of primate handlers. J. of Zoo and Wildl. Med. 37(3): 219–233, 2006
3. National Research Counsel. Occupational health and safety in the care and use of nonhuman primates. The National Academies Press. Washington, D.C. USA. 2003.

Table 1. Preventative Health: Vaccinations Differ Depending on the Age and Type of NHP (Old World vs. New World).

Disease	Vaccination Schedule	Severity	Efficacy	Adverse Reactions	Vaccination Recommendations
Tetanus	2 mo, 4 mo, 6 mo, 18 mo, 4–6 yrs, 14–16 yrs, every 10 yrs after	Can be fatal	High	Numerous	All species
Poliomyelitis	2 mo, 4 mo, 6 mo, 18 mo, 4–6 yrs, 14–16 yrs	Inapparent to fatal	High	None reported	Great apes
Measles	15 mo, 10–12 yrs	Inapparent to fatal	High	None reported	All species if exposure risks
Hemophilus	2 mo, 4 mo, 6 mo, 18 mo	Mild to fatal	Unknown	Few	Limited
Rabies	16 weeks, annually after that	Fatal	High	Few	All in endemic areas
Hepatitis B	2 mo, 4 mo, 6 mo	Mild to fatal	Unknown	Few	Great apes
Mumps	15 mo, 10–12 yrs	Mild to fatal	Unknown	Few	Great apes

AAZV EXOTIC ANIMAL EUTHANASIA GUIDELINES

Hayley Weston Murphy, DVM
Zoo New England
Boston, MA

The *Guidelines for Euthanasia of Nondomestic Animals* is an official publication of the American Association of Zoo Veterinarians (AAZV) published in 2006 and is endorsed by the American Association of Wildlife Veterinarians, the American Association of Zoo Veterinarians, the American Board of Veterinary Toxicology, the American College of Zoological Medicine, the Association of Avian Veterinarians, the Association of Reptilian and Amphibian Veterinarians, the Canadian Association of Zoo and Wildlife Veterinarians, and the Wildlife Disease Association.

It is provided by the AAZV as a reference to provide accurate and authoritative information regarding euthanasia methods that mitigate pain and distress and provide for humane euthanasia in captive nondomestic species and free-ranging wildlife. The guidelines are edited by Charlotte Kirk Baer and incorporate the expertise of 28 contributing authors and 57 reviewers with varied experiences and knowledge in the field of nondomestic animals, toxicology, and related regulatory agencies.

Part One of the guidelines provides a comprehensive overview of issues such as the criteria for humane euthanasia and associated concerns; the physiology of euthanasia; personnel safety; regulatory oversight and wildlife issues.

Part Two provides taxon specific recommendations. Taxa discussed include invertebrates, fish, amphibians, reptiles, birds, monotremes, marsupials, bats, nonhuman primates, rodents and small mammals, marine mammals, sea otters, carnivores, hoofstock, swine and megavertebrates.

Part Three provides a summary of euthanasia methods discussed with a chart of all methods and taxa given in guidelines.

These guidelines should be utilized as a reference of comprehensive recommendations to minimize pain and distress and provide humane euthanasia to numerous taxa of captive nondomestic species and free-ranging wildlife. The guidelines can be purchased from the AAZV by going to www.aazv.org.

REFERENCES

1. American Association of Zoo Veterinarians (AAZV). Guidelines for Euthanasia of Nondomestic Animals. 2006, 111 pp.

THEY'RE RETRO, CAMPY, FOAMY, AND RUNNY— GETTING TO KNOW YOUR PRIMATE ZOONOSES

Hayley Weston Murphy, DVM
Zoo New England, Boston, MA,

It is beyond the scope of this report to cover all of the zoonotic diseases transmissible from nonhuman primates (NHP) to humans. It is imperative to state that keeping NHP as pets should be strongly discouraged, both from an animal health and welfare point of view, as well as a human health concern. It should also be pointed out that seeing NHPs in a private veterinary clinical setting should be approached with caution. Only a well-equipped practice, with staff that have been properly trained in occupational health and hazard prevention and NHP handling, and have been informed about and screened for zoonotic disease, should take on this challenge. Even then, the occupational health and safety hazards and ethical and legal ramifications can be significant. Training programs for people who work with NHP should include zoonoses education, safe job practices, personnel protective equipment use, injury treatment and reporting protocols, as well as primate behavior and husbandry needs.

Some of the zoonotic diseases of NHP can be devastating to humans. Therefore, the prevention of disease transmission is absolutely essential to any training programs. Any facility that works with NHP needs to review, understand and comply with the elements of the OSHA blood-borne pathogen standard (www.osha.gov/SLTC/bloodbornepathogens/standrads.html). Staff needs to be trained in the use of personal protective equipment, effective restraint, and anesthesia of NHPs; proper training for bite wound management and disease exposure and should participate in an ongoing staff health program. This program should include serum screening and storage, as well as vaccination programs including vaccinations for rabies, measles, hepatitis A, hepatitis B, and tetanus. A disease surveillance program must also be included in any NHP facility including TB screening for NHP and staff, fecal examination of NHP and staff, serologic testing (B virus, retroviruses, measles, filoviruses), fecal examinations and complete necropsies on any animal that dies.

NON-HUMAN PRIMATE VIRAL ZOONOSES
Hepatitis Viruses

Viral infectious hepatitis virus (Hepatitis A) has been identified in macaques, baboons, apes, guenons, patas, wooley monkey, cebus, aotus, and some tamarins. Many species of NHPs are susceptible to hepatitis A viruses of human origin and outbreaks in captive colonies have been attributed to human strains. Only chimpanzees have been implicated in retransmission of the hepatitis A virus back to humans. Clinical disease in NHP is rare and may include anorexia, diarrhea and elevated liver enzymes. Illness in humans is primarily acquired through fecal-oral routes and disease is usually self-limiting.

Hepatitis B infection can occur in chimpanzees, gibbons, and macaques. A chronic carrier status with little or mild clinical signs can exist and no transmission has been documented of primate origin HBV to humans. Hepatitis C has been reported in chimpanzees and produces a chronic active hepatitis, cirrhosis and hepatocellular carcinoma.

Herpes Viruses

The family Herpesviridae is divided into three distinct subfamilies: Alphaherpesvirinae, Betaherpesvirinae, and Gammaherpesvirinae. Herpes infections are responsible for a wide range of symptoms ranging from inapparent infections to fatal disease.

Herpes B

Cercopithecine herpesvirus 1 or *herpesvirus simiae* is a disease of macaque species and may be fatal in several non-macaque species of monkeys when they are exposed. Only a small percentage of infected macaques will present with clinical signs of ulcers and white plagues on lips, nares, tongue, genitalia, and palate and they may have conjunctivitis. Disseminated, fatal disease may occur in macaques but is rare. Like herpes simplex virus infections in humans, B-virus infections in macaques can be characterized by life long infections with periodic activation and viral shedding in saliva and genital secretions. The primary mode of transmission between monkeys is by sexual activity and bites, while transmission to humans may be through bites, scratches, needle stick injuries, or contact with infected blood or urinary secretions to mucus membranes or broken skin. Likelihood of B virus infection is not correlated with the severity of the injury/ exposure and post-exposure wound cleansing and antiviral prophylaxis is crucial if exposure is suspected. Although symptomatic human infections from exposure to herpes B virus are rare, when symptomatic infection does occur, the infection is usually severe and often fatal. The incubation period in man is variable and can occur from 3 to 5 days post exposure to 2 to 3 weeks or longer with clinical signs starting out as pain, fever, numbness, vesicles, and neurasthesia or parestheia at site of exposure. In the exposed extremity there may be a regional lymphadenopathy, fever, muscle weakness or paralysis and conjunctivitis, often accompanied by generalized malaise and flu-like symptoms. The disease then may progress to cause persistent hiccups, sinusitis, neck stiffness, headache, flu-like symptoms, nausea, vomiting, confusion, brain stem damage and fatal meningoencephalitis in humans. Antiviral treatments given early in the course of the disease may prevent progression of the disease and has proven to be life saving in some patients. Rapid diagnosis and treatment is essential in preventing permanent disability and death in patients that are symptomatic. It should be remembered when screening animals that a negative antibody test or viral culture result does not exclude the possibility of B-virus infection or viral shedding and it is safest to assume that all macaques are carrying and capable of transmitting Herpes B infection.

Other Herpes Viruses

Other herpes viruses that can be of concern, either because of zoonotic risks or transmission between susceptible species of monkeys are *Herpesvirus Hominis (Herpes simplex)*, *Herpesvirus tamerinus*, *Epstein-Barr virus*, *Spider-monkey herpesvirus*, *Simian varicellalike herpesviruses*, and *Simian Cytomegalovirus*.

Paramyxoviruses

Measles is an RNA paramyxovirus related to canine distemper and rinderpest. Although measles is not considered a naturally occurring disease in NHPs, it is one of the most frequently reported viral diseases. Infection in NHPs occurs as a result of human contact, and then the infected primate can shed the virus, and re-infect man. Clinical signs in NHP can range from fever, conjunctivitis, coryza, bronchitis and Koplik spots on oral mucosa. A skin rash may appear on the third to seventh day and leukopenia is common. Measles infection in New World primates (marmosets, tamarins, and owl monkeys) is usually fatal and can be easily avoided by good husbandry practices and a vaccination program using an attenuated vaccine for both animals and staff.

Lymphocytic Choriomeningitis Virus (LCMV)

This rodent virus has been determined to be the cause of Callitrichid hepatitis. It presents as acute onset of lethargy, anorexia and elevated liver enzymes. There is high mortality associated with this infection in captive collections of marmosets and tamarins. The animals are thought to get this infection from mice in the exhibit, or from being fed pinkie mice as treats in their diet. This practice should be avoided. The mode of transmission from NHP to humans is unknown but may occur through oral and respiratory exposures. The incubation period in humans is 8 to 13 days and disease may start as flu-like symptoms but progress to symptoms of meningitis or encephalitis. The disease is rarely fatal but may be in immunocompromised individuals and also may be a fetal teratogen so caution is needed when exposure concerns involve women of childbearing age.

Retroviruses

There are two groups of retroviruses that are endemic in human populations, the human T-cell leukemia/lymphotropic viruses (HTLV) types I and II and the human immunodeficiency viruses (HIV) types 1 and 2. Non-human primates are the natural hosts for several retroviruses including simian immunodeficiency virus (SIV), simian spumaviruses (simian foamy viruses SFV), simian T-lymphotropic viruses (STLV), and/or simian type D retroviruses. All of these viruses cause life-long infections in NHPs and may be transmissible through sexual contact, blood, bodily fluids or breast milk. The risk of transmission of simian retroviruses to humans following occupational exposure to NHP is not totally understood, but is being studied. In 1993, the CDC and the National Institutes of Health implemented a voluntary testing and counseling surveillance program for SIV following detection of SIV in a worker at a primate facility. This study was later expanded to include voluntary testing and counseling for exposures to SFV, STLV, and simian type D retroviruses. There are significant implications for laboratory workers and zoo personnel that work with NHPs.

Simian Immunodeficiency Virus (SIV)

SIV is a lentivirus, morphologically similar and biologically related to HIV-1 and HIV-2. SIV can cause acquired immunodeficiency syndrome (AIDS)-like illnesses in susceptible macaque monkeys and when it crosses from host-specific species to non-host specific species. SIV strains are not usually pathogenic in their natural host species. Presently monkeys with SIV are used extensively in the study of AIDS. SIV is genetically and antigenically related to HIV-2, resulting in substantial serological cross-reactivity. All of the simian viral isolates have characteristics in common with HIV, including some serological cross reactivity and suspected immune suppression resulting in clinical disease. Two of the SIV viruses, SIV_{cpz} from chimpanzees and SIV_{sm} from sooty mangabeys, have been shown to be the source of HIV1 and HIV2 and AIDS in humans. The relationship between simian retroviruses and the disease in humans is a great concern, especially with the recent increase in the poaching and consuming of primate meat. Blood donation and organ donation research is also concerned with possible transmission of these viruses. In a study conducted by the CDC, 0.06% of zoo and laboratory workers were positive for antibodies cross-reactive to SIV with no associated clinical disease.

Foamy Viruses (Spumavirus Genus of Retroviridae: SFV or Simian Spumaviruses)

SFV has been found to be prevalent in more than 50% of the captive NHP colonies of New and Old world origin. SFV can be readily isolated from infected animal's saliva or from peripheral blood lymphocytes and it has been isolated in approximately 3% of tested laboratory and zoo workers with NHP exposure. To date, there have been no ill effects to health in either the humans that are positive for SFV or the positive NHP.

Simian Retrovirus (Type D)

A simple retrovirus and an oncovirus, SRV may be prevalent in up to 90% of some populations of wild and captive macaques. SRV has been associated with syndromes including opportunistic infections, fibromatosis, necrotizing stomatitis with osteomyelitis, acute death, fever, anemia, neutropenia, lymphopenia, thrombocytopenia, hypoproteinemia, persistent diarrhea, lymphadenopathy, splenomegaly, weight loss, thymic atrophy and fibroproliferative disorders. Disease has only been associated with macaques. The virus has been isolated from blood, saliva, urine, and other body fluids and latent infections may occur. Serosurveys have described partial serologic reactivity against SRV in human sera, but additional evidence of infection has been lacking. Antibodies to type D retrovirus have been reported in 2 of 418 persons (0.48%) who were occupationally exposed to macaques at research centers.

Simian T-Cell Lymphotropic Virus (STLV)

STLVs are complex retroviruses and are composed of three major groups termed types 1, 2, and 3. STLV has been found in more than 33 species of Old World primates. The close genetic relationship between STLV-1 and HTLV-1 strongly indicates that STLV-1 has crossed over into humans from NHPs. Likewise; the finding of similar STLV-1 genotypes in sympatric primates or captive animals indicates that cross-species transmissions between different primate species can also occur. STLV-1 may be asymptomatic or may be associated with the development of lymphoproliferative disease in affected NHPs. Despite evidence that STLV can enter into humans, screenings of sera from 418 persons working with NHPs in zoos and research institutions were all found to be negative for antibodies to HTLV/STLV. These results indicate that the risk for infection with STLV in the work place may be low. The absence of STLV-1 infection in primate workers may be explained by a lower prevalence of this virus in captive animals as a result of the inclusion of STLV-1 in pathogen-free breeding programs at many research institutions.

Rabies

NHPs housed in rabies endemic areas are as susceptible to rabies as humans. Killed vaccines have unknown efficacy, although they have been used extensively in zoos housing NHP in rabies endemic areas.

Ebola/Marburg/Filoviruses

Filoviruses belong to the family Filoviridae, one of several groups of viruses that can cause hemorrhagic fever in animals and humans. Imported macaques have been implicated in outbreaks of Ebola subtype Reston in the US since 1989. The three subtypes that are known to cause disease in humans are Ebola-Zaire, Ebola-Sudan and Ebola-Ivory Coast. The disease is called Ebola Virus Hemorrhagic Fever and clinical signs in both humans and NHP are: fever, chills, headaches, muscle aches, and anorexia. As the disease progresses, vomiting, diarrhea, abdominal pain, sore throat, and chest pain may develop. A coagulopathy then develops and bleeding may occur from injection sites as well as into the gastrointestinal tract, skin, and internal organs. Because of the high mortality rate from human filovirus infections, the CDC has updated regulations and inspections of imported primates. Knowledge of filovirus modes of transmission and preventability are particularly important in primate import stations, field researchers and when performing field necropsies in outbreak areas.

Pox Viruses

There are five types of poxviruses that infect NHP and three of these are zoonotic to humans. They can infect numerous species of NHP, usually presenting as typical cutaneous lesions, which can be severe enough to cause death. Monkeypox, caused by Monkeypox virus, is serologically related to smallpox virus in humans. The disease is characterized by proliferate dermal ulcerations and vesicles. Adult monkeys may get fevers but death is rare except in infants. Because Monkeypox is serologically related to smallpox, it has the potential to be devastating in unvaccinated human populations. Benign epidermal Monkeypox is a nonfebrile disease seen in macaques and is serologically related to Yaba tumor virus and is known as Yaba pox or Yaba like pox. The virus is identical to the agent that produces Tanapox in children in Africa. Yaba virus disease is seen in rhesus monkeys, baboons and rarely man. It appears as large subcutaneous, tumor like lesions.

Several Other Viral Zoonoses of NHP have been documented including yellow fever virus (arbovirus group B flavivirus) and Denque fever viruses (flavivirues), and several that are questionable as far as zoonoses but worth considering including SV40, simian parvo virus and Molluscum contagiosum.

NON-HUMAN PRIMATE BACTERIAL ZOONOSES
Mycobacterium Tuberculosis

Historically, the three major species of *Mycobacteria—avium, bovis,* and *tuberculosis—*have been incriminated as causing disease in NHPs. Recently; there have also been reports of atypical mycobacteria in immunocompromised NHPs. The primary route of transmission is through inhalation or ingestion. Tuberculosis can be transmitted from humans to NHPs and then spread from NHP to NHP and secondarily spread back to humans again. All species of NHP are susceptible, although Old World species of primates appear to be more susceptible than New World species. Clinical disease can be hard to detect until the disease is in advanced stages. Clinical tuberculosis causes severe weight loss, lethargy, draining tracts of skin and vertebral bone and coughing and is almost always fatal in NHP. In both humans and NHPs the skin test detects only TB exposure, not active disease and both false positives and negatives may occur. Active disease is diagnosed either by recovery of the organisms in culture or at necropsy or by thoracic radiographic lesions consistent with active TB. A valuable ancillary test is the use of a rapid whole blood interferon- γ (WB-IFN-γ test – Primagam). This test measures cell mediated immune responses in non-human primates. The test kit also contains tuberculosis antigens (Bovine PPD, Avian PPD and Nil antigen control). Primagam® is available from Prionics AG Wagistrassa 27A. 8952 Schlieren-ZU Rich. Switzerland Phone +41 44 200 20 00; Fax +41 44 200 20 10 or www.info@prionics.com. Other diagnostic tests may include radiographs, sputum, fecal and blood cultures, gastric lavage for cytology and culture, and comparative TB tests. All owners of NHP and others having contact with them, including veterinary staff, should be TB tested annually. Prevention of contact of actively infected persons with NHP is essential.

Pseudotuberculosis

Pseudotuberculosis caused by either *Yersinia pseudotuberculosis* or *Y. enterocolitica* is a zoonotic, infectious bacterial agent that has a worldwide distribution. The infection can affect a wide range of host species but in particular has caused numerous deaths in tamarins, marmosets and Goeldi's monkeys in captivity. Clinical signs of infection can range from asymptomatic animals that shed the bacteria, to nonspecific signs of systemic or enteric diseases and wasting or sudden death that may be difficult to diagnose. Birds and rodents are thought to be the primary reservoir, but NHP may be carriers and present a threat to humans. The organism can live in the soil for long periods of time and asymptomatic animals, combined with the difficulties in culturing the organism from rectal or fecal swabs, can all lead to difficulties in controlling the organism. Preventative measures such as quarantine, good sanitation, good hygiene, and pest control, together with a vaccination program in endemic areas, are all recommended in preventing infection.

Enteric Bacterial Pathogens

Diarrhea is the most common medical problem seen in NHP.[2] Some of the etiological agents involved in diarrhea outbreaks includes *Salmonella* sp, *Shigella* sp, enteropathic *Escheria coli*, *Klebsiella* sp, and *Campylobacter* sp. Most of these agents in captive NHP probably occur from infected people to NHP then back again. Severity of disease in NHP depends on species affected and immune status at the time of infection. Diagnosis is typically through stool cultures and biochemical markers.

Protozoal Infections

Giardia lamblia, *Cryptosporidium*, *Enterocytozoan bieneusi*, *Balantidium coli*, malarial sporozoans and *Entamoeba histolytica* are all protozoa that can infect monkeys and humans. Clinical signs usually include diarrhea in both monkeys and humans that can range from mild to severe. There have been a few documented cases of fatalities in neonatal and juvenile monkeys due to these protozoa.

Metazoan Parasites

Metazoan parasites such as *Hymenolepis nana*, *Oesophagostomum apiostomum* and *O. bifurcum*, *Enetrobius vermicularis* (pinworm), *Strongyloides*, and *Trichuris sp.* have all been reported in NHP species and transmission to humans is usually through the fecal-oral route. Preventative anthelmintics as well as diligent fecal screens and vector / intermediate host control are critical in maintaining these animals.

REFERENCES

1. Bennett BT, Abee CR, Henrickson R. Nonhuman Primates in Biomedical Research—Diseases. San Diego: Academic Press, 1998.
2. Fowler ME. Zoo and Wild Animal Medicine Current Therapy 3. Philadelphia: WB Saunders, 1993.
3. Murphy HW, Miller M, Ramer J, et al. Implications of simian retroviruses for captive primate population management and the occupational safety of primate handlers. J Zoo Wildl Med. 2006; 219–233.
4. National Research Counsel. Occupational Health and Safety in the Care and Use of Nonhuman Primates. The National Academies Press. Washington, DC, 2003.

NO SMALL FEAT: LAPAROSCOPIC ELEPHANT VASECTOMIES IN SOUTH AFRICA

Mark Stetter, DVM, Diplomate ACZM
Disney's Animal Programs
Lake Buena Vista, FL

Elephant population control is a significant animal welfare and habitat conservation issue facing southern Africa. Elephant populations, which have exceeded the parks' carrying capacity, are associated with habitat destruction. In South Africa, wildlife officials have used both culling and translocation as their primary methods of population control. Humane concerns prompted the park service to discontinue culling in the 1990s and elephant numbers have risen to such an extent that translocation is no longer a viable alternative. New options for population management are needed, and our goal is to develop a safe and effective technique that can be used to humanely manage elephant populations.

Vasectomy is one of the most common methods of birth control in humans. For free-ranging animals, a vasectomy has the advantage of maintaining normal hormone levels and thus breeding and natural social behaviors are preserved. Elephants that have been vasectomized will continue to go into musth, breed (without being fertile), and maintain their social status among other elephants.

It is important to note that elephant testes are intra-abdominal and are located just caudal to the kidneys. To access the testes and spermatic cord, the abdomen must be entered. Routine abdominal surgery in elephants is rarely attempted and rarely successful. Laparoscopy allows this abdominal surgery to be carried out in a safe and effective way. Advances in laparoscopy have allowed an elephant-size, portable, laparoscopic unit to be built and used in field conditions. Laparoscopy is well suited for free-ranging wildlife since small incisions reduce the chance of infection and allow much faster healing times. The surgery can be completed in a couple of hours and the animals do not require postoperative care.

IMMOBILIZATION

Using a helicopter, the male elephant is darted with a combination of etorphine (M99®, Wildlife Pharmaceuticals, Inc., Fort Collins, CO) and azaperone (Stresnil®, Wildlife Pharmaceuticals, Inc.). After induction, an endotracheal tube is placed and respirations are assisted using a portable ventilator system. Throughout anesthesia, the elephant's blood pressure, oxygen saturation, end total carbon dioxide, body temperature, heart rate, respiratory rate and blood gas analysis are all monitored. Additional small boluses of intravenous etorphine and azaperone are administered as required. At the completion of surgery, the elephants are reversed with intravenous naltrexone hydrochloride (Trexonil®, Wildlife Pharmaceuticals Inc.) and diprenorphine (M5050®, Wildlife Pharmaceuticals Inc.). Animals recover and are ambulatory in 5 to 10 minutes.

PATIENT POSITIONING

A crane truck is utilized to assist patient positioning and suspend the animal in an upright standing position throughout the surgery. This enhances the safety of the anesthesia and allows improved abdominal insufflation and laparoscopic visualization. The crane positions the elephant so that each foot rests squarely on the ground, and then wooden splints are attached to the legs and are used to lock each limb in extension. This allows the legs to support the majority of the elephant's weight and places minimal pressure on the suspension ropes.

After the elephant has been placed in a standing position, surgical equipment is moved into place. A 14-inch flat screen monitor is placed in a specialized cradle on the elephant's caudal dorsum for laparoscopic viewing. A mobile surgical laparoscopic suite is set up next to the elephant with tables and electrical equipment powered by a portable generator.

SURGICAL PROCEDURE

The paracostal areas on left and right sides of the elephant are cleaned and scrubbed for surgery. After the surgical scrub, each site is sterily draped. The primary incision is approximately 15 cm long and is located just cranial to the tuber coxae. A human chest Finnochetto retractor is utilized to separate the sides of the incision and provide visualization of the fibro-elastic peritoneum. Tumor forceps are utilized to grasp the fatty connective tissue that covers the peritoneum and withdraw it through the incision. A portion of this fatty connective tissue is resected and an incision is made through the peritoneum. The abdomen is insufflated with ambient air using a specifically designed device capable of rapid and regulated air flow (Dean Hendrickson, Colorado State University, Ft. Collins, CO). In general, a high intra-abdominal pressure of 1 psi (52 mmHg) is required to provide operating space and enhance visualization during surgery. A specially designed operating laparoscope has been made for pachyderms by Karl Storz Endoscopy (Goleta, CA). The telescope has an instrument port into which a laparoscopic scissor or grasping forceps can be inserted and used. A second instrument cannula is placed approximately 15- to 20-cm from the primary incision. The testes can be visualized just caudal to the kidney with the epididymus and deferent ductus trailing off its caudal pole. A 6- to 10-cm portion of duct is resected using a hook-shaped laparoscopic scissor. Samples are initially confirmed grossly to be appropriate and also placed in formalin for histopathologic evaluation

While the laparoscopic surgeons are working, a second set of surgeons make an incision on the contralateral side. Once the vasectomy is complete on side one, the elephant is lifted in its standing position and rotated 180 degrees. The laparoscopic surgeons will now complete the vasectomy on the second side while the other surgical team closes the incision from the completed side. The peritoneum and muscle layers are closed separately with an absorbable suture in a single continuous pattern. The skin is then closed with #2 nylon in a modified far-far-near-near (tension relieving) suture pattern. During the procedure the elephant receives a long-acting penicillin injection and a single dose of a nonsteroidal anti-inflammatory drug. After the closure is complete, the animal is rinsed with water and lowered from the crane for anesthetic reversal.

POSTOPERATIVE MONITORING

During the surgery, each animal is fitted with a VHF biotelemetry collar. On-site elephant researchers, along with ranger staff, follow the elephants after their surgery. Digital photographs are taken to document wound healing and any change in body condition. Other behavioral data is collected including activity, appetite, and social interactions.

CONCLUSION

Laparoscopic vasectomy of free ranging bull elephants is a viable surgical option for reproductive sterilization. This management tool is probably not realistic for very large elephant populations (>10,000), but should be considered for small and medium size elephant populations. In 2006 and 2007 laparoscopic vasectomies were conducted at the Welgevonden Game Reserve and with the Mpumalanga Parks Board in Songimvelo, South Africa. Surgical times are approximately 2 hours, and total anesthetic time approximately 3 to 3.5 hours. Elephants heal well after surgery and show no observable long-term problems from the procedure. Vasectomized bulls have been seen breeding and continue to exert dominance and prevent less dominant bulls from breeding. Further research is currently underway to make this a more efficient and practical field technique and to fully understand any potential negative impact this procedure may have on the individual elephant, the elephant population, or the ecosystem.

This is an international collaborative effort which brings together conservation organizations, universities, government entities and private industry to address this complex problem. It is our hope that this work may provide a useful management tool which balances ecosystem health and animal welfare concerns.

ACKNOWLEDGMENTS

We are indebted to the Karl Storz Company for the design and manufacture of the elephant laparoscopic equipment. We thank the following individuals for their participation and support of our work through the years: Beth Ament, LVT, Nancy Boedeker, DVM, Michael Briggs, DVM, Lidia Castro, LVT, Greg Fleming, DVM, ACZM, Don Neiffer, VMD, ACZM, Mark Penning, BVSc, MSc, PK Robbins, MRCVS, Anne Savage, PhD, Cora Singleton, DVM, Julia Sweet, LVT, Kelly Stetter, LVT, Scott Terrell, DVM, ACVP, and Laura Wheeler, LVT. This work would not have been possible without key partnerships with conservation groups in Africa, including Catchco Africa (Douw Grobler, Li-Ann Small and JJ Van Altena), CC Africa/Phinda (Kevin Pretorius and Helene Druce), the Makalali Game Reserve (Audrey Delsink and Ross Kettle), and the Welgevonden Game Reserve (David Powrie and Hanno Kilian).